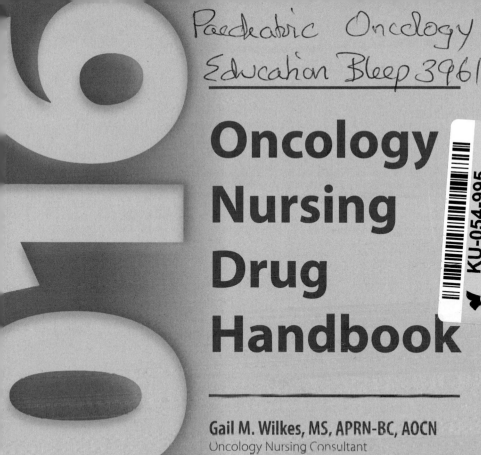

Oncology Nursing Drug Handbook

2016

Gail M. Wilkes, MS, APRN-BC, AOCN
Oncology Nursing Consultant
Kilauea, Hawaii

Margaret Barton-Burke, PhD, RN, FAAN
Director of Nursing Research
Memorial Sloan Kettering Cancer Center
New York, New York

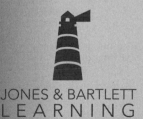

JONES & BARTLETT
LEARNING

World Headquarters
Jones & Bartlett Learning
5 Wall Street
Burlington, MA 01803
978-443-5000
info@jblearning.com
www.jblearning.com

Jones & Bartlett Learning books and products are available through most bookstores and online booksellers. To contact Jones & Bartlett Learning directly, call 800-832-0034, fax 978-443-8000, or visit our website, www.jblearning.com.

Substantial discounts on bulk quantities of Jones & Bartlett Learning publications are available to corporations, professional associations, and other qualified organizations. For details and specific discount information, contact the special sales department at Jones & Bartlett Learning via the above contact information or send an email to specialsales@jblearning.com.

Production Credits
VP, Executive Publisher: David Cella
Executive Editor: Amanda Martin
Acquisitions Editor: Teresa Reilly
Editorial Assistant: Danielle Bessette
Senior Production Editor: Amanda Clerkin
Marketing Communications Manager: Katie Hennessy

VP, Manufacturing and Inventory Control:
  Therese Connell
Composition: S4Carlisle Publishing Services
Cover Design: Kristin E. Parker
Rights & Media Specialist: Wes DeShano
Printing and Binding: Edwards Brothers Malloy
Cover Printing: Edwards Brothers Malloy

6048

Printed in the United States of America
19 18 17 16 15   10 9 8 7 6 5 4 3 2 1

Contents

Chapter 2   Biologic Response Modifier Therapy   361

Chapter 5   Chemobiotherapy for Noncancer Diseases   909

Section 2 Symptom Management   947

Chapter 6   Pain   948

Chapter 11 **Infection** **1227**

Chapter 12 **Constipation   1481**

Chapter 13 **Diarrhea   1498**

Key to Abbreviations

ABV	doxorubicin (doxorubicin HCl Adriamycin) bleomycin vincristineac
ac	*ante cibum*; before meals
ADH	antidiuretic hormone
Afib	atrial fibrillation
AIDS	acquired immunodeficiency syndrome
ALL	acute lymphocytic leukemia
ALT	alanine aminotransferase (formerly SGPT)
AML	acute myelocytic leukemia
ANC	absolute neutrophil count
ANLL	acute nonlymphocytic leukemia
APC	adenomatous polyposis coli gene
APL	acute promyelocytic leukemia
aPTT	activated partial thromboplastin time
ARDS	adult respiratory distress syndrome
ASA	acetylsalicylic acid
AST	aspartate aminotransferase (formerly SGOT)
AUC	area under curve
BBB	blood–brain barrier
BCR-ABL	mutation resulting in the formation of the Philadelphia chromosome, found in 90% of patients with CML
bid	*bis in die*; twice a day
bili	bilirubin
BMT	bone marrow transplant
BP	blood pressure
BRM	biologic response modifier
BTP	breakthrough pain
BUN	blood urea nitrogen
Ca	calcium
CAPD	continuous ambulatory periotoneal dialysis
CBC	complete blood count
CFU-GEM	colony-forming unit–granulocyte, erythrocyte, megakaryocyte, and macrophage
CHF	congestive heart failure
CLL	chronic lymphocytic leukemia
CML	chronic myelogenous leukemia
CPK	creatinine phosphokinase
CR	complete response, e.g., disappearance of all detectable tumor cells
creat	creatinine

CSF	colony-stimulating factor
CTZ	chemoreceptor trigger zone
CVA	cerebrovascular accident
CXR	chest X-ray
D_5W	5% dextrose in water
DEHP	diethylhexlphthalate
DHFR	difolate reductase
DIC	disseminated intravascular coagulation
DLCO	diffusion capacity of the lung for carbon monoxide, which reflects rate of gas transfer across the alveolar-capillary membrane
DLT	dose-limiting toxicity
DMSO	dimethyl sulfoxide
DTIC	dacarbazine
DVT	deep vein thrombosis
EBV	Epstein-Barr virus
ECHO	echocardiogram
EDTA	edetic acid, one of several salts of edetic acid used as a chelating agent
EGFRI	epidermal growth factor receptor inhibitor
EPS	extra pyramidal side effects
FAC	fluorouracil-adriamycin-cytoxan combination chemotherapy
FOLFIRI	combination chemotherapy of folinic acid (leucovorin), 5-fluorouracil, and irinotecan
FOLFOX	combination chemotherapy of folinic acid (leucovorin), 5-fluorouracil, and oxaliplatin
FSH	follicle-stimulating hormone
FUDR-MP	5-fluoro-23-deoxyuridine-53-monophosphate
FVC	forced vital capacity
G6PD	glucose-6-phosphate dehydrogenase
GABA	gamma-aminobutyric acid
GBPS	gated blood pool scan
G-CSF	granulocyte-colony stimulating factor
GFR	glomerular filtration rate
GGT	(SGGT) gamma-glutamine transferase
GU	genitourinary
HACA	human antichimeric antibody
HAMA	human antimurine antibody
HCC	hepatocellular cancer
HCl	hydrochloride
HCT	hematocrit
Hgb	hemoglobin
5-HIAA	5-hydroxyindoleacetic acid
HIV	human immunodeficiency virus
$5\text{-}HT_2$	5-hydroxytryptamine 2
$5\text{-}HT_3$	5-hydroxytryptamine 3
Hs	*hora somni*; at bedtime

HSV	herpes simplex virus
HUS	hemolytic uremic syndrome
ICP	intracranial pressure
ICU	intensive care unit
IFN	interferon
IL	interleukin
I/O	intake/output
IOP	intraocular pressure
IT	intrathecal
IVB	intravenous bolus
IVP	intravenous push; intravenous pyelogram
LAK	lymphocyte activated killer cells
LDH	lactate dehydrogenase
LFTs	liver function tests
LH	luteinizing hormone
LHRH	luteinizing hormone-releasing hormone
LVEF	left ventricular ejection fraction
lytes	electrolytes
MAb	monoclonal antibody
MAC	mycobacterium avium complex
MAO	monoamine oxidase
MAOI	monoamine oxidase inhibitor
MAPK	mitogen-activated protein kinase pathway, aka Ras-Raf-MEK-ERK pathway
MCV	mean corpuscular volume
MI	myocardial infarction
MIU	milli international units
MOPP	mustard-oncovin-prednisone-procarbazine combination chemotherapy for Hodgkin's disease
mTOR	mammalian target of rapamycin, which coordinates cell growth, nutrient use, and angiogenesis
MTX	methotrexate
MU	milli units
NCI	National Cancer Institute
NHL	non-Hodgkin's lymphoma
NK	natural killer cells
NK1	neurokinin 1 receptor for substance P
NMDA	N-methyl-D-aspartate pain receptor
NS	normal saline
NSAIDs	nonsteroidal anti-inflammatory drugs
n/v	nausea/vomiting
OS	overall survival
OTC	over-the-counter
PACs	premature atrial contractions
PBPCs	packed red blood cells for transfusion
PCA	patient controlled analgesia
PCP	*Pneumocystis (carinii) jiroveci* pneumonia

PFS	progression-free survival
PFTs	pulmonary function tests
phos	phosphorus
plts	platelets
PDGFR	platelet-derived growth factor receptor
PI3K	phosphatidylinositol 3-kinase pathway, most frequently mutated pathway in cancer
PML	polymorphonuclear leukocyte
PR	partial response, e.g., reduction in tumor mass by 50% lasting for 3 months or longer
PRN	*pro re nata*; as needed
PSA	prostate-specific antigen
PT	prothrombin time
PTEN	phosphatase and tensin homolog
PTH	parathyroid hormone
PTT	partial thromboplastin time
PVCs	premature ventricular contractions
qid	*quater in die*; four times a day
QT	measure of the interval of time between the start of the Q wave and end of T wave; if prolonged, it can increase risk of fatal ventricular arrhythmias
RAS	protein that activates a number of pathways, such as MAPK pathway
REMS	risk evaluation and management strategy
RFTs	renal function tests
RT	radiation therapy
RUQ	right upper quadrant
SBP	systolic blood pressure
sed rate	sedimentation rate
SGOT	serum glutamic-oxalacetic transaminase
SGPT	serum glutamic-pyruvic transferase
SIADH	syndrome of inappropriate antidiuretic hormone
SOB	shortness of breath
SPF	skin protection factor
SQ	subcutaneous
SSRI	selective serotonin reuptake inhibitor
STAT	signal transducers and activators of transcription protein pathway, which carries a message from the cell surface to the cell nucleus and then activates transcription of specific genes
Sx	symptom
T	temperature
T_3	triiodothyronine
T_4	thyroxine
TCA	tricyclic antidepressants
TFT	thyroid function tests
TGF$\updownarrow$	transforming growth factor beta
THC	tetrahydrocannabinol

tid	*ter in die*; three times a day
TIL	tumor-infiltrating lymphocytes
TKI	tyrosine kinase inhibitor
TLS	tumor lysis syndrome
TMP-SMX	trimethoprim-sulfamethoxazole
TNF	tumor necrosis factor
TTP/HUS	thrombotic thrombocytopenic purpura/hemolytic anemia syndrome
UA	urinalysis
ULN	upper limit of normal
US	ultrasound
UTI	urinary tract infection
VC	vomiting center
VEGF	vascular endothelial growth factor
Vfib	ventricular fibrillation
VOD	veno-occlusive disease
VS	vital signs
VSCC	voltage-sensitive calcium channel
VZV	varicella zoster virus
WHO	World Health Organization
XRT	radiation therapy

Preface

Oncology nurses provide expert nursing care to patients with cancer and their families as the patient moves along the disease trajectory from diagnosis to primary treatment and cure, or to remission, then possible relapse, and death. The nurse uses the nursing process to assess patient and family needs in the 14 high-incidence problem areas identified in the Oncology Nursing Society (ONS) standards: health promotion, patient/family education, coping, comfort, nutrition, complementary and alternative medicine, protective mechanisms, mobility, GI and urinary function, sexuality, cardiopulmonary function, oncologic emergencies, palliative and end-of-life care, and survivorship (Brandt and Wickham, 2013).

In 2003, Andrew von Eschenbach, MD, set the NCI challenge goal as the elimination of suffering and death due to cancer. He identified seven major initiatives to accomplish this goal, including development of more effective strategies for prevention and screening; early detection as well as improvement of our understanding of the molecular processes of carcinogenesis; and refinement of molecular targeted therapy (von Eschenbach, 2003). In this view, cancer becomes a chronic disease characterized by periods of exacerbations and remissions. As has been demonstrated in work on angiogenesis, malignant tumors must establish a blood supply when they reach a size of 1–2 mm in order to obtain oxygen and glucose, and to remove cellular waste products. Mortality is caused by metastasis in most people with cancer, and if a malignancy is confined to 1–2 mm with a combination of chemotherapy, anti-angiogenesis drugs, other signal transduction inhibitors, along with immune checkpoint inhibitors, then indeed, people can "live with cancer." Today, more and more is being revealed about genetic tumor-typing and identifying tumor targets that individualize cancer care, much like doing blood cultures to identify an infectious organism and tailoring antimicrobial therapy to the infectious microbe. Together, the nurse and patient, along with other members of the healthcare team, develop a plan of care. Because cancer, for many, is a chronic illness with periods of remission and relapse, nursing goals center around promoting self-care and empowering the patient and family to live a high-quality, meaningful life outside the hospital or office practice.

Nurses are involved in the pharmacologic management of disease (e.g., chemotherapy, including targeted molecular and biological therapy) and of symptoms that arise during the course of illness (e.g., pain, anxiety, constipation, nausea, vomiting). In addition, as patients receive more aggressive treatment, nurses are deeply involved in the management of complications of disease or treatment, such as infection. As new technologies emerge, such as molecular and biological-/immune-targeted therapies, nurses need to stay abreast of newly approved agents, their mechanisms of action, potential side effects, and issues of cost. Knowledge of cancer biology and metastases is evolving and offers potential targets. Nurses must keep up with understanding the fundamental molecular flaws, both to teach patients and their families, as well as to understand the mechanism of action and potential toxicities. As the paradigm moves to multitargeted oral agents, the nurse must be creative in developing strategies to promote adherence with treatment regimens and individualize patient care to enhance adherence. For example, nurses are working to establish the evidence base for minimization of toxicity and distress related to EGFR inhibitor rash. In addition, as the cost of cancer therapy—targeted and biological/immune therapies, in particular—skyrockets, the nurse must be able either to access resources or to refer patients and their families to resources for help. Finally, oncology nurses have long said that much of symptom management is in the domain of nursing practice, and they continue to advocate for effective management and symptom resolution. Knowledge of the drugs used in cancer care is critical for today's practicing nurse. In the past, pharmacists wrote drug books for nurses that did not address the application of the nursing process to potential drug toxicities. Today, as the science of cancer treatment is rapidly exploding, it is imperative to keep current with new, emerging therapies.

This book is divided into sections addressing broad areas of nursing practice; individual chapters within each section present an introductory overview. Included in *Chapter 1* of this edition is lanreotide (Somatuline Depot Injection). Other drugs included in *Chapter 1* were updated for new indications, postmarketing side effects, or warnings. *Chapter 2* agents were reviewed and updated, and the first biosimilar product, filgrastim-sndz (Zarxio) added. *Chapter 3* addresses cytoprotective agents. *Chapter 4* addresses targeted molecular and biologic/immune therapies, and new information was added about how tumors evade the immune system, the resurgence of immunotherapies, including immune checkpoint inhibitors and adoptive therapies. *Chapter 4*, Molecularly Targeted Therapies, discusses basic cell biology, carcinogenesis, malignant flaws resulting in abnormal cell division and cell death, immune escape, invasiveness, and metastases. This is intended to provide a framework for understanding the new agents that target molecular flaws. Many of these agents inhibit steps in the processes of carcinogenesis and metastases in the areas of signal transduction (growth receptor over expression, and mutation of proteins in major signaling pathways), cell-cycle movement (cyclin-dependent kinases, apoptosis), angiogenesis, invasion, and metastases. In addition, the processes of apoptosis and ubiquitination are further explored. All chapter drugs were reviewed and updated to reflect new indications or prescribing information. As most tyrosine kinase inhibitors have significant drug interactions, the P450 microenzyme system and drug interactions are discussed in more detail. A table has been included that shows drug interactions for targeted therapies. In addition, as some drugs prolong the QTc on ECG, this is discussed in greater detail. Finally, as more attention is focused on immune checkpoint inhibitors, such as ipilumumab (Yervoy), the immune-related adverse effects and management are highlighted, as they differ from those adverse effects of other agents. The following new drugs were added: blinatumomab (Blincyto), dinutuximab (Unituxin), gefitinib (Iressa), levatinib (Lenvima), nivolumab (Opdivo), olaparib (Lynparza), palbociclib (Ibrance), panobinostat (Farydak), and sonidegib (Odomzo).

Because oncology nurses are often asked to administer monoclonal antibodies and other unusual drugs to patients with autoimmune diseases, a new chapter was added. *Chapter 5*, Chemobiotherapy for Noncancer Diseases appears in *Section 1*. Drugs in this section are abatacept (Orencia), adalimumab (Humira), certolizumab pegol (Cimzia), etanercept (Enbrel), golimumab (Simponi), infliximab (Remicade), tocilizumab (Actemra), and tofacitinib (Xeljanz), a JAK inhibitor.

In *Sections 2* (Symptom Management) and *3* (Complications), *Chapters 6, 7, 8, 9, 10, 12,* and *13* have been updated. In Chapter 7, netupitant/palonosetron (Akynzeo), a combination substance P/Neurokinin 1 receptor antagonist with a serotonin-3 (5-HT3) receptor antagonist, has been added. The following drugs were added to *Chapter* 11: ceftazidime/avibactam (Avycaz), isavuconazonium sulfate (Cresemba), oritavancin (Orbactiv), tedizolid phosphate (Sivextro), ceftolozane/tazobactam (Zerbaxa), dalbavancin (Dalvance). Naloxegol (Movantik) was added to Chapter 12. In order to make more space, *Appendix 2* is abridged and referenced to indicate how to locate the NCI Common Toxicity Criteria of Adverse Events (CTCAE) 4.03.

All agents were updated to reflect newly approved indications. Specific drugs are described in terms of their mechanism of action, metabolism, FDA indications, dosage/range, administration, drug interactions, laboratory effects/interference, special considerations, and application of the nursing process to manage potential adverse effects. The most important and common drug side effects are discussed.

Nursing priorities in the assessment and management of EGFRI skin toxicity are discussed in terms of pathophysiology and consensus management strategies. As more targeted therapies are used that have prolongation of the QT interval in the cardiac cycle as side effects, this is discussed in detail with nursing implications. Standards may change as new scientific knowledge becomes available and as dictated by governmental regulations that affect practice. This book will be updated regularly with new drugs and nursing management strategies to reflect those changes.

The authors, editor, and publisher have made every effort to provide accurate information. However, they are not responsible for errors, omissions, or for any outcomes related to the use of the contents of this book and take no responsibility for the use of the products and procedures described. Treatment and side effects described in this book may not be applicable to all people; likewise, some people may require a dose or experience a side effect that is not described herein. Drugs and medical devices are discussed that may have limited availability, controlled by the Food and Drug Administration (FDA) for use only in a research study or clinical trial. Research, clinical practice, and government regulations often change the accepted standards in this field. When consideration is being given for use of any drug in the clinical setting, the healthcare provider or reader is responsible for determining FDA status of the drug, reading the package insert, and reviewing prescribing information for the most up-to-date recommendations on dose, precautions, and contraindications, and determining the appropriate usage for the product. This is especially important in the case of drugs that are new or seldom used.

DRUG INFORMATION sections reflect current prescribing practices in the United States, which may differ from clinical practices in Europe and the United Kingdom.

References

Brandt JM, Wickham R. Statement on the scope and standards of oncology nursing practice, Generalist and advanced practice. Pittsburgh, PA: Oncology Nursing Society, 2013, pp. 21–35.
von Eschenbach. Keynote presentation: *Summit series on cancer clinical trials. Executive Summary VIII: Retooling the System: Implementing Solution.* September 29–October 1, 2003.

Contributors

Catherine K. Bean, BSN, RN, BA
Tampa, FL

Deborah Berg, BSN, RN
North Londonderry, NH

Karen Ingwersen, MS, RN
Belmont, MA

Section 1
Cancer Treatment

Chapter *1*
Introduction to Chemotherapy Drugs

Traditional chemotherapy drugs interfere with cell division, leading to cell kill, called *cytocidal effects*, or failure to replicate, called *cytostatic effects* (see Figure 1.1). Unfortunately, drugs cannot discriminate between frequently dividing cells that are normal and those that are malignant. Consequently, normal cells as well as malignant cells are injured. Thus, anticipated acute side effects are found also in normal cell populations that divide frequently, i.e., bone marrow, gastrointestinal (GI) mucosa, gonads, and hair follicles. Since normal cells are better able to repair themselves, these side effects are usually reversible. Depending on drug properties, delayed, longer-term toxicities may occur, which may be irreversible. Properties to be aware of include route of administration, dose, excretion, and predilection for uptake by specific organ cells. Examples of toxicities are:

- Lung toxicity from bleomycin, busulfan, and the nitrosoureas (BCNU, CCNU)
- Cardiomyopathy from the anthracyclines doxorubicin and daunorubicin, the anthracenedione mitoxantrone, as well as from the mitotic inhibitor paclitaxel
- Renal dysfunction from cisplatin and high-dose methotrexate
- Hemorrhagic cystitis (bladder) from ifosfamide and cyclophosphamide
- Neurotoxicity from the platinums, taxanes, and vinca alkaloids
- Development of second malignancies from melphalan and cyclophosphamide, either alone or when certain drugs are combined with radiotherapy

Nurses play a critical role in patient assessment, education, drug administration, and minimization of toxicities. See Table 1.1 for prechemotherapy nursing assessment guidelines. Table 1.2 describes classifications of antineoplastic drugs. Table 1.3 highlights the newly updated 2013 American Society of Clinical Oncology (ASCO)/Oncology Nursing Society (ONS) chemotherapy administration safety standards. The new standards also describe standards for the safe prescription and management of patients receiving oral antineoplastic drugs.

This 2015 edition has been updated to include newly approved drugs, as well as important investigational agents, that may be approved in the near future. This section examines antineoplastic agents and classifies them by their mechanism(s) of action. As knowledge of cancer and its treatment emerge, drugs may be reclassified, such as the anthracycline antitumor antibiotics, which now appear to work by inhibiting topoisomerase II.

As an example, the topoisomerase inhibitors cause protein-linked DNA single-strand breaks and block DNA and RNA synthesis in dividing cells, thus preventing cells from entering mitosis. To better understand the topoisomerase inhibitors, it is important to go back to the DNA helix. The entire DNA genome consists of two strands wound into a double helix, which measures more than 3 feet long. In order to fit into a tiny cell, it is condensed into chromosomes by torsion of the helix. During cell replication, the DNA strands that are coiled in the double helix need to unwind so that they can separate and be copied. This is made possible by the topoisomerase I and II enzymes (Chen and Liu, 1994).

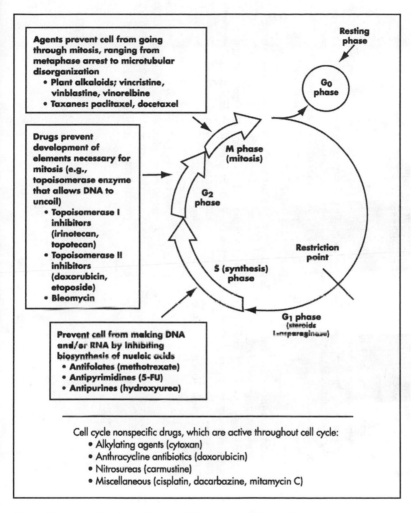

Figure 1.1　Mechanism of Action of Major Chemotherapy Drugs

Topoisomerase I relaxes tension in the DNA helix torsion by causing a transient single-strand break or nick in the DNA when it covalently bonds to the end of one of the DNA strands. The other, intact strand then passes through the break, and relaxation of the DNA helix occurs as the strands swivel at the strand break.

The topoisomerase I enzyme then reseals the cleaved strand (religation step), and the enzyme is released from the DNA strand. Transcription (copying of the strands) is then initiated. Interestingly, topoisomerase I is found in greater concentrations in patients with cancers of the colon, non-Hodgkin's lymphoma, and some leukemias. Drugs such as topotecan and irinotecan work by inhibiting the religation or repair of the single-strand break by binding to topoisomerase I, and cells are arrested in the G_2 phase.

Table 1.1   Prechemotherapy Nursing Assessment Guidelines

Potential Problems/Nursing Diagnoses	Physical Status: Assessment Parameters/ Signs and Symptoms	Drug and Dose-Limiting Factors/ Nursing Implications
Hematopoietic System		
1. Impaired tissue perfusion related to chemotherapy-induced anemia, leading to activity intolerance, changes in cardiopulmonary status due to compensatory changes	• Hgb (norms women, 12–14; men, 14–16) • HCT% (norms women, 36–46; men, 42–54) • Vital signs (↓BP, ↑pulse, ↑ or ↓respiration) • Pallor (face, palms, conjunctiva) • Fatigue or weakness • Vertigo	Hgb < 8 g HCT < 20% and blood transfusions not initiated • Consider erythropoietin growth factor support when Hgb < 10 g/dL when receiving anemia-causing chemotherapy; e.g., cisplatin for palliation; do not exceed an Hgb of 12 g/dL (FDA, 2007)
2. Impaired immunocompetence and potential for infection related to chemotherapy-induced neutropenia, lymphopenia	• WBC (norm 4,500–9,000/mm^3); ANC > 2,000/mm^3 • Lymphocyte count >500/mm^3 • Pyrexia/rigor, erythema, swelling, pain any site • Abnormal discharges, draining wounds, skin/mucous membrane lesions • Productive cough, SOB, rectal pain, urinary frequency	WBC ≤ 3,000/mm^3; ANC < 1,000/mm^3–1,500/mm^3; Fever > 38°C or 100.4°F • Hold all myelosuppressive agents (exceptions may include leukemia, lymphoma, and/or situations in which there is neoplastic marrow infiltration) • Consider growth factor support to prevent febrile neutropenia if risk > 20% • Febrile neutropenia is a medical emergency • Severe risk of infection ANC < 500 cells/mm^3 • Protective precautions if actual or potential ANC < 500 cells/mm^3

Table 1.1 *(Continued)*

Potential Problems/Nursing Diagnoses	Physical Status: Assessment Parameters/ Signs and Symptoms	Drug and Dose-Limiting Factors/ Nursing Implications
3. Potential for injury (bleeding) related to chemotherapy-induced thrombocytopenia	Platelet count (150,000–400,000/mm³) • Spontaneous gingival bleeding or epistaxis • Presence of petechiae or easy bruisability • Hematuria, melena, hematemesis, hemoptysis • Hypermenorrhea • Signs and symptoms of intracranial bleeding (irritability, sensory loss, unequal pupils, headache, ataxia)	Platelet count ≤ 100,000/mm³ • Hold all myelosuppressive agents (exceptions may include leukemia, lymphoma, and/or situations in which there is neoplastic marrow infiltration) • Platelet transfusion if bleeding • Platelet precaution: platelet count < 20,000 cells/mm³
Integumentary System		
1. Potential for injury related to severe sterile inflammatory rash 2. Alteration in skin integrity related to alopecia	• EGFR inhibitor rash • Assess for risk of infection, itching, open areas *Anthracyclines such as doxorubicin *May be partial or total alopecia	• Teach patient self-care to avoid infection, maintain hydration and skin integrity; use sunscreens and hat when outside • Discuss topical and/or systemic preventive or treatment of evolving rash • Consider doxycycline 100 mg PO bid, topical clindamycin gel, and/or steroid tapper *Explore effect of hair loss on patient, and encourage verbalization of feelings *Discuss ways to facilitate coping, such as cranial prosthesis prior to losing hair, *Look Good Feel Better* American Cancer Society programs

(continued)

5

Table 1.1 *(Continued)*

Potential Problems/Nursing Diagnoses	Physical Status: Assessment Parameters/ Signs and Symptoms	Drug and Dose-Limiting Factors/ Nursing Implications
3. Anorexia	• Lab values: Albumin and total protein • Normal weight/present weight and % of body weight loss • Normal diet pattern/changes in diet pattern • Alterations in taste sensation, dysgeusia • Early satiety	• Manage nutrition impact symptoms • Dietary teaching • Appetite stimulants as needed
4. Nausea and vomiting	• Lab values: Electrolytes • Pattern of n/v (incidence, duration, severity); hydration status • Hydration status • Antiemetic plan: Drug(s), dosage(s), schedule, efficacy; Other (dietary adjustments, relaxation techniques, environmental manipulation)	Intractable n/v × 24 h: IV hydration if unable to take oral fluids • Aggressive combination antiemesis (serotonin and NK$_1$ antagonists and dexamethasone; palonostron for severe with delayed nausea and/or vomiting; addition of aprepitant to serotonin-antagonist for highly emetogenic, moderately emetogenic with delayed nausea and vomiting)
5. Bowel disturbances A. Diarrhea	• Normal pattern of bowel elimination • Consistency (loose, watery/bloody stools) • Assess hydration status and ability to take fluids in • Frequency and duration (no./day and no. of days) • Antidiarrheal drug(s), dosage(s), efficacy	Diarrheal stools × 3/24 h above baseline • Hold antimetabolites (esp. methotrexate, 5-FU); irinotecan • Teach patient self-administration of antidiarrheal medicine • Assess electrolytes, need for parenteral hydration • Antibiotic therapy for unresolved diarrhea per MD as mucositis may occur during nadir, with resulting sepsis.

Table 1.1 *(Continued)*

Potential Problems/Nursing Diagnoses	Physical Status: Assessment Parameters/ Signs and Symptoms	Drug and Dose-Limiting Factors/ Nursing Implications
B. Constipation	• Normal pattern of bowel elimination • Consistency (hard, dry, small stools) • Frequency (hours or days beyond normal pattern) • Stool softener(s), laxative(s), efficacy • Assess medication profile for opioids, antiemetics	No BM × 48 h past normal bowel patterns • Hold vinca alkaloids (vinblastine, vincristine) • Teach patient to take stool softener with serotonin-antagonist antiemetic or opioids to prevent constipation from the drug

4. Hepatotoxicity	• Lab values: LDH, ALT, AST, alk phos, bili
	• Pain/tenderness over liver; feeling of fullness
	• Increase in n/v or anorexia
	• Changes in mental status
	• Jaundice
	• High-risk factors:
	  • Hepatic metastasis
	  • Concurrent hepatotoxic drugs
	  • Viral hepatitis
	  • Graft-vs-host disease
	  • Abdominal XRT
	  • Blood transfusions
		Evidence of chemical hepatitis:
		• Hold hepatotoxic agents (esp. methotrexate, 6-MP), until differential dx established
		• Hold oxaliplatin if venous occlusive disease suspected
		• Hold or dose-reduce drugs metabolized by liver if severe liver dysfunction (e.g., docetaxel, doxorubicin)
		• Hold imatinib mesylate if lab thresholds exceeded

(continued)

Table 1.1 *(Continued)*

Potential Problems/Nursing Diagnoses	Physical Status: Assessment Parameters/ Signs and Symptoms	Drug and Dose-Limiting Factors/ Nursing Implications
Respiratory System		

Impaired gas exchange or ineffective breathing pattern related to chemotherapy-induced pulmonary fibrosis	• Lab values: PFTs CXR
	 • Respirations (rate, rhythm, depth)
	 • Chest pain
	 • Nonproductive cough
	 • Progressive dyspnea
	 • Wheezing/stridor
	 • High-risk factors:
	   • Total cumulative dose of bleomycin
	   • Age > 60 years
	   • Preexisting lung disease
	   • Concomitant use of other pulmonary toxic drugs
	   • Prior/concomitant XRT
	   • Smoking hx
		• Acute unexplained onset respiratory symptoms, or worsening beyond baseline
		 • Hold all antineoplastic agents until differential dx established (e.g., bleomycin, busulfan, oxaliplatin, gemcitabine)
		 • Interstitial lung disease (ILD) is a class effect of EGFR antagonists (rare), e.g., cetuximab, erlotinib
		 • Chemotherapy drug may be combined with EGFR antagonists (e.g., gemcitabine and erlotinib). If pulmonary symptoms develop, hold drug until ILD can be ruled out

Cardiovascular System		
Decreased cardiac output related to chemotherapy-induced: 1. Cardiac arrhythmias 2. Cardiomyopathy 3. Hypertension 4. QTc Prolongation	• Lab values: cardiac enzymes, electrolytes, ECG, ECHO, MUGA, QTc interval measurement • Vital signs • Presence of arrhythmia (irregular radial/apical pulse) • Signs sx CHF (dyspnea, ankle edema, PND, decrease in LVEF, S_3 gallop, nonproductive cough, rales, cyanosis)	Acute sx CHF and/or cardiac arrhythmia • Hypertension: risk increased in combination with bevacizumab • Hold all antineoplastic agents until differential dx established • Total dose doxorubicin > 350–550 mg/m²; also assess epirubicin, daunorubicin cumulative dose and compare to drug threshold • Risk of CHF increased when chemotherapy given with trastuzumab; hold anthracyclines, trastuzumab, paclitaxel; monitor LVEF closely and hold drug per standard

Table 1.1 *(Continued)*

Potential Problems/Nursing Diagnoses	Physical Status: Assessment Parameters/ Signs and Symptoms	Drug and Dose-Limiting Factors/ Nursing Implications

	• History of Congenital Long QT Syndrome, CAD, medications which prolong QTc
	• High-risk factors:
	  • Total cumulative dose anthracyclines
	  • Preexisting cardiac disease
	  • Prior/concurrent mediastinel XRT
	  • Combined anthracycline, cyclophosphamide, trastuzumab, and paclitaxel
	  • LV EF < 50%; QTc > 500 msec
		• Trastuzumab should never be given **concomitantly** with doxorubicin
		• Monitor baseline and serial ejection fractions (LVEF) while receiving treatment with potentially cardiotoxic drugs; evaluate any significant ↓ in LVEF > 10% from baseline, or lower than LLN (e.g., 50%), drug is usually held
		• Severe hypertension: hold bevacizumab until hypertension controlled
		• Hold drug if QTc ≥ 500 msec, or > 50 msec longer than baseline QTc

Genitourinary System
 	
1. Alteration in fluid volume (excess) related to chemotherapy-induced:
  A. Glomerular or renal tubule damage
  B. Hyperuricemic nephropathy
2. Alteration in comfort related to chemotherapy-induced hemorrhagic cystitis
	• Lab values: BUN, creatinine clearance, serum creatinine, uric acid, electrolytes, urinalysis, magnesium, calcium, phosphate
	• Color, odor, clarity of urine
	• 24-hour fluid intake and output (estimate/actual)
	• Hematuria; proteinuria
	• Development of oliguria or anuria
	• High-risk factors:
	  • Preexisting renal disease
	  Concurrent treatment with nephrotoxic drugs (esp. aminoglycoside antibiotics)
	  • Bevacizumab: rare nephrotic syndrome
		• Hold cyclophosphamide, ifosfamide, cisplatin
		• Serum creatinine > 2.0 and/or
		• Creatinine clearance < 70 mL/min
		  Hematuria
		• Hold cisplatin, streptozotocin Anuria × 24 h
		• Hold bevacizumab if patient develops nephrotic syndrome or 24-hour urine shows protein more than 2 g
		• Check BUN/creatinine before treatment
		• 24-hour urine for protein if spilling protein

(continued)

Table 1.1 *(Continued)*

Potential Problems/Nursing Diagnoses	Physical Status: Assessment Parameters/ Signs and Symptoms	Drug and Dose-Limiting Factors/ Nursing Implications
Nervous System		
1. Impaired sensory/motor function related to chemotherapy-induced A. Peripheral neuropathy (PN) B. Cranial nerve neuropathy C. Acute oxaliplatin neurotoxicity D. Chemotherapy-induced cognitive changes	• Paresthesias (numbness, tingling in feet, fingertips) • Trigeminal nerve toxicity (severe jaw pain) • Jaw or muscle spasm • Diminished or absent deep tendon reflexes (ankle and knee jerks) • Motor weakness/slapping gait/ataxia • Visual and auditory disturbances • Cold-induced paresthesias and dysesthesias lasting < 14 days (oxaliplatin) • Cognitive changes may be influenced by genetics, comorbidities; incidence estimated at 20% of patients receiving standard-dose chemotherapy	• Presence of any neurologic signs and symptoms or worsening: • Perform brief nursing neuro exam before each treatment focusing on symptom analysis and functional impairment; consult MD for full neuro exam if signs/symptoms or worsening of existing signs/symptoms • For progressive chronic PN (grade 2 or higher), hold vinca alkaloids, cisplatin, examethylmelamine, oxaliplatin, procarbazine and discuss treatment plan with physician or midlevel • Acute oxaliplatin neurotoxicity: increase length of infusion time to 6 h (decreases peak serum level by 32%); teach patient to avoid cold exposure to hands/feet, oral mucosa for 1–3 days after oxaliplatin drug administration • Assess for motor/sensory changes, impact on function and ability to do ADLs prior to oxaliplatin, taxane, or cisplatin administration; hold for grades 3 and 4 toxicity (see *Appendix 2*)

Table 1.1 *(Continued)*

Potential Problems/Nursing Diagnoses	Physical Status: Assessment Parameters/ Signs and Symptoms	Drug and Dose-Limiting Factors/ Nursing Implications
		• Teach avoidance of cold for 1–3 days after oxaliplatin administration • Cognitive changes may appear after adjuvant therapy; assess for changes in memory, concentration, effect on work or school performance; reinforce teaching if slower ability to learn new information, following directions

2. Impaired bowel and bladder elimination related to chemotherapy-induced autonomic nerve dysfunction	• Urinary retention
	• Constipation/abdominal cramping and distension
	• High-risk factors:
	  • Changes in diet or mobility
	  • Frequent use of opioid analgesics
	  • Obstructive disease process
		Presence of any neurologic signs and symptoms
		• Hold vinca alkaloids until differential dx established

ALT = alanine aminotransferase; AST = aspartate aminotransferase; bili = bilirubin; BM = bowel movement; CHF = congestive heart failure; CXR = chest X-ray; dx = diagnosis; ECG = electrocardiogram; ECHO = echocardiogram; EGFR = epidermal growth factor receptor; 5-FU = 5-fluorouracil; hx = history; LDH = lactate dehydrogenase; LVEF = left ventricular ejection fraction; MUGA = multigated acquisition (MUGA heart scan); n/v = nausea and vomiting; PFT = pulmonary function test; 6-MP = 6-mercaptopurine; SOB = shortness of breath; sx = symptoms; XRT = radiation therapy. Modified from: Engleking C. Prechemotherapy Nursing Assessment in Outpatient Settings. *Outpatient Chemotherapy* 3(1) 10–11.

Table 1.2   Classifications of Antineoplastic Drugs

Classification	Mechanism of Action	Examples
Cell-Cycle Specific Agents		
Antimetabolites	Interfere with DNA and RNA synthesis by acting as false metabolites, which are incorporated into the DNA strand or block essential enzymes, so that DNA synthesis is prevented	Pemetrexate (Alimta) Cytosine arabinoside (ara-C, Cytosar-U) Eniluracil5-Fluorouracil (5-FU) Floxuridine (FUDR, 5-FUDR) Hydroxyurea (Hydrea) 6-Mercaptopurine (6-MP, purinethol) Methotrexate (amethopterin, Mexate, Folex) 6-Thioguanine (6-TG) Gemcitabine (Gemzar®) Fludarabine (Fludara®) Capecitabine (Xeloda®) Pralatrexate (Folotyn®)
Vinca Alkaloids	Crystallize microtubules of mitotic spindle causing metaphase arrest (vincristine, vinblastine, vindesine), role in blocking DNA and preventing cell division in M phase (vinorelbine)	Vincristine (VCR, Oncovin) Vinblastine (VLB, Velban) Vinorelbine (Navelbine®)
Epipodophyllotoxins	Damage the cell prior to mitosis, late S and G_2 phase; inhibit topoisomerase II	Etoposide (VP-16, Vepesid) Teniposide (VM-26, Vumon)
Taxanes	Promote early microtubule assembly; prevent depolymerization, causing cell death (paclitaxel); enhance microtubule assembly and inhibit tubulin depolymerization, thus arresting cell division in metaphase (docetaxel)	Paclitaxel (Taxol®) Docetaxel (Taxotere®) Paclitaxel protein bound Cabazitaxel (Jevtana®)
Epothilones	Naturally occurring microstabilizing agents similar to taxanes; bind tubulin and cause apoptotic cell death	Ixabepilone (Ixempra®) Investigational: Patupilone
Camptothecins *Miscellaneous*	Act in S phase to inhibit topoisomerase I and cause cell death	Topotecan (Hycamtin®) Irinotecan (CPT-11, Camptosar®) G_1 phase: L-asparaginase (ELSPAR), prednisone G_2 phase: Bleomycin (Bleo, Blenoxane)

Table 1.2 *(Continued)*

Classification	Mechanism of Action	Examples
	Cell Cycle-Nonspecific Agents	
Alkylating Agents	Substitute alkyl group for H⁺ ion causing single- and double-strand breaks in DNA, as well as crosslinkages; thus DNA strands are unable to separate during DNA replication	Bendamustine (Treanda) Busulfan (Myleran®, oral; Busulfex®, IV) Carboplatin (Paraplatin) *Carmustine (BiCNU, BCNU) Chlorambucil (Leukeran) Cisplatin (*Cis*-Platinum, CDDP, Platinol) Cyclophosphamide (Cytoxan, CTX, Neosar) Dacarbazine (DTIC-Dome, imidazole) Estramustine phosphate (Estracyte, Emcyt) Oxaliplatin (Eloxatin®) Ifosfamide (IFEX) *Lomustine (CCNU) Mechlorethamine hydrochloride (nitrogen mustard, mustargen, HN₂) Melphalan (Alkeran, 1-PAM, phenylala-nine mustard) Oxaliplatin (Eloxatin) *Streptozocin (streptozotocin, Zanosar) Thiotepa (triethylene thiophosphoramide, TSPA)
Antibiotics	Use a variety of mechanisms to prevent cell division and death (DNA strand breakage, intercalation of base pairs, inhibition of RNA and DNA synthesis)	Dactinomycin (actinomycin D, Cosmegan) Daunorubicin hydrochloride (daunomy-cin, cerubidine) Doxorubicin hydrochloride (Adria, adriamycin) Epirubicin HCl (Ellenee) Idarubicin (Idamycin) Mithramycin (mithramycin, plicamycin) Mitomycin C (Mito, mutamycin) Mitoxantrone (Novantrone)

*Nitrosoureas (cross blood–brain barrier).

Topoisomerase II is also involved in the relaxation of the helix torsion, but it causes a double-strand break to allow crossing of two double-stranded DNA segments. It then causes the closing of the two DNA strand breaks. This permits assembly of chromatin, as well as condensation and decondensation of the chromosomes, and separation of the DNA in the daughter cells during mitosis. Drugs that are well known to interfere with topoisomerase II are etoposide (non-intercalator and cell cycle specific for M phase) and doxorubicin (intercalator of base pairs and cell cycle nonspecific) (Eber, 1996).

Descriptions of the drugs in the chapter have been updated to reflect new indications. Agents that have now been approved by the Food and Drug Administration (FDA) for use in cancer treatment have been updated.

Table 1.3   ASCO/ONS Chemotherapy Administration Safety Standards and Management of Oral Chemotherapy (*See Document for Full Details)

Standard	Content
1.	Staffing-related standards: policies and procedures and/or guidelines for verification of training and continuing education for clinical staff
2.	Chemotherapy planning: chart documentation standards (e.g., diagnosis confirmation, staging, full medical history and PE, allergies, patient comprehension, psychosocial assessment and plan, chemotherapy treatment plan, assessment of patient's ability to obtain an oral agent, and frequency of outpatient follow-up for patients on oral agents)
3–8.	General chemotherapy practice standards (e.g., defines regimens, recommends lab evaluations, quality control of drug preparation)
9–14.	Chemotherapy order prescription standards (e.g., no verbal orders, complete chemotherapy order, procedure for notifying team and patient about discontinuation of oral agents)
15–17.	Drug preparation (e.g., independent double check prior to drug preparation, labeling, preparation, and isolation of intrathecal drug(s) separately from parenteral chemotherapy)
18–20.	Patient consent and education, for all chemotherapy, including oral chemotherapy. Education appropriate to the patient's and caregiver's reading/literacy level
21–23.	Chemotherapy administration (e.g., confirmation with patient planned treatment/drug(s), double check of chemotherapy, defined chemotherapy extravasation guidelines, a licensed independent practitioner is on site)
24–36.	Monitoring and assessment (e.g., protocol for life-threatening emergencies, policy/procedure to complete initial assessment of patient adherence to oral chemotherapy, patient assessment before chemotherapy, medication reconciliation)
	*Reference: Neuss MN, Polovich M, McNiff K et al. (2013) 2013 Updated American Society of Clinical Oncology/Oncology Nursing Society chemotherapy administration safety standards including standards for the safe administration and management of oral chemotherapy. Oncol Nurs Forum 40(3): 225–233
	Chemotherapy is defined as all antineoplastic agents, parenteral and oral, and includes traditional chemotherapy and targeted agents.

Data from: Neuss MN, Polovich M, McNiff K et al. (2013) ASCO/ONS Chemotherapy Safety Standards. Journal of Oncology Practice (Supplement to March 2013), DOI: 10.1200/JOP.2013.000874

EMERGING FRONTIERS

As our knowledge of genomics and proteogenomics grows, the possibility of individualized cancer therapy increases. Although the human genome was decoded in 2003, this only opened the door to understanding each of the 35,000 different genes. As each individual—except for identical twins—has a unique genetic makeup, so too each individual with cancer has individual genetic features of the tumor. Genetic signatures have emerged showing the different types and responses of colon/rectal, breast, and lung cancers to therapy (Allen and Johnston, 2005; Chen et al., 2007; Marsh and McLeod, 2006; O'Shaughnessy, 2006). Already, microarray technology is used to identify genetic signatures within tumors that are likely to respond to given drug therapy and those that are not. For example, a recent review of genomic markers in colorectal cancer revealed that tumors that overexpress thymidylate synthase (TS) and the 3*R/3*R TS gene polymorphism are resistant to 5-FU, whereas those with low TS gene expression have a response with increased survival (Allen and Johnston, 2005). Potti et al. (2006) reported that by using in vitro drug-sensitivity data, together with microarray gene-expression data, they were able to develop gene-expression signatures and predict sensitivity to individual chemotherapy drugs with 80% accuracy. This also allows prediction of effective chemotherapy and targeted therapy combinations.

A question that has recently been answered is which women with node-negative, estrogen receptor-positive breast cancer should receive adjuvant chemotherapy. A report by the National Surgical Adjuvant Breast and Bowel Project revealed that a 21-gene recurrence assay is able to quantify and predict the magnitude of benefit from chemotherapy (tamoxifen compared with tamoxifen plus chemotherapy). Women with a low recurrence risk (< 18%) derived minimal if any benefit from chemotherapy, whereas women with high-risk tumors (> 31%) derived a large benefit (an absolute decrease in 10-year distant recurrence rate) of 27.6% (mean). Women with intermediate recurrence did not appear to derive a large benefit, but the study could not say there was no benefit to receiving chemotherapy (Paik et al., 2006). As no two people have identical genetic makeups, their ability to metabolize drugs may also differ. Proteogenomics can help predict toxicity based on certain polymorphisms or different variations in a gene that is responsible for drug metabolism. Patients receiving irinotecan with a specific polymorphism have an increased risk of bone marrow suppression. For example, tamoxifen is a prodrug, which is metabolized into its active metabolite in the liver via the cytochrome P450 CYP2D6 microenzyme system. In a recent study, women who were poor metabolizers of tamoxifen were 2.5 times more likely to have breast cancer recurrence or death than women with normal CYP2D6 (Goetz et al., 2012).

New technology has permitted a reduction in toxicity and/or increasing dosing from a number of drugs. For instance, nanotechnology to manufacture liposomal delivery vehicles for docetaxel, doxorubicin, daunorubicin, cytarabine, amphotericin, paclitaxel, and camptothecins is currently available or is being studied. The liposomal "wrapping" of water-soluble or -insoluble drugs permits the drug to be preferentially delivered to sites of infection, inflammation, or tumor. Liposomes may pass through gaps in the endothelial lining of blood capillaries within the tumor, where the drug may be unpackaged and released within the tumor. Healthy tissues, on the other hand, have capillary walls that prevent the leakage of liposomes into the tissues, so that toxicity is reduced. The targeting of liposomes for specific tissues or disease sites is accomplished by variation in the number of lipid layers, and the size, charge, and permeability of the layers (Bangham, 1992). The future of nanotechnology has never been brighter, as seven national centers continue their study of different agents in nanotechnology-crafted devices (Jones, 2007). Efforts are being made to try to find agents offering equal efficacy that can improve quality of life, such as new oral antineoplastic agents, by minimizing trips to the hospital or intrusive administration techniques.

Within the last few years, interest and clinical testing of new approaches to old drugs has occurred. 5-Fluorouracil (5-FU) is an old drug that has good efficacy in colorectal cancer and other gastrointestinal cancers. However, it is limited, and increased doses are not necessarily more effective. Also, given by continuous infusion, 5-FU is often more effective because, being cell cycle specific for the S phase, more malignant cells are likely to be exposed to continuous infusion of chemotherapy than if the drug is given by bolus injection.

In an effort to improve the efficacy, new oral fluoropyrimidines have been developed, along with other agents that decrease the breakdown of 5-FU, so that serum drug levels are higher and more sustained, mimicking a continuous infusion. An example of a prodrug is capecitabine (Xeloda). In an effort to reduce the toxicity of bolus 5FU/LV, de Gramont et al. (1997) showed that infusional 5FU/LV was equivalent or, in one study, superior, in efficacy but significantly less toxic. This has become the standard way to administer 5FU/LV in the United States at this time. Capecitabine is preferentially taken up by tumor cells. The drug has been approved for both the adjuvant treatment of patients with colon cancer, as well as patients with advanced metastatic breast and colorectal cancers. Capecitabine has been shown to be equivalent to 5FU/LV and is being used as a replacement in combination with oxaliplatin, irinotecan, or alone during radiotherapy.

As the cancer treatment paradigm shifts toward the administration of oral chemotherapy as well as targeted agents, nurses must focus on patient safety, strategies to enhance adherence to prescribed therapy, and teaching patient/family to provide self-care, including notifying the provider of early toxicity. Successful treatment requires meticulous assessment of patient/family learning needs and styles, in addition to close telephone monitoring and triage of telephone calls. Other strategies may be useful in monitoring patient adherence, such as (1) giving the patients a detailed calendar showing the pill(s) to take each day/time, with small check boxes that they can check off as the dose is taken, (2) asking the patients to maintain a diary of dose administration and side effects, or (3) asking the patients to bring their pill bottles with them to each visit for a pill count. Studies are underway using electronic methods to monitor patient adherence (Goodin et al., 2007).

Planned drug holidays in patients with advanced cancers are another changing paradigm. A number of studies in patients with advanced colorectal cancer (CRC) showed that more aggressive therapy with 5-FU, leucovorin (LV), and oxaliplatin (FOLFOX) for 6 cycles, followed by maintenance using 5-FU/LV only for 12 cycles, and then returning to FOLFOX compared with FOLFOX4 continuously resulted in similar overall survival, but with less neurotoxicity in the group receiving a period of maintenance (OPTIMOX1) (Tournigand et al., 2006); however, completely halting chemotherapy for a period of time resulted in earlier onset of progression. A similar study by Labianca et al. (2006) of patients with metastatic CRC looked at intermittent 5-FU, LV, and irinotecan (FOLFIRI) and found similar survival with less toxicity and cost in patients receiving intermittent FOLFIRI compared with those receiving continuous FOLFIRI.

Finally, national evidence-based treatment guidelines based on randomized clinical trials for patients with specific types of cancer have been promulgated, and studies are beginning to document patients who receive therapy based on these guidelines compared with those that do not have lower mortality. Cronin et al. (2006) demonstrated that in the year 2000, patients with stage III rectal cancer were less likely to receive guideline-recommended treatment, whereas patients with stage III colon and stage II rectal cancer did, with a consequent decrease in their mortality regardless of their comorbidities. Although there did not appear to be any race/ethnicity bias, there were age disparities. There is compelling evidence in the treatment of patients with colon and rectal cancer that older patients derive the same benefit from chemotherapy without greater toxicity (Cronin et al., 2006). Nurses need to advocate for older patients to consider carefully all treatment options to derive the maximal benefit.

Oncology nurses work very hard to prevent or minimize toxicity from chemotherapy agents in their patients. It is now apparent that certain patients have different abilities to metabolize certain drugs, called polymorphisms, or variability in the genes that are responsible for metabolizing the drug. For example, if a patient does not metabolize the drug as well due to a genetic factor, that patient will have more toxicity, such as neutropenia. Pharmacogenetics is an emerging field that will allow the use of knowledge of polymorphisms and drug-metabolizing enzymes to maximize the benefit and minimize the risk to patients. For example, 10% of the US population expresses the UGT1A1*28 polymorphism, which reduces the metabolism of SN-38, the active metabolite of irinotecan. This results in higher serum levels with more grades 3 and 4 neutropenia in those patients who should receive lower doses of irinotecan. Patients can be tested for this allele, or any patient who has a high bilirubin should be suspected, and a lower dose of the drug should be used initially. In addition, genetic profiling will assist in predicting responses to certain chemotherapy agents such as 5-FU/cisplatin combinations, 5-FU, oxaliplatin, and other agents.

Stimulated by the success of taxanes, epothilones were discovered, and the first, ixabepilone (Ixempra), is now FDA-approved for patients with advanced breast cancer who have progressed on paclitaxel. Epothilones are a class of natural substances that cause tubulin polymerization and stabilization similar to paclitaxel. However, these substances have activity in tumor cell lines that are resistant to paclitaxel due to mutations in beta-tubulin (Altmann, 2003). Another agent that interferes with the tumor cell in mitosis is Eribulin mesylate (Halaven), a non-taxane microtubular dynamics inhibitor, a product of a sea sponge. Although fewer chemotherapy agents are being developed that have collateral damage in normal, frequently dividing organ systems, many more targeted agents are being developed and are presented in *Chapter 5*.

Antineoplastic agents are classified by mechanism of action (see Table 1.2). Cell cycle-specific agents are most active during specific phases of the cell cycle and include antimetabolites (S or synthesis phase), vinca alkaloids (M or mitotic phase), and miscellaneous drugs. Examples of these include L-asparaginase and prednisone (G_1 phase) and bleomycin and etoposide (G_2 phase). In addition, effective drugs such as the taxanes, which have a clear mechanism of action at therapeutic doses, may in fact have an antiangiogenic effect at lower, more frequent dosing. Endothelial cells appear to be very sensitive to the taxanes.

Cell cycle-nonspecific agents can damage cells in all phases of the cell cycle and include alkylating agents (cyclophosphamide, cisplatin), antitumor/antibiotics (doxorubicin, mitomycin-C), the nitrosoureas (carmustine, lomustine), and others (dacarbazine, procarbazine) (see Table 1.2).

Antineoplastic agents are effective because they interfere with cellular metabolism and replication, resulting in cell death. When malignant cells mutate and develop mechanisms to evade programmed cell death, the tumor cells are no longer sensitive to the drug(s), and resistance emerges. Because of their mechanism of action, it is critical that nurses protect themselves when handling these drugs so that they are not exposed to the potential drug hazards. These drugs can be:

- **Mutagenic**: capable of causing a change in the genetic material within a cell that can be passed on to future cell generations
- **Teratogenic**: capable of causing damage to a developing fetus exposed to the drug; the greatest risk is during the first trimester of pregnancy when the fetal organ systems are developing
- **Carcinogenic**: capable of causing malignant change in a cell

In 1985, the Occupational Safety and Health Administration (OSHA) developed guidelines for the safe handling of antineoplastic agents. These guidelines were revised in 1995 and then again in 2004 to include all hazardous drugs (see *Appendix I*). NIOSH has updated recommendations as of March 2004.

Hormones are used in the management of hormonally sensitive cancers, such as breast and prostate cancers. The hormone changes the hormonal environment, probably affecting growth factors, so that the stimulus for tumor growth is suppressed or removed (see Table 1.4). New selective estrogen receptor modulators (SERMs) and aromatize inhibitors are being developed to improve on the demonstrated success of tamoxifen.

Lastly, as obesity becomes a national health problem, the question arises about calculating dosages accurately. Thompson et al. (2010) conducted a survey of oncologists and board-certified oncology pharmacists, via the Association of Community Cancer Centers and Board of Pharmaceutical Specialties, to determine current practices of empiric chemotherapy dose adjustments in obese patients. Of the 174 responses, 95% were returned

Table 1.4   Common Hormonal Agents

Classification	Examples
Adrenocorticoids	cortisone
	hydrocortisone
	dexamethasone
	methylprednisone
	methylprednisolone
	prednisone
	prednisolone
Androgens	testosterone propionate (Neo-hombreol, Oreton)
Anti-androgens (nonsteroidal)	bicalutamide (Casodex)
	flutamide (Eulexin)
	nilutamide (Nilandron)
Androgen receptor inhibitors	enzalutamide (Xtandi)
Androgen biosynthesis inhibitors: CYP17 enzyme inhibitor (blocks other sources of androgen)	abiraterone (Zytiga)

Table 1.4 *(Continued)*

Classification	Examples
Lutenizing hormone-releasing hormone analog (LHRH analog), LH-RH agonist	Goserelin acetate (Zoladex) Histrelin (Vantas implant) leuprolide acetate (Lupron, Lupron depot) Triptorelin (Trelstar)
Gonadatropic-releasing hormone antagonist (suppresses lutenizing hormone (LH) and follicle-stimulating hormone (FSH) and thereby decreases testes production of testosterone	abarelix (Plenaxis) Degarelix (Firmagon)
Estrogens	chlorotrianisene (TACE) diethylstilbestrol (DES) diethylstilbestrol diphosphate (Stilphostrol) ethinyl estradiol (Estinyl) conjugated estrogen (Premarin) Stradiol
Selective estrogen receptormodulators (SERMs) (Anti-estrogen, nonsteroidal)	tamoxifen citrate (Nolvadex) toremifene citrate (Fareston) raloxifene (Evista)
Selective aromatase inhibitors (Anti-estrogen, nonsteroidal) • Reversible	anastrozole (Arimidex) letrozole (Femara)
Selective aromatase inhibitor Anti-estrogen (steroidal) • Irreversible	exemestane (Aromasin)
(Anti-estrogen)	Fulvestrant (Faslodex)
Progesterones	medroxyprogesterone acetate (Provera, Depo-Provera) megestrol acetate (Megace, Pallace)

by pharmacists, and of them, 50% practiced in academic medical centers. The most common methods used were (1) adjusted body weight in calculating BSA and (2) capping BSA. They found that indeed there was no standard of practice, but that decisions were determined based on intent to treat, degree of obesity, performance status, age, and type of medication. The American Society of Clinical Oncology (ASCO) developed clincial practice guidelines (2012) recommending that full weight-based cytotoxic chemotherapy doses be used, as they found no data to show increased toxicity at full weight-based dosing. They recommended further research into pharmacogenetics and the role of pharmacokinetics in obese patients.

COMPLICATIONS OF DRUG ADMINISTRATION

Complications include hypersensitivity reactions (HSRs) and extravasation. HSRs are mediated by an immune mechanism, IgE, and involve the release of vasoactive agents (e.g., histamine, leukotrienes, prostaglandins) by the mast cells in tissue and basophils in the blood *when exposed to a drug a second time, after prior exposure,* and thus, when the immune cells are sensitized. This results in contraction of smooth muscle and dilation of capillaries (Lenz, 2007). Patient response depends on the severity of the HSR, and ranges from rash to frank anaphylaxis. See Table 1.5.The systemic response is characterized by degrees of urticaria, rash, hypotension, more severe grade 3 bronchospasm (symptomatic, with angioedema), and grade 4 anaphylaxis, with profound vasomotor collapse. In contrast, some patients have a reaction, which may be severe, *on first exposure* to the drug. This reaction is not an immune reaction and is not mediated by IgE, but rather an *anaphylactoid* reaction, in which the drug or vehicle (e.g., Cremophor with paclitaxel) interacts with the mast cells and basophils, causing a release of the vasoactive agents; however, the end result is the same, and the nursing/medical interventions are the same whether the reaction is immune related or not. Thus, the nurse must be vigilant at all times when administering chemotherapy. Patients who have had hypersensitivity reactions to certain chemotherapy agents may be successfully desensitized and go on to complete their therapy (Feldweg et al., 2005).

All drugs can cause hypersensitivity reactions including anaphylaxis, but only a few drugs cause severe problems. These include the following:

- Paclitaxel (related to carrier vehicle solution Cremaphor)
- Docetaxel (related to delivery vehicle solution Tween)
- Cisplatin
- Carboplatin, oxaliplatin (delayed HSR, occurring around cycle 7)
- Teniposide (VumoM-26)
- Bleomycin (less common; 2% incidence in lymphoma patients)
- Cetuximab (Erbitux, discussed in *Chapter 4*), 3% incidence with most occurring on the first treatment, geographically related; may be fatal
- Rituximab (Rituxan, discussed in *Chapter 4*)
- Infliximab (Remicade discussed in *Chapter 5*)

In addition, certain drugs can cause delayed hypersensitivity, such as carboplatin and oxaliplatin, where the patient develops a range of signs and symptoms of hypersensitivity after receiving a number of cycles of the drug, such as 7 cycles of carboplatin. For nursing management of patients experiencing hypersensitivity or anaphylaxis, as recommended by the Oncology Nursing Society Practice Committee, see Table 1.5.

Table 1.5   Management of Hypersensitivity (HSR), Anaphylactic Reaction, Cytokine Release Syndrome (CRS), and Anaphylactoid Reaction

1. Review the patient's allergy history. Patients with preexisting allergies are at increased risk.
2. Review drug(s) to be administered and risk for a reaction.
   A. **HSR (chemotherapy):** L-asparaginase, bleomycin (5% incidence in lymphoma patients) paclitaxel, docetaxel, cisplatin, carboplatin, oxaliplatin, etoposide.
   B. **HSR, CRS (biotherapy):** interferons, interleukin-2, denileukin diftitox, murine and chimeric MAbs; recognize that patients can still react to humanized and human MAbs.
3. Consider prophylactic medications with hydrocortisone and/or an antihistamine in atopic/allergic individuals. (This requires a physician's order.)

Table 1.5   *(Continued)*

4. *Patient and family education*: Assess the patient's readiness to learn. Inform patient of the potential for an allergic reaction and instruct to report any unusual symptoms such as:
   A. Uneasiness or agitation
   B. Abdominal cramping
   C. Itching
   D. Chest tightness
   E. Light-headedness or dizziness
   F. Chills
5. Ensure that emergency equipment and medications are readily available.
6. Obtain baseline vital signs and note patient's mental status.
7. As appropriate, perform a scratch test, intradermal skin test, or test dose before administering the full dosage (this requires a physician's order). If there is no reaction, the remaining dose can be administered. If an allergic response is suspected, discontinue the test dose (unless it has been completed), maintain the intravenous line, and notify the physician.
8. For a *localized allergic response*:
   A. Evaluate symptoms; observe for urticaria, wheals, localized erythema.
   B. Administer diphenhydramine and/or hydrocortisone as per physician's order.
   C. Monitor vital signs every 15 minutes for 1 hour.
   D. Continue subsequent dosing or desensitization program according to a physician's order.
   E. If a "flare" reaction appears along the vein with doxorubicin (Adriamycin) or daunorubicin, flush the line with saline.
      a. Ensure that extravasation has not occurred.
      b. Administer hydrocortisone or diphenhydramine 25–50 mg intravenously with a physician's order, followed by a 0.9% NS flush. This may be adequate to resolve the "flare" reaction.
      c. Once the "flare" reaction has resolved, continue slow infusion of the drug.
      d. Monitor for repeated "flare" episodes. It is preferable to change the intravenous site if possible. Consider premedication with an antihistamine for subsequent cycles.
      e. Document specific observations, intervention, and patient response.
9. For a generalized allergic response, assess for the following signs or symptoms (these usually occur within the first 15 minutes of the start of the infusion or injection). Reaction can be either an *anaphylactoid (has never been exposed to the drug before) or anaphylaxis (severe hypersensitivity reaction after having received the drug before)*.
   A. Subjective signs and symptoms:
      a. Generalized itching
      b. Chest tightness
      c. Agitation
      d. Uneasiness
      e. Dizziness
      f. Nausea
      g. Crampy abdominal pain
      h. Anxiety
      i. Sense of impending doom
      j. Desire to urinate or defecate
      k. Chills
   B. Objective signs:
      a. Flushed appearance (edema of face, hands, or feet)
      b. Localized or generalized urticaria

(continued)

Table 1.5   (Continued)

   c. Respiratory distress with or without wheezing
   d. Hypotension
   e. Cyanosis
   f. Difficulty speaking
10. For a *generalized allergic response*:
   A. Stop the infusion immediately and notify the physician.
   B. Maintain the intravenous line with appropriate solution to expand the vascular space, e.g., NS.
   C. If not contraindicated, ensure maximum rate of infusion if the patient is hypotensive.
   D. Position the patient to promote perfusion of the vital organs; the supine position is preferred.
   E. Monitor vital signs every 2 minutes until stable, then every 5 minutes for 30 minutes, then every 15 minutes as ordered.
   F. Reassure the patient and the family.
   G. Maintain the airway and anticipate the need for cardiopulmonary resuscitation.
   H. All medications must be administered with a physician's order.
   I. Anticipate administering the following medications for the following effects:
     a. Vasoconstriction to increase cardiac output and blood pressure, as well as bronchodilation to open the airway:
       1) epinephrine (1:1,000, 0.3–0.5 mL or 0.3–0.5 mg IM or subcutaneous q 10–15/min; or if hypotensive, 1:10,000 concentration giving 0.5–1.0 mL [0.1 mg] IVP in adults; in pediatrics, 1:1,000 0.01 mL/kg [up to 0.3 mL])
       2) dopamine 2–20 micrograms/kg/min (adults)
     b. Antihistamines to stop allergic release of histamines:
       1) diphenhydramine: 25–50 mg IVP (adults), 1 mg/kg (max 50 mg), pediatrics
       2) ranitidine 50 mg IV or famotidine 20 mg IV (adults)
     c. Bronchodilation: aminophylline 5 mg/kg IV over 30 min (adults)
     d. Anti-inflammation/bronchodilation: steroids. Hydrocortisone 100–500 mg IV (peds 1–2 mg/kg), or methylprednisolone 30–50 mg IV (peds 0.3–0.5 mg/kg), or dexamethasone 10–20 mg IVP (peds 1–2 mg/kg), or hydrocortisone 100–500 mg IV (peds 1–2 mg/kg)
11. Document the incident in the medical record according to institution policy and procedures.
12. Physician-guided desensitization may be necessary for subsequent dosing.

Source: Data from Polovich M, Olsen M, LeFebvre KB. (eds), *Chemotherapy and Biotherapy Guidelines and Recommendations for Practice.* 4th ed. Pittsburgh, PA: ONS 2014; 163–168;. Ellis AK, Day JH. Diagnosis and Management of Anaphylaxis. *Canadian Medical Association Journal* 2003; 169(4) 307–312. Sheperd GM. Hypersensitivity Reactions to Chemotherapeutic Drugs. *Allergy and Immunology* 2003; 24 253–262.

EXTRAVASATION

Specific chemotherapeutic drugs called *vesicants* may cause severe tissue necrosis if extravasated or inadvertently administered outside the vein. Some of these drugs have antidotes that will minimize or prevent local tissue damage. These are shown in Table 1.6. For a Standardized Nursing Care Plan for management of patients experiencing extravasation, see Table 1.7. It is imperative that the nurse be very careful when administering vesicant chemotherapy to minimize the chance of this occurring. The nurse carefully assesses the patient's response, the administration site, and patency of the IV site throughout the

Table 1.6   Vesicants and Irritants

Chemotherapeutic Agents	Antidote	Antidote Preparation	Antidote and Local Care	Comments, Patient Monitoring, and Follow-Up
			Vesicants	
Alkylating agents				

Mechlorethamine (nitrogen mustard, Mustargen®)	Isotonic sodium (Na) thiosulfate	Prepare 1/6 molar solution
		
		1. **10% Na thiosulfate** solution, mix 4 mL with 6 mL sterile water for injection.
		2. **25% Na thiosulfate** solution, mix 1.6 mL with 8.4 mL sterile water.
		3. Store at room temperature (15°C–30°C or 59°F–86°F).
			1. Inject antidote (2 mL sodium thiosulfate solution for each mg of mechlorethamine extravasated) into subcutaneous (SC) tissue of the area of extravasation, using a 25- or 27-gauge needle (change needle with each injection).
			2. Teach patient to
			  a. apply ice for 6–12 hrs after antidote administration.
			  b. elevate arm and hand, and to report swelling right away (peripheral extravasation).
				1. Na thiosulfate neutralizes nitrogen mustard, forming thioesters, which are excreted via the kidneys.
				2. Time is essential in treating extravasation.
				3. Apply ice for 6–12 hours after antidote administered to minimize local reaction (Lundbeck, 2012).
				4. Assess the extravasation area the next day for pain, blister formation, and desquamation; then in accordance with policy and clinical judgment.
				5. Teach the patient/caregiver to monitor the extravasation site and call the practice right away if fever, chills, worsening pain, blistering, desquamation, swelling.

(continued)

23

Table 1.6 *(Continued)*

Vesicants

Chemotherapeutic Agents	Antidote	Antidote Preparation	Antidote and Local Care	Comments, Patient Monitoring, and Follow-Up
Antitumor antibiotics				
Anthracyclines Doxorubicin (Adriamycin®) Daunorubicin (Cerubidine) Epirubicin (Ellence) Idarubicin (Idamycin)	Dexrazoxane	Drug may cause fetal harm if used during pregnancy; nursing mothers should discontinue nursing or discontinue the drug (Topotarget, 2011). Dexrazoxane **must be started within 6 hours of the extravasation.** Dose: Day 1: 1,000 mg/m² Day 2: 1,000 mg/m² Day 3: 500 mg/m²; Maximum dose per day: days 1, 2 is 2g and on day 3 is 1g. Dose-reduce 50% for impaired renal function (cr cl < 40 mL/min). Mix each 500 mg drug vial with 50 mL diluent, and further dilute in 1L NS.	1. Apply cold pad with circulating ice water, ice pack, or Cryogel pack for 15–20 min at least 4 times a day until able to start antidote. 2. Remove ice at least 15 min prior to starting dexrazoxane. 3. DO NOT give with DMSO as this may worsen injury. 4. Use safe chemotherapy, safe handling, and administration precautions. 5. Administer IV over 1–2 hr in a large vein in the opposite arm unless contraindicated (e.g., lymphedema); in that case, use large vein distal to the extravasation site. 6. Give at about the same time each day × 3. 7. Teach patient about self-care measures and side effects of dexrazoxane: nausea, vomiting, stomatitis, BMD, elevated LFTs, burning at the infusion site.	1. Dexrazoxane is a free-radical scavenger so protects tissue from free radical damage caused by anthracycline extravasation. Totect™ is FDA-approved for anthracycline extravasation; however, dexrazoxane (generic or Zinecard®) has been shown to be effective (Arroyo et al., 2010). 2. Extravasations of less than 1–2 cc often will heal spontaneously. If greater than 3 cc, ulceration often results. 3. Assess the extravasation each day of dexrazoxane treatment: presence or worsening of pain, blister formation, desquamation; then in accordance with policy and clinical judgment. 4. Teach the patient/caregiver to elevate the affected arm/hand, to monitor the extravasation site, and to call the practice right away if fever, chills, worsening pain, blistering, desquamation, or arm/hand stiffening or swelling occurs. 5. Teach patient to protect the extravasation site from sunlight and heat. 6. Discuss frequency of assessing cbc/plt, LFTs after administering dexrazoxane (Totect™) with physician or NP/PA.

Table 1.6 *(Continued)*

Vesicants

Chemotherapeutic Agents	Antidote	Antidote Preparation	Antidote and Local Care	Comments, Patient Monitoring, and Follow-Up
		Use PPE in handling and administration of drug as it is hazardous (e.g., chemo gown and gloves). Store at room temperature (15°C–30°C or 59°F–86°F).		7. Most common adverse effects of dexrazoxane are nausea, pyrexia, injection-site pain, and vomiting. 8. If drug is given in a clinic setting, anticipate how and where dexrazoxane will be administered if the extravasation occurs on a Thursday or Friday as the drug must be given 3 days in a row.
Other Antitumor Antibiotics Mitomycin (mitomycin-C, Mutamycin®)	None known		1. Apply ice pack 15–20 min at least 4 times a day, for the first 24 hours, to increase comfort at the site. 2. Elevate for 48 hours, then resume normal activity.	1. Protect from sunlight. 2. Delayed skin reactions have occurred in areas far from original IV site. 3. Assess the extravasation area the next day for pain, blister formation, desquamation, then in accordance with policy and clinical judgment. 4. Teach the patient/caregiver to elevate the affected arm/hand, to monitor the extravasation site, and to call the practice right away if fever, chills, worsening pain, blistering, desquamation, or arm/hand stiffening or swelling occurs. 5. Discuss with physician or NP/PA referral to specialists as needed (e.g., plastic/hand surgeon, OT/PT, pain management).

(continued)

25

Table 1.6 *(Continued)*

			Vesicants	
Chemotherapeutic Agents	Antidote	Antidote Preparation	Antidote and Local Care	Comments, Patient Monitoring, and Follow-Up
Anthracenedione Mitoxantrone (concentrated dose) [Novantrone]	Unknown		1. Apply ice pack 15–20 min at least 4 times a day, for the first 24 hours, to increase comfort at the site. 2. Teach patient to elevate arm/hand.	1. Antidote and local care measures unknown. 2. Ulceration rare unless concentrated dose infiltrates. 3. Drug is blue and causes blue skin discoloration. 4. Assess the extravasation area for pain, blister formation, desquamation, arm or hand stiffening or swelling the next day, then in accordance with policy and clinical judgment. 5. Teach the patient/caregiver to monitor the extravasation site and call the practice right away if fever, chills, worsening pain, blistering, desquamation, or hand stiffening or swelling occurs. 6. Discuss with physician or NP/PA referral to specialists as needed (e.g., plastic/hand surgeon, OT/ PT, pain management).

Vinca alkaloids/microtubular inhibiting agents

Vincristine (Oncovin®e) Vinblastine (Velban®e) Vinorelbine (Navelbine®f)	Hyaluronidase	Hyaluronidase: Amphadase (bovine): Vial contains 150 units per 1 mL: use undiluted; store in refrigerator at 2–8°C (36–46°F).	1. Administer 1 mL of hyaluronidase solution as five separate injections, each containing 0.2 mL of hyaluronidase into the area of extravasation, using a 25- or 27-gauge needle (change needle with each injection).	1. Hyaluronidase is an enzyme that degrades hyaluronic acid so that extravasated drug diffuses away from site of injury and is absorbed. 2. Assess the extravasation area for pain, blister formation, desquamation, hand/arm swelling the next day, then in accordance with policy and clinical judgment.

Table 1.6 *(Continued)*

		Vesicants	
Chemotherapeutic Agents	**Antidote**	**Antidote Preparation**	**Antidote and Local Care**	**Comments, Patient Monitoring, and Follow-Up**
		Hydase: Vial contains 150 units per 1 mL: use undiluted; store in refrigerator at 2–8°C (36–46°F). Hylenex: Vial contains 150 units per 1 mL: use undiluted; store in refrigerator at 2–8°C (36–46°F). Vitrase (bovine): Vial contains 200 units per 1 mL: Dilute 0.75 mL solution with 0.25 mL 0.9% sodium chloride (final concentration is 150 units per 1 mL); store in refrigerator at 2–8°C (36–46°F).	2. Apply warm pack for 15–20 min at least four times per day for the first 24–48 hours and elevate arm/hand.	3. Teach the patient/caregiver to monitor the extravasation site and call the practice right away if fever, chills, worsening pain, blistering, desquamation, arm/hand swelling or stiffness occurs.

(continued)

Table 1.6 *(Continued)*

		Vesicants		
Chemotherapeutic Agents	Antidote	Antidote Preparation	Antidote and Local Care	Comments, Patient Monitoring, and Follow-Up

Taxanes

Chemotherapeutic Agents	Antidote	Antidote Preparation	Antidote and Local Care	Comments, Patient Monitoring, and Follow-Up
Paclitaxel (Taxol®a) Docetaxel (Taxotere®) Paclitaxel protein-bound particles for injectable suspension (albumin-bound) [Abraxane].	None	None known	Apply ice pack for 15–20 min at least four times per day for the first 24 hours.	1. Paclitaxel: injection-site reactions, including those following extravasation: – are usually mild (erythema, tenderness, skin discoloration, swelling at injection site). Recall of skin reactions can occur. – more severe events have been reported (phlebitis, cellulitis, induration, skin exfoliation, necrosis, fibrosis), which may be delayed up to 7–10 days from date of extravasation (Teva, 2012). 2. Docetaxel infusion-site reactions are generally mild (hyperpigmentation, inflammation, erythema, skin dryness, extravasation, phlebitis or swelling of the arm) [Sanofi-Aventis, 2014]. 3. Abraxane® may cause phlebitis, cellulitis, induration, necrosis, and fibrosis during or up to 7–10 days after a prolonged infusion. Recall may occur at a prior site of paclitaxel injection. Abraxane infusion should be infused over 30 minutes to reduce infusion-related adverse reactions (Celgene, 2013). 4. Assess the extravasation area the next day for pain, blister formation, desquamation, hand/arm swelling and stiffness, then in accordance with policy and clinical judgment.

Table 1.6 *(Continued)*

Chemotherapeutic Agents	Vesicants			Comments, Patient Monitoring, and Follow-Up
	Antidote	Antidote Preparation	Antidote and Local Care	

				5. Teach the patient/caregiver to
				  a. apply ice pack (per local care above)
				  b. monitor the extravasation site and call the practice right away if fever, chills, worsening pain, blistering, desquamation, arm/hand swelling or stiffness occurs.

	Irritants			

Alkylating agents

Chemotherapeutic Agents				Comments, Patient Monitoring, and Follow-Up
Bendamustine hydrochloride (Treanda®)				1. May cause erythema, marked swelling and pain; dilution in 500mL and infusion over 1–2 hours reduces venous irritation (Watanabe et al., 2013).
Dacarbazine (DTIC)				1. May cause phlebitis. 2. Protect drug from sunlight.
Ifosfamide Carboplatin				1. May cause phlebitis. 2. Antidote or local care measures unknown.
Melphalan (Alkeran®)				1. Consider using a CL if the patient has poor venous access (GlaxoSmithKline, 2010).

(continued)

Table 1.6 *(Continued)*

Chemotherapeutic Agents	Irritants			
	Antidote	Antidote Preparation	Antidote and Local Care	Comments, Patient Monitoring, and Follow-Up
Oxaliplatin (however, has vesicant potential)				1. Oxaliplatin has vesicant potential, so is best given via CL, although care must be taken as it can still extravasate from a CL. If oxaliplatin given via peripheral line, drug can be diluted in 500 mL D5W (Sanofi-Aventis, 2014) and infused over 6 hours to decrease discomfort. 2. High-dose dexamethasone can reduce inflammation in the event of extravasation (Kretzschman et al, 2003). Topical heat may reduce discomfort.
Antitumor antibiotics				
Daunorubicin citrate (DaunoXome®)				1. May cause pain or burning at IV site. 2. Antidote or local care measures unknown.
Nitrosoureas				
Carmustine (BCNU)				1. Diluent is absolute alcohol and may cause phlebitis. Local care measures are unknown. 2. Antidote or local care measures unknown.
Antitumor antibiotics				
Doxorubicin liposome (Doxil®)				1. May produce redness and tissue edema. 2. Low ulceration potential. 3. If ulceration begins or pain, redness, or swelling persist, treat like doxorubicin.

Table 1.6 *(Continued)*

Chemotherapeutic Agents	Antidote	Antidote Preparation	Antidote and Local Care	Comments, Patient Monitoring, and Follow-Up
			Irritants	
Bleomycin (Blenoxane®)				1. May cause irritation to tissue. 2. Little information known.
Epipodophyllotoxin				
Etoposide (VP-16)			Apply warm pack.	1. Treatment necessary only if large amount of a concentrated solution extravasates. In this case, treat like vincristine or vinblastine. 2. May cause phlebitis, urticaria, and redness.

[a] Bristol-Myers-Squibb Oncology, Princeton, NJ

[b] Pharmacia & Upjohn Co, Kalamazoo, MI

[c] Chiron Therapeutics, Emeryville, CA

[d] Andria Laboratories, Dublin, OH

[e] Eli Lilly and Co., Indianapolis. IN

[f] Glaxo Wellcome Oncology/HIV, Research Triangle Park, NC

Data from: Lundbeck ILC. Mustargen [package insert]. Deerfield, IL. 2012; Polovich M, Olsen M, LeFebvre KB. (eds), *Chemotherapy and Biotherapy Guidelines and Recommendations for Practice.* 4th ed. Pittsburgh, PA: ONS 2014; 155–163; Polovich M, White JM, & Kelleher LO. *Chemotherapy and Biotherapy Guidelines and Recommendations for Practice*, 2nd ed. Pittsburgh, PA: Oncology Nursing Society; 2005: 34; Griffin-Sobel JP. *Clin J Oncol Nurs* 2005; 9(5) 510; Sanofi-Aventis US, LLC. Taxotere [package insert]. Bridgewater, NJ, May 2014; Teva Parenteral Medicines, Inc. Paclitaxel Injection [package insert]. Sellersville, PA, August 2012; Totect [package insert]. Rockaway, NJ: TopoTarget USA, October 2007.

Table 1.7   Standardized Nursing Care Plan for Management of the Patient Experiencing Extravasation

Nursing Diagnosis	Defining Characteristics	Expected Outcomes	Nursing Interventions

I. Potential alteration in skin integrity related to extravasation.	I. Vesicant drugs may cause erythema, burning, tissue necrosis, tissue sloughing.	I. Extravasation, if it occurs, is detected early with early intervention to minimize severity and extent of injury.	I. Careful technique is used during venipuncture.
			  A. Select venipuncture site away from underlying tendons and blood vessels.
			  B. Secure IV so that catheter/needle site is visible at all times.
			  C. Administer vesicant through freely flowing IV, constantly monitoring IV site, blood return, and patient response. Nurse should be thoroughly familiar with institutional policy and procedure for administration of a vesicant agent, and management of extravasation.
			  D. If vesicant drug is administered as a continuous infusion, drug must be given through a patent central line and monitored closely.

II. Potential pain at site of extravasation.	II. Vesicant drugs include:
	  A. Commercial agents
	    1. dactinomycin
	    2. daunorubicin
	    3. doxorubicin
	    4. mitomycin C
	    5. estramustine
	    6. mechlorethamine
	    7. vinblastine
	    8. vincristine
	    9. vinorelbine
	    10. idarubicin
		II. Skin and underlying tissue damage is minimized.	II. If extravasation is suspected:
			  A. Stop drug administration.
			  B. Aspirate any residual drug and blood from IV tubing, IV catheter/needle, IV site if possible.
			  C. Instill antidote, if one exists, through needle if able to remove remaining drug in previous step. If standing orders are not available, notify MD and obtain order.
			  D. Remove needle.
			  E. Inject antidote into area of apparent infiltration, if antidote is recommended, using 25-gauge needle into subcutaneous tissue.

32

Table 1.7 *(Continued)*

Nursing Diagnosis	Defining Characteristics	Expected Outcomes	Nursing Interventions

	11. vindesine
	12. epirubicin
	13. esorubicin
	14. cisplatin
	    (if concentrated)
	15. mitoxantrone
	16. paclitaxel
	    (if concentrated)
	17. fluorouracil
	    (if concentrated)
	B. Investigational
	   agents
	   1. amsacrine
	   2. maytansine
	   3. bisantrene
	   4. pyrazofurin
	   5. adozelesin
	   6. anti-B4-blocked
	     ricin
			F. Apply topical cream if recommended.
			G. Cover lightly with occlusive sterile dressing.
			H. Apply warm or cold applications as prescribed.
			I. Elevate arm.
			J. Assess site regularly for pain, progression of erythema, induration, and for evidence of necrosis:
			   1. If outpatient, arrange to assess site or teach patient to and to notify provider if condition worsens. Arrange next visit for assessment of site depending on drug, amount infiltrated, extent of potential injury, and patient variables.
			   2. Discuss with MD the need for plastic-surgical consult if erythema, induration, pain, tissue breakdown occurs.
			   3. Assess the extravasation area the next day for pain, blister formation, and desquamation; then in accordance with policy and clinical judgment.
			   4. Teach the patient/caregiver to monitor the extravasation site and call the practice right away if fever, chills, worsening pain, blistering, desquamation.
			   5. Document monitoring plan and follow up concisely.
			K. When in doubt about whether drug is infiltrating, treat as an infiltration.
			L. Document precise, concise information in patient's medical record:
			   1. Date, time
			   2. Insertion site, needle size, and type

(continued)

Table 1.7 *(Continued)*

Nursing Diagnosis	Defining Characteristics	Expected Outcomes	Nursing Interventions
			3. Drug administration technique, drug sequence, and approximate amount of drug extravasated
			4. Appearance of site, patient's subjective response
			5. Nursing interventions performed to manage extravasation, and notification of MD
			6. Photo documentation if possible
			7. Follow-up plan
			8. Nurse's signature
			9. Institutional policy and procedure for documentation should be adhered to

III. Potential loss of function of extremity related to extravasation.

IV. Potential infection related to skin breakdown.

Data from Polovich M, Whitford JM, Olsen M (eds). Chemotherapy and Biotherapy Guidelines and Recommendations for Practice. 3rd ed. Pittsburgh, PA: ONS; 2009: 105–110.

administration of the vesicant agent. If ever in doubt whether or not a drug is extravasating, treat it as an extravasation to minimize potential tissue damage to the patient; then, start another IV in the patient's other arm, and continue the drug administration.

When vesicants are administered as a continuous infusion, a central line (CL) is required. In addition, it is imperative that the CV insertion site be checked for signs/symptoms of extravasation regularly, and that the patient be instructed to tell the nurse immediately if stinging or burning is felt. As many continuous infusions of vesicant chemotherapy occur when the patient is at home, it is again imperative to instruct the patient to pay attention to any changes in sensation at the site, and to call the nurse if any discomfort, stinging, or burning is felt. A number of patients have had extravasation of drug from a huber needle dislodged from an implanted port, onto or under the surrounding skin, which then caused a necrotic ulcer and necessitated explantation of the subcutaneous port. Dexrazoxane for injection (Totect™) was approved for the treatment of doxorubicin extravasations. It works as a free radical scavenger and may inhibit topoisomcrase II irreversibly (Mouridsen et al., 2007; Schulmeister, 2007); however, the drug in itself is cytotoxic, expensive, and must be administered within 6 hours of the extravasation. The drug is given as an infusion daily for 3 days.

Within the last decade, oncology nurses have been humbled by the reports of significant and lethal errors that have occurred during the chemotherapy prescription, admixing, and administration processes. It is clear that institutional and physician office practices must have systematic review of the entire linked process and take steps to prevent the occurrence of these errors and tragic consequences through competent checks and balances. Fortunately, the series of well-publicized errors has been a "wake-up" call, and oncology nurses, pharmacists, and physicians have worked together to develop safe environments for clinical practice. The Oncology Nursing Society position paper, "Regarding the Preparation of the Professional Registered Nurse Who Administers and Cares for the Individual Receiving Chemotherapy," states that the nurse administering chemotherapy and caring for patients receiving chemothcrapy should complete a chemotherapy course and clinical practicum to deliver chemotherapy safely and competently. The course topics should include history of cancer chemotherapy; drug development; principles of cancer chemotherapy; chemotherapy preparation, storage, and transport; nursing assessment; chemotherapy administration; safety precautions during chemotherapy administration; disposal/accidental exposure and spills; and, finally, institutional considerations (ONS Position Paper, revised 6/99: ONS Safe Handling of Hazardous Drugs, 2003; NIOSH Safe Handling of Hazardous Drugs, June 2004).

In an effort to recognize and encourage quality in the care of oncology patients, ASCO and ONS have joined together to issue "Chemotherapy Administration Safety Standards," which specify for the first time in 2008 the expected standards in providing chemotherapy to patients in the outpatient setting. These guidelines are now being applied to inpatient settings, and in 2013, updated guidelines include the administration of oral chemotherapy (antineoplastic therapy). See Table 1.3. Further, ASCO's Quality Oncology Practice Initiative (QOPI) ensures that these standards are supported in the oncologist-led, practice-based quality improvement program.

Finally, in the last decade, we have seen new challenges. As the frequency of cancer chemotherapy treatments has increased, so has the demand for these drugs, leading to drug shortages. In 2013, up to 83% of oncologists have experienced a drug shortage (Gogineri et al., 2013). In the study, 78% of oncologists reported treating the patient with a different drug or drug regimen, 77% substituted different drugs partway through therapy, 43% had to delay treatment, 37% had to choose among patients who need a particular drug, 29% omitted doses, 20% gave reduced doses, and 17% referred patients to another practice. Clearly, the drug shortage is interfering with high-quality cancer care in the United States.

In the past, a Drug Shortages Summit was convened by ASHP, the Institute for Safe Medication Practices (ISMP), the American Society of Anesthesiologists, and the American Society of Clinical Oncology (ASCO). The group found that in addition to increased demand for some of the drugs, fewer manufacturers are producing sterile injectables, and most are generic. Not only does this decrease the manufacture of some of the drugs, but two of the largest manufacturers of sterile injectables were forced to shut down some production lines in 2010 due to inadequate quality-control standards, further reducing supply of the products (Drug Shortages Summit Summary Report, 2010). The ASHP has been instrumental in monitoring drugs in short supply, identifying those that have been resolved, and providing guidance for hospitals and health systems (Fox et al., 2009). Today, the shortage is often of common generic chemotherapy drugs, forcing physicians to substitute more expensive brand name drugs or similar drugs that may not have the supporting clinical trial evidence to support it. In addition, supportive medications such as antiemetics may also be in short supply. The Government Accountability Office conducted an investigation of the causes of the shortages which was released in a report in February 2014. Finally, ASCO has asked Congress to convene a panel that will bring together providers, manufacturers, suppliers, the FDA, and patients to discuss how to control this issue.

References

Abbott Laboratories. Lupron Depot 45 mg 6-month depot [package insert]. Abbott Laboratories: North Chicago, IL, June 2011.

Ahles TA, Saykin AJ. Candidate Mechanisms for Chemotherapy-Induced Cognitive Changes. *Nat Rev Cancer* 2007; 7 192−201.

Ajani JA, Dodd LS, Daughtery K, et al., Taxol-Induced Soft-Tissue Injury Secondary to Extravasation: Characterization by Histo-Pathology and Clinical Course. *JNCI* 1994; 86 51−53.

Anova Rx Distribution LLC. Purixan (mercaptourine suspension) [package insert]. Memphis, TN, April 2014.

Astra Zeneca. Arimidex (anastrazole) [package insert]. Wilmington, DE, May 2014.

Aubert RE, Stanek EJ, Yao J, et al. 2009 Risk of Breast Cancer Recurrence in Women Initiating Tamoxifen with CYP2D6 Inhibitors. *J Clin Oncol* 27:18s, (suppl; abst CRA 508).

Baylin SB, Herman JG, Graff JR, et al. Alterations in DNA Methylation-A Fundamental Aspect of Neoplasia. *Adv Cancer Res* 1998; 72 141−196.

Bedford Laboratories. VinBLAStine sulfate [package insert]. Bedford, OH, April 2014.

Camp-Sorrell D. Chemotherapy Toxicities and Management. *Chapter 17* in Yarbro CH, Frogge MH, Goodman M. *Cancer Nursing: Principles and Practice,* 6th ed. Sudbury, MA: Jones and Bartlett Publishers; 2005: 412−458.

Celgene Corporation. Abraxane (protein-bound paclitaxel particles for injectable suspension) [package insert]. Summit, NJ, October 2013.

Celgene Corporation. Vidaza (azacitidine for injection) [package insert]. Summit, NJ, Jan 2014.

Centocor Ortho Biotech Inc. Zytiga [package insert]. Centocor Ortho Biotech Inc: Horsham, PA, April 2011.

Chen HY, et al. 5 Gene Pattern Predicts NSCLC Outcome. *New Engl J Med* 2007; 356 11–20.

Chiron Therapeutics. *Depocyt* [package insert]. Emeryville, CA, Chiron Therapeutics; 2007.

Ciuleanu TE, Brodowicz T, Belani CP, et al. Maintenance Pemetrexed Plus Best Supportive Care (BSC) Versus Placebo Plus BSC: A Phase III Study. *J Clin Oncol* 2008; 26 (May 20 suppl; abstr 8011).

Clinical Trials. *Colorectal Cancer Trials Involving Irinotecan and the Saltz Regimen Are Temporarily Suspended* 2001; http://www.cancer.gov/clinicaltrials. Accessed October 16, 2009.

Cortes J, Baselga J. Targeting the Microtubules in Breast Cancer Beyond Taxanes: The Epothilones. *Oncologist* 2007; 12 271–280.

Cronin DP, Harlan LC, Potosky AL, et al. Patterns of Care for Adjuvant Therapy in a Random Population-Based Sample of Patients Diagnosed with Colorectal Cancer. *Am J Gastroenterol* 2006; 101(10) 2308–2318.

Dang C, Smith K, Fornier M, et al. Updated Cardiac Safety Results with Dose-Dense (DD) Doxorubicin and Cyclophosphamide (AC) Followed by Paclitaxel (T) with Trastuzumab (H) in HER2/neu Overexpressed/Amplified Breast Cancer (BCA). *J Clin Oncol* 2006; 24(18S) 582 (abstract).

Davies C, Pan H, Goodwin J, and et al. (2013). Long-term effects of continuing adjuvant tamoxifen to 10 years versus stopping at 5 years after diagnosis of oestrogen receptor-positive breast cancer: ATLAS, a randomized trial. *Lancet* 381(9869): 805–816.

deGramont A, Boni C, Navarro M, et al. Oxaliplatin/5FU/LV in the Adjuvant Treatment of Stage II and Stage III Colon Cancer: Efficacy Results with a Median Follow-up of 4 years. Oral Abstract Presented at: ASCO 2005 Gastrointestinal Cancers Symposium; January 27–29, 2005; Hollywood, FL.

deGramont A, Bossett JF, Milan C, et al. Randomized Trial Comparing Monthly Low-Dose Leucovorin and Fluorouracil Bolus with Bimonthly High-Dose Leucovorin and Fluorouracil Bolus Plus Continuous Infusion for Advanced Colorectal Cancer: A French Intergroup Study. *J Clin Oncol* 1997; 15 808–815.

Deshmane V, Krishnamurthy S, Melemed AS, et al. Phase III Double Blind Trial of Arzoxifene Compared with Tamoxifen for Locally Advanced or Metastatic Breast Cancer. *Clin J Oncol* 2007; 25(31) 4967–4973.

Drug Shortages Summit Members. Drug Shortages Summit Summary Report, November 5, 2010. Available at http://www.ashp.org/drugshortages/summitreport. Accessed July 4, 2011.

Eisai Inc. *Havalan (eribulin mesylate)* [package insert]. Woodcliff Lake, NJ: Eisai Inc, August 2014.

Ellis AK, Day JH. Diagnosis and Management of Anaphylaxis. *Can Med Assoc J* 2003; 169(4) 307–312.

Emanuel EJ, Shuman K, Chinn D et al. (2013). Impact of oncology drug shortages. *J Clin Oncol 31*, 2013 (suppl; abstr CRA6510). Presented at ASCO Annual Meeting, Chicago, IL, June 3, 2013.

Federal Drug Administration. 2007; FDA Advisory Committee Suggests Changes to ESA Use. *NCI Cancer Bulletin* 4(17), available at http://www.fda.gov/drugs/drugsafety/postmarketdrugsafety informationforpatientsandproviders/ucm126481.htm. Accessed June 3, 2014.

Federal Drug Administration: Safety update leustatin (Cladribine injection). October 4, 2012. Available at http://www.fda.gov/Safety/MedWatch/SafetyInformation/ucm318760.htm. Accessed June 3, 2014.

Federal Drug Administration. FDA Drug safety podcast for healthcare professionals: Safety review update on reports of hepatosplenic T-cell lymphoma in adolescents and young adults receiving tumor necrosis factor (TNF) blockers, azathioprine and/or mercaptopurine. Available at http://www.fda.gov/Drugs/DrugSafety/DrugSafetyPodcasts/ucm251809.htm. Accessed April 29, 2014.

Federal Drug Administration Safety Update CeeNu (lomustine) capsules. Available at http://www.fda.gov/Safety/MedWatch/SafetyInformation/Safety-RelatedDrugLabelingChanges/ucm155122.htm. Accessed June 6, 2014.

Feldweg AM, Lee CW, Matulonis UA, Castells M. Rapid Desensitization for Hypersensitivity Reactions to Paclitaxel and Docetaxel: A New Standard Protocol Used in 77 Successful Treatments. *Gynecol Oncol* 2005; 96(3) 824–829.

Fox ER, Birt A, James KB, et al. ASHP Guidelines on Managing Drug Product Shortages in Hospitals and Health Systems. *Am J Health-Syst Pharm*, 2009; 66: 1399–1406.

Gianni L, Dombernowsky P, Sledge G, et al. Cardiac Function Following Combination Therapy with Taxol (T) and Doxorubicin (D) for Advanced Breast Cancer (ABC). *Proc Am SocClin Oncol* 1998; 17 115a.

GlaxoSmithKline Alkeran (melphalan) [package insert]. Research Triangle Park, NC, 2010.

Goetz MP, Suman V, Hoskin TL et al. (2012) CYP2D6 metabolism and patient outcome in the Austrian Breast and Colorectal Cancer Study Group Trial (ABCSG) 8 Clin Cancer Res published online 12.3.12; doi: 10.1158/1078-0432.CCR-12-2153.

Goss PE, Ingle JN, Ales-Martinez J, et al. Exemestane for primary prevention of breast cancer in postmenopausal women: NCIC CTG MAP.3-A randomized, placebo-controlled clinical trial. *J Clin Oncol* 29: 2011 (suppl; abstr LBA504).

Griffin-Sobel JP. Correction: Paclitaxel Is Not a Vesicant. *Clin J Oncol Nurs* 2005; 9(5) 510.

Griggs JJ, Mangu PB, Anderson H, et al. Appropriate chemotherapy dosing for obese adult patients with cancer: American Society of Clinical Oncology practice guideline. *J Clin Oncol* 3099: 2012 available online at http://jco.ascopubs.org/cgi/doi/10.1200/JCO.2011.39.9436. Accessed June 16, 2012.

Hospira, Inc. Vincristine sulfate injection [package insert]. Lake Forest, IL, January 2014.

Jones D. Cancer Nanotechnology: Small but Heading for the Big Time. *Nat Rev Drug Disc* 2007; 6(3) 174–175.

Labianca R, Floriani I, Cortesi E, et al. Alternating Versus Continuous "FOLFIRI" in Advanced Colorectal Cancer (ACC): A Randomized "GISCAD" Trial. *J Clin Oncol* 2006; 24(18S) 3505.

Lee W, Lockhart AC, Kim RB, Rothenberg ML. Cancer Pharmacogenomics: Powerful Tools in Cancer Chemotherapy and Drug Development. *Oncologist* 2005; 10 104–111.

Lenz HL. Resistance to therapy: Molecular Markers in GI Oncology State of the Science: GI Oncology, http://www.webtie.org/SOTS/Meetings/Gastrointestinal/March62001/lectures/htm. Accessed May 2006.

Lenz HL. Management and Preparedness for Infusion and Hypersensitivity Reactions. *Oncologist* 2007; 12 601–609.

Marsh S, McLeod HL. Pharmacogenomics: From Bedside to Clinical Practice. *Hum Mol Genet* 2006; 15 R89–R93.

Minotti G, Saponiero A, Licata S, et al. Paclitaxel and Docetaxel May Enhance the Metabolism of Doxorubicin to Toxic Species in Human Myocardium. *Clin CA Res* 2001; 7 1511–1515.

Molinski TF, Dalisay DS, Lievens SL, Saludes JP. Drug Development from Marine Natural Products. *Nature Rev Drug Discov* 2009; 8 69–85.

Moore HCF, Phillips K-A, Boyle FM et al. Phase III trial (Prevention of early menopause study [POEMS]-SWOG S0230) of LHRH analog during chemotherapy (CT) to reduce ovarian failure in early-stage, hormone receptor-negative breast cancer: An international intergroup trial of SWOG, IBCSG, ECOG, and CALGB (Alliance). *J Clin Oncol* 2014; 32:5s (suppl); abstr LBA505.

Mouridsen HT, et al. Treatment of Anthracycline Extravasation with Savene (Dexrazoxane). Results from Two Prospective Clinical Multicentre Studies. *Ann Oncol* 2007; 18 546–550.

Neuss MN, Polovich M, McNiff K, et al. (2013). 2013 updated American Society of Oncology/ Oncology Nursing Society chemotherapy administration safety standards including standards for the safe administration and management of oral chemotherapy. *Oncol Nurs Forum,* 40(3): 225–233.

O'Shaughnessy JA. Molecular Signatures Predict Outcomes of Breast Cancer. *New Engl J Med* 2006; 355 615–617.

Occupational Safety and Health Administration. *Controlling Occupational Exposure to Hazardous Drugs* 1995 Washington (OSHA Instruction CPL 2-2.20B).

Oncology Nursing Society Board of Directors. Pittsburgh, PA: *ONS Position Paper: Regarding the Preparation of the Professional Registered Nurse Who Administers and Cares for the Individual Receiving Chemotherapy.* Oncology Nursing Society; 2012.

Onoda S, Masuda N, Seto T, et al. Phase II Trial of Amrubicin for Treatment of Refractory or Relapsed Small-Cell Lung Cancer: Thoracic Oncology Research Group Study 0301. *J Clin Oncol* 2006; 24(34) 5448–5453.

Overk CR, Peng KW, Asghodom RT, et al. Structure-activity Relationships for a Family of Benzothiophene Selective Estrogen Receptor Modulators Including Raloxifene and Arzoxifene. *Chem Med Chem* 2007; 2(10) 1520–1526. doi:10.1002/cmdc.200700104.

Paik S, Tang G, Shak S, et al. Gene Expression and Benefit of Chemotherapy in Women with Node-Negative Estrogen Receptor-Positive Breast Cancer. *J Clin Oncol* 2006; 24(23) 3726–3734.

Perry MC. *The Chemotherapy Source Book,* 4th ed. Philadelphia, PA: Lippincott, Williams & Wilkins; 2008.

Polovich M, Olsen M, LeFebvre KB. *Chemotherapy and Biotherapy Guidelines and Recommendations for Practice,* Oncology Nursing Society; 4th ed. Pittsburgh, PA: ONS, 2014, pp.158–162.

Polovich M, Whitford JM, Olsen M, *Chemotherapy and Biotherapy Guidelines and Recommendations for Practice,* 3rd ed. Pittsburgh, PA: ONS, 2009. 105–110.

Posner MR, Haddad RI, Wirth LJ. The Evolution of Induction Chemotherapy and Sequential Therapy for Locally Advanced Squamous Cell Cancer of the Head and Neck. *2006 American Society of Clinical Oncology Educational Book,* Alexandria, VA: American Society of Clinical Oncology, 2006, pp 346–352.

Potti A, Dressman HK, Bild A, et al. Genomic Signatures to Guide the Use of Chemotherapeutics. *Nat Med* 2006; 12(11) 1294–3000.

Sanofi-Aventis US LLC. *Jevtana (*cabazitaxel) [package insert]. Bridgewater, NJ, June 2010.

Sanofi-Aventis US LLC. *Taxotere* (docetaxel) [package insert]. Bridgewater, NJ, May 2014.

Sanofi Synthelabo. *Eloxatin* (oxaliplatin) [package insert]. Bridgewater NJ, February 2014.

Schulmeister L. Totect™: A New Agent for Treating Anthracycline Extravasation. *Clin J Oncol Nurs* 2007; 11(3) 387–395.

Sheperd GM. Hypersensitivity Reactions to Chemotherapeutic Drugs. *Allergy Immunol* 2003; 24 253–262.

Taplin M-E, Montgomery RB, Logothetis C, et al. 2012; Effect of neo-adjuvant abiraterone acetate (AA) plus leuprolide acetate (LHRHa) on PSA, pathological complete response (pCR), and near pCR in localized high-risk prostate cancer (LHRPC): Results of a randomized phase II study. *J Clin Onco,* 30 supplement abstract 4521.

Teva Pharmaceuticals USA, Inc. Paclitaxel [package insert]. Sellersville, PA, August 2012.

Teva Pharmaceuticals USA, Inc. Synribo (omacetaxine mepesuccinate) for injection [package insert]. North Wales, PA, April 2014.

Thompson LA, Lawson AP, Sutphin SD, et al. Description of Current Practices of Empiric Chemotherapy Dose Adjustment in Obese Adult Patients. *J Oncol Pract* 2010; 6(3) 141–145.

Topotarget A/S. Totect (dexrazoxane) [package insert]. Copenhagen, Denmark. May 2011.

Tournigand C, Cervantes A, Figer A, et al. OPTIMOX1: A Randomized Study of FOLFOX4 or FOLFOX7 with Oxaliplatin in a Stop-and-Go Fashion in Advanced Colorectal Cancer: A GERCOR Study. *J Clin Oncol* 2006; 24(3) 394–400.

Trissel LA, Saenz CA, Ingram DS, Ogundele AB. Compatibility Screening of Oxaliplatin During Simulated Y-site Administration with Other Drugs. *J Oncol Pharm Practice* 2002; 8(1) 33–37.

Twelves C, Loesch D, Blum JL, et al. A Phase III Study (EMBRACE) of Eribulin Mesylate Versus Treatment of Physician's Choice in Patients with Locally Recurrent or Metastatic Breast Cancer Previously Treated with an Anthracycline and a Taxane. *J Clin Oncol* 2010; 28 18s (suppl; abstr CRA1004).

Vahdat L, Gopalakrishna P, Garcia AA, et al. 2011; Comparison of the incidence of peripheral neuropathy with eribulin mesylate versus ixabepilone in metastatic breast cancer patients: A randomized phase II study. *Proceedings of the San Antonio Breast Cancer Symposium*. San Antonio, TX, December 6–10, 2011, Abstract P5-19-02.

Vahdat LT, Pruitt B, Fabian CJ, et al. Phase II Study of Eribulin Mesylate, a Halichondrin B Analog, in Patients with Metastatic Breast Cancer Previously Treated with an Anthracycline and a Taxane. *Clin J Oncol* April 2009; online pub: 10.1200/JCO.2008.17.7618.

Watanabe H, Ikesue H, Tsujikawa T, et al. Decrease in venous irritation by adjusting the concentration of injected bendamustine. *Biological and Pharmaceutical Bulletin* 2013; 36:574–578 [doi:10.1248/bpb.b12-0090].

Zhang ZY, King BM, Pelletier RD, Wong YN. Delineation of the Interactions between the Chemotherapeutic Agent Eribulin Mesylate (E7389) and Human CYP3A4. *Cancer Chemother Pharmacol* 2008; 62(4) 707–716.

Drug: abarelix for injectable suspension (Plenaxis)

Class: Gonadotropin-releasing hormone (GnRH) antagonist.

Mechanism of Action: Directly and competitively blocks GnRH receptors in the pituitary: suppresses luteinizing hormone (LH) and follicle-stimulating hormone (FSH) secretion, and thereby reduces the secretion of testosterone by the testes. There is no initial increase in serum testosterone concentrations.

Metabolism: Following IM administration, drug is slowly absorbed with a mean peak concentration 3 days after injection, and distributes extensively within the body. Drug is highly protein-bound (96–99%), and is excreted in the urine, with 13% of drug unchanged.

Indication: Drug is indicated for the palliative treatment of men with advanced symptomatic prostate cancer, in whom LHRH agonist therapy is not appropriate, who refuse surgical castration, and who have one or more of the following:

- Risk of neurologic compromise due to metastases,
- Ureteral or bladder outlet obstruction due to local encroachment of metastatic disease, or
- Severe bone pain from skeletal metastases persisting in opioid analgesia.

Dosage/Range:
- Drug is restricted due to risk of immediate-onset systemic allergic reactions. Only physicians enrolled in the Plenaxis User Safety Program, Plenaxis PLUS, may prescribe the drug.
- 100 mg IM in the buttock on days 1, 15, 29 (week 4), and every 4 weeks thereafter.

Drug Preparation:
- Reconstitute drug following manufacturer's recommendations to yield 50 mg/mL.
- Administer in the buttock, and rotate sites.

Drug Administration:
- 100 mg IM in the buttock on days 1, 15, 29 (week 4), and every 4 weeks thereafter. Rotate IM sites.
- Observe patient for 30 minutes in the office/clinic and assess for immediate-onset systemic allergic reactions, sometimes resulting in hypotension and syncope.
- Assess efficacy by monitoring serum testosterone levels baseline, day 29, and then every 8 weeks thereafter.

Drug Interactions:
- None known.

Lab Effects/Interference:
- LFTs: transaminases may become elevated.
- Serum testosterone levels should decrease to < 50 ng/dL. Slight decrease in Hgb.
- Increase in serum triglycerides by 10%.

Special Considerations:
- Drug is restricted and can be prescribed only by physicians approved by the Plenaxis PLUS program.
- Drug achieves castration levels of testosterone 24 hours after IM injection.
- The effectiveness of abarelix in suppressing serum testosterone to castration levels decreases with continued dosing in patients weighing > 225 lbs, and effectiveness beyond 12 months has not been established. Assess total serum testosterone levels just prior to drug administration on day 29, and every 8 weeks thereafter, to assure continued response in all patients. Periodic measurement of serum PSA will assist in assessing response.
- Immediate-onset systemic allergic reactions, with hypotension and syncope, may occur; risk increases with increased cumulative dose so patients should be observed for at least 30 minutes following the injection.
- Drug may cause QT interval prolongation in 20% of patients (changes from baseline of > 30 msec, or end-of-treatment QTc values > 450 msec); use cautiously, if at all, in patients taking class IA (quinidine, procainamide) or class III (amiodarone, sotalol) antiarrhythmic medications.

- Drug is not indicated for women or children; drug may cause fetal harm if administered to a pregnant woman.
- Transaminase levels became clinically significantly elevated in some patients, so levels should be assessed bascline, and periodically during treatment.
- Bone mineral density may decrease with extended treatment with GnRH antagonists and LHRH agonists.

Potential Toxicities/Side Effects and the Nursing Process

I.   POTENTIAL FOR INJURY related to HYPERSENSITIVITY REACTION

Defining Characteristics: Allergic reactions can occur immediately after injection, and may result in hypotension and syncope, starting with the initial dose, or occurring later in the course of treatment. Risk increases with the duration of treatment.

Nursing Implications: Assess baseline VS and mental status prior to drug administration, and observe patient for 30 minutes following injection. Recall signs/symptoms of anaphylaxis, and if these occur, notify physician, and assess patient's vital signs. Subjective symptoms are generalized itching, nausea, chest tightness, crampy abdominal pain, difficulty speaking, anxiety, agitation, sense of impending doom, uneasiness, desire to urinate/defecate, dizziness, and chills. Objective signs are flushed appearance; angioedema of face, neck, eyelids, hands, and feet; localized or generalized urticaria; respiratory distress with or without wheezing; hypotension; and cyanosis. Review standing orders or nursing procedures for patient management of anaphylaxis, and be prepared to administer ordered medications, which may include epinephrine 1:1,000, hydrocortisone sodium succinate, and diphenhydramine. Teach patient to report any unusual symptoms.

II.   ALTERATION IN COMFORT related to HOT FLUSHES, SLEEP DISTURBANCES, PAIN, BREAST ENLARGEMENT/TENDERNESS, HEADACHE, EDEMA, AND DIZZINESS

Defining Characteristics: Signs and symptoms of androgen deprivation are: hot flushes (79%), sleep deprivation (44%), breast enlargement (30%), breast pain/nipple tenderness (20%). Pain in general occurs in about 31% of patients, as well as back pain (17%).

Nursing Implications: Teach patient that symptoms may occur. Encourage patient to report symptoms early. Develop symptom management plan with patient and physician.

III. ALTERATION IN BOWEL AND BLADDER ELIMINATION related to HORMONAL CHANGES

Defining Characteristics: Diarrhea occurs in about 11% of patients, while constipation occurs in 15%. 10% of patients develop dysuria, micturition frequency, urinary retention, or urinary tract infection.

Nursing Implications: Assess baseline bowel and bladder elimination pattern, and teach patient to report any changes. Teach patient to modify diet to minimize either diarrhea or constipation. Discuss need for referral to urologist if dysuria, urinary retention, or urinary tract infections persist.

Drug: abiraterone acetate (Zytiga)

Class: CYP17 inhibitor.

Mechanism of Action: Abiraterone is an androgen biosynthesis inhibitor that inhibits the enzyme CYP17, which is expressed in testicular, adrenal, and prostatic tumor tissues. CYP17 is required for androgen biosynthesis. CYP17 catalyzes 2 sequential reactions: (1) conversion of pregnenolone and progesterone to derivatives, and (2) formation of DHEA (dehydroepiandrosterone) and androstenedione, which are androgen precursors of testosterone. CYP17 inhibition by abiraterone can cause increased adrenal mineralocorticoid production. Androgen-sensitive prostate cancer is sensitive to agents that decrease androgen serum levels. Androgen deprivation therapies (e.g., GnRH agonists or orchiectomy) decrease androgen production by the testes, but not the adrenals or in the tumor. It is not necessary to monitor testosterone levels, and although PSA levels may change, it does not necessarily correlate to clinical benefit.

Metabolism: Following oral administration, abiraterone acetate is hydrolyzed to abiraterone, the active metabolite. Median time to reach maximum plasma abiraterone concentrations is 2 hours. Food affects systemic exposure of the drug. Low-fat meals result in 5-fold higher levels, and high-fat meals result in 17-fold higher levels of abiraterone. Therefore, drug should be taken on an empty stomach. Drug is highly protein-bound (> 99%) to human plasma proteins, albumin, and alpha-1 acid gycoprotein. Neither prodrug nor drug is a substrate of P-glycoprotein (P-gp), but abiraterone acetate is an inhibitor of P-gp. No studies have been performed with other transporter proteins. There are two inactive metabolites that involve CYP3A4 and SULT2A1. The mean terminal half-life of abiraterone in plasma is 12±5 hrs. After oral administration, 88% is recovered in feces (55% abiraterone acetate, 22% abiraterone), and 5% in urine. Hepatic dysfunction increases systemic exposure: 1.1-fold with mild (Child-Pugh Class A), and 3.6-fold in moderate (Child-Pugh Class B), prolonging mean half-life of abiraterone to 18 hours and 19 hours respectively. Drug has not been studied in patients with severe (Class C) hepatic dysfunction. There is no increase in systemic exposure in patients with severe renal dysfunction.

Indication: Drug is FDA-approved in combination with prednisone for the treatment of patients with metastatic castration-resistant prostate cancer.

Dosage/Range: 1,000 mg (4 tablets) orally once daily on an empty stomach, with prednisone 5 mg orally twice daily.

- Dose-reduce to 250 mg PO once daily in patients with baseline moderate hepatic impairment (Child-Pugh class B). Monitor ALT, AST, and bilirubin before starting therapy, then weekly for the 1st month, every 2 weeks for the next 2 months of treatment, then monthly. If ALT and/or AST > 5X ULN or total bilirubin is > 3X ULN, discontinue drug and do not retreat with abiraterone.

- Do not administer to patients with baseline severe hepatotoxicity.
- Hold drug in patients who develop hepatotoxicity during treatment until recovery to baseline or AST and/or ALT ≤ 2.5 ULN and total bilirubin ≤ 1.5X ULN; then re-treatment may be started at a reduced dose of 750 mg once daily; if hepatotoxicity occurs at this dose, interrupt until recovery and dose-reduce to 500 mg orally. If hepatotoxicity occurs at this dose, discontinue treatment with abiraterone.
- Discontinue drug in patients who develop severe hepatotoxicity.
- Drug is contraindicated in women who are or may become pregnant.

Drug Preparation:
- Oral, available as 250-mg tablets.

Drug Administration:
- Take once daily with water, swallow whole, and do not chew or crush tablet.
- Teach patient to avoid food for 2 hours prior to the dose of abiraterone, and for 1 hour after the dose of abiraterone. They should also take one tablet of prednisone 5 mg PO twice a day, ideally with food at a different time from the abiraterone (more than 2 hours before, or more than 1 hour after taking abiraterone).
- If one dose is missed of either abiraterone acetate or prednisone, take the normal dose the next day and do not make up; patient should tell the physician if he or she misses more than one dose.
- Teach patient and family that drug can harm a developing fetus, so women who are or may be pregnant should not handle the drug unless wearing gloves. Men receiving the drug should use a condom if having sex with a pregnant woman. The patient should use both a condom and another effective method of birth control if he is having sex with a woman of child bearing potential. Use these precautions during and for one week after treatment with abiraterone.

Drug Interactions: Drug is a strong inhibitor of CYP1A2 and CYP2D6, and a moderate inhibitor of CYP2C9, CYP2C19, and CYP3A4/5. Drug is also a substrate of CYP3A4.

- Dextromethorphan (CYP2D6 substrate): 2.8-fold increase in systemic exposure.
- Strong CYP3A4 inhibitors or inducers: AVOID or use with caution, and monitor the patient closely.
- CYP2D6 substrates with a narrow therapeutic index (e.g., all tricyclic antidepressants, most SSRI antidepressants, tramadol, oxycodone, antipsychotics, beta-blockers). Avoid coadministration; if must coadminister, use together cautiously and consider a dose reduction of the concomitant CYP2D6 substrate.

Lab Effects/Interference:
- Decreased testosterone and PSA levels.
- Increased ALT, AST, bilirubin.
- Hypokalemia.

Special Considerations:
- Mineralocorticoid excess may occur; use drug cautiously in patients with a history of cardiovascular disease. Safety in patients with LVEF < 50%, or NYHA class III or IV heart

failure, has not been established. Correct HTN and hypokalemia before treatment. Monitor BP, serum potassium, and symptoms of fluid retention at least monthly. Use drug cautiously and monitor closely patients with heart failure, recent MI, or ventricular arrhythmia.

- **Adrenocortical insufficiency:** Monitor for signs and symptoms of adrenal insufficiency (fatigue, lightheadedness with position change, muscle weakness, fever, weight loss, nausea/vomiting/diarrhea, changes in mood/personality, myalgias, arthralgias, headache, low BP when standing, but high BP when supine, increased bronze pigmentation of skin, urinary frequency), and discuss management with physician or midlevel practitioner. Assess patients at times when risk of adrenocortical insufficiency may be high: patients withdrawn from prednisone, who have prednisone dose reductions, or who have unusual stress. Patients may require increased corticosteroid doses before, during, and after stressful situations.
- Hepatotoxicity
  - Assess LFTs (ALT, AST, direct BR) baseline, then every 2 weeks for the first 3 months, then monthly thereafter. Increases in liver enzymes may require dose interruption, dose modification, and/or dose discontinuation. Promptly assess LFTs if patient develops signs/symptoms of hepatotoxicity.
  - Patients with moderate hepatic impairment should have ALT, AST, bilirubin assessed baseline, then every week for the first month, every 2 weeks for the following 2 months of treatment, and monthly thereafter.
  - If ALT and/or AST are elevated > 5 × ULN or total bilirubin is greater than 3 × ULN, discontinue abiraterone and do not re-treat patients with the drug.
  - Patients who develop hepatotoxicity (ALT ±AST > 5 × ULN or total bilirubin > 3 × ULN) should have abiraterone stopped. Drug can be restarted at a reduced dose of 750 mg once daily following return of LFTs to patient's baseline or to AST/ALT < 2.5 × ULN and total bilirubin < 1.5 × ULN. Once drug is restarted, monitor the patient's LFTs at a minimum every 2 weeks for 3 months, then monthly thereafter.
- Reinforce patient teaching that drug MUST be taken on an empty stomach, as drug systemic exposure (AUC) is 10-fold higher when taken with meals.
- Most common side effects occurring in ≥ 10% of patients are joint swelling/discomfort, hypokalemia, edema, myalgia, hot flush, diarrhea, UTI, cough, HTN, arrythmia, urinary frequency, nocturia, dyspepsia, URI.
- Drug is contraindicated in women who are or may become pregnant; drug should not be used in patients with baseline severe hepatic impairment (Child-Hugh Class C).

Potential Toxicities/Side Effects and the Nursing Process

I. POTENTIAL FOR INJURY related to MINERALOCORTICOID EXCESS-INDUCED EDEMA, HYPOKALEMIA, AND STEROID-INDUCED IMMUNOSUPPRESSION

Defining Characteristics: Water retention may occur and lead to CHF, hypertension, and edema; hypokalemia may occur due to increased excretion of potassium. Osteoporosis may occur with long-term corticosteroid therapy. Steroids increase susceptibility to infections, may mask or aggravate infection, and may prolong or delay healing of injuries.

Nursing Implications: Identify patients at risk for complications associated with fluid/ sodium retention (i.e., patients with preexisting cardiac, renal, hepatic dysfunction); monitor fluid and electrolyte balance and assess for imbalance. Document baseline cardiac status and monitor through therapy. Teach patients to report the following right away: dizziness, fast heartbeats, feeling faint or lightheaded, confusion, muscle weakness, pain in the legs, and swelling in legs or feet. Instruct patient to report signs/symptoms of hypokalemia (anorexia, muscle twitching, tetany, polyuria, polydipsia); monitor electrolytes regularly and discuss abnormal values with physician. Encourage high-potassium diet, and instruct patient in safety measures as needed, such as taking prednisone with food 2 hours prior to or 1 hour after abiraterone. Teach patient to report slow healing of wounds, signs/symptoms of infection (erythema, warmth, purulence) of skin areas, as well as cough, dyspnea, signs/ sympoms of URI, and burning on urination. Reinforce/teach patient hygiene measures for mouth, perineum, and skin.

II.   ALTERATION IN COMFORT related to MYALGIAS, ARTHRALGIAS, FEVER, HOT FLUSH, DYSPEPSIA

Defining Characteristics: Signs and symptoms of adrenocortical insufficiency may occur: fatigue, lightheadedness with position change, muscle weakness, fever, weight loss, nausea/ vomiting/diarrhea, changes in mood/personality, myalgias, arthralgias, headache, low BP when standing but high BP when supine, increased bronze pigmentation of skin, amd urinary frequency. Severity and incidence is reduced with coadministration of prednisone.

Nursing Implications: Teach patient that arthralgias, myalgias, fever, discomfort may occur, and strategies to reduce discomfort. Monitor for signs and symptoms of adrenal insufficiency, and discuss management with physician or midlevel practitioner. Assess patients at times when risk of adrenocortical insufficiency may be high: patients withdrawn from prednisone, who have prednisone dose reductions, or who have unusual stress. Patients may require increased corticosteroid doses before, during, and after stressful situations.

Drug: adrenocorticoids (cortisone, dexamethasone, hydrocortisone, methylprednisolone, prednisolone, prednisone)

Class: Hormones.

Mechanism of Action: Cause lysis of lymphoid cells, which leads to their use against lymphatic leukemia, myeloma, malignant lymphoma. May also recruit malignant cells out of G_0 phase, making them vulnerable to damage caused by cell cycle phase-specific agents.

Metabolism: Metabolized by the liver, excreted in urine. Prednisone is activated by the liver in its active form, prednisolone.

Dosage/Range:
- Varies according to which preparation is used. Dexamethasone is 25 times the potency of hydrocortisone.
- Cortisone 25 mg.

* Dexamethasone 0.75 mg
* Hydrocortisone 20 mg
* Methylprednisolone 4 mg
* Prednisone, prednisolone 5 mg

Drug Preparation:
* None

Drug Administration:
* Oral

Drug Interactions:
* May increase K+ loss and hypokalemia when combined with amphotericin B or potassium-depleting diuretics.
* Warfarin (Coumadin) dose may need to be increased.
* Insulin or oral hypoglycemia dose may need to be increased.
* Oral contraceptives may inhibit steroid metabolism.

Lab Effects/Interference:
* Increased Na, decreased K with hypokalemic alkalosis.
* Decreased ^{131}I uptake and protein-bound iodine concentration. May cause difficulty monitoring therapeutic response of patients treated for thyroid conditions.
* False-negative results in nitroblue tetrazolium test for systemic bacterial infections.
* May suppress reactions to skin tests.

Special Considerations:
* Chronic steroid use is associated with numerous side effects. Intermittent therapy is safer and, under some conditions, just as effective as daily therapy.

Potential Toxicities/Side Effects and the Nursing Process

I.   ALTERATION IN NUTRITION, LESS THAN BODY REQUIREMENTS, related to GASTRIC IRRITATION, DECREASED CARBOHYDRATE METABOLISM, AND HYPERGLYCEMIA

Defining Characteristics: Steroids can cause increased secretion of hydrochloric acid and decreased secretion of protective gastric mucus, which can exacerbate an existing gastric ulcer. They are insulin antagonists and may cause gluconeogenesis. In addition, steroids may increase appetite and cause weight gain.

Nursing Implications: Administer drugs with meals or an antacid. Instruct patient to report evidence of gastric distress immediately; teach patient to take steroids prior to a meal or with milk or food. Obtain baseline glucose levels and monitor periodic blood sugars throughout therapy. Teach patient to recognize signs/symptoms of hyperglycemia (polyuria, polydipsia, polyphagia), and to report these to the doctor or nurse.

II.   POTENTIAL FOR INJURY related to SODIUM AND WATER RETENTION, ALTERATIONS IN FLUID AND ELECTROLYTE BALANCE, AND STEROID-INDUCED IMMUNOSUPPRESSION

Defining Characteristics: Sodium and water retention may occur and lead to CHF, hypertension, and edema in susceptible individuals; hypokalemia and hypocalcemia may occur due to increased excretion of potassium and calcium. Osteoporosis may occur with long-term therapy. Steroids increase susceptibility to infections and tuberculosis, may mask or aggravate infection, and may prolong or delay healing of injuries.

Nursing Implications: Identify patients at risk for complications associated with fluid/sodium retention (i.e., patients with preexisting cardiac, renal, hepatic dysfunction); monitor fluid and electrolyte balance and assess for imbalance. Document baseline cardiac status and monitor through therapy. Instruct patient to report signs/symptoms of hypokalemia (anorexia, muscle twitching, tetany, polyuria, polydipsia) and of hypocalcemia (leg cramps, tingling in fingertips, muscle twitching); monitor electrolytes regularly and discuss abnormal values with physician. Encourage high-potassium, high-calcium diet, and instruct patient in safety measures as needed. Teach patient to report slow healing of wounds, signs/symptoms of infection (erythema, warmth, purulence) of skin areas, as well as sore throat and burning on urination. Reinforce/teach patient hygiene measures for mouth, perineum, and skin.

III.   POTENTIAL FOR INJURY related to RAPID WITHDRAWAL OF THERAPY

Defining Characteristics: Long-term therapy leads to suppression of normal adrenal function. Rapid cessation of therapy will lead to adrenal insufficiency, characterized by anorexia, nausea, orthostatic hypotension, dizziness, depression, dyspnea, hypoglycemia, and rebound inflammation (fever, myalgias, arthralgia, malaise). It can be fatal.

Nursing Implications: Discuss with physician the taper of steroids and instruct patient and family carefully. Teach patient to report symptoms of rapid withdrawal to nurse or physician.

IV.   POTENTIAL FOR BODY IMAGE DISTURBANCE related to CUSHINGOID CHANGES

Defining Characteristics: Cushingoid state may occur with prolonged use and may be diminished by every-other-day dosing. Changes include moonface, striae, purpura, acne, and hirsutism. In addition, increased appetite from steroids may lead to weight gain.

Nursing Implications: Teach patient about potential changes and provide reassurance that they will resolve once therapy ceases; encourage patient to verbalize feelings, and provide emotional support.

V. POTENTIAL FOR SENSORY/PERCEPTUAL ALTERATIONS related to CATARACTS OR GLAUCOMA, AND OCULAR INFECTIONS (increased risk)

Defining Characteristics: Cataracts or glaucoma may develop with prolonged steroid use; risk of ocular infections from virus or fungi is increased.

Nursing Implications: Teach patient to report signs/symptoms of eye infection, such as discharge, erythema, or visual changes; ophthalmologic exams are recommended every 2–3 months.

VI. INEFFECTIVE COPING related to AFFECTIVE/BEHAVIORAL CHANGES

Defining Characteristics: Emotional lability, insomnia, mood swings, euphoria, and psychosis may occur, causing ineffective coping and role-relationship problems if unprepared.

Nursing Implications: Teach patient and family that affective/behavioral changes may occur and that they will resolve once therapy is discontinued. Encourage patient and family to report these changes, especially if troublesome.

VII. IMPAIRED PHYSICAL MOBILITY related to MUSCULOSKELETAL CHANGES

Defining Characteristics: With chronic, high-dose usage, loss of muscle mass, muscle weakness (steroid myopathy), tendon rupture, osteoporosis, pathologic fractures, and aseptic necrosis of the heads of the humerus and femur can occur.

Nursing Implications: Teach patient that muscle weakness and other effects can occur with therapy and that muscle cramping may occur with discontinuation of therapy. Teach patient to report weakness, cramping, and any musculoskeletal changes. If weakness occurs, therapy may be discontinued.

Drug: altretamine (Hexalen, Hexamethylmelamine)

Class: Alkylating agent.

Mechanism of Action: The exact mechanism of action is unknown. May inhibit incorporation of thymidine and uridine into DNA and RNA, respectively, inhibiting DNA and RNA synthesis. Altretamine is believed not to act as an alkylating agent in vitro, but it may be activated to an alkylating agent in vivo. Also may act as an antimetabolite with activity in S phase.

Metabolism: Well absorbed orally, although bioavailability is variable. Protein-bound with peak plasma concentration in 1 hour. Metabolized extensively in the liver, with majority excreted in the urine. Some of the drug is excreted as respiratory CO_2. Half-life of the parent compound is 4.7–10.2 hours.

Indication: For use as a single agent in the palliative treatment of patients with recurrent ovarian cancer following 1st-line therapy with a cisplatin and/or alkyating agent-based combination.

Dosage/Range:
- 260 mg/m^2 daily in four equally divided doses × 14 or 21 consecutive days, repeated every 28 days.
- Discontinue for 14 or more days and restart at 200 mg/m^2 daily if any of the following occur: refractory GI intolerance, WBC < 2,000 cells/mm^3 or ANC < 1,000 cells/mm^3, platelet count < 75,000/mm^3, or progressive neurotoxicity.

Drug Preparation:
- Available in 50-mg capsules.

Drug Administration:
- Oral. Administer dose after meals and at bedtime.

Drug Interactions:
- Concurrent administration of drug with monoamine oxidase (MAO) inhibitor antidepressants may cause severe orthostatic hypotension.

Lab Effects/Interference:
- Decreased CBC.
- Increased BUN, creatinine.

Special Considerations:
- Nausea and vomiting can be minimized if patient takes dose 2 hours after meals and at bedtime.
- Nadir 3–4 weeks after treatment.

Potential Toxicities/Side Effects and the Nursing Process

I.   INFECTION AND BLEEDING related to BONE MARROW DEPRESSION

Defining Characteristics: Causes mild to moderate bone marrow suppression, with nadir occurring 21–28 days after beginning treatment, and rapid recovery within 1 week of cessation of drug. Anemia occurs in 33% of patients and is moderate to severe in 9% of patients.

Nursing Implications: Assess CBC, WBC, differential, and platelet count before each cycle of drug administration, as well as for signs/symptoms of infection or bleeding. Teach patient signs/symptoms of infection and bleeding, and instruct to report them immediately. Teach self-care measures to minimize risk of infection and bleeding, including avoidance of OTC aspirin-containing medications. Assess energy and activity tolerance; discuss blood transfusion with physician as appropriate. Discuss with physician dose interruption and reduction if WBC < 2,000/mm^3, ANC < 1,000/mm^3, or platelet count < 75,000/mm^3.

II. SENSORY/PERCEPTUAL ALTERATIONS related to PERIPHERAL NEUROPATHY AND CNS EFFECTS

Defining Characteristics: Peripheral sensory neuropathy occurs in 31% of patients and is moderate to severe in 9% of patients. Paresthesia, hyperesthesia, hyperreflexia, and numbness may occur; they are reversible. CNS effects of agitation, confusion, hallucinations, depression, mood disorders, and Parkinson-like symptoms may occur, and usually are reversible. Neurologic effects are more common with continuous dosing > 3 months, rather than pulse dosing.

Nursing Implications: Assess baseline neurologic status. Teach patient that possible side effects may occur, and instruct to report them. If nerologic toxicity is severe, drug should be dose reduced, then discontinued if symptoms do not improve.

III. ALTERATION IN NUTRITION, LESS THAN BODY REQUIREMENTS, related to NAUSEA AND VOMITING, DIARRHEA, ABDOMINAL CRAMPS, ANOREXIA

Defining Characteristics: Nausea occurs in 33% of patients and is dose related. Tolerance may develop after 3 weeks of drug administration. Diarrhea and cramps may be dose-limiting. Anorexia may occur.

Nursing Implications: Premedicate with antiemetics (phenothiazines are usually effective) at least initially, then as needed. Divide dose into four doses, and give 1−2 hours after meals and at bedtime. Instruct patient to report nausea/vomiting, diarrhea, abdominal cramping. Teach self-administration of prescribed antidiarrheals and self-care techniques to manage cramps, e.g., heat pads or position change. If GI side effects are refractory to symptom management, discuss interrupting dose and then dose reduction with physician.

IV. ALTERATION IN SKIN INTEGRITY related to SKIN RASHES

Defining Characteristics: Skin rashes, pruritus, eczematous skin lesions may occur but are rare.

Nursing Implications: Assess for changes in skin color, texture, and integrity. Teach patient to report any changes in skin, and discuss measures to minimize discomfort.

V. ALTERATION IN ELIMINATION related to RENAL DYSFUNCTION

Defining Characteristics: Elevations in BUN (9% of patients) or creatinine (7%) can occur.

Nursing Implications: Assess baseline renal status and monitor renal function studies throughout treatment.

VI.   POTENTIAL SEXUAL DYSFUNCTION related to DRUG EFFECTS

Defining Characteristics: Drug is mutagenic, carcinogenic, and teratogenic. Drug causes testicular atrophy and decreased spermatogenesis. It is unknown whether drug is excreted in human milk.

Nursing Implications: Discuss with patient and partner normal sexual patterns and anticipated dysfunction resulting from drug or disease. Provide information, emotional support, and referral for counseling as appropriate.

Drug: aminoglutethimide (Cytadren, Elipten)

Class: Adrenal steroid inhibitor.

Mechanism of Action: Causes "chemical adrenalectomy." Blocks adrenal production of steroids, reducing levels of glucocorticoids, mineralocorticoids, and estrogens. Also inhibits peripheral aromatization of androgens to estrogens.

Metabolism: Well absorbed orally. Hydroxylated in liver; undergoes enterohepatic circulation. Most of drug is excreted in urine.

Indication: For the suppression of adrenal function in selected patients with Cushing's syndrome. It does not affect the underlying disease process.

Dosage/Range:
- 750–2,000 mg PO daily in divided doses.
- 40 mg hydrocortisone daily given to replace glucocorticoid deficiencies.

Drug Preparation:
- None. Available in 250-mg tablets.

Drug Administration:
- Oral.

Drug Interactions:
- Drug enhances dexamethasone metabolism, so hydrocortisone should be used for glucocorticoid replacement.
- Warfarin (Coumadin) dose may need to be increased.
- Alcohol potentiates drug side effects.
- May need to increase doses of theophylline, digitoxin, or medroxyprogesterone.

Lab Effects/Interference:
- Hypothyroidism: monitor TFT.
- Elevated LFTs, especially SGOT, alk phos, bili.

Special Considerations:
- Skin rash may develop within 5–7 days, lasting 8 days, often with malaise and fever (37.7–39°C [100–102°F]). If not resolved in 7–14 days, drug should be discontinued.
- Adjuvant corticosteroids need to be administered.

Potential Toxicities/Side Effects and the Nursing Process

I. ALTERATION IN ENDOCRINE FUNCTION related to ADRENAL INSUFFICIENCY

Defining Characteristics: Drug causes reversible chemical adrenalectomy by blockade of steroid hormone production. Patient will experience signs/symptoms of adrenal insufficiency if enough replacement glucocorticoid steroids are not received. Signs/symptoms of adrenal insufficiency include hyponatremia, hypoglycemia, dizziness, and postural hypotension. In addition, possible ovarian blockade may result in virilization.

Nursing Implications: Teach patient about self-administration of hydrocortisone replacement therapy (i.e., administer in AM with breakfast), potential side effects, and tapering schedule; refer to section on adrenocorticoids. Teach patient side effects of hormone replacement and self-assessment techniques, including weekly weights and signs/symptoms of infection. Monitor electrolytes, especially Na+, K+, and Ca++. Assess for signs/symptoms of adrenal insufficiency (fatigue, anorexia, nausea, vomiting, diarrhea, weight loss, weakness, dizziness, and low blood sugar). As appropriate, explore with patient's significant other reproductive and sexuality patterns and the impact chemotherapy may have. Recognize that patient may need increased hydrocortisone and mineralocorticoid support if surgery is needed (increased stress requirement).

II. IMPAIRED SKIN INTEGRITY related to DRUG RASH

Defining Characteristics: Area of erythema, pruritus, and unexplained dermatitis may appear within 1 week of treatment and disappear in 5–8 days. May be accompanied by malaise and low-grade fever.

Nursing Implications: Teach patient to report symptoms and to avoid scratching involved areas if rash develops. Assess skin for any changes and rash development. Consider use of Sarna cream, and use of OTC diphenhydramine.

III. SENSORY/PERCEPTUAL ALTERATIONS related to TRANSIENT SYMPTOMS

Defining Characteristics: Transient symptoms such as drowsiness, lethargy, somnolence, visual blurring, vertigo, and ataxia may occur, as may nystagmus. Lethargy may be severe in elderly patients.

Nursing Implications: Document baseline neurologic function and general health assessment. Teach patient possible side effects, self-assessment, and to report symptoms. Discuss with physician possible dose reduction for significant symptoms.

IV. ALTERATION IN NUTRITION related to NAUSEA/VOMITING AND ANOREXIA

Defining Characteristics: Nausea/vomiting and anorexia occur in approximately 10–13% of patients and are mild.

Nursing Implications: Initially, premedicate (and teach patient to) with antiemetics prior to drug administration. Usually symptoms subside within 2 weeks. Encourage small, frequent feedings.

V.   ALTERATION IN OXYGENATION/PERFUSION related to HYPOTENSION

Defining Characteristics: Drug may block aldosterone production leading to orthostatic or persistent hypotension. This is not usually a problem when hydrocortisone replacement is given.

Nursing Implications: Monitor BP regularly. Instruct patient to change position slowly and to report dizziness.

Drug: anastrozole (Arimidex)

Class: Nonsteroidal aromatase inhibitor.

Mechanism of Action: Inhibits the enzyme aromatase. Aromatase is one of the P450 enzymes and is involved in estrogen biosynthesis. Circulating estrogen in postmenopausal women (mainly estradiol) arises from the aromatase-mediated conversion of androstenedione (made by the adrenals) to estrone, then estrone to estradiol, in the peripheral tissues, such as adipose tissue. Anastrozole is highly selective for this enzyme and does not affect steroid synthesis, so that estradiol synthesis is potently suppressed (to undetectable levels) while cortisol and aldosterone levels are unchanged.

Metabolism: Extensively metabolized, with 85% of the drug metabolized by the liver. About 10% of the unchanged drug and 60% of the drug as metabolites are excreted in the urine within 72 hours of drug administration.

Indication: Anastrozole is an aromatase inhibitor indicated for
- Adjuvant treatment of postmenopausal women with hormone receptor-positive early breast cancer.
- First-line treatment of postmenopausal women with hormone receptor-positive or hormone receptor unknown, locally advanced, or metastatic breast cancer.
- Treatment of advanced breast cancer in postmenopausal women with disease progression following tamoxifen therapy. Patients with ER-negative disease and patients who did not respond to previous tamoxifen therapy rarely responded to anastrozole.

Contraindications: (1) women of premenopausal endocrine status, including pregnant women; (2) patients with demonstrated hypersensitivity to anastrozole or any excipient.

Dosage/Range:
- 1 mg PO daily. No dosage adjustment required for mild to moderate hepatic impairment. In the ATAC adjuvant study, the treatment duration was 5 years. The optimal duration of

treatment is unknown in adjuvant patients. In patients with metastatic disease, continue until disease progression.

Drug Preparation:
• None. Available as 1-mg tablet.

Drug Administration:
• Take orally with or without food, at approximately the same time daily.

Drug Interactions:
• Tamoxifen: coadministration with anastrozole decreases anastrozole serum levels by 27%.
• Estrogen: coadministration with anastrozole may decrease anastrozole activity; do not use concurrently.
• Herbal estrogen-containing supplements: may decrease drug effect.

Lab Effects/Interference:
• Elevated GGT, especially in patients with liver metastases.
• Decreased total hip and lumbar spine bone mineral density (BMD) compared with baseline.
• Total cholesterol may be increased.

Special Considerations:
• In the large Arimidex Tamoxifen Alone or in Combination (ATAC) clinical trial, anastrozole was shown to reduce the relative risk of breast cancer recurrence by 17% over tamoxifen in hormone receptor-positive patients in the adjuvant setting.
• Well tolerated with low toxicity profile.
• Coadministration of corticosteroids is not necessary.
• Absolutely contraindicated during pregnancy. The drug showed no benefit in ER-negative women.
• Most common (≥10%) adverse reactions in patients with (1) early breast cancer: hot flashes, asthenia, arthritis, pain, arthralgia, pharyngitis, HTN, depression, nausea and vomiting, rash, osteoporosis, fractures, back pain, insomnia, headache, peripheral edema, lymphedema; (2) advanced breast cancer: hot flashes, nausea, asthenia, pain, headache, back pain, bone pain, increased cough, dyspnea, pharyngitis, peripheral edema.

Warnings and Precautions:
• Ischemic cardiovascular events: Increased incidence of ischemic events was seen in the ATAC trial in anastrozole arm (17%) compared to tamoxifen (10%). Consider risks and benefits of anastrozole in patients with preexisting ischemic heart disease.
• Bone effects: Patients in the anastrozole arm had a mean decrease in both LS spine and total hip bone mineral density (BMD) compared to baseline, while patients in the tamoxifen arm had a mean increase in both measures compared to baseline. Monitor BMD in patients receiving anastrozole.
• Cholesterol: More patients receiving anastrozole had elevated serum cholesterol (9%) compared to 3.5% in the tamoxifen arm.

Potential Toxicities/Side Effects and the Nursing Process

I.   SEXUAL DYSFUNCTION related to DECREASED ESTROGEN LEVELS

Defining Characteristics: Hot flashes (12%), asthenia or loss of energy (16%), and vaginal dryness may occur.

Nursing Implications: As appropriate, explore with patient and partner patterns of sexuality and impact therapy may have. Discuss strategies to preserve sexual health. Teach patient that the vaginal dryness may be from menopause rather from the drug, and that the patient SHOULD NOT use estrogen creams. Teach patient to use lubricants.

II.   POTENTIAL ALTERATION IN CARDIAC OUTPUT related to THROMBOPHLEBITIS, ISCHEMIC CARDIOVASCULAR EVENTS

Defining Characteristics: Thrombophlebitis may occur, but is uncommon. In the ATAC trial, patients in the anastrozole arm had increased incidence of ischemic events (17%) compared to tamoxifen (10%).

Nursing Implications: Identify patients at risk. Teach patients to report/come to emergency room for pain, redness, or marked swelling in arms or legs, or if shortness of breath or dizziness occurs. Assess patient for prior ischemic heart disease, and teach patient to report any changes (such as chest pain, difficulty breathing, dizziness) immediately.

III.   ALTERATION IN COMFORT related to HEADACHES, WEAKNESS, JOINT DISORDERS

Defining Characteristics: Headaches are mild and occur in about 13% of patients. Decreased energy and weakness is common. Mild swelling of arms/legs may occur and is mild. Patients receiving anastrozole had more arthrosis, arthralgias, and arthritis.

Nursing Implications: Teach patient that headache and joint disorders are usually relieved by nonprescription analgesics and to report headaches that are unrelieved. Teach patient to elevate extremities when at rest, as needed.

IV.   POTENTIAL ALTERATION IN NUTRITION, LESS THAN BODY REQUIREMENTS, related to NAUSEA

Defining Characteristics: Nausea is mild, with a 15% incidence.

Nursing Implications: Determine baseline weight, and monitor at each visit. Teach patient that nausea may occur, and to report this. Discuss strategies to minimize nausea, including diet and dosing time.

V. POTENTIAL ALTERATION IN BOWEL ELIMINATION related to DIARRHEA

Defining Characteristics: Diarrhea is uncommon (9% incidence) and mild.

Nursing Implications: Assess for change in bowel patterns and teach patient to report diarrhea. If diarrhea occurs, teach patient that diarrhea is usually relieved by nonprescription medications, such as loperamide HCl and Kaopectate, and to report unrelieved diarrhea.

Drug: androgens: testosterone propionate (Testex), fluoxymesterone (Halotestin), testolactone (Teslac)

Class: Hormones.

Mechanism of Action: Has stimulatory effect on red blood cells that results in an increased HCT. Other mechanism of action unknown.

Metabolism: Metabolized by the liver; excreted in the urine and feces.

Dosage/Range:
- Fluoxymesterone: 10–30 mg PO daily (3–4 divided doses).
- Testolactone: 100 mg IM 3 × weekly or 250 mg PO 4 × daily.
- Testosterone propionate: 50–100 mg IM 3 × weekly.

Drug Preparation:
- Drug comes in ready-to-use vials or tablets.

Drug Administration:
- Before IM administration, shake vial vigorously and give injection immediately to avoid solution settling.

Drug Interactions:
- Pharmacologic effects of oral anticoagulants may be enhanced; monitor patient and adjust dose.

Lab Effects/Interference:
- LFTs: possible hepatic dysfunction with long-term use.
- Increased serum Ca.
- May cause decreased total serum thyroxine (T_4) concentrations and increased T_3 and T_4.

Special Considerations:
- Fluoxymesterone may increase sensitivity to oral anticoagulants. Should be administered in divided doses because of its short action.

Potential Toxicities/Side Effects and the Nursing Process

I.   POTENTIAL FOR INJURY related to SODIUM AND WATER RETENTION, HYPERCALCEMIA, AND OBSTRUCTIVE JAUNDICE

Defining Characteristics: Sodium and water retention may occur, necessitating dose reduction or diuretic use; hypercalcemia may occur initially in patients with bony metastases and needs to be distinguished from disease progression. Obstructive jaundice has occurred with methyltesterone, fluoxymesterone, and oxymetholone.

Nursing Implications: Identify patients most at risk for injury related to sodium and water retention: patients with cardiac, renal, or hepatic dysfunction, as well as patients with low serum albumin. Teach patient about potential side effects and instruct to report any changes to physician or nurse; assess patient at each visit for signs/symptoms of fluid and electrolyte imbalance. Identify patients at risk for hypercalcemia (those with bony metastases) and monitor serum calcium during first few weeks of therapy; hypercalcemia is an indication to discontinue therapy. Teach patient and family signs/symptoms of hypercalcemia (drowsiness, increased thirst, constipation, polyuria) and to notify physician. Monitor LFTs and instruct patient and family to report signs/symptoms of GI distress, diarrhea, jaundice.

II.   POTENTIAL FOR SEXUAL DYSFUNCTION related to MASCULINIZATION

Defining Characteristics: Commonly occurs in women receiving drug for > 3 months; with prolonged use, masculinization may be irreversible. Symptoms include increased libido, deepening of voice, excessive growth of body (face) hair, acne, and clitoral hypertrophy. In men, priapism (sustained and often painful erections) and reduced ejaculatory volume may occur.

Nursing Implications: Instruct patient to report symptoms of changes in sexual health. Discuss strategies to preserve sexual health; if unacceptable, discuss alternative medications with physician.

III.   ALTERATION IN NUTRITION, LESS THAN BODY REQUIREMENTS, related to NAUSEA AND VOMITING

Defining Characteristics: Nausea may occur.

Nursing Implications: Teach patient about possible side effects and administer antiemetics as ordered. Encourage small, frequent feedings and dietary modifications as appropriate.

Drug: arsenic trioxide (Trisenox)

Class: Miscellaneous antineoplastic agent.

Mechanism of Action: Not completely understood, but drug appears to cause changes in DNA with fragmentation typical of apoptosis or programmed cell death. Drug also damages and causes degradation of the fusion protein PML/RAR alpha characteristic of acute promyelocytic leukemia. The gene responsible for the fusion protein is corrected in many cases (cytogenetic complete response), so that immature malignant myelocytic cells mature into normal white blood cells.

Metabolism: Pharmacokinetics continues to be characterized. Drug is metabolized by methylation, primarily in the liver. Arsenic is stored primarily in the liver, kidney, heart, lung, hair, and nails. Drug appears to be excreted in the urine.

Indication: Drug is indicated for induction of remission and consolidation in patients with acute promyelocytic leukemia (APL) who are refractory to, or have relapsed from, retinoid and anthracycline chemotherapy, and whose APL is characterized by the presence of the t(15;17) translocation or PML/RAR-alpha gene expression.

Dosage/Range:
Adult:
- Induction dose of 0.15 mg/kg/d IV until bone marrow remission, not to exceed 60 doses.
- Consolidation begins 3–6 weeks after induction therapy is completed, at a dose of 0.15 mg/kg/d IV for 25 doses over a period of up to 5 weeks.

Drug Preparation:
- Drug is available in 10 mL, single-use ampules containing 10 mg of arsenic trioxide, with a concentration of 1 mg/mL, preservative-free.
- Further dilute prescribed dose immediately in 100–250 mL 5% dextrose injection, USP, or 0.9% sodium chloride injection, USP.
- Administer IV over 1–2 hours, or up to 4 hours if acute vasomotor reactions occur (does not require a central line).
- Drug is chemically and physically stable for 24 hours at room temperature and 48 hours when refrigerated.
- Drug does not contain any preservatives, so unused portions should be discarded.
- **Overdosage:** If symptoms of serious acute arsenic toxicity appear (seizures, muscle weakness, confusion), discontinue drug immediately and chelation therapy should be considered: dimercaprol 3 mg/kg IM q 4 hours until immediate life-threatening toxicity has subsided, then give penicillamine 250 mg PO up to qid ($\leq$ 1 g/day).

Drug Interactions:
- Unknown; do not mix with any other medications.
- Drugs that can prolong the QT interval (e.g., certain antiarrhythmics or thioridazine) or lead to electrolyte abnormalities (e.g., diuretics or amphotericin B) should be avoided if possible; otherwise, scrupulous monitoring and correction of abnormalities is critical.

Lab Effects/Interference:
- Hyperkalemia or hypokalemia.
- Hypomagnesemia.
- Hyperglycemia or hypoglycemia.
- Hypocalcemia.
- Increased hepatic transaminases ALT and AST.

- Leukocytosis.
- Anemia.
- Thrombocytopenia.
- Neutropenia.
- Disseminated intravascular coagulation (DIC).

Special Considerations:
- Drug may cause APL differentiation syndrome similar to the retinoic acid acute promyelocytic leukemia (RA-APL), which is characterized by fever, dyspnea, weight gain, pulmonary infiltrates, and pleural or pericardial effusions, with or without leukocytosis. This syndrome can be fatal, and, at the first suggestion, high-dose steroids should be instituted (dexamethasone 10 mg IV bid) for at least 3 days or longer until signs and symptoms abate. The drug manufacturer states that the majority of patients do not require termination of arsenic trioxide therapy during treatment of the syndrome (Cephalon Oncology, Trisenox package insert, June 2010).
- Drug can cause QT interval prolongation and complete atrioventricular block. Prolonged QT interval can progress to a torsades de pointes-type fatal ventricular arrhythmia. Risk factors for development of torsades de pointes are significant QT prolongation; concomitant administration of drugs that prolong the QT interval; history of torsades de pointes; preexisting QT prolongation; CHF; administration of potassium-wasting diuretics; conditions resulting in hypokalemia or hypomagnesemia, such as concurrent administration of amphotericin B.
- Prior to treatment with arsenic trioxide, the patient should have a baseline 12-lead EKG, as well as serum electrolytes and renal function tests. Electrolyte abnormalities should be corrected. Any drugs that prolong the QT interval should be discontinued. If the QT interval prolongation is > 500 msec, this should be corrected prior to drug administration. During arsenic trioxide therapy, serum potassium should be kept > 4.0 mEq/dL and serum magnesium > 1.8 mg/dL. If the QT interval exceeds 500 msec, reassessment and correction of risk factors should occur. The patient should be hospitalized for monitoring if syncope, or rapid or irregular heart rate occurs, and serum electrolytes assessed and any abnormalities corrected. Drug should be stopped until QT interval falls below 460 msec, electrolyte abnormalities are corrected, and symptoms resolve.
- Drug is a human carcinogen. Drug should not be used by pregnant or breastfeeding women.
- Standard monitoring: At least 2 times a week, the patient should have electrolyte, hematologic, and coagulation assessed; more frequently if abnormal during the induction phase, and at least weekly during the consolidation phase. EKGs should be done weekly; more frequently if abnormal.
- Most common side effects include leukocytosis, nausea, vomiting, diarrhea, abdominal pain, fatigue, edema, hyperglycemia, dyspnea, cough, rash, itching, headaches, and dizziness.
- Use with caution in patients with renal and hepatic insufficiency.

Potential Toxicities/Side Effects and the Nursing Process

I. ALTERATION IN OXYGENATION, POTENTIAL, related to APL DIFFERENTIATION SYNDROME

Defining Characteristics: Drug may cause APL differentiation syndrome similar to the retinoic acid acute promyelocytic leukemia (RA-APL), which is characterized by fever, dyspnea, weight gain, pulmonary infiltrates, and pleural or pericardial effusions, with or without leukocytosis. This syndrome develops in response to the differentiation of immature malignant cells into mature normal white blood cells and the increased white blood cell count. The body's response is an inflammatory reaction with fluid retention in the lining of the lungs and heart. This syndrome can be fatal, and at the first suggestion, high-dose steroids should be instituted (dexamethasone 10 mg IV bid) for at least 3 days or longer until signs and symptoms abate. The drug manufacturer states that the majority of patients do not require termination of arsenic trioxide therapy during treatment of the syndrome. The reported incidence is approximately 22%. Leucocytosis, if it occurs, at levels > 10 × 10³/μL is unrelated to baseline or peak white blood cell counts. Leukocytosis was not treated with chemotherapy, and levels were lower during consolidation than during induction.

Nursing Implications: Assess temperature and VS, oxygen saturation, cardiopulmonary status baseline and at each visit. Assess weight daily, and teach patient to report any SOB, fever, or weight gain immediately. If signs or symptoms develop, notify physician immediately and discuss obtaining CXR, cardiac echo, and focused exam. Discuss CXR, ECHO, and laboratory findings with physician. Be prepared to administer high-dose steroids (e.g., dexamethasone 10 mg IV bid 3 days or longer depending on symptom resolution). Provide pulmonary and hemodynamic support as necessary. Assess CBC, with focus on white blood cell count and presence of leukocytosis.

II. POTENTIAL ALTERATION IN CARDIAC FUNCTION related to QT PROLONGATION AND ARRHYTHMIA

Defining Characteristics: Drug can cause QT interval prolongation and complete atrioventricular block. Prolonged QT interval can progress to a torsades de pointes–type fatal ventricular arrhythmia. Risk factors for development of torsades de pointes are significant QT prolongation, concomitant administration of drugs that prolong the QT interval, history of torsades de pointes, preexisting QT prolongation, CHF, administration of potassium-wasting diuretics, and conditions resulting in hypokalemia or hypomagnesemia, such as concurrent administration of amphotericin B.

Nursing Implications: Assess baseline risk, cardiovascular status, EKG-determined QT interval, electrolyte and renal blood studies, and medications the patient is taking that may prolong QT interval, such as serotonin antagonist antiemetics. At least 2 times a week, the patient should have electrolyte, hematologic, and coagulation assessed; more frequently if abnormal during the induction phase, and at least weekly during the consolidation phase. EKGs should be done weekly and more frequently if abnormal. Discuss correction of any electrolyte abnormalities, as well as other risk factors, with physician. Any drugs that prolong the QT interval should be discontinued. If the QT interval prolongation is > 500 msec, this should be corrected prior to drug administration. During arsenic trioxide therapy, serum potassium should be kept > 4.0 mEq/dL and serum magnesium > 1.8 mg/dL. If the QT interval exceeds 500 msec, reassessment and correction of risk factors should occur. The patient should be hospitalized for monitoring if syncope or rapid or irregular heart rate occurs, and serum electrolytes assessed and any abnormalities corrected. Drug should be stopped until QT interval falls below 460 msec, electrolyte abnormalities corrected, and symptoms resolve.

III.   ALTERATION IN NUTRITION, LESS THAN BODY REQUIREMENTS, related to GI DYSFUNCTION

Defining Characteristics: Nausea is most common (incidence 75%), followed by vomiting (58%), abdominal pain (58%), diarrhea (53%), constipation (28%), anorexia (23%), dyspepsia (10%), abdominal tenderness or distention (8%), and dry mouth (8%).

Nursing Implications: Assess GI, nutrition status, and presence of GI dysfunction baseline, and with each visit, administer antiemetics and teach patient self-administration. Discuss risk of serotonin antagonists to prolong QT interval, and contraindication with physician. Teach patient to report signs and symptoms, and evaluate symptom-management plan based on effectiveness of symptom control. Assess presence of pain, and discuss pharmacologic and nonpharmacologic analgesic plan with physician.

IV.   ALTERATION IN PROTECTIVE MECHANISMS, related to FEVER, ANEMIA, DIC, BLEEDING

Defining Characteristics: Fever affects 63% of patients (13% febrile neutropenia), with 38% of patients having rigors. In clinical studies, 8% of patients had hemorrhage, 20% anemia, 18% thrombocytopenia, 10% neutropenia, and 8% DIC. Patients may develop infections, and in clinical studies, most commonly these were sinusitis 20%, herpes simplex 13%, upper respiratory tract infection 13%, nonspecific bacterial 8%, herpes zoster 8%, oral candidiasis 5%, and (rarely) sepsis 5%.

Nursing Implications: At least twice a week, the patient should have electrolyte, hematologic, and coagulation assessed; more frequently if abnormal during the induction phase, and at least weekly during the consolidation phase. Monitor laboratory results, and discuss abnormalities with physician. Assess patient for fever, signs and symptoms of infection, rigors, and bleeding, and implement management plan to assure patient safety. Transfuse patient as ordered, and monitor closely.

V. ALTERATION IN COMFORT related to HEADACHE, CHEST PAIN, AND INJECTION-SITE CHANGES

Defining Characteristics: Headache occurred in approximately 60% of patients, while chest pain occurred in 25%. Injection-site reactions of pain, erythema, and edema occurred in 20%, 13%, and 10% of patients, respectively.

Nursing Implications: Assess level of comfort, and develop plan for comfort, including pharmacologic and nonpharmacologic measures. Assess effectiveness, and revise plan as needed. Assess patency of IV site and need for IV catheter change. Assess need for central line. Although not necessary for drug delivery, if patient venous access is limited, this may provide enhanced patient comfort.

VI. ALTERATION IN ACTIVITY TOLERANCE related to FATIGUE, MUSCULOSKELETAL PROBLEMS

Defining Characteristics: 63% of patients reported fatigue. In clinical studies, musculoskeletal events were arthralgias (33%), myalgias (25%), bone pain (23%), back pain (18%), neck pain (13%), and pain in limbs (13%).

Nursing Implications: Assess baseline energy and activity level, and level of comfort. Assess need for assistance with ADL and home assistance. Assess need for analgesics or local measures to relieve pain and discomfort. Teach patient self-care strategies to minimize exertion and maximize activity, such as clustering activity during shopping, alternating rest and activity periods, diet, gentle exercise. Evaluate success of plan and need for revisions.

VII. ALTERATION IN FLUID AND ELECTROLYTE BALANCE related to HYPOKALEMIA, HYPOMAGNESEMIA, HYPERGLYCEMIA, EDEMA

Defining Characteristics: Hypokalemia occurs in about 50% of patients, hypomagnesemia (45%), hyperglycemia (45%), and edema (40%). Other electrolyte abnormalities are hyperkalemia (18%), hypocalcemia (10%), hypoglycemia (8%), acidosis (5%), and increased transaminases (13–20%).

Nursing Implications: At least twice a week, the patient should have electrolyte, hematologic and coagulation assessed; more frequently if abnormal during the induction phase, and at least weekly during the consolidation phase. EKGs should be done weekly and more frequently if abnormal. Teach patient that edema may occur, and to report it. Assess patient baseline and before each treatment for weight and presence of edema. Discuss abnormalities with physician, correct as ordered, and monitor closely for signs and symptoms of imbalance.

VIII. SENSORY/PERCEPTUAL ALTERATIONS, POTENTIAL, related to PARESTHESIA, DIZZINESS, TREMOR, INSOMNIA

Defining Characteristics: Insomnia occurs in 43% of patients, paresthesia (33%), dizziness (23%), tremor (13%), seizures (8%), somnolence (8%), and (rarely) coma (5%).

Nursing Implications: Assess baseline mental and neurologic status, and monitor frequently during therapy. Assess sensory function, and teach patient to report numbness, tingling, dizziness, tremor, seizure, decrease in alertness, and changes in sleep. Assess presence of paresthesias, and motor and sensory function prior to each treatment; discuss presence or worsening with physician. Teach patient self-care strategies, including maintaining safety when walking, getting up, taking a bath, or washing dishes if unable to feel temperature changes. Teach self-care measures to manage sleep problems, and discuss possible need for sleeping medication.

IX. ALTERATION IN GAS EXCHANGE, POTENTIAL, related to COUGH, DYSPNEA, HYPOXIA, PLEURAL EFFUSION

Defining Characteristics: Cough is common, affecting 65% of patients, followed by dyspnea (53%), epistaxis (25%), hypoxia (23%), pleural effusion (20%), postnasal drip (13%), wheezing (13%), decreased breath sounds (10%), crepitations (10%), rales (crackles) (10%), hemoptysis (8%), tachypnea (8%), and rhonchi (8%).

Nursing Implications: Assess baseline pulmonary status, including breath sounds and oxygen saturation, and monitor at least daily during treatment. Teach patient that symptoms may occur and to report them. Discuss management of patients experiencing cough, dyspnea, and other symptoms with physician, and develop individualized management plan.

X. ALTERATION IN SKIN INTEGRITY, POTENTIAL, related to SKIN IRRITATION

Defining Characteristics: Dermatitis affects about 43% of patients, pruritus (33%), ecchymosis (20%), dry skin (13%), erythema (13%), hyperpigmentation (8%), and urticaria (8%).

Nursing Implications: Assess baseline skin integrity and monitor at each visit. Teach patient to report any skin changes or itching. Teach patient symptomatic local measures to manage dermatitis, itch, or other changes. If plan is ineffective, discuss other measures with physician.

Drug: asparaginase (Elspar, Erwinaze, L-asparaginase)

Class: Miscellaneous agents (enzyme).

Mechanism of Action: Hydrolyzes serum asparagine, which deprives leukemia cells of the required amino acid. Normal cells are spared because they generally have the ability to synthesize their own asparagine. Cell cycle-specific for G_1 postmitotic phase. Some leukemic cells are unable to synthesize asparagine. These cells must obtain asparagine from an exogenous source, the patient's serum. Administration of the enzyme L-asparaginase causes hydrolysis of asparagine to aspartate, resulting in rapid depletion of the asparagine concentration in the patient's serum. The leukemic cells cannot synthesize protein or proliferate.

Metabolism: Metabolism of L-asparaginase is independent of renal and hepatic function. The drug is not recovered in the urine and does not appear to cross the blood–brain barrier.

Indication: For the therapy of patients with acute lymphocytic leukemia, primarily in combination with other chemotherapeutic agents in the induction of disease remissions in pediatric patients. Drug should not be used as the sole induction agent unless combination therapy is inappropriate. Drug is not recommended for maintenance therapy.

Contraindications: History of hypersensitivity to the type of asparaginase, (e.g., Erwinaze, *E. coli*); history of serious pancreatitis, thrombosis, or hemorrhagic events with prior L-asparaginase therapy.

Dosage/Range:
- Indicated as a component of a multi-agent chemotherapeutic regimen for treatment of patients with acute lymphoblastic leukemia (ALL).
- Erwinaze (asparaginase Erwinia chrysanthem) is indicated for patients who have developed hypersensitivity to E. coli–derived asparaginase.
- IM or IV varies with protocol.
- **Erwinaze:**
- To substitute for pegaspargase: 25,000 IU/m² IM 3 times a week (M/W/F) for 6 doses for each planned dose of pegaspargase.
- To substitute for a dose of native *E coli* asparaginase: 25,000 IU/m² IM for each scheduled dose of native *E. coli* asparaginase.

Drug Preparation:
- Erwinaze: available as vials containing 10,000 IU lyophylized powder per vial. Limit the volume of reconstituted Erwinaze as a single injection to 2 mL; if reconstituted dose to be administered is > 2 mL, use multiple injection sites.
- IV injection: reconstitute with sterile water for injection or 0.9% sodium chloride injection (without preservative), and use within 8 hours of restoration.
- IV infusion: dilute with 0.9% sodium chloride injection or 5% dextrose injection and use within 8 hours, only if clear; if gelatinous particles develop, filter through a 5.0-μm filter.
- IM: 6,000–12,000 units/m² dose as a single agent: reconstitute to 10,000 units/mL.
- The lyophilized powder must be stored under refrigeration. The reconstituted solution must also be stored under refrigeration if it is not used immediately. The solution must be discarded 8 hours after preparation.

Drug Administration:
- Erwinaze is administered IM.
- Test dose: often ordered before first dose or after restarting drug after a break; 0.1–0.2 mL of a 20- to 250-units/mL dose (2–50 units) intradermally and observe patient for 15–30 minutes.

• Use in a hospital setting. Make preparations to treat anaphylaxis at each administration of the drug and have epinephrine, diphenhydramine, and hydrocortisone nearby. Ensure that patent IV is available before giving drugs IM.

Drug Interactions:
• Prednisone: potential additive hyperglycemic effect; monitor blood glucose levels.
• Cyclophosphamide, vincristine, 6-mercaptopurine: may increase or decrease drug's effect (CTX, VCR, 6-MP).
• 6-mercaptopurine: enhanced hepatotoxicity; monitor LFTs closely.
• Methotrexate: antagonism if administered immediately prior to methotrexate; when administered some time after methotrexate, may enhance methotrexate activity.
• Synergy with cytosine arabinoside.
• Increased hyperglycemia when given together with prednisone.
• Reduced hypersensitivity when given with 6-mercaptopurine or prednisone.
• Additive neurotoxicity when given with vincristine.
• Asparaginase, when given before vincristine, will decrease vincristine excretion, with resulting increased neurotoxicity; give vincristine 12–24 hours before asparaginase.
• Live vaccines may enhance viral replication and toxicity.

Lab Effects/Interference:
• Increased LFTs.
• Increased pancreatic enzymes.
• Decreased hepatically derived clotting factors.
• Interferes with thyroid function tests after first 2 days of therapy: effect lasts 4 weeks.

Special Considerations:
• Discontinue the drug if serious hypersensitivity, including anaphylaxis, or serious hemorrhagic pancreatitis occurs.
• Glucose intolerance may occur, and in some cases is irreversible; perform glucose monitoring as appropriate and treat hyperglycemia with insulin as necessary.
• Thrombosis, hemorrhage may rarely occur; discontinue drug until this is resolved.
• Potential reduction in antineoplastic effect of methotrexate when given in combination.
• Anaphylaxis is associated with the administration of this drug.
• Intravenous administration of L-asparaginase concurrently with or immediately before prednisone and vincristine administration may be associated with increased toxicity.
• Drug is derived from purified *E. coli* or *Erwinia chrysanthemi,* and if an allergic reaction occurs, the patient may try the other drug. Also, pegylated asparaginase is also available.

Potential Toxicities/Side Effects and the Nursing Process

I.   POTENTIAL FOR INJURY related to HYPERSENSITIVITY
      OR ANAPHYLACTIC REACTIONS

Defining Characteristics: Occurs in 20–30% of patients. Increased incidence after several doses administered, but may occur with first dose. Occurs less often with IM route of administration. May be life-threatening reaction, but is usually mild.

Nursing Implications: Discuss with physician use of test dose prior to drug administration. Assess baseline vital signs and mental status prior to drug administration. Review standing orders or nursing procedure for management of anaphylaxis and be prepared to stop drug immediately if signs/symptoms occur; keep IV line open with 0.9% sodium chloride, notify physician, monitor vital signs, and administer ordered medications, which may include epinephrine 1:1,000, hydrocortisone sodium succinate, and diphenhydramine. Teach patient the potential of a hypersensitivity or anaphylactic reaction and to report any unusual symptoms immediately. *Escherichia coli* preparation of L-asparaginase and *Erwinia carotovora* preparation are non-cross-resistant, so if an anaphylactic reaction occurs with one, the other preparation may be used. HSR with Erwinaze is 17% incidence.

II. POTENTIAL FOR INJURY related to PANCREATITIS, HEPATIC DYSFUNCTION OR THROMBOEMBOLISM

Defining Characteristics: Pancreatitis occurred in 4% of patients receiving Erwinaze. Two-thirds of patients have elevated LFTs starting within the first 2 weeks of treatment: e.g., SGOT, bili, and alk phos. Hepatically derived clotting factors may be depressed, resulting in excessive bleeding or blood clotting. Relatively uncommon.

Nursing Implications: Monitor SGOT, bili, alk phos, albumin, and clotting factors CPT, PTT, fibrinogen. Teach patient of the potential of excessive bleeding or blood clotting, and instruct to report any unusual symptoms. Serious thrombotic events have been described, including sagittal sinus thrombosis. After a two-week course of Erwinase therapy, fibrinogen, protein C activity, protein S activity, and anti-III thrombin coagulation points were decreased. Assess patient for signs/symptoms of thrombosis or bleeding. Discontinue Erwinase for a thrombotic or hemorrhagic event until symptoms resolve, and then drug may be resumed. Assess patients receiving Erwinaze for signs/symptoms of severe or hemorrhagic pancreatitis: abdominal pain > 72 hr, amylase elevations > 2.0 × ULN, and stop drug. Drug should be discontinued if severe or hemorrhagic pancreatitis; if only moderate, drug can be reintroduced after serum amylase returns to normal levels, and signs/symptoms resolve.

III. ALTERED NUTRITION, LESS THAN BODY REQUIREMENTS, related to NAUSEA/VOMITING, ANOREXIA, HYPERGLYCEMIA

Defining Characteristics: 50–60% of patients experience mild to severe nausea and vomiting, starting within 4–6 hours after treatment. Anorexia commonly occurs. Hyperglycemia is a transient reaction caused by effects on the pancreas with decreased insulin synthesis. Pancreatitis occurs in 5% of patients.

Nursing Implications: Premedicate with antiemetics and continue prophylactically for 24 hours to prevent nausea and vomiting. Encourage small, frequent meals of cool, bland foods and liquids, as well as favorite foods, especially high-calorie, high-protein foods. Encourage use of spices and do weekly weights. Teach patient about the potential of hyperglycemia and pancreatitis, and instruct to report any unusual symptoms, e.g., increased thirst, urination, and appetite. Monitor serum glucose, amylase, and lipase levels periodically during treatment. Report any laboratory elevations to physician. Treat hyperglycemia issues with diet or insulin as ordered by physician. Treat pancreatitis per physician orders.

IV. SENSORY/PERCEPTUAL ALTERATIONS related to CHANGES IN MENTAL STATUS

Defining Characteristics: 25% of patients experience some changes in mental status—commonly, lethargy, drowsiness, and somnolence; rarely coma. Predominantly seen in adults. Malaise (feeling "blah") occurs in most patients, and generally gets worse with subsequent doses. Drug does not cross BBB.

Nursing Implications: Teach patient about the potential of CNS toxicity, and instruct to report any unusual symptoms. Obtain baseline neurologic and mental function. Assess patient for any neurologic abnormalities and report changes to physician. Discuss with patient the impact of malaise on his/her general sense of well-being and strategies to minimize the distress.

V. POTENTIAL FOR SEXUAL DYSFUNCTION related to REPRODUCTION HAZARD

Defining Characteristics: Drug is teratogenic.

Nursing Implications: As appropriate, explore with patient and partner issues of reproductive and sexual patterns and impact chemotherapy will have. Discuss strategies to preserve sexuality and reproductive health (e.g., sperm banking, contraception).

VI. INFECTION, BLEEDING, AND FATIGUE related to BONE MARROW DEPRESSION

Defining Characteristics: Bone marrow depression is not common. Mild anemia may occur. Serious leukopenia and thrombocytopenia are rare.

Nursing Implications: Monitor CBC, platelet count prior to drug administration, as well as signs/symptoms of infection, bleeding, or anemia. Instruct patient in self-assessment of signs/symptoms of infection, bleeding, or anemia and to report immediately.

Drug: azacytidine for injection (Vidaza)

Class: Nucleoside metabolic inhibitor (antimetabolite).

Mechanism of Action: Azacitidine is a pyrimidine nucleoside analogue of cytidine. It is believed to cause hypomethylation of DNA and to directly kill abnormal hematopoietic cells in the bone marrow (direct cytotoxicity). Hypomethylation may restore normal function to genes critical for cell differentiation and proliferation. Direct cytotoxicity causes the death of rapidly dividing cells, including cancer cells no longer responsive to normal growth control mechanisms, and it spares non-proliferating cells that are insensitive to the drug.

Metabolism: Rapidly absorbed following subcutaneous administration, with peak plasma level in 30 minutes. Bioavailability of subcutaneously administered drug is 89% of IV dose. 85% of the total administered dose is excreted in the urine, and < 1% in feces. Mean elimination half-life is about 4 hours in both subcutaneous and IV-administered drug.

Indication: Azacytidine is indicated for treatment of patients with myelodysplastic subtypes: (1) refractory anemia (RA), or (2) refractory anemia with ringed sideroblasts (RARS) (if accompanied by neutropenia or thrombocytopenia or requiring transfusions), (3) refractory anemia with excess blasts (RAEB), (4) refractory anemia with excess blasts in transformation (RAEB-T), and (5) chronic myelomonocytic leukemia (CMMoL).

Contraindication:
• Drug is contraindicated in patients with hypersensitivity to mannitol and in patients with advanced malignant hepatic tumors.

Dosage/Range:
Initial cycle: 75 mg/m² subcutaneous injection *or* IV infusion daily for 7 days, repeated every 4 weeks for at least 4 cycles. Premedicate for nausea and/or vomiting.
• Dose may be increased to 100 mg/m² after 2 cycles if initial dose ineffective and toxicity manageable (no toxicity except nausea and vomiting). A minimum of 4–6 cycles is recommended.
• Monitor patients for hematologic response and renal toxicities.

Dosage Adjustment:
• If baseline WBC ≥ 3,000/mm³, ANC ≥ 1,500/mm³, and platelets ≥ 75,000/mm³, modify dose based on nadir counts.
  • ANC < 500/mm³, platelets < 25,000/mm³—give 50% of dose next course.
  • ANC 500–1,500/mm³, platelets 25,000–50,000/mm³—give 67% of dose next course.
  • ANC > 1,500/mm³, platelets > 50,000/mm³—give 100% of dose.
• If baseline WBC < 3,000/mm³, ANC < 1,500/mm³, or platelets < 75,000/mm³, dose adjustments should be based on nadir and bone marrow biopsy cellularity at time of nadir, unless there is clear improvement in differentiation (% mature granulocytes is higher with ANC, higher than at onset of treatment) at the time of the next cycle—see package insert.
• Dose modification based on renal function and serum electrolytes.
  • If unexplained decreases in serum bicarbonate < 20 mEq/L, dose-reduce 50% in next cycle.
  • If elevations of BUN or serum creatinine occur, delay next dose until values return to normal or baseline, and reduce dose by 50% in next cycle.

Drug Preparation:
- Drug is a lyophilized powder in 100-mg single-use vials.
- Reconstitute aseptically with 4 mL sterile water for injection, adding diluent slowly into the vial.
- Vigorously shake or roll the vial until a uniform suspension is achieved, which will be cloudy and contain 25 mg/mL. Do not filter the suspension after reconstitution, as this may remove active substance.
- Divide doses greater than 4 mL into 2 syringes and administer within 1 hour of reconstitution at room temperature.
- Reconstituted solution may be kept in the vial or drawn in a syringe(s) and refrigerated immediately for later use. It may be stored for up to 8 hours if reconstituted with unrefrigerated sterile water for injection, and up to 22 hours if reconstituted with refrigerated sterile water for injection. After removal from the refrigerator, the suspension may be allowed to equilibrate to room temperature for up to 30 minutes prior to administration.
- IV preparation: Reconsititute with 10 mL sterile water for injection, and vigorously shake vial until dissolved. Resulting solution should be a clear concentration of 10 mg/mL. Withdraw the ordered amount, and inject into a 50- to 100-mL infusion bag of either 0.9% sodium chloride injection or Lactated Ringer's Injection. Drug is INCOMPATIBLE with 5% dextrose solutions, Hespan, or solutions containing bicarbonate.

Drug Administration:
- Contraindicated in patients with advanced malignant hepatic tumors and in patients who have had a prior hypersensitivity reaction to azacitidine or mannitol.
- To provide a homogenous suspension, the contents of the dosing syringe must be resuspended immediately prior to administration. To resuspend, vigorously roll the syringe between the palms until a uniform, cloudy suspension is achieved.
- Rotate sites for each subcutaneous injection (thigh, abdomen, or upper arm), and give new injection at least 1 inch from old site, and never into areas where site is tender, bruised, red, or hard. Doses > 4 mL should be divided equally into 2 syringes and injected into 2 separate sites.
- Administer IV solution over 10–40 minutes, so that administration is completed within 1 hour of reconstitution.
- Monitor hematologic response as well as for renal toxicity; delay or reduce drug dose as appropriate. Continue treatment as long as the patient continues to benefit.

Drug Interactions:
- IV solution: incompatible with 5% dextrose, Hespan, solutions containing bicarbonate.

Lab Effects/Interference:
- Decreased ANC, platelets, red blood cell counts.
- Renal tubular acidosis.
- Increased BUN and creatinine.
- Hypokalemia.

Special Considerations:
- Patients with hepatotoxicity or preexisting hepatic impairment are at higher risk for toxicity. Use cautiously in patients with preexisting hepatic disease, as patients with extensive liver metastases have been reported to develop coma and death. Teach patients to inform their physician if they have any underlying liver or renal disease.
- Drug is fetotoxic and embryotoxic. Women of childbearing age must use effective contraception methods; men should be advised not to father a child while receiving treatment with azacitidine. Nursing mothers should discontinue nursing or discontinue use of azacitidine, taking into consideration the importance of the drug to the mother.
- Monitor CBC/ANC frequently, as anemia, neutropenia, and thrombocytopenia are common. Monitor CBC/ANC for response and/or toxicity, at least prior to each dosing cycle. After cycle 1, adjust doses for subsequent cycles based on nadir counts and hematologic response.
- Monitor liver chemistries and serum creatinine, baseline and prior to each cycle of therapy. Azacitidine and its metabolites are primarily excreted by the kidney. Patients with renal impairment should be closely monitored for renal function and toxicity.
- Monitor renal function closely in the elderly.

Potential Toxicities/Side Effects and the Nursing Process

I.   INFECTION AND BLEEDING related to BONE MARROW DEPRESSION

Defining Characteristics: In clinical studies 1 and 2, incidence of leukopenia was 48.2%, neutropenia 32.3%, and febrile neutropenia 16.4%. Thrombocytopenia and anemia occurred in 65.5% and 69.5% of patients, respectively.

Nursing Implications: Monitor CBC, neutrophil, and platelet count baseline and prior to cycle, then as needed postchemotherapy; assess for signs/symptoms of infection, bleeding, and anemia. Teach patient and family signs/symptoms of infection, bleeding, and anemia, and instruct to report them to nurse or physician immediately. Teach patient to avoid aspirin-containing OTC medications.

II.   ALTERATION IN NUTRITION, LESS THAN BODY REQUIREMENTS, related to NAUSEA AND VOMITING, ANOREXIA, STOMATITIS, CONSTIPATION, AND DIARRHEA

Defining Characteristics: Nausea/vomiting is dose-related, and occurs in about 70.5%/54.1% of patients, respectively. This tends to be worse in the first 1–2 cycles, and increases in incidence with increasing doses. Diarrhea develops in 36.4% of patients, with incidence increasing as dose increases. Constipation occurs in about 33.6% of patients and is worse during the first 2 cycles of therapy. Anorexia affects 20% of patients, and stomatitis occurs in 7.7% of patients.

Nursing Implications: Assess nutritional and elimination status baseline, and periodically at visits. Premedicate with antiemetics before injection, and teach patient self-administration of antiemetics at home; encourage small, frequent feedings as tolerated; if severe vomiting occurs, treat with alternative antiemetics and assess for signs/symptoms of fluid and electrolyte imbalance. Monitor serum potassium, as hypokalemia may be a side effect of treatment. Assess baseline bowel elimination status. Instruct patient to report onset of diarrhea and administer antidiarrheals as ordered. If diarrhea is protracted, ensure adequate hydration, monitor total body fluid balance, and teach/reinforce perineal hygiene. Instruct patient to monitor for constipation and to use measures to prevent constipation if that is a problem. If patient has anorexia, teach patient to identify nutrient-dense foods and to eat small frequent meals, including a bedtime snack. Teach patient strategies to increase appetite, depending upon an individualized assessment. Teach patient to self-assess oral mucosa and to use a systematic cleansing of teeth/mouth after meals and at bedtime. Monitor LFTs periodically during therapy and discuss abnormalities with physician.

III.   ALTERATION IN COMFORT related to PYREXIA, FATIGUE, ARTHRALGIAS, HEADACHE, AND INJECTION-SITE IRRITATION

Defining Characteristics: Pyrexia occurred in 51.8% of patients, arthralgias in 22.3%, headache in 21.8%, injection-site erythema in 35%, injection-site pain in 22.7%, injection-site bruising in 14.1%, and injection-site reaction in 13.6%. Injection-site discomfort was more pronounced during the first and second cycles of therapy.

Nursing Implications: Monitor temperature and teach patient to self-assess temperature. Teach patient that pyrexia may occur and how to self-administer antipyretics. Teach measures to reduce discomfort related to myalgias if they occur, such as application of heat and NSAIDs. Teach patient strategies to conserve energy, such as alternating activity with rest. Teach patient to rotate sites used for injection, as well as local measures to increase comfort.

Drug: bendamustine hydrochloride (Treanda)

Class: Alkylating agent; nitrogen mustard derivative.

Mechanism of Action: Bifunctional with both alkylating and purine-like (antimetabolite) action. It causes sustainable double-strand DNA breaks and induces apoptosis, resulting in cell death. It appears to also cause apoptosis-independent cell death. It differs from nitrogen mustard by a benzimidazole ring, which helps to explain why the drug is active in patients who are refractory to other alkylating agents. Drug is active in dividing as well as resting cells. The exact MOA is unknown.

Metabolism: It undergoes biotransformation in the liver into an active compound; drug's active minor metabolites gamma-hydroxybendamustine and N-desmethyl-bendamustine are formed via cytochrome P450 CYP1A2. Low plasma protein binding; terminal half-life is 3.5 hours. Excreted via the kidneys as active drug and metabolites. No clinically significant differences in gender, or in geriatric patients, were seen in the adverse reaction profile.

Indication: FDA-indicated for the treatment of patients with (1) indolent B-cell non-Hodgkin's lymphoma that has progressed during or within 6 months of treatment with rituximab or a rituximab-containing regimen, as well as (2) patients with chronic lymphocytic leukemia (CLL). Comparative efficacy to first-line therapies in CLL other than chlorambucil unknown.

Contraindications: Patients with a known hypersensitivity to bendamustine.

CLL: 100-mg/m^2 IV infusion over 30 minutes on days 1 and 2 of a 28-day cycle, for up to 6 cycles.
- Grades 3 or higher hematologic toxicity: Dose-reduce to 50 mg/m^2 on days 1 and 2; if grades 3 or higher toxicity recurs, dose-reduce to 25 mg/m^2 on days 1 and 2.
- For nonhematologic toxicity, grades 3 or higher, dose-reduce to 50 mg/m^2 on days 1 and 2.

Indolent B-cell NHL: 120 mg/m^2 IV infusion over 60 minutes on days 1 and 2 of a 21-day cycle, for up to 8 cycles.
- Grade 4 hematologic toxicity: Dose-reduce to 90 mg/m^2 on days 1 and 2 of each cycle; if grade 4 toxicity recurs, dose-reduce to 60 mg/m^2 on days 1 and 2 of each cycle.
- Non-hematologic grades 3–4 toxicity: Dose-reduce to 90 mg/m^2 on days 1 and 2 of each cycle; if grade 3–4 toxicity recurs, dose-reduce to 60 mg/m^2 on days 1 and 2 of each cycle.

General Dosing Considerations:
- Delay treatment for grade 4 hematologic toxicity or clinically significant grade 2 or higher non-hematologic toxicity.
- Discontinue for severe skin reactions (as Stevens-Johnson syndrome may occur), severe infusion reactions, or anaphylactic reactions.
- Assess patient for tumor lysis syndrome, especially during cycle 1 of treatment and maintain adequate volume status with close monitoring of blood chemistry (i.e., potassium and uric acid levels).

Drug Preparation:
- Drug is available in two formulations:
  - (1) Solution (Treanda Injection) and (2) lyophilized powder (Treanda for Injection). Do NOT mix or combine the two formulations, as they have different drug concentrations.
  - If Treanda Injection solution is used, *do not* use devices containing polycarbonate or acrylo-nitrile-butadiene-styrene (ABS), including closed-system transfer devices (CSTDs), adapters, or syringes. ONLY USE polypropylene syringe (translucent) with a metal needle and polypropylene hub to withdraw and transfer Treanda Injection. Rationale: Treanda Injection contains *N,N*-dimethylacetamide (DMA), which is incompatible with polycarbonate and ABS, causing CSTDs, adaptors, and syringes containing polycarbonate or ABS to dissolve. This may lead to leaking, breaking of CSTD components, product contamination, and injury to patient and practitioner.

- Select formulation to administer.
  - If a closed-system transfer device or adaptor is to be used as supplemental protection during preparation, or the preparation area does not have polypropylene syringes with metal needles, *only use Treanda for Injection,* the lyophilized formulation.
  - **Preparing Treanda Injection** (45 mg/0.5 mL or 180 mg/2 mL solution; prepare only a single dose):
    - Use only a *polypropylene* syringe with a metal needle and polypropylene hub to withdraw and transfer the drug solution.
    - Aseptically withdraw the volume needed using a **polypropylene syringe with a metal needle and polypropylene hub**, for the calculated dose from the 90 mg/mL solution; **immediately** transfer solution to a 500-mL infusion bag of 0.9% sodium chloride injection, USP (an alternative of a 500-mL infusion bag of 2.5% dextrose/0.45% sodium chloride injection USP may be considered; no other diluents are compatible); the resulting bendamustine HCl concentration in the 500-mL bag should be within 0.2–0.7 mg/mL.
    - Visually inspect the filled syringe and the prepared infusion bag to ensure there is no visible particulate matter prior to administration. The prepared solution should be clear, colorless to yellow.
  - **Preparing Treanda for Injection** (25 mg/vial or 100 mg/vial lyophilized powder; each vial is single use only).
    - Aseptically reconstitute each Treanda for Injection vial as follows:
      - 25-mg vial: add 5 mL sterile water for injection, USP.
      - 100-mg vial: add 20 mL sterile water for injection, USP.
    - Shake well to completely dissolve the lyophilized powder; the result should be a clear, colorless to pale yellow solution with bendamustine HCl concentration of 5 mg/mL. Visibly inspect for particulate matter, and if found, do not use. *Transfer to the infusion bag must occur within 30 min of preparation.*
    - Aseptically withdraw the ordered dose and **immediately** transfer it to a 500-mL infusion bag of 0.9% sodium chloride injection, USP (an alternative 500-mL infusion bag of 2.5% dextrose/0.45% sodium chloride injection USP may be considered; no other diluents are compatible); the resulting concentration of bendamustine HCl in the bag should be within 0.2–0.6 mg/mL. Thoroughly mix the contents of the infusion bag, and again inspect for any particulate matter before administration. The solution should be clear, colorless to slightly yellow in color. Discard any unused drug.
  - **Admixture Stability:** Neither formulation contains an antimicrobial preservative, so the drug admixture should be prepared as close to the time of drug administration as possible.
    - **Treanda Injection** (45 mg/0.5 mL or 180 mg/2 mL solution): Once diluted in the infusion bag (either 0.9% sodium chloride USP or 2.5% dextrose/0.45% sodium chloride injection USP), the final admixture is stable for 24 hours when refrigerated at 2–8°C (36–47°F) or for 2 hours when stored at room temperature (15–30°C [59–86°F]) and room light.
    - **Treanda for Injection** (25 mg/vial or 100 mg/vial lyophilized powder): Once diluted in the infusion bag (either 0.9% sodium chloride USP or 2.5% dextrose/0.45% sodium chloride injection USP), the final admixture is stable for

24 hours when refrigerated at 2–8°C (36–47°F) or for **3 hours** when stored at room temperature (15–30°C [59–86°F]) and room light.

Drug Administration:
* Assess: ANC $\geq 1 \times 10^9$/L and platelets $\geq 75 \times 10^9$/L.
* Administer as an IV infusion over 30–60 minutes.
* Assess for rare allergic reactions.

Drug Interactions:
* Decrease bendamustine drug exposure: CYP1A2 inducers (e.g., omeprazole); smoking may decrease plasma concentrations of bendamustine and increase plasma concentrations of the active metabolites; consider alternative drugs to avoid CYP1A2 inducers.
* Increase bendamustine drug exposure: CYP1A2 inhibitors (e.g., ciprofloxacin, fluvoxamine), which may increase plasma concentrations of bendamustine and decrease concentration of active metabolites; consider alternative drugs to avoid CYP1A2 inhibitors.

Lab Effects/Interference:
* Decreased WBC, platelet counts, hemoglobin.

Special Considerations:
* Renal impairment: Do not use if Cr Cl is < 40 mL/min. Use with caution in lesser degrees of renal impairment. Hepatic impairment: Do not use in moderate to severe hepatic impairment. Use with caution in lesser degrees of hepatic impairment.
* Infusion reactions and anaphylaxis have occurred.
* Drug is carcinogenic and mutagenic. Women should use effective birth control measures to avoid pregnancy while receiving the drug. Alkylating drugs impair spermatogenesis with azoospermia and total germinal aplasia in men; spermatogenesis may return in several years. Depending on the patient's age, sperm banking may be recommended.
* If overdose is experienced, provide supportive care including monitoring of hematologic parameters and EKGs (QTc prolongation, tachycardia, ST and T-wave deviations).
* Premalignant and malignant diseases have been reported following bendamustine therapy.
* The most common non-blood-related side effects are nausea, fatigue, vomiting, diarrhea, fever, constipation, anorexia, cough, headache, weight decreased, dispend, rash, and stomatitis.
* The most common blood-related side effects are lymphopenia, anemia, leukopenia, thrombocytopenia, and neutropenia.

Potential Toxicities/Side Effects and the Nursing Process

I.   INFECTION AND BLEEDING related to BONE MARROW DEPRESSION

Defining Characteristics: Myelosuppression is major toxicity, with nadir occurring during the third week after drug administration, and recovery by day 28. Grades 3–4 neutropenia affects 24% with 3% febrile neutropenia. Thrombocytopenia is less common with 3% grades 3–4 and < 1% of patients requiring platelet transfusions. Decreased hemoglobin affects 89% of patients with 13% grades 3–4, and 20% requiring red cell transfusions.

Nursing Implications: Monitor CBC, neutrophil, and platelet count before drug administration and postchemotherapy. Subsequent treatments require ANC ≥ 1 × 10^9/L and platelets > 75 × 10^9/L; assess for signs/symptoms of infection, bleeding, and anemia. Teach patient/family signs/symptoms of infection, bleeding, and anemia, and instruct to report them to nurse or physician immediately. Teach patient to avoid aspirin-containing OTC medications. Teach patient to report increasing fatigue, signs of severe anemia (shortness of breath, chest pain/angina, headaches). Monitor hemoglobin/hematocrit; discuss transfusion or erythrocyte growth factor support with physician if signs/symptoms develop or hematocrit falls < 25 mg/dL. Teach patient about diet high in iron.

II.   POTENTIAL FOR INJURY related to INFUSION REACTION AND ANAPHYLAXIS

Defining Characteristics: Infusion reactions occur commonly and are characterized by fever, chills, pruritus, and rash. Fever occurs in 24% of patients and chills in 6%. Rarely, anaphylactoid and anaphylactic reactions may occur, especially on the second and subsequent cycles of therapy. Two percent of patients withdrew from therapy for hypersensitivity reactions.

Nursing Implications: Assess baseline VS and mental status before drug administration. Review standing orders or nursing procedure for patient management of anaphylaxis, and be prepared to stop drug immediately if signs/symptoms occur. Keep IV line open with 0.9% sodium chloride; notify physician, monitor VS, and administer ordered medications, which may include epinephrine 1:1,000, hydrocortisone sodium succinate, and diphenhydramine. If patients develop a grade 1 or grade 2 reaction, premedicate with antihistamines, antipyretics, and corticosteroids before subsequent cycles. Do not rechallenge, and discontinue therapy for grades 3 or 4 infusion reactions.

III.   POTENTIAL FOR INJURY related to TUMOR LYSIS SYNDROME (TLS)

Defining Characteristics: May develop with initial therapy if patient has a large tumor burden; results from rapid lysis of tumor cells. This usually begins 1 to 5 days after initiation of therapy and causes elevations in serum uric acid, potassium, phosphorus, creatinine.

Nursing Implications: For patients with a high tumor burden, expect medical orders to include oral allopurinol and vigorous oral hydration prior to beginning first cycle of therapy, together with IV hydration with the first cycle of therapy. Reinforce teaching about allopurinol and the importance of adhering to therapy as directed for the first few weeks after cycle 1 therapy. Monitor baseline and daily BUN, creatinine, phosphorus, uric acid, and calcium. Monitor for renal, cardiac, neuromuscular signs/symptoms of TLS.

TREATMENT

IV. ALTERATION IN NUTRITION, LESS THAN BODY REQUIREMENTS, related to NAUSEA AND VOMITING, DIARRHEA

Defining Characteristics: Nausea and/or vomiting are dose related and occur in 20% and 16% of patients, respectively. Grades 3–4 occur in < 1% of patients. Diarrhea occurs in 9% of patients and is generally mild. Dry mouth, mucositis, stomatitis, and constipation may also occur less commonly.

Nursing Implications: Assess nutritional status baseline and before each treatment. Premedicate with antiemetics before injection, and teach patient self-administration of antiemetics at home; encourage small, frequent feedings as tolerated. If severe vomiting occurs, treat with alternative antiemetics and assess for signs/symptoms of fluid and electrolyte imbalance. Monitor serum potassium, as hypokalemia may be a side effect of treatment. Assess baseline bowel elimination status. Instruct the patient to report the onset of diarrhea and to administer antidiarrheals as ordered. If diarrhea is protracted, ensure adequate hydration, monitor total body fluid balance, and teach/reinforce perineal hygiene. Teach patient dietary modifications, such as the BRAT (bananas, rice, applesauce, toast) diet if diarrhea develops.

V. POTENTIAL FOR IMPAIRED SKIN INTEGRITY related to RASH

Defining Characteristics: Rash occurs in 8% and pruritus in 5% of patients. Rarely, toxic skin reactions and bullous exanthema can occur. Skin reactions may be progressive and increase in severity with further treatment; if this occurs, drug should be withheld or discontinued.

Nursing Implications: Teach patient about possible side effects and self-care measures. Teach patient to report rash, and then monitor patient closely for signs of increase in severity or extent. Discuss with physician symptomatic treatment of skin changes and holding or discontinuing drug if rash is progressive or more severe.

Drug: bicalutamide (Casodex)

Class: Nonsteroidal antiandrogen [androgen receptor inhibitor].

Mechanism of Action: Binds to androgen receptors in the prostate, preventing normal androgen stimulation; affinity is four times greater than that of flutamide.

Metabolism: Extensively metabolized in the liver. Decreased drug excretion in patients with moderate to severe hepatic dysfunction.

Indication: Bicalutamide (Casodex) 50 mg is indicated for use in combination therapy with a lutenizing hormone-releasing hormone (LHRH) analog for the treatment of Stage D2 metastatic prostate cancer. Casodex 150 mg daily is not approved for use alone or with other treatments.

Contraindications: Hypersensitivity, women, and pregnancy.

Dosage/Range:
• 50 mg PO daily.

Drug Preparation:
• None.

Drug Administration:
• Orally. Given with luteinizing hormone-releasing hormone (LHRH) analogue or as a single agent after surgical castration. Teach patient to take pill at the same time each day.

Drug Interactions:
• R-bicalutamide is an inhibitor of CYP3A4; if bicalutamide is administered with a CYP 3A4 substrate, caution should be used. For example, when coadministered with midazolam, a CYP3A4 substrate, midazolam Cmax was increased 1.5 fold, and AUC 1.9 fold.
• Warfarin: Bicalutamide may increase anticoagulant effect; monitor PT, INR closely in patients who have been on coumarin anticoagulants who have started on bicalutamide, and adjust dose as needed.

Lab Effects/Interference:
• Increased LFTs.
• Increased BUN, WBC, Hgb.

Special Considerations:
• Use cautiously in patients with moderate to severe hepatic dysfunction. Observe closely for toxicity, as dosage adjustment may be required.
• No dose modification needed for renal dysfunction.

Warnings and Precautions:
• Hepatitis: post-marketing reports of patients with severe liver injury resulting in death have occurred, generally within the first 3–4 months of therapy.
  • Assess serum transaminase levels baseline, then at regular intervals for the first 4 months of therapy, and then periodically thereafter.
  • Teach patient to report signs/symptoms of liver dysfunction (e.g., nausea, vomiting, abdominal pain, fatigue, anorexia, flulike symptoms, dark urine, jaundice, RUQ tenderness).
  • If signs/symptoms occur, assess LFTs immediately, especially the ALT. If patient develops jaundice, or his ALT > 2 × ULN, immediately discontinue drug and closely follow liver function.
• Gynecomastia and breast pain: when drug given at 150-mg dose in clinical trials, gynecomastia and breast pain was reported in 38% and 39% of patients, respectively.
• Decreased glucose tolerance: has occurred, manifested by diabetes or loss of glycemic control in patients with preexisting diabetes. Assess baseline serum glucose and monitor it during drug therapy.

- Lab tests: regular assessment of PSA may be helpful in monitoring response to bicalutamide. If PSA levels rise on therapy, the patient should be evaluated for disease progression. If patient has progressed, continuing the LHRH analog and witholding antiandrogen therapy may be considered.
- Most common adverse events (> 10% incidence): hot flashes, pain (general, back, pelvic, abdominal), as thenia, constipation, infection, nausea, peripheral edema, dyspnea, diarrhea, hematuria, nocturia, anemia.

Potential Toxicities/Side Effects and the Nursing Process

I. ALTERATION IN COMFORT, POTENTIAL, related to GYNECOMASTIA AND HOT FLASHES

Defining Characteristics: Gynecomastia occurs in 23% of patients, breast tenderness in 26%, and hot flashes in 9.3%.

Nursing Implications: Teach patient that these side effects may occur, and discuss measures that may offer symptomatic relief.

II. ALTERATION IN NUTRITION, LESS THAN BODY REQUIREMENTS, related to NAUSEA, POTENTIAL

Defining Characteristics: Nausea may occur in 6% of patients.

Nursing Implications: Teach patient that nausea may occur, and instruct to report nausea. Determine baseline weight, and monitor at each visit. Discuss strategies to minimize nausea, including diet modification and time of dosing.

III. ALTERATION IN ELIMINATION, POTENTIAL, related to CONSTIPATION OR DIARRHEA

Defining Characteristics: Incidence of constipation is 6%, while that of diarrhea is 2.5%.

Nursing Implications: Assess baseline elimination pattern. Teach patient that alterations may occur, and instruct to report them if changes do not respond to usual nonprescription management strategies (OTC medications, dietary modifications).

Drug: bleomycin sulfate (Blenoxane)

Class: Antitumor action of bleomycin; isolated from fungus *Streptomyces verticullus*. Possesses both antitumor and antimicrobial actions.

Mechanism of Action: Induces single-strand and double-strand breaks in DNA. DNA synthesis is inhibited.

Metabolism: Excreted via the renal system. About 70% is excreted unchanged in urine; 30–60 minutes after IV infusion, urine levels are 10 times the serum level.

Indication: Initial indication is for palliative therapy useful in managing cancer of the head and neck (squamous cell carcinoma), Hodgkin's Disease, NHL, testicular cancer (embryonal cell, choriocarcinoma, and teratocarcinoma); useful as a sclerosing agent for managing malignant pleural effusion and preventing recurrent pleural effusions.

Dosage/Range:
- 5–20 units/m² once a week.
- 10–20 units/m² twice a week.
- **Continuous infusion:** 15 units/m²/day × 4 days.
- Pleural space (for pleurodesis): 50–60 units in 50- to 100-mL diluent, infused into pleural space and followed by change in position every 15 minutes. Give lidocaine 100–200 mg before infusion or mix with bleomycin to maximize comfort.
- Frequency and schedule may vary according to protocol and age.

Drug Preparation:
- Dilute powder in 0.9% sodium chloride or sterile water to prepare 15- or 30-unit vials.

Drug Administration:
- IV, IM, or subcutaneous doses may be administered. Some clinical trial protocols may use 24-hour infusions. There is a risk for anaphylaxis in lymphoma patients and hypotension with higher doses of drug. It may be recommended that a test dose be given before the first dose to detect hypersensitivity in patients with lymphoma.
- Dose-reduce if renal insufficiency: creatinine clearance 10–50 mL/min, decrease dose by 25%; creatinine clearance < 10 mL/min, give 50% of dose.
- Maximum lifetime dose is 400 units.

Drug Interactions:
- Cisplatin: may decrease bleomycin excretion with increased toxicity due to renal dysfunction.
- Oxygen: increased risk of pulmonary toxicity; do not use FiO₂ 100% oxygen.
- Bleomycin decreases the oral bioavailability of digoxin, so digoxin dose may need to be increased.
- Bleomycin decreases the pharmacologic effect of phenytoin when given in combination, so phenytoin dose may need to be increased.

Lab Effects/Interference:
- None.

Special Considerations:
- Because of pulmonary toxicities with increasing dose, pulmonary function tests (PFTs) and CXR should be obtained before each course or as outlined by protocol.
- Maximum cumulative lifetime dose: 400 units.
- Oxygen (FiO₂) increases risk of pulmonary toxicity.
- Reduce dose for impaired renal function (urinary creatinine clearance < 40–60 mL/min).

- Risk of pulmonary toxicity increased in elderly (age > 70 years old); renal impairment; pulmonary disease or prior chest XRT; exposure to high oxygen concentration (i.e., surgery); cumulative doses > 400 units lifetime.
- May cause chemical fevers up to 39.4–40.5°C (103–105°F) in up to 60% of patients. May need to administer premedications such as acetaminophen, antihistamines, or, in some cases, steroids.
- Watch for signs/symptoms of hypotension and anaphylaxis with high drug doses; physician may order test dose in patients with lymphoma.
- May cause irritation at site of injection (is considered an irritant, not a vesicant).
- Drug is being studied in novel administration routes, such as electrical pulse delivery.

Potential Toxicities/Side Effects and the Nursing Process

I. POTENTIAL FOR IMPAIRED GAS EXCHANGE related to PULMONARY TOXICITY

Defining Characteristics: Pneumonitis occurs in 10% of patients and is characterized by rales, dyspnea, infiltrate on CXR; in 1% may progress to irreversible pulmonary fibrosis. Risk factors include age > 70, dose > 400 units (but may occur at much lower doses), and concurrent or prior radiotherapy to the chest. Slower, continuous infusion may lower the risk.

Nursing Implications: Discuss with physician the need for PFTs and CXR prior to initiating therapy and monthly during therapy. Assess pulmonary status prior to each treatment (early symptom is dyspnea, and earliest sign is fine crackles). Instruct patient to report cough, dyspnea, shortness of breath. If patient needs surgery, discuss with physician the need to use low FiO_2 during surgery, since the lung tissue has been sensitized to bleomycin, and high concentrations of oxygen will cause further lung damage.

II. POTENTIAL FOR INJURY related to ANAPHYLAXIS

Defining Characteristics: Anaphylactoid reaction may occur in 1% of lymphoma patients, characterized by hypotension, confusion, tachycardia, wheezing, and facial edema. Reaction may be immediate or delayed for several hours and may occur after the first or second drug administration.

Nursing Implications: Discuss with physician the use of test dose prior to drug administration in lymphoma patients. Assess baseline VS and mental status prior to drug administration. Review standing orders or nursing procedure for patient management of anaphylaxis, and be prepared to stop drug immediately if signs/symptoms occur. Keep IV line open with 0.9% sodium chloride; notify physician, monitor VS, and administer ordered medications, which may include epinephrine 1:1,000, hydrocortisone sodium succinate, and diphenhydramine.

III. POTENTIAL ALTERATION IN COMFORT related to FEVER AND CHILLS,
AND PAIN AT TUMOR SITE

Defining Characteristics: Fever (up to 39.4–40.5°C [103–105°F]) and chills, occurring in up to 60% of patients, begin 4–10 hours after drug administration and may last 24 hours. There appears to be tolerance with successive doses of bleomycin. Pain may occur at tumor site due to chemotherapy-induced cellular damage.

Nursing Implications: Teach patient that these side effects may occur, and assess patient during and after administration. If fever occurs, notify physician and administer ordered acetaminophen, antihistamine, or steroid. If tumor pain occurs, reassure patient and discuss with physician the use of acetaminophen as analgesic.

IV. POTENTIAL FOR IMPAIRED SKIN INTEGRITY related to ALOPECIA,
SKIN CHANGES, AND NAIL CHANGES

Defining Characteristics: Dose-related alopecia begins 3–4 weeks after first dose and is reversible. Skin changes occur in 50% of patients and include erythema, rash, striae, hyperpigmentation, skin peeling of fingertips, and hyperkeratosis; these are dose-related and begin after 150–200 units have been administered. Skin eruptions include a macular rash over hands and elbows, urticaria, and vesiculations. Pruritus may occur. Nail changes and possible nail loss may occur. Phlebitis at the IV site may occur.

Nursing Implications: Teach patient about possible side effects and self-care measures, including obtaining a wig or cap as appropriate prior to hair loss. Encourage patient to verbalize feelings and provide patient emotional support. Discuss with physician symptomatic treatment of skin changes. Assess IV site for phlebitis and restart IV at alternate site if phlebitis develops.

V. POTENTIAL ALTERATION IN NUTRITION, LESS THAN BODY
REQUIREMENTS, related to NAUSEA AND VOMITING, ANOREXIA
AND WEIGHT LOSS, AND STOMATITIS

Defining Characteristics: Nausea with or without vomiting may occur; anorexia and weight loss may occur and may continue after treatment is completed; stomatitis may occur and decrease ability and desire to eat.

Nursing Implications: Administer antiemetic prior to initial treatment and revise plan for successive treatments if no nausea/vomiting. Teach patient about possible anorexia and encourage patient to eat high-calorie, high-protein foods. Assess oral mucosa prior to drug administration; teach patient self-assessment and instruct to notify nurse or physician if stomatitis develops. Teach patient oral care prior to drug administration.

VI. POTENTIAL FOR SEXUAL DYSFUNCTION related to REPRODUCTIVE HAZARDS

Defining Characteristics: Drug is mutagenic and probably teratogenic.

Nursing Implications: Discuss with patient and partner both sexuality and reproductive goals, as well as possible impact of chemotherapy. Discuss contraception and sperm banking if appropriate.

Drug: busulfan (Myleran)

Class: Alkylating agent.

Mechanism of Action: Forms carbonium ions through the release of a methane sulfonate group, resulting in the alkylation of DNA. Acts primarily on granulocyte precursors in the bone marrow and is cell cycle phase nonspecific.

Metabolism: Well absorbed orally; almost all metabolites are excreted in the urine. Has a very short half-life.

Indications: (Initial) Treatment of chronic granulocytic leukemia; also produces prolonged remission in polycythemia vera.

Dosage/Range:
Chronic myelogenous leukemia:
- 4–8 mg/day PO for 2–3 weeks initially, then maintenance dose of 1–3 mg/m² PO daily or 0.05 mg/kg orally daily. Dose titrated based on leukocyte counts. Drug withheld when leukocyte count reaches 15,000/µL; resume when total leukocyte count is 50,000/µL; maintenance dose of 1–3 mg daily used if remission lasts > 3 months.

High doses with bone marrow transplantation:
- See *busulfan for injection.*

Drug Preparation:
- None.

Drug Administration:
- Available in 2-mg scored tablets given orally.

Drug Interactions:
- Combination treatment with thioguanine may cause hepatic dysfunction and the development of esophageal varices in a small number of patients.

Lab Effects/Interference:
- Decreased CBC.
- Increased LFTs.

Special Considerations:
Regular dose:
- If WBC is high, patient is at risk for hyperuricemia. Allopurinol and hydration may be indicated.
- Follow weekly CBC and platelet count initially, then monthly. Dose is decreased to maintenance level when leukocyte count falls below 50,000 mm³.
- Hyperpigmentation of skin creases may occur due to increased melanin production.
- If given according to accepted guidelines, patients should have minimal side effects.

High dose:
- See *busulfan for injection.*

Potential Toxicities/Side Effects and the Nursing Process

I.   **POTENTIAL FOR INFECTION, BLEEDING, AND FATIGUE related to BONE MARROW DEPRESSION**

Defining Characteristics: The nadir is at 11–30 days following initial drug administration, with recovery in 24–54 days; however, delayed, refractory pancytopenia has occurred.

Nursing Implications: Monitor CBC, WBC differential, and platelets, initially weekly, then at least monthly. Expect drug will be interrupted if counts fall rapidly or steeply. Teach patient to self-assess for signs/symptoms of infection, bleeding, or severe fatigue, and to notify nurse or physician immediately. Teach patient to avoid aspirin-containing OTC medications.

II. **POTENTIAL FOR IMPAIRED GAS EXCHANGE related to INTERSTITIAL PULMONARY FIBROSIS**

Defining Characteristics: Rarely, bronchopulmonary dysplasia progressing to pulmonary fibrosis can occur, beginning 1 to many years posttherapy. Symptoms are usually delayed (occurring after 4 years) and include anorexia, cough, dyspnea, and fever. High-dose corticosteroids may be helpful, but condition may be fatal due to rapid, diffuse fibrosis.

Nursing Implications: Assess pulmonary status routinely in all patients receiving long-term therapy. Discuss plan for regular pulmonary function studies with physician.

III. **POTENTIAL FOR SEXUAL AND REPRODUCTIVE DYSFUNCTION related to REPRODUCTIVE HAZARDS**

Defining Characteristics: Premenopausal female patients commonly experience ovarian suppression and amenorrhea with menopausal symptoms; men experience sterility, azoospermia, and testicular atrophy. Although successful pregnancies have occurred following busulfan therapy, the drug is potentially teratogenic.

Nursing Implications: Assess patient's/partner's sexual patterns and reproductive goals. Provide information, supportive counseling, and referral as needed. Teach importance of birth control measures as appropriate.

Drug: busulfan for injection (Busulfex)

Class: Alkylating agent.

Mechanism of Action: Forms carbonium ions through the release of a methane sulfonate group, resulting in the alkylation of DNA. Acts primarily on granulocyte precursors in the bone marrow, and is cell cycle phase nonspecific.

Metabolism: After IV administration, drug achieves equal concentrations in the plasma and CSF. Drug is 32% protein-bound, metabolized in the liver, and excreted in the urine (30%). Appears metabolites may be long lived.

Indication: For use in combination with cyclophosphamide as a conditioning regimen prior to allogeneic hematopoietic progenitor cell transplantation for chronic myelogenous leukemia.

Dosage/Range:
Conditioning regimen:
- Indicated in combination with cyclophosphamide prior to allogeneic hematopoietic progenitor cell transplantation for chronic myelogenous leukemia.
- 0.8 mg/kg (IBW or actual weight, whichever is lower, or adjusted IBW) IV q 6 h × 4 days (total of 16 doses).
- Cyclophosphamide dose is given on each of 2 days as a 1-hour infusion at a dose of 60 mg/kg beginning on BMT day-3, 6 hours following the 16th dose of IV busulfan.

Drug Preparation:
- Aseptically open ampule, and using the 25-mm, 5-micron nylon membrane syringe filter provided, remove the ordered, calculated drug dose.
- Remove the syringe/filter, replace with a new needle, and dispense the syringe contents into a bag or syringe containing 10 times the volume of the drug, either 0.9% NS injection or 5% dextrose injection. The final concentration of drug should be ≥ 0.5 mg/mL. For example, a 70-kg patient at a dose of 0.8 mg/kg given a concentration of 6 mg/mL would require 9.3 mL (56 mg) busulfan total dose. 9.3 mL of drug × 10 = 93 mL. Adding 0.9% NS inj or D_5W inj, the total volume is 9.3 mL + 93 mL = 102.3 mL.
- Mix contents thoroughly.
- Ensure that this meets the recommended drug concentration, e.g., (9.3 mL × 6 mg/mL)/ 102.3 mL = 0.54 mg/mL.
- Unopened ampules must be refrigerated at 2–8°C (36–46°F).
- Diluted drug is stable at room temperature (25°C) for up to 8 hours, but infusion must be completed within this time. Drug diluted in 0.9% NS inj, USP, is stable refrigerated (2–8°C) for up to 12 hours, but the infusion must be completed within that time.

Drug Administration:
- Available in a 10-mL, single-use ampule containing 60 mg (6 mg/mL).
- Dilute in 0.9% NS injection or 5% dextrose injection to 10 times volume of drug (see example in Drug Preparation) prior to IV infusion.
- Infuse dose over 2 hours via infusion pump.
- Drug should be administered through a central line.
- All patients should be premedicated with phenytoin, as drug crosses BBB and causes seizures (see Drug Interactions).

Drug Interactions:
- CYP3A4 inducers: Phenytoin decreases busulfan AUC by 15%, resulting in the target dose. Use carbamazepine, nafcillin, and phenobarbital cautiously.
- Other anticonvulsants may increase busulfan AUC, increasing the risk of veno-occlusive disease or seizures. Monitor busulfan exposure and toxicity closely.
- CYP3A4 inhibitors: Itraconazole decreases busulfan clearance by up to 25% with potential significant increases in serum busulfan levels. Use ciprofloxacin, clarithromycin, erythromycin, imatinib, and verapamil cautiously.
- Acetaminophen prior to (< 72 hours) or concurrent with busulfan may result in decreased drug clearance and increased serum busulfan levels.
- St. John's wort: may decrease busulfan serum level; do not use concomitantly.
- Grapefruit juice: may enhance busulfan toxicity as inhibits CYP3A4 enzymes.

Lab Effects/Interference:
- Profound myelosuppression/aplasia with decreased WBC, neutrophils, Hgb/HCT, and platelet counts.
- If liver veno-occlusive disease develops, increased serum transaminases, alk phos, and bili.
- Creatinine is elevated in 21% of patients.

Special Considerations:
- Drug clearance in obese patients may be best predicted when the busulfan dose is based on adjusted ideal body weight (AIBW).
  - Ideal body weight (IBW in kg): men = 50 + 0.91 × (height in cm − 152); women = 45 + 0.91 × (height in cm − 152).
  - AIBW = IBW + 0.25 × (actual body weight − IBW).
- No known antidote if overdose occurs; one report says that drug is dialyzable.
- Drug is metabolized by conjugation with glutathione, so consider administration of same. Drug should only be given in combination with hematopoietic progenitor cell transplantation, as expected toxicity is profound myelosuppression.
- CNS effects including seizures, hepatic veno-occlusive disease (VOD), cardiac tamponade, bronchopulmonary dysplasia with pulmonary fibrosis 4 months to 10 years after therapy.
- Contraindicated in patients with a history of hypersensitivity to drug or its components.
- Women of childbearing age should use effective birth control measures; nursing mothers should interrupt breastfeeding during therapy.

- Drug is for adult use, and has not been studied in patients with hepatic insufficiency.
- Drug may cause cellular dysplasia in many organs (characterized by giant, hyperchromatic nuclei in lymph nodes, pancreas, thyroid, adrenal glands, liver, lungs, and bone marrow), which may cause difficult interpretation of subsequent cytologic examinations in lungs, bladder, and uterine cervix.
- Factors that may increase risk of veno-occlusive disease are history of XRT, more than 3 cycles of chemotherapy, prior progenitor cell transplantation, or Busulfex dose AUC concentrations of > 1,500 μm/min.

Potential Toxicities/Side Effects and the Nursing Process

I. POTENTIAL FOR INFECTION, BLEEDING, AND ANEMIA related to BONE MARROW DEPRESSION

Defining Characteristics: Myelosuppression is profound in 100% of patients. ANC < 500 cells/mm³ occurred a median of 4 days posttransplant in 100% of patients. Following progenitor cell infusion, the median recovery of neutrophil count to ≥ 500 cells/mm³ was day 13 when prophylactic G-CSF was given. 51% of patients experienced 1 + episodes of infection; fever occurred in 80% of patients, with chills in 33%. Thrombocytopenia (< 25,000/mm³ or requiring platelet transfusion) occurred in 5–6 days in 98% of patients. There was a median of six platelet transfusions per patient in clinical trials. Anemia affected 50% of patients, and the median number of red blood cell transfusions on clinical trials was 4 per patient.

Nursing Implications: Assess WBC, with differential, Hgb/HCT, and platelet count prior to drug administration, and at least daily during treatment. Discuss any abnormalities with physician. Monitor continuously for signs/symptoms of infection or bleeding. Teach patient signs/symptoms of infection and bleeding, self-assessment, and to report signs/symptoms immediately. Teach self-care measures to minimize infection and bleeding, including avoidance of OTC aspirin-containing medications. Discuss with physician use of granulocyte-colony stimulating factor (G-CSF) to prevent febrile neutropenia. Transfuse platelets and red blood cells per physician order.

II. ALTERATION IN CARDIAC OUTPUT, POTENTIAL, related to TACHYCARDIA, THROMBOSIS, HYPERTENSION, VASODILATION

Defining Characteristics: Mild-to-moderate tachycardia has been noted in 44% of patients (11% during drug infusion), and, less commonly, other rhythm disturbances such as arrhythmia (5%), atrial fibrillation (2%), ventricular extrasystoles (2%), and third-degree heart block (2%). Mild-to-moderate thrombosis may occur in 33% of patients, usually associated with a central venous catheter. Hypertension has been seen in 36% of patients and grade 3–4 in 3%. Mild vasodilation (flushing and hot flashes) occurs in 25% of patients. In clinical trials, most commonly in the postcyclophosphamide phase, other less common events were cardiomegaly (5%), mild EKG changes (2%), grades 3 and 4 CHF (2%), and moderate pericardial effusion (2%).

Nursing Implications: Assess baseline cardiac status frequently during shift/care depending upon patient condition, including HR, BP, EKG, and total body fluid balance. Monitor patient for changes in cardiac function throughout treatment course, and report changes immediately. Monitor central venous lines for patency, and use scrupulous care in maintaining catheters; assess for signs/symptoms of venous thrombosis, and discuss management with physician as soon as it is discovered.

III. ALTERATION IN FLUID AND ELECTROLYTE BALANCE, POTENTIAL, related to TREATMENT, CARDIAC RESPONSE

Defining Characteristics: 79% of patients develop edema, hypervolemia, or weight increase, mild or moderate.

Nursing Implications: Assess baseline fluid volume status, weight, orthostatic vital signs, and presence/absence of edema, and assess at least daily, especially after fluid or blood product infusion. Closely monitor I/O and daily total body balance, and discuss abnormalities with physician. Assess renal status, as BUN and creatinine can become elevated in 21% of patients. Assess patient for signs/symptoms of dysuria, oliguria, and hematuria, as hemorrhagic cystitis may occur with cyclophosphamide.

IV. POTENTIAL FOR IMPAIRED GAS EXCHANGE related to DYSPNEA AND INTERSTITIAL PULMONARY FIBROSIS

Defining Characteristics: Mild or moderate dyspnea was seen in 25% of study patients, and was severe in 2% (severe hyperventilation). 5% of patients in the study developed alveolar hemorrhage and died. One patient developed nonspecific interstitial fibrosis and died from respiratory failure on BMT day +98. Other reported pulmonary events were mild or moderate, including pharyngitis (18%), hiccup (18%), asthma (8%), atelectasis (2%), pleural effusion (3%), hypoxia (2%), hemoptysis (3%), and sinusitis (3%). As with oral busulfan, pulmonary fibrosis can occur 1 to many years posttherapy, with the average onset of symptoms 4 years after therapy (range 4 months to 10 years).

Nursing Implications: Assess pulmonary status, including breath sounds, rate, and oxygen saturation, at baseline and regularly during care. Assess for any underlying problems, such as infection, effusions, and leukemic infiltrates. Teach patient to report any dyspnea, SOB, or other change, and monitor closely. Provide oxygen and support and discuss management plan with physician and implement promptly. After therapy is completed, remind patient that pulmonary fibrosis may develop as a late effect. The patient should have long-term follow-up, and report any dyspnea or SOB, especially in the cold.

V. POTENTIAL FOR ALTERATION IN NUTRITION, LESS THAN BODY REQUIREMENTS, related to NAUSEA/VOMITING, ANOREXIA, STOMATITIS, DIARRHEA, AND ELECTROLYTE ABNORMALITIES

Defining Characteristics: The incidence of GI toxicities is high, but manageable: nausea 98%, vomiting 95%, stomatitis 97%, diarrhea 84%, anorexia 85%, dyspepsia 44%, and mild-to-moderate constipation 38%. Grade 3–4 stomatitis occurred in 26% of patients, severe anorexia in 21%, and grade 3–4 diarrhea in 5%. Additionally, hyperglycemia was seen in 67% of patients, with grade 3–4 in 15%. Hypomagnesemia was mild/moderate in 62%, and severe in 2%; hypokalemia was mild/moderate in 62% and severe in 2%; hypocalcemia was mild/moderate in 46% and severe in 3%; hypophosphatemia was mild/moderate in 17%, and hyponatremia occurred in 2%.

Nursing Implications: Assess baseline weight, usual weight, and any changes. Assess appetite, and favorite foods. Assess baseline glucose, electrolytes, and minerals, and monitor throughout therapy. Premedicate with aggressive antiemetics (serotonin antagonist) and continue protection throughout treatment. Assess efficacy and modify regimen as needed. Assess oral mucosa and teach patient self-care strategies, including assessment, what to report, oral hygiene regimen. Encourage dietary modifications as needed. Assess bowel elimination pattern baseline and daily during therapy. Teach patient to report diarrhea, and discuss management with physician. Provide comfort measures, and teach patient scrupulous hygiene to prevent infection. Discuss abnormal lab values with physician, correct hyperglycemia, and replete magnesium, potassium, phosphate, calcium, and sodium as ordered.

VI. POTENTIAL FOR SENSORY/PERCEPTUAL ALTERATIONS related to NEUROLOGIC TOXICITY

Defining Characteristics: Drug crosses BBB, achieving levels equivalent to plasma concentration. Neurologic changes observed in clinical testing were insomnia (84%), anxiety (75%), headaches (65%), dizziness (30%), depression (23%), confusion (11%), lethargy (7%), and hallucinations (5%). Less commonly, delirium occurred in 2%, agitation in 2%, encephalopathy in 2%, and somnolence in 2%. Despite prophylaxis with phenytoin, one patient developed seizures while receiving cyclophosphamide. Special caution should be used when patients with a history of seizure disorder or head trauma receive the drug.

Nursing Implications: Assess baseline neurologic status and continue to monitor status throughout. Closely monitor patients who have a history of seizure disorder, or head trauma for the development of seizures (seizure precautions). Teach patient to report any changes in usual patterns. Discuss any abnormalities with physician, and develop collaborative symptom-management strategies, including medications. Assess patient interest in relaxation exercises or imagery, or other techniques, and teach self-care strategies. Be prepared to manage seizures as needed.

VII.   ALTERATION IN HEPATIC FUNCTION, POTENTIAL, related to VENO-OCCLUSIVE DISEASE (VOD) AND GRAFT-VERSUS-HOST DISEASE (GVHD)

Defining Characteristics: Increased bilirubin occurred in 49% of patients, and grade 3–4 hyperbilirubinemia occurred in 30% within 28 days of transplantation. This was associated with GVHD in 6 patients in clinical studies, and with VOD in 8% of patients (5). Severe increases in SGPT occurred in 7%, while mild increases in alkaline phosphatase occurred in 15% of patients. Jaundice occurred in 12%, while hepatomegaly developed in 6%. VOD is a complication of conditioning therapy prior to transplant and occurred in 8% of patients (fatal in 2 of the 5 patients).

Factors that may increase risk of veno-occlusive disease are history of XRT, more than 3 cycles of chemotherapy, prior progenitor cell transplantation, or Busulfex dose AUC concentrations of > 1,500 µm/min. Use Jones' criteria to diagnose VOD hyperbilirubinemia, and two of the following: painful hepatomegaly, weight gain > 5%, or ascites. GVHD developed in 18% of patients (severe 3%, mild/moderate 15%, fatal in 3 patients).

Nursing Implications: Assess hepatic function baseline and daily during treatment. Discuss any abnormalities with physician. Teach the patient to report RUQ pain, weight gain, increasing girth, or yellowing of eyes or skin.

VIII.   ALTERATION IN COMFORT, POTENTIAL, related to ASTHENIA, PAIN, INJECTION SITE INFLAMMATION, ARTHRALGIAS

Defining Characteristics: Symptoms leading to discomfort include: abdominal pain (mild/moderate 69%, severe 3%), asthenia (mild/moderate 49%, severe 2%), general pain (45%), injection-site inflammation or pain (25%), chest or back pain (23–26%), and arthralgia (13%).

Nursing Implications: Assess baseline comfort, and usual strategies to promote comfort. Teach patient to report any pain, weakness, listlessness, injection-site discomfort, or any other changes. Discuss strategies to promote comfort, such as use of heat or cold. If discomfort persists, discuss pharmacologic management to reduce symptom distress.

IX.   POTENTIAL SEXUAL DYSFUNCTION related to DRUG EFFECTS

Defining Characteristics: Similar to oral busulfan: premenopausal female patients commonly experience ovarian suppression and amenorrhea with menopausal symptoms; men experience sterility, azoospermia, and testicular atrophy. The drug is potentially teratogenic.

Nursing Implications: Assess patient's signs/symptoms and partner's patterns of sexuality and reproductive goals. Teach patient/partner about need for effective contraception and provide other information as appropriate. Provide emotional support, supportive counseling, and referral as needed.

X. ALTERATION IN SKIN INTEGRITY, POTENTIAL, related to SKIN RASH, ALOPECIA

Defining Characteristics: Rash is common (57%) and pruritus less so (28%). Alopecia occurred in 15% of patients. Character of rash ranged from mild vesicular rash (10%), mild/moderate maculopapular rash (8%), vesiculobullous rash (10%), and exfoliative dermatitis (5%). Other skin abnormalities described were erythema nodosum (2%).

Nursing Implications: Assess baseline skin integrity, presence of rashes, itching, and repeat daily. Teach patient that skin changes may occur, and to report them. Discuss use of topical agents and antipruritic medications with physician.

Drug: cabazitaxel (Jevtana injection)

Class: Taxoid, mitotic spindle poison.

Mechanism of Action: Drug binds to tubulin and promotes its assembly into microtubules (making the structure for mitotis) while simultaneously inhibiting its disassembly. This leads to stabilization of the microtubules so that cell division is halted because the mitotic and interphase cellular functions are inhibited. Thus, tumor cell proliferation is halted.

Metabolism: Following an IV dose of 25 mg/m^2 every 3 weeks, the mean peak serum concentration (C_{max}) was reached at the end of the 1-hour infusion. The drug binds to human serum proteins (89–92%), mainly to serum albumin and lipoproteins, and the drug is equally distributed into blood and plasma. Drug is extensively metabolized in the liver (> 95%) mainly by the CYP3A4/5 isoenzymes and to a lesser extent, CYP2C8. The potential for the drug to inhibit drugs that are substrates of other isoenzymes is low, and the drug does not induce CYP isoenzymes. The drug has multiple metabolites that are excreted into the urine and feces (primary route). 2.3% of the drug is excreted intact in the urine. 80% of the drug is eliminated within 2 weeks of a dose. Mild to moderate renal dysfunction does not affect the pharmacokinetics of the drug significantly. Although not studied, hepatic impairment is likely to increase cabazitaxel concentrations. Therefore, patients with hepatic impairment should not receive the drug.

Indication: Microtubule inhibitor indicated in combination with prednisone for treatment of patients with hormone-refractory metastatic prostate cancer previously treated with a docetaxel-containing regimen.

Drug should not be given to patients with hepatic impairment (total bilirubin ≥ ULN, or AST and/or ALT ≥ 1.5 ULN).

Dosage/Range:
Following premedication, 25 mg/m^2 IV over 1 hour, every 3 weeks in combination with prednisone 10 mg PO administered daily throughout cabazitaxel therapy. Dose modifications of cabazitaxel for adverse reactions (Jevtana, 2010) follow:

Toxicity	Dose Modification
Prolonged grade ≥ 3 neutropenia (> 1 week) despite G-CSF	Delay treatment until neutrophil count is > 1,500 cells/mm^3, then reduce dose to 20 mg/m^2. Use G-CSF for secondary prophylaxis.
Febrile neutropenia	Delay treatment until improvement or resolution and until neutrophil count is > 1,500 cells/mm^3, then reduce dose to 20 mg/m^2. Use G-CSF for secondary prophylaxis.
Grade ≥ 3 diarrhea or persisting diarrhea despite appropriate medication, fluid, and electrolyte replacement	Delay treatment until improvement or resolution; reduce dose to 20 mg/m^2.

Discontinue drug if toxicity recurs despite dose reduction to 20 mg/m^2.

Drug Preparation:
Requires double dilution:
- Drug contains polysorbate 80. DO NOT USE PVC infusion containers or polyurethane infusion sets for preparation or administration of cabazitaxel (use same tubing and filter as with paxitaxel).
- Drug is supplied as a kit containing one single-use vial of cabazitaxel injection 60 mg/1.5 mL polysorbate 80, and one vial of diluent 5.7 mL (13% w/w ethanol in water). Both vials contain an overfill to compensate for liquid loss during preparation. The overfill ensures that after dilution with the **entire contents** of the supplied diluent, there is an initial diluted solution containing 10 mg/mL of cabazitaxel. Store at 25°C (77°F). Excursions permitted at 15–30°C (59–86°F). Do not refrigerate.

First dilution:
- Aseptically add the **entire contents** of the supplied diluent into the vial of cabazitaxel 60 mg/1.5 mL; the resulting solution contains 10 mg/mL of cabazitaxel. Inject the diluent along the wall of the drug vial slowly to decrease foaming. Remove syringe/needle and gently mix the solution followed by repeated inversions for at least 45 sec. Do not shake. Let the solution stand so the foam will dissipate, although if a little foam remains, can continue to second dilution.
- Proceed to second dilution right away, or at least within 30 minutes of initial dilution.

Second dilution:
- Aseptically withdraw the ordered dose from drug vial (10 mg/mL) into a sterile 250 mL PVC-free container of either 0.9% sodium chloride solution or 5% dextrose solution for infusion. If the dose is > 65 mg of cabazitaxel, use a larger volume so that a concentration of 0.26 mg/mL cabazitaxel is not exceeded. The resulting concentration of the second dilution should be between 0.10 mg/mL and 0.26 mg/mL. Once the drug is added to the infusion bag, gently invert the bag or bottle to assure mixing.
- Inspect the bag for any particles or precipitation. If precipitation occurs, discard the solution.
- Use fully prepared solution (in 0.9% sodium chloride or 5% dextrose) within 7 hours at ambient temperature (8 hours including 1-hour infusion time), or 24 hours (including 1-hour infusion time) if refrigerated. If refrigerated and crystals appear, do not use solution.

Drug Administration:
- Assess patient: Neutrophil count must be > 1,500 cells/mm^3.
- Premedication:
  - Antihistamine (e.g., diphenhydramine 25 mg or dexchlorpheniramine 5 mg)
  - Corticosteroid (e.g., dexamethasone 8 mg or equivalent)
  - H$_2$ antagonist (e.g., ranitidine 50 mg or equivalent)
  - Antiemetic regimen
  - Administer cabazitaxel IV over 1 hour, using an inline filter of 0.22-μm nominal pore size. Assess for signs/symptoms of hypersensitivity reactions, especially during cycles 1 and 2.

Drug Interactions:
- Strong CYP3A inducers (e.g., phenytoin, carbamazepine, rifampin, rifabutin, rifapentin, phenobarbital, St. John's wort) probably decrease cabazitaxel concentrations; avoid coadministration.
- Strong CYP3A inhibitors (e.g., ketoconazole, itraconazole, clarithromycin, atazanavir, indinavir, nefazodone, nelfinavir, ritonavir, saquinavir, telithromycin, voriconazole) are expected to raise cabazitaxel serum concentration. Avoid coadministration.
- Moderate CYP3A inhibitors: use together cautiously and monitor closely for cabazitaxel adverse effects.

Lab Effects/Interference:
- Neutropenia, thrombocytopenia, anemia common.
- Hematuria (17%).

Special Considerations:
- Cabazitaxel is FDA-approved for treatment of patients with hormone-refractory metastatic prostate cancer previously treated with a docetaxel-containing regimen, in combination with oral prednisone 10 mg.
- Drug is contraindicated in patients with (1) neutrophil count ≤ 1,500 cells/mm^3 or (2) history of severe hypersensitivity to cabazitaxel or polysorbate 80 (detergent used to dissolve

and keep cabazitaxel in solution). Polysorbate 80 is also used to dilute docetaxel, so if the patient had a hypersensitivity reaction to docetaxel, the patient should not receive this drug. In addition, patients with hepatic insufficiency (total bilirubin ≥ ULN or AST and/ or ALT ≥ 1.5 ULN) should not receive the drug.

- Most common all-grade toxicities were neutropenia, anemia, leukopenia, thrombocytopenia, diarrhea, fatigue, nausea, vomiting, constipation, asthenia, abdominal pain, hematuria, back pain, anorexia, peripheral neuropathy, pyrexia, dyspnea, dysgeusia, cough, arthralgia, and alopecia. The most common grades 3–4 adverse reactions were neutropenia, leukopenia, anemia, febrile neutropenia, diarrhea, fatigue, and asthenia. Alopecia occurs in 10% of patients.

- Deaths within 30 days of the last dose not due to disease progression were 5% in the cabazitaxel-treated patients, compared to < 1% in the mitoxantrone-treated patients. Causes of death were infections, renal failure, diarrhea-induced dehydration, and electrolyte imbalance. Patients in the United States had a mortality of < 1%, compared to 4.9% for European patients.

- FDA approval based on a randomized, open-label, international trial of 755 patients with metastatic hormone-resistant prostate cancer (mHRPC) previously treated with docetaxel-containing regimens. Median survival for the cabazitaxel group was 15.1 months compared to 12.7 months for the mitoxantrone-treated group (HR 0.70, $p < .0001$). No complete responses were seen in either arm.

Warnings and Precautions:

- Neutropenic deaths have been reported related to sepsis, so the patient's CBC/differential should be monitored weekly for the first cycle, and before each treatment thereafter so that the dose can be modified as needed.
  - The patient should receive the drug only if the neutrophil count is > 1,500/cells mm^3.
  - Determine if the patient should receive G-CSF and/or dose modification as primary (at high-risk) or secondary (along with dose reduction) prophylaxis.
  - Patients with high-risk clinical features should receive G-CSF as primary prophylaxis (e.g., age > 65 years, poor performance status, previous episodes of febrile neutropenia, extensive prior radiation ports, poor nutritional status, or other serious comorbidities).
  - If the patient experiences febrile neutropenia or prolonged (> 1 week) neutropenia despite G-CSF, the cabazitaxel dose should be decreased to 20 mg/m$_2$ when the patient's ANC is > 1,500/mm^3.

- Severe hypersensitivity can occur within minutes after starting the infusion and may be characterized by generalized rash/erythema, hypotension, and bronchospasm.
  - All patients should be premedicated prior to starting the drug infusion.
  - Drug should be stopped immediately if severe reaction occurs and appropriate emergency care instituted.
  - The patient should be monitored closely during the infusion, especially cycles 1 and 2, and emergency equipment and medications should be readily available.

- Cabazitaxel should be discontinued if the patient has a severe hypersensitivity reaction, and appropriate therapy instituted. Do not rechallenge the patient.
- Gastrointestinal toxicity can be severe, and patients on clinical trials have died from diarrhea and electrolyte imbalance. The trial was multi-institutional (146 institutions) and involved 26 countries.
  - Patients should receive aggressive correction and management of severe diarrhea and fluid and electrolyte imbalance. Rehydration, anti-diarrheal, or antiemetic therapy should be instituted promptly. Patients may require a treatment delay or dose reduction if patient develops grade 3 or higher diarrhea.
  - GI hemorrhage, perforation, Ileus, enterocolitis, neutropenic enterocolitis, including fatal outcome, have been reported. Risk may be increased with neutropenia, age, steroid use, concomitant use of NSAIDs, anti-platelet therapy, anti-coagulation, and prior history of pelvic radiotherapy, adhesions, and GI bleeding.
  - Assess and evaluate promptly patients who develop abdominal pain and tenderness, fever, persistent constipation, diarrhea with or without neutropenia, which may be early signs/symptoms of serious GI toxicity. Treatment delay or discontinuation may be necessary.
- Renal failure with fatal outcome has been reported in the clinical trials, so patients with new-onset renal failure should be evaluated and treated aggressively, with efforts made to determine the etiology.
  - Hematuria was reported in 17% of patients.
  - Most cases occurred in association with sepsis, dehydration, obstructive uropathy.
- Elderly patients had increased adverse reactions, including neutropenia, febrile neutropenia, fatigue, asthenia, pyrexia, dizziness, UTI, and dehydration.
  - Elderly patients should be monitored closely during therapy to identify side effects and manage them aggressively.
  - Telephone calls to the patient to assess tolerance between cycles, as well to reinforce patient teaching to minimize toxicity and to encourage calling the provider if problems occur, will help identify problems early.
- Hepatic impairment: drug is extensively metabolized in the liver, and hepatic impairment increases the risk of severe and life-threatening complications, especially in patients receiving other drugs of the same class as cabazitaxel. Drug should not be administered to patients with hepatic impairment (total bilirubin ≥ ULN, or AST and/ or ALT ≥ 1.5 ULN).
- Drug is fetotoxic, embryotoxic, and abortifacient.
  - If the drug is used during pregnancy, or if the patient becomes pregnant while receiving the drug, the patient should be told of the potential risk to the fetus.
  - If used in women, teach women of childbearing age to use effective contraception to avoid pregnancy. Drug crosses placental barrier in rodents, so mothers receiving the drug should not nurse their infants. A decision should be made whether to discontinue nursing or to discontinue the drug.

Potential Toxicities/Side Effects and the Nursing Process

I.   POTENTIAL FOR INJURY related to HYPERSENSITIVITY OR ANAPHYLAXIS REACTIONS

Defining Characteristics: Severe hypersensitivity reactions characterized by generalized rash/erythema, hypotension, and/or bronchospasm can occur, especially during the first or second infusions. If patient experiences a severe hypersensitivity reaction, patient should not be rechallenged and drug should be discontinued. Polysorbate 80 (Tween 80) is an emulsifier that is water-soluble, which is the vehicle by which cabazitaxel is soluble in the blood. Polysorbate 80 serves a similar purpose for docetaxel. However, it may cause hypersensitivity reactions. Patients who have had a hypersensitivity reaction to polysorbate 80 should not receive the drug. If the patient had a hypersensitivity reaction to docetaxel, it is likely the patient reacted to polysorbate 80 and should not receive cabazitaxel. Cardiac arrhythmias may occur in 5% of patients; hypotension may occur in 5% of patients as well.

Nursing Implications: Ensure that patient has received premedication (e.g., antihistamine, corticosteroid, H2 receptor antagonist). Assess baseline VS and mental status prior to drug administration, especially first and second doses of the drug. Monitor VS every 15 minutes, and remain with patient during first 15 minutes of drug infusion, as most reactions occur during the first 10 minutes. Continue to monitor closely for the duration of the 1-hour infusion. Stop drug if cardiac arrhythmia (irregular apical pulse) or hypo- or hypertension occur and discuss continuance of infusion with physician. Recall signs/symptoms of anaphylaxis, and if these occur, stop drug immediately and notify physician. Subjective symptoms are generalized itching, nausea, chest tightness, crampy abdominal pain, difficulty speaking, anxiety, agitation, sense of impending doom, uneasiness, desire to urinate/defecate, dizziness, chills. Objective signs are flushed appearance; angioedema of face, neck, eyelids, hands, feet; localized or generalized urticaria; respiratory distress with or without wheezing, hypotension, cyanosis. Review standing orders or nursing procedure for patient management of anaphylaxis, and be prepared to stop drug immediately if signs/symptoms occur. Keep IV line open with 0.9% sodium chloride, notify physician, monitor VS, and administer ordered medications, which may include epinephrine 1:1,000, hydrocortisone sodium succinate, and diphenhydramine. Teach patient the potential of a hypersensitivity or anaphylactic reaction and to report any unusual symptoms immediately. The drug should be permanently discontinued in patients who have a hypersensitivity reaction.

II.   POTENTIAL FOR INFECTION AND BLEEDING related to BONE MARROW DEPRESSION

Defining Characteristics: Neutropenia is common (94%), with 82% grades 3–4, and is the dose-limiting toxicity. Febrile neutropenia occurred in 7% of patients. Anemia occurs in almost all patients (98%), while thrombocytopenia is less common (48%). Pyrexia was reported by 12% of patients.

Nursing Implications: Assess baseline CBC and differential to ensure that ANC is > 1,500/mm^3 and platelet count is > 100,000/mm^3 prior to chemotherapy, as well as for signs/symptoms of infection or bleeding. Patients should have weekly CBC/differential and assessment for neutropenia for the first cycle. Assess need for G-CSF with cycle 1 in high-risk patients (e.g., age > 65 years, poor performance status, previous episodes of febrile neutropenia, extensive prior radiation ports, poor nutritional status, or other serious comorbidities), and discuss with physician to ensure that patient receives primary prophylaxis. Teach patient signs/symptoms of infection or bleeding and to report these immediately, and teach patient self-care measures to minimize risk of infection and bleeding. This includes avoidance of crowds, proximity to people with infections, and avoidance of OTC aspirin-containing medications. Teach patient self-administration of G-CSF as ordered to prevent severe neutropenia. Instruct patient to alternate rest and activity periods and to report increased fatigue, shortness of breath, or chest pain that might herald severe anemia. If the patient is elderly, monitor more closely both at the time of treatment and between cycles, assessing for tolerance and need for additional support.

III. ALTERED NUTRITION, LESS THAN BODY REQUIREMENTS, related to NAUSEA AND VOMITING, DIARRHEA, CONSTIPATION, DYSGEUSIA, ANOREXIA

Defining Characteristics: Diarrhea is common (47%) and may be severe and life-threatening. Nausea and vomiting occur in 34% and 22% of patients, respectively, but are mild and preventable with antiemetics. Constipation occurs in 20% of patients, while other symptoms are less common: dyspepsia (10%), anorexia (16%), dehydration (5%), dysgeusia (11%), and weight loss (9%). Mucosal inflammation affected 6% of patients.

Nursing Implications: Premedicate patient with antiemetic. If patient develops nausea and/or vomiting, encourage small, frequent intake of cool, bland foods. Instruct patient to report nausea, and teach self-administration of antiemetic medications. If nausea/vomiting occur and are severe, assess for signs/symptoms of fluid/electrolyte imbalance. Encourage patient to report onset of diarrhea. Teach patient to self-administer antidiarrheal medications if needed. If the patient has diarrhea, ensure it is well controlled and that potential complications of dehydration and electrolyte imbalance are avoided. Give special attention to the elderly patient and follow more closely between cycles as to tolerance and remaining hydrated. Involve dietitian as needed.

IV. POTENTIAL ALTERATION IN ACTIVITY TOLERANCE related to ASTHENIA, FATIGUE, ARTHRALGIA, ANEMIA

Defining Characteristics: Fatigue affects about 37% of patients, and 20% experience asthenia. Back pain (16%), arthralgia (11%), and muscle spasms (7%) may also occur.

Nursing Implications: Assess Hgb/HCT prior to each treatment and at nadir counts. Assess patient activity tolerance and ability to do ADLs. Teach patient self-care strategies to minimize exertion and maximize activity, such as clustering activity during shopping, alternating rest and activity periods, diet, gentle exercise. Instruct patient to alternate rest and activity periods and to report increased fatigue, shortness of breath, or chest pain that might herald severe anemia.

V.   SENSORY/PERCEPTUAL ALTERATIONS related to SENSORY NEUROPATHY

Defining Characteristics: Grade 1–4 peripheral neuropathy may affect up to 13% of patients (grades 3–4 < 1%). All patients previously received docetaxel, which may cause peripheral neuropathy. Dizziness occurs in 8% of patients, as does headache.

Nursing Implications: Assess baseline neurologic status. Instruct patient to report signs/symptoms of pins-and-needle sensation, numbness, pain, increased discomfort with certain sensations, especially in the extremities, or motor weakness. Identify patients at risk: those with history of docetaxel use or with preexisting neuropathies (ethanol- and diabetes mellitus-related). Assess sensory and motor function prior to each treatment, and if abnormality found, assess impact on patient's function, safety, independence, and quality of life. Test patient's ability to button a shirt or pick up a dime from a flat surface. If severely impacting safety or quality of life, discuss with patient and physician drug discontinuance or use of cytoprotective agent. Teach self-care strategies, including maintaining safety when walking, getting up, taking a bath, or washing dishes; discuss risk of inability to sense temperature and the need to keep extremities warm in cold weather. If peripheral neuropathy affects function, discuss impact on quality of life with patient and physician.

Drug: capecitabine (Xeloda, N4-pentoxycarbonyl-5-deoxy-5-fluorocytidine)

Class: Nucleoside metabolic inhibitor (fluoropyrimidine carbamate).

Mechanism of Action: Metabolites bind to thymidylate synthetase, inhibiting the formation of uracil from thymidylate, and reducing the cell's ability to produce DNA. It also prevents cell division by hindering the formation of RNA, by causing nuclear transcription enzymes to mistakenly incorporate its metabolites in the process of RNA transcription.

Metabolism: Absorbed from the intestinal mucosa as an intact molecule, metabolized in the liver to intermediary metabolite, and then in the liver and tumor tissue to 5-FU precursor. It is then converted through catalytic activation to 5-FU at the tumor site. Metabolites are cleared in the urine.

Indications: Capecitabine in indicated for:
- Adjuvant treatment of patients with Duke's C colon cancer.
- Metastatic colorectal cancer (mCRC) as first-line monotherapy when treatment with fluoropyrimidine therapy alone is preferred.
- Metastatic breast cancer, in combination with docetaxel after failure of prior anthracycline-containing therapy, or as monotherapy in patients resistant to both paclitaxel and an anthracycline-containing regimen.

Contraindications: Patients with
- Dihydropyrimidine dehydrogenase (DPD) deficiency.
- Severe renal impairment.
- Hypersensitivity.

Dosage/Range:
- Monotherapy: 1250 mg/m^2 twice daily orally for 2 weeks followed by a one-week rest period in 3-week cycles.
- Adjuvant treatment is recommended for a total of 6 months (8 cycles).
- Breast cancer in combination with docetaxel, the recommended dose of capecitabine is 1250 mg/m^2 twice daily for 2 weeks followed by a 7-day rest period, combined with docetaxel at 75 mg/m^2 as a 1-hour infusion every 3 weeks.
- Capecitabine dosage may need to be individualized to optimize patient management treatment. Toxicity due to capecitabine may be managed symptomatically, by dose interruptions and dose adjustment. Once the dose has been reduced, it should not be increased at a later time.
- Doses of capecitabine omitted for toxicity should not be replaced or restored; rather, resume planned treatment cycle.
- Reduce the dose of capecitabine by 25% in patients with moderate renal impairment (CrCl 30–50 mL/min) when used as monotherapy, or when combined with docetaxel from 1250 mg/m^2 to 950 mg/m^2 twice daily.
- Package insert has Xeloda dose calculation, according to BSA reference.
- See package insert for toxicity directed dose levels/modifications for toxicity, and docetaxel dose reductions in combination with capecitabine.

Drug Preparation:
- Available in 150- and 500-mg tablets.

Drug Administration:
- Administer within 30 min of a meal with a full glass of water.
- Divide daily dose in half; take 12 hours apart.

Drug Interactions:
- Warfarin: INR, monitor closely and adjust warfarin dose as needed.
- Phenytoin: monitor phenytoin serum level closely and decrease phenytoin dose as needed.
- Leucovorin: increases the concentration of 5-FU, so synergy and enhanced toxicity; monitor closely.
- CYP2C9 substrates: coadminister carefully and monitor patient closely.
- Food: reduces rate and extent of capecitabine absorption.

Lab Effects/Interference:
- Increased bili, alk phos.
- Decreased WBCs.

Special Considerations:
- Monitor bilirubin baseline and before each cycle, as dose modifications are necessary with hyperbilirubinemia.

- Folic acid should be avoided while taking drug.
- Contraindicated in patients hypersensitive to 5-fluorouracil or patients with creatinine clearance < 30 mL/mm.
- There are reports that patients on capecitabine who develop hand-foot syndrome involving the fingers may lose their fingerprints, which can cause problems for patients who travel internationally.
- Most common adverse reactions (≥ 30%) were diarrhea, hand-foot syndrome, nausea, vomiting, abdominal pain, fatigue/weakness, and hyperbilirubinemia.
- Nursing mothers should discontinue nursing when receiving capecitabine.

Warnings and Precautions:

- Diarrhea: can be severe; monitor patient closely and replace fluid and electrolytes to prevent dehydration. Dose interrupt and dose-reduce for reoccurrence of grade 2 or occurrence of any grade 3 or 4 diarrhea (see package insert). Necrotizing enterocolitis (typhlitis) has been reported.
- Coagulopathy: Patients taking warfarin or oral coumarin-derivative anticoagulants may develop altered coagulation parameters and/or bleeding.
  - Assess and monitor INR or PT closely, and make dose adjustments based on laboratory results.
  - Occurs several days to up to several months after starting capecitabine therapy; may also be seen within 1 month after drug stopped.
  - Predisposing factors: age > 60, diagnosis of cancer.
- Cardiotoxicity: MI, myocardial ischemia, angina, dysrhythmias, cardiac arrest, cardiac failure, sudden death, ECG changes, and cardiomyopathy have occurred, and patients with prior history of coronary heart disease may be at higher risk.
- Dihydropyrimidine dehydrogenase deficiency (DPD) increases risk of 5-FU toxicity (e.g., stomatitis, diarrhea, neutropenia, and neurotoxicity).
- Renal insufficiency: patients with baseline moderate renal impairment require dose reduction; carefully monitor patients for adverse effects. If toxicity occurs (grade 2–4), immediately interrupt therapy and adjust dose when toxicity resolves (see package insert).
- Pregnancy: drug can cause fetal harm. If capecitabine is used during pregnancy, or if a patient becomes pregnant while receiving capecitabine, apprise the patient of the potential hazard to the fetus.
- Hand-foot syndrome (HFS, palmar-plantar erythrodysesthesia, chemotherapy-induced acral erythema) has occurred. Median time to onset was 79 days.
  - Grade 1 = numbness, dysesthesia/paresthesia, tingling, painless swelling or erythema of the hands and/or feet and/or discomfort that does not disrupt normal activities.
  - Grade 2 = painful erythema and swelling of hands and/or feet and/or discomfort affecting patient's ADLs.
  - Grade 3 = moist desquamation, ulceration, blistering or severe pain of hand and/or feet, and/or severe discomfort that causes the patient to be unable to work or perform ADLs.
  - Interrupt capecitabine for grade 2 or 3 HFS until it resolves or decreases to a grade 1.
  - Grade 3 HFS: decrease dose of capecitabine when event/HFS resolves to grade 1.

- Hyperbilirubinemia: may occur, and patients with liver metastases are at risk. If drug-related grade 3–4 elevations in bilirubin occur, interrupt capecitabine immediately until bilirubin decreases to ≤ 3.0 × ULN (see package insert for dose modifications).
- Hematologic: do not administer drug to patients with a baseline ANC < 1,500/mm³ and/ or platelet count of < 100,000/mm³. If unscheduled lab assessments during a treatment cycle show grade 3 or 4 neutropenia or thrombocytopenia occurs, hematologic toxicity, interrupt capecitabine therapy until recovery. See package insert.
- Geriatric patients: patients 80 years of age and older may experience a greater incidence of grade 3–4 adverse events. Take extra care with the elderly, monitoring the patient closely and intervening promptly to minimize toxicity.
- Hepatic insufficiency: monitor patients with mild to moderate hepatic dysfunction related to liver metastases closely for toxicity, and intervene promptly.

Potential Toxicities/Side Effects and the Nursing Process

I. POTENTIAL FOR INFECTION AND BLEEDING related to BONE MARROW DEPRESSION

Defining Characteristics: Commonly causes anemia, neutropenia, and thrombocytopenia.

Nursing Implications: Assess baseline CBC, WBC with differential, and platelet count prior to chemotherapy, as well as for signs/symptoms of infection or bleeding. Teach patient signs/symptoms of infection and bleeding and instruct to report these immediately; teach patient self-care measures to minimize risk of infection and bleeding. This includes avoidance of crowds, proximity to people with infections, and avoidance of OTC aspirin-containing medications.

II. ALTERED NUTRITION, LESS THAN BODY REQUIREMENTS, related to NAUSEA AND VOMITING, STOMATITIS, AND DIARRHEA

Defining Characteristics: Nausea and vomiting occur in 30–50% of patients. Stomatitis and diarrhea also occur in about 50% of patients. Less common with reduced doses. Abdominal pain (35%), constipation (14%), anorexia (26%), dehydration (7%) also occur. Side effects are increased in the elderly (≥ 80 yrs old). The median time to first occurrence of grade 2–4 diarrhea was 34 days, and the median duration of grade 3–4 diarrhea was 5 days.

Nursing Implications: Premedicate patient with antiemetics (phenothiazines usually effective), and continue for 24 hours, at least for first cycle. Encourage small, frequent meals of cool, bland foods. Assess oral mucosa prior to drug administration and teach patient to report changes. Teach patient oral hygiene measures and self-assessment. Instruct patient to report diarrhea, to self-administer prescribed antidiarrheal medications, and to drink adequate fluids. Moderate to severe stomatitis, diarrhea, or nausea and vomiting are indications to interrupt therapy. If grade 2, 3, or 4 diarrhea occurs, capecitabine should be interrupted immediately until diarrhea resolves or decreases in intensity to grade 1. If grade 2 diarrhea reoccurs, or occurrence of any grade 3 or 4 diarrhea, capecitabine dose should be reduced.

III.   ALTERATION IN SKIN INTEGRITY/COMFORT related to HAND-FOOT SYNDROME

Defining Characteristics: Hand-foot syndrome occurs in more than half of patients and is characterized by tingling, numbness, pain, erythema, dryness, rash, swelling, and/or pruritus of hands and feet. Less common with reduced doses.

Nursing Implications: Teach patient about the possibility of this side effect and instruct him or her to stop drug use and inform the physician/nurse immediately should it occur. If patient has pain, expect dose interruption, with dose reduction if this is second or subsequent episode at current dose. Teach patient self-assessment of soles of feet and palms of hands daily for erythema, pain, dry desquamation, and to report pain right away. Teach patients to avoid hot showers, whirlpools, paraffin treatments of nails, vigorous repetitive movements of hands, feet, as well as other body areas; avoid tight-fitting shoes and clothes. Teach patients to take cool showers, keep skin surfaces intact and soft with skin emollients. Studies ongoing establishing evidence base for prophylaxis or treatment: vitamin B_6, urea moisturizers, nicotine patch.

IV.   ALTERATION IN COMFORT related to FATIGUE, WEAKNESS, DIZZINESS, HEADACHE, FEVER, MYALGIAS, INSOMNIA, AND TASTE PROBLEMS

Defining Characteristics: Fatigue affects approximately 43% of patients, while 42% of patients complained of weakness. Fever was reported in 18% of patients, headache 10%, dizziness 8%, insomnia 7%, and taste problems 6%. Eye irritation was reported by 13% of patients and is related to the drug's excretion via tears.

Nursing Implications: Assess baseline comfort, and teach patient that these symptoms may occur. Teach patient strategies to manage fatigue, such as alternating rest and activity periods, and consolidating tasks. Teach patient to report fever, headache, and eye irritation, and discuss management plan with physician.

Drug: carboplatin (Paraplatin)

Class: Alkylating agent (heavy metal complex).

Mechanism of Action: A second-generation platinum analog. The cytotoxicity is identical to that of the parent, cisplatin, and it is cell cycle phase nonspecific. It reacts with nucleophilic sites on DNA, causing predominantly intrastrand and interstrand crosslinks rather than DNA-protein crosslinks. These crosslinks are similar to those formed with cisplatin but are formed later.

Metabolism: At 24 hours postadministration, approximately 70% of carboplatin is excreted in the urine. The mean half-life is roughly 100 minutes.

Indication:

- Initial treatment of advanced ovarian carcinoma in established combination with other approved chemotherapy agents.
- Secondary, palliative treatment of patients with ovarian carcinoma recurrent after prior chemotherapy, including patients previously treated with cisplatin.

Dosage/Range:

- Dose usually given as a function of area under the curve (AUC). Since carboplatin has predictable pharmakinetics based on the drug's excretion by the kidneys, AUC dosing is recommended for this drug. This allows tailoring the drug dose precisely to the individual patient's excretion of the drug (renal function). The Calvert formula is used where total dose (mg) = target AUC × glomerular filtration rate (GFR) + 25. The GFR is approximated by the urine creatinine clearance, either estimated or actual, and can be calculated by hand. The target AUC is determined by the treatment plan depending on the type of malignancy, such as an AUC of 6 for cancer of unknown primary. Then the dose calculation can be done by hand. Additionally, the manufacturer (Bristol-Myers Squibb Oncology) distributes a calculator to determine the dose.
- As a single agent, 360 mg/m^2 every 4 weeks, or 300 mg/m^2 when combined with cyclophosphamide for advanced ovarian cancer. Delay drug for neutrophil count < 2,000/mm^2 or platelets < 100,000/mm^3.
- Drug dose reduction for urine creatinine clearance < 60 mL/minute.
- Autologous bone marrow transplantation: 1600 mg/m^2 IV in divided doses over 4 days (creatinine clearance must be more than 50 mL/min).
- Intraperitoneal: 200–650 mg/m^2 in 2-L IP (ovarian cancer).

Drug Preparation:

- Available as a white powder in amber vial in 50-, 150-, and 450-mg vials.
- Reconstitute with sterile water for injection, 5% dextrose, or 0.9% sodium chloride solution.
- Dilute further in 5% dextrose or 0.9% sodium chloride.
- Injection solution available (10 mg/mL) in 50-, 150-, 450-, and 600-mg vials.
- The solution is chemically stable for 24 hours; discard solution after 8 hours because of the lack of bacteriostatic preservative.

Drug Administration:

- Administered by IV bolus over 15 minutes to 1 hour.
- May also be given as a continuous infusion over 24 hours.
- May be administered intraperitoneally in patients with advanced ovarian cancer.

Drug Interactions:

- Increases renal toxicity when combined with cisplatin.
- Increases bone marrow depression when combined with myelosuppressive drugs.
- Avoid aluminum needles in drug handling.
- Paclitaxel, docetaxel: administer carboplatin after taxane to maximize cell kill and to minimize the risk of myelosuppression caused by decreased drug excretion.

- Phenytoin: may decrease phenytoin serum levels; monitor levels, and increase drug dose as needed.
- Warfarin: may increase warfarin effect; monitor INR frequently, and dose modify as needed.

Lab Effects/Interference:
- Increased LFTs, RFTs.

Special Considerations:
- Does not have the renal toxicity seen with cisplatin.
- Thrombocytopenia is dose-limiting toxicity and correlates with GFR.
- Monitor urine creatinine clearance.

Potential Toxicities/Side Effects and the Nursing Process

I.   POTENTIAL FOR INFECTION AND BLEEDING related to BONE MARROW DEPRESSION

Defining Characteristics: Myelosuppression is dose-limiting toxicity; platelet nadir is 14–21 days, with usual recovery by day 28; WBC nadir follows 1 week later, but recovery may take 5–6 weeks. The risk of thrombocytopenia is severe, especially when the drug is combined with other myelosuppressive drugs, or if the patient has renal compromise. Anemia may occur with prolonged treatment.

Nursing Implications: Assess CBC, WBC, with differential, and platelet count prior to drug administration. Monitor for signs/symptoms of infection or bleeding. Drug dosage should be reduced if urine creatinine clearance is < 60 mL/min. Drug should be held or dose reduced if absolute neutrophil count (ANC) and/or platelet count is low. Teach the patient signs/symptoms of infection and bleeding, and instruct to report them immediately if they occur. Teach self-care measures to minimize infection and bleeding. Discuss with physician use of granulocyte-colony stimulating factor (G-CSF) to prevent neutropenia in heavily pretreated patients.

II.   POTENTIAL FOR ALTERED URINARY ELIMINATION related to NEPHROTOXICITY

Defining Characteristics: The drug does not have the renal toxicity seen with cisplatin (Platinol), so that only minimal hydration is needed. However, the drug is excreted by the kidneys, and concomitant treatment with drugs causing nephrotoxicity (i.e., aminoglycoside antibiotics) can alter renal function studies. Nephrotoxicity does occur at high doses, and patients with renal dysfunction are at risk. In addition, serum electrolyte loss can occur (potassium, magnesium, rarely calcium). Monitor serum electrolytes prior to treatment and periodically after treatment. Replete electrolytes as ordered.

Nursing Implications: Assess renal function studies (i.e., urine creatinine clearance, serum blood urea nitrogen [BUN], and creatinine) prior to drug administration. Discuss drug dose modification if creatinine clearance < 60 cc/min, or if other values are abnormal.

III. POTENTIAL FOR ALTERATION IN NUTRITION, LESS THAN BODY REQUIREMENTS, related to NAUSEA/VOMITING, ANOREXIA, STOMATITIS, DIARRHEA, AND HEPATIC DYSFUNCTION

Defining Characteristics: Nausea and vomiting begin 6+ hours after administration and last for < 24 hours, but may be easily prevented by available antiemetics. Anorexia occurs in 10% of patients but is usually mild, lasting 1–2 days. Diarrhea occurs in 10% of patients and is mild. Reversible hepatic dysfunction is mild to moderate, as evidenced by changes in alk phos and SGOT and, rarely, serum glutamic pyruvic transaminase (SGPT) and bili.

Nursing Implications: Premedicate with antiemetics and continue protection for 24 hours, at least for the first cycle. Encourage dietary modifications as needed. Monitor LFTs prior to and periodically during treatment.

IV. POTENTIAL FOR SENSORY/PERCEPTUAL ALTERATIONS related to NEUROLOGIC CHANGES

Defining Characteristics: Neurologic dysfunction is infrequent, but there is increased risk in patients > 65 years old, or if previously treated with cisplatin and receiving prolonged carboplatin treatment.

Nursing Implications: Assess baseline neurologic status and continue to monitor status throughout treatment, looking for dizziness, confusion, peripheral neuropathy, ototoxicity, visual changes, and changes in taste. Teach patient the potential for side effects, and to report any changes.

V. POTENTIAL SEXUAL DYSFUNCTION related to DRUG EFFECTS

Defining Characteristics: Drug is mutagenic and probably teratogenic. It is unknown whether drug is excreted in breastmilk.

Nursing Implications: Assess patient's signs/symptoms and partner's patterns of sexuality and reproductive goals. Teach patient/partner about need for contraception and provide other information as appropriate. Provide emotional support.

VI. POTENTIAL FOR INJURY related to HYPERSENSITIVITY REACTIONS

Defining Characteristics: Drug may cause allergic reactions, ranging from rash, urticaria, erythema, and pruritus to anaphylaxis; they can occur within minutes of drug administration.

Nursing Implications: Assess baseline VS. During drug administration, observe for signs/symptoms of hypersensitivity reaction. If signs/symptoms of anaphylaxis (tachycardia, wheezing, hypotension, facial edema) occur, stop drug immediately. Keep IV patent with 0.9% sodium chloride, notify physician, monitor VS, and be prepared to administer ordered drugs (i.e., steroid, epinephrine, or antihistamines).

Drug: carmustine (BCNU, BiCNU)

Class: Nitrosourea.

Mechanism of Action: Alkylates DNA by causing crosslinks and strand breaks in the same manner as classic mustard agents; it also carbamylates cellular proteins, thus inhibiting DNA repair. Cell cycle phase nonspecific.

Metabolism: Rapidly distributed and metabolized with a plasma half-life of 1 hour; 70% of IV dose is excreted in urine within 96 hours. Significant concentrations of drug remain in cerebrospinal fluid for 9 hours due to lipid solubility of drug.

Indications: Palliative therapy as a single agent or in established combination therapy with other chemotherapy agents in the following:
- Brain tumors.
- Multiple myeloma, in combination with prednisone.
- Hodgkin's disease, as secondary therapy with other approved drugs for patients who relapse while being treated with primary therapy, or who fail to respond to primary therapy.
- NHL: as secondary therapy in combination with other approved drugs for patients who relapse while being treated with primary therapy, or who fail to respond to primary therapy.

Dosage/Range:
Usual:
- 75–100 mg/m^2 IV/day × 2 day OR
- 150–200 mg/m^2 every 6 week OR
- 40 mg/m^2/day on 5 successive days, repeating cycle every 6–8 weeks.
- Polifeprosan 20 with carmustine (BCNU) implant: see *polifeprosan*.

High dose with autologous BMT (investigational):
- 450–600 mg/m^2 IV; however, doses of 900 mg/m^2 (in combination with cyclophosphamide) or 1200 mg/m^2 as single agent have been reported.
- These doses are fatal and require AUTOLOGOUS BMT after drug administration.
- Refer to protocol for exact dosages.

Drug Preparation:
- Add sterile alcohol (provided with drug) to vial, then add sterile water for injection.
- May be further diluted with 100–250 mL 5% dextrose or 0.9% sodium chloride.

High dose (investigational):
- IV bolus in at least 500 mL of 5% dextrose over 2 hours; can also divide dose into two equal fractions administered 12 hours apart. Refer to protocol for exact information.
- When given for gliomas as a single agent, administer with dexamethasone or mannitol infusion to reduce cerebral edema.
- Usually given in combination with other cytotoxic agents in BMT protocols.

Mycosis fungoides:
- Carmustine topical solution 0.5–3.0 mg/mL may be painted on body after showering, daily × 14 days (investigational).

Drug Interactions:
- Cimetidine may increase myelosuppression when given concurrently. AVOID IF POSSIBLE.
- Possible increased cellular uptake of drug when administered in combination with amphotericin B.
- Carmustine may decrease the pharmacologic effects of phenytoin.
- Avoid concomitant administration of renally or hepatically toxic drugs, as these may increase carmustine-induced renal or hepatic dysfunction.

Lab Effects/Interference:
- Pulmonary, hepatic, and renal function tests.

Special Considerations:
- Drug is an irritant; avoid extravasation.
- Pain at the injection site or along the vein is common. Treat by applying ice pack above the injection site and decreasing the infusion flow rate.
- Patient may act inebriated related to the alcohol diluent and may experience flushing.

High dose:
- Pulmonary toxicity related to higher systemic levels (higher AUC).

Potential Toxicities/Side Effects and the Nursing Process

I. POTENTIAL FOR INFECTION AND BLEEDING related to BONE MARROW DEPRESSION

Defining Characteristics: Delayed myelosuppression is dose-limiting toxicity and is cumulative. WBC nadir 3–5 weeks after dose and persists 1–2 weeks; platelet nadir at 4 weeks, persisting 1–2 weeks. Drug should not be dosed more frequently than once every 6 weeks.

Nursing Implications: Assess baseline CBC, WBC with differential, and platelet count prior to chemotherapy and at least weekly postchemotherapy for the first cycle. Discuss dose reductions with physician for subsequent cycles if counts are lower than normal since bone marrow depression is cumulative. Teach patient and family self-assessment for signs/symptoms of infection and bleeding, and instruct to report them immediately. Teach self-care measures to minimize risk of infection and bleeding, including avoidance of aspirin-containing medicines.

II. POTENTIAL FOR IMPAIRED GAS EXCHANGE related to PULMONARY FIBROSIS

Defining Characteristics: Pulmonary toxicity appears to be dose-related, with risk greatest in patients receiving total doses > 1400 mg (although it can occur at lower doses).

Other risk factors include patients with abnormal PFTs prior to drug administration—i.e., baseline forced vital capacity (FVC) < 70% of predicted; carbon monoxide diffusion capacity (DLCO) < 70% of predicted; or if patient is receiving concurrent cyclophosphamide or thoracic radiation. Presents as insidious cough and dyspnea, or may be the sudden onset of respiratory failure. CXR shows interstitial infiltrates. Incidence is 20–30% of patients, with a mortality of 24–80%.

Nursing Implications: Assess patient's risk and baseline pulmonary function prior to chemotherapy, as well as the results of pulmonary function testing periodically during treatment, for evidence of pulmonary dysfunction. Teach patient to report any changes in respiratory pattern.

III.   ALTERATION IN NUTRITION, LESS THAN BODY REQUIREMENTS, related to NAUSEA/VOMITING AND LIVER DYSFUNCTION

Defining Characteristics: Severe nausea and vomiting may occur 2 hours after administration and last 4–6 hours. Reversible liver dysfunction, although rare, is related to subacute hepatitis and is characterized by abnormal LFTs, painless jaundice, and (rarely) coma.

Nursing Implications: Premedicate with antiemetics and continue antiemetic protection for 24 hours, at least for the first treatment. Encourage small, frequent feedings of cool, bland foods, and liquids. Infuse drug over 60–120 minutes. Monitor LFTs (SGOT, SGPT, lactic dehydrogenase [LDH], alk phos, bili) during treatment and discuss any abnormalities with physician.

IV.   ALTERATION IN COMFORT related to DRUG ADMINISTRATION

Defining Characteristics: Drug diluent is absolute alcohol, so irritation may result in pain along the vein path. Thrombosis is rare, but venospasms and flushing of skin or burning of the eyes can occur with rapid drug infusion.

Nursing Implications: Administer drug only through patent IV and dilute drug in 250 mL of 5% dextrose or 0.9% sodium chloride and infuse over 1–2 hours. If pain along vein occurs, use ice packs above injection site, decrease infusion rate, or further dilute drug. If patient will receive ongoing therapy, consider venous access device.

V.   ALTERED URINARY ELIMINATION related to NEPHROTOXICITY

Defining Characteristics: Increase in BUN occurs in 10% of patients and is usually reversible. However, decreased kidney size, progressive azotemia, and renal failure have occurred in patients receiving large cumulative doses over long periods.

Nursing Implications: Assess baseline renal function and monitor BUN and creatinine prior to each successive cycle. Since drug is excreted by the kidneys, drug dosage should be reduced if renal dysfunction exists. If abnormalities occur and persist, discuss discontinuing drug with physician.

VI. POTENTIAL SEXUAL DYSFUNCTION related to DRUG EFFECTS

Defining Characteristics: Drug is mutagenic and teratogenic.

Nursing Implications: Assess patient's and partner's pattern of sexuality and reproductive goals. Teach patient and partner the need for contraception as appropriate. Provide emotional support and counseling, or referral as appropriate.

VII. SENSORY/PERCEPTUAL ALTERATIONS related to OCULAR TOXICITY

Defining Characteristics: Infarcts of optic nerve fiber, retinal hemorrhage, and neuroretinitis have been associated with high-dose therapy.

Nursing Implications: Assess baseline vision and appearance of eyes. Instruct patient to report any visual changes to physician or nurse.

Drug: chlorambucil (Leukeran)

Class: Alkylating agent.

Mechanism of Action: Alkylates DNA by causing strand breaks and crosslinks in the DNA. The drug is a derivative of a nitrogen mustard.

Metabolism: Pharmacokinetics are poorly understood. It is well absorbed orally, with a plasma half-life of 1.5 hours. Degradation is slow; it appears to be eliminated by metabolic transformation, with 60% excreted in urine in 24 hours.

Indication: For the treatment of patients with chronic lymphatic (lymphocytic) leukemia, malignant lymphomas including lymphosarcoma, giant follicular lymphoma, and Hodgkin's disease.

Dosage/Range:
- 0.1–0.2 mg/kg/day (equals 4–8 mg/m^2/day) to initiate treatment for 3–6 weeks OR
- 14 mg/m^2/day × 5 days with a repeat every 21–28 days, depending on platelet count and WBC.

Drug Preparation:
- 2-mg tablets.

Drug Administration:
- Oral.

Drug Interactions:
- None significant.
- Simultaneous administration of barbiturates may increase toxicity of chlorambucil due to hepatic drug activation.

Lab Effects/Interference:
- BUN, uric acid.
- LFTs, especially alk phos and AST (SGOT).
- CBC, especially WBC with differential.

Special Considerations:
- None.

Potential Toxicities/Side Effects and the Nursing Process

I.   POTENTIAL FOR INFECTION related to BONE MARROW DEPRESSION

Defining Characteristics: Neutropenia after third week of treatment lasting for 10 days after the last dose. Neutropenia and thrombocytopenia occur with prolonged use and may be irreversible occasionally (especially if high total doses are given; i.e., > 6.5 mg/kg). Increased toxicity may occur with prior barbiturate use.

Nursing Implications: Assess baseline CBC, including WBC with differential, and platelet count prior to dosing, as well as weekly for the first cycle of therapy. Discuss dose reduction with physician if blood values are abnormal. Teach patient self-assessment of signs/symptoms of infection and bleeding and instruct to report them immediately. Teach self-care measures to minimize risk of infection and bleeding, including avoidance of OTC aspirin-containing medications.

II.   POTENTIAL FOR SEXUAL DYSFUNCTION related to REPRODUCTIVE HAZARD

Defining Characteristics: Drug is mutagenic, teratogenic, and suppresses gonadal function with consequent temporary or permanent sterility. Amenorrhea occurs in females, and oligospermia/azoospermia occurs in males.

Nursing Implications: Assess patient's and partner's sexual patterns and reproductive goals. Provide teaching and emotional support; encourage birth control measures as appropriate.

III.   POTENTIAL FOR ALTERATION IN NUTRITION, LESS THAN BODY REQUIREMENTS, related to NAUSEA/VOMITING, ANOREXIA/WEIGHT LOSS, AND HEPATIC DYSFUNCTION

Defining Characteristics: Nausea and vomiting are rare. Anorexia and weight loss may occur and be prolonged. Hepatotoxicity with jaundice is rare, but abnormal LFTs may occur.

Nursing Implications: Administer antiemetics as needed and instruct patient in self-administration. Suggest weekly weights and dietary instruction if patient develops anorexia and weight loss. Monitor LFTs baseline and periodically during treatment. Discuss any abnormalities with physician and consider dose modification.

IV. POTENTIAL FOR IMPAIRED GAS EXCHANGE related to PULMONARY FIBROSIS

Defining Characteristics: Bronchopulmonary dysplasia and pulmonary fibrosis may occur rarely with long-term use.

Nursing Implications: Assess patients at risk: increased risk with cumulative dose > 1 g/m², preexisting lung disease, concurrent treatment with cyclophosphamide or thoracic radiation. Assess pulmonary status prior to chemotherapy and at each visit, notifying physician of dyspnea. Monitor PFTs periodically for evidence of pulmonary dysfunction. Teach patient to report any changes in pulmonary pattern, such as dyspnea.

V. POTENTIAL FOR SENSORY/PERCEPTUAL ALTERATIONS related to OCULAR DISTURBANCES, CNS ABNORMALITIES

Defining Characteristics: Ocular disturbances may occur, e.g., diplopia, papilledema, retinal hemorrhage. Tremors, muscular twitching, confusion, agitation, ataxia, flaccid paresis, and hallucinations have been described. Seizures, although uncommon, have occurred in adults and children during normal dosing, as well as with overdosing.

Nursing Implications: Assess baseline neurologic status prior to treatment and at each visit. Instruct patient to report any abnormalities.

Drug: cisplatin (Platinol)

Class: Heavy metal that acts like alkylating agent.

Mechanism of Action: Inhibits DNA synthesis by forming inter- and intrastrand crosslinks and by denaturing the double helix, preventing cell replication. Cell cycle phase nonspecific; the chemical properties are similar to those of bifunctional alkylating agents.

Metabolism: Rapidly distributed to tissues (predominately the liver and kidneys) with less than 10% in the plasma 1 hour after infusion. Clearance from plasma proceeds slowly after the first 2 hours due to platinum's covalent bonding with serum proteins; 20–74% of administered drug is excreted in the urine within 24 hours.

Indication: Indicated for the treatment of patients with:
- Metastatic testicular tumors, with other approved chemotherapy agents, after appropriate surgical and/or radiotherapeutic procedures.
- Metastatic ovarian tumors, with other approved chemotherapy agents, after appropriate surgical and/or radiotherapeutic procedures. An established combination is cisplatin

plus cyclophosphamide. Cisplatin as a single-agent is indicated as secondary therapy in patients with metastatic ovarian tumors refractory to standard chemotherapy who have not previously received cisplatinum.

- Advanced bladder cancer (transitional cell), which is no longer amenable to local treatment (e.g., surgery and/or radiotherapy), as a single agent.

Contraindicated in patients with preexisting renal impairment; also should not be used in myelosuppressed patients, or patients with a hearing impairment.

Dosage/Range:
- 50–100 mg/m² every 3–4 weeks, OR
- 15–30 mg/m² × 5 days repeated every 3–4 weeks.
- **Radiosensitizing effect:** Administer 1–3 times per week at doses of 15–50 mg/m² (total weekly dose 50 mg/m²) with concomitant radiotherapy.
- Intraperitoneal: 100 mg/m² every 3 weeks for ovarian cancer.

Drug Preparation:
- 10-mg and 50-mg vials. Add sterile water to develop a concentration of 1 mg/mL.
- Further dilute solution with 250 mL or more of 0.9% sodium chloride (recommended) or 5% dextrose (D₅ ½ NS) sodium chloride.
- Never mix with 5% dextrose, as a precipitate will form. Drug stability increased in 0.9% sodium chloride.
- Available as an aqueous solution.
- Do not refrigerate.

Drug Administration:
- Avoid aluminum needles when administering, as precipitate will form. Ensure adequate urinary output prior to administration.

Drug Interactions:
- Decreases pharmacologic effect of phenytoin, so dose may need to be increased.
- Possible increase in ototoxicity when combined with loop diuretics.
- Increased renal toxicity with concurrent use of aminoglycosides, amphotericin B.
- Cisplatin reduces drug clearance of high-dose methotrexate (MTX) and standard-dose bleomycin by increasing the drugs' half-life; enhances toxicity of ifosfamide (myelosuppression) and etoposide.
- Synergy when cisplatin is combined with etoposide.
- Radiosensitizing effect.
- Sodium thiosulfate and mesna: Each directly inactivates cisplatin.
- Taxanes: Administer cisplatin *after* taxanes (paclitaxel, docetaxel) to prevent delayed taxane excretion with subsequent increased bone marrow depression.

Lab Effects/Interference:
- Decreased Mg, Ca, phos.
- Increased creatinine, uric acid.

Special Considerations:
- Administer cautiously, if at all, to patients with renal dysfunction, hearing impairment, peripheral neuropathy, or prior allergic reaction to cisplatin.
- Hydrate vigorously before and after administering drug. Urine output should be at least 100–150 mL/hour. Mannitol or furosemide diuresis may be needed to ensure this output.
- Hypersensitivity reactions have occurred, manifested by wheezing, flushing, hypotension, tachycardia. Usually occurs within minutes of starting infusion. Treat with epinephrine, corticosteroids, antihistamines.
- Drug causes potassium and magnesium wasting. Add magnesium and potassium to hydration IV prior to and following cisplatin administration. Other ideas to help increase magnesium follow:
- To help increase absorption, it is recommended that excessive milk, cheese, or other high-calcium products be limited when eating foods high in magnesium. Calcium and magnesium compete to gain entrance to the body in the intestines, so a high-calcium diet increases requirements for dietary magnesium. Foods high in magnesium are those with 100 mg or greater per 100 grams, including:

Nuts:
Almonds
Brazil nuts
Cashews
Peanut butter
Peanuts
Pecans
Walnuts
Peas and beans:
Red beans
Split peas
White beans
Other good sources:
Blackstrap molasses
Brewer's yeast
Chocolate (bitter)
Cocoa (dry breakfast)
Cornmeal
Instant coffee and tea
Oatmeal
Shredded wheat
Wheat germ
Whole wheat breads and cereals
- Phase I studies are ongoing, evaluating an oral platinum (JM-216) agent in small-cell lung cancer.
- Amifostine has been shown to be renally protective in patients at risk for renal toxicity from cisplatin; in addition, drug offers protection from neurotoxicity. Other agents are being studied, e.g., BNP7787.

Potential Toxicities/Side Effects and the Nursing Process

I.   POTENTIAL ALTERATION IN URINARY ELIMINATION related to DRUG-INDUCED RENAL DAMAGE

Defining Characteristics: Dose-limiting toxicity, which may be cumulative. The drug accumulates in the kidneys, causing necrosis of proximal and distal renal tubules. Damage to renal tubules prevents reabsorption of magnesium, calcium, potassium, with resultant decreased serum levels. Renal damage becomes most obvious 10–20 days after treatment, is reversible, and can be prevented by adequate hydration and diuresis, as well as slower infusion time. Hyperuricemia may occur due to impaired tubular transport of uric acid, but it is responsive to allopurinol. Concurrent administration of nephrotoxic agents is not recommended.

Nursing Implications: Assess renal function studies prior to administration (BUN, creatinine, 24-hour creatinine clearance) and discuss any abnormalities with physician. Assess cardiac and pulmonary status in terms of tolerance of aggressive hydration. Anticipate vigorous hydration regimen with or without forced diuresis (i.e., mannitol, lasix). The typical hydration schedule is 0.9% sodium chloride or D_5 ½ NS at 250 mL/hr × 3–5 hours prechemotherapy and 3–5 hours postchemotherapy (total hydration 3 L). Outpatient hydration of 1–2 L over 1–2 hours prechemotherapy and 1 L postchemotherapy is typical. Strictly monitor I/O and total body fluid balance. Assess for signs/symptoms of fluid overload and notify physician for supplemental furosemide or other diuretic as needed. Monitor serum electrolytes (sodium, potassium, magnesium, calcium, PO_4) and replete electrolytes as ordered by physician. Teach patient and family the need for increased oral fluids on discharge—up to 3 L or more for 5 days posttherapy.

II.   ALTERATION IN NUTRITION, LESS THAN BODY REQUIREMENTS, related to SEVERE NAUSEA AND VOMITING, TASTE ALTERATIONS

Defining Characteristics: Nausea and vomiting may be severe and will occur in 100% of patients if antiemetics are not given. They begin 1 or more hours postchemotherapy and last 8–24 hours. Since the drug is slowly excreted over 5 days, delayed nausea and vomiting may occur 24–72 hours after dose. Taste alterations and anorexia occur with long-term use.

Nursing Implications: Premedicate with combination antiemetics (i.e., serotonin antagonist plus dexamethasone), especially for high-dose cisplatin, and continue antiemetics for up to 5 days with dopamine antagonist. Encourage small, frequent intake of cool, bland foods as tolerated. Infuse cisplatin over at least 1 hour to minimize emesis, since slower infusion rates decrease emesis. Taste alterations may be improved with the use of spices and zinc dietary supplementation. Refer the patient for dietary consultation as needed.

III.   POTENTIAL FOR INJURY related to ANAPHYLAXIS

Defining Characteristics: Anaphylaxis has occurred, characterized by wheezing, bronchoconstriction, tachycardia, hypotension, and facial edema, in patients who have previously received the drug.

Nursing Implications: Assess baseline VS and continue to assess patient during infusion. Prior to drug administration, review standing orders or protocols for nursing management of anaphylaxis: stop infusion; keep line open with 0.9% sodium chloride; notify physician; monitor VS; be prepared to administer epinephrine, antihistamines, corticosteroids.

IV. POTENTIAL FOR SENSORY/PERCEPTUAL ALTERATIONS related to NEUROLOGIC TOXICITY

Defining Characteristics: Severe neuropathy may occur in patients receiving high doses or prolonged treatment and may be irreversible, and is seen in stocking-and-glove distribution, with numbness, tingling, and sensory loss in arms and legs. Areflexia, loss of proprioception and vibratory sense, and loss of motor function can occur. Ototoxicity, beginning with loss of high-frequency hearing, affects > 30% of patients. It may be preceded by tinnitus, is dose related, and can be unilateral or bilateral. The damage results from destruction of hair cells lining the organ of Corti and is cumulative and may be permanent. Rarely, ocular toxicity has occurred, but it is reversible (optic neuritis, papilledema, cerebral blindness).

Nursing Implications: Assess baseline neurologic, motor, and sensory functions prior to drug administration. Discuss use of neuroprotector in high-risk patients. Discuss baseline audiogram with physician as appropriate. Instruct patient to report changes in function or sensation, as well as diminished hearing. Discuss with physician risks versus benefits of continuing therapy if/when symptoms develop. If severe neuropathies develop, provide teaching related to activity, emotional support, and referral to physical/occupational therapy as appropriate. Discuss use of neuroprotector in high-risk patients.

V. POTENTIAL FOR ACTIVITY INTOLERANCE related to ANEMIA

Defining Characteristics: Drug may interfere with renal erythropoietin production, resulting in late development of anemia.

Nursing Implications: Teach patient to report increasing fatigue, signs of severe anemia (shortness of breath, chest pain/angina, headaches). Monitor hemoglobin/hematocrit; discuss transfusion with physician if signs/symptoms develop or hematocrit falls < 25 mg/dL or symptoms (e.g., angina). Teach patient about diet high in iron. Exogenous erythropoietin (epoetin alpha) may be helpful if treatment goal is palliation.

VI. INFECTION AND BLEEDING related to BONE MARROW DEPRESSION

Defining Characteristics: Bone marrow depression is mild with low to moderate doses, but may be significant when high doses are used, or when drug is given in combination with radiation as a radiation-sensitizer. Nadir is in 2–3 weeks, with recovery in 4–5 weeks.

Nursing Implications: Assess CBC, WBC, differential, and platelet count, as well as any signs/symptoms of infection or bleeding, prior to drug administration. Teach patient to self-assess for signs/symptoms of infection and bleeding. Teach self-care measures to minimize infection and bleeding, including avoidance of aspirin-containing medications.

VII. POTENTIAL SEXUAL DYSFUNCTION related to DRUG EFFECTS

Defining Characteristics: Drug is mutagenic and probably teratogenic.

Nursing Implications: Assess patient's and partner's sexual patterns and reproductive goals. Provide emotional support and discuss strategies to preserve sexual and reproductive health (i.e., contraception and sperm banking).

VIII. POTENTIAL FOR ALTERATIONS IN CARDIOVASCULAR FUNCTION related to CISPLATIN-CONTAINING COMBINATION CHEMOTHERAPY

Defining Characteristics: Angina, myocardial infarction, cerebrovascular accident, thrombotic microangiopathy, cerebral arteritis, and Raynaud's phenomenon have occurred, although they are uncommon. Combination drugs include bleomycin, vinblastine, vincristine, and etoposide.

Nursing Implications: Assess cardiopulmonary status, especially if patient has preexisting cardiac disease, both prior to and throughout treatment.

Drug: cladribine (Leustatin, 2-CdA)

Class: Antimetabolite.

Mechanism of Action: Selectively damages normal and malignant lymphocytes and monocytes that have large amounts of deoxycytidine kinase but small amounts of deoxynucleotidase. The drug, a chlorinated purine nucleoside, enters passively through the cell membrane, is phosphorylated into the active metabolite 2-CdATP, and accumulates in the cell. 2-CdATP interferes with DNA synthesis and prevents repair of DNA strand breaks in both actively dividing and normal cells. The process may also involve programmed cell death (apoptosis).

Metabolism: Drug is 20% protein-bound and is cleared from the plasma within 1–3 days after cessation of treatment.

Indication: Treatment of hairy-cell leukemia (as defined by clinically significant anemia, neutropenia, thrombocytopenia, or disease-related symptoms).

Dosage/Range:
- 0.09 mg/kg/day IV as a continuous infusion for 7 days for one course of therapy of hairy-cell leukemia.

Drug Preparation:
- Available in 10 mg/10 mL preservative-free, single-use vials (1 mg/mL), which must be further diluted in 0.9% sodium chloride injection. Diluted drug is stable at room temperature for at least 24 hours in normal light. Once prepared, the solution may be refrigerated up to 8 hours prior to use.
- Single daily dose: add calculated drug dose to 500 mL of 0.9% sodium chloride injection, and administer over 24 hours; repeat daily for a total of 7 days.
- 7-day continuous infusion by ambulatory infusion pump: add calculated drug dose for 7 days to infusion reservoir using a sterile 0.22-μm hydrophilic syringe filter. Then add, again using 0.22-μm filter, sufficient sterile bacteriostatic 0.9% sodium chloride injection containing 0.9% benzyl alcohol to produce 100 mL in the infusion reservoir.
- Do not use 5% dextrose, as it accelerates degradation of drug.

Drug Administration:
- Dilute in minimum of 100 mL. DO NOT use 5% dextrose, as unstable.
- Administer as continuous infusion over 24 hours for 7 days.

Drug Interactions:
- Bone marrow-suppressing drugs: increased bone marrow suppression.
- Live attenuated vaccines: increased risk of infection; do not administer when receiving leustatin.

Lab Effects/Interference:
- Decreased CBC, platelets.
- Increased LFTs, RFTs.

Special Considerations:
- Unstable in 5% dextrose; should not be used as diluent or infusion fluid.
- Store unopened vials in refrigerator and protect from light.
- Drug may precipitate when exposed to low temperatures. Allow solution to warm to room temperature and shake vigorously. DO NOT HEAT OR MICROWAVE.
- Drug is structurally similar to pentostatin and fludarabine.
- Contraindicated in patients who are hypersensitive to the drug.
- Administer with caution in patients with renal or hepatic insufficiency.
- Embryotoxic; women of childbearing age should use effective contraception to avoid pregnancy.
- May cause impairment of fertility in men.

Potential Toxicities/Side Effects and the Nursing Process

I.   INFECTION AND BLEEDING related to BONE MARROW DEPRESSION

Defining Characteristics: Neutropenia occurs in 70% of patients with nadir 1–2 weeks after infusion, recovery by weeks 4–5. Incidence of infection 28%, with 40% caused by bacterial infection of lungs and venous access sites. Prolonged hypocellularity of bone marrow occurs in 34% of patients, and may last for at least 4 months. Infections most common in patients with pancytopenia and lymphopenia due to hairy-cell leukemia. Lymphopenia is common with decreased CD4 (helper T cells) and CD8 (suppressor T cells), with recovery by weeks 26–34. Common infectious agents are viral (20%) and fungal (20%). Thrombocytopenia occurs commonly, along with purpura (10%), petechiae (8%), and epistaxis (5%). Platelet recovery occurs by day 12, but 14% of patients require platelet support.

Nursing Implications: Monitor CBC, platelet count prior to therapy, and periodically post-therapy at expected time of nadir. Monitor for, and teach patient self-assessment of signs/symptoms of infection, bleeding. Instruct patient to call physician or nurse or go to emergency room if temperature is greater than 101°F (38.3°C) or bleeding. Transfuse platelets per physician order. DO NOT give live attenuated vaccines to patients receiving leustatin due to increased risk of infection in the setting of immunosuppression (FDA, 2012).

II.   ALTERATION IN COMFORT related to FEVER, HEADACHES

Defining Characteristics: Fever (> 100°F [37.5°C]) occurs in 66% of patients during the month following treatment due either to infection (47%) or the release of endogenous pyrogen from lysed lymphocytes. Other symptoms include chills (9%), diaphoresis (9%), malaise (7%), dizziness (9%), insomnia (7%), myalgia (7%), arthralgias (5%). Headaches occur in 22% of patients.

Nursing Implications: Assess patient for fever, chills, diaphoresis during visits; assess signs/symptoms of infection. Teach patient self-assessment, how to report this, and measures to reduce fever. Anticipate laboratory and X-ray tests to rule out infection and perform according to physician order.

III.   POTENTIAL IMPAIRMENT OF SKIN INTEGRITY related to RASH

Defining Characteristics: Rash occurs in 27–50% of patients. Other symptoms include pruritus (6%), erythema (6%), injection-site reactions (erythema, swelling, pain, phlebitis).

Nursing Implications: Assess skin for any cutaneous changes, such as rash or changes at injection site, and any associated symptoms such as pruritus; discuss with physician. Instruct patient in self-care measures, including avoiding abrasive skin products and clothing; avoiding tight-fitting clothing; use of skin emollients appropriate to specific skin alteration; measures to avoid scratching involved areas. Consider venous access device if skin is at risk for reaction.

IV.   FATIGUE related to ANEMIA

Defining Characteristics: Fatigue occurs in 45% of patients. Red cell recovery is by week 8, but 40% of patients require red cell transfusion.

Nursing Implications: Monitor Hgb and HCT and transfuse per physician order. Administer erythropoietin per physician order and teach patient self-administration. Teach patient about diet and instruct to alternate rest and activity; stress reduction/relaxation techniques may improve energy level.

V. ALTERATION IN ELIMINATION related to DIARRHEA, CONSTIPATION

Defining Characteristics: Diarrhea occurs in 10% of patients, while constipation occurs in 9%. Abdominal pain affects 6% of patients.

Nursing Implications: Encourage patient to report onset of change in bowel habits (diarrhea or constipation), and assess factors contributing to changes. Administer or teach patient self-administration of antidiarrheal medication or cathartic as ordered. Teach patient diet modification regarding foods that minimize diarrhea or constipation.

VI. POTENTIAL FOR IMPAIRED GAS EXCHANGE related to COUGH

Defining Characteristics: Cough affects 10%, while abnormal breath sounds occur in 11%, and shortness of breath in 7%.

Nursing Implications: Assess baseline pulmonary status, including breath sounds, presence of cough, shortness of breath. Instruct patient to report symptoms of cough, shortness of breath, other abnormalities.

VII. ALTERATION IN NUTRITION, LESS THAN BODY REQUIREMENTS, related to NAUSEA, VOMITING

Defining Characteristics: Nausea is mild and occurs in 28% of patients, while vomiting may occur in 13%. If antiemetics are required, nausea/vomiting is easily controlled by phenothiazines. Renal and hepatic function studies are rarely affected.

Nursing Implications: Premedicate with antiemetics. If nausea and/or vomiting occur, teach patient to self-administer antiemetics per physician order. Encourage small, frequent feedings of cool, bland foods and liquids. Teach patient to record diet history for 2–3 days and weekly weights. If patient has decreased appetite, assess food preferences (encourage or discourage) and suggest use of spices.

VIII. POTENTIAL ALTERATION IN CARDIAC OUTPUT related to TACHYCARDIA

Defining Characteristics: Occurs rarely, with edema and tachycardia each affecting 6% of patients.

Nursing Implications: Assess baseline cardiac status, including apical heart rate, presence of peripheral edema. Instruct patient to report rapid heartbeat or swelling of ankles.

Drug: clofarabine (Clolar)

Class: Purine nucleoside antimetabolite.

Mechanism of Action: Drug inhibits DNA and DNA repair, causing cell death of both cycling and quiescent cancer cells. In addition, it breaks down the mitochondrial membranes, releasing cytochrome C and apoptosis-inducing factor, leading to programmed cell death.

Metabolism: Drug is 47% protein-bound (mostly to albumin), with a terminal half-life of 5.2 hours. 49–60% of the dose is excreted unchanged in the urine. Other nonrenal excretion is unknown.

Indication: For the treatment of pediatric patients 1–21 years old with relapsed or refractory acute lymphoblastic leukemia after at least 2 prior regimens. Indication is based on response rate.

Dosage/Range: 52 mg/m² IV over 2 h daily × 5, to be repeated after recovery of all baseline organ function, about q 2–6 weeks. IV hydration should be continued during the 5 days of treatment.
- Patient should receive IV hydration thoughout the 5 days of treatment to prevent tumor lysis syndrome (TLS). For first cycle, discuss with physician need for allopurinol if hyperuricemia is likely.
- Renal and hepatic function studies should be monitored during the 5 days of drug treatment.

Drug Preparation: Drug is supplied as a 20 mg in 20-mL vial. Withdraw drug using a sterile 0.2-µm syringe filter and then further dilute with 5% dextrose injection USP or 0.9% sodium chloride injection USP prior to IV infusion. This admixture may be stored at room temperature but must be used within 24 hours of preparation.

Drug Administration: Administer IV over 2 hours; if hyperuricemia (tumor lysis syndrome), patient should receive allopurinol, and may need urine alkalinization and aggressive hydration as well.

Drug Interactions: Concurrent administration with other renally cleared drugs may alter drug levels so should be avoided during the 5 days of treatment; avoid other hepatotoxic drugs, as well as those affecting blood pressure or cardiac function if possible during drug administration.

Lab Effects/Interference:
Drug may cause
- Severe bone marrow depression with decreased white blood cells, neutrophils, red blood cells, and platelets.
- Tumor lysis syndrome with increased levels of potassium, phosphate, uric acid, creatinine, and changes in other electrolyte values.
- Increased hepato-biliary enzyme serum levels.

Special Considerations:
- Treatment results in the rapid lysis of peripheral leukemia cells, increasing the risk of tumor lysis syndrome (TLS). Discuss TLS prophylaxis with physician or NP/PA to prevent TLS.
- Drug is fetotoxic, so all patients (male and female) should be taught to use effective contraceptive measures to prevent pregnancy; female patients should be cautioned not to breastfeed during treatment.

- Drug may cause dehydration, hypotension, systemic inflammatory response syndrome (SIRS), capillary leak syndrome.
- Patients who have previously received a hematopoietic stem cell transplant may be at higher risk for hepatotoxicity.

Potential Toxicities/Side Effects and the Nursing Process

I.   INFECTION AND BLEEDING related to BONE MARROW DEPRESSION

Defining Characteristics: Bone marrow depression is dose-limiting. Febrile neutropenia occurs in some patients. Pyrexia affects some patients, others experience rigors. Infections include bacteremia, cellulitis, herpes simplex, oral candidiasis, pneumonia, sepsis, and staphylococcal infections.

Nursing Implications: Assess WBC, neutrophil, and platelet count, and discuss any abnormalities with physician prior to drug administration; assess for signs/symptoms of skin infections (all mucosal surfaces, body orifices) and bleeding; instruct patient in signs/symptoms of infection and bleeding, as well as to report them or come to emergency room. Teach patient self-care measures to minimize risk of infection and bleeding, including avoidance of OTC aspirin-containing medications. Assess patient's Hgb/HCT and signs/symptoms of fatigue; teach patient self-assessment and to alternate rest and activity as needed.

II.   ALTERED NUTRITION, LESS THAN BODY REQUIREMENTS, related to NAUSEA AND VOMITING, ANOREXIA, DIARRHEA, AND HEPATOTOXICITY

Defining Characteristics: Nausea and vomiting occur in some patients, and can be successfully prevented with combination antiemetics. Anorexia can occur. Diarrhea is frequent, affecting some patients. Constipation affects some patients. Hepatotoxicity and jaundice occur in some patients.

Nursing Implications: Premedicate with antiemetics depending on dose, using aggressive, combination antiemetics, and continue throughout chemotherapy. If patient develops nausea/vomiting, assess fluid and electrolyte balance and the need for replacements. Assess oral mucosa prior to chemotherapy and teach patient oral hygiene regimen and self-assessment; encourage patient to report diarrhea, discuss use of antidiarrheals with physician, and teach self-care PRN. Because patients become neutropenic, all mucosal surfaces need to be assessed for infection, and patients must be taught scrupulous perineal hygiene. Monitor LFTs prior to, during, and following therapy.

III.   IMPAIRED SKIN/MUCOSAL INTEGRITY related to RASH, ANAL INFLAMMATION/ULCERATION, ALOPECIA

Defining Characteristics: Maculopapular rash, with or without fever, myalgia, bone pain, occasional chest pain, conjunctivitis, and malaise (cytarabine syndrome) may occur. Syndrome is not common, but occurs 6–12 hours after drug administration; corticosteroids have been helpful in treating/preventing syndrome. Mucosal inflammation and ulceration of anus/rectum may occur, especially in patients with prior hemorrhoids or history of abscesses. Alopecia occurs less frequently.

Nursing Implications: Assess baseline skin and mucous membranes prior to chemotherapy and identify patients at risk for problems. Consider including corticosteroid in antiemetic regimen, especially for high-dose therapy, and discuss with physician prophylactic use of dexamethasone eye drops to prevent conjunctivitis. Teach patient scrupulous perineal hygiene, instruct to report any rectal discomfort, and assess rectal mucosa daily with high-dose therapy. Discuss with patient potential coping strategies if alopecia occurs (i.e., wig, scarves).

IV.   ALTERATION IN COMFORT, POTENTIAL, related to EDEMA, FATIGUE, LETHARGY, PAIN

Defining Characteristics: In clinical studies, frequently occurring symptoms were: edema, fatigue, injection site pain, pain, arthralgia, back pain, myalgia, pain in limb, dermatitis, erythema, pruritus, palmar plantar erythrodysesthesia syndrome (PPE), and flushing.

Nursing Implications: Teach patient that these symptoms may occur and to report them. Teach patient self-care measures to reduce discomfort, such as application of heat or cold for pain, arthralgias, and myalgias. Teach patient to report redness and pain on palms of hands or soles of feet as this may be PPE, and would require close monitoring and follow-up to prevent moist desquamation. Instruct patient to report any symptoms that do not resolve or improve with self-care measures.

Drug: cyclophosphamide (Cytoxan)

Class: Alkylating agent.

Mechanism of Action: Causes cross-linkage in DNA strands, thus preventing DNA synthesis and cell division. Cell cycle phase nonspecific.

Metabolism: Inactive until converted by microsomes in liver and serum enzymes (phosphamidases). Both cyclophosphamide and its metabolites are excreted by the kidneys. Plasma half-life: 6–12 hours, with 25% of drug excreted after 8 hours. Prolonged plasma half-life in patients with renal failure results in increased myelosuppression.

Indications (initial): For the treatment of patients with the following, as a single agent, or in combination with other chemotherapy:
- Malignant lymphomas
- Multiple myeloma
- Leukemias
- Mycosis fungoides (advanced disease)
- Neuroblastoma (disseminated disease)

- Adenocarcinoma of the ovary
- Retinoblastoma
- Breast cancer

Dosage/Range:
- 400 mg/m^2 IV × 5 days.
- 100 mg/m^2 PO × 14 days every 4 weeks.
- 500–1,500 mg/m^2 IV every 3–4 weeks.

High dose with BMT (investigational):
- 1.8–7 g/m^2 in combination with other cytotoxic agents.

Drug Preparation:
- Available in 25- and 50-mg tablets; powder for injection: 100-mg, 200-mg, 500-mg, 1-g, and 2-g vials.
- Dilute vials with sterile water. Shake well. Allow solution to clear if lyophilized preparation is not used. Do not use solution unless crystals are fully dissolved.

Drug Administration:
- Oral use: Administer in morning or early afternoon to allow adequate excretion time. Should be taken with meals.
- IV use: for doses > 500 mg, pre- and posthydration to total 500–3,000 mL is needed to ensure adequate urine output and to avoid hemorrhagic cystitis. Administer drug over at least 20 minutes for doses > 500 mg.
- Mesna given with high-dose cyclophosphamide to prevent hemorrhagic cystitis.
- Solution is stable for 24 hours at room temperature, 6 days if refrigerated.
- Rapid infusion may result in dizziness, nasal stuffiness, rhinorrhea, sinus congestion during or soon after infusion.

Drug Interactions:
- Increases chloramphenicol half-life.
- Increases duration of leukopenia when given with thiazide diuretics.
- Increases effect of anticoagulant drugs.
- Decreases digoxin level, so dose may need to be increased.
- Potentiation of doxorubicin-induced cardiomyopathy.
- Increased succinylcholine action with prolonged neuromuscular blockage.
- Increased drug action of barbiturates; induction of hepatic microsomes.

Lab Effects/Interference:
- Increased K, uric acid secondary to tumor lysis.
- Monitor electrolytes for symptoms of SIADH.
- Decreased CBC, platelets.

Special Considerations:
- Metabolic and leukopenic toxicity is increased by simultaneous administration of barbiturates, corticosteroids, phenytoin, and sulfonamides.
- Activity and toxicity of both cyclophosphamide and the specific drug may be altered by allopurinol, chloroquine, phenothiazides, potassium iodide, chloramphenicol, imipramine, vitamin A, warfarin, succinylcholine, digoxin, thiazide diuretics.

- Test urine for occult blood.
- High-dose cyclophosphamide therapy may require catheterization and constant bladder irrigation. Mesna should be given, either as a continuous infusion or in bolus doses, around drug administration. Consult protocol. See *Chapter 4*.
- Monitor patients with hepatic dysfunction closely for toxicity.

Potential Toxicities/Side Effects and the Nursing Process

I.   INFECTION AND BLEEDING related to BONE MARROW DEPRESSION

Defining Characteristics: Leukopenia nadir occurs days 7–14, with recovery in 1–2 weeks; thrombocytopenia is less frequent and anemia is mild. Drug is a potent immunosuppressant.

Nursing Implications: Assess CBC, WBC with differential, platelet count, and signs/symptoms of infection and bleeding prior to treatment. Teach patient signs/symptoms of infection and instruct to report them if they occur. Teach patient self-care measures to minimize infection and bleeding. Increased risk of bone marrow depression in patients with prior radiation or chemotherapy.

II.   ALTERED URINARY ELIMINATION related to HEMORRHAGIC CYSTITIS

Defining Characteristics: Metabolites of drug, if allowed to accumulate in the bladder, irritate bladder wall capillaries, causing hemorrhagic cystitis. This occurs in 7–40% of patients, is evidenced by microscopic or gross hematuria, is common with high doses, and is preventable. Long-term drug exposure may lead to bladder fibrosis.

Nursing Implications: Monitor BUN and creatinine prior to drug dose and as drug is excreted by the kidneys. Assess for signs/symptoms of hematuria, urinary frequency, or dysuria; instruct patient to report these if they occur. Instruct patient to take in at least 3 L of fluid per day and to empty bladder every 2–3 hours, as well as at bedtime. If patient is receiving a high dose, ensure vigorous hydration prior to drug administration. Bladder irrigation per protocol. Instruct patient to take oral cyclophosphamide early in the day to prevent drug accumulation in bladder during the night.

III.   ALTERATION IN NUTRITION, LESS THAN BODY REQUIREMENTS, related to NAUSEA AND VOMITING, ANOREXIA, STOMATITIS, DIARRHEA, AND HEPATOTOXICITY

Defining Characteristics: Nausea and vomiting are dose-related and begin 2–4 hours after dose, peak in 12 hours, and may last 24 hours. Anorexia is common; stomatitis, if it occurs, is mild; and diarrhea is mild and infrequent. Hepatotoxicity is rare.

Nursing Implications: Premedicate with antiemetics prior to drug administration and continue prophylactically for 24 hours, at least for the first cycle. Encourage small feedings of bland foods and liquids. Encourage favorite foods and consult dietitian regarding anorexia if needed. Assess oral mucosa prior to drug administration; teach patient self-assessment techniques and oral care. Monitor LFTs before, during, and after therapy.

IV. ALTERED BODY IMAGE related to ALOPECIA, CHANGES IN NAILS AND SKIN

Defining Characteristics: Alopecia occurs in 30–50% of patients, especially with IV dosing, but some degree of hair loss occurs in all patients. Hair loss begins after 3+ weeks; hair may grow back while on therapy, but will grow back after therapy is discontinued (may be softer in texture). Hyperpigmentation of nails and skin, as well as transverse ridging of nails (banding), may occur.

Nursing Implications: Teach patient about potential hair loss and other changes. Discuss impact of hair loss on patient and strategies to minimize it (i.e., wig, scarf, cap) prior to drug administration. Assess ongoing coping during treatment. If nail changes are distressing, discuss the use of nail polish or other measures.

V. POTENTIAL SEXUAL DYSFUNCTION related to DRUG EFFECTS

Defining Characteristics: Drug is mutagenic and teratogenic. Amenorrhea often occurs in females, and testicular atrophy, possibly with reversible oligospermia/azoospermia, occurs in males. Drug is excreted in breastmilk.

Nursing Implications: Assess patient's/partner's sexual patterns and reproductive goals. Discuss strategies to preserve sexual and reproductive health, including contraception and sperm banking, as appropriate. Mothers receiving cyclophosphamide should not breastfeed.

VI. POTENTIAL FOR INJURY related to ACUTE WATER INTOXICATION (SIADH) AND SECOND MALIGNANCY

Defining Characteristics: SIADH may occur with high-dose administration (> 50 mg/kg). Prolonged therapy may cause bladder cancer and acute leukemia.

Nursing Implications: Assess patients receiving high-dose cyclophosphamide: monitor serum Na+, osmolality, and urine osmolality and electrolytes; strictly monitor I/O, total body fluid balance, and daily weight. Screen patients who are receiving prolonged cyclophosphamide therapy for secondary malignancies.

VII. ALTERATION IN CARDIAC OUTPUT related to HIGH-DOSE CYCLOPHOSPHAMIDE

Defining Characteristics: Cardiomyopathy may occur with high doses as well as hemorrhagic cardiac necrosis, transmural hemorrhage, and coronary artery vasculitis at doses of 120–240 mg/kg. The mechanism is endothelial injury with subsequent hemorrhagic necrosis. The incidence is 22%, with 11% mortality, which may be decreased by dividing the dose into two split daily infusions. The risk at standard doses is increased by coadministration of doxorubicin (Adriamycin).

Nursing Implications: Assess cardiac status, especially if patient is receiving a high dose. Discuss baseline cardiac function test (GBPS) and assess for signs/symptoms of cardiomyopathy as treatment continues. Instruct patient to report dyspnea, shortness of breath, or other changes.

VIII. POTENTIAL FOR IMPAIRED GAS EXCHANGE related to PULMONARY TOXICITY

Defining Characteristics: Rare, but may occur with prolonged, high-dose therapy or continuous, low-dose therapy. Onset is insidious and appears as interstitial pneumonitis, which may progress to fibrosis. May respond to steroids.

Nursing Implications: Assess patients receiving high-dose or continuous low-dose cyclophosphamide for signs/symptoms of pulmonary dysfunction. Discuss pulmonary function studies with physician. Assess lung sounds prior to drug administration and periodically during treatment. Teach patient to report dyspnea, cough, or any abnormalities.

Drug: cytarabine, cytosine arabinoside (ara-C, Cytosar-U)

Class: Antimetabolite.

Mechanism of Action: Incorporated into DNA, slowing its synthesis and causing defects in the linkages to new DNA fragments. Also, cells exposed to cytarabine in the S phase reinitiate DNA synthesis when the drug, a pyrimidine analogue, is removed, resulting in erroneous duplication of the early portions of the DNA strands. Most effective when cells are undergoing rapid DNA synthesis.

Metabolism: Inactivated by liver enzymes in biphasic manner: half-lives 10–15 minutes and 2–3 hours. Crosses the BBB with cerebrospinal fluid concentration of 50% that of plasma; 70% of dose excreted in urine as ara-U; 4–10% excreted 12–24 hours after administration.

Indication:
- In combination with other approved anticancer drugs for remission induction in acute nonlymphocytic leukemia of adults and pediatric patients.
- Treatment of patients with acute lymphochytic or chronic myelocytic leukemia in blast phase.
- Meningeal leukemia prophylaxis and treatment by IT administration.
- NHL and Hodgkin's lymphoma.

Dosage/Range:
- Varies depending on disease.
- Leukemia: 100 mg/m^2/day IV continuous infusion × 5–10 days; 100 mg/m^2 every 12 h × 1–3 weeks IV or subcutaneously.
- Head and neck: 1 mg/kg every 12 h × 5–7 days IV or subcutaneously.
- High dose: 1–3 g/m^2 IV every 12 h × 4–12 doses to treat refractory acute leukemia.
- Differentiation: 10 mg/m^2 subcutaneously every 12 h × 15–21 days.
- Intrathecal: 5–75 mg/m^2 every 2–7 days until CSF is clear.
- Bone marrow transplant conditioning regimen: 1.5 mg/m^2 IV as continuous infusion over 48 hours.

Drug Preparation:
- 100-mg vials: add water with benzyl alcohol, then dilute with 0.9% sodium chloride or 5% dextrose.
- 500-mg vials: add water with benzyl alcohol, then dilute with 0.9% sodium chloride or 5% dextrose.
- For intrathecal use and high dose: use preservative-free diluent.
- Reconstituted drug is stable 48 hours at room temperature and 7 days refrigerated.

Drug Administration:
- Doses of 100–200 mg can be given subcutaneously.
- Doses less than 1 g: administer via pump over 10–20 minutes.
- Doses over 1 g: administer over 2 hours or longer.

Drug Interactions:
- May be a decreased bioavailability of digoxin when given in combination.

Lab Effects/Interference:
- Decreased CBC (neutropenia, thrombocytopenia, anemia).
- Increased LFTs, RFTs.
- Increased uric acid due to tumor lysis.

Special Considerations:
- Thrombophlebitis, pain at the injection site, should be treated with warm compresses.
- Dizziness has occurred with too-rapid IV infusions.
- Use with caution if hepatic dysfunction exists.
- Drug is excreted in tears, requiring protection of eye conjunctiva (corticosteroid eye drops such as dexamethasone 0.1% ophthalmic drops) with high-dose therapy.

Potential Toxicities/Side Effects and the Nursing Process

I. INFECTION AND BLEEDING related to BONE MARROW DEPRESSION

Defining Characteristics: Bone marrow depression is related to dose and duration of therapy. WBC depression is biphasic. After a 5-day continuous infusion at doses of 50–600 mg/m^2, WBC begins to fall within 24 hours, reaching nadir in 7–9 days, briefly rises around day 12, and begins to fall again, reaching nadir at days 15–24, with recovery within 10 days. Platelet drop begins day 5, reaching nadir at days 12–15, with recovery within 10 days. Anemia is seen frequently, with megaloblastic changes common in the bone marrow. Potent but transient suppression of primary and secondary antibody responses occur.

Nursing Implications: Assess WBC, neutrophil, and platelet count, and discuss any abnormalities with physician prior to drug administration; assess for signs/symptoms of skin infections (all mucosal surfaces, body orifices) and bleeding; instruct patient in signs/symptoms of infection and bleeding, as well as to report them or come to emergency room. Teach patient self-care measures to minimize risk of infection and bleeding, including avoidance of OTC aspirin-containing medications. Assess patient's Hgb/HCT and signs/symptoms of fatigue; teach patient self-assessment and to alternate rest and activity as needed.

II.   ALTERED NUTRITION, LESS THAN BODY REQUIREMENTS, related to NAUSEA AND VOMITING, ANOREXIA, STOMATITIS, DIARRHEA, HEPATOTOXICITY

Defining Characteristics: Nausea and vomiting occurs in 50% of patients, is dose related, and lasts for several hours. Can be successfully prevented with combination antiemetics. Anorexia commonly occurs. Stomatitis occurs 7–10 days after therapy is initiated, occurs in 15% of patients, and is dose related. May be preceded by angular stomatitis (reddened area at juncture of lips). Diarrhea is infrequent and mild. Hepatotoxicity is usually mild and reversible, but drug should be used cautiously in patients with impaired hepatic function.

Nursing Implications: Premedicate with antiemetics depending on dose, using aggressive, combination antiemetics for high-dose therapy, and continue throughout chemotherapy. If patient develops nausea/vomiting, assess fluid and electrolyte balance and the need for replacements. Assess oral mucosa prior to chemotherapy and teach patient oral hygiene regimen and self-assessment; encourage patient to report diarrhea, discuss use of antidiarrheals with physician, and teach self-care PRN. Since patients become neutropenic, all mucosal surfaces need to be assessed for infection, and patients must be taught scrupulous perineal hygiene. Monitor LFTs prior to, during, and posttherapy.

III.   IMPAIRED SKIN/MUCOSAL INTEGRITY related to RASH, ANAL INFLAMMATION/ULCERATION, ALOPECIA

Defining Characteristics: Maculopapular rash, with or without fever, myalgia, bone pain, occasional chest pain, conjunctivitis, and malaise (cytarabine syndrome) may occur. Syndrome is not common, but occurs 6–12 hours after drug administration; corticosteroids have been helpful in treating/preventing syndrome. Mucosal inflammation and ulceration of anus/rectum may occur, especially in patients with prior hemorrhoids or history of abscesses. Alopecia occurs less frequently.

Nursing Implications: Assess baseline skin and mucous membranes prior to chemotherapy and identify patients at risk for problems. Consider including corticosteroid in antiemetic regimen, especially for high-dose therapy, and discuss with physician prophylactic use of dexamethasone eye drops to prevent conjunctivitis. Teach patient scrupulous perineal hygiene, instruct to report any rectal discomfort, and assess rectal mucosa daily with high-dose therapy. Discuss with patient potential coping strategies if alopecia occurs (i.e., wig, scarves).

IV.   POTENTIAL FOR INJURY related to NEUROTOXICITY

Defining Characteristics: Neurotoxicity can occur at high doses. If cerebellar toxicity (characterized by nystagmus, dysarthria, ataxia, slurred speech, and/or dysdiadochokinesia or inability to make fine, coordinated movements) develops, it is an indication to terminate therapy. Onset usually 6–8 days after first dose, lasts 3–7 days. Lethargy and somnolence have resulted from rapid infusion of the drug. Incidence of CNS toxicity is 10% and may be related to total cumulative drug dose, impaired renal function, and/or age > 50 years old. Ocular toxicity may occur, characterized by injection of conjunctive, corneal opacities, decreased visual acuity. This may be a result of inhibition of DNA synthesis of corneal epithelium. Conjunctivitis occurs due to excretion of drug in lacrimal tearing and can be prevented by corticosteroid eye drops. Other visual symptoms that may occur are increased lacrimation, blurred vision, photophobia, eye pain.

Nursing Implications: Assess baseline neurologic status and cerebellar function (coordinated movements such as handwriting and gait) prior to and during therapy. Teach patient to self-assess and report changes in coordination, control of eye movement, handwriting. Monitor patient for somnolence and lethargy during infusion, and infuse drug according to established guidelines. With high-dose therapy, discuss with physician use of prophylactic corticosteroid eye drops. Assess and teach patient self-assessment of eyes and instruct to report increased lacrimation, blurred vision, photophobia, eye pain.

V.   POTENTIAL FOR INJURY related to TUMOR LYSIS SYNDROME (TLS)

Defining Characteristics: May develop with initial therapy if patient has a large tumor burden; results from rapid lysis of tumor cells. This usually begins 1–5 days after initiation of therapy and causes elevations in serum uric acid, potassium, phosphorus, BUN, creatinine.

Nursing Implications: If this is induction therapy for a patient with acute leukemia or high tumor burden, expect medical orders to include IV hydration at 150 mL/hour with or without alkalinization, oral allopurinol, strict monitoring of I/O, daily weight, and total body fluid balance determination. Monitor baseline and daily BUN, creatinine, K+, phosphorus, uric acid, and calcium. Monitor for renal, cardiac, neuromuscular signs/symptoms of TLS.

VI.   POTENTIAL SEXUAL DYSFUNCTION related to DRUG EFFECTS

Defining Characteristics: Drug is mutagenic and probably teratogenic. Although normal babies have been delivered by mothers receiving drug in first trimester, other babies have had congenital defects. It is unknown whether the drug is excreted in breastmilk.

Nursing Implications: Discuss with patient and partner sexuality and reproductive goals and possible impact of chemotherapy. Discuss contraception and sperm banking if appropriate. Discourage breastfeeding if the mother is receiving chemotherapy.

Drug: cytarabine, liposome injection (DepoCyt)

Class: Antimetabolite.

Mechanism of Action: Drug is converted to the metabolite ara-CTP intracellularly. Ara-CTP is thought to inhibit DNA polymerase, thereby affecting DNA synthesis. Incorporation into DNA and RNA may also contribute to cytarabine cellular toxicity.

Metabolism: With systemically administered cytarabine, the drug is metabolized to an inactive compound, ara-U, and is then renally excreted. In the CSF, however, conversion to the ara-U is negligible, because CNS tissue and CSF lack the enzyme necessary for the conversion to occur. Liposomal formulation gives sustained effect over 2 weeks, with a half-life in the CSF of 100–263 hours.

Indication: For the intrathecal treatment of lymphomatous meningitis.

Dosage/Range: Indicated for the intrathecal treatment of lymphomatous meningitis only. To be given as follows:
- **Induction therapy:** DepoCyt, 50 mg, administered intrathecally (intraventricular or lumbar puncture) every 14 days for 2 doses (weeks 1 and 3).
- **Consolidation therapy:** DepoCyt, 50 mg, administered intrathecally (intraventricular or lumbar puncture) every 14 days for 3 doses (weeks 5, 7, and 9) followed by 1 additional dose at week 13.
- **Maintenance therapy:** DepoCyt, 50 mg, administered intrathecally (intraventricular or lumbar puncture) every 28 days for 4 doses (weeks 17, 21, 25, and 29).
- If drug-related neurotoxicity develops, the dose should be reduced to 25 mg. If toxicity persists, treatment with DepoCyt should be terminated.
- Dexamethasone 4 mg PO twice daily × 5 days should begin on day of liposomal cytarabine injection.

Drug Preparation:
- Drug is supplied in single-use vials containing 10 mg/mL and comes as a white to off-white suspension in 5 mL of fluid, preservative-free.
- Drug is to be withdrawn immediately before use and should not be used later than 4 hours from the time of withdrawal from vial.

- DepoCyt should be administered directly into the CSF over 1–5 minutes. Patients should lie flat for 1 hour after administration.
- Patients should be started on dexamethasone 4 mg bid either PO or IV for 5 days beginning on the day of DepoCyt injection.

Drug Interactions:
- No formal drug interaction studies of DepoCyt and other drugs have been done.
- Expect increased neurotoxicity if drug is administered at same time as other intrathecal, cytotoxic agents.

Lab Effects/Interference:
- DepoCyt particles are similar in size and appearance to white blood cells, so care must be taken when interpreting CSF samples.

Special Considerations:
- Do not use inline filters with DepoCyt; administer directly into CSF.
- Must be administered with concurrent dexamethasone as described above.
- Granted full FDA approval in 2007 based on two RCTs showing significantly more patients treated with DepoCyt had absence of neurologic progression of disease and significantly higher complete cytologic response (clearing of malignant cells from CSF) compared with standard intrathecal cytarabine.

Potential Toxicties/Side Effects and the Nursing Process

I. ALTERATION IN NUTRITION, LESS THAN BODY REQUIREMENTS, related to NAUSEA AND VOMITING

Defining Characteristics: Nausea, vomiting, and headache are common, and are physical manifestations of chemical arachnoiditis.

Nursing Implications: Administer dexamethasone throughout treatment course as described above. Observe patient for at least 1 hour after administration for toxicity. Administer antiemetics as ordered. Encourage small, frequent feedings of cool, bland foods. Instruct patient to report nausea and vomiting and to self-administer antiemetics as ordered.

II. ALTERATION IN COMFORT related to HEADACHE, NECK AND/OR BACK PAIN, FEVER, NAUSEA, AND VOMITING

Defining Characteristics: Some degree of chemical arachnoiditis is expected in about one-third of patients: incidence approaches 100% of patients when dexamethasone is NOT given with DepoCyt. Causes headache, neck pain, and/or rigidity, back pain, fever, nausea, and vomiting, which are reversible.

Nursing Implications: Instruct patient in dexamethasone self-administration and to report to physician if oral doses are not tolerated. Patients should lie flat for 1 hour after lumbar puncture and should be observed for immediate toxic reactions. Administer medications to treat pain.

Drug: dacarbazine (DTIC-Dome, dimethyl-triazeno-imidazole carboxamide)

Class: Alkylating agent.

Mechanism of Action: Appears to methylate nucleic acids (particularly DNA) causing cross-linkage and breaks in DNA strands, which inhibits RNA and DNA synthesis. Also interacts with sulfhydryl groups to inhibit protein synthesis. Generally, cell cycle phase nonspecific.

Metabolism: Thought to be activated by liver microsomes; 15% of the drug crosses the blood–brain barrier. Undergoes metabolism in liver and biliary excretion, with 18–63% of drug excreted unchanged in the urine. Plasma half-life of 0.65 hour, and terminal half-life of 5 hours.

Indication: (1) For the treatment of patients with metastatic malignant melanoma, as well as for (2) second-line treatment of patients with Hodgkin's disease when used in combination with other effective agents.

Dosage/Range:
- 375 mg/m^2 every 2 weeks OR
- 150–250 mg/m^2/day × 5 days, repeat every 3–4 weeks.

Drug Preparation:
- Available in 100-, 200-, or 500-mg vials.
- Add sterile water or 0.9% sodium chloride to vial.

Drug Administration:
- Administer via pump over 20 minutes or give via IV push over 2–3 minutes.
- Stable for 8 hours at room temperature, for 72 hours if refrigerated. Store lyophilized drug in refrigerator and protect from light. Drug decomposition is denoted by a change in color from yellow to pink.

Drug Interactions:
- Increased drug metabolism with concurrent administration of Dilantin, phenobarbital; potential increased toxicity with Imuran and 6-MP.

Lab Effects/Interference:
- Decreased CBC.
- Increased LFTs.

Special Considerations:
- Irritant—avoid extravasation.
- Pain may occur above site: usually unrelieved by slowing IV, but may be relieved by applying ice to painful area. May cause venospasm; slow rate if this occurs.
- Anaphylaxis has occurred with infusion of dacarbazine.

Potential Toxicities/Side Effects and the Nursing Process

I. INFECTION AND BLEEDING related to BONE MARROW DEPRESSION

Defining Characteristics: Nadir occurs days 14–28 following drug administration; anemia may occur with long-term treatment.

Nursing Implications: Evaluate WBC, neutrophil, and platelet count and discuss any abnormalities with physician prior to drug administration; assess for signs/symptoms of infection or bleeding; instruct patient in identifying signs/symptoms of infection and bleeding, and to report them. Teach patient self-care measures to minimize risk of infection and bleeding, including avoidance of OTC aspirin-containing medications. Assess patient's Hgb/HCT and signs/symptoms of fatigue; teach patient self-assessment and instruct to alternate rest and activity as needed.

II. ALTERATION IN NUTRITION, LESS THAN BODY REQUIREMENTS, related to NAUSEA AND VOMITING, DIARRHEA, ANOREXIA, HEPATOTOXICITY

Defining Characteristics: Nausea/vomiting occurs in 90% of patients and is moderate to severe, beginning 1–3 hours after dose. Nausea and vomiting decrease with each consecutive day the drug is given. Preventable by aggressive combination antiemetics. Diarrhea is uncommon. Anorexia is common, occurring in 90% of patients; drug may also cause a metallic taste. Hepatotoxicity is rare, but hepatic veno-occlusive disease has been described (hepatic vein thrombosis and hepatocellular necrosis).

Nursing Implications: Premedicate with combination antiemetics and continue protection during infusions. Administer drug over at least 1 hour. Use relaxation exercises, imagery, or other techniques; teach patient exercises prior to drug treatment. Teach patient to report diarrhea and administer antidiarrheal medication as ordered, or teach patient self-administration as appropriate. Encourage small, frequent feedings of favorite foods; teach patient/caregiver to make foods ahead of time so patient will have them ready for snacks when hungry; encourage use of spices if food tastes bland; encourage patient to weigh self on a weekly basis. Monitor LFTs and discuss abnormalities with physician.

III. ALTERATION IN COMFORT related to FLU-LIKE SYNDROME, PAIN AT INJECTION SITE

Defining Characteristics: Flu-like syndromes may occur, characterized by malaise, headache, myalgia, hypotension; may occur up to 7 days after first dose, lasting 7–21 days, and may recur with subsequent doses of drug. Drug is an irritant and may cause phlebitis of vein.

Nursing Implications: Teach patient that flu-like symptoms may occur; suggest symptom management using acetaminophen as needed; encourage fluid intake of > 3 L/day and rest, as determined by healthcare team. Assess patient vein selection prior to drug administration and suggest venous access device early on if patient is to receive ongoing treatment with dacarbazine (DTIC). Administer drug in 100- to 250-mL IV fluid and infuse slowly over 1 hour. Consider premedications when drug is given peripherally and discuss with physician: hydrocortisone IVP (DTIC forms precipitate with hydrocortisone sodium succinate [Solu-Cortef] but not with hydrocortisone), lidocaine 1–2% IVP, or heparin IVP to minimize vein trauma prior to DTIC infusion. Apply heat or ice above injection site to reduce venous burning.

IV.   IMPAIRED SKIN INTEGRITY related to ALOPECIA, FACIAL FLUSHING, ERYTHEMA, URTICARIA

Defining Characteristics: Alopecia occurs in 90% of patients. Facial flushing occurs rarely and is self-limiting; erythema and urticaria may occur around injection site. High dose-related photosensitization may occur, with resulting severe reaction to sunlight, e.g., burning, pain.

Nursing Implications: Teach patient about expected hair loss; encourage patient to verbalize feelings regarding anticipated/actual hair loss and discuss strategies to minimize impact of alopecia. Encourage female patients to obtain wig prior to hair loss; ask male patients to identify how they will manage hair loss. Provide emotional support. In cold climates, encourage patient to wear cap at night to prevent loss of body heat. Teach patient receiving high-dose therapy to cover body, head, and hands when exposed to sunlight, or to avoid direct sunlight. Patient should also use sunblock.

V.   POTENTIAL FOR SENSORY/PERCEPTUAL ALTERATIONS related to FACIAL PARESTHESIA, PHOTOSENSITIVITY

Defining Characteristics: Photosensitivity may occur in bright sunlight or ultraviolet light. Facial paresthesias may occur.

Nursing Implications: Instruct patient to report facial paresthesias and in self-care measures if sensory changes occur; wear sunglasses in strong sunlight; wear sunscreens when out in the sun, as well as protective clothing, including a hat; avoid UV or strong sunlight exposure if possible.

VI.   POTENTIAL SEXUAL DYSFUNCTION related to DRUG EFFECTS

Defining Characteristics: Drug is teratogenic. It is unknown whether drug is excreted in breastmilk. Drug is probably carcinogenic.

Nursing Implications: Assess patient's and partner's patterns of sexuality and reproductive goals. Teach need for contraception and provide information and referral as appropriate.

Encourage verbalization of feelings and provide emotional support. Discourage breast-feeding if patient is a lactating mother.

Drug: dactinomycin (Actinomycin D, Cosmegen)

Class: Antitumor antibiotic isolated from *Streptomyces* fungus.

Mechanism of Action: Binds to guanine portion of DNA and blocks the ability of DNA to act as a template for both DNA and RNA. At lower drug doses, the predominant action inhibits RNA, whereas at higher doses both RNA and DNA are inhibited. Cell cycle specific for G_1 and S phases.

Indication:
1. As part of combination chemotherapy and/or multi-modality treatment regimen, indicated for the treatment of patients with Wilms' tumor, childhood rhabdomyosarcoma, Ewing's sarcoma, and metastatic, nonseminomatous testicular cancer.
2. As a single agent or as part of combination chemotherapy for the treatment of patients with gestational trophoblastic neoplasia.
3. As a component of regional perfusion, for the palliative and/or adjunctive treatment of locally recurrent or locoregional solid malignancies.

Metabolism: Most of drug is excreted unchanged in bile and urine. There is a rapid clearance of drug from plasma (approximately 36 hours). Dose reduction in the presence of liver or renal failure may be needed.

Dosage/Range:
- 10–15 µg/kg/day × 5 days q 3–4 weeks.
- 15–30 µg/kg/week, OR 15 µg/kg/day for 5 days IV.
- Frequency and schedule may vary according to protocol and age.

Drug Preparation:
- Add sterile water for a concentration of 500 µg/mL. Use preservative-free water, as precipitate may develop otherwise.

Drug Administration:
- IV: Drug is a vesicant and should be given through a running IV to avoid extravasation, which can lead to ulceration, pain, and necrosis. Be sure to check the nursing policy and procedure for administration of vesicants.

Drug Interactions:
- None significant.

Lab Effects/Interference:
- Decreased CBC.
- Increased LFTs.
- Decreased calcium.

Special Considerations:
- Drug is a vesicant. Give through a running IV to avoid extravasation, which may develop into ulceration, necrosis, and pain.
- Nausea and vomiting are moderate to severe. Usually occurs 2–5 hours after administration; may persist up to 24 hours.
- Potent myelosuppressive agent: Severity of nadir is dose-limiting toxicity.
- GI toxicity: Mucositis, diarrhea, and abdominal pain.
- Skin changes: Radiation recall phenomenon. Skin discoloration along vein used for injection.
- Alopecia.
- Malaise, fatigue, mental depression.
- Contraindicated in patients with chickenpox or herpes zoster, as life-threatening systemic disease may develop.

Potential Toxicities/Side Effects and the Nursing Process

I.   POTENTIAL FOR INFECTION AND BLEEDING related to BONE MARROW DEPRESSION

Defining Characteristics: Myelosuppression often dose-limiting toxicity. Onset of decreasing WBC and platelets in 7–10 days, with nadir 14–21 days after dose and recovery in 21–28 days. Delayed anemia.

Nursing Implications: Assess CBC, WBC, differential, and platelet count prior to drug administration, as well as for signs/symptoms of infection and bleeding, and discuss any abnormalities with physician prior to drug administration. Instruct patient in signs/symptoms of infection and bleeding, and instruct to report this; teach patient self-care measures to minimize risk of infection and bleeding, including avoidance of OTC aspirin-containing medications. Assess patient's Hgb/HCT and signs/symptoms of fatigue; teach patient self-assessment and instruct to alternate rest and activity as needed.

II.   ALTERATION IN NUTRITION, LESS THAN BODY REQUIREMENTS, related to NAUSEA/VOMITING, DIARRHEA, ANOREXIA

Defining Characteristics: Nausea/vomiting may be severe and begins 2–5 hours after dose, lasting 24 hours. Diarrhea with/without cramps occurs in 30% of patients. Anorexia occurs frequently.

Nursing Implications: Use combination antiemetics to prevent nausea and vomiting. Nausea/vomiting may be prevented by aggressive, combination antiemetics, such as serotonin antagonist plus dexamethasone. Encourage small, frequent feedings of bland foods. Encourage patient to eat favorite foods and use seasonings on foods if anorexia persists; refer to dietitian as needed.

III. ALTERATION IN MUCOUS MEMBRANES related to STOMATITIS, ESOPHAGITIS, AND PROCTITIS

Defining Characteristics: Irritation and ulceration may occur along the entire GI mucosa.

Nursing Implications: Assess baseline oral mucosa and presence of irritation along GI tract. Instruct patient in self-assessment and teach patient to report irritation; instruct regarding oral hygiene regimen.

IV. POTENTIAL IMPAIRED SKIN INTEGRITY related to RADIATION RECALL, RASH, ALOPECIA, AND DRUG EXTRAVASATION

Defining Characteristics: Recalls damage to skin from previous radiation, resulting in erythema or increased pigmentation at the radiation site. Acne-like rash and alopecia can occur in 47% of patients. Drug is a potent vesicant.

Nursing Implications: Conduct baseline skin, hair assessment. Discuss with patient impact of potential changes on body image, as well as possible coping/adaptive strategies (e.g., obtain wig prior to hair loss). When administering the drug, ensure use of a patent vein to avoid extravasation; consider the use of venous access device early. Be familiar with institution's policy and procedure for administration of a vesicant and management of extravasation.

V. ALTERATION IN COMFORT related to FLU-LIKE SYMPTOMS

Defining Characteristics: Flu-like symptoms can occur, including symptoms of malaise, myalgia, fever, depression.

Nursing Implications: Inform patient this may occur. Assess for occurrence during and after treatment. Discuss with physician symptomatic management.

VI. POTENTIAL FOR ALTERATION IN METABOLISM related to HEPATOTOXICITY AND RENAL TOXICITY

Defining Characteristics: Hepatotoxicity is related to drug metabolism in liver; renal toxicity is related to drug excretion by kidneys.

Nursing Implications: Monitor LFTUN and creatinine. Discuss abnormalities with physician, as drug doses may need to be reduced.

VII. POTENTIAL FOR SEXUAL DYSFUNCTION

Defining Characteristics: Drug is carcinogenic, mutagenic, and teratogenic. It is unknown if drug is excreted in breastmilk.

Nursing Implications: Assess patient's/partner's sexual patterns and reproductive goals. Provide information, supportive counseling, and referral as needed. Teach importance of birth control measures as appropriate. Discourage breastfeeding if patient is a lactating mother.

Drug: daunorubicin citrate liposome injection (DaunoXome)

Class: Anthracycline antibiotic that is isolated from streptomycin products, in particular the rhodomycin products, and encapsulated in a liposome.

Mechanism of Action: No clearly defined mechanism. Intercalates DNA, therefore blocking DNA, RNA, and protein synthesis. Binds to DNA and inhibits DNA replication and DNA-dependent RNA synthesis. Drug is encapsulated within liposomes (lipid vesicles) and is preferentially delivered to solid tumor sites. The liposomal encapsulated drug is protected from chemical and enzymatic degradation, protein binding, and uptake by normal tissues while circulating in the blood. The exact mechanism for selective targeting of tumor sites is unknown but is believed to be related to increased permeability of the tumor neovasculature. Once delivered to the tumor, the drug is slowly released and exerts its antineoplastic action.

Metabolism: Cleared from the plasma at 17 mL/min with a small steady-state volume of distribution. As compared to standard IV daunorubicin, the liposomal encapsulated daunorubicin has higher daunorubicin exposure (plasma AUC). The elimination half-life (4.4 hours) is shorter than standard daunorubicin.

Indication: Indicated as first-line cytotoxic chemotherapy for advanced HIV-associated Kaposi's sarcoma (KS). Drug is not recommended for patients with less than advanced HIV-related KS.

Dosage/Range:
- 20–40 mg/m^2/day IV bolus over 60 minutes every 2 weeks.
- Dosage adjustment if hepatic dysfunction or renal dysfunction.

Drug Preparation:
- Drug is available as 50 mg of daunorubicin base in a total volume of 25 mL (2 mg/mL).
- Visually inspect for particulate matter and discoloration (drug appears as a translucent dispersion of liposomes that scatters light, but should not be opaque or have precipitate or foreign matter present).
- Withdraw the calculated volume of drug and add to an equal volume of 5% dextrose to deliver a 1:1, or 1 mg/mL solution.
- Administer immediately, or may be stored in the refrigerator at 2–8°C (36–46°F) for 6 hours.
- Use ONLY 5% dextrose, NOT 0.9% sodium chloride or any other solution.
- Drug contains no preservatives.
- Unopened drug vials should be stored in the refrigerator at 2–8°C (36–46°F), but should not be frozen. Protect from light.

Drug Administration:
- IV bolus over 60 minutes, repeated every 2 weeks.
- Do not use an inline filter.
- Drug is an irritant, not a vesicant.
- Dose should be reduced in patients with renal or hepatic dysfunction.
- Hold dose if absolute granulocyte (neutrophil) count is < 750 cells/mm^3.

Drug Interactions:
- Colchicine, allopurinol, other antigout medications: may have increased effects.
- Bone marrow suppressant agents: increased bone marrow depression.

Lab Effects/Interference:
- Increased LFTs, RFTs (especially if elevated prior to administration).
- Increased uric acid secondary to tumor lysis.

Special Considerations:
- Drug is embryotoxic, so female patients should use contraceptive measures as appropriate.
- Back pain, flushing, and chest tightness may occur during the first 5 minutes of drug administration and resolve with cessation of the infusion. Most patients do not experience recurrence when the infusion is restarted at a slower rate.
- Drug activity reported to be equivalent to treatment with ABV (doxorubicin, vincristine, bleomycin) but with less alopecia, cardiotoxicity, and neurotoxicity.

Potential Toxicities/Side Effects and the Nursing Process

I. POTENTIAL FOR INFECTION AND BLEEDING related to BONE MARROW DEPRESSION

Defining Characteristics: Myelosuppression can be severe and affects the granulocytes primarily. Incidence of neutropenia of 36% is similar to that of patients receiving ABV (doxorubicin, vincristine, bleomycin), which is 35%. Neutropenia with < 500 cells/mm^3 occurs in 15% of patients (versus 5% in patients receiving ABV). Fever incidence is 47%. Concurrent antiretroviral and antiviral agents received for HIV infection may enhance this. Patients are immunocompromised; therefore, monitoring for opportunistic infection is essential. Platelets and RBCs are less affected.

Nursing Implications: Monitor CBC, WBC, differential, and platelet count prior to drug administration, and discuss any abnormalities with physician. Drug should not be given if ANC is < 750 cells/mm^3. Assess for signs/symptoms of infection or bleeding, and instruct patient in self-assessment and to report signs/symptoms immediately. Teach patient self-care measures to minimize risk of infection and bleeding, including avoidance of OTC aspirin-containing medications. Drug dosage must be reduced if patient has hepatic dysfunction: 75% of drug dose if serum bili 1.2–3.0 mg/dL, 50% reduction if bili is > 3.0 mg/dL. Drug dosage must be reduced if patient has renal impairment: creatinine > 3 mg/dL, give 50% of normal dose.

II.   ALTERATION IN COMFORT related to TRIAD OF BACK PAIN, FLUSHING, CHEST TIGHTNESS

Defining Characteristics: This occurs in 13.8% of patients and is mild to moderate. The syndrome resolves with cessation of the infusion, and does not usually recur when the infusion is resumed at a slower infusion rate.

Nursing Implications: Infuse drug at prescribed rate over 60 minutes. Assess for, and teach patient to report, back pain, flushing, and chest tightness. Stop infusion if this occurs, and once symptoms subside, resume infusion at a slower rate.

III.   POTENTIAL FOR ALTERATION IN SKIN INTEGRITY related to ALOPECIA, CHANGES IN SKIN

Defining Characteristics: Mild alopecia occurs in 6% of patients and moderate alopecia in 2% of patients, as compared to 36% of patients receiving ABV chemotherapy. The drug is considered an irritant, NOT a vesicant. Folliculitis, seborrhea, and dry skin occur in about 5% of patients.

Nursing Implications: Teach patient that hair loss is unlikely, and to report this or any skin changes.

IV.   POTENTIAL FOR ALTERATION IN NUTRITION, LESS THAN BODY REQUIREMENTS, related to NAUSEA AND VOMITING, ANOREXIA, DIARRHEA

Defining Characteristics: Mild nausea occurs in 35% of patients, moderate nausea in 16% of patients, and severe nausea in 3% of patients. Vomiting is less common, with 10% experiencing mild, 10% experiencing moderate, and 3% experiencing severe vomiting. Anorexia may occur (21%) or increased appetite may occur in < 5% of patients. Diarrhea may occur in 38% of patients. Other GI problems, occurring about 5% of the time, are dysphagia, gastritis, hemorrhoids, hepatomegaly, dry mouth, and tooth caries.

Nursing Implications: Premedicate with antiemetics. Encourage small, frequent feedings of bland foods. If patient has anorexia, teach patient or caregiver to make foods ahead of time, use spices, and encourage weekly weights. Instruct patient to report diarrhea and to use self-management strategies (medications as ordered, diet modification). Instruct patient to report other GI problems.

V.   POTENTIAL FOR ALTERATION IN CARDIAC OUTPUT related to CARDIAC CHANGES

Defining Characteristics: Daunorubicin may cause cardiotoxicity and CHF, but studies with liposomal daunorubicin show rare clinical cardiotoxicity at cumulative doses > 600 mg/m². However, especially in patients with preexisting cardiac disease or prior anthracycline treatment, assessment of cardiac function (history and physical) should be performed prior to each dose. In addition, testing of cardiac ejection fraction and echocardiogram should be performed at cumulative doses of 320 mg/m², 480 mg/m², and every 160 mg/m² thereafter.

Nursing Implications: Assess cardiac status prior to chemotherapy administration: signs/ symptoms of CHF, quality/regularity and rate of heartbeat, results of prior tests of left ventricular ejection fraction (LVEF) or echocardiogram, if performed. Instruct patient to report dyspnea, palpitations, swelling in extremities. Maintain accurate records of total dose, and expect GBPS to be repeated periodically during treatment and the drug to be discontinued if there is a significant drop in heart function.

VI.   POTENTIAL FOR ACTIVITY INTOLERANCE related to FATIGUE

Defining Characteristics: Fatigue occurs in 49% of patients.

Nursing Implications: Assess baseline activity level. Instruct patient to report fatigue and activity intolerance. Teach self-management strategies, including alternating rest and activity periods, and stress reduction.

Drug: daunorubicin hydrochloride (Cerubidine, Daunomycin HCl, Rubidomycin)

Class: Anthracycline antibiotic isolated from streptomycin products, in particular therhodomycin products.

Mechanism of Action: No clearly defined mechanism. Intercalates DNA, therefore blocking DNA, RNA, and protein synthesis. Binds to DNA and inhibits DNA replication and DNA-dependent RNA synthesis.

Metabolism: Site of significant metabolism is in the liver. Doses need to be modified in presence of abnormal liver function. Excreted in urine and bile.

Indication: In combination with other approved anticancer drugs, (1) for remission induction in adult patients with acute nonlymphocytic leukemia (myelogenous, monocytic, erythroid), and (2) for remission induction in children and adults with acute lymphocytic leukemia.

Dosage/Range:
- 30–60 mg/m²/day IV for 3 consecutive days.
- **AML induction:** 45 mg/m²/day IV × 3 days with cytosine arabinoside 100 mg/m²/day IV continuous infusion × 7 days.
- Adjust dose for hepatic dysfunction (25% dose reduction [DR]), BR 1.2–3 mg/dL; 50% DR BR > 3.0 mg/dL.

Drug Preparation:
- Available in 20- and 50-mg vials for injection or 20- and 50-mg vials containing lyophilized powder.
- Add sterile water to produce liquid. Drug will form a precipitate when mixed with heparin and is incompatible with dexamethasone.

Drug Administration:
- IV: This drug is a potent vesicant. Give through a running IV to avoid extravasation, which can lead to ulceration, pain, and necrosis. Check individual hospital policy and procedure on administration of a vesicant.

Drug Interactions:
- Incompatible with heparin (forms a precipitate).
- Other bone marrow suppressive drugs: increased bone marrow depression.
- Trastuzumab: may increase cardiotoxicity.

Lab Effects/Interference:
- Increased bili, AST, alk phos.
- Increased uric acid secondary to tumor lysis.

Special Considerations:
- Drug is a potent vesicant. Give through running IV to avoid/minimize risk of extravasation.
- Moderate to severe nausea and vomiting occur in 50% of patients within first 24 hours.
- Causes discoloration of urine (pink to red for up to 48 hours after administration).
- Potent myelosuppressive agent. Nadir occurs within 10–14 days.
- Alopecia.
- Cardiac toxicity: Dose limit at 400–550 mg/m² in adults, and 300 mg/m² in children > 2 years old. Patients may exhibit irreversible CHF. Acute toxicity may be seen within hours after administration. This is unrelated to cumulative dose and may manifest symptoms of pump or conduction dysfunction. Rarely, transient ECG abnormalities, CHF; pericardial effusion (whole syndrome referred to as myocarditis-pericarditis syndrome) may occur, which may lead to death.
- Dose reduction necessary in patients with impaired liver function.
- Available in liposomal encapsulated vehicle (Daunoxome) that has less myelosuppression and cardiotoxicity. Drug is currently approved for therapy of Kaposi's sarcoma.

Potential Toxicities/Side Effects and the Nursing Process

I.   POTENTIAL FOR INFECTION AND BLEEDING related to BONE MARROW DEPRESSION

Defining Characteristics: WBC and platelet counts begin to decrease in 7 days, with nadir 10–14 days after drug dose; recovery in 21–28 days. Dose reduction indicated with renal or hepatic dysfunction as drug is excreted by these routes.

Nursing Implications: Evaluate WBC, neutrophil, and platelet count and discuss any abnormalities with physician prior to drug administration; assess for signs/symptoms of infection and bleeding; instruct patient in signs/symptoms of infection and bleeding and to report these immediately. Teach patient self-care measures to minimize risk of infection and bleeding, including avoidance of OTC aspirin-containing medications.

II. POTENTIAL FOR ALTERATION IN CARDIAC OUTPUT related to ACUTE AND CHRONIC CARDIAC CHANGES

Defining Characteristics: Acute effects (i.e., EKG changes, atrial arrhythmias) occur in 6–30% of patients 1–3 days after dose and are not life-threatening. Chronic myofibril damage resulting in irreversible cardiomyopathy is life-threatening and dose-related. Cumulative dose should not exceed 550 mg/m^2 or 450 mg/m^2 if patient is receiving/has received radiation to chest or with concurrent administration of cyclophosphamide or other cardiotoxic agent. CHF may develop 1–16 months after therapy ceases if cumulative dose is exceeded.

Nursing Implications: Assess baseline cardiac status, quality and regularity of heartbeat, and baseline EKG. Patient should have baseline GBPS or other measure of left ventricular ejection fraction at baseline, and periodically during treatment. If there is a significant drop in ejection fraction, then drug should be stopped. Maintain accurate documentation of doses administered so that cumulative dose is known. Instruct patient to report dyspnea, shortness of breath, edema, orthopnea.

III. ALTERATION IN NUTRITION, LESS THAN BODY REQUIREMENTS, related to NAUSEA AND VOMITING, STOMATITIS

Defining Characteristics: Mild nausea and vomiting on the day of therapy occur in 50% of patients and can be prevented with antiemetics. Stomatitis is infrequent but may occur 3–7 days after dose.

Nursing Implications: Premedicate with antiemetics, and continue for 24 hours for protection. Assess oral mucosa prior to chemotherapy, teach patient oral hygiene regimen and self-assessment, and encourage patient to report burning or oral irritation. Assess pain in mouth, and administer analgesics as needed and ordered.

IV. POTENTIAL FOR IMPAIRED SKIN INTEGRITY related to ALOPECIA, HYPERPIGMENTATION OF FINGERNAILS AND TOENAILS, RADIATION RECALL, AND DRUG EXTRAVASATION

Defining Characteristics: Reversible total alopecia occurs 3–4 weeks after treatment begins; nail beds become hyperpigmented. Drug is a potent vesicant and will result in severe soft tissue damage if extravasated. Damage to skin from prior irradiation may be reactivated (radiation recall). Rash may occur, as may onycholysis (nail loosening from nail bed).

Nursing Implications: Teach patient that alopecia will occur and discuss impact hair loss will have on body image. Discuss coping strategies, including obtaining wig or cap prior to hair loss. Encourage patient to verbalize feelings and provide patient with emotional support. Drug dose may be decreased with prior irradiation; assess for skin changes from radiation recall. Hyperpigmentation of nail beds may cause body image problem; discuss with patient and identify measures to minimize distress. Ensure that drug is administered only through a patent IV and that nurse is familiar with institution's policy for vesicant administration and management of extravasation. Manufacturer recommends aspiration of any remaining drug from IV tubing, discontinuing IV, and applying ice. Assess need for venous access device early.

V.   POTENTIAL SEXUAL DYSFUNCTION related to DRUG EFFECTS

Defining Characteristics: Drug is mutagenic and teratogenic. Drug may cause testicular atrophy and azoospermia. It is unknown whether drug is excreted in breastmilk.

Nursing Implications: Assess patient's and partner's sexual patterns and reproductive goals. Provide information, supportive counseling, and referral as needed. Male patients may wish to try sperm banking. Teach importance of birth control measures as appropriate. Women receiving the drug should not breastfeed.

VI.   POTENTIAL FOR ALTERATION IN COMFORT related to ABDOMINAL PAIN, FEVER, CHILLS

Defining Characteristics: Abdominal pain may occur but is uncommon. Fever and chills, with or without rash, occur rarely.

Nursing Implications: Assess patient for occurrence and provide symptomatic management.

Drug: decitabine (Dacogen, 5-aza-2-deoxycytidine)

Class: Nucleoside metabolic inhibitor (antimetabolite); molecular/genetic modulator.

Mechanism of Action: Drug is a pyrimidine analogue and prevents DNA synthesis in the S phase, leading to cell death. Drug is incorporated into DNA and inhibits DNA methyltransferase, causing hypomethylation and cellular differentiation or apoptosis (programmed cell death). Methyltransferase is an enzyme necessary for the expression of cellular genes. The cells in tumors that have progressed or that are resistant to therapy, characteristically have DNA *hyper*methylation. Decitabine "traps" DNA methyltransferase, thus greatly reducing its activity, which results in the synthesis of DNA that is *hypo*methylated.

DNA hypomethylation results in activating genes that have been silent, causing the cell to differentiate, and then to die (cell death through disorganized gene expression or extinction of clones of cells that were terminally differentiated). Research has shown that the drug modulates tumor suppressor genes, the expression of tumor antigens, other genes, and overall cell differentiation. Non-proliferating cells are relatively insensitive to the drug.

Metabolism: Biphasic distribution, with mean terminal phase elimination half-life of 0.5 ± 0.31 hours. Drug is not plasma-bound to serum proteins. Metabolism not fully characterized, but appears to involve deamination in the liver, granulocytes, intestinal epithelium, and whole blood.

Indication: Treatment of patients with myelodysplastic syndromes (MDS), including: Previously treated and untreated, *de novo* and secondary MDS of all French-American-British subtypes

- Refractory anemia
- Refractory anemia with ringed sideroblasts
- Refractory anemia with excess blasts in transformation
- Chronic myelomonocytic leukemia
- Intermediate-1, Intermediate-2, and high-risk International Prognostic Scoring System groups

Dosage/Range:
- MDS recommended treatment for at least 4 cycles of therapy; however, a CR or PR may take more than 4 cycles.

Option 1:
- Decitabine 15 mg/m² IV continuous infusion over 3 hours, repeated every 8 hours for 3 days.
- Subsequent treatment cycles: Repeat initial cycle every 6 weeks for a minimum of 4 cycles.
- Dose modification: Delay next cycle until ANC is 1,000/μL and platelets are 50,000/μL, and dose-reduce as follows:
  - Recovery requiring more than 6 but less than 8 weeks: Delay drug up to 2 weeks and then temporarily reduce dose to 11 mg/m² every 8 hours (33/m² per day, 99 mg/m² per cycle) upon restarting therapy.
  - Recovery requiring more than 8 but less than 10 weeks: Assess bone marrow for disease progression; if no progression, delay dose up to 2 more weeks and reduce dose to 11 mg/m² every 8 hours (33 mg/m² per day, 99 mg/m² per cycle) upon restarting therapy; maintain or dose increase in subsequent cycles as clinically indicated.

Option 2:
- Decitabine 20 mg/m² IV infusion over 1 hour, repeated daily × 5 days. Repeat cycle every 4 weeks. Premedicate with antiemetic therapy.
- Dose modification: If myelosuppression is present, subsequent treatment cycles of decitabine should be delayed until there is hematologic recovery (ANC = 1,000/μL, platelets = 50,000 μL).

Dose modifications:
- Delay next cycle until ANC ≥ 1,000/μL and platelets ≥ 50,000 μL, and dose-reduce as follows:
  - Recovery requiring more than 6 but less than 8 weeks: Delay drug up to 2 weeks and then temporarily reduce dose to 11 mg/m^2 every 8 hours (33mg/m^2 per day, 99 mg/m^2 per cycle) upon restarting therapy.
  - Recovery requiring more than 8 but less than 10 weeks: Assess BM for disease progression; if no progression, delay dose up to 2 more weeks and reduce dose to 11 mg/m^2 every 8 hours (33 mg/m^2 per day, 99 mg/m^2 per cycle) upon restarting therapy; maintain or dose increase in subsequent cycles as clinically indicated.
  - If any of the nonhematologic toxicities are present, do not restart until toxicity has resolved: serum creatinine ≥ 2 mg/dL, SGPT ≥ 2 times ULN; total bilirubin > 2 times ULN; active or uncontrolled infection.

Drug Preparation:
- Drug supplied for injection as a sterile lyophilized white to almost-white powder in a single-dose vial containing 50 mg of decitabine. Store vials at 25°C (77°F) with excursions up to 15–30°C (59–86°F) permitted.
- Aseptically add 10 mL sterile water for injection (USP); upon reconstitution, each mL contains approximately 5.0 mg of decitabine at pH 6.7–7.3. Immediately after reconstitution, further dilute with 0.9% sodium chloride injection, 5% dextrose injection, or lactated Ringer's injection to a final drug concentration of 0.1–1.0 mg/mL. Use within 15 min of reconstitution, or prepare diluted solution with cold infusion fluids (2–8°C) to further dilute the drug, then store at 2–8°C (36–46°F) for up to a maximum of 7 hours until administration. Inspect for clarity, and do not use if discolored or particulate matter present.

Drug Administration:
- IV continuous infusion over 3 hours repeated every 8 hours for 3 days.
  - Option 1: IV continuous infusion over 3 hours repeated every 8 hours for 3 days, repeated every 6 weeks.
  - Option 2: IV continuous infusion over 1 hour daily for 5 days, repeat cycle every 4 weeks.
- Assess CBC/differential at a minimum, before each treatment cycle.

Drug Interactions:
- Appears to be synergistic with biologic agents, such as interferons and retinoids (retinoic acid).
- Synergistic cytotoxic effects when given together with each of the following: cisplatin, 4-hydroperoxycyclophosphamide, 3-deazauridine, cyclopentenyl cytosine, cytosine arabinoside, topotecan, and thymidine.
- Does not appear to affect P450 hepatic microenzymes.

Lab Effects/Interference:
- Neutropenia, thrombocytopenia, anemia.
- Hyperglycemia, hyperbilirubinemia, hypo- or hyperkalemia, hypomagnesemia.
- Increased creatinine, AST.

Special Considerations:

- Contraindicated in patients with a history of hypersensitivity reactions to the drug or any of its components.
- Neutropenia and thrombocytopenia may be severe. CBC and platelet counts should be performed before each dosing cycle and as indicated. Consider early institution of growth factors and/or antimicrobial agents for the prevention or treatment of infections in patients with MDS.
- Drug alters DNA synthesis, and may cause fetal harm; women of childbearing potential should be advised to avoid pregnancy during treatment and for one month following completion of therapy; if pregnancy occurs, the patient should be apprised of the potential hazard to the fetus. Men should be advised not to father a child while receiving decitabine, and for 2 months following completion of treatment. Men with female partners of childbearing potential should use effective contraception during this time.
- Rarely, serious adverse events that occurred in patients receiving decitabine, regardless of causality, included cardiac events (MI, CHF, cardiopulmonary arrest, cardiomyopathy, atrial fibrillation, supraventricular tachycardia); fungal infection, bronchopulmonary aspergillosis, mycobacterium avium complex infection; intracranial hemorrhage.
- Women of childbearing potential should be taught to use effective contraception during treatment, and for 1 month after treatment ends, to avoid pregnancy. If the drug is used during pregnancy or if the patient becomes pregnant while receiving the drug, the mother should be apprised of the risk to the fetus, as drug can cause fetal harm.
- Men should be advised not to father children during treatment and for 2 months afterward.
- Nursing mothers should make a decision whether to stop nursing or discontinue decitabine, taking into account the importance of the drug to the mother's health.
- Cases of Sweet's Syndrome (acute febrile neutrophilic dermatosis) have been described in post-marketing reports.

Potential Toxicities/Side Effects and the Nursing Process

I. POTENTIAL FOR INFECTION AND BLEEDING related to BONE MARROW DEPRESSION

Defining Characteristics: Dose-limiting factor is bone marrow suppression. In MDS studies, the incidence of neutropenia was 90%, with 29% of patients developing febrile neutropenia. Thrombocytopenia occurred in 89% of patients. Drug is extensively metabolized in the liver, and partially excreted by the kidneys. Anemia occurs in 82% of patients.

Nursing Implications: Assess baseline CBC and differential, and platelet count, renal and hepatic function tests, prior to initial and subsequent cycles of chemotherapy. Drug should be held if ANC < 1,000/μL platelets, 50,000/μL, BR > 2.0 times ULN, AST > 2 times ULN, creatinine > 2.0 mg/dL (see Dosage). Discuss with physician early use of growth factor and/or antimicrobials for prevention of infection. Assess for signs/symptoms of infection, bleeding, and fatigue. Teach patient signs/symptoms of infection or bleeding, to report these immediately, and to come to the emergency room or clinic if febrile or bleeding. Teach patient self-care measures to minimize risk of infection and bleeding. This includes avoidance of crowds and proximity to people with infections, and avoidance of OTC aspirin-containing medications.

II. ALTERED NUTRITION, LESS THAN BODY REQUIREMENTS, related to NAUSEA AND VOMITING, STOMATITIS

Defining Characteristics: Nausea and vomiting may occur, are mild to moderate, and are preventable by antiemetic medicines. Nausea occurs in 42% of patients and vomiting in 25% of patients. Stomatitis and dyspepsia occurs in 12% of patients.

Nursing Implications: Premedicate patient with antiemetic. If patient develops nausea and/or vomiting, encourage small, frequent intake of cool, bland foods. Instruct patient to report nausea, and teach self-administration of antiemetic medications. If nausea/vomiting occur and are severe, assess for signs/symptoms of fluid/electrolyte imbalance. Teach patient to self-administer antidiarrheal medications if needed. Assess baseline oral mucous membranes. Teach patient oral assessment, hygiene measures, and to report any alterations.

III. ALTERATION IN COMFORT related to LETHARGY, FEVER, EDEMA, PAIN, RIGORS, ARTHRALGIAS

Defining Characteristics: Pyrexia affects 53% of patients, with rigors in 22% of patients, and fatigue occurred in 46%. Peripheral edema affects 25%, arthralgias 20%, and pain 13%. Catheter-site pain, erythema, and injection site swelling occurred in 5% of patients.

Nursing Implications: Assess comfort level, symptoms experienced at baseline and prior to each dose, then prior to each cycle. Teach patient to alternate rest and activity periods. Teach patient to report fevers > 100.5°F, rigors right away, and to come to the clinic or ED. Teach patient symptomatic management of pain. Assess catheter and injection sites to rule out infection and to manage comfort.

Drug: degarelix (Firmagon)

Class: Gonadotropin-releasing hormone (GnRH) antagonist.

Mechanism of Action: Drug binds irreversibly to GnHR receptors in the pituitary gland and reduces the release of gonadotropins, thus reducing the serum levels of luteinizing hormone (LH) and follicle-stimulating hormone (FSH); this decreases the production of testosterone by the Leydig cells in the male testes. A 240-mg dose of degarelix achieves and maintains testosterone suppression below the castration level of 50 ng/dL.

Metabolism: Administered subcutaneously, degarelix forms a depot, which slowly releases the drug. The peak serum concentration (C_{max}) occurs 2 days after administration. The drug is widely distributed in body water and is 90% serum protein-bound. Drug undergoes protein hydrolysis as it passes through the hepatobiliary system, with about 70–80%

metabolized and excreted in the feces and 20–30% excreted in the urine. Drug is not a substrate, inducer, or inhibitor of the P450 microenzyme system, or of the P-glycoprotein transport system. Elimination is biphasic, and the median terminal half-life of the drug is 53 days.

Indication: Drug is indicated for the treatment of patients with advanced prostate cancer.

Contraindication: Patients with known hypersensitivity to degarelix or to any product components; and women who are or may become pregnant (as drug can cause fetal harm).

Long-term androgen deprivation therapy prolongs the QTc interval; a risk-benefit analysis should precede use of degarelix in patients with congenital long QT syndrome, electrolyte abnormalities, CHF, or those who are taking Class IA or Class III antiarrhythmic drugs.

Drug Preparation:
- Available in 80-mg and 120-mg vials.
- Initial: The drug pack contains 2 sets of degarelix 120-mg vial, 2–3 mL prefilled syringes containing sterile water for injection USP, syringe, vial adapter, and administration needle. Uncap vial and use alcohol swab to wipe the rubber stopper; remove vial adapter and attach to the vial until the spike pushes through the rubber stopper and snaps into place.
- Prepare the prefilled syringe, and attach the syringe to the vial by screwing it on to the adapter. Transfer all sterile water for injection USP to the vial. With syringe still attached, swirl gently until liquid is clear. If powder adheres to side of vial above liquid surface, tilt vial slightly but do not shake, as foam will form. Reconstitution may take up to 15 minutes but usually takes a few minutes.
- Turn vial upside down and draw up to the 3mL mark on the syringe for injection. Always withdraw the precise volume and expel air bubbles.
- Detach syringe from vial adapter, and aseptically attach administration needle to syringe.
- Immediately after reconstitution, inject 3 mL of degarelix 120 mg slowly as a deep subcutaneous injection. Repeat reconstitution procedure for the second 120-mg vial to complete the 240-mg starting dose and choose a different injection site for the second dose.
- Maintenance dose: the pack contains 1 set of degarelix 80-mg vial, 1 prefilled syringe containing 4.2 mL sterile water for injection USP, vial adapter, and administration needle. Use same procedure as above, but withdraw 4 mL of prepared drug into administration syringe. Administer immediately as a single 4-mL deep subcutaneous injection.
- Drug should be used within 1 hour of reconstitution.

Drug/Dose Administration:
- Starting dose is 240 mg, and is administered subcutaneously as two injections of 120 mg each; administer deep subcutaneously in the abdomen in two separate areas.
- Maintenance dose is 80 mg given starting 28 days after initial dose and repeated every 28 days as a deep subcutaneous injection in the abdomen.
- Pinch abdominal skin to achieve a deep subcutaneous injection, and insert the needle at a 45 degree angle; gently pull back the plunger to assess if needle is in vein; if blood aspirated into the syringe, product cannot be used and a new vial should be prepared.

- AVOID areas of abdominal pressure such as under belt or waistband, or near the ribs.
- Assess for hypersensitivity reactions (HSRs), including anaphylaxis, urticaria, and angioedema. Discontinue the injection immediately if not yet completed, and provide emergency support and intervention as ordered.
- Therapeutic effect should be monitored by baseline and periodic PSA testing. If the PSA rises, serum level of testosterone should be measured.

Lab Effects/Interference:
- Decreased serum LH, FSH, testosterone levels.
- Hypercholesterolemia (3–6% of patients).
- Increased liver transaminases and GGT.
- Prolonged QTc Interval.

Drug Interactions:
- Not tested, unknown.
- Clinically significant CYP450 drug-drug interactions are unlikely.

Special Considerations:
- Use with caution in patients with severe liver or renal dysfunction.
- Drug is contraindicated in patients who are hypersensitive to the drug, and in pregnant women because the drug is fetotoxic; women should not breastfeed while receiving the drug.
- Drug is at least as effective as leuprolide in sustaining castration testosterone levels, and achieves this reduction significantly faster.
- Drug is a new-generation GnHR receptor antagonist with low histamine-release properties, without an initial testosterone surge seen in prior-generation GnHR receptor antagonists. Direct biochemical suppression of testosterone begins on day 1 of therapy.
- Long-term androgen suppression can cause QTc prolongation, so patients with risk factors such as CHF, or who are on other drugs that prolong the QTc interval, should be monitored closely with baseline and frequent ECG and QTc measurements during treatment. Monitor serum potassium, magnesium, and calcium, and ensure values are WNL.
- Hypertension occurs rarely in 6–7% of patients; monitor BP baseline and periodically during treatment.
- Most common adverse reactions occurring in 10% or more patients: injection-site reaction (pain, erythema, swelling, induration), hot flashes, increased weight, fatigue, and increased serum levels of transaminases and gamma glutamyltransferase. Most reactions were grade 1 or 2.

Potential Toxicities/Side Effects and the Nursing Process

I.   POTENTIAL ALTERATION IN COMFORT related to CHILLS, HOT FLUSHES, INJECTION SITE PAIN, ARTHRALGIAS, ASTHENIA, INSOMNIA, COUGH

Defining Characteristics: Constitutional symptoms such as chills occur in 3–5% of patients, dizziness (9–11%), fatigue (3–23%), hot flushes (25–48%), injection site pain

(3–18%), injection site reactions (35–44%), arthalgias (3–6%), asthenia (5–6%), back pain (3–9%), insomnia (3–8%), and cough (3–10%). Injection-site reactions were primarily transient, mild to moderate in intensity, occurred with the starting dose, and led to few discontinuations (<1%).

Nursing Implications: Assess baseline comfort, and tell patient these symptoms may occur. Discuss self-care strategies, and teach patient to report side effects that do not resolve. Assess abdominal subcutaneous injection sites for irritation, and teach patient that warm or cold compresses following drug administration may reduce discomfort. Ensure that drug is administered in abdominal sites that are NOT under belt lines, close to the ribs, or in areas that will be under pressure.

II. POTENTIAL ALTERATION IN NUTRITION related to CONSTIPATION, DIARRHEA, WEIGHT GAIN

Defining Characteristics: Weight gain occurs in 6–13% of patients, constipation in 3–6%, and diarrhea in 3–9% of patients.

Nursing Implications: Assess baseline nutritional status, weight, and elimination status. Teach patient that these side effects may occur and to report them.

III. POTENTIAL ALTERATION IN SEXUALITY related to ERECTILE DYSFUNCTION

Defining Characteristics: Erectile dysfunction occurs in 3–9% of patients, nocturia in 2–11%, and urinary tract infections in 1–7%.

Nursing Implications: Assess baseline sexuality and teach patient that these side effects may occur and to report them. Discuss possible management strategies with physician, and revise plan as needed.

Drug: docetaxel (Taxotere)

Class: Taxoid, mitotic spindle poison.

Mechanism of Action: Enhances microtubule assembly and inhibits disassembly. Disrupts microtubule network that is essential for mitotic and interphase cellular function. Drug binds to free tubulin and promotes the assembly of tubulin into stable microtubules and also prevents their disassembly. Stabilization of microtubules inhibits mitosis. At low weekly doses, drug may have antiangiogenic properties.

Metabolism: Drug is extensively protein-bound (94–97%). Triphasic elimination. Metabolism involves P450 3A (CYP3A4) isoenzyme system (in vitro testing). Fecal elimination is main route, accounting for excretion of 75% of the drug and its metabolites within 7 days;

80% of the fecal excretion occurs during the first 48 hours. Mild to moderate liver impairment (SGOT and/or SGPT > 1.5 times normal and alk phos > 2.5 times normal) results in decreased clearance of drug by an average of 27%, resulting in a 38% increase in systemic exposure (AUC).

Indications: Docetaxel is a microtubule inhibitor indicated for the treatment of
- Breast cancer: (1) as a single agent in the treatment of locally advanced or metastatic breast cancer after chemotherapy failure, and (2) with doxorubicin and cyclophosphamide as adjuvant treatment of operable, node-positive breast cancer.
- NSCLC: (1) as a single agent for the treatment of locally advanced or metastatic NSCLC after platinum therapy failure, and (2) with cisplatin for the treatment of unresectable, locally advanced, or metastatic untreated NSCLC.
- Hormone refractory prostate cancer: with prednisone, in androgen-independent (hormone refractory) metastatic prostate cancer.
- Gastric adenocarcinoma: with cisplatin and fluorouracil for untreated advanced gastric adenocarcinoma, including the gastroesophageal junction.
- Squamous cell carcinoma of the head and neck cancer (SCCHN): with cisplatin and fluorouracil for induction treatment of locally advanced SCCHN.

Dosage/Range:
- Adjuvant breast cancer: docetaxel 75 mg/m² IV 1 hour after doxorubicin 50 mg/m² IVP and cyclophosphamide 500 mg/m² IV q 3 weeks × 6 courses, with G-CSF support PRN.
- Locally advanced or metastatic breast cancer: 60–100 mg/m² IV as a 1-hour infusion every 3 weeks.
- NSCLC: (1) after platinum therapy failure: 75 mg/m² single agent, every 3 weeks; (2) chemotherapy-naive: 75 mg/m² followed by cisplatinum 75 mg/m² IV over 30–60 min every 3 weeks.
- Hormone refractory prostate cancer: docetaxel 75 mg/m² IV infusion repeated q 21 days, in combination with prednisone 5 mg PO bid continuously.
- Advanced gastric cancer: 75 mg/m² as a 1-hour infusion followed by cisplatin 75 mg/m² over 1–3 hours (both on day 1 only), followed by fluorouracil 750 mg/m² per day as a 24-hour IV infusion (days 1–5), starting at the end of cisplatin infusion. Cycle is repeated every 3 weeks. Patients must receive premedication with antiemetics and hydration prior to cisplatin.

SCCHN
- All patients must receive premedication with antiemetics, as well as appropriate hydration (prior to and after cisplatin).
- **Induction therapy followed by RT**: 75 mg/m² IV over 1 hr (day 1), followed by cisplatin 75 mg/m² (IV over 1 hour, day 1) followed by fluorouracil 750 mg/m² per day as a 24-hr IV infusion (days 1–5), starting at end of cisplatin infusion, for 4 cycles.
- **Induction therapy followed by chemoradiation**: 75 mg/m² IV over 1 hr (day 1), followed by cisplatin 100 mg/m² IV over 30 min–3 hr, day 1, followed by fluorouracil 1,000 mg/m² per day as a 24-hr IV infusion (days 1–4), starting at end of cisplatin infusion, repeated every 3 weeks for 3 cycles.

Premedication regimen with corticosteroids:
- e.g., dexamethasone 8 mg PO bid × 3 days, starting 1 day prior to docetaxel to reduce the incidence and severity of fluid retention and hypersensitivity reactions.
- For patients with prostate cancer receiving prednisone, the doses of oral dexamethasone are 8 mg at 12 hours, 3 hours, and 1 hour prior to docetaxel dose.

Dose reductions: See package insert.
- (1) Patients with **breast cancer** dosed initially at 100 mg/m^2 who experience either febrile neutropenia, ANC < 500/mm^3 for > 1 week, or severe or cumulative cutaneous reactions, or other grade 3–4 nonhematologic toxicity, should have dose reduced to 75 mg/m^2. If reactions continue at the reduced dose, further reduce to 55 mg/m^2 or discontinue drug. Patients dosed initially at 60 mg/m^2 who do not experience febrile neutropenia, ANC < 500/mm^3 for > 1 week, nadir platelets < 25,000 cells/mm^3, severe cutaneous reactions, or severe peripheral neuropathy during drug therapy may tolerate higher drug doses and may be dose-escalated. Patients who develop ≥ grade 3 peripheral neuropathy should have drug discontinued.
- (2) Patients receiving **adjuvant treatment of breast cancer who** experience febrile neutropenia should receive G-CSF in all subsequent cycles; if febrile neutropenia recurs, continue G-CSF and dose-reduce docetaxel to 60 mg/m^2. Patients who develop grade 3–4, severe or cumulative cutaneous reactions, or moderate neurosensory signs and/or symptoms should have docetaxel dose reduced to 60 mg/m^2. If patient continues to experience these reactions on the reduced dose, treatment should be discontinued.
- (3) Patients with **NSCLC receiving monotherapy**, dosed initially at 75 mg/m^2, who experience febrile neutropenia, ANC < 500 mg/m^2 for > 1 week, nadir platelets < 25,000 cells/mm^3, severe or cumulative cutaneous reactions, or other nonhematologic toxicity grades 3 or 4 should have treatment withheld until toxicity resolves and then have dose reduced to 55 mg/m^2; patients who develop grade 3 or greater peripheral neuropathy should discontinue docetaxel chemotherapy.
- (4) Patients with **NSCLC receiving combination therapy** who are initially dosed at 75 mg/m^2 in combination with cisplatin and whose platelet nadir count during the previous course of therapy is < 25,000 cells/mm^3, or who develop febrile neutropenia, or serious nonhematologic toxicities should have a docetaxel dose reduction to 65 mg/m^2 in subsequent cycles. If a further dose reduction is necessary, reduce dose to 50 mg/m^2.
- (5) Patients with **prostate cancer** who experience febrile neutropenia, ANC < 500/mm^3 for > 1 week, or severe or cumulative cutaneous reactions, or moderate neurosensory signs and/or symptoms during docetaxel therapy should have dose reduced from 75 mg/m^2 to 60 mg/m^2. If the same symptoms arise at the reduced dosage, the drug should be discontinued.
- (6) Patients with **gastric or SCCHN** receiving docetaxel in combination with cisplatin and fluorouracil must receive antiemetics and appropriate hydration.
  - G-CSF is recommended for second and subsequent cycles if the patient develops febrile neutropenia, neutropenic infection, or neutropenia lasting more than 7 days. If neutropenic fever, infection, or prolonged neutropenia occur despite G-CSF, reduce

docetaxel dose from 75 mg/m² to 60 mg/m²; if neutropenic complications continue to occur despite dose reduction and G-CSF, reduce dose to 45 mg/m². In the case of grade 4 thrombocytopenia, dose-reduce docetaxel from 75 mg/m² to 60 mg/m².
* Retreatment with docetaxel requires that neutrophils recover to > 1,500 cells/mm³ and platelets recover to > 100,000 cells/mm³. Drug should be discontinued if toxicities persist.
* Dose modifications of fluorouracil (5-FU): Grade 3 diarrhea, reduce 5-FU dose by 20%; if it occurs a second time, reduce docetaxel dose by 20% as well. If grade 4 diarrhea occurs, reduce 5-FU and docetaxel doses by 20%. If it occurs again, discontinue treatment. Grade 3 stomatitis/mucositis: first episode, reduce 5-FU dose by 20%; second episode, stop 5-FU only in this and all subsequent cycles; third episode, dose-reduce docetaxel by 20%. Grade 4 stomatitis/mucositis: first episode, stop 5-FU only in this and all subsequent cycles; second episode, dose-reduce docetaxel by 20%. See package insert for docetaxel dose modifications for abnormal LFTs, as well as those for cisplatin and HFS from 5-FU.

Drug Preparation (requires two dilutions prior to administration):
* Vials available as 80-mg and 20-mg concentrate as single-dose blister packs with diluent. Do not reuse single-dose vials. Drug contains polysorbate 80.
* Unopened vials require protection from bright light. May be stored at room temperature or in refrigerator (36–77°F). Allow to stand at room temperature for at least 5 minutes prior to reconstitution.
* Reconstitute 20-mg and 80-mg vials with the entire contents of accompanying diluent vial (13% ethanol in water for injection). Reconstituted vials contain 10 mg/mL docetaxel (initial diluted solution).
* Gently invert repeatedly, but do not shake the initial diluted solution for approximately 45 seconds.
* Reconstituted vials (10 mg/mL initial diluted solution) are stable for 8 hours at either room temperature or under refrigeration.
* Use only glass or polypropylene or polyolefin plastic (bag) IV containers.
* Withdraw ordered dose, and further dilute in 250 mL volume of 5% dextrose or 0.9% sodium chloride to a final concentration of 0.3–0.74 mg/mL. Thoroughly mix by manual rotation.
* Inspect for any particulate matter or discoloration, and if found, discard.
* Use infusion solution immediately; solution is stable under the following conditions:
  * Docetaxel final dilution for infusion, if stored between 2°C–25°C (36°F–77°F), is stable for 6 hours, using either 0.9% Sodium Chloride or 5% Dextrose solution and should be used within 6 hours, including the 1 hour IV administration time;
  * Infusion solution prepared as recommended in non-PVC bags is physically and chemically stable for 48 hours when stored between 2°C–8°C (36°F–46°F).

Drug Administration:
* ANC ≥ 1,500 cells/m³; BR must be < ULN; SGOT and/or SGPT < 1.5 × ULN concomitant with alkaline phosphatase < 2.5 × ULN. Assess patient's ANC and liver function studies, and if abnormal, discuss with physician. See Special Considerations.

- Use only glass or polypropylene bottles, or polypropylene or polyolefin plastic bags for drug infusion, and administer infusion ONLY through polyethylene-lined administration sets.
- Patient should receive corticosteroid premedication (e.g., dexamethasone 8 mg bid) for 3 days beginning 1 day before drug administration to reduce the incidence and severity of fluid retention and hypersensitivity reactions.
- Infuse drug over 1 hour.
- Assess for severe hypersensitivity reactions (HSRs), as generalized rash/erythema, hypotension, bron chospasm or, very rarely, fatal anaphylaxis have been described, despite premedication. Immediately stop drug and provide emergency management.

Drug Interactions:
- Radiosensitizing effect.
- Theoretically, CYP3A4 inhibitors, such as ketoconazole, erythromycin, troleandomycin, cyclosporine, terfenadine, and nifedipine, can inhibit docetaxel metabolism and result in elevated serum levels of docetaxel; use together with caution or not at all.
- Theoretically, CYP3A4 inducers, such as anticonvulsants and St. John's wort, may increase metabolism and decrease serum levels of docetaxel.
- Calcitriol (high dose, DN-101): suggested increase in patient survival without added toxicity in patients with prostate cancer (Beer et al., 2007).

Lab Effects/Interference:
- Decreased CBC.

Special Considerations:
- Contraindicated in patients with history of severe hypersensitivity reactions to docetaxel or to other drugs formulated with polysorbate 80; drug should not be used in patients with neutrophil counts of < 1,500 cells/mm^3. Drug should not be used in pregnant or breastfeeding women; women of childbearing age should use effective birth control measures.
- Treatment-related mortality increases with abnormal liver function, at higher doses, and in patients with NSCLC and prior platinum-based therapy receiving docetaxel at 100 mg/m^2.
- Docetaxel generally should not be administered to patients with bilirubin > upper limit of normal (ULN) or to patients with SGOT and/or SGPT > 1.5 × ULN concomitant with alkaline phosphatase > 2.5 × ULN.
  - Patients treated with elevated bilirubin or abnormal transaminases plus alkaline phosphatase have an increased risk of grade 4 neutropenia, febrile neutropenia, severe stomatitis, infections, severe thrombocytopenia, severe skin toxicity, and toxic death.
  - Assess serum bilirubin, SGOT or SGPT, and alkaline phosphatase before each cycle of docetaxel treatment.
  - Patients should receive dexamethasone premedication (such as 8 mg bid × 3 days starting 1 day prior to Taxotere) to reduce fluid accumulation.

- Nursing mothers should make a decision to discontinue nursing or to discontinue the drug, taking into account the importance of the drug to the mother's health.
- Administration of docetaxel in Europe is not subject to US Federal Drug Administration recommendations; non-PVC containers and tubing are not required.

Warnings and Precautions:
- Toxic deaths have occurred; monitor patients closely.
- Hepatic impairment: patients with combined transaminase and alkaline phosphatase abnormalities should not receive the drug.
- Hematologic effects: monitor CBC/differential frequently and dose-interrupt or dose-reduce per package insert. Patients should not receive subsequent treatment cycles until ANC recovers to > 1,500 cells/mm^3 and platelet count > 100,000cells/mm^3.
- Severe hypersensitivity reactions (HSRs) have occurred, including very rare fatal anaphylaxis, despite premedication with 3 days of corticosteroids. Monitor patients closely during the first and second infusions for signs and symptoms, e.g., generalized rash/erythema, hypotension, and/or bronchospasm. Discontinue drug immediately for severe HSRs and provide aggressive medical intervention as ordered by physician or NP/PA. Do not rechallenge patients who have had a severe HSR.
- Fluid retention may be severe, and this is reduced in incidence and severity by the administration of corticosteroids prior to drug infusion. If the patient has preexisting effusions, closely monitor the patient for possible exacerbation of effusions. If fluid retention occurs, it begins in the lower extremities, may become generalized, and patients gain a median of 2 kg.
- Acute myeloid leukemia or MDS may rarely occur after treatment with the drug.
- Cutaneous reactions (severe skin toxicity): localized erythema of extremities with edema, followed by desquamation, has occurred. Severe skin toxicity did not occur in clinical trials in patients who received premedication with 3-day corticosteroids.
- Neurologic reactions: severe neurosensory symptoms (e.g., paresthesia, dysesthesia, pain) may occur and requires a dose adjustment (see package insert). If symptoms persist, the drug should be discontinued. Patients for whom follow-up data was available in clinical trials had spontaneous reversal of symptoms with a median of 9 weeks from onset. Severe peripheral motor neuropathy occurred in 4.4% of patients and was mainly distal extremity weakness.
- Eye disorders: cystoid macular edema (CME) has been reported. If a patient has impaired vision while on treatment, a comprehensive ophthalmologic exam should be done promptly. If CME is diagnosed, docetaxel should be discontinued, and visual impairment treated per the ophthamologist. Alternative nontaxane therapy should be considered.
- Asthenia may be severe (reported in 14.9% of metastatic breast cancer patients), lasting a few days to several weeks.
- Drug is fetotoxic. Women of childbearing potential should use effective contraception to avoid pregnancy. If the drug is used during pregnancy or if the patient becomes pregnant while receiving the drug, the patient should be apprised of the potential hazard to the fetus.

Potential Toxicities/Side Effects and the Nursing Process

I. POTENTIAL FOR INJURY related to HYPERSENSITIVITY OR ANAPHYLAXIS REACTIONS

Defining Characteristics: Severe hypersensitivity reactions characterized by hypotension, dyspnea and/or bronchospasm, or generalized rash/erythema occurred in 2.2% (2 of 92) of patients who received 3-day dexamethasone premedication. If patient experiences a severe hypersensitivity reaction, patient should not be rechallenged with docetaxel (e.g., patients with bronchospasm, angioedema, systolic BP < 80 mm Hg, generalized urticaria). Minor allergic reactions are characterized by flushing, chest tightness, or low back pain.

Nursing Implications: Ensure that patient has taken premedication (e.g., dexamethasone 8 mg bid starting 1 day prior to chemotherapy). Assess baseline VS and mental status prior to drug administration, especially first and second doses of the drug. Monitor VS every 15 minutes, and remain with patient during first 15 minutes of drug infusion, as most reactions occur during the first 10 minutes. Stop drug if cardiac arrhythmia (irregular apical pulse) or hypo- or hypertension occur and discuss continuance of infusion with physician. Recall signs/symptoms of anaphylaxis, and if these occur, stop drug immediately and notify physician. Subjective symptoms are generalized itching, nausea, chest tightness, crampy abdominal pain, difficulty speaking, anxiety, agitation, sense of impending doom, uneasiness, desire to urinate/defecate, dizziness, chills. Objective signs are flushed appearance, angioedema of face, neck, eyelids, hands, feet; localized or generalized urticaria; respiratory distress with or without wheezing, hypotension, cyanosis. Review standing orders or nursing procedure for patient management of anaphylaxis, and be prepared to stop drug immediately if signs/symptoms occur, keep IV line open with 0.9% sodium chloride, notify physician, monitor VS, and administer ordered medications, which may include epinephrine 1:1,000, hydrocortisone sodium succinate, and diphenhydramine. Teach patient the potential of a hypersensitivity or anaphylactic reaction and to report any unusual symptoms immediately. Depending upon severity of reaction, when planning subsequent treatment discuss with physician administration of antihistamine prior to docetaxel and also gradual increase in infusion rate, e.g., starting at 8-hour rate × 5 minutes, then increasing to 4-hour rate × 5 minutes, then 2-hour rate × 5 minutes, and finally 1-hour infusion rate.

II. POTENTIAL FOR INFECTION AND BLEEDING related to BONE MARROW DEPRESSION

Defining Characteristics: Neutropenia may be severe, is dose-related, is the dose-limiting toxicity, and is noncumulative. Nadir is day 7, with recovery by day 15. There have been some incidences of grade 4 neutropenia (ANC < 500 mm^3) in 2045 patients (any tumor type) with normal hepatic function. There have also been incidences of febrile neutropenia requiring IV antibiotics and/or hospitalization in some patients, and a small percentage of incidences of septic deaths. Severe thrombocytopenia was less common. However, fatal GI bleeding has been reported in patients with severe hepatic impairment who received docetaxel.

Nursing Implications: Assess LFTs, as dose generally should not be given if SGOT, SGPT, alk phos, or bili suggest moderate to severe hepatic dysfunction (see Special Considerations section). Assess baseline CBC and differential to ensure that ANC is > 1,500/mm³, and platelet count is > 100,000/mm³ prior to chemotherapy, as well as for signs/symptoms of infection or bleeding. Teach patient signs/symptoms of infection or bleeding and to report these immediately, and teach patient self-care measures to minimize risk of infection and bleeding. This includes avoidance of crowds and proximity to people with infections, and avoidance of OTC aspirin-containing medications. Teach patient self-administration of G-CSF as ordered to prevent severe neutropenia, and EPO as ordered to prevent severe anemia/transfusion requirements. Instruct patient to alternate rest and activity periods, and to report increased fatigue, shortness of breath, or chest pain that might herald severe anemia.

III.   POTENTIAL ALTERATION IN ACTIVITY TOLERANCE related to ASTHENIA, FATIGUE, MYALGIA, ANEMIA

Defining Characteristics: Fatigue, weakness, and malaise may last from a few days to several weeks, but is rarely severe enough to be dose-limiting. There is some incidence of asthenia (all grades) and some incidence of anemia, with grades of 3 and 4 occurring in some at doses of 100 mg/m² and in doses of 75 mg/m².

Nursing Implications: Assess Hgb/HCT prior to each treatment and at nadir counts. Assess patient activity tolerance and ability to do ADLs. Teach patient self-care strategies to minimize exertion, and maximize activity, such as clustering activity during shopping, alternating rest and activity periods, diet, gentle exercise. Teach self-administration of EPO, if ordered, to prevent severe anemia/transfusion requirements. Instruct patient to alternate rest and activity periods, and to report increased fatigue, shortness of breath, or chest pain that might herald severe anemia.

IV.   POTENTIAL ALTERATION IN FLUID BALANCE related to FLUID RETENTION

Defining Characteristics: Fluid retention is a cumulative toxicity that may occur in docetaxel-treated patients. Peripheral edema usually begins in the lower extremities and may become generalized with weight gain (2 kg average). Fluid retention is not associated with cardiac, renal, or hepatic impairment and may be minimized by use of dexamethasone 8 mg bid for 3 days beginning the day prior to therapy. Severe fluid retention may occur in up to 6.5% of patients despite premedication, and is characterized by generalized edema, poorly tolerated peripheral edema, pleural effusion requiring drainage, dyspnea at rest, cardiac tamponade, or abdominal distention (due to ascites). Fluid retention usually resolves completely within 16 weeks of last docetaxel dose (range, 0–42 weeks).

Nursing Implications: Ensure that patient takes corticosteroids as ordered to minimize risk of developing fluid retention. Assess baseline weight and skin turgor, especially in the extremities. Assess respiratory status, including breath sounds. Instruct patient to report any alterations in breathing patterns, swelling in the extremities, and weight gain. If patient has preexisting effusion, monitor effusion closely during treatment. If fluid retention occurs, instruct patient to elevate extremities while at rest. Teach patient not to use added salt when eating or cooking. Discuss with physician use of diuretics for new-onset edema, progression of edema, and weight gain, e.g., ≥ 2 lb.

V. POTENTIAL IMPAIRMENT OF SKIN INTEGRITY related to RASH, ALOPECIA, NAIL CHANGES

Defining Characteristics: Maculopapular, violaceous/erythematous, and pruritic rash may occur, usually on the feet and/or hands, but may also occur on arms, face, or thorax. These localized eruptions usually occur within 1 week of last docetaxel treatment, and are reversible and usually resolve prior to next treatment. Overall, there are some patients who do experience skin problems. Palmar-plantar erythrodysesthia (hand-foot syndrome) may occur but can be minimized by adherence to 3-day corticosteroid premedication. Drug extravasation may cause skin discoloration, but no necrosis. Most patients on every-3-week schedules experience alopecia. Changes in nails may occur in some of patients, and may be severe in a small percentage of patients (hypo- or hyperpigmentation, onycholysis [loss of nail]).

Nursing Implications: Assess skin for any cutaneous changes, such as rash, and any associated symptoms, such as pruritus, and discuss management with physician. If patient develops severe or cumulative skin toxicity, docetaxel dose should be reduced (see Special Considerations). Instruct patient in self-care measures such as avoidance of abrasive skin products and clothing, avoidance of tight-fitting clothes, use of skin emollients appropriate for skin problem, and measures to prevent itching. Discuss potential impact of hair loss prior to drug administration, coping strategies, and plan to minimize body image distortion (e.g., wig, scarf, cap). Assess patient for signs/symptoms of hair loss. Assess patient's response and use of coping strategies; help patient to build on effective strategies. Teach patient self-care measures to preserve hair, such as washing hair with warm water, use of a gentle shampoo and conditioner, use of a soft-bristle brush, cutting hair short to reduce pressure on hair shaft, and use of a satin pillowcase to minimize friction on hair shaft. Teach patient to wear a wide-brimmed hat and sunglasses when outside, and to use sunscreen (at least SPF 15) on scalp when outdoors without a hat. Assess nails baseline, and teach patient to report changes. Teach patient to keep nails clean and trimmed, not to wear nail polish or imitation nails, and to wear protective gloves when doing house cleaning and gardening. Teach patient to use a nail hardener if nails appear soft, and to use Lotrimin cream if ordered. Severe skin problems require a dose reduction.

VI. SENSORY/PERCEPTUAL ALTERATIONS related to SENSORY NEUROPATHY

Defining Characteristics: Grade 1–4 peripheral neuropathy may affect many patients, a small percentage severe. Sensory alterations are paresthesias in a glove-and-stocking distribution, and numbness. There may be loss of sensation symmetrically, of vibration, and of proprioception. Risk is increased in patients receiving both docetaxel and cisplatin, or in patients with prior neuropathy from diabetes mellitus or alcohol. Extremity weakness or transient myalgia may also occur. Patients described spontaneous reversal of symptoms in a median of 9 weeks from onset (range 0–106 weeks).

Nursing Implications: Assess baseline neurologic status. Instruct patient to report signs/ symptoms of pins-and-needle sensation, numbness, pain, increased discomfort with certain sensations, especially in the extremities, or motor weakness. Identify patients at risk: those with history of cisplatin use or with preexisting neuropathies (ethanol- and diabetes mellitus-related). Assess sensory and motor function prior to each treatment, and if abnormality found, assess impact on patient's function, safety, independence, and quality of life. Test patient's ability to button a shirt or pick up a dime from a flat surface. If severely impacting safety or quality of life, discuss with patient and physician drug discontinuance or use of cytoprotective agent. Teach self-care strategies, including maintaining safety when walking, getting up, taking bath, or washing dishes; discuss inability to sense temperature and the need to keep extremities warm in cold weather. Docetaxel should be discontinued if patient develops grades 3 or 4 peripheral neuropathy (see NCI Common Toxicity Criteria of Adverse Effects, *Appendix II*). Grade 3 motor = objective weakness, interfering with ADLs; grade 3 sensory = sensory loss or paresthesia interfering with ADLs; grade 4 motor = paralysis; grade 4 sensory = permanent sensory loss that interferes with function.

VII. ALTERED NUTRITION, LESS THAN BODY REQUIREMENTS, related to NAUSEA AND VOMITING, DIARRHEA, CONSTIPATION, DYSGEUSIA, ANOREXIA, STOMATITIS

Defining Characteristics: Nausea and vomiting may occur, but are mild and preventable with antiemetics. Diarrhea occurs and is mild; incidence of any grade of nausea is 33–42%, vomiting 22%, and diarrhea 22–42%. Incidence of stomatitis is 26–51% (severe 5.5%). Only 1.1% of breast cancer patients who received 3-day corticosteroid treatment developed severe mucositis.

Nursing Implications: Premedicate patient with antiemetic. If patient develops nausea and/or vomiting, encourage small, frequent intake of cool, bland foods. Instruct patient to report nausea, and teach self-administration of antiemetic medications. If nausea/vomiting occur and are severe, assess for signs/symptoms of fluid/electrolyte imbalance. Encourage patient to report onset of diarrhea. Teach patient to self-administer antidiarrheal medications if needed. Assess baseline oral mucous membranes. Ensure that patient takes 3-day corticosteroid regimen. Teach patient oral assessment, hygiene measures, and to report any alterations.

VIII. ALTERATION IN VISION, POTENTIAL, related to HYPERLACRIMATION

Defining Characteristics: Epiphora or hyperlacrimation occurs as a result of lacrimal duct stenosis. There is inflammation of the conjunctiva and ductal epithelium, which occurs chronically, especially with weekly docetaxel therapy. This appears related to cumulative dose, usually about 300 mg/m^2 and resolves after treatment is stopped. Stenosis of tear ducts is reversible.

Nursing Implications: Assess baseline vision and function of tear ducts. Teach patient that this may occur, and to report it. If this occurs, teach patient to use "artificial tears" frequently throughout day, or saline eyewash. Discuss with physician use of prophylactic steroid ophthalmic solution, such as prednisolone acetate 2 gtt bid × 3 days, beginning the day before docetaxel treatment, if patient does not have a history of herpetic eye infection. If the patient is on weekly therapy, discuss with physician treatment break × 2 weeks for symptoms to resolve, and resumption of therapy on a 3-week-on, 1-week-off schedule.

Drug: doxorubicin hydrochloride (Adriamycin)

Class: Anthracycline antibiotic isolated from streptomycin products, in particular from the rhodomycin products.

Mechanism of Action: Topoisomerase-II inhibitor; antitumor antibiotic binds directly to DNA base pairs (intercalates) and inhibits DNA and DNA-dependent RNA synthesis, as well as protein synthesis; also binds to lipid cellular membrane and disrupts cellular functions, as well as creating hydroxyl free radicals (causes cardiotoxicity in heart cells). Both actions result in programmed cell death (apoptosis). Cell cycle-specific for S phase.

Metabolism: Excretion of drug predominates in the liver; renal clearance is minor. Alteration in liver function requires modification of doses, whereas with renal failure there is no need to alter doses. Terminal half-life is 20–48 hours. Drug does not cross the blood–brain barrier. Drug is excreted through urine and may discolor urine from 1 to 48 hours after administration.

Indication: (initial): Use in acute lymphoblastic leukemia, acute myeloblastic leukemia, Wilms' tumor, neuroblastoma, soft tissue and bone sarcomas, Hodgkin's disease, malignant lymphoma, and cancers of the breast, ovary, transitional cell bladder, thyroid, stomach (gastric), bronchus including small cell lung cancer. Also, a component of adjuvant therapy in women with axillary lymph node involvement after resection of primary breast cancer.

Contraindications: Patients with baseline ANC < 1,500 cells/mm^3, severe hepatic impairment, recent MI, severe myocardial insufficiency, severe arrhythmias, previous treatment with complete cumulative doses of doxorubicin, daunorubicin, idarubicin, and/or other anthracyclines and anthracenediones, or hypersensitivity to doxorubicin or any of its excipients, or other anthracyclines or anthracenediones.

Dosage/Range:
- 60–75 mg/m^2 IV every 2 weeks (dose dense) or 20 mg/m^2 IV weekly.
- 30–75 mg/m^2 IV every 3–4 weeks; most common is 60–75 mg/m^2 IV every 21 days.
- 40–60 mg/m^2 when combined with other antineoplastics, every 21–28 days.

- AC adjuvant breast cancer: doxorubicin 60 mg/m² plus cyclophosphamide 600 mg/m² every 21 days for 4 cycles. (NSABP B-15)
- 20–30 mg/m² IV for 3 consecutive days.
- For bladder instillation: 3–60 mg/m².
- For intraperitoneal instillation: 40 mg in 2 L dialysate (no heparin).
- Continuous infusion: varies with individual protocol.
- Dose-reduce for hepatic dysfunction (50% DR BR 1.2–3 mg/dL; 75% DR BR > 3.0 mg/dL).

Drug Preparation:

- Available powder for injection (RDF, 10-, 20-, 50-, or 150-mg vials), lyophilized powder (Rubex, 50- or 100-mg vials), solution for injection (PFS, 2 mg/mL), and preservative-free solution (PFS, 2 mg/mL).
- Drug will form a precipitate if mixed with heparin or 5-FU. Dilute with 0.9% sodium chloride (preservative-free) to produce 2-mg/mL concentration.

Drug Administration:

- This drug is a potent vesicant. Give through a patent, running IV to avoid extravasation, which may lead to ulceration, pain, and necrosis. Be sure to check nursing procedure for administration of a vesicant. ANC must be ≥ 1,500 cells/m³.
- Assess baseline ECHO or MUGA scan results and know LVEF, and discuss with provider frequency of retesting while patient is receiving doxorubicin.

Drug Interactions:

- Barbiturates: increased plasma clearance of doxorubicin.
- Phenytoin: reduced phenytoin levels.
- Cyclophosphamide: risk of hemorrhage and increased cardiotoxicity.
- Mitomycin: increased risk of cardiotoxicity.
- Trastuzumab: increased risk of cardiotoxicity, avoid concomitant administration.
- Paclitaxel: increased risk of cardiotoxicity; give sequentially.
- Digoxin: decreased serum levels of digoxin; avoid concomitant administration.
- Mercaptopurine: increased risk of hepatotoxicity.
- Incompatible with heparin, forming a precipitate.
- Progesterone (high doses): increased neutropenia and thrombocytopenia.
- Verapamil: in mice, increased cardiotoxicity.
- Cyclosporine: increased toxicity, coma; do not use concurrently.

Lab Effects/Interference:

- Decreased CBC.
- Increased LFTs.
- Increased uric acid secondary to tumor lysis.

Special Considerations:

- Drug is a potent vesicant. Give through patent, running IV to avoid extravasation and tissue necrosis.
- Give through central line if drug is to be given by continuous infusion.
- Nausea and vomiting are dose-related, occur in 50% of patients, and begin 1–3 hours after administration.

- Causes discoloration of urine (from pink to red for up to 48 hours).
- Skin changes: May cause radiation recall phenomenon—recalls reaction in previously irradiated tissue.
- Potent myelosuppressive agent causes GI toxicities: mucositis, esophagitis, and diarrhea.
- Vein discoloration.
- Increased pigmentation in black patients.
- Drug dosage reductions necessary for hepatic dysfunction: 50% dose given for serum bili 1.2–2.9 mg/dL, 25% dose given for serum bili 3 mg/dL.
- Dexrazoxane available for patients at risk for cardiotoxicity but for whom doxorubicin continues to be effective. See *Chapter 3*.
- Secondary acute myelocytic leukemia (AML) or myelodysplastic syndrome (MDS); often refractory when results from combination chemotherapy or radiation therapy.

Cardiac Toxicity:
- Dose lifetime limit at 550 mg/m^2 and less if receiving another potentially cardiotoxic drug (e.g., cyclophosphamide) or chest RT. Patients may exhibit irreversible CHF.
- Prior chest radiation therapy (XRT): reduce total lifetime dose to 300–350 mg/m^2.
- Concomitant cyclophosphamide administration: may limit to 450 mg/m^2.
- Acute toxicity may be seen within hours after administration. This is unrelated to cumulative dose and may manifest symptoms of pump or conduction dysfunction. Rarely, transient ECG abnormalities, CHF, pericardial effusion (whole syndrome referred to as *myocarditis- pericarditis syndrome*) may occur, which may lead to death of patient.
- Delayed cardiotoxicity when used in children.

Potential Toxicities/Side Effects and the Nursing Process

I.   POTENTIAL FOR INFECTION AND BLEEDING related to BONE MARROW DEPRESSION

Defining Characteristics: WBC and platelet nadir 10–14 days after drug dose, with recovery from days 15–21. Myelosuppression may be severe but is less severe with weekly dosing.

Nursing Implications: Monitor CBC, WBC, differential, and platelet count prior to drug administration; discuss any abnormalities with physician. Assess for signs/symptoms of infection or bleeding; instruct patient in self-assessment and to report signs/symptoms immediately. Teach patient self-care measures to minimize risk of infection and bleeding, including avoidance of OTC aspirin-containing medications. Drug dosage must be reduced if patient has hepatic dysfunction: 50% reduction of drug dose if bili is 1.2–3.0 mg/dL; 75% reduction if bili is > 3.0 mg/dL.

II.   POTENTIAL FOR ALTERATION IN CARDIAC OUTPUT related to ACUTE AND CHRONIC CARDIAC CHANGES

Defining Characteristics: Acutely, pericarditis-myocarditis syndrome may occur during infusion or immediately after (non–life-threatening EKG changes of flat T waves, ST-segment changes, PVCs). With high cumulative doses > 550 mg/m^2 (450 mg/m^2 if concurrent treatment with cardiotoxic drugs or radiation to the chest), cardiomyopathy may occur. Risk is decreased if drug given as continuous infusion.

Nursing Implications: Assess cardiac status prior to chemotherapy administration: signs/symptoms of CHF, quality/regularity and rate of heartbeat, results of prior GBPS or other test of LVEF (stop drug if 10% decrease below LLN, LVEF of 45%, or decrease in LVEF of 20% at any level). Instruct patient to report dyspnea, palpitations, swelling in extremities. Maintain accurate records of total dose; expect GBPS to be repeated periodically during treatment and the drug to be discontinued if there is a significant drop in heart function.

III. POTENTIAL FOR ALTERATION IN NUTRITION, LESS THAN BODY REQUIREMENTS, related to NAUSEA AND VOMITING, ANOREXIA, STOMATITIS

Defining Characteristics: Nausea/vomiting occurs in 50% of patients, is moderate to severe, and is preventable with combination antiemetics. Onset 1–3 hours after drug dose and lasts 24 hours. Anorexia occurs frequently, and stomatitis occurs in 10% of patients.

Nursing Implications: Premedicate with combination antiemetics and continue protection for 24 hours. If patient has a central line, slower infusion of drug over 1 hour decreases nausea/vomiting. Encourage small, frequent feedings of bland foods. Anorexia occurs frequently: teach patient or caregiver to make foods ahead of time and use spices; encourage taking weight weekly. Stomatitis occurs in 10% of patients, and esophagitis may occur in patients who have received prior radiation to the chest. Perform oral assessment prior to drug administration and during posttreatment visits. Teach patient oral hygiene and self-assessment techniques.

IV. POTENTIAL ALTERATION IN SKIN INTEGRITY related to ALOPECIA, RADIATION RECALL, NAIL AND SKIN CHANGES, AND DRUG EXTRAVASATION

Defining Characteristics: Complete alopecia occurs with doses > 50 mg/m², occurring after therapy begins. Regrowth usually begins a few months after drug is stopped. Hyperpigmentation of nail beds and dermal creases of hands is greatest in dark-skinned individuals. Skin damage from prior radiation may be reactivated. Adriamycin "flare" may occur during peripheral drug administration, often with urticaria and pruritus, and is due to local allergic reaction. Drug is a potent vesicant and causes SEVERE tissue destruction if drug extravasates.

Nursing Implications: Discuss with patient hair loss, anticipated impact, and strategies to decrease distress, e.g., obtaining wig prior to hair loss. Assess body disturbance from hyperpigmentation and discuss strategies to minimize this, e.g., nail polish for dark nail beds. Drug must be administered via patent IV. If flare occurs, this must be distinguished from extravasation, where there is leakage of drug into the perivascular tissue. Stop or slow drug injection and flush with plain IV solution. Wait to see whether reaction will resolve. If confirmed flare, consider diphenhydramine 25 mg IVP to resolve pruritus and/or urticaria, and then resume administration of drug slowly into freely flowing IV. Assess need for venous access device early. If drug is administered as a continuous infusion, IT MUST BE GIVEN VIA A CENTRAL LINE.

V. POTENTIAL SEXUAL DYSFUNCTION related to DRUG EFFECT

Defining Characteristics: Drug is teratogenic, mutagenic, and carcinogenic.

Nursing Implications: Assess patient's/partner's sexual patterns and reproductive goals. Provide information, supportive counseling, and referral as needed. Teach importance of birth control measures as appropriate. Male patients may wish to use a sperm bank prior to therapy.

Drug: doxorubicin hydrochloride liposome injection (Doxil)

Class: Anthracycline antibiotic isolated from streptomycin products wrapped in a STEALTH liposome.

Mechanism of Action: Topoisomerase-inhibitor; antitumor antibiotic binds directly to DNA base pairs (intercalates) and inhibits DNA and DNA-dependent RNA synthesis, as well as protein synthesis. Cytotoxic in all phases of cell cycle but maximally in S phase. Cell cycle nonspecific. Drug is encapsulated in STEALTH liposomes, which have surface-bound methoxypolyethylene glycol to protect the liposome from detection by blood phagocytes, and thus prolong circulation time. It is believed that the liposomal-encapsulated drug is able to penetrate the tumor through abnormal capillaries (tumor neovasculature) and then, once inside the tumor, accumulates and the drug is released.

Metabolism: Slower clearance from the body than doxorubicin (0.041 L/h/m^2 vs 24–35 L/h/m^2) with resulting larger AUC than a similar dose of doxorubicin. Half-life is approximately 55 hours. Has preferential uptake in Kaposi's sarcoma tumors.

Indication: Treatment of patients with (1) ovarian cancer after failure of platinum-based chemotherapy, (2) AIDS-related Kaposi's sarcoma (KS) after failure of prior systemic chemotherapy or intolerance to such therapy, (3) multiple myeloma in combination with bortezomib in patients who have not previously received bortezomib and have received at least one prior therapy.

Dosage/Range:

- Metastatic carcinoma of the ovary: 50 mg/m^2 IV every 4 weeks for a minimum of 4 cycles, or until disease progression or toxicity.
- Multiple myeloma in combination with bortezomib: 30 mg/m^2 IV over 1 hour on day 4 (after bortezomib dose) of a 21-day treatment cycle. Bortezomib 1.3 mg/m^2 IV on days 1, 4, 8, and 11 of a 21-day cycle.
- AIDS KS: 20 mg/m^2 IV over 30 minutes once every 3 weeks.
- Dose-reduce for palmar-plantar erythrodysesthesia, hematologic toxicity, or stomatitis.

Drug Preparation:
* Drug is available as vials containing 20 mg/10 mL and 50 mg/25 mL doxorubicin HCl in a 2-mg/mL concentration.
* Inspect drug for any particulate matter or discoloration; drug is translucent, with red liposomal dispersion.
* Further dilute drug (dose up to 90 mg) in 250 mL 5% dextrose USP ONLY; use 500 mL 5% dextrose USP for doses > 90 mg.
* Administer at once or store diluted drug for 24 hours refrigerated at 2–8°C (36–46°F).

Drug Administration:
* Administer IV at an initial rate of 1 mg/min to minimize risk of infusion reaction; if no reaction, increase rate to complete administration over 1 hour.
* Treat if ANC ≥ 1,500 cells/mm³ and platelets > 75,000/mm³.
* Dose-reduce for hepatic dysfunction: 50% dose reduction for bilirubin 1.2–3.0 mg/dL; 75% dose reduction if bilirubin > 3.0 mg/dL.
* Delay next dose and dose-reduce for grade 3–4 hand-foot syndrome, hematologic toxicity.
* Do not use inline filter.
* Monitor for infusion reactions during infusion, and stop drug if reaction; discuss management with physician or NP/PA, as drug may be resumed at a slower infusion rate if symptoms are minor.
* DO NOT ADMINISTER as bolus injection, or undiluted solution. DO NOT administer IM OR SUBCUTANEOUSLY. DO NOT SUBSTITUTE for doxorubicin (nonliposomal).

Drug Interactions:
* Doxorubicin may potentiate the toxicity of (1) cyclophosphamide-induced hemorrhagic cystitis; (2) hepatotoxicity of 6-mercaptopurine; (3) radiation toxicity to heart, mucous membranes, skin, liver.

Lab Effects/Interference:
* Decreased CBC.

Special Considerations:
* Drug is an irritant, not a vesicant.
* Acute, infusion-associated reactions may occur (10% incidence) during drug infusion, characterized by flushing, shortness of breath, facial swelling, headache, chills, back pain, chest or throat tightness, and/or hypotension.
* Infusion should be stopped. If symptoms are minor, infusion may be resumed at a slower rate, but discontinue if symptoms reoccur.
* Serious and sometimes fatal allergic/anaphylactoid-like infusion reactions have been reported.
* Emergency medications and equipment should be readily available in infusion area when drug is administered, and physician or NP/PA available to give orders for management during/after infusion.
* Assessment for cardiac toxicity similar to that for doxorubicin should be done, since limited information is available as to cardiotoxicity of liposomal doxorubicin at high cumulative doses.

- Myocardial damage may lead to CHF and may occur as the total cumualtive dose of doxorubicin approaches 550 mg/m^2.
- Cardiac toxicity may also occur at lower cumulative doses with mediastinal irradiation or concurrent cardiotoxic agents.
- Contraindicated in patients who are hypersensitive to doxorubicin, or the components of liposomal doxorubicin.
- Most common adverse reactions (20% or higher): asthenia, fatigue, fever, anorexia, nausea, vomiting, stomatitis, diarrhea, constipation, hand-foot syndrome, rash, neutropenia, thrombocytopenia, anemia.
- Drug can cause fetal harm when used during pregnancy. Teach women of childbearing potential to use effective contraception.
- Nursing mothers should decide whether to discontinue nursing or discontinue the drug, taking into consideration the importance of the drug to the mother's health.

Potential Toxicities/Side Effects and the Nursing Process

I. POTENTIAL FOR INFECTION AND BLEEDING related to BONE MARROW DEPRESSION

Defining Characteristics: Leukopenia occurs in 91% of patients, with anemia and thrombocytopenia (< 150,000/mm^3) less common (55% and 60%, respectively). Neutropenia (< 2,000/mm^3) occurred in 85% and ANC (< 500/mm^3) occurred in 13% of patients. In ovarian cancer patients, incidence of neutropenia (< 2,000 cells/mm^3) was 51%, but ANC < 500 cells/mm^3 was only 8.3%. Thrombocytopenia (< 150,000/mm^3) occurred in 24%, while severe (< 25,000/mm^3) occurred in 1.1% of patients with ovarian cancer. Myelosuppression is the dose-limiting toxicity in the treatment of HIV-infected patients, possibly because of HIV disease and/or concomitant medications. Anemia may also occur.

Nursing Implications: Monitor CBC, WBC, differential, and platelet count prior to drug administration, and discuss any abnormalities with physician. Assess for signs/symptoms of infection or bleeding, and instruct patient in self-assessment and to report signs/symptoms immediately. Teach patient self-care measures to minimize risk of infection and bleeding, including avoidance of OTC aspirin-containing medications. See drug dosage reductions in Special Considerations section.

II. POTENTIAL FOR ALTERATION IN CARDIAC OUTPUT related to ACUTE AND CHRONIC CARDIAC CHANGES

Defining Characteristics: Experience and data are limited in the cardiotoxicity of liposomal doxorubicin at high cumulative doses. Therefore, the manufacturer recommends the adoption of cardiotoxicity warnings made for doxorubicin HCl. With high cumulative doses > 550 mg/m^2 (400 mg/m^2 if concurrent treatment with cardiotoxic drugs such as cyclophosphamide, or radiation to the chest), cardiomyopathy may occur. In clinical trials, the incidence of "possibly or probably related" cardiac-related adverse events, including cardiomyopathy, arrhythmia, heart failure, pericardial effusion, and tachycardia, was

1–5% in patients with AIDS/Kaposi's sarcoma and < 1% in ovarian cancer patients. In patients with multiple myeloma, the incidence of heart failure events is similar in treatment arms (3%), with decreases in LVEF 13% in combination arm compared with 8% in the bortezomib arm alone.

Nursing Implications: Assess patient risk (history of prior anthracycline chemotherapy, history of cardiovascular disease). Assess cardiac status prior to chemotherapy administration: signs/symptoms of CHF, quality/regularity and rate of heartbeat, results of prior GBPS or other test of LVEF. Instruct patient to report dyspnea, palpitations, swelling in extremities. Maintain accurate records of total dose. Expect GBPS to be repeated periodically during treatment and the drug to be discontinued if there is a significant drop in heart function.

III.   POTENTIAL FOR INJURY related to ALLERGIC INFUSION REACTION TO LIPOSOMAL COMPONENT(S)

Defining Characteristics: During the initial infusion, patients may experience an acute reaction characterized by flushing, shortness of breath, facial swelling, headache, chills, back pain, chest or throat tightness, and/or hypotension. Incidence is 5–6%. Reactions generally resolve after the immediate termination of the infusion in several hours to a day, or in some patients, after slowing of the infusion rate. Of those patients who experienced reactions, many were able to tolerate subsequent treatment without problem; however, some patients terminated therapy with liposomal doxorubicin because of the reaction.

Nursing Implications: Assess baseline comfort, vital signs, general condition. Infuse liposomal doxorubicin at 1 mg/min to minimize risk of acute reaction. Teach patient to report signs/symptoms of reaction immediately during infusion, and assess patient frequently during initial infusion. If signs/symptoms occur, stop infusion immediately. Discuss with the physician, but anticipate that if signs/symptoms are mild, infusion will resume at slower rate, and if signs/symptoms are severe, patient may not receive additional liposomal doxorubicin.

IV.   POTENTIAL ALTERATIONS IN COMFORT AND ACTIVITY related to PALMAR-PLANTAR ERYTHRODYSESTHESIA (HAND-FOOT SYNDROME)

Defining Characteristics: Incidence is approximately 3.4% in patients receiving a dose of 20 mg/m² and 37% in patients with ovarian cancer (16% grades 3 and 4). Toxicity becomes dose-limiting in clinical studies at doses of 60 mg/m², or when treatment is administered more frequently than every 3 weeks. Signs/symptoms are swelling, pain, erythema, possibly progressing to desquamation of the skin on hands and feet, and usually occur after 6 weeks of treatment. Reaction is generally mild, not requiring treatment delays. However, in some patients, reaction can be severe and debilitating, necessitating discontinuance of treatment.

Nursing Implications: Assess baseline skin of patients' hands and feet, and in women with ovarian cancer, skin under areas of pressure, such as under the breasts of women with large breasts or skin folds, before each treatment. Teach patient to report signs/symptoms of reaction (e.g., tingling or burning, redness, flaking of skin in areas of pressure such as soles of feet, under breasts in large-breasted women, small blisters, or small sores on the palms of hands or soles of feet). If signs/symptoms occur, discuss treatment, treatment delays, or discontinuance. Do not use hydrocortisone cream, as this will cause greater desquamation of skin.

V. POTENTIAL FOR ALTERATION IN NUTRITION, LESS THAN BODY REQUIREMENTS, related to NAUSEA AND VOMITING, STOMATITIS, DIARRHEA, ANOREXIA

Defining Characteristics: Nausea and/or vomiting occur in 17% and 8% of patients, respectively, are mild to moderate, and are preventable with antiemetics. Stomatitis occurs in 7% of patients. Incidence of diarrhea is 8%. Anorexia may affect 1–5% of patients.

Nursing Implications: Premedicate with antiemetic (dopamine antagonist or serotonin antagonist). Encourage small, frequent feeding of bland foods. Stomatitis occurs in 7% of patients. Perform oral assessment prior to drug administration, and during posttreatment visits. Dose reductions or delay necessary for grades 2–4 stomatitis. Teach patient oral hygiene and self-assessment techniques. Instruct patient to report diarrhea, and teach self-management strategies for diarrhea

VI. POTENTIAL FOR ALTERATION IN SKIN INTEGRITY related to ALOPECIA, RASH, PRURITUS, AND RADIATION RECALL

Defining Characteristics: Incidence of alopecia significantly less with liposomal delivery of doxorubicin, and is about 9% in AIDS/Kaposi's sarcoma patients and 15% in women with ovarian cancer. Skin damage from prior radiation may be reactivated. Rash and itching occur in 1–5% of the patients. Rarely, significant skin reactions may occur, such as exfoliative dermatitis. Drug is an irritant, but extravasation should be avoided.

Nursing Implications: Discuss with patient low incidence of hair loss, and to report hair thinning if it occurs. At that time, discuss impact and strategies to decrease distress. Instruct patient to report skin rash or itching, and discuss significance and management with physician. Teach patient to assess for skin changes in prior irradiated sites, including mucous membranes, and to report this immediately. Assess and develop management strategies depending on site and extent. Use caution to avoid drug extravasation; if infiltration occurs, stop infusion, apply ice for 30 minutes, and restart a new IV elsewhere.

VII. POTENTIAL ALTERATION IN NUTRITION related to NAUSEA AND/OR VOMITING, STOMATITIS

Defining Characteristics: Nausea occurs in 37% (severe, grade 3–4 in 8%) of ovarian cancer patients and 17% of AIDS/Kaposi's sarcoma patients. Vomiting occurs in 22% of ovarian cancer patients and 7.8% of patients with AIDS/Kaposi's sarcoma. Stomatitis occurs in 37% of women with ovarian cancer and is severe in 7.7%; overall incidence in AIDS/Kaposi's sarcoma patients is 6.8%.

Nursing Implications: Assess baseline nutritional status. Teach patient that these side effects may occur and teach self-care measures, including self-assessment, oral hygiene regimen, and to report occurrence of symptoms. Administer antiemetic prior to chemotherapy, especially in ovarian cancer patients, and assess efficacy after treatment. Revise antiemetic regimen as needed to provide complete protection from nausea and/or vomiting. Assess oral mucosa prior to each treatment. If stomatitis develops, dose reduction should be considered.

VIII.   POTENTIAL SEXUAL DYSFUNCTION related to DRUG EFFECTS

Defining Characteristics: Drug is embryotoxic. Doxorubicin has been shown to be carcinogenic and mutagenic.

Nursing Implications: Assess patient's/partner's sexual pattern and reproductive goals. Provide information, supportive counseling, and referral as needed. Teach importance of birth control measures for female patients of childbearing age. Mothers who are nursing should discontinue nursing during treatment.

IX.   ACTIVITY INTOLERANCE related to ASTHENIA AND FATIGUE

Defining Characteristics: Anemia is the most common hematologic event, affecting 52.6% of women with ovarian cancer, but only 25% experienced severe anemia (Hgb < 8 g/dL). Incidence for patients with AIDS/Kaposi's syndrome overall is 55%, with 4% experiencing severe anemia. Asthenia is more common in women with ovarian cancer, affecting 33%, while patients with AIDS/Kaposi's syndrome had an incidence of 9.9%.

Nursing Implications: Assess activity tolerance and HCT/Hgb baseline and prior to each treatment. Teach patients to report any changes in energy and activity level. Teach patients self-care strategies to maximize energy use and conservation. Evaluate efficacy of strategies at each visit, and if ineffective, assist patient to problem solve other alternative solutions, such as friends, volunteers, to help with activities such as shopping, food preparation.

Drug: enzalutamide (Xtandi)

Class: Androgen receptor inhibitor.

Mechanism of Action: Drug competitively inhibits androgen binding to androgen receptors, thus stopping the androgen receptor nuclear translocation and interaction with DNA. The drug acts on different steps in the androgen receptor signaling pathway, and *in vitro,* decreases prostate cancer cell proliferation and induces cell death. This results in decreased tumor volume. The major metabolite N-desmethyl enzalutamide has similar activity *in vitro*, to enzalutamide. Enzalutamide has higher affinity to the androgen receptor than bicalutamide.

Metabolism: The drug is well absorbed following either a fasting or high-fat meal. Enzalutamide is 97% to 98% bound to plasma proteins (primarily albumin), while the metabolite N-desmethyl enzalutamide is 95% protein bound. Following oral administration, median time to reach maximal plasma concentration (C_{max}) is 1 hour (range 0.5 to 3 hours), and with daily dosing, enzalutamide steady state is reached by day 28, with the drug accumulation approximately 8.3-fold compared to a single daily dose. Enzalutamide is metabolized in the liver by the P450 microenzyme system (CYP2C8 and CYP3A4); CYP2C8 is primarily responsible for the formation of the active metabolite N-desmethyl enzalutamide. Following a single dose of radiolabeled enzalutamide, 85% of the radioactivity is recovered by 77 days post dose, with 71% excreted in the urine, and 14% in the feces. The mean terminal half-life of enzalutamide given as a single dose of 160 mg is 5.8 days (range 2.8 to 10.2 days), while that of the active metabolite is 7.8 to 8.6 days. Renal and hepatic clearance of the drug and active metabolite in healthy patients and in patients with mild to moderate renal or hepatic impairment are similar; patients with severe renal (CrCl < 30 mL/min) or hepatic (Child-Pugh Class C) impairment were not studied. Bone density remains stable.

Indication: Treatment of patients with metastatic castration-resistant prostate cancer who have previously received docetaxel.

Contraindication: Pregnancy. Drug is not indicated for use in women, and is contraindicated in women who are or may become pregnant. Teach patients to use a condom if having sex with a pregnant woman, and to use a condom and another effective method of birth control if the patient is having sex with a woman of child bearing potential. These precautions should be used during and for 3 months after treatment with enzalutamide.

Dosage/Range:
• 160 mg (four-40 mg capsules) orally once daily at the same time each day, with or without food.

Dose Modifications:
• If a patient experiences a grade 3 or higher toxicity or intolerable side effect: hold dose for 1 week or until symptoms improve to < grade 2, then resume at the same or reduced dose (120 mg or 80 mg), if warranted.
• Concomitant administration of a strong CYP2C8 inhibitor (e.g., gemfibrozil): avoid if possible, but if unavoidable, reduce initial dose of enzalutamide to 80 mg once daily. If the strong inhibitor is discontinued, resume enzalutamide at the dose used prior to initiation of the strong CYP2C8 inhibitor.

Drug Preparation: None (available as 40-mg capsules, in a bottle of 120 capsules).

Drug Administration: Oral, with or without food. Patient should be instructed to take the dose at about the same time each day, and to swallow capsules whole; do not chew, dissolve, or open the capsule. If the patient forgets a dose, it should be taken when remembered unless it is at the end of the day, in which case, the normal dose should be taken the next day. The patient should not take more than the normal dose per day.

Drug Interactions:

- Drugs that induce CYP2C8 (e.g., rifampin): may decrease serum enzalutamide level; avoid coadministration.
- Drugs that inhibit CYP2C8 (e.g., gemfibrozil is a strong inhibitor): increase area under the plasma curve of enzalutamide and its active metabolite, thus increasing risk of toxicity; avoid coadministration if possible, and if unavoidable, reduce dose of enzalutamide.
- Drugs that inhibit CYP3A4 (e.g., itraconazole) increase area under the curve of enzalutamide and its active metabolite by 1.3-fold in healthy volunteers, potentially increasing toxicity. Teach patient to avoid grapefruit and grapefruit juice.
- Drugs that induce CYP3A4 (e.g., strong inducers: carbamazepine, phenobarbital, phenytoin, rifabutin, rifampin, rifapentine; moderate inducers: bosentan, efavirenz, etravirine, modafinil, nafcillin, St. John's wort) may decrease plasma level of enzalutamide, and should be avoided by selecting another drug that does not induce CYP3A4; teach patients to avoid St. John's wort.
- Effect on drug metabolizing enzymes: enzalutamide is a strong CYP3A4 inducer and a moderate CYP2C9 and CYP2C19 inducer; enzalutamide reduces plasma levels of midazolam (CYP3A4 substrate), warfarin (CYP2C9 substrate), and omeprazole (CYP2C19 substrate). Avoid concomitant administration with drugs having a narrow therapeutic window, as enzalutamide may decrease drug serum level: drugs metabolized by CYP3A4 (e.g., alfentanil, cyclosporine, dihydroergotamine, ergotamine, fentanyl, pimozide, quinidine, sirolimus, and tacrolimus), CYP2C9 (e.g., phenytoin, warfarin), and CYP2C19 (e.g., S-mephenytoin). If coadministration with warfarin is unavoidable, increase INR monitoring.

Lab Effects/Interference:

- Neutropenia (15% grades 1–4; 1% grades 3–4).
- Hematuria (6.9%).

Special Considerations:

- In clinical trials, seizure occurred rarely (0.9%) in patients receiving enzalutamide 160 mg once daily, occurring from 31 to 603 days after drug initiation. All seizures resolved, and as patients were removed from the clinical trial, there is no experience re-administering the drug to these patients. Eligibility for the trials excluded patients with a history of seizure, underlying brain injury with loss of consciousness, transient ischemic attack within the last 12 months, CVA, brain metastases, brain arteriovenous malformation or the use of concomitant medications that may lower seizure threshold. Thus, the safety of enzalutamide in patients with predisposing factors for seizure is unknown.
- Monitor patients with increased risk for seizures closely, including those taking medication that may lower seizure threshold.

- Teach patients to avoid activities where a sudden loss of consciousness could cause serious harm to themselves or others, and to report loss of consciousness or seizure right away.
- Most common adverse reactions (>5%) are asthenia/fatigue (50.6%), back pain (26.4%), diarrhea (21.8%), arthralgia (20.5%), hot flush (20.3%), peripheral edema (15.4%), musculoskeletal pain (15%), headache (12.1%), upper respiratory tract infection (URI) (10.9%), muscular weakness (9.8%), dizziness (9.5%), insomnia (8.8%), lower respiratory tract and lung infection (8.5%), spinal cord compression and cauda equina syndrome (7.4%), hematuria (6.9%), paresthesia (6.6%), anxiety (6.5%), and hypertension (6.4%).

Potential Toxicities/Side Effects and the Nursing Process

I. POTENTIAL FOR SENSORY/PERCEPTUAL ALTERATIONS related to DIZZINESS, SPINAL CORD COMPRESSION AND CAUDA EQUINA SYNDROME, PARESTHESIA

Defining Characteristics: Although most symptoms are not common, these symptoms increase the risk for falls. The incidence of falls was 4.6% in the enzalutamide group, compared with 1.3% in the placebo group. Dizziness occurred in 9.5%, spinal cord compression/cauda equina syndrome in 7.4% (compared with 4.5% in the placebo group), paresthesia in 6.6%, mental impairment disorders (amnesia, memory impairment, cognitive disorder, attention disturbance) in 4.3%, and hypoesthesia in 4%. Seizure occurred in 0.9%. Hallucinations (visual, tactile, or undefined) occurred in 1.6% (grades 1 or 2), compared with 0.3% in the placebo group, and most occurred in patients receiving opioid analgesics. Insomnia occurred in 8.8% of patients. Asthenia/fatigue occurred in 50.6%, which also increases the risk of falls.

Nursing Implications: Assess neurologic and mental status, baseline and at visits during drug administration. Assess risk for seizures (e.g., history of seizure, medications that may lower seizure threshold, brain metastases), and advise patient to avoid any activity where sudden loss of consciousness could cause serious harm to self or others. Assess for spinal cord compression or cauda equina syndrome, as these are oncologic emergencies. Assess for back pain (e.g., constant, dull, aching, radiating, may wax and wane (crescendo pain), exacerbated by movement, unrelieved by lying down), motor weakness, and sensory impairment. Teach patient to report radicular back pain right away, change in bowel or bladder patterns, or change in sensation in lower extremities. Discuss assessment with physician, nurse practitioner (NP), or physician assistant (PA) immediately, as IV dexamethasone should be administered emergently once diagnosis is confirmed. Teach patients that although these side effects may occur uncommonly, any alterations in behavior, sensation, or perception should be reported to the physician or nurse right away. Develop a plan of care with patient and family if side effects develop to manage distress, and promote safety. Drug should be stopped if a seizure occurs, and then once resolved, the patient should discuss the risks and benefits of resuming the drug with the physician. Assess patient for insomnia, and if present, discuss strategies to promote sleep, and if ineffective, discuss with physician, NP, or PA medication to promote sleep.

II.   ALTERATION IN COMFORT related to BACK PAIN, ARTHRALGIA, MUSCULOSKELETAL PAIN AND WEAKNESS, HEADACHE, HOT FLUSHES, PERIPHERAL EDEMA

Defining Characteristics: Back pain occurred in 26.4% of patients, arthralgias in 20.5%, musculoskeletal pain 15% and weakness 9.8%; headache in 12.1%, and peripheral edema in 15.4% of patients. Vasodilation or hot flushes occurred in 20.3% of patients.

Nursing Implications: Assess baseline comfort, and self-care measures used. Teach patient these symptoms may occur and to report them. If back pain occurs, assess for possible spinal cord compression or cauda equina syndrome (see I). Discuss self-care strategies to improve comfort if symptoms occur, such as use of heat and cold for musculoskeletal discomfort, acetaminophen for headache, leg elevation for peripheral edema. If hot flashes are severe, review common hot flash management, including wearing loose, layered clothing that can be removed when the patient becomes hot, sipping cold beverages throughout the day, sleeping with light nightclothes and a window open, avoiding triggers such as caffeine or alcohol. If the patient has peripheral edema, assess for skin integrity. Teach patient self-assessment of peripheral edema, to wear loose stockings and shoes, to keep skin moisturized to prevent cracking, and comfort measures. Teach patient to report increasing edema or related problems.

III.   POTENTIAL FOR INFECTION related to NEUTROPENIA

Defining Characteristics: Grades 1–4 neutropenia occurred in 15% of patients during clinical trials, with 1% grades 3–4, compared to 6% all grades in the placebo group. URI occurred in 10.9% and lower respiratory infection in 8.5% of patients receiving enzalutamide compared to 6.5% and 4.8% respectively in the placebo group.

Nursing Implications: Assess baseline CBC, WBC, and ANC baseline and at visits during therapy, as well as for signs/symptoms of infection. Teach patient signs/symptoms of infection and instruct to report these immediately. Teach patient self-care measures to minimize risk of infection, such as avoidance of crowds, and frequent hand washing.

IV.   ALTERATION IN ELIMINATION, POTENTIAL, related to DIARRHEA

Defining Characteristics: Diarrhea occurred in 21.8% of patients.

Nursing Implications: Assess baseline bowel elimination pattern and use of laxatives or stool softeners. Teach patient that diarrhea may occur, and self-care measures to minimize diarrhea, such as to modify diet, to avoid laxatives and stool softeners, to use over-the-counter antidiarrheal medicine, and to report diarrhea that persists. If these are ineffective, discuss further pharmacological management with physician.

V. ALTERATION IN BOWEL ELIMINATION PATTERN related to DIARRHEA

Defining Characteristics: Diarrhea occurred in 21.8% of patients and was grade 3–4 in 1.1%.

Nursing Implications: Assess baseline bowel elimination status, and teach patient that diarrhea may occur and to report it. Teach patient to manage diarrhea with loperamide if needed, and to modify diet as needed (increased fluids, BRAT diet). Teach patient that if diarrhea persists, to report it as well. Discuss management (e.g., pharmacological, assessing electrolytes, IV hydration) as needed with physician/NP/PA.

VI. ALTERATION IN ACTIVITY related to ASTHENIA, FATIGUE

Defining Characteristics: Asthenia and fatigue were the most common side effects, affecting 50.6% of patients in clinical trials.

Nursing Implications: Assess baseline activity tolerance, weakness, and level of fatigue. Teach patient that these side effects may occur and to report them. Teach patient to alter nate rest and activity periods. Teach fatigue self-care measures, such as strategies to maximize energy use and conservation while shopping, interacting with friends, and other activities.

Drug: epirubicin hydrochloride (Ellence, Farmorubicin[e], Farmorubicina, Pharmorubicin)

Class: Anthracycline antitumor antibiotic analogue (topoisomerase II inhibitor).

Mechanism of Action: Drug complexes with DNA by intercalation of planar rings between DNA base pairs; this inhibits nucleic acid (DNA and RNA) and protein synthesis. This also causes cleavage of DNA by topoisomerase II, causing cell death. Drug also prevents enzymatic separation of DNA, interfering with replication and transcription. Drug also causes the production of cytotoxic free radicals.

Metabolism: Following IV administration, drug rapidly disperses into body tissues and into red blood cells; drug is 77% bound to plasma proteins. Drug is rapidly and extensively metabolized in the liver, excreted primarily through the biliary system, and to a lesser extent in the urine. Drug clearance is reduced in elderly women (35% lower in women aged > 70 years old). Drug clearance is reduced 30% in mild hepatic dysfunction, and 50% in moderate hepatic dysfunction. Drug clearance is reduced (50%) in patients with severe renal impairment (serum creatinine > 5 mg/dL). Dose reductions should be made for patients with hepatic dysfunction and patients with severe renal dysfunction.

Indication: As a component of adjuvant therapy in breast cancer patients with evidence of axillary node involvement following resection of primary breast cancer.

Contraindications: Patients with ANC < 1,500 cells/mm³, severe myocardial insufficiency, recent MI, severe arrhythmias, previous treatment with an anthracycline up to the maximum cumulative dose, hypersensitivity to epirubicin, other anthracyclines, or anthracenediones, or severe hepatic dysfunction.

Dosage/Range:
Starting dose as part of adjuvant therapy in patients with axillary node-positive breast cancer: 100 mg/m² to 120 mg/m² IV every 3–4 weeks.
- CEF-120: cyclophosphamide 75 mg/m² PO days 1–14, epirubicin 60 mg/m² IV days 1, 8; 5-FU 500 mg/m² IV days 1–8; repeat every 28 days for 6 cycles.
- FEC-100: 5-FU 500 mg/m² IV day 1, epirubicin 100 mg/m² IV day 1; cyclophosphamide mg/m² IV day 1; repeated every 21 days for 6 cycles.

Dose Modifications:
- Bone marrow dysfunction: Consider dose of 75–90 mg/m² if patient heavily pretreated (e.g., with existing BMD or bone marrow infiltration by tumor).
- Hepatic dysfunction: Bilirubin 1.2–3 mg/dL or AST 2–4 × upper limit of normal (ULN) give 50% of recommended starting dose; bilirubin > 3 mg/dL or AST > 4 × ULN give 25% of recommended starting dose.
- Renal dysfunction: Consider lower doses if serum creatinine > 5 mg/dL.

Dosage adjustment after first treatment cycle based on nadir counts:
- Platelet count < 50,000/mm³, ANC < 250/mm³, neutropenic fever, or grades 3–4 nonhematologic toxicity: day 1 dose should be 75% of prior day 1 dose.
- Delay day 1 chemo until platelet count ≥ 100,000/mm³, ANC ≥ 1,500/mm³, and nonhematologic toxicities have recovered to ≤ grade 1.
- If patient is receiving dose divided into day 1 and 8, day 8 dose should be 75% of day 1 dose if platelet counts are 75,000–100,000/mm³ and ANC is 1,000–1,499/mm³. If day 8 platelet counts are < 75,000/mm³, ANC < 1,000, or grade 3–4 nonhematologic toxicity has occurred, omit the day 8 dose.
- **Patients receiving dose of 120 mg/m² regimen** should also receive prophylactic antibiotic therapy with trimethoprim-sulfamethoxazole or a fluoroquinolone.

Drug Preparation:
- Drug is provided as a preservative-free, ready-to-use solution of 2 mg/mL concentration (50-mg/25-mL and 200-mg/100-mL single-use vials). Product may become gelled in the refrigerator, and will return to a slightly viscous to modile solution after 2–4 hours equilibrium at controlled room temperature (59°–77°F or 15°–25°C).
- Use within 24 hours of penetration of rubber stopper; discard any unused drug.
- Store unopened vials in refrigerator at 36–46°F (2–8°C).

Drug Administration:
- Drug is a vesicant, so vesicant precautions should be used (check nursing procedure for administration of a vesicant).
- ANC must be > 1,500 cells/mm³, platelets > 100,000/mm³.
- Administer via slow IVP into the tubing of a freely flowing IV infusion of 0.9% NS or 5% dextrose solution over 3–5 minutes, checking blood return every few milliliters of drug. Administration time is 15–20 minutes. If drug dose is reduced, administer drug slowly over at least 3 minutes.
- Assesss LFTs, serum creatinine, and CBC/differential baseline before each cycle, as well as during epirubicin treatment as needed.
- Assess results of baseline ECHO or GBPS, and discuss with physician or NP/PA frequency of monitoring during epirubicin therapy.
- Epirubicin should not be administered with other cardiotoxic agents unless cardiac function is closely monitored. Do not give epirubicin-based therapy for up to 24 weeks after stopping trastuzumab (long half-life of trastuzumab).
- Administer antiemetics prior to drug administration, as drug is emetogenic.

Drug Interactions:
- Cytotoxic drugs: Additive toxicity (hematologic and gastrointestinal).
- Cardioactive drugs (e.g., calcium channel blockers): May increase risk of congestive heart failure; use together cautiously, and monitor cardiac function closely during treatment.
- Radiation therapy: Tissue sensitization to cytotoxic effects of radiation therapy; when drug is given after prior radiation therapy, a radiation recall inflammatory reaction may occur at site of prior radiation.
- Cimetidine: Increases drug AUC by 50%, DO NOT use together. Hold cimetidine during treatment with epirubicin.
- Other drugs extensively metabolized by the liver: Changes in hepatic function caused by concomitant therapies may affect clearance of epirubicin; use together with caution, if at all, and monitor for hematologic and gastrointestinal toxicity closely during treatment.
- Bone marrow-suppressing drugs: Increased bone marrow depression.
- Taxanes: Separate administration by at least 24 hours to minimize risk of toxicity.

Lab Effects/Interference:
- Decreased white blood and neutrophil cell counts, platelet counts.

Special Considerations:
Warnings:
- Drug is a vesicant, and severe local tissue necrosis will occur if drug infiltrates; avoid IV sites over joints, into small veins, or in veins on arms that have compromised venous or lymphatic drainage.
  - Venous sclerosis may occur if injections used in the same vein.
  - Extravasation may cause local pain, severe tissue lesions, and necrosis. Be careful to avoid extravasation.

- Facial flushing, as well as local erythema/streaking along vein path, may indicate excessively rapid administration. This may precede local phlebitis or thrombophlebitis.
- Myocardial toxicity (e.g., CHF) may occur during therapy or months to years after cessation of therapy, and risk increases according to dose (acute or late/delayed).
  - Cumulative doses > 900 mg/m^2 should generally not be exceeded.
  - Risk increases with prior anthracycline or anthracenedione therapy, past or concurrent radiation therapy to mediastinal/pericardial area, active or history of cardiovascular disease, or concomitant use of other cardiotoxic drugs.
  - Do not administer epirubicin in combination with other cardiotoxic agents unless the patient's cardiac function is closely monitored.
- Rarely, secondary cancers (e.g., acute myelogenous leukemia) have been reported, and risk is increased when given in combination with other cytotoxic drugs or when doses of anthracycline chemotherapy have been escalated. The estimated risk is 0.2% at 3 years and 0.8% at 5 years.
- Doses must be reduced in patients with hepatic dysfunction. Assess bilirubin and AST levels before and during epirubicin treatment. If values are elevated, drug clearance is slowed, raising risk of toxicity. Epirubicin dose should be reduced.
- Myelosuppression is the dose-limiting toxicity, and severe myelosuppression may occur.
- Assess serum creatinine baseline and during therapy. If value is > 5mg/dL, dose should be reduced.
- Rapid lysis of tumor cells may result in hyperuricemia (tumor lysis syndrome). Discuss TLS prevention treatment in patients at high risk at initial treatment.
- Do not give patient live or live-attenuated vaccines, as serious or fatal infections may occur.
- Administration of epirubicin after previous RT may induce an inflammatory recall reaction at the site or irradiation.
- Thrombophlebitis and thromboembolism (including pulmonary embolism) have been reported.
- Drug should never be given intramuscularly or subcutaneously.
- Drug is mutagenic, carcinogenic, and genotoxic. Men and women of childbearing age should use effective birth control measures to avoid pregnancy.
- Nursing mothers should not breastfeed during chemotherapy treatment.
- Teach patients that urine will be pink-red for the first 1–2 days following drug administration.
- Most common adverse effects in early breast cancer patients, occurring in 10% or more patients, were leucopenia, neutropenia, anemia, thrombocytopenia, amenorrhea, lethargy, nausea/vomiting, mucositis, diarrhea, infection, conjunctivitis/keratitis, alopecia, local toxicity, and rash/itch.
- Long-term adverse effects with an incidence of 1–2% were asymptomatic drops in LVEF, CHF, secondary leukemia.
- Geriatric use: administer drug carefully with close monitoring in patients who are 70 years or older.

Potential Toxicities/Side Effects and the Nursing Process

I. POTENTIAL FOR INFECTION, BLEEDING, FATIGUE related to BONE MARROW DEPRESSION

Defining Characteristics: WBC and platelet nadir 10–14 days after drug dose, with recovery by day 21. Leukopenia and neutropenia may be severe, especially when given with other myelosuppressive chemotherapy. Thrombocytopenia may be severe, and anemia may occur.

Nursing Implications: Monitor CBC, WBC, differential, and platelet count prior to drug administration; discuss any abnormalities with physician. Assess for signs/symptoms of infection or bleeding; instruct patient in self-assessment and to report signs/symptoms immediately. Teach patient self-care measures to minimize risk of infection and bleeding, including avoidance of company of people with colds and OTC aspirin-containing medications. Dose reduction necessary in patients with hepatic dysfunction, as decreased metabolism of drug results in increased serum levels of drug and hematologic toxicity. Patients receiving 120 mg/m^2 dose should also receive prophylactic antibiotic therapy with trimethoprim-sulfamethoxazole or a fluoroquinolone antibiotic.

II. POTENTIAL FOR ALTERATION IN CARDIAC OUTPUT related to ACUTE AND CHRONIC CARDIAC CHANGES

Defining Characteristics: Cardiotoxicity is dose-related, cumulative, and may occur during or months to years after cessation of therapy. The estimated probability of developing clinically evident CHF is 0.9% at a cumulative dose of 500 mg/m^2, 1.6% at 700 mg/m^2, and 3.3% at a cumulative dose of 900 mg/m^2. The risk of CHF increases rapidly with cumulative doses in excess of 900 mg/m^2. Risk of developing cardiotoxicity is increased by history of cardiovascular disease, prior anthracycline or anthracenedione therapy, prior or concomitant radiation therapy to mediastinum and/or pericardial area, and concomitant use of other cardiotoxic drugs. Cardiotoxicity may be acute (early) or delayed (late). Signs/symptoms of early toxicity are not usually of clinical significance, do not predict late cardiotoxicity, and usually do not require change in epirubicin therapy. These include sinus tachycardia and EKG abnormalities (nonspecific ST and T-wave changes, and, rarely, PVCs, VT, bradycardia, atrioventricular, and bundle branch block). Delayed cardiotoxicity is related to cardiomyopathy, characterized by decreased left ventricular ejection fraction (LVEF) and classic signs/symptoms of CHF (tachycardia, dyspnea, pulmonary edema, dependent edema, hepatomegaly, ascites, pleural effusion, gallop rhythm). If late cardiotoxicity occurs, it is in the late stages of treatment or within months following treatment, and is cumulative dose-related.

Nursing Implications: Assess cardiac status prior to chemotherapy administration: risk factors and signs/symptoms of CHF, quality/regularity and rate of heartbeat, results of baseline and periodic prior gated blood pool scan (GBPS), multigated radionuclideangiography (MUGA), echocardiogram (ECHO), or other test of LVEF. Instruct patient to report dyspnea, palpitations, and swelling in extremities. Maintain accurate records of total dose; expect GBPS or measure of LVEF to be repeated periodically during treatment and the drug to be discontinued if there is a significant drop in heart function as evidenced by LVEF falling below normal range.

III. POTENTIAL FOR ALTERATION IN NUTRITION, LESS THAN BODY REQUIREMENTS, related to NAUSEA AND VOMITING, DIARRHEA, STOMATITIS

Defining Characteristics: Nausea/vomiting occurs in > 90% of patients, can be moderate to severe especially when drug is given together with other emetogenic chemotherapy, and is preventable with combination antiemetics. Onset 1–3 hours after drug dose and lasts 24 hours. Mucositis may occur; stomatitis is most common. Esophagitis is less common but may occur, especially if patient has had prior radiotherapy to the chest. Drug dose must be reduced in patients with hepatic dysfunction; otherwise, increased gastrointestinal toxicity will occur.

Nursing Implications: Assess baseline LFTs, and discuss with physician dose reduction if abnormal. Premedicate with combination antiemetics and continue protection for 24 hours. If patient has a central line, slower infusion of drug over 1 hour decreases nausea/vomiting. Encourage small, frequent feedings of bland foods. Perform oral assessment prior to drug administration and during posttreatment visits. Teach patient oral hygiene and self-assessment techniques. Teach patient to report pain, burning sensation, erythema, erosions, ulcerations, bleeding, or oral infections.

IV. POTENTIAL ALTERATION IN SKIN INTEGRITY related to ALOPECIA, RADIATION RECALL, FACIAL FLUSHING, FLARE REACTION, NAIL/ SKIN/ORAL MUCOUS MEMBRANE HYPERPIGMENTATION, AND DRUG EXTRAVASATION

Defining Characteristics: Alopecia is universal, but is reversible, with hair regrowth in 2–3 months following cessation of therapy. Skin damage and inflammation from prior radiation may be reactivated when drug is given. Drug may cause "flare" reaction or streaking along vein during peripheral drug administration, often with facial flushing, and may be related to excessively rapid drug administration. If it occurs, slow drug administration time, flush line with plain IV solution, and slowly complete therapy. This must be distinguished from extravasation, where there is leakage of drug into the perivascular tissue. Skin and nail hyperpigmentation may occur.

Nursing Implications: Discuss with patient hair loss, anticipated impact, and strategies to decrease distress, e.g., obtaining wig prior to hair loss. Assess body disturbance from hyperpigmentation and discuss strategies to minimize this, e.g., nail polish for dark nail beds. Drug must be administered via patent IV. Local phlebitis or thrombophlebitis may follow a flare reaction, so assess vein path closely, and teach patient to report any pain, erythema, or swelling following drug administration. Drug is a potent vesicant and causes SEVERE tissue destruction if drug extravasates. Teach patient to report any stinging or burning during drug administration, and stop administration if there is any question at all. Assess need for venous access device early.

V. POTENTIAL FOR SEXUAL DYSFUNCTION related to REPRODUCTIVE HAZARD

Defining Characteristics: Drug is genotoxic, mutagenic, and carcinogenic. In laboratory animals receiving very high doses of the drug, testicular atrophy occurred. Drug may cause irreversible amenorrhea in premenopausal women (premature menopause).

Nursing Implications: Assess patient's/partner's sexual patterns and reproductive goals. Provide information, supportive counseling, and referral as needed. Teach importance of birth control measures as appropriate. Male patients may wish to use a sperm bank, and women may wish to investigate cryopreservation of oocytes prior to therapy.

Drug: eribulin mesylate injection (Havalen)

Class: Non-taxane microtubular dynamics inhibitor, synthetic analogue of the marine natural product halichondrin B.

Mechanism of Action: Drug is a synthetic analogue of halichondrin B, a natural product found in the rare marine sponge Halichondria okadai. The drug has a unique mechanism of action to suppress microtubule growth, without shortening; it also sequesters tubulin into nonfunctional aggregates to prevent (irreversibly) the formation of the mitotic spindle during mitosis so that the cell undergoes mitotic arrest at the G_2–M phase resulting in apoptosis (programmed cell death). Drug has activity in taxane-resistant cell lines.

Metabolism: Unchanged eribulin is the major circulating species in the plasma, and eribulin is negligibly metabolized by CYP3A4 in vitro. However, it does not induce or inhibit hepatic CYP3A4 activity at clinically relevant concentrations. In addition, it does not affect the metabolism of other therapeutic agents metabolized by CYP3A4. Drug is excreted primarily unchanged in the feces (82%) and the urine (9%).

Indication: treatment of patients with metastatic breast cancer who have previously received at least 2 chemotherapeutic regimens for the treatment of metastatic disease. Prior therapy should have included an anthracycline and a taxane in either the adjuvant or metastatic setting.

Dosage/Range: 1.4 mg/m^2 IV over 2–5 minutes on days 1 and 8 of a 21-day cycle.
• Do not administer drug on day 1 or 8 if ANC < 1,000/mm^3, platelets < 75,000/mm^3, or patient has grade 3 or 4 non-hematologic toxicities.

- Day 8 dose may be delayed for a maximum of 1 week; if toxicities do not resolve or improve to ≤ grade 2 severity by day 15, omit the dose; if toxicities have resolved or improved to ≤ grade 2 severity by day 15, administer drug at a reduced dose and initiate the next cycle no sooner than 2 weeks later.
- Reduce dose in patients with hepatic impairment and moderate renal impairment.
- Do not mix with other drugs or administer with dextrose-containing solutions.
- If a dose has been delayed for toxicity and toxicities have recovered to grade 2 or less, resume eribulin mesylate at a reduced dose as showing in the table below.
- Do not re-escalate eribulin mesylate after it has been dose reduced.
- Recommended dose modifications:

Event Description	Recommended Dose (eribulin mesylate)
Permanently reduce the 1.4 m^2 dose for any of the following:	1.1 mg/m^2
- ANC < 500/mm^3 for >7 days - ANC < 1,000/mm^3, with fever or infection - Platelets < 25,000/mm^3 - Platelets < 50,000/mm^3, requiring transfusion - Non-hematologic grade 3 or 4 toxicities - Omission or delay of day 8 dose in previous cycle for toxicity	
Occurrence of any event requiring permanent dose reduction while receiving 1.1 mg/m^2	0.7 mg/m^2
Occurrence of any event requiring permanent dose reduction while receiving 0.7 mg/m^2	Discontinue eribulin mesylate injection
Hepatic Impairment	
Mild hepatic impairment (Child-Hugh A)	1.1 mg/m^2
Moderate hepatic impairment (Child-Hugh B)	0.7 mg/m^2
Severe hepatic impairment (Child-Hugh C)	Eribulin mesylate injection was not studied in this population
Renal Impairment	
Mild renal impairment (CrCl 50–80 mL/min)	No modification necessary
Moderate renal impairment (CrCl 30–50 mL/min)	1.1 mg/m^2
Severe renal impairment (CrCl < 30 mL/min)	Eribulin mesylate injection was not studied in this population

Halaven package insert. Woodcliffe, NJ: Eisai Inc, August 2014.

Drug Preparation: Available as 1 mg per 2 mL (0.5 mg per mL).
- Aseptically withdraw ordered dose from the single-use vial and administer, either undiluted or diluted in 100 mL 0.9% sodium chloride USP.
- Do NOT dilute in or administer drug through IV line containing dextrose solutions.
- Do NOT administer in the same IV line concurrent with other medicines.
- Store undiluted drug in the syringe for up to 4 hours at room temperature or for up to 24 hours under refrigeration (40°F or 4°C).
- Store diluted solutions containing the drug for up to 4 hours at room temperature or up to 24 hours under refrigeration (40°F or 4°C).
- Discard any unused drug remaining in the vial.
- Store vial in its original carton at 25°C (77°F); excursions permitted to 15–30°C (59–86°F); do not freeze.

Drug/Administration:
- Assess for CBC/differential before each dose, and assess for signs and symptoms of peripheral neuropathy.
- Administer IV over 2–5 minutes on days 1 and 8 of a 21-day cycle.
- Do not mix with other drugs or administer with dextrose-containing solutions.

Drug Interactions:
- Minimal risk of drug–drug interactions in the clinical setting (Zhang et al., 2008).
- Dextrose containing solutions; do not use.

Lab Effects/Interference:
- Neutropenia, leukopenia, anemia, thrombocytopenia.
- Hypokalemia.
- Increased LFTs.

Special Considerations:
- Most commonly reported adverse events (> 25%): neutropenia, anemia, asthenia/fatigue, alopecia, peripheral neuropathy, nausea, and constipation.
- Eribulin showed a significant survival benefit in heavily pretreated women with metastatic breast cancer (13.12 months vs 10.65 months, p < .04), in the global EMBRACE phase III study (Twelves et al., 2010). The study was composed of 672 patients who had been heavily pretreated with previous chemotherapy regimens (median of 4) including an anthracycline and a taxane. The 1-year survival is 53.9% in the eribulin arm compared to 43.7% in the physician's treatment choice arm, where women were treated with vinorelbine, gemcitabine, or capecitabine, as none chose best supportive care.
- Drug is embryo-fetotoxic. Women of childbearing age should use effective contraception to avoid pregnancy. Nursing mothers should discontinue drug or nursing, taking into account the importance of the drug to the mother. Testicular toxicity occurs in men.
- Neutropenia: monitor peripheral blood cell counts and adjust dose as needed.
- Peripheral neuropathy (PN): monitor for signs of motor and sensory PN, and manage with dose delay and adjustment (withhold dose for grades 3 or 4 PN until resolution to grade 2 or less).

• QT prolongation occurs rarely, and was observed at day 8 in a small number of patients. Monitor for prolonged QT intervals in patients with CHF, bradyarrhythmias, taking drugs known to prolong QT interval and electrolyte abnormalities. Do not administer drug to patients with congenital long QT syndrome. Correct hypokalemia and hypomagnesemia before starting drug, and monitor serum levels during treatment.

Potential Toxicities/Side Effects and the Nursing Process

I.   POTENTIAL FOR INFECTION, BLEEDING, FATIGUE related to BONE MARROW DEPRESSION

Defining Characteristics: Neutropenia affected 82% of patients (all grades). Incidence of grades 3–4 neutropenia was 57%, with 5% febrile neutropenia. Neutropenia (ANC < 500/mm³) lasting > 1 week occurred in 12% of patients, leading to discontinuation in < 1% of patients. Mean time to nadir was 13 days, and mean time to recovery from severe neutropenia (ANC < 500/mm³) was 8 days. Patients with elevated LFTs > 3 × ULN and bilirubin > 1.5 × ULN experienced a higher incidence of grade 4 neutropenia and febrile neutropenia. G-CSF was used in 19% of patients. Two patients died of complications of febrile neutropenia in clinical trials. Grade 3 or higher thrombocytopenia occurred in 1% of patients. Asthenia/fatigue occurred in 54%. Incidence of anemia is 58%, and thrombocytopenia 12%.

Nursing Implications: Monitor CBC, WBC, differential, and platelet count prior to each drug administration, and increase frequency in patients who develop grade 3 or 4 cytopenias. Delay administration and reduce subsequent doses in patients who experience febrile or grade 4 neutropenia lasting > 7 days. Discuss utility of G-CSF in high-risk patients with physician. Ensure that patients with hepatic dysfunction are dosed according to the Child-Pugh Class grading scale. Assess for signs/symptoms of infection or bleeding; instruct patient in self-assessment and to report signs/symptoms immediately. Teach patient self-care measures to minimize risk of infection and bleeding, including avoidance of company of people with colds and avoidance of OTC aspirin-containing medications. Teach patient energy-conserving activities, gentle exercise, and to report fatigue. Refer to ONS Putting Evidence into Practice (PEP) cards on fatigue. Assess and manage according to clinical trial protocol.

II.   SENSORY/PERCEPTUAL ALTERATIONS related to SENSORY AND MOTOR NEUROPATHY

Defining Characteristics: Peripheral neuropathy occurred in 31–35% of patients (8% grades 3, 0.4% grade 4). Neuropathy lasting > 1 year occurred in 5% of patients. 22% developed new or worsening neuropathy that had not recovered within a median follow-up duration of 269 days (range 25–662 days). When compared to patients receiving ixabepilone, PN, and it occurred later in the course of disease treatment, PN was the most common adverse reaction resulting in discontinuation. Dizziness, dysgeusia, and headache may also occur.

Nursing Implications: Assess baseline neurologic status. Instruct patient to report signs/ symptoms of pins-and-needles sensation, numbness, burning sensation, pain, increased discomfort with certain sensations, especially in the extremities, or motor weakness. Identify patients at risk: those with history of cisplatin use or with preexisting neuropathies (ethanol- and diabetes mellitus-related). Assess sensory and motor function prior to each treatment, and if abnormality found, assess impact on patient function, safety, independence, ability to do activities of daily living (ADLs), and quality of life. Test patient's ability to button a shirt or pick up a dime from a flat surface. If impacting ability to do ADLs, safety, or quality of life, discuss with physician/midlevel. Drug should be held for grade 3 or 4 PN until resolution to grade 2 or less, then with dose reduction.

III. POTENTIAL ALTERATION IN COMFORT related to JOINT PAIN, DYSPNEA, ALOPECIA, PYREXIA

Defining Characteristics: Mild or moderate joint pain occurred in 22% of patients, back pain in 16%, bone pain in 12%, and extremity pain in 11%. Alopecia occurred in 45% of patients.

Nursing Implications: Teach patient that these side effects may occur and to report them. Assess patient for occurrence of symptoms and discuss measures for symptomatic relief with physician or midlevel practitioner.

IV. POTENTIAL FOR ALTERATION IN NUTRITION, LESS THAN BODY REQUIREMENTS, related to NAUSEA AND VOMITING, DIARRHEA, CONSTIPATION, STOMATITIS

Defining Characteristics: Nausea and vomiting occur in 35% and 18% of patients, respectively, in clinical trials. Constipation occurred in 25%, and diarrhea in 18%. Mucosal inflammation occurred in 9%, anorexia in 20%, and decreased weight in 21%. Dry mouth, dyspepsia, and stomach pain may also occur. Hypokalemia occurs rarely. Increased LFTs (in patients with normal baseline LFTs) occurred in 18% of patients.

Nursing Implications: Assess baseline nutritional, fluid, and electrolyte status and monitor throughout treatment. Premedicate with antiemetics prior to drug administration and continue through treatment. Monitor daily or weekly weights. Teach patient to report unrelieved nausea, vomiting, or inability to take oral fluids.

Drug: estramustine (Estracyte, Emcyt)

Class: Alkylating agent.

Mechanism of Action: Acts as a weak alkylator at usual therapeutic concentrations. A chemical combination of mechlorethamine and estradiol phosphate, estramustine is believed to selectively enter cells with estrogen receptors, where the drug acts as an alkylating agent due to bischloroethyl side-chain and liberated estrogens. Believed to have antimicrotubule activity. Cell cycle nonspecific.

Metabolism: Well absorbed orally, metabolized in liver, partly excreted in urine. Induces a marked decline in serum calcium and phosphate levels.

Indication: For the palliative treatment of patients with metastatic and/or progressive carcinoma of the prostate.

Contraindication: Not to be taken by patients with (1) known hypersensitivity to either estradiol or to nitrogen mustard, and (2) active thrombophlebitis or thromboembolic disorders, except when the actual tumor mass is the cause of the thromboembolic phenomenon and the physician believes the benefits outweigh the risks.

Dosage/Range:
- 14 mg/kg (or one 140-mg capsule for each 22 lbs or 10 kg of body weight) orally daily in 3 or 4 divided doses. Following treatment for 30–90 days, the physician should evaluate response. Drug continues as long as the favorable response lasts. Some patients have been maintained on therapy for > 3 years, at doses ranging from 10–16 mg/kg/day.
- IV: Available for investigational use; 150 mg IV initially, then may increase to 300 mg/day per protocol.

Drug Preparation:
- Available in 140-mg capsules.
- Store in refrigerator (2–8°C [36–46°F]); may be stored at room temperature for 24–48 hours.
- IV: Dissolve in at least 10 mL sterile water.

Drug Administration:
- Oral with water, at least 1 hour before or 2 hours after meals. DO NOT take with milk, milk products, or calcium-rich foods or drugs (e.g., calcium-containing antacids).
- IV (investigational): Slow IVP via IV containing 5% dextrose.

Drug Interactions:
- Drug/food: milk, milk products, and Ca^{2+}-rich foods may decrease drug absorption.
- Calcium-containing antacids: may impair drug absorption; take 1 hour before, or 2 hours after drug dose.
- Synergy with vinblastine.

Lab Effects/Interference:
- Changes in Ca.
- Increased serum glucose, LDH, triglyceride levels.
- Increased LFTs, RFTs.
- May affect certain endocrine (e.g., thyroid function tests, prolactin, cortisol) and LFTs because it contains estrogen.

Special Considerations:
- Avoid taking drug with milk, milk products, and calcium-rich foods (e.g., antacids), as this will delay or impair drug absorption.
- Contraindicated or to be used with great caution in patients who are children or who have thrombophlebitis or thromboembolic disorders, peptic ulcers, severe hepatic dysfunction, cardiac disease, hypertension, or diabetes. Drug may increase the risk of embolic events; physician may recommend prophylactic warfarin or aspirin.
- IV preparation is a vesicant; avoid extravasation.
- Transient perineal itching and pain after IV administration.

Potential Toxicities/Side Effects and the Nursing Process

I. POTENTIAL ALTERATION IN TISSUE PERFUSION related to THROMBOPHLEBITIS, THROMBOSIS

Defining Characteristics: Increased risk of clot formation, with risk for development of thrombophlebitis, pulmonary emboli, myocardial infarction, and cerebrovascular accident.

Nursing Implications: Assess patient risk; drug is contraindicated in patients with thrombophlebitis or thromboembolic disorders, unless caused by the malignancy. Should be used cautiously in these patients, and in those patients with coronary artery disease. Drug may worsen CHF. Assess baseline cardiac and peripheral vascular status, including signs/symptoms of CHF. Monitor blood pressure and glucose tolerance during therapy. Instruct patient to report immediately any signs/symptoms, e.g., dyspnea, edema, pain, and erythema in legs.

II. BODY IMAGE DISTURBANCE related to GYNECOMASTIA

Defining Characteristics: Mild to moderate breast enlargement may occur, with nipple tenderness initially.

Nursing Implications: Teach patient about potential side effects; discuss potential impact on body image and comfort. Encourage patient to verbalize feelings; provide information and emotional support.

III. POTENTIAL ALTERATION IN COMFORT related to PERINEAL SYMPTOMS, HEADACHE, RASH, URTICARIA, TRANSIENT PARESTHESIAS (IV)

Defining Characteristics: Perineal itching and pain, as well as transient paresthesias of the mouth, may occur after IV administration (investigational). Other symptoms that may accompany oral dosing are rash, pruritus, dry skin, peeling skin of fingertips, thinning hair, night sweats, lethargy, pain in eyes, and breast tenderness.

Nursing Implications: Assess patient for occurrence of symptoms and discuss measures for symptomatic relief.

IV. POTENTIAL FOR ALTERATION IN NUTRITION, LESS THAN BODY REQUIREMENTS, related to NAUSEA AND VOMITING, DIARRHEA, HEPATIC DYSFUNCTION

Defining Characteristics: Nausea and vomiting occur at higher dosing; tolerance may develop, but dose may need to be reduced. Nausea and vomiting may be delayed but become intractable and necessitate discontinuance of the drug. Diarrhea occurs occasionally. Mild elevations in liver function tests may occur (LDH, SGOT, bili) with or without jaundice, but are usually self-limiting. Abnormal Ca++ and P levels may occur.

Nursing Implications: Assess baseline nutritional fluid and electrolyte status. Premedicate with antiemetics prior to drug administration and continue through treatment. Assess baseline LFTs and Ca++ and P levels; monitor during therapy and discuss any abnormalities with physician. Monitor daily or weekly weights.

Drug: estrogens: diethylstilbestrol (DES), ethinyl estradiol (Estinyl), conjugated estrogen (Premarin), chlorotrianisene (Tace)

Class: Hormones.

Mechanism of Action: Unknown; estrogens change the hormonal milieu of the body.

Metabolism: Metabolized mainly in the liver. Undergoes enterohepatic recirculation. DES is metabolized more slowly than natural estrogens.

Dosage/Range:
- DES: Prostate cancer: 1–3 mg PO daily; breast cancer: 5 mg PO tid.
- Diethylstilbestrol diphosphate: Prostate cancer: 50–200 mg PO tid, 0.5–1.0 g IV daily × 5 days, then 250–1,000 mg each week.
- Chlorotrianisene: 1–10 mg PO tid.
- Ethinyl estradiol: 0.5–1.0 mg PO tid.

Drug Preparation:
- None.

Drug Administration:
- Oral.

Drug Interactions:
- None significant.

Lab Effects/Interference:
- Increased Ca.
- Increased T_4 levels.
- Increased clotting factors.
- Decreased serum folate.

Special Considerations:
- Long-term dosage of DES in men has been associated with cardiovascular deaths. Maximum dose should be 1 mg tid for prostate cancer.
- Can cause inaccurate laboratory results (liver, adrenal, thyroid).
- Causes rapid rise in serum calcium in patients with bony metastases; watch for symptoms of hypercalcemia.

Potential Toxicities/Side Effects and the Nursing Process

I. POTENTIAL FOR INJURY related to THROMBOEMBOLIC COMPLICATIONS, HYPERCALCEMIA, SODIUM AND WATER RETENTION, AND CARDIOTOXICITY

Defining Characteristics: Thromboembolic complications are infrequent but serious, and increased risk occurs with long-term use and higher doses. Hypercalcemia occurs in 5–10% of women with breast cancer metastatic to bone, appears in first 2 weeks of therapy, and is aggravated by preexisting renal disease. There is an increased risk of cardiovascular-related deaths, especially in men on high-dose estrogens for prostate cancer. Drug should be used cautiously, if at all, in patients with underlying cardiac, renal, or hepatic disease.

Nursing Implications: Assess risk (preexisting cardiac, hepatic, and renal disease), baseline cardiac, and vascular status; discuss abnormalities with physician. Monitor status during therapy. Teach patient to report signs/symptoms of edema, dyspnea, localized swelling, pain, tenderness, erythema, and CNS changes. Teach female patient signs/symptoms of hypercalcemia (drowsiness, increased thirst, constipation, increased urine output) and to report this. Monitor Ca++ level in women with metastatic breast cancer closely during first few weeks of therapy.

II. ALTERATION IN NUTRITION, LESS THAN BODY REQUIREMENTS, related to NAUSEA AND VOMITING

Defining Characteristics: Occurs in 25% of patients; intensity is related to specific drug and dose. Tolerance occurs after a few weeks of therapy.

Nursing Implications: Inform patient that this may occur; teach self-administration of antiemetics prior to drug administration per physician order, and to take drug at bedtime to decrease nausea. Discuss with physician starting patient at low dose, with increase as tolerated.

III. ALTERATION IN MALE SEXUAL FUNCTION related to GYNECOMASTIA, LOSS OF LIBIDO, IMPOTENCE, AND VOICE CHANGE

Defining Characteristics: Gynecomastia may be prevented by pretreatment of breast with low dose of radiotherapy. Feminine characteristics disappear when therapy is stopped.

Nursing Implications: Explore with patient and partner reproductive and sexual patterns and impact that chemotherapy may have. Provide information, supportive counseling, and referral as indicated. Since alternative, superior hormonal manipulative drugs are available, discuss these with physician.

IV.   POTENTIAL FOR FEMALE SEXUAL DYSFUNCTION related to BREAST TENDERNESS/ENGORGEMENT, UTERINE PROLAPSE, AND URINARY INCONTINENCE

Defining Characteristics: Breast engorgement may occur in postmenopausal women; uterine prolapse and exacerbation of preexisting uterine fibroids with possible uterine bleeding may occur, as may urinary incontinence.

Nursing Implications: Explore with patient sexual and reproductive patterns, and any impact the drug may have. Provide information, supportive counseling, and referral as needed. Discuss with physician alternative hormonal manipulative drugs as needed.

Drug: etoposide (VP-16, VePesid, Etopophos)

Class: Plant alkaloid, a derivative of the mandrake plant (mayapple plant).

Mechanism of Action: Inhibits DNA synthesis in S and G_2 so that cells do not enter mitosis. Causes single-strand breaks in DNA. Cell cycle specific for S and G_2 phases.

Metabolism: Etoposide is rapidly excreted in the urine and, to a lesser extent, in the bile. About 30% of drug is excreted unchanged. Binds to serum albumin (94%) and then becomes extensively tissue-bound.

Indications: Management of (1) refractory testicular tumors, in combination with other approved chemotherapy agents in patients who have already received appropriate surgical, chemotherapeutic, and radiotherapeutic therapy, (2) small cell lung cancer, in combination with other approved chemotherapy agents as first-line treatment.

Dosage/Range:
- 50–100 mg/m^2 IV daily × 5 days (testicular cancer) every 3–4 weeks.
- 75–200 mg/m^2 IV daily × 3 days (small-cell lung cancer) every 3–4 weeks.
- Many other doses based on tumor type being treated (e.g., lymphomas, ANLL, bladder, prostate, uterus, Kaposi's sarcoma).
- Oral dose is twice the intravenous dose, rounded to the nearest 50 mg; can take with or without food.
- High dose (bone marrow transplantation): 750–2400 mg/m^2 IV, or 10–60 mg/kg over 1–4 hours to 24 hours, usually combined with other cytotoxic agents or total body irradiation.
- Dose modification if renal or hepatic dysfunction (see Special Considerations section).

Drug Preparation:
- Available in 5-cc (100-mg) vial as VePesid; the 100-mg Etopophos vial is reconstituted with 5 mL or 10 mL normal saline, D_5W, sterile water, bacteriostatic sterile water, or bacteriostatic normal saline with benzyl alcohol to 20 mg/mL or 10 mg/mL, respectively. May be further diluted with NS or D_5W to 0.1 mg/mL final concentration.
- Oral capsules are available in 50-mg and 100-mg capsules, and should be stored in the refrigerator.

Drug Administration:
- IV infusion: VePesid over 30–60 minutes to minimize risk of hypotension and bronchospasm (wheezing). In some instances, a test dose may be infused slowly (0.5 mL in 50 mL 0.9% sodium chloride) and the remaining drug infused if no untoward reaction after 5 minutes. Etopophos: IVB over 5 minutes as drug is significantly less likely to cause hypotension.
- Stability: Drug must be diluted with either 5% dextrose injection USP or 0.9% sodium chloride solution and is stable 96 hours in glass and 48 hours in plastic containers at room temperature (25°C [77°F]) under normal fluorescent light at a concentration of 0.2 mg/mL.
- Inspect for clarity of solution prior to administration.
- Oral administration: may give as a single dose up to 400 mg; otherwise, divide dose into 2–4 doses.

Drug Interactions:
- Enhances warfarin action by increasing prothrombin time (PT); need to monitor closely.
- Increased toxicity of methotrexate when given concurrently.
- Cyclosporin: additive cytotoxicity when given concurrently.
- CYP3A4 inducers (e.g., phenytoin) may decrease etoposide level, while CYP3A4 inhibitors (e.g., ketoconazole) may increase etoposide level.
- St. John's wort: may decrease etoposide level, do not use concurrently.

Lab Effects/Interference:
- Increased PT with patients on warfarin.
- Increased LFTs, metabolic acidosis with higher doses.

Special Considerations:
- Nadir 7–14 days after treatment.
- Dose modifications: reduce drug dose by 50% if bili > 1.5 mg/dL, by 75% if bili > 3.0 mg/dL. Reduce drug 25% if creatinine clearance 10–50 mL/min; reduce by 50% if creatinine clearance < 10 mL/min.
- Synergistic drug effect in combination with cisplatin.
- Radiation recall may occur when combined therapies are used.
- Patients receiving high-dose therapy are at risk for the development of second malignancy or ethanol intoxication (injection contains polyethylene glycol with absolute alcohol).
- VePesid: drug stability is concentration-dependent, while Etopophos is prepared as a phosphate ester, which negates the need for concentration-dependent stability (equally stable for 24 hours at concentrations of 20 mg/mL to 0.1 mg/mL).

Etoposide Concentration (mg/mL)	5% Dextrose	0.9% Sodium Chloride
2	0.5 hour*	0.5 hour*
1	2 hours	2 hours
0.6	8 hours	8 hours
0.4	48 hours	48 hours
0.2	96 hours	96 hours

*Check for fine precipitate.
Source: Data from Dorr RT, Von Hoff DD. *Cancer Chemotherapy Handbook,* 2nd ed. Norwalk, CT: Appleton & Lange; 1994: 462.

Potential Toxicities/Side Effects and the Nursing Process

I.   POTENTIAL FOR INJURY related to ALLERGIC REACTION, HYPOTENSION, ANAPHYLAXIS DURING DRUG INFUSION

Defining Characteristics: Bronchospasm (wheezing) may occur, with or without fever, chills; hypotension may occur during rapid infusion. Anaphylaxis may occur, but is rare.

Nursing Implications: Infuse drug over at least 30–60 minutes in correct amount of IV solution (stability related to volume). Monitor temperature, vital signs prior to drug administration, and periodically during treatment. Remain with patient during first 15 minutes of infusion and assess for signs/symptoms of bronchospasm. Discontinue drug and notify physician if bronchospasm or signs/symptoms of anaphylactic-like reaction occur. Maintain patent IV, monitor VS, and have ready epinephrine, diphenhydramine, and hydrocortisone, as well as emergency equipment. Be familiar with institution's practice guidelines for management of anaphylaxis.

II.   POTENTIAL FOR INFECTION AND BLEEDING related to BONE MARROW DEPRESSION

Defining Characteristics: Nadir 10–14 days after drug dose, with recovery on days 21–22. Neutropenia may be severe. Profound bone marrow suppression when given in high doses for bone marrow/stem cell rescue.

Nursing Implications: Monitor CBC, WBC, differential, and platelet count prior to chemotherapy and at expected nadir. Assess for signs/symptoms of infection or bleeding prior to drug administration; instruct patient in self-assessment and to report signs/symptoms immediately. Teach patient self-care measures to minimize risk of infection and bleeding, including avoidance of OTC aspirin-containing medications.

III.   ALTERED NUTRITION, LESS THAN BODY REQUIREMENTS, related to NAUSEA AND VOMITING, ANOREXIA

Defining Characteristics: Nausea and vomiting are usually mild, occurring soon after infusion. Oral dosing has higher incidence of nausea/vomiting. Anorexia is mild but may be severe with oral dosing. Severe nausea and vomiting when given in high doses, requires aggressive, maximal antiemesis. In addition, hepatitis, stomatitis, and metabolic acidosis may occur with high-dose therapy.

Nursing Implications: Premedicate with antiemetics and continue prophylactically for at least 4–6 hours after drug administration. Encourage small feedings of bland, cool foods and liquids; encourage spices as desired. Consult dietitian if anorexia is severe. Patients receiving high-dose therapy should have baseline and periodic assessment of laboratory parameters (e.g., LFTs and chemistries), as well as assessment of oral mucosa. Teach patients self-care, including oral assessment, use of oral hygiene regimen, and to report pain, burning, oral lesions.

IV.   BODY IMAGE DISTURBANCE related to ALOPECIA

Defining Characteristics: Incidence is 20–90% and is dose-dependent; regrowth may occur between drug cycles.

Nursing Implications: Discuss with patient possible hair loss and potential coping strategies, including obtaining wig or cap. If hair loss is complete, instruct patient to wear cap or scarf at night to prevent loss of body heat in cold climates.

V.   POTENTIAL SEXUAL DYSFUNCTION related to DRUG EFFECTS

Defining Characteristics: Drug is mutagenic and teratogenic.

Nursing Implications: Explore with patient and partner sexual patterns and reproductive goals. Teach about need for contraception as appropriate. Provide information, emotional support, and referral as needed.

VI.   ALTERED SKIN INTEGRITY related to RADIATION RECALL, PERIVASCULAR IRRITATION IF DRUG INFILTRATES, AND SKIN LESIONS WITH HIGH-DOSE THERAPY

Defining Characteristics: Drug is a radiosensitizer and an irritant. Patients receiving high-dose therapy may develop bullae on the skin (similar to Stevens-Johnson syndrome).

Nursing Implications: Assess skin in area of prior radiation when combined therapies are given as well as mucous membranes. Drug may need to be withheld until skin healing occurs if radiation recall results in skin breakdown. Teach patient wound-management techniques.

Use careful venipuncture and infuse drug through patent IV over 30–60 minutes, diluted according to manufacturer's specifications. Teach patients receiving high-dose therapy to report any skin changes.

VII. ALTERATION IN CARDIAC OUTPUT related to RARE MYOCARDIAL INFARCTION, ARRHYTHMIAS

Defining Characteristics: Rare myocardial infarction has been reported after prior mediastinal XRT in patients receiving etoposide-containing regimens. Arrhythmias are uncommon but may occur, especially in patients with preexisting coronary artery disease.

Nursing Implications: Monitor patient during infusion and instruct patient to report any unusual sensations. Discuss any abnormalities with physician.

VIII. SENSORY/PERCEPTUAL ALTERATION related to NEUROTOXICITY

Defining Characteristics: Peripheral neuropathies may occur but are uncommon and mild.

Nursing Implications: Assess motor and sensory function prior to drug administration. Instruct patient to report any changes in sensation or function. Discuss any abnormalities with physician. Encourage patient to verbalize feelings about discomfort and sensory loss, and discuss alternative coping strategies.

Drug: exemestane (Aromasin)

Class: Steroidal aromatase inactivator.

Mechanism of Action: Aromatase converts adrenal and ovarian androgens into estrogen, peripherally, in postmenopausal women. Exemestane acts as a false substrate (looks like androstenedione) and binds irreversibly to the aromatase enzyme, making it inactive ("suicide inhibition"). This results in a significant decrease (up to 95%) in circulating estrogen levels in postmenopausal women without affecting other adrenal enzymes. In the absence of estrogen, the stimulus for breast cancer growth is removed.

Metabolism: Oral drug is rapidly absorbed from the GI tract, with plasma levels increased by about 40% if taken after a high-fat breakfast. Drug is extensively distributed into the tissues, and is highly protein-bound (90%). Drug is extensively metabolized in the liver by the P450 3A4 (CYP3A4) isoenzyme system, and excreted equally in urine and feces. After a single dose of 25 mg, maximal suppression of circulating estrogen occurs 2–3 days after the dose, and lasts for 4–5 days. In patients with either hepatic or renal insufficiency, the dose of exemestane was three times higher than in patients with normal liver or renal function. This does not require dosage adjustment, but studies looking at the safety of chronic dosing in these groups of patients have not been done.

Indication: For (1) adjuvant treatment of postmenopausal women with estrogen-receptor positive early breast cancer who have received 2–3 years of tamoxifen and are switched to exemestane for completion of a total of 5 consecutive years of adjuvant hormonal therapy, and (2) treatment of advanced breast cancer in postmenopausal women whose disease has progressed following tamoxifen therapy.

Contraindication: Patients with a known hypersensitivity to the drug or to its excipients, and premenopausal women, including pregnant women.

Dosage/Range:
- 25 mg tab PO daily.

Drug Preparation:
- None. Store tablets at 77°F (25°C).

Drug Administration:
- Oral, once daily, after a meal.
- Assess 25-hydroxyvitamin D levels prior to the start of aromatase inhibitor treatment.
- Assess bone mineral density (BMD) results baseline and during therapy, as BMD decreases with treatment over time.

Drug Interactions:
- CYP3A4 inhibitors: significant drug interactions unlikely.
- CYP3A4 inducers (rifampin, phenytoin, carbamazepine, phenobarbital, St. John's wort): may significantly lower exemestane serum levels; do not use concurrently.

Lab Effects/Interference:
- Lymphopenia (20% incidence).
- Elevated LFTs (AST, ALT, alk phos, GGT) rarely.

Special Considerations:
- Drug is excreted in maternal milk so mothers should make a decision to stop nursing or stop the drug, taking into account the importance of the drug to the mother's health.
- Drug is well tolerated, with mild to moderate side effects.
- Differs from other selective aromatase inhibitors in that drug irreversibly binds to aromatase, and androgens cannot displace drug from this enzyme. Body must synthesize new aromatase to start estrogen production again.
- Drug similar to or superior to megestrol acetate after tamoxifen failure in metastatic breast cancer (Kaufmann et al., 2000).
- Exemestane has been shown to reduce the risk for breast cancer by 65% in high-risk women, adding the drug to the breast cancer preventive agent armamentarium. In addition, the study showed a 60% reduction in invasive breast cancer plus pre-invasive ductal carcinoma in situ and fewer cases to cancer precursor lesions, including atypical ductal hyperplasia and atypical lobular hyperplasia, compared to the placebo group (Goss et al., 2011).
- Drug causes decreases in bone mineral density (BMD) over time, so bone density should be monitored during treatment.

Most common adverse events:
- Early breast cancer: hot flashes, fatigue, arthralgia, headache, insomnia, increased sweating.
- Advanced breast cancer: hot flashes, nausea, fatigue, increased sweating, increased appetite.

Potential Toxicities/Side Effects and the Nursing Process

I.   ALTERATION IN ACTIVITY related to FATIGUE

Defining Characteristics: Overall incidence in studies is 22%, while incidence considered drug-related or of indeterminate cause is 8%.

Nursing Implications: Assess baseline activity tolerance and self-care ability. Teach patient that fatigue may occur but is usually mild to moderate. Teach patient to alternate rest and activity. Teach patient to manage activities of daily living using energy-saving strategies, e.g., shopping, cooking. Teach patient to accept assistance from friends and family as needed.

II.   ALTERATION IN COMFORT related to HOT FLASHES, INCREASED SWEATING, PAIN

Defining Characteristics: Incidence of events attributable to exemestane were hot flashes (13%) and increased sweating (4%). In total evaluation of all adverse events, all patients, pain was reported in 13%.

Nursing Implications: Assess patient baseline comfort, and incidence and tolerance of hot flashes and increased sweating. Assess whether patient has any pain, as well as effectiveness of current pain-management regimen. Teach patient self-care strategies to maximize comfort, to keep cool (e.g., light, loose clothing; fans; cool drinks) and dry (e.g., use of cornstarch after bathing, fan), and to minimize any painful discomfort (e.g., depending upon type and location of pain, OTC analgesics, application of heat, cold, Tiger Balm).

III.   ALTERATION IN NUTRITION, POTENTIAL, related to NAUSEA, INCREASED APPETITE

Defining Characteristics: Nausea appeared drug-related or of indeterminate cause in 9% of patients, and 3% of patients noted an increased appetite. 8% of patients receiving drug complained of weight gain (greater than 10% of baseline). These side effects are mild to moderate if they occur.

Nursing Implications: Assess baseline nutritional status, optimal and desired weight, and any changes. Teach patient to report nausea or weight gain. Teach patient strategies to minimize nausea (e.g., dietary modification, taking drug after meals) if it occurs, and discuss with physician antiemetic medication if dietary modification not effective. If patient experiences weight gain, discuss patient interest in gentle exercising, such as progressive muscle resistance, which would encourage weight gain as lean body mass rather than fat.

IV.   SENSORY/PERCEPTION ALTERATIONS, POTENTIAL, related to DEPRESSION, INSOMNIA

Defining Characteristics: While not reported as side effects considered drug-related or of indeterminate cause, depression and insomnia occurred in 13% and 11%, respectively, of patients participating in the clinical trials.

Nursing Implications: Assess baseline effect, use of effective coping strategies in dealing with disease and treatment, and usual sleep patterns. Teach patient to report changes in mood, such as depression, and difficulty falling asleep, or early awakening. If this occurs, further assess symptom, and suggest self-care strategies to minimize symptom. If nonpharmacologic measures are ineffective, discuss use of antidepressant or sleeping medication with physician, depending upon assessment.

Drug: floxuridine (FUDR, 2'-deoxy-5-fluorouridine)

Class: Antimetabolite.

Mechanism of Action: Antimetabolite (fluorinated pyrimidine) that is metabolized to 5-FU when given by IV bolus, or metabolized to 5-FUDR-MP 5-fluoro-2'-deoxyuridine-5'-monophosphate when smaller doses are given, by continuous infusion intra-arterially. FUDR-MP is four times more effective in inhibiting the enzyme thymidine synthetase than 5-FU. The inhibition prevents the synthesis of thymidine, an essential component of DNA, resulting in interruption of DNA synthesis and cell death. Other FUDR metabolites inhibit RNA synthesis. Drug is cell cycle specific, with activity during the S phase.

Metabolism: When given IV, drug is transformed to 5-FU; 70–90% of drug is extracted by liver on first pass. Metabolites are excreted by kidneys and lungs. Continuous infusion decreases metabolism of drug with more of the drug being converted to the active metabolite FUDR-MP.

Indication: FDA-approved for intrahepatic arterial infusion only.

Dosage/Range:
* Intra-arterially (hepatic) by slow infusion pump: 0.1–0.6 mg/kg/day × 7–14 days.

Drug Preparation:
* Reconstitute 500-mg vial of lyophilized powder with 5-mL sterile water (100 mg/mL), then dilute with 0.9% sodium chloride or D_5W to volume appropriate for intra-arterial pump.

Drug Administration:
- Usually administered by slow intra-arterial infusion using a surgically placed catheter or percutaneous catheter in a major artery.
- H_2 antagonist antihistamine (i.e., ranitidine 150 mg PO bid) administered concurrently during intra-arterial infusion to prevent development of peptic ulcer disease.

Drug Interactions:
- None significant.

Lab Effects/Interference:
- Decreased WBC, platelets.
- PT, total protein, sedimentation rate (abnormal values).
- Increased LFTs.

Special Considerations:
- Higher doses of the drug increase the risk of biliary sclerosis and fibrosis.
- Drug usually given for 14 days, then heparinized saline for 14 days to maintain line patency.
- Dose reductions or infusion breaks may be necessary depending on toxicity.

Potential Toxicities/Side Effects and the Nursing Process

I.   ALTERED NUTRITION, LESS THAN BODY REQUIREMENTS, related to NAUSEA/VOMITING, ANOREXIA, STOMATITIS/ESOPHOPHARYNGITIS, DIARRHEA, GASTRITIS, HEPATIC DYSFUNCTION

Defining Characteristics: Nausea and vomiting occur infrequently and are mild; anorexia is common. Mucositis is milder than 5-FU when administered intrahepatically, but more severe when given via carotid artery. Diarrhea is mild to moderately severe. Gastritis may occur, with abdominal cramping and pain. Incidence is greater in patients receiving hepatic artery infusion. Duodenal ulcers may occur in 10% of patients, be painless, and lead to gastric outlet obstruction and vomiting. Chemical hepatitis may be severe, with increased alk phos in patients receiving drug via hepatic artery infusions.

Nursing Implications: Premedicate with antiemetics as ordered and teach patient in self-administration of prescribed antiemetics. Encourage small, frequent feedings of cool, bland foods. If intractable nausea and vomiting, severe diarrhea, or severe cramping occurs, notify physician, stop drug, and infuse heparinized saline. Teach patient oral assessment and oral hygiene regimen, and instruct to report any signs/symptoms of stomatitis, esophopharyngitis. Instruct patient to report diarrhea. Teach self-care measures, including diet modification and self-administration of prescribed antidiarrheal medication. Assess for signs/symptoms of abdominal stress, cramping prior to and during infusion. Discuss with physician use of antacids and antisecretory medications. Catheter placement should be verified prior to each infusion cycle, and inadvertent drug infusion into gastric/ duodenal-supplying arteries should be investigated. Monitor LFTs prior to drug initiation, during treatment, and at end of 14-day cycle. Discuss abnormalities and dose reductions with physician. Assess patient for signs/symptoms of liver dysfunction: lethargy, weakness, malaise, anorexia, fever, jaundice, icterus.

II. POTENTIAL FOR INJURY related to INTRA-ARTERIAL CATHETER PROBLEMS

Defining Characteristics: Catheter problems that may occur include leakage, arterial ischemia or aneurysm, bleeding at catheter site, catheter occlusion, thrombosis or embolism of artery, vessel perforation or dislodged catheter, infection, and biliary sclerosis.

Nursing Implications: Assess catheter carefully prior to each cycle of therapy for patency, signs/symptoms of infection. Ensure that catheter position and patency are determined prior to each cycle of therapy; do not force flushing solution—reassess and try again. If still unsuccessful, notify physician.

III. SENSORY/PERCEPTUAL ALTERATIONS related to HAND-FOOT SYNDROME AND OTHER CNS SYMPTOMS

Defining Characteristics: Hand-foot syndrome occurs in 30–40% of patients (numbness, sensory changes in hands and feet). Uncommonly, cerebellar ataxia, vertigo, nystagmus, seizures, depression, hemiplegia, hiccups, lethargy, and blurred vision may occur.

Nursing Implications: Assess baseline neurologic status prior to and during therapy. Teach patient that hand-foot syndrome may occur and instruct to report signs/symptoms. Discuss with physician use of pyridoxine 50 mg tid to prevent hand-foot syndrome. Assess ability to do activities of daily living and level of comfort.

IV. ALTERATION IN SKIN INTEGRITY related to LOCALIZED ERYTHEMA, DERMATITIS, NONSPECIFIC SKIN TOXICITY, OR RASH

Defining Characteristics: Erythema, dermatitis, pruritus, or rash may occur.

Nursing Implications: Assess for skin changes. Assess impact on comfort and body image. Teach patient self-care.

V. POTENTIAL FOR INFECTION AND BLEEDING related to BONE MARROW DEPRESSION

Defining Characteristics: Occurs rarely when FUDR is given as a single agent via continuous intra-arterial infusion.

Nursing Implications: Assess baseline WBC, neutrophil count, and platelets, during treatment and at completion of 14-day infusion. Discontinue drug infusion if WBC < 3,500/mm^3 or if platelet count < 100,000/mm^3, or per established physician orders; refill pump with heparinized saline.

Drug: fludarabine phosphate (Fludara)

Class: Antimetabolite.

Mechanism of Action: Inhibits DNA synthesis, probably by inhibiting DNA-polymerase-alpha, ribonucleotide reductase, and DNA primase.

Metabolism: Drug is rapidly converted to the active metabolite 2-fluoro ara-A when given intravenously. The drug's half-life is about 10 hours. The major route of elimination is via the kidneys, and approximately 23% of the active drug is excreted unchanged in the urine.

Indication: Indicated for the treatment of adult patients with B-cell chronic lymphocytic leukemia (CLL) who have not responded to treatment with at least one standard alkylating agent-containing regimen, or who have progressed on prior treatment.

Dosage/Range:
- IV: 25 mg/m^2 IV over 30 minutes daily × 5 days, repeated every 28 days.
- Oral: 40 mg/m^2 PO daily for 5 days, repeated every 28 days.
- PO/IV: Dose-reduce 20% for creatinine clearance 30–70 mL/min; IV: hold drug if creatinine clearance < 30 mL/min; Oral: reduce dose by 50% for creatinine clearance < 30 mL/min.
- Delay or discontinue drug if neurotoxicity develops.

Drug Preparation:
- IV: Aseptically add 2 mL sterile water for injection USP to the 50-mg vial, resulting in a final concentration of 25 mg/mL. The drug may then be diluted further in 100 mL of 5% dextrose or 0.9% sodium chloride. Once reconstituted, the drug should be used within 8 hours.
- Oral: none, available in 10-mg tablets in blister packs of 5 tablets, in 10- or 20-tablet boxes.

Drug Administration:
- IV infusion over 30 minutes.
- Oral: swallow tablet whole with water; may take with or without food; do not chew or crush.

Drug Interactions:
- Pentostatin: increased risk for severe, potentially fatal pulmonary toxicity; do not administer concomitantly.

Lab Effects/Interference:
- Decreased CBC.
- Tumor lysis syndrome.

Special Considerations:
- Dose-dependent toxicity: overdosage (four times recommended dose) has been associated with delayed blindness, coma, and death.
- Do not administer in combination with pentostatin, as fatal pulmonary toxicity can occur.

- Administer cautiously in patients with renal insufficiency.
- Drug is teratogenic; patients should use effective contraceptions to avoid pregnancy.
- Drug may cause severe bone marrow depression.
- Dose-dependent irreversible neurotoxicity has been observed; discontinue or delay treatment if neurotoxicity develops.
- Postmarketing adverse reactions include progressive multifocal leukoencephalopathy, trilineage bone marrow hypoplasia or aplasia resulting in pancytopenia, and severe pulmonary toxicity.

Potential Toxicities/Side Effects and the Nursing Process

I.   INFECTION AND BLEEDING related to BONE MARROW DEPRESSION

Defining Characteristics: Severe and cumulative bone marrow depression may occur; nadir, 13 days (range, 3–25 days).

Nursing Implications: Monitor CBC, platelet count prior to drug administration, as well as signs/symptoms of infection and bleeding. Instruct patient in self-assessment of signs/symptoms of infection and bleeding as well as self-care measures, including avoidance of OTC aspirin-containing medication.

II.   POTENTIAL FOR ACTIVITY INTOLERANCE related to ANEMIA-INDUCED FATIGUE

Defining Characteristics: Bone marrow depression often includes red cell line.

Nursing Implications: Monitor Hgb/HCT; discuss transfusion with physician if HCT does not recover postchemotherapy. Teach patient high-iron diet as appropriate.

III.   SENSORY/PERCEPTUAL ALTERATIONS related to CNS EFFECTS, PERIPHERAL NEUROPATHIES

Defining Characteristics: Agitation, confusion, visual disturbances, and coma have occurred. Objective weakness has been reported (9–65%), as have paresthesias (4–12%).

Nursing Implications: Assess baseline neurologic status; monitor neurologic vital signs. Teach patient signs/symptoms and instruct to report them if they occur. Evaluate these changes with physician and discuss continuation of therapy.

IV.   POTENTIAL FOR IMPAIRED GAS EXCHANGE related to PULMONARY TOXICITY

Defining Characteristics: Pneumonia occurs in 16–22% of patients. Pulmonary hypersensitivity reaction characterized by dyspnea, cough, interstitial pulmonary infiltrate has been observed. Fatal pulmonary toxicity has occurred when drug is given in combination with pentostatin (Deoxycoformycin).

Nursing Implications: Instruct patient in possible side effects and to report dyspnea, cough, signs of breathlessness following exertion. Assess lung sounds prior to chemotherapy administration. DO NOT administer drug in combination with pentostatin.

V.   POTENTIAL FOR SEXUAL DYSFUNCTION related to TERATOGENICITY

Defining Characteristics: Drug is teratogenic; may cause testicular atrophy. It is unknown whether drug is excreted in breastmilk.

Nursing Implications: As appropriate, explore with patient and partner issues of reproduction and sexuality patterns, and impact that chemotherapy may have. Discuss strategies to preserve sexual and reproductive health (sperm banking, contraception). Mothers receiving drug should not breastfeed.

VI.   ALTERED NUTRITION, LESS THAN BODY REQUIREMENTS, related to NAUSEA/VOMITING, DIARRHEA

Defining Characteristics: Nausea/vomiting occurs in about 30% of patients and can be prevented with standard antiemetics; diarrhea occurs in 15% of patients.

Nursing Implications: Premedicate with antiemetics; evaluate response to emetic protection. Encourage small, frequent meals of cool, bland foods and liquids. If vomiting occurs, assess for signs/symptoms of fluid/electrolyte imbalance; monitor I/O and daily weights, lab results. Encourage patient to report onset of diarrhea; teach patient to administer antidiarrheal medication as ordered.

Drug: fluorouracil, adrucil, 5-FU, 5-fluorouracil (Fluorouracil, Adrucil, 5-FU, Efudex [topical])

Class: Pyrimidine antimetabolite.

Mechanism of Action: Acts as a "false" pyrimidine, inhibiting the formation of an enzyme (thymidine synthetase) necessary for the synthesis of DNA. Also incorporates into RNA, causing abnormal synthesis. Methotrexate given prior to 5-FU results in synergism and enhanced efficacy.

Metabolism: Metabolized by the liver; most is excreted as respiratory CO_2, remainder is excreted by the kidneys. Plasma half-life is 20 minutes.

Indication: In the palliative treatment of carcinoma of the colon, rectum, breast, stomach, and pancreas.

Contraindicated: In the treatment of patients in a poor nutritional state, with depressed bone marrow function, with potentially serious infections, or those with a known hypersensitivity to the drug.

Dosage/Range:
- 12–15 mg/kg IV once per week, OR
- 12 mg/kg IV every day × 5 days every 4 week, OR
- 500 mg/m^2 every week or every week × 5 weeks.
- **Hepatic infusion:** 22 mg/kg in 100 mL 5% dextrose infused into hepatic artery over 8 hours for 5–21 consecutive days.
- Head and neck: 1,000 mg/m^2 day × 4–5 days as continuous infusion.
- **Colon cancer:** Adjuvant:
  - Roswell Park: 5-FU 500 mg/m^2 IVB 1 hour into 2-hour infusion of leucovorin 500 mg/m^2, weekly for 6 weeks, repeated q 8 weeks for a total of 3 cycles (6 months).
  - De Gramont (LV5-FU2): Day 1: Leucovorin 200 mg/m^2 IV over 2 hours d 1, 2; 5-FU 400 mg/m^2 IVB followed by 600 mg/m^2 IV infusion × 22 hours d 1, 2.
  - FLOX and FOLFOX regimens: See oxaliplatin.
- **Metastatic CRC:** A variety of regimens, together with leucovorin, in combination with oxaliplatin, irinotecan, bevacizumab.
- Topical: multiple actinic or solar keratoses: apply twice daily.

Drug Preparation:
- No dilution required. Can be added to 0.9% sodium chloride or 5% dextrose.
- Store at room temperature; protect from light. Solution should be clear: if crystals do not disappear after holding vial under hot water, discard vial.

Drug Administration:
- Given via IV push or bolus (slow drip), or as continuous infusion.
- Topical: As cream.

Drug Interactions:
- Warfarin: may increase anticoagulant effect; monitor INR closely and dose warfarin based on result.
- When given with cimetidine, there are increased pharmacologic effects of fluorouracil.
- When given with thiazide diuretics, there is increased risk of myelosuppression.
- Leucovorin causes increased 5-fluorouracil cytotoxicity.

Lab Effects/Interference:
- Decreased CBC.

Special Considerations:
- Cutaneous side effects occur, e.g., skin sensitivity to sun, splitting of fingernails, dry flaky skin, and hyperpigmentation on face, palms of hands.
- Patients who have had adrenalectomy may need higher doses of prednisone while receiving 5-FU, or dose of 5-FU may be reduced in postadrenalectomy patients.
- Reduce dose in patients with compromised hepatic, renal, or bone marrow function and malnutrition.
- Inspect solution for precipitate prior to continuous infusion.

Potential Toxicities/Side Effects and the Nursing Process

I.   POTENTIAL FOR INFECTION AND BLEEDING related to BONE MARROW DEPRESSION

Defining Characteristics: Nadir 10–14 days after drug dose; neutropenia, thrombocytopenia are dose-related. Toxicity is enhanced when combined with leucovorin calcium.

Nursing Implications: Assess baseline CBC, WBC, differential, and platelet count prior to chemotherapy, as well as for signs/symptoms of infection or bleeding. Teach patient signs/symptoms of infection or bleeding, and instruct to report these immediately; teach patient self-care measures to minimize risk of infection and bleeding. This includes avoidance of crowds and proximity to people with infections, and avoidance of OTC aspirin-containing medications.

II.   ALTERED NUTRITION, LESS THAN BODY REQUIREMENTS, related to NAUSEA AND VOMITING, STOMATITIS, AND DIARRHEA

Defining Characteristics: Nausea and vomiting occur in 30–50% of patients and severity is dose-dependent. Stomatitis can be severe, with onset in 5–8 days, and may herald severe bone marrow depression. Diarrhea can be severe, and in combination with leucovorin, calcium is the dose-limiting toxicity.

Nursing Implications: Premedicate patient with antiemetics (phenothiazines are usually effective), and continue for 24 hours, at least for the first cycle. Encourage small, frequent meals of cool, bland foods. Assess oral mucosa prior to drug administration and instruct patient to report changes. Teach patient oral hygiene measures and self-assessment. Instruct patient to report diarrhea, to self-administer prescribed antidiarrheal medications, and to drink adequate fluids. Moderate to severe stomatitis or diarrhea is an indication to interrupt therapy.

III.   ALTERATION IN SKIN INTEGRITY related to ALOPECIA, CHANGES IN NAILS AND SKIN

Defining Characteristics: Alopecia is more common with 5-day course and involves diffuse thinning of scalp hair, eyelashes, and eyebrows. Brittle nail cracking and loss may occur. Photosensitivity occurs. Chemical phlebitis may occur during continuous infusion with higher doses (pH > 8.0).

Nursing Implications: Teach patient about possible hair loss and skin changes; discuss possible impact on body image. Assess patient's risk for hair loss and skin changes during the therapy and discuss with patient strategies to minimize distress (wig, scarf, nail polish). Instruct patient to use sunblock when outdoors. Suggest implanted venous access device for continuous infusion of 5-FU, especially if patient will receive ongoing therapy.

IV. SENSORY/PERCEPTUAL ALTERATIONS related to PHOTOPHOBIA, CEREBELLAR ATAXIA, OCULAR CHANGES

Defining Characteristics: Photophobia may occur. Occasional cerebellar ataxia may occur and will disappear once drug is stopped. Drug is excreted in tears. Ocular changes that may occur are conjunctivitis, increased lacrimation, photophobia, oculomotor dysfunction, and blurred vision.

Nursing Implications: Assess baseline neurologic status, including vision. Instruct patient to report any changes. Teach patient safety precautions as needed.

Drug: flutamide (Eulexin)

Class: Antiandrogen (nonsteroidal).

Mechanism of Action: Inhibits androgen uptake or inhibits nuclear binding of androgen in target tissues or both.

Metabolism: Rapidly and completely absorbed. Excreted mainly via urine. Biologically active metabolite reaches maximum plasma levels in approximately 2 hours. Plasma half-life is 6 hours. Largely plasma-bound.

Indication: For the treatment of men with locally confined Stage B2-C, and Stage D2 metastatic prostate cancer in combination with an LHRH agonist.
* Stage B2-C: Treatment with flutamide and the LHRH agonist should start 8 weeks prior to initiating R, and continue through RT.
* Stage D2: Combination therapy should continue until progression.
* Contraindicated in patients with severe hepatic dysfunction.

Dosage/Range:
* 250 mg every 8 hours (total daily dose of 750 mg).

Drug Preparation:
* None (available in 125-mg tablets).

Drug Administration:
* Oral.

Drug Interactions:
* Alcohol: increased facial flushing.
* Warfarin: may increase risk of bleeding; monitor INR closely.

Lab Effects/Interference:
* Increased LFTs.
* Increased BUN, creatinine.
* Monitor PSA for changes.

Special Considerations:

- Drug may cause acute hepatic failure within the first 3 months of treatment and is reversible after discontinuation. Teach patient to report jaundice, nausea, vomiting, abdominal (RUQ) tenderness, fatigue, and anorexia and to have liver function evaluated.
- Drug should not be used by pregnant women, as fetal harm may occur.

Potential Toxicities/Side Effects and the Nursing Process

I.   POTENTIAL SEXUAL DYSFUNCTION related to DRUG EFFECTS

Defining Characteristics: Decreased libido and impotence can occur in 33% of patients; gynecomastia occurs in 10% of patients.

Nursing Implications: Assess patient's sexual pattern, any alterations, and patient response. Encourage patient to verbalize feelings; provide information, emotional support, and referral for counseling as available and appropriate.

II.   ALTERATION IN COMFORT related to HOT FLASHES

Defining Characteristics: Hot flashes occur commonly.

Nursing Implications: Teach patient that this may occur, and encourage patient to report symptoms. Provide symptomatic support.

III.   ALTERED NUTRITION, LESS THAN BODY REQUIREMENTS, related to DIARRHEA, NAUSEA, AND VOMITING

Defining Characteristics: Diarrhea and nausea/vomiting occur in 10% of patients.

Nursing Implications: Teach patient that these may occur, and instruct to report them. Assess for occurrence; teach patient self-administration of prescribed antidiarrheal or antiemetic medications.

Drug: fulvestrant injection (Faslodex)

Class: Estrogen receptor antagonist (down regulator).

Mechanism of Action: Fulvestrant is an estrogen receptor antagonist that binds to the estrogen receptor of cells that are dependent upon estrogen for growth, including breast cancer cells that are hormone positive. There is no agonist effect as with other antiestrogens, such as tamoxifen. In addition, the estrogen receptor is also degraded so that it is lost from the cell. Because of this, there is no chance that the hormone receptor can be stimulated by low concentrations of estrogen, as with other antiestrogens, and this theoretically reduces the development of resistance.

Metabolism: When given IM, it takes 7 days for the drug to reach maximal plasma levels, which are maintained for at least 1 month. Half-life is about 40 days, and after 3–6 monthly doses, steady-state plasma area under the curve levels are reached at 2.5 times that of a single-dose injection. Drug undergoes biotransformation similar to endogenous steroids (oxidation, aromatic hydroxylation, conjugation), and oxidative pathway is via cytochrome P450 (CYP3A4). Drug is metabolized by the liver and rapidly cleared from the plasma via the hepatobiliary route. 90% is excreted via the feces; renal excretion is < 1%. There were no pharmacokinetic differences found in the elderly and younger adults, men and women, different races, patients with renal impairment, and patients with mild hepatic impairment. However, patients with moderate to severe liver dysfunction have not been studied.

Indication: For the treatment of hormone receptor positive metastatic breast cancer in postmenopausal women with disease progression following antiestrogen therapy.

Dosage/Range:
- 500 mg given IM, into the buttock on days 1, 15, 29, and once monthly thereafter.
- 250 mg IM is recommended for patients with moderate hepatic impairment, into the buttock on days 1, 15, 29, and once monthly thereafter.

Drug Preparation:
- Drug available in refrigerated 5 mL prefilled syringes containing 50 mg/mL.
- Unopened vials should be stored in the refrigerator at 2–8°C (36–46°F), but do not freeze. Drug can be left at room temperature for a short period of time prior to injection to increase patient comfort.
- Remove glass syringe barrel from tray and ensure it is undamaged.
- Open safety glide needle and attach to Luer lock end of the syringe.
- Expel any air.

Drug Administration:
- Administer IM slowly (1–2 minutes per injection) into the buttocks as two 5 mL injections, one in each buttock, on days 1, 15, 29, and once monthly thereafter.
- Z-track administration is recommended to prevent drug leakage into subcutaneous tissue.
- Following drug injection, activate needle protection device when withdrawing needle from patient by pushing lever arm completely forward until needle tip is fully covered.
- If unable to activate, drop into sharps disposal container.

Drug Interactions:
- None significant, as drug does not significantly inhibit the major CYP isoenzymes, including rifampin.
- Herbals that contain estrogen may decrease the drug effect.

Lab Effects/Interference:
- None.

Special Considerations:
Warnings and precautions:
- Blood disorders: use with caution in patients with bleeding diathesis, thrombocytopenia, or anticoagulant use.
- Hepatic impairment: dose reduction for patients with moderate hepatic impairment. Drug has not been studied in patients with severe hepatic impairment.

- Drug should not be used during pregnancy: teach women of childbearing potential to use effective contraception to avoid pregnancy. If patient becomes pregnant while receiving the drug, the patient should be apprised of the potential hazard to the fetus.
- Nursing mothers should decide whether to discontinue nursing or discontinue the drug, taking into account the importance of the drug to the mother's health.
- Injection-site reactions more common when drug is given in two divided doses.

Potential Toxicities/Side Effects and the Nursing Process

I.   ALTERATION IN COMFORT related to INJECTION-SITE REACTION, ABDOMINAL PAIN, BACK PAIN

Defining Characteristics: Injection-site reactions (pain and inflammation) occurred in 7% of patients receiving a single 5-mL injection (European trial) as compared to 27% of patients (North American trial) receiving two 2.5-mL injections, one in each buttock. Back and bone pain occurred in 15.8% of patients, while abdominal pain occurred in 11.8% of patients and often was associated with other gastrointestinal symptoms.

Nursing Implications: Teach patient this may occur and to report it. Consider using Z-track method, and if using two separate injections of 2.5 mL, try a single-dose injection to see if discomfort is reduced. Teach patient to report bone and/or back pain. Teach patient to use OTC analgesics such as acetaminophen or nonsteroidal anti-inflammatory drugs as appropriate to bleeding history or risk factors. Discuss alternatives with physician if ineffective in symptom management.

II.   ALTERATION IN NUTRITION, POTENTIAL, related to NAUSEA, VOMITING, CONSTIPATION, DIARRHEA

Defining Characteristics: Nausea occurs in 26%, vomiting 13%, constipation 12.5%, diarrhea 12.3%, and anorexia 9%.

Nursing Implications: Assess baseline appetite, presence of nausea and/or vomiting, and bowel elimination pattern. Teach patient that these side effects may occur, self-care measures to minimize nausea and vomiting such as dietary modification, and to report these side effects. Discuss antiemetics with physician if dietary modification is ineffective. Teach patient to use dietary modification to relieve constipation or diarrhea and, if ineffective, to use OTC laxatives or antidiarrheal medicine. If ineffective, discuss pharmacologic management with physician.

III.   ALTERATION IN SKIN INTEGRITY, POTENTIAL, related to HOT FLASHES AND PERIPHERAL EDEMA

Defining Characteristics: Vasodilation or hot flashes occurred in 17.7% of patients, and peripheral edema in 9% of patients.

Nursing Implications: Assess baseline skin integrity, history of hot flashes in postmenopausal patients, and presence of peripheral edema. Teach patient these side effects may occur and to report them. If hot flashes are severe, review common hot flash management including wearing loose, layered clothing that can be removed when the woman becomes hot, sipping cold beverages throughout the day, sleeping with light nightgown and window open, avoiding triggers such as caffeine or alcohol, and if ineffective, discuss use of venlafaxine (Effexor) or fluoxetine (Paxil) to reduce intensity and frequency of hot flashes (Loprinski et al., 2000). Teach patient self-assessment of peripheral edema, to wear loose stockings and shoes, to keep skin moisturized to prevent cracking, and comfort measures. Teach patient to report increasing edema or related problems.

Drug: gemcitabine hydrochloride (Gemzar, difluorodeoxycytidine)

Class: Nucleoside metabolic inhibitor (Antimetabolite).

Mechanism of Action: Inhibits DNA synthesis by inhibiting DNA polymerase activity through a process called masked chain termination. It is a prodrug, structurally similar to ara-C, needing intracellular phosphorylation. It then inhibits DNA synthesis. Cell cycle-specific for S phase, causing cells to accumulate at the G_1–S boundary.

Metabolism: Pharmacokinetics varies by age, gender, and infusion time. Half life for short infusions ranges from 32–94 minutes, while that of long infusions ranges from 245–638 minutes. Following short infusions (< 70 minutes), the drug is not extensively tissue-bound; following long infusions (70–285 minutes), the drug slowly equilibrates within tissues. The terminal half-life of the parent drug, gemcitabine, is 17 minutes. There is negligible binding to serum proteins. Drug and metabolites are excreted in the urine, with 92–98% of the drug dose recovered in the urine within 1 week. Mean systemic clearance is 90 L/h/m^2. Clearance is about 30% lower in women than in men, and also reduced in the elderly, but this does not necessarily require a dose reduction.

Indications:
- In combination with carboplatin, for the treatment of advanced ovarian cancer that has relapsed at least 6 months after completion of platinum-based therapy.
- In combination with paclitaxel, for the first-line treatment of metastatic breast cancer after failure of prior anthracycline-containing adjuvant chemotherapy, unless anthracyclines were clinically contraindicated.
- In combination with cisplatin for the treatment of NSCLC.
- As a single agent for the treatment of pancreatic cancer.

Dosage/Range:
Adults:
- **Breast cancer:** 1250 mg/m^2 IV over 30 minutes d 1, 8 q 21 days, in combination with paclitaxel 175 mg/m^2 IV over 3 hours administered prior to gemcitabine, day 1 repeated q 21 days.
  - Day 1 ANC must be ≥ 1,500 × 10^6/L and a platelet count of ≥ 100,000 × 10^6/L prior to each cycle. If ANC < 1,500/mm3 or platelets < 100,000, delay treatment cycle.

- Dose-reduce 25% day 8 dose for ANC 1,000–1,199/mm^3 or platelets 50,000–75,000 × 10^6/L.
- Dose-reduce for ANC 799-999/mm^3 and platelets ≥ = 50,000/mm^3 × 10^6/L, but hold drug if ANC < 700/mm^3 or platelets < 50,000/mm^3 × 10^6/L.
- Hold drug if ANC < 500/mm^3 or platelets < 50,000 × 10^6/L.
- **Pancreatic cancer:** 1,000 mg/m^2 IV infusion over 30 min every week for up to 7 weeks (or until toxicity necessitates dose reduction or delay), then followed by 1-week break. Weeks 8+: weekly dosing on Days 1, 8, 15 of a 28-day cycle.
  - Dose-reduce 25% if ANC 500–999/mm^3 or platelets 50–99,000 × 10^6/L, and hold if ANC < 500/mm^3 or platelets < 50,000 × 10^6/L.
- **Non–small-cell lung cancer** (inoperable, locally advanced stage IIIA and IIIB or meta-static) in combination with cisplatin: **4-week cycle**: 1,000 mg/m^2 IV over 30 minutes on days 1, 8, and 15, repeat q 28 days, with cisplatin 100 mg/m^2 IV on day 1 after the gemcitabine infusion; or as a **3-week cycle**, with gemcitabine 1250 mg/m^2 IV over 30 minutes on days 1 and 8; cisplatin 100 mg/m^2 IV is given following gemcitabine infu-sion on day 1, repeated q 3 weeks.
  - Dose-reduce 25% if ANC 500–999/mm^3 or platelets 50–99,000 × 10^6/L, and hold if ANC < 500/mm^3 or platelets < 50,000 × 10^6/L.
  - Dose-reduce 50% for grade 3–4 nonhematologic toxicities when gemcitabine given with cisplatin.
- **Ovarian cancer:** 1,000 mg/m^2 IV over 30 minutes on days 1 and 8 of each 21-day cycle, together with carboplatin (AUC 4) IV on day 1 after gemcitabine administration.
  - Day 1: ANC must be ≥ 1,500 × 10^6/L and a platelet count of ≥ 100,000 × 10^6/L prior to each cycle. If ANC < 1,500/mm3 or platelets < 100,000, delay treatment cycle.
  - Dose modify day 8 if ANC 1,000–1,499/mm^3/or platelets 75–99,999 × 10^6/L by giving 50% of dose; hold dose if values are lower than this.
  - See package insert for dose modification for myelosuppression in previous cycles.
- **Grade 3-4 Nonhematologic Toxicity.** Hold or 50% dose reduction (except alopecia, nausea or vomiting). Permanently discontinue gemcitabine for:
  - Unexplained dyspnea or other evidence of severe pulmonary toxicity,
  - Severe hepatic toxicity,
  - Hemolytic-uremic syndrome,
  - Capillary leak syndrome,
  - Posterior reversible encephalopathy syndrome.

Drug Preparation:
- Drug available in single-use vials of 200 mg/10 mL and 1 g/50 mL.
- Use 0.9% sodium chloride USP and reconstitute the 200-mg vial with 5 mL, and the 1-g vial with 25 mL.
- Shake to dissolve the powder. This results in a concentration of 38 mg/mL.
- Withdraw recommended dose and further dilute in 0.9% sodium chloride injection.
- Discard unused portion. Inspect solution for particulate matter or discoloration and do not use if these occur.

- Stable 24 hours at room temperature (20–25°C [68–77°F]). DO NOT refrigerate, as drug crystallization may occur.

Drug Administration:
- ANC ≥ 1,500/mm^3 and platelets ≥ 100,000 × 10^6/L for day 1 treatment; assess CBC/differential, LFTs, and renal function before each cycle.
- Administer IV over 30 minutes. Infusion time > 60 minutes or dosing more frequently than weekly is associated with greater toxicity.
- Administer gemcitabine before cisplatin.
- Administer gemcitabine after paclitaxel.

Drug Interactions:
- Administer cisplatin after gemcitabine to enhance renal drug clearance; paclitaxel should be administered before gemcitabine.

Lab Effects/Interference:
- Decreased CBC.
- Increased LFTs.

Special Considerations:
- Monitor liver and renal function at baseline and throughout therapy; use cautiously in patients with renal or hepatic dysfunction and monitor closely; drug may aggravate hepatic dysfunction. Discontinue drug for severe hepatic toxicity.
- Dose reduction or delay required for hematologic toxicity.
- Drug can rarely cause severe pulmonary toxicity (interstitial pneumonitis, pulmonary fibrosis, pulmonary edema, adult respiratory distress syndrome), occurring up to 2 weeks following the last gemcitabine infusion. If patient develops new onset dyspnea, with or without bronchospasm, stop gemcitabine until further pulmonary evaluation can proceed; discontinue drug if related to gemcitabine.
- Hemolytic uremic syndrome (HUS) and/or renal failure have been reported rarely.
- Drug is a radiosensitizer, and radiation recall may occur.
- Monitoring labs: hepatic and renal function baseline and periodically during treatment; CBC/differential before each dose; serum creatinine, potassium, calcium, magnesium during combination with cisplatin.
- Use with caution in patients with impaired renal function or hepatic dysfunction. (Studies have not been done to identify risks in this population.)
- Rarely, HUS (hemolytic uremic syndrome) has occurred. Discontinue drug if signs/symptoms occur (rapid decrease in hemoglobin and thrombocytopenia, together with elevated BUN/creatinine). Observe for elevation of serum bili or LDH.
- Drug may cause sedation in 10% of patients; caution patient not to drive or operate heavy machinery until it is determined whether patient develops this side effect.
- Drug is embryotoxic; women of childbearing age should use effective contraception to avoid pregnancy while receiving the drug.
- Drug may be irritating to the vein, requiring local heat; may require a central line for (long-term) administration.

- Drug can exacerbate radiation therapy toxicity, and it may cause severe or life-threatening toxicity if given during or within 7 days of RT.
- Capillary leak syndrome has been described. Discontinue gemcitabine if this occurs.
- Posterior reversible encephalopathy syndrome (PRES) may occur; if so, discontinue gemcitabine.
- The most common adverse reactions for drug as a single agent (incidence ≥ 20%) are nausea/vomiting, anemia, hepatic transaminitis, neutropenia, increased alkaline phosphatase, proteinuria, fever, hematuria, rash, thrombocytopenia, dyspnea, and peripheral edema.

Potential Toxicities/Side Effects and the Nursing Process

I. POTENTIAL FOR INFECTION AND BLEEDING related to BONE MARROW DEPRESSION

Defining Characteristics: Myelosuppression is dose-limiting toxicity. Incidence of leukopenia is 63%, thrombocytopenia 36%, and anemia 73%. Dose reductions required are shown in the Special Considerations section. Grades 3–4 thrombocytopenia are more common in the elderly, and grades 3–4 neutropenia and thrombocytopenia are more common in women (especially older women). Older women were less able to complete subsequent courses of therapy. Myelosuppression is usually short-lived with recovery within 1 week. Approximately 19% of patients require RBC transfusions.

Nursing Implications: Assess baseline CBC, WBC, differential, and platelet count prior to chemotherapy, as well as for signs/symptoms of infection or bleeding. Discuss dose reductions or delay based on neutrophil and platelet counts. Teach patient signs/symptoms of infection or bleeding, and instruct to report these immediately. Teach patient self-care measures to minimize risk of infection and bleeding. This includes avoidance of crowds, proximity to people with infections, and OTC aspirin-containing medications. Transfuse red blood cells and platelets as needed per physician order.

II. POTENTIAL ALTERATION IN NUTRITION, LESS THAN BODY REQUIREMENTS, related to NAUSEA AND VOMITING, DIARRHEA, STOMATITIS, AND ALTERATIONS IN LFTS

Defining Characteristics: Nausea and vomiting occur in 69% of patients, and of these, < 15% are severe. Nausea and vomiting are usually mild to moderate and are easily prevented or controlled by antiemetics. Diarrhea may occur (19% incidence), as may stomatitis (11% incidence). Abnormalities in liver transaminases occur in two-thirds of patients; rarely does this require drug discontinuance.

Nursing Implications: Premedicate patient with antiemetics (phenothiazides are usually effective). Encourage small, frequent meals of cool, bland foods. Teach patient self-administration of prescribed antiemetic medications, and to drink adequate fluids. Assess oral mucosa prior to drug administration, and instruct patient to report changes. Teach patient oral hygiene measures and self-assessment. Instruct patient to report diarrhea, to self-administer prescribed antidiarrheal medications, and to drink adequate fluids. Monitor LFTs baseline and periodically during therapy. Notify physician of any abnormalities and discuss implications. Drug should be used cautiously in any patient with hepatic dysfunction.

III. POTENTIAL ALTERATION IN COMFORT related to FLU-LIKE SYMPTOMS

Defining Characteristics: Flu-like symptoms occur in 20% of patients with first treatment dose. Transient febrile episodes occur in 41% of patients.

Nursing Implications: Encourage patient to report flu-like symptoms. Treat fevers with acetaminophen per physician. Assess for alterations in comfort, and discuss symptomatic measures. If severe, discuss drug discontinuance with physician.

IV. IMPAIRED SKIN INTEGRITY related to ALOPECIA, RASH, PRURITUS, EDEMA

Defining Characteristics: Skin rash occurs in about 30% of patients, often within 2–3 days of starting drug. The rash is erythematous, pruritic, and/or maculopapular, and may occur on the neck and extremities. Edema occurs in about 30% of patients, and is primarily peripheral but can rarely be facial or pulmonary. Edema is reversible after drug is discontinued, and appears unrelated to cardiac, renal, or hepatic impairment. Edema is usually mild to moderate. Minimal hair loss occurs in 15% of patients, and is reversible.

Nursing Implications: Assess skin integrity and presence of rash, pruritus, alopecia, and edema prior to dosing. Assess impact of these alterations on patient, and develop plan to manage symptom distress and promote skin integrity. Instruct patient to report rash, itching; discuss treatment of rash with topical corticosteroids. Teach patient self-assessment of signs/symptoms of edema, and instruct to notify healthcare provider if swelling occurs. If severe, discuss drug discontinuance with physician.

Drug: goserelin acetate (Zoladex)

Class: Gonadotropin Releasing Hormone (GnRH).

Mechanism of Action: Inhibits pituitary gonadotropin, achieving a chemical orchiectomy in 2–4 weeks. Sustained-release medication provides continuous drug diffusion from the depot into subcutaneous tissue. This permits monthly injection instead of daily.

Metabolism: Absorbed slowly for first 8 days, then more rapid and constant absorption for remaining 28 days. Time to peak concentration 12–15 days for males and 8–22 days for females.

Indication: Indicated for (1) palliative treatment of advanced prostate cancer; (2) treatment of locally confined prostate cancer in combination with flutamide; drug also indicated for 3) use as an endometrial thinning agent prior to endometrial ablation for dysfunctional uterine bleeding; and 4) palliative treatment of advanced breast cancer in pre-and perimenopausal women.

Contraindication: (1) Hypersensitivity; (2) pregnancy, unless used for the treatment of advanced breast cancer.

Dosage/Range:
Adults:
- Subcutaneous: 3.6-mg dose into the anterior upper abdominal wall below the navel line every 28 days or the 10.8-mg implant every 3 months.

Drug Preparation:
- Inspect package for damage. Open package and inspect drug in translucent chamber.
- Select site on upper abdomen.
- Prepare site with alcohol swab, cleansing from center outward.
- Administer local anesthetic as ordered.
- Aseptically, stretch skin at site with nondominant hand, and insert needle into subcutaneous tissue with dominant hand at 45-degree angle.
- Redirect needle so it is parallel to the abdominal wall. Advance needle forward until hub touches skin. Withdraw needle 1 cm (approximately ½ inch).
- Depress plunger fully, expelling depot into prepared site.
- Withdraw needle carefully. Apply gentle pressure bandage to site. Confirm that tip of plunger is visible within needle tip.
- Document in chart.

Drug Interactions:
- None.

Lab Effects/Interference:
- Hypercalcemia in patients with bone metastases.
- Tests of pituitary/gonadal function may be inaccurate while on therapy due to suppression of pituitary/gonadal system.
- Hyperglycemia.

Special Considerations:
- Compliance to 28-day injection schedule is important.
- Initially, there is transient increase in serum testosterone levels, with flare of symptoms during the first few weeks of treatment, which may include ureteral obstruction and spinal cord compression. Closely monitor patients at risk for complications of tumor flare. Tumor flare may also occur in women with breast cancer on initiation of goserlin acetate.
- Hypersensitivity (systemic) has been reported in patients receiving implants. Monitor closely.
- Hyperglycemia and increased risk of developing diabetes have been reported in patients receiving GnRH analogues. Monitor blood glucose baseline and during treatment, and manage using current clinical guidelines.

- Cardiovascular diseases, including risk of MI, sudden cardiac death, and stroke have been reported in men receiving GnRH analogues. Monitor patients for cardiovascular disease and manage current clinical guidelines.
- Hypercalcemia has been reported in patients with bone metastases; monitor and treat appropriately.
- The most common clinically significant adverse reactions occurring in >10% of men: hot flashes, sexual dysfunction, decreased erections, and lower urinary symptoms. Tumor flare can occur on goserlin acetate initiation. The most common adverse events for women treated with breast cancer, dysfunctional uterine bleeding or endometiosis (>20% of patients) were: hot flushes, headache, sweating, acne, emotional lability, depression, decreased libido, vaginitis, breast atrophy, seborrhea, and peripheral edema.
- Premenopausal women must use effective contraception during and for 12 weeks after treatment with the drug.
- Nursing mothers should decide whether to discontinue nursing or to discontinue the drug, taking into account the importance of the drug to the mother.
- New data shows drug used with cyclophosphamide (which induces ovarian failure) minimizes risk of early menopause and loss of fertility (Moore et al., 2014).

Potential Toxicities/Side Effects and the Nursing Process

I.   SEXUAL DYSFUNCTION related to DECREASED TESTOSTERONE LEVELS

Defining Characteristics: Hot flashes, sexual dysfunction, and decreased erections can occur.

Nursing Implications: Assess normal sexual pattern. Refer as needed for sexual counseling.

II.   POTENTIAL ALTERATION IN CARDIAC OUTPUT related to ARRHYTHMIA, CARDIOVASCULAR DYSFUNCTION

Defining Characteristics: Arrhythmia, cerebrovascular accident (CVA), hypertension, myocardial infarction, peripheral vascular disease, chest pain may occur in 1–5% of patients.

Nursing Implications: Assess heart rate, blood pressure, peripheral pulses. Teach patient to report palpitations, shortness of breath, chest pain, or leg pain immediately. Evaluate abnormalities with physician.

III.   SENSORY/PERCEPTUAL ALTERATION related to ANXIETY, DEPRESSION, HEADACHE

Defining Characteristics: Anxiety, depression, headache may occur (< 5%).

Nursing Implications: Assess baseline effect, comfort. Instruct patient to report mood disorder. Encourage patient to verbalize feelings, provide patient with emotional support, assess efficacy of supportive care, and if needed, discuss pharmacologic management of symptoms with physician.

IV.   ALTERATION IN NUTRITION, LESS THAN BODY REQUIREMENTS, related to VOMITING, HYPERGLYCEMIA

Defining Characteristics: Vomiting may occur (< 5%); also increased weight, ulcer, hyperglycemia.

Nursing Implications: Teach patient to report GI disturbances. Assess severity and discuss management with physician. Assess serum glucose, and if abnormal, discuss dietary or pharmacologic management, depending upon severity, with physician.

V.   ALTERATION IN BOWEL ELIMINATION related to CONSTIPATION OR DIARRHEA

Defining Characteristics: Constipation or diarrhea may occur (< 5%).

Nursing Implications: Instruct patient to report problems in elimination. Teach symptomatic management.

VI.   ALTERATION IN URINARY ELIMINATION related to OBSTRUCTION OR INFECTION

Defining Characteristics: Urinary obstruction, urinary tract infection, renal insufficiency may occur.

Nursing Implications: Monitor baseline urinary elimination pattern, baseline kidney function tests, and continue to monitor through therapy. Instruct patient to report signs/ symptoms of urinary tract infection (UTI).

VII.   ALTERATION IN COMFORT related to FEVER, CHILLS, TENDERNESS

Defining Characteristics: Chills, fever, breast swelling, and tenderness. Also, discomfort may result from injection, as a 16-gauge needle is used to inject depot.

Nursing Implications: Instruct patient to report discomfort. Discuss strategies to increase comfort. Administer local anesthetic prior to injection of medication (per physician's order).

Drug: histrelin implant (Vantas)

Class: Synthetic analogue of gonadotropin-releasing factor (GnRH).

Mechanism of Action: Histrelin inhibits pituitary gonadotropin, achieving a chemical orchiectomy.

Metabolism: Implant delivers histrelin continuously for 12 months at 50–60 micrograms per day. Drug serum concentration 50% higher in patients with severe renal dysfunction, but this is not considered clinically significant.

Indication: Palliative treatment of patients with advanced prostate cancer.

Contraindication: Known hypersensitivity; pregnancy.

Dosage/Range:
Adults:
- Histrelin implant (50 mg) is aseptically inserted subcutaneously under skin on upper, inner arm using implant tool; at 12 months, implant must be removed before new one is implanted.

Drug Preparation:
- Keep implant refrigerated until implanted.
- Select site on upper inner arm, and follow guidelines in package insert using aseptic technique and implant tool.
- Implant is NOT radio-opaque, so care must be given to carefully secure the implant as directed.

Drug Interactions:
- Unknown.

Lab Effects/Interference:
- Hypercalcemia in patients with bone metastases.
- Tests of pituitary/gonadal function may be inaccurate while on therapy due to suppression of pituitary/gonadal system.
- Decreased serum testosterone to below castrate levels.

Special Considerations:
- Initially (1st week of treatment), there is transient increase in serum testosterone levels, with flare of symptoms or onset of new symptoms such as bone pain, neuropathy, hematuria, or ureteral/bladder outlet obstruction. If severe (rarely spinal cord compression, ureteral obstruction), these should be managed immediately.
- Patients with metastatic vertebral and/or urinary tract obstruction should be monitored very closely during the first few weeks of treatment.
- The most common adverse reactions observed in >5% of men: hot flashes, fatigue, implant-site reactions, testicular atrophy.
- Response to the drug should be monitored using serum concentrations of testosterone and PSA periodically, especially if the anticipated clinical or biochemical response has not been achieved.

Warnings and Precautions:
- Transient increase in serum testosterone levels, with flare of symptoms or onset of new symptoms such as bone pain, neuropathy, hematuria, or ureteral/bladder outlet obstruction.

- Rarely spinal cord compression and ureteral obstruction may occur: these should be managed immediately.
- Patients with metastatic vertebral and/or urinary tract obstruction should be monitored very closely during the first few weeks of treatment.
- Difficulty locating or removing implant has been reported. Caution is recommended.
- Hyperglycemia and increased risk of developing diabetes have been reported in patients receiving GnRH analogues. Monitor blood glucose baseline and during treatment, and manage using current clinical guidelines.
- Cardiovascular diseases, including risk of MI, sudden cardiac death, and stroke have been reported in men receiving GnRH analogues. Monitor patients for cardiovascular disease and manage current clinical guidelines.

Potential Toxicities/Side Effects and the Nursing Process

I.   SEXUAL DYSFUNCTION related to DECREASED TESTOSTERONE LEVELS

Defining Characteristics: Hot flashes (66% with 2.3% severe), testicular atrophy (5.3%), gynecomastia (4.1%), decreased libido (2.3%), and erectile dysfunction (3.5%) can occur.

Nursing Implications: Assess normal sexual pattern. Encourage patient to verbalize feelings to assess impact of symptoms on sexual function; refer as needed for sexual counseling. Teach patient self-care strategies to reduce distress of hot flashes.

II.   ALTERATION IN BOWEL ELIMINATION related to CONSTIPATION

Defining Characteristics: Constipation may occur (< 5%).

Nursing Implications: Instruct patient to report problems in elimination. Teach symptomatic management.

III.   ALTERATION IN URINARY ELIMINATION related to OBSTRUCTION OR INFECTION

Defining Characteristics: Urinary obstruction, urinary tract infection, renal insufficiency may occur. Renal impairment occurs in 4.7% of patients.

Nursing Implications: Monitor baseline urinary elimination pattern, baseline kidney function tests, and continue to monitor through therapy. Instruct patient to report signs/symptoms of urinary tract infection (UTI).

IV.   ALTERATION IN COMFORT related to IMPLANT SITE IRRITATION, ASTHENIA, AND INSOMNIA

Defining Characteristics: Implantation site reactions occur in at least 5.8% of patients: these include bruising, pain/soreness/tenderness after insertion or removal; rarely, erythema and swelling may occur. Asthenia occurs in about 10% of patients, and insomnia in 2.9% of patients.

Nursing Implications: Instruct patient to report discomfort. Discuss strategies to increase comfort. Teach patient to self-assess and reassure local effects will resolve. Teach patient to report any signs/symptoms of infection.

Drug: hydroxyurea (Hydrea, Droxia)

Class: Antimetabolite.

Mechanism of Action: Prevents conversion of ribonucleotides to deoxyribonucleotides by inhibiting the converting enzyme ribonucleoside diphosphate reductase. DNA synthesis is thus inhibited. Cell cycle phase specific for S phase. May also sensitize cells to the effects of radiation therapy, although the process is not clearly understood.

Metabolism: Rapidly absorbed from GI tract. Peak plasma level reached in 2 hours, with plasma half-life of 3–4 hours. About half the drug is metabolized in the liver and half is excreted in urine as urea and unchanged drug. Some of the drug is eliminated as respiratory CO_2. Crosses BBB.

Indication: Significant tumor response to hydroxyurea capsules has been demonstrated in melanoma, CML, and recurrent, metastatic, or inoperable carcinoma of the ovary. Drug is used concommitantly with RT in the local control of primary squamous cell carcinomas of the head and neck, excluding the lip.

Contraindication: (1) Patients with WBC < 2,500 or thrombocytopenia (platelets < 100K), or severe anemia; (2) patients hypersensitve to drug or its components.

Dosage/Range:
- 500–3,000 mg PO daily (dose reduced in renal dysfunction).
- 20–30 mg/kg/day PO as a continuous dose.
- 100 mg/kg IV daily × 3 days.
- Dose modification in renal dysfunction: Reduce dose by 50% if creatinine clearance 10–50 mL/ min; reduce dose 80% (give only 20% of dose) if creatinine clearance <10 mL/min.
- **Radiation sensitization:** 80 mg/kg as a single dose every third day, starting at least 7 days before initiation of radiation.
- **Sickle cell disease**: To prevent painful crises, initial 15 mg/kg/day, increased by 5 mg/kg every 12 weeks to a maximum dose of 35 mg/kg/day as tolerated.

Drug Preparation:
- None. Hydrea available in 500-mg capsules or Droxia in 200-mg, 300-mg, and 400-mg tablets.

Drug Administration:
- Oral.
- High-dose IV continuous infusions are being studied with doses of 0.5–1 $g/m^2/day$ × 5–12 weeks (investigational).

Drug Interactions:
- None significant.

Lab Effects/Interference:
- Decreased CBC.
- Increased BUN, creatinine, uric acid.
- Increased hepatic enzymes.

Special Considerations:
- Hydroxyurea has a side effect of dramatically lowering the WBC in a relatively short period of time (24–48 hours). In leukemia patients endangered by the potential complication of leukostasis, this is the desired effect.
- May need to pretreat with allopurinol to protect patient from tumor lysis syndrome.
- Dermatologic radiation recall phenomena may occur.
- In combination with radiation therapy, mucosal reactions in the radiation field may be severe and require dose interruption.
- Drug used in the treatment of chronic myelogenous leukemia (CML) in chronic phase, as a radiosensitizer (primary brain tumors, head and neck cancer, cancer of the cervix or uterus, non–small-cell lung cancer), and in sickle cell anemia.
- Drug should not be used during pregnancy or by breastfeeding mothers, as drug is excreted in breastmilk.

Potential Toxicities/Side Effects and the Nursing Process

I.   INFECTION AND BLEEDING related to BONE MARROW DEPRESSION

Defining Characteristics: WBC begins to decrease 24–48 hours after beginning therapy, with nadir in 10 days and recovery within 10–30 days. Leukopenia more common than thrombocytopenia and anemia, and is dose-related.

Nursing Implications: Assess CBC, WBC with differential, and platelet count prior to drug administration, as well as for signs/symptoms of infection or bleeding. Doses may need to be reduced if patient has undergone prior radiotherapy or chemotherapy. Dose must be reduced if patient has renal dysfunction. Discuss any abnormalities with physician prior to drug administration. Teach patient signs/symptoms of infection and bleeding, and instruct to report them immediately. Teach self-care measures to minimize risk of infection and bleeding, including avoidance of OTC aspirin-containing medications.

II.   ALTERED NUTRITION, LESS THAN BODY REQUIREMENTS, related to NAUSEA AND VOMITING, DIARRHEA, STOMATITIS, ANOREXIA, HEPATIC DYSFUNCTION

Defining Characteristics: Nausea and vomiting are uncommon, anorexia is mild to moderate, stomatitis is uncommon, diarrhea is uncommon, and hepatic dysfunction is rare, although abnormal LFTs may occur.

Nursing Implications: Premedicate with antiemetics as needed. Teach self-administration of prescribed medications. Instruct patient to report nausea/vomiting, diarrhea, anorexia, and stomatitis. Teach patient oral hygiene regimen and assess baseline oral mucosa. Monitor baseline LFTs, and monitor them periodically during therapy.

III. POTENTIAL ALTERATION IN FLUID/ELECTROLYTES/RENAL ELIMINATION STATUS related to TUMOR LYSIS SYNDROME

Defining Characteristics: When drug is first started in patients with high tumor burden (e.g., CML with high WBC), this often results in rapid death of a large number of malignant cells. The lysis or breakdown of these cells results in the release of intracellular contents into the systemic circulation. The resulting metabolic abnormalities are hyperkalemia, hyperphosphatemia, hypocalcemia, and hyperuricemia. If these persist, renal failure with oliguria can result.

Nursing Implications: Assess baseline chemistries, including metabolic panel, renal function. Expect that if the patient is at risk for the development of tumor lysis syndrome, the patient will begin allopurinol 200–300 mg/m^2/day prior to therapy, and receive hydration with alkalization (e.g., 50–100 mEq bicarbonate added per liter) to deliver 3 liters/m^2/day. Assess serum potassium, phosphate, calcium, uric acid, and BUN and creatinine at least daily, and discuss any abnormalities with physician to revise current regimen. Monitor I/O, weights, and total body balance carefully, and at least daily.

IV. SENSORY/PERCEPTUAL ALTERATIONS related to DROWSINESS, HALLUCINATIONS, OTHER CNS EFFECTS

Defining Characteristics: Drug crosses the BBB, so CNS effects may occur, such as drowsiness, confusion, disorientation, headache, vertigo; symptoms last < 24 hours.

Nursing Implications: Assess baseline mental status and neurologic functioning. Instruct patient to report signs/symptoms, and reassure that they will resolve. If symptoms persist, discuss interrupting drug with physician.

V. POTENTIAL SEXUAL/REPRODUCTIVE DYSFUNCTION related to DRUG EFFECTS

Defining Characteristics: Drug is mutagenic and teratogenic. Drug is excreted in breastmilk.

Nursing Implications: Assess patient's sexual patterns and reproductive goals. Discuss with patient and partner potential toxicity and impact on sexuality. Provide information, emotional support, and referral as needed. Patient should use contraceptive measures; a mother receiving the drug should not breastfeed.

Drug: idarubicin (Idamycin, 4-demethoxydaunorubicin)

Class: Antitumor antibiotic.

Mechanism of Action: Cell cycle phase specific for S phase. Analogue of daunorubicin. Has a marked inhibitory effect on RNA synthesis.

Metabolism: Excreted primarily in the bile and urine, with approximately 25% of the intravenous dose accounted for over 5 days. The half-life is 6–9.4 hours.

Indication: In combination with other approved anti-leukemic drugs, for the treatment of acute myeloid leukemia (AML) in adults.

Dosage/Range:
- Induction: 12 mg/m^2 daily slow IVP × 3 days in combination with ara-C 100 mg/m^2 continuous infusion × 7 days, with consolidation using 10–12 mg/m^2/day × 2 days.
- Dose-reduce for renal dysfunction.
- Dose-reduce for hepatic dysfunction: give 50% of dose if serum bili is ≥ 2.5 mg/dL; do not give dose if serum bili is > 5 mg/dL.

Drug Preparation:
- Available as a red powder.
- The drug is reconstituted with 0.9% sodium chloride injection to give a final concentration of 1 mg/1 mL.

Drug Administration:
- Drug is a vesicant. Administer IV over 10 to 15 minutes into the sidearm of a patent, freely running IV.
- Dose reduction (25%) recommended if renal dysfunction (serum creatinine > 2 mg/dL) or for severe mucositis.

Drug Interactions:
- Other myelosuppressive drugs: additive bone marrow suppression; monitor patient closely.
- Incompatible with heparin—causes precipitant.

Lab Effects/Interference:
- Decreased CBC.
- Increased LFTs, RFTs.

Special Considerations:
- Vesicant.
- Discolored urine (pink to red) may occur up to 48 hours after administration.
- Cardiomyopathy is less common and less severe than with doxorubicin and daunorubicin.
- Drug is light-sensitive.

Potential Toxicities/Side Effects and the Nursing Process

I.   INFECTION AND BLEEDING related to BONE MARROW DEPRESSION

Defining Characteristics: Hematologic toxicity is dose limiting. Leukopenia nadir 10–20 days with recovery in 1–2 weeks. Thrombocytopenia usually follows leukopenia and is mild. Bone marrow toxicity is not cumulative.

Nursing Implications: Evaluate WBC, neutrophil, and platelet count and discuss any abnormalities with physician prior to drug administration. Assess for signs/symptoms of infection or bleeding and instruct patient in signs/symptoms of infection and bleeding and to report them immediately. Suggest strategies to minimize risk of infection and bleeding, including avoidance of OTC aspirin-containing medications.

II.   ALTERATION IN CARDIAC OUTPUT related to CUMULATIVE DOSES OF IDARUBICIN

Defining Characteristics: Cardiac toxicity is similar characteristically but less severe than that seen with daunorubicin and doxorubicin; CHF due to cardiomyopathy seen after large cumulative doses.

Nursing Implications: Assess cardiac status prior to chemotherapy administration: signs/symptoms of CHF, quality/regularity and rate of heartbeat, results of prior GBPS or other test of LVEF. Teach patient to report dyspnea, palpitations, swelling in extremities. Maintain accurate records of total dose; expect GBPS to be repeated periodically during treatment and the drug to be discontinued if there is a significant drop in heart function.

III.   ALTERED NUTRITION, LESS THAN BODY REQUIREMENTS, related to NAUSEA/VOMITING, ANOREXIA, STOMATITIS, DIARRHEA, AND HEPATIC DYSFUNCTION

Defining Characteristics: Nausea/vomiting is usually mild to moderate, although it is seen to some degree in most patients; anorexia commonly occurs; stomatitis is mild; diarrhea is infrequent and mild; hepatitis is rare but may occur, and there are also disturbances in LFTs.

Nursing Implications: Premedicate with combination antiemetics and continue protection for 24 hours. If patient has a central line, slower infusion of drug over 1 hour decreases nausea/vomiting. Encourage small, frequent meals of bland foods. Anorexia occurs frequently: teach patient or caregiver to make foods ahead of time and use spices; encourage weekly weights. Stomatitis and esophagitis may occur in patients who have received prior radiation and during posttreatment visits. Teach patient oral hygiene regimen and self-assessment techniques. Encourage patient to report onset of diarrhea; administer or teach patient to self-administer antidiarrheal medications. Monitor SGOT, SGPT, LDH, alk phos, and bili periodically during treatment. Notify physician of any elevations.

IV.   ALTERATION IN SKIN INTEGRITY related to ALOPECIA, SKIN CHANGES

Defining Characteristics: Alopecia occurs in about 30% of patients after oral drug and can be partial after IV drug; begins after 3 or more weeks of starting therapy, and hair may grow back while on treatment; may be slight-to-diffuse thinning. Skin changes include darkening of nail beds, skin ulcer/necrosis, sensitivity to sunlight, skin itching at irradiated areas, radiation recall, and potential necrosis with extravasation.

Nursing Implications: Discuss with patient hair loss, anticipated impact, and strategies to decrease distress, e.g., obtaining wig prior to hair loss. Assess disturbance of body image from hyperpigmentation and discuss strategies to minimize this, e.g., nail polish. Drug must be administered via patent IV. Assess need for venous access device early. If drug administered as continuous infusion, IT MUST BE GIVEN VIA A CENTRAL LINE.

V.   POTENTIAL SEXUAL/REPRODUCTIVE DYSFUNCTION related to DRUG EFFECTS

Defining Characteristics: Gonadal function and fertility may be affected (may be permanent or transient). Reported to be excreted in breastmilk.

Nursing Implications: As appropriate, explore with patient and partner issues of reproductive and sexuality patterns and impact chemotherapy will have; discuss strategies to preserve sexuality and reproductive health (e.g., contraception, sperm banking).

Drug: ifosfamide (Ifex)

Class: Alkylating agent.

Mechanism of Action: Destroys DNA throughout the cell cycle by binding to protein and by DNA crosslinking and causing chain scission, as well as inhibition of DNA synthesis. Analogue of cyclophosphamide and is cell cycle phase nonspecific. Ifosfamide has been shown to be effective in tumors previously resistant to cyclophosphamide. Activated by microsomes in the liver.

Metabolism: Only about 50% of the drug is metabolized, with much of the drug excreted in the urine almost completely unchanged. Up to 70–86% of the drug dose is recoverable in the urine. Half-life is 13.8 hours for high doses vs 3–10 hours for lower doses.

Indication (FDA): In combination with certain other approved antineoplastic agents, for the third-line treatment of germ cell testicular cancer, together with mesna.

Drug active in cancers of lung, breast, ovary, pancreas, and stomach; Hodgkin's and NHL, acute and chronic lymphocytic leukemias.

Contraindication: (1) Patients with severely depressed bone marrow function; (2) patients hypersensitive to the drug.

Dosage/Range:
- All doses given with 2-L hydration/day and mesna.
- 700 mg–2 grams/m^2/day × 5 days, every 3 weeks.
- Continuous infusion: 1200 mg/m^2/day × 5 days.
- Dose-reduce by 25–50% if serum creatinine is 2.1–3.0 mg/dL and hold if creatinine > 3.0 mg/dL.
- High dose (bone marrow transplant/stem cell rescue): 7.5–16 grams/m^2 IV in divided doses over several days.

Drug Preparation:
- Available as a powder in 1- and 3-g vials and should be reconstituted with sterile water for injection.
- Solution is chemically stable for 7 days, but discard after 8 hours due to lack of bacteriostatic preservative in the solution.
- May be diluted further in either 5% dextrose or 0.9% sodium chloride.

Drug Administration:
- IV bolus: Administer over 30 minutes. Mesna (20% of ifosfamide dose) should be administered with ifosfamide: mesna is begun 15 minutes prior to ifosfamide and repeated at 4 and 8 hours after the ifosfamide (see drug sheet on mesna). Mesna, ascorbic acid, and mucomycin have been used to protect the bladder. Pre- and posthydration (1,500–2,000 mL/day) or continuous bladder irrigations are recommended to prevent hemorrhagic cystitis.
- **Continuous infusion:** Administer intravenously for 5 days. Mesna is mixed with ifosfamide in equal amounts (1:1 mix). Prior to initiating continuous infusion, mesna is given IVB (10% of total ifosfamide dose). Following completion of the infusion, mesna alone should be infused for 12–24 hours to protect from delayed drug excretion activity against the bladder.

Drug Interactions:
- Activity/toxicity affected by allopurinol, chloroquine, phenothiazides, potassium iodide, chloramphenicol, imipramine, vitamin A, corticosteroids, succinylcholine.
- Bone marrow-depressant drugs: additive bone marrow depression.
- Mesna binds to and inactivates ifosfamide metabolite, thus preventing bladder toxicity.

Lab Effects/Interference:
- Decreased CBC.
- Increased RFTs, LFTs (AST and ALT).

Special Considerations:
- Metabolic toxicity is increased by simultaneous administration of barbiturates.
- Renal function: BUN, serum creatinine, and creatinine clearance must be determined prior to treatment.
- Therapy requires the concomitant administration of a uroprotector such as mesna and pre- and posthydration; may also require catheterization and constant bladder irrigation, and/or ascorbic acid.
- Test urine for occult blood.

- Dose-limiting toxicity has been renal and bladder dysfunction.
- Increased risk for toxicity in patients who have received prior or concurrent radiotherapy or other antineoplastic agents.

Potential Toxicities/Side Effects and the Nursing Process

I. ALTERED URINARY ELIMINATION related to HEMORRHAGIC CYSTITIS AND RENAL TOXICITY

Defining Characteristics: Symptoms of bladder irritation; hemorrhagic cystitis with hematuria, dysuria, urinary frequency; preventable with uroprotection and hydration. Symptoms of renal toxicity; increased BUN and serum creatinine, decreased urine creatinine clearance (usually reversible); acute tubular necrosis, pyelonephritis, glomerular dysfunction; metabolic acidosis.

Nursing Implications: Assess presence of RBC in urine prior to successive doses, especially if symptoms are present, as well as BUN and creatinine. Administer drug with concomitant uroprotector (e.g., mesna). Encourage prehydration: oral intake of 2–3 L/day prior to chemotherapy; posthydration: increase oral fluids to 2–3 L for 2 days after chemotherapy. If possible, administer drug in morning to minimize drug accumulation in bladder during sleep. Instruct patient to empty bladder every 2–3 hours, before bedtime, and during night when awake. Monitor urinary output and total body balance. Assess urinary elimination pattern prior to each drug dose. If rigorous regimen is adhered to, minimal renal toxicity will result. Monitor BUN and creatinine.

II. ALTERED NUTRITION, LESS THAN BODY REQUIREMENTS, related to NAUSEA AND VOMITING, HEPATOTOXICITY

Defining Characteristics: Nausea and vomiting occur in 58% of patients; dose- and schedule-dependent, with increased severity with higher dose and rapid injection. Occurs within a few hours of drug administration and may last 3 days. Elevations of serum transaminase and alk phos may occur; usually transient and resolve spontaneously without apparent sequelae.

Nursing Implications: Premedicate with antiemetics and continue prophylactically to prevent nausea and vomiting for 24 hours at least for the first treatment. Encourage small, frequent feedings of cool, bland foods and liquids. Refer to section on nausea and vomiting. Monitor LFTs during treatment.

III. INFECTION AND BLEEDING related to BONE MARROW DEPRESSION

Defining Characteristics: Leukopenia is mild to moderate. Thrombocytopenia and anemia are rare. Dosage adjustment may be necessary when ifosfamide is combined with other chemotherapy agents. Patients at risk for bone marrow depression include patients with impaired renal function and decreased bone marrow reserve (bone marrow metastases, prior XRT).

Nursing Implications: Evaluate WBC, with neutrophil, and platelet count and discuss any abnormalities with physician prior to drug administration. Assess for signs/symptoms of infection or bleeding and instruct patient in signs/symptoms of infection and bleeding, and to report them immediately; discuss strategies to minimize risk of infection and bleeding, including avoidance of OTC aspirin-containing medications. Assess patient's Hgb/HCT and signs/symptoms of fatigue; teach patient self-assessment and to alternate rest and activity as needed.

IV. ALTERATION IN SKIN INTEGRITY related to ALOPECIA, STERILE PHLEBITIS, SKIN CHANGES

Defining Characteristics: The incidence of alopecia is 83%, with 50% experiencing severe hair loss in 2–4 weeks. Sterile phlebitis may occur at injection site; irritation occurs with extravasation. Hyperpigmentation, dermatitis, and nail ridging may occur.

Nursing Implications: Discuss with patient anticipated impact of hair loss; suggest wig, as appropriate, prior to actual hair loss. Explore with patient response to hair loss and alternative strategies to minimize distress. Carefully monitor injection site during drug administration for signs/symptoms of phlebitis, irritation, vein patency. Assess skin integrity. Assess impact of skin changes on body image. Discuss strategies to minimize distress.

V. POTENTIAL SEXUAL/REPRODUCTIVE DYSFUNCTION related to DRUG EFFECTS

Defining Characteristics: Drug is carcinogenic, mutagenic, and teratogenic. Drug is excreted in breastmilk.

Nursing Implications: As appropriate, explore with patient and partner issues of reproductive and sexual patterns, and impact chemotherapy will have. Discuss strategies to preserve sexuality and reproductive health (e.g., sperm banking, contraception).

VI. SENSORY/PERCEPTUAL ALTERATIONS related to CONFUSION, ACTIVITY INTOLERANCE, FATIGUE

Defining Characteristics: Intact drug passes easily into CNS; however, active metabolites do not. Lethargy and confusion may be seen with high doses, lasting 1–8 hours, usually spontaneously reversible. CNS side effects occur in about 12% of patients treated, including somnolence, confusion, depressive psychosis, hallucinations. Less frequent side effects: dizziness, disorientation, cranial nerve dysfunction, seizures, and coma. Incidence of CNS side effects may be higher in patients with compromised renal function, as well as in patients receiving high doses. In most instances, CNS changes are reversible.

Nursing Implications: Identify patients at risk (decreased renal function) and observe closely. Assess neurologic and mental status prior to and during drug administration and on follow-up. Instruct patient to report any alterations in behavior, sensation, perception. Develop a plan of care with patient and family if side effects develop to manage distress and promote safety. Drug should be stopped if confusion, hallucinations, and coma occur.

Drug: irinotecan (Camptosar, Camptothecan-11, CPT-11)

Class: Topoisomerase I inhibitor.

Mechanism of Action: Induces protein-linked DNA single-strand breaks and blocks DNA and RNA synthesis in dividing cells, thus preventing cells from entering mitosis. The active metabolite, SN-38, prevents repair (relegation) of previous, reversible single-strand breaks in DNA by binding to topoisomerase I. Topoisomerase I is an enzyme that relaxes tension in the DNA helix torsion by initially causing this single-strand break in DNA so that DNA replication can occur. Topoisomerases I and II then work together to bring about replication, transcription, and recombination of DNA material. Topoisomerase I is found in higher-than-normal concentrations in certain malignant cells, such as colon adenocarcinoma cells and non-Hodgkin's lymphoma cells.

Metabolism: Metabolized to its active metabolite SN-38 in the liver; 11–20% of the drug is excreted in the urine, and 5–39% in the bile over a 48-hour period. Mean terminal half-life is 6 hours, while that of SN-38 is 10 hours. Drug is moderately protein-bound (30–68%), while SN-38 is highly protein-bound (95%).

Indication: Patients with metastatic cancer of the colon or rectum, whose disease has recurred or progressed following initial fluorouracil-based therapy.

Dosage/Range:
Metastatic colorectal cancers
- FOLFIRI day 1: Irinotecan 180 mg/m² IV over 90 minutes, at the same time as leucovorin 200 mg/m² IV over 2 hours through separate arms of a Y-tubing, followed by 5-FU 400 mg/m² IVB and then 23-hour 5-FU 1200 mg/m² IV continuous infusion (CI), days 1 and 2. Total 5-FU CI dose is 2400 mg/m² over 46–48 hours. Repeat q 2 weeks.
- Douillard day 1: Irinotecan 180 mg/m² IV over 90 minutes, at the same time as leucovorin 200 mg/m² IV over 2 hours through separate arms of a Y-tubing, followed by 5-FU 400 mg/m² IVB and then 22-hour 5-FU 600 mg/m² IV continuous infusion (CI). Day 2: Leucovorin 200 mg/m² IV over 2 hours and then 5-FU 400 mg/m² IVB and then 22-hour 5-FU 600 mg/m² IV continuous infusion (CI). Repeat q 2 weeks.
- IFL regimen: Metastatic colorectal cancer (in combination with 5-FU and leucovorin): irinotecan 125 mg/m² IV over 90 minutes (days 1, 8, 15, and 22); leucovorin 20 mg/m² IVB immediately after irinotecan (days 1, 8, 15, and 22); 5-FU 500 mg/m² IVB immediately after leucovorin (days 1, 8, 15, and 22), followed by 2-week rest period (total, 6-week cycle). Requires very close monitoring and supportive care, and thus, bolus 5-FU/LV (IFL) is rarely used in favor of infusional 5-FU/LV; see FOLFIRI or Douillard regimen.

- 350-mg/m^2 IV day 1 repeated every 21 days (300 mg/m^2 for patients > 70 years old, those who have received prior pelvic/abdominal radiotherapy, or those with an ECOG performance status of 2).
- CapIri: Capecitabine 1,000 mg/m^2 po bid days 1–14; irinotecan 80 mg/m^2 IV days 1 and 8. Repeat q 22 days.

Drug Preparation:
- Store unopened vials at room temperature and protect from light.
- Dilute and mix drug in 5% dextrose (preferred) or 0.9% sodium chloride to a final concentration of 0.12–1.1 mg/mL. Commonly, the drug is diluted in 500 mL 5% dextrose.
- Diluted drug is stable 24 hours at room temperature. If diluted in 5% dextrose, the drug is stable for 48 hours if refrigerated (2–8°C [36–46°F]) and protected from light.

Drug Administration:
- Administer IV bolus over 90 minutes.
- Do not administer irinotecan if ANC < 1,000/mm^3.

Drug Interactions:
- Vinorelbine, St. John's wort: inhibits SN38 catabolism by CYP3A4 with increased serum levels and subsequent toxicity of irinotecan.
- 5-FU: additive or synergistic effect.

Lab Effects/Interference:
- Decreased CBC.
- UGT1A1*28* allele polymorphism occurs in 10% of population; results in decreased metabolism of SN38 and subsequent increased risk of neutropenia, other toxicities.

Special Considerations:
- IFL (Saltz) regimen may result in increased deaths. Use cautiously and monitor patients closely, especially patients with ↓ performance status (2), elderly, or patients with prior pelvic/abdominal radiation, or with hepatic dysfunction. Assess for signs/symptoms of dehydration, febrile neutropenia, diarrhea. Modify dose per manufacturer's guidelines.
- Independent expert panel reviewed clinical trial data and did not recommend changes in starting doses; potential life-threatening toxicity was highlighted, especially severe myelosuppression, and both early and late diarrhea.
- Patient must have weekly assessment for toxicity.
- Patient must have dose reduction as recommended; drug should not be administered if the patient is neutropenic or has diarrhea.
- Patient must be taught to notify provider if toxicity develops, and how to manage diarrhea, nausea, vomiting, potential infection.
- Drug is indicated for first-line treatment of metastatic colon or rectal cancer in combination with 5-FU and leucovorin, and as a single agent for colorectal cancer recurring or progressing after treatment with 5-FU.
- Dose-limiting toxicities are diarrhea and severe myelosuppression.
- Drug is teratogenic and thus contraindicated in pregnant women; women of childbearing age should be taught and encouraged to use birth control.

- Drug is an irritant. If extravasation occurs, the manufacturer recommends flushing the IV site with sterile water, and then applying ice.
- All patients should receive self-care instructions on management of diarrhea, self-administration of loperamide for delayed diarrhea, and assessment of the patient's ability to purchase loperamide, and ability to comply with instructions.
- Patient response to treatment is usually apparent within two courses of therapy (12 weeks).
- Flushing (vasodilation) may occur during drug infusion, and usually does not require intervention.
- Patient educational material is available from Pharmacia/Upjohn Co.
- Rarely, patients may lack an enzyme necessary for drug metabolism, resulting in increased toxicity (Gilbert's syndrome, abnormal glucuronidation of bilirubin).
- Dose reductions must be made for neutropenia and severe diarrhea, and are different for combination therapy (irinotecan/5-FU/leukovorin) and irinotecan as a single agent.
- Contraindications: serum BR > 2.0 mg/dL although no studies done, grades 3–4 neutropenia occurred in patients with BR 1–2 mg/dL.

Potential Toxicities/Side Effects and the Nursing Process

I.   ALTERATION IN ELIMINATION related to DIARRHEA

Defining Characteristics: Diarrhea may be early or late. Early diarrhea is characterized by onset within 24 hours of drug dose and is mediated by cholinergic pathway(s), as the metabolite SN-38 inhibits acetylcholinesterase; diaphoresis and abdominal cramping may precede diarrhea, and may be prevented by atropine. Other cholinergic effects that may appear are salivation, lacrimation, visual disturbances, piloerection, and bradycardia. This can be managed effectively with atropine 0.25–1.0 mg IV or scopolamine. Late diarrhea occurs > 24 hours after the drug dose, can be severe, prolonged, and lead to dehydration and electrolyte imbalance; the etiology appears related to changes in intestinal mucosal epithelium that prevent the reabsorption of water and electrolytes, which are then lost during diarrhea. 88% of patients may experience late diarrhea, and 31% have severe, or grade 3–4 diarrhea. Loperamide is effective in halting late diarrhea. Irinotecan should be held for grade 3 diarrhea (7–9 stools/day, incontinence, or severe cramping) and grade 4 (> 10 stools/day, grossly bloody stool, or need for parenteral support). Once recovered, decrease drug dose at next treatment per manufacturer's guidelines and per physician's order.

Nursing Implications: Acute diarrhea: teach patient to report diarrhea, sweating, and abdominal cramping during or after drug administration. Administer atropine 0.25–1 mg IVP per physician order, unless contraindicated, to prevent diarrhea. Delayed diarrhea: teach patient self-management of diarrhea (diet, fluids, avoidance of laxatives), and to notify nurse or physician of vomiting, fever, or if signs/symptoms of dehydration occur (fainting, light-headedness, dizziness). Teaching about diet should include drinking 8–10 large glasses of fluid/day, including soup/broth, soda, Gatorade; avoiding dairy products; eating small meals often; using BRAT diet (bananas, rice, applesauce, toast);

and adding other foods as tolerated, such as bland, low-fiber foods, white chicken meat without skin, scrambled eggs, crackers, or pasta without sauce. Also, teach patient to avoid foods that worsen diarrhea (fatty, fried, or greasy foods, high-fiber foods with bran, raw fruits and vegetables, popcorn, beans, nuts, chocolate). Review patient's medication profile, including OTC medicines, and teach patient to stop taking any laxatives. Teach patient to avoid cigarette smoking to promote comfort. Instruct patient to record stools, and to take loperamide, not as indicated on the medication package, but as instructed: At the first episode of late-onset diarrhea, take 4 mg (two 2-mg capsules) of loperamide, then 2 mg (1 capsule) every 2 hours until free of diarrhea for at least 12 hours. Take a 4-mg dose (two 2-mg capsules) at bedtime (Camptosar recommendations). Patient should notify doctor or nurse if diarrhea is unrelieved by loperamide taken as instructed. Assess patient's ability to purchase loperamide if impoverished, and identify other sources that can provide the medication prior to patient's discharge from clinic after drug therapy. Review patient's medication profile to ensure that the patient is not taking any cathartics. Diarrhea must be monitored closely and managed aggressively to prevent morbidity and mortality.

II.   POTENTIAL FOR INFECTION, ANEMIA related to BONE MARROW DEPRESSION

Defining Characteristics: Leukopenia has been noted in 63% of patients on single-dose schedules, with an overall neutropenia incidence of 54%, and grade 3–4 neutropenia occurring in 26% of patients. Thrombocytopenia is uncommon, occurring in about 3% of patients. Anemia is common (61%). Nadir is commonly on day 6–9.

Nursing Implications: Evaluate WBC, with neutrophil, and platelet count, and discuss any abnormalities with physician prior to drug administration. Refer to Special Considerations section for dosage modifications based on hematologic toxicity. Assess patient tolerance of chemotherapy and nadir blood counts, especially cycle 1. Assess for signs/symptoms of infection or bleeding; instruct patient in signs/symptoms of infection and bleeding, and to report them immediately. If febrile neutropenia develops, assess and begin antibiotic therapy ASAP. Instruct in measures to minimize risk of infection and bleeding, including avoidance of OTC aspirin-containing medications. Assess patient's Hgb/HCT and signs/symptoms of fatigue; teach patient self-assessment and to alternate rest and activity as needed.

III.   POTENTIAL ALTERATION IN NUTRITION, LESS THAN BODY REQUIREMENTS, related to NAUSEA AND VOMITING, DEHYDRATION

Defining Characteristics: Moderate to severe nausea and vomiting occur in 35–60% of patients, with 17% experiencing NCI grade 3–4 nausea and 13% experiencing NCI grade 3–4 vomiting. Aggressive combination antiemetics are effective in preventing nausea/vomiting.

Nursing Implications: Premedicate with aggressive combination antiemetics, such as serotonin antagonist (dolasetron, granisetron, or ondansetron) plus dexamethasone 10 mg IV 30 minutes prior to chemotherapy to prevent nausea and vomiting. Encourage small, frequent meals of cool, bland foods and liquids. Teach patients to monitor their fluid intake, and take daily weights if nausea/vomiting occurs. Assess for signs/symptoms of fluid and electrolyte imbalance. Teach patients self-assessment, and instruct to notify doctor or nurse if these occur. Late-onset nausea and vomiting may occur, and dopamine antagonists such as prochlorperazine are then recommended. If dehydration develops, replace fluid and electrolytes to prevent worsening dehydration and cardiovascular complications.

IV.   POTENTIAL FOR IMPAIRED GAS EXCHANGE related to DYSPNEA, PULMONARY INFILTRATES, FEVER

Defining Characteristics: Pulmonary effects may occur in up to 22% of patients, ranging from transient dyspnea to pulmonary infiltrates, fever, increased cough, and decreased DLCO in a small number of patients.

Nursing Implications: Assess baseline pulmonary status, and teach patient to report any changes. Assess pulmonary status prior to each treatment and at visits between treatment. If patient develops dyspnea, discuss patient having PFTs with physician, and evaluating whether related to drug. Teach patient to manage dyspnea if it occurs, including alternating activity and rest periods.

Drug: ixabepilone (Ixempra)

Class: Microtubule inhibitor; Epothilone B analogue.

Mechanism of Action: Normally, cells need to have flexibility in making the structures for mitosis, such as tubulin and the microtubules; the tubulin needs to be able to polymerize and then depolymerize. Ixabepilone binds to the beta-tubulin subunits on microtubules, and strongly promotes tubulin polymerization and stabilization, similar to paclitaxel but at a different binding site; the drug causes the cell to stop cycling (mitotic arrest) at the G_2/M phase of the cell cycle and to die (cytotoxicity). The drug avoids multiple tumor-resistance mechanisms, including efflux transporters and P-glycoprotein; thus, it has effectiveness against tumors that possess these mechanisms resulting in refractoriness to taxanes, anthracyclines, and vinca alkaloids. Ixabepilone also has antiangiogenic activity.

Metabolism: Drug is a semisynthetic analogue of epothilone B. It is a macrolide fermentation product of the myxobacterium Sorangium cellulosum. Drug has linear pharmacokinetics, with 67–77% binding to serum proteins. Drug is extensively metabolized in the liver, primarily via oxidative metabolism by CYP3A4/5 microenzyme system (hepatic microsomes). This produces > 30 inactive metabolites, which are then excreted in the urine (65%) and feces (21%). Eighty-six percent of the dose is eliminated in 7 days. The terminal half-life of the drug is 52 hours, with no accumulation in the plasma when given every 3 weeks. It is unlikely that ixabepilone affects serum levels of drugs that are substrates of CYP enzymes.

Indication:
- In combination with capecitabine for the treatment of patients with metastatic or locally advanced breast cancer resistant to treatment with an anthracycine and a taxane, or whose cancer is resistant and for whom furter anthracycline therapy is contraindicated.
  - Anthracycline resistance is defined as progression while on therapy or within 6 months in the adjuvant setting or 3 months in the metastatic setting.
  - Taxane resistance is defined as progression while on therapy or within 12 months in the adjuvant setting or 4 months in the metastatic setting.
- As monotherapy, for the treatment of patients with metastatic or locally advanced breast cancer after failure of an anthracycline, a taxane and capecitabine.

Contraindication: Ixabepilone in combination with capecitabine in patients with AST or ALT >2.5 × ULN or bilirubin >1 × ULN due to increased risk of toxicity and neutropenia-related death.

Dosage/Range:
- 40 mg/m^2 IV over 3 hours every 21 days.
- In breast cancer, given with capecitabine 1,000 mg/m^2 PO twice daily × 14 days, repeated every 3 weeks.
- Do not exceed maximum dose calculated at BSA 2.2 m^2.
- Dose-reduce for mild hepatic dysfunction, severe neutropenia, or severe thrombocytopenia; contraindicated in severe hepatic dysfunction (see Special Considerations).
- Hematologic (ixabepilone): When recovered (ANC ≥ 1,500 cells/mm^3 and platelets ≥ 100,000 cells/mm^3), decrease dose by 20% for neutrophils < 500 cells/mm^3 for > 7 days, febrile neutropenia, or platelets < 25,000 cells/mm^3 or platelets < 50,000 cells/mm^3 with bleeding.
- Hematologic (capecitabine): For platelets < 25,000 cells/mm^3 or < 50,000 cells/mm^3 with bleeding, hold capecitabine for concurrent diarrhea or stomatitis until platelet count > 50,000 cells/mm^3 then continue at same dose; for neutrophils < 500 cells/mm^3 for > 7 days or febrile neutropenia, hold capecitabine for concurrent diarrhea or stomatitis until ANC > 1,000 cells/mm^3, then continue at same dose.
- Nonhematologic (ixabepilone): When toxicity improved to grade 1, decrease by 20% for moderate grade 2 neuropathy (moderate) lasting ≥ 7 days; grade 3 neuropathy (severe) lasting < 7 days; any grade 3 toxicity (severe) other than neuropathy. Discontinue drug for grade 3 neuropathy (severe) lasting ≥ 7 days or any grade 4 toxicity (disabling).
- Nonhematologic (capecitabine): Follow capecitabine label.
- Hepatic impairment (ixabepilone monotherapy): **Mild** (AST and ALT ≤ 2.5 × ULN and bilirubin ≤ 1 × ULN), give full dose; AST or ALT ≤ 10 × ULN and bili ≤ 1.5 × ULN give 32 mg/m^2; **moderate** (AST and ALT ≤ 10 × ULN and bilirubin > 1.5 × ULN but less than or equal to 3 × ULN), give 20–30 mg/m^2.

Drug Preparation:
- Available as Ixempra 15 mg for injection supplied with 8-mL diluent and Ixempra 45 mg with 23.5-mL diluent. Reconstituted solution delivers ixabepilone concentration of 2 mg/mL. This must be further diluted with lactated Ringer's injection USP to a final concentration of 0.2–0.6 mg/mL. Drug is stable only in solution with a pH in the range of 6–7.5.

- Reconstituted solution is stable for 1 hour in a syringe at room temperature and light but should be further diluted as soon as possible following reconstitution. After further diluted in lactated Ringer's, the infusion must be completed within 6 hours of preparation.
- Ixempra kit contains two vials (vial containing 16 mg drug powder [labeled 15 mg] or 47 mg [labeled 45 mg] and vial of diluent containing dehydrated alcohol). Kit must be stored in a refrigerator (2–8°C [36–46°F]) in original packaging to protect from light. Remove from refrigerator 30 minutes before mixing; this will also give time for any white precipitate in the diluent to dissolve.
- Reconstitute by aseptically withdrawing diluent and slowly injecting into vial containing Ixempra drug; gently swirl and invert vial until completely dissolved. Aspirate ordered dose (2 mg/mL).
- Further dilute in 250-mL lactated Ringer's (or larger if needed to deliver a final concentration of 0.2–0.6 mg/mL)—bag must be DEHP-free (e.g., non-PVC). Gently invert bag to mix (manual rotation).
- Administer via DEHP-free tubing with DEHP-free final filter 0.2–1.2 microns.
- The drug infusion must be completed within 6 hours of preparation.

Drug Administration:
- ANC must be $\geq$ 1,500 cells/mm^3 and platelets $\geq$ cells/mm^3.
- Administer as IV infusion over 3 hours. Premedicate with an H$_1$ antagonist (e.g., diphenhydramine 50 mg PO) and H$_2$ antagonist (e.g., ranitidine 150–300 mg PO) 1 hour before chemotherapy to minimize hypersensitivity reaction.
- If patient has had a hypersensitivity reaction to ixabepilone in the prior cycle, add a corticosteroid (e.g., dexamethasone 20 mg IV 30 minutes or PO 60 minutes before chemotherapy) to premedications.
- Drug contains dehydrated alcohol; thus, assess patient's neurologic status during and after infusion.

Drug Interactions:
- Capecitabine: synergy, so used together to increase tumor cell kill.
- Strong CYP3A4 inhibitors decrease the metabolism, thus increasing plasma level of ixabepilone and thus should be avoided (ketoconazole, itraconazole, clarithromycin, atazanavir, nefazodone, saquinavir, telithromycin, ritonavir, amprenavir, indinavir, nelfinavir, delavirdine, voriconazole, grapefruit juice); if a strong CYP3A4 inhibitor must be given concurrently, reduce ixabepilone dose to 20 mg/m^2; after the strong inhibitor is discontinued, wait 1 week (washout period) before increasing the ixabepilone dose to indicated dose.

Lab Effects/Interference:
- Neutropenia, thrombocytopenia, anemia.

Special Considerations:
- Drug is 3–20 times more potent than paclitaxel.
- Drug is able to overcome p-glycoprotein–related drug resistance.
- Drug is indicated in the treatment of patients with metastatic or locally advanced breast cancer.

- Drug is contraindicated in patients who are hypersensitive to Cremophor EL or its derivatives (polyoxyethylated castor oil), patients with a baseline ANC < 1,500 cells/mm³ or platelet count < 100,000 cells/mm³, or when given in combination with capecitabine, in patients with hepatic dysfunction (AST or ALT > 2.5 × ULN or bilirubin > 1 × ULN due to increased risk of neutropenia-related death and other toxicity).
- As a single agent, use cautiously in patients with hepatic dysfunction (AST or ALT > 5 × ULN); do not use in patients with AST or ALT > 10 × ULN or bilirubin > 3 × ULN.
- Use cautiously and assess frequently in patients with preexisting moderate to severe peripheral neuropathy or diabetes mellitus.
- Drug is fetotoxic: Teach women of reproductive potential to use effective contraception.
- Toxicity profile similar to paclitaxel.
- A randomized phase III trial in patients with refractory breast cancer showed that patients who received ixabepilone and capecitabine had significantly longer progression-free survival (5.8 months) compared with patients receiving capecitabine alone (4.2 months, p < .0003). The objective response rate was 35% in the combination group compared with 14% in the single-agent group (Vahdat et al., 2007).

Potential Toxicities/Side Effects and the Nursing Process

I. POTENTIAL FOR INFECTION AND BLEEDING related to BONE MARROW DEPRESSION

Defining Characteristics: Myelosuppression is dose-dependent, expressed primarily as neutropenia. Incidence of neutropenia is 68% with grades 3–4 54% (incidence of febrile neutropenia 3% as monotherapy and 5% when given with capecitabine, with infection occurring in 5–6% of patients, respectively). Neutropenic deaths occurred in 1.9% of patients receiving ixabepilone in combination with capecitabine, with normal hepatic function or mild hepatic dysfunction, and in 0.4% in patients receiving monotherapy. Drug is contraindicated in patients with severe hepatic dysfunction (see Special Considerations), and in patients with ANC < 1,500 cells/mm³ or platelets < 100,000 cells/mm³. Grades 3–4 thrombocytopenia occur in 7% (monotherapy) and 8% (combination therapy) of patients, and anemia in 8% (mono) and 10% (combination). Fatigue is common, affecting 56% (mono) and 60% (combination).

Nursing Implications: Assess baseline CBC, WBC, differential, and platelet count prior to chemotherapy, as well as signs/symptoms of infection or bleeding, and assure ANC ≥ 1,500 cells/mm³ and platelet count ≥ 100,000 cells/mm³. If patient experienced severe neutropenia or thrombocytopenia, discuss dose reduction with physician. Teach patient the signs/symptoms of infection or bleeding, and to report these immediately, such as temperature ≥ 100.5°F. Teach patient self-care measures to minimize risk of infection and bleeding. This includes avoidance of crowds, proximity to people with infections, and OTC aspirin-containing medications. Assess baseline activity and energy level. Teach patient that fatigue may occur, and ways to minimize exertion and energy expenditure by alternating rest and activity, and organizing chores so that they are done as efficiently as possible.

II.   POTENTIAL FOR INJURY related to HYPERSENSITIVITY REACTIONS

Defining Characteristics: In studies, 1% of patients had severe hypersensitivity reactions (HSRs), including anaphylaxis. The risk of HSRs is reduced by premedication with H_1 and H_2 antagonists.

Nursing Implications: Assess baseline VS and mental status before drug administration. Administer H_1 antagonist (e.g., diphenhydramine 50 mg PO) and H_2 antagonist 30–60 minutes before starting drug. If patient has had a prior reaction, administer ordered corticosteroid (e.g., dexamethasone 20-mg IV or PO) in addition. Remain with patient during first 15 minutes of infusion, and monitor frequently during infusion. Teach patient to report any itching, rash, any new sensations or symptoms. Recall signs/symptoms of HSR. If these occur, stop drug immediately, and notify physician. Subjective symptoms are generalized itching, nausea, chest tightness, crampy abdominal pain, difficulty speaking, anxiety, agitation, sense of impending doom, uneasiness, desire to urinate/defecate, dizziness, chills. Objective signs are flushed appearance; fever, chills, bronchospasm, angioedema of face, neck, eyelids, hands, feet; localized or generalized urticaria; respiratory distress with or without wheezing, hypotension, cyanosis. Review standing orders or nursing procedure for patient management of anaphylaxis and be prepared to stop drug immediately. Notify physician. Monitor VS, and administer ordered medications, which may include epinephrine 1:1,000, hydrocortisone sodium succinate, and diphenhydramine.

III.   SENSORY/PERCEPTUAL ALTERATIONS related to SENSORY NEUROPATHY

Defining Characteristics: Peripheral neuropathy is common, with sensory neuropathy affecting 62–65% of patients, and motor neuropathy affecting 10–16% of patients. It occurs early with 75% of new onset and worsening neuropathy occurring during first three cycles. Dose reduction results in improvement or no worsening in neuropathy in most patients. About 10% of patients receiving monotherapy and 23% of patients receiving combination with capecitabine developed grade 3–4 peripheral neuropathy. Median number of cycles to onset of grade 3–4 neuropathy was four cycles in both groups, with a median time to improvement of grade 3–4 to baseline or grade 1 of 4–6 weeks for patients receiving monotherapy and 6 weeks for patients receiving combination. Neuropathy is cumulative and reversible (Vahdat et al., 2007).

Nursing Implications: Assess baseline neurologic status. Instruct patient to report signs/ symptoms of pins-and-needles sensation, numbness, burning sensation, pain, increased discomfort with certain sensations, especially in the extremities, or motor weakness. Identify patients at risk: those with history of cisplatin use or with preexisting neuropathies (ethanol- and diabetes mellitus-related). Assess sensory and motor function prior to each treatment, and if abnormality found, assess impact on patient function, safety, independence, ability to do activities of daily living (ADLs), and quality of life. Test patient's ability to button a shirt, or pick up a dime from a flat surface. If impacting ability to do ADLs, safety, or quality of life, discuss with patient and physician drug reduction (20% for grade 2 lasting > 7 days or grade 3 lasting < 7 days). If grade 3 neuropathy lasts ≥ 7 days, the drug should be discontinued. Teach self-care strategies, including maintaining safety when walking, getting up, taking a bath, or washing dishes; discuss inability to sense temperature, and the need to keep extremities warm in cold weather. See NCI Common Toxicity Criteria Adverse Events in *Appendix II*: grade 2 motor = symptomatic weakness interfering with function but not ADLs; grade 2 sensory = sensory alteration or paresthesia interfering with function but not ADLs; grade 3 motor = objective weakness, interfering with ADLs; grade 3 sensory = sensory loss or paresthesia interfering with ADLs; grade 4 motor = paralysis; grade 4 sensory = permanent sensory loss that interferes with function.

IV.   ALTERATION IN SKIN INTEGRITY related to ALOPECIA, NAIL CHANGES

Defining Characteristics: Alopecia affects 31–48% of patients in clinical trials and is reversible; 9–24% of patients developed nail changes during clinical trials. Palmar-plantar erythrodysesthesia (hand-foot syndrome) occurred in 64% of patients receiving capecitabine with ixabepilone.

Nursing Implications: Discuss potential impact of hair loss prior to drug administration. Discuss coping strategies and a plan to minimize body image distortion (e.g., wig, scarf, cap). Assess patient for signs/symptoms of hair loss. Assess patient's response and use of coping strategies, and help patient to build on effective strategies. Assess patient's fingernails and toenails, and teach patients changes may occur and to report them. Develop plan of care with patient if changes are severe. Refer to capecitabine drug sheet for the assessment, prevention, and management of palmar-plantar erythrodysesthesia.

V.   ALTERATION IN COMFORT related to ARTHRALGIAS AND MYALGIAS

Defining Characteristics: Arthralgias and myalgias affect about 39–49% of patients, and musculoskeletal pain affects 20–23% of patients.

Nursing Implications: Arthralgias and myalgias may be troublesome, and can be managed with NSAIDs, application of warmth, and other comfort measures. Some patients report that swimming is helpful in minimizing discomfort. Studies of gabapentin, glutamine, and steroids have been disappointing. Opioids may be needed if severe.

VI.   ALTERATION IN NUTRITION, LESS THAN BODY REQUIREMENTS, related to NAUSEA, VOMITING, DIARRHEA

Defining Characteristics: Nausea and vomiting occur in approximately 42–53% and 29–39% of patients, respectively. It is mild and preventable with antiemetics. Diarrhea occurs in 22–44% of patients and is mild. Drug appears to cause diarrhea by direct injury to the intestinal mucosa (necrosis of cells), causing inflammation of the bowel wall and decreased absorption. Stomatitis and mucositis occur in 29–31% of patients. Constipation occurs in 16–22% of patients.

Nursing Implications: Assess patient's nutritional status, as well as elimination status. Premedicate patient with antiemetic prior to chemotherapy and give antiemetic to take at home if needed. Encourage small, frequent meals of cool, bland foods. Instruct patient to report nausea unrelieved with antiemetics, and teach self-administration of antiemetics, as most patients will receive the drug as an outpatient. If nausea/vomiting occur and are severe, assess for signs/symptoms of fluid/electrolyte imbalance and bring to clinic for aggressive antiemesis. Encourage patient to report onset of diarrhea and to self-administer antidiarrheal medications; review dietary changes to reduce bowel irritation (e.g., avoid spicy, high-fat, high-insoluble fiber foods and increase fluids to 3 L/day). If patient develops constipation, review measures and dietary changes to relieve constipation. Assess baseline oral mucous membranes. Teach patient oral assessment and to report any alterations. Assess LFTs prior to drug administration and periodically during treatment.

Drug: lanreotide (Somatuline depot injection)

Class: Somatostatin analogue.

Mechanism of Action: As a synthetic somatostatin analogue, lanreotide has a high affinity for human somatostatin receptors, so it blocks the binding of human somatostatin to the receptors, most significantly 2 and 5. This inhibits growth hormone (GH) and insulin-like growth factor (IGF-1), as well as other endocrine, neuroendocrine, exocrine, and paracrine functions.

Metabolism: Lanreotide passively diffuses from the depot into the tissues, and enters the bloodstream. Steady state is reached after 4–5 injections (4–5 months). In renal failure, drug excretion is slowed, with a twofold increase in AUC and drug half-life. Less than 5% of the drug is excreted in the urine, and less than 0.5% in the feces; instead, the major route of excretion is believed to be biliary.

Indication: (1) Long-term treatment of patients with acromegaly who have had an inadequate response to surgery and/or radiotherapy, or are not candidates for this treatment; (2) treatment of patients with unresectable, well- or moderately differentiated, locally advanced, or metastatic gastroenteropancreatic neuroendocrine tumors (GEP-NETs) to improve progression-free survival.

Dosage/Range:
- **GEP-NETS:** 120 mg deep SQ in superior external quadrant of buttock, every 4 weeks. No effect on drug clearance was seen in patients with mild to moderate renal impairment. The effect of hepatic dysfunction on drug clearance in GEP-NETS patients has not been studied. Use lanreotide in these patients cautiously and monitor closely.
- **Acromegaly:** 60–120 mg SQ every 4 weeks, starting at a dose of 90 mg every 4 weeks for 3 months. Adjust the dose thereafter based on GH and/or IGF-1 levels. If patient has moderate to severe renal or hepatic dysfunction, the initial dose should be 60 mg every 4 weeks for 3 months; adjust the dose thereafter based on GH and/or IGF-1 levels.

Drug Preparation/Administration:
- Available in 60 mg/0.2 mL, 90 mg/0.3 mL, and 120 mg/0.5 mL single-use, prefilled syringes.
- Administer monthly by deep subcutaneous injection in the superior external quadrant of the buttock; rotate injection sites.

Drug Interactions:
- Hypoglycemic agents: May result in hypoglycemia or hyperglycemia. Monitor glucose closely, and adjust antidiabetic treatment accordingly.
- Cyclosporine: Concomitant administration may decrease the bioavailability of cyclosporine, necessitating adjustment of the cyclosporine dose.
- Drugs affecting heart rate (e.g., beta blockers): Lanreotide may decrease heart rate. If given with another drug causing a similar effect, dose adjustment of the coadministered drugs may be needed.
- Drugs metabolized by the CYP3A4 liver microenzyme system, which have a narrow therapeutic window: Use cautiously; lanreotide may slow the metabolism of the coadministered drug, resulting in increased toxicity. This reaction may be the result of interference with GH.

Lab Effects/Interference:
- Hyperglycemia or hypoglycemia
- Changes in GH and IGF-1 levels

Special Considerations:
- Warnings and precautions:
  - Lanreotide slows down gallbladder motility; monitor patients for the development of cholelithiasis and gall bladder sludge. Incidence in studies was 14%.
  - Lanreotide inhibits the secretion of insulin and glucagon; some patients may develop hypoglycemia or hyperglycemia. Assess blood glucose at baseline and when the dose is altered, and adjust antidiabetic medicine as needed.
  - Thyroid function may undergo slight decreases in patients with acromegaly.
  - Lanreotide may cause sinus bradycardia; in all three studies, the incidence was 5.5%. Teach patients which signs and symptoms to report, and manage symptomatic bradycardia. If the patient has baseline bradycardia, use lanreotide cautiously and monitor closely. The drug may cause hypertension in patients with acromegaly.
- Lanreotide is embryocidal in animals. It should be used during pregnancy only if the potential benefit justifies the risk to the fetus. Nursing mothers should make a decision whether to discontinue nursing or the drug, taking into account the importance of the drug to the mother.
- Most common adverse reactions (≥10%) in GEP-NET patients are abdominal pain, musculoskeletal pain, vomiting, headache, injection-site reaction, hyperglycemia, hypertension, and cholelithiasis. Most common reactions in patients with acromegaly are diarrhea, cholelithiasis, abdominal pain, nausea, and injection-site reactions.
- Dizziness may occur (incidence 9%); teach patient to change position slowly. If dizziness does occur, teach the patient not to drive a car or operate machinery.

Potential Toxicities and the Nursing Process:

I.   ALTERATION IN COMFORT related to ABDOMINAL PAIN, MUSCULOSKELETAL PAIN, HEADACHE, AND INJECTION-SITE REACTION

Defining Characteristics: In study 3 with GEP-NET patients, 34% had abdominal pain, 19% musculoskeletal pain, 16% headache, and 15% injection-site reactions.

Nursing Considerations: Assess baseline comfort, and teach patient about potential side effects. Teach patient self-assessment and management, and how to contact the provider if symptoms persist or worsen. Assess the prior injection site each month, and document site rotation. Ensure that the SQ injection is deep in the superior external quadrant of the buttock. Teach patient to report persistent discomfort, formation of induration, or mass if it develops.

II.   ALTERATION IN NUTRITION, POTENTIAL related to NAUSEA, VOMITING, CHOLELITHIASIS, OR HYPERGLYCEMIA OR HYPOGLYCEMIA

Defining Characteristics: In study 3 with GEP-NET patients, 19% had vomiting and 14% had hyperglycemia. Cholelithiasis occurred in 14% of patients.

Nursing Considerations: Assess baseline nutritional status, presence of nutritional impact symptoms, and blood glucose. Teach patient about potential side effects, self-care management strategies, and reporting persistent or unrelieved vomiting. Teach patient the signs and symptoms of hypoglycemia and hyperglycemia, and how to report them if they occur. If the patient is diabetic, assess blood glucose more frequently (e.g., at the beginning of therapy and with any dose change, and during therapy), and have patient monitor it at home with fingersticks. Discuss adjustments to antidiabetic agents as needed based on blood sugar results. Teach patient signs and symptoms of cholelithiasis, and how to report them if they occur: severe abdominal pain; pain extending beneath the right shoulder or to the back; pain that worsens after a meal (e.g., fatty or greasy foods); pain that feels sharp or dull, and crampy; pain that increases when the patient takes a deep breath; and chest pain.

Drug: letrozole (Femara)

Class: Aromatase inhibitor, nonsteroidal.

Mechanism of Action: Inhibits estrogen synthesis. Drug is a highly selective, potent agent that significantly suppresses (90%) serum estradiol levels within 14 days, without interfering with other steroid hormone synthesis. Binds to the heme group of aromatase, a cytochrome P450 enzyme necessary for the conversion of androgens to estrogens. Aromatase is thus inhibited, leading to a significant reduction in plasma estradiol, estrone, and estrone sulfate. After 6 weeks of therapy, there is 97% suppression of estradiol.

Metabolism: Rapidly and completely absorbed after oral administration, with a terminal half-life of 2 days. Steady state reached in 2–6 weeks. Metabolized in the liver and excreted in the urine.

Patients with cirrhosis and severe hepatic impairment had double the drug exposure, so dose must be reduced 50% in these patients.

Indication: (1) Adjuvant treatment of postmenopausal women with hormone receptor positive early breast cancer; (2) extended adjuvant treatment of postmenopausal women with early breast cancer who have received prior standard adjuvant tamoxifen therapy; (3) first- and second-line treatment of postmenopausal women with hormone receptor positive or unknown advanced breast cancer.

Contraindication: Premenopausal women, including pregnant women.

Dosage/Range:
- 2.5 mg PO daily, without regard to meals.
- 50% dose reduction recommended in patients with cirrhosis and severe hepatic dysfunction (2.5 mg letrozole every other day).
- No dosage adjustment in patients with impaired renal function unless creatinine clearance is < 10 mL/min.

Drug Preparation:
- Oral; available in 2.5 mg tablets.

Drug Interactions:
- Tamoxifen: coadministration with tamoxifen decreased letrozole plasma levels by 38% but was not significant when letrozole was administered immediately after tamoxifen.
- Estrogen: may decrease drug effect.

Lab Effects/Interference:
- Liver transaminases may be transiently elevated.
- Increase in total cholesterol (nonfasting, adjuvant studies).
- Rare, mild ↓ in lymphocyte and/or platelet count.

Special Considerations:
- About 200 times more potent than aminoglutethimide.
- Letrozole may cause fetal harm when administered to pregnant women, as drug is embryotoxic and fetotoxic in lab animals. If there is exposure to letrozole during pregnancy, the patient should be apprised of the potential hazard to the fetus.
- Discuss need for effective contraception in women who have the potential to become pregnant until their postmenopausal status is fully established.
- Teach patients to use caution when driving or using machinery, because letrozole can cause dizziness, fatigue, and uncommonly, somnolence.
- Monitor bone mineral density (BMD), because drug may cause a decrease in BMD. Teach patient to take calcium and vitamin D daily.
- Monitor serum cholesterol because increases in total cholesterol may occur.
- Most common adverse reactions (>20%): hot flashes, arthragia, flushing, asthenia, edema, arthralgia, headache, dizziness, hypercholesterolemia, increased sweating, bone pain, musculoskeletal pain.

Potential Toxicities/Side Effects and the Nursing Process

I.   ALTERATION IN COMFORT related to HOT FLASHES, ARTHRALGIAS, MYALGIA, ARTHRITIS, SWEATING, ASTHENIA, DIZZINESS, HEADACHE, BONE PAIN, EDEMA

Defining Characteristics: Most common side effects were hot flashes/flushes (33%) and arthralgia/arthritis (25%). Less commonly myalgia, back pain, fatigue/asthenia, and dizziness can occur.

Nursing Considerations: Assess baseline comfort levels, and teach patient that this discomfort may occur. Teach patient symptomatic measures, instruct to report if symptoms are unrelieved.

II.   ALTERATION IN NUTRITION, LESS THAN BODY REQUIREMENTS, related to NAUSEA/VOMITING, HYPERCHOLESTEROLEMIA

Defining Characteristics: Nausea may occur, with vomiting less common. Hypercholesterolemia may occur in up to 52% of patients.

Nursing Implications: Determine baseline weight, and monitor at each visit. Teach patient that these side effects may occur, and instruct to report this. Discuss strategies to minimize nausea, including diet and dosing time.

Discuss baseline and periodic monitoring of total cholesterol with physician or mid-level practitioner, while patient is on therapy.

III.   POTENTIAL FOR THROMBOEMBOLIC EVENT, ENDOMETRIAL HYPERPLASIA/CANCER, FRACTURES

Defining Characteristics: Updated safety data with follow-up for 73 months showed that letrozole had lower incidences of thromboembolism (2.9% vs 4.5%), and endometrial hyperplasia/cancer (0.4% vs 2.9%) when compared to tamoxifen.

In the adjuvant trial, the incidence of bone fractures at any time after randomization was 13.8% for letrozole and 10.5% for tamoxifen. The incidence of osteoporosis was 5.1% for letrozole and 2.7% for tamoxifen. In the extended adjuvant trial, the incidence of bone fractures at any time after randomization was 13.3% for letrozole and 7.8% for placebo. The incidence of new osteoporosis was 14.5% for letrozole and 7.8% for placebo.

Nursing Implications: Discuss plan to monitor and minimize bone loss with physician, and reinforce teaching with patient, such as baseline and periodic bone mineral density testing, as well as exercise, and daily nutritional supplementation of vitamin D and calcium. Although rare, teach patient that thromboembolism and endometrial changes may occur. Teach patient to report any new onset pain or tenderness in the calf or difficulty breathing, and to discuss annual endometrial monitoring (e.g., biopsy) with patient's gynecologist.

Drug: leuprolide acetate for depot suspension (Lupron, Viadur)

Class: GnRH agonist, inhibits gonadotropin secretion.

Mechanism of Action: Leuprolide acetate is a gonadotropin-releasing hormone (GnRH) agonist that potently suppresses the secretion of gonadotropins, including follicle-stimulating hormone (FSH) and luteinizing hormone (LH) from the pituitary gland, when given continuously and in therapeutic doses. There is an initial increase in circulating LH, FSH which leads to a transient rise in gonadal steroids (testosterone and dihydrotestosterone in males, and estrone and estradiol in premenopausal females), and then a significant decrease. Continuous administration of the drug results in decreased levels of LH and FSH and, in men, testosterone is reduced to castrate levels (decrease in LH causes the Leydig cells to reduce testosterone production to castrate levels).

Metabolism: Ninety-five percent of the drug is absorbed after subcutaneous injection, with 85–100% of the drug being absorbed after IM or subcutaneous injection. Drug is slightly protein-bound (43–49%). Following administration, < 5% of the drug (parent or metabolite) is recovered in the urine.

Indication: Palliative treatment of patients with advanced prostate cancer.

Contraindication: Drug is contraindicated in patients hypersensitive to the GnRH, GnRH agonists, or any of the excipients in Lupron Depot; pregnancy.

Dosage/Range:
- For palliative treatment of prostate cancer: Depot suspension 22.5 mg IM every 3 months; OR 30 mg IM every 4 months; OR 45 mg IM every 6 months; OR Viadur implant 65 mg every 12 months; OR 1 mg/day subcutaneous injection.

Drug Preparation:
See package insert.
- Use syringes, diluent, kit provided by manufacturer. Inspect depot powder, and syringe should not be used if clumping or caking. A thin layer of powder on the syringe wall is normal; diluent should appear clear. To prepare for injection:
- Screw the white plunger into the end stopper until the stopper begins to turn.
- Hold the syringe upright. Release the diluent by SLOWLY PUSHING (6–8 sec) the plunger until the first stopper is at the blue line in the middle of the syringe barrel.
- Keep the syringe upright. Gently mix the powder thoroughly to form a uniform suspension (appears milky). If the powder adheres to the stopper or caking/clumping is present, tap the syringe with your finger to disperse. DO NOT USE if any of the powder has not gone into suspension.
- Hold the syringe upright. With the opposite hand, pull the needle cap upwards without twisting.
- Keep the syringe upright. Advance the plunger to expel the air from the syringe. Inject the entire contents of the syringe IM right after reconstitution. The suspension settles very quickly following reconstitution; therefore, the drug should be mixed and used immediately.

- Injection: 5 mg/mL; kit 5 mg/mL for 7.5-mg, 22.5-mg doses.
- Lupron Depot injection kit contains the following for the 7.5-mg kit: one prefilled dual chambered syringe containing sterile lyophilized microspheres of leuprolide acetate in a biodegradable lactic acid polymer; needle with LuproLoc safety device; one plunger; two alcohol swabs; prescribing information. Mix with 1.0 mL of accompanying diluent. Store at controlled room temperature (25° C, 77°F), with excursions 15–30°C, 59–86°F permitted.
- Lupron Depot injection kit contains the following for the 22.5-mg depot (3 months), 30 mg (4 months), 45 mg (6 months): one prefilled dual chambered syringe containing sterile lyophilized microspheres of leuprolide acetate in a biodegradable lactic acid polymer; needle with LuproLoc safety device; one plunger; two alcohol swabs; prescribing information. Mix with 1.5 mL of accompanying diluent. Store at controlled room temperature (25°C, 77°F), with excursions 15–30°C, 59–86°F permitted.
- Viadur implant kit contains implant, implanter, and sterile field/supplies. Sterile gloves must be added. Procedure is sterile and uses a special implant technology.

Drug Administration:
- Depot is administered IM (see reconstitution above; drug should be given immediately after mixing): 7.5 mg once every month, 22.5 mg once every 3 months, 30 mg once every 4 months, 45 mg once every 6 months. Rotate sites. When administering IM, any aspirated blood would be visible just below the luer lock connection (transparent LuproLoc safety device) if a blood vessel is accidently penetrated. After injection, immediately activate the LuproLoc safety device by pushing the arrow forward with the thumb or finger until the device is fully extended and you hear or feel a click.
- Viadur: Kit contains specific directions for insertion of implant, removal, and reinsertion of subsequent dose after 1 year.

Drug Interactions:
- None reported.

Lab Effects/Interference:
- Decreased PSA, testosterone levels; increased calcium, decreased WBC, decreased serum total protein.
- Injection: Increased BUN and creatinine.
- Depot: Increased LDH, alk phos, AST, uric acid, cholesterol, LDL, triglycerides, glucose, WBC, phosphate; decreased potassium, platelets.

Special Considerations:
- Ensure patient is given return appointment for next injection, e.g., 1 month, 3 months, 4 months, 6 months. Sites should be rotated. For Viadur, patient has implant inserted by MD/RN once yearly.
- Initially, drug causes increased LH secretion, resulting in increased testosterone secretion and tumor flare. Usually disappears after 2 weeks.
- Drug has been studied in the treatment of breast and islet cell cancers.
- Studies on Viadur show that implant delivers 120 micrograms of leuprolide acetate per day over 12 months, reducing testosterone levels to castration levels within 2–4 weeks after insertion.

- Increased serum testosterone (~50% above baseline) during first week of treatment; monitor serum testosterone and PSA. Patient may experience a transient worsening of symptoms, or additional signs/symptoms of prostate cancer in the first few weeks of treatment. Some patients may experience a temporary increase in bone pain, which can be treated symptomatically. Isolated cases of ureteral obstruction and spinal cord compression have been reported with GnRh agonists, which may contribute to paralysis.
- Hyperglycemia and new onset diabetes have been reported. Monitor blood glucose level and manage medically.
- Cardiovascular disease may be exacerbated with increased risk of MI, sudden cardiac death, and stroke in men. Assess for cardiovascular risk and monitor closely if at risk.
- Long-term androgen deprivation therapy prolongs the QT interval. Consider the risks and benefits, and monitor during therapy. Adverse reactions by formulation (> 10%):
  - 22 mg (3 months): general pain, injection-site reaction, hot flashes/sweats, GI disorders, joint disorders, testicular atrophy, urinary disorders.
  - 30 mg (4 months): asthenia, flu syndrome, general pain, headache, injection-site reaction, hot flashes/sweats, GI disorders, edema, skin reaction, urinary disorders.
  - 45 mg (6 months): hot flush, injection-site pain, URI, fatigue.
- In postmarketing experience, mood swings, depression, rare suicidal ideation, and rare pituitary apoplexy (presenting as sudden headache, vomiting, visual changes, ophthalmoplegia, change in mental status, sometimes cardiovascular collapse) have been reported. Patients with pituitary apoplexy may have a pituitary adenoma, and symptoms arise within 2 weeks of the first dose, sometimes within the first hour.
- Monitor bone density in patients as chronic androgen suppression may decrease bone density. Men should be encouraged to take calcium and vitamin D supplementation, in addition to monitoring of bone density studies.

Potential Toxicities/Side Effects and the Nursing Process

I.   ALTERATION IN COMFORT related to HOT FLASHES, TUMOR FLARE, EDEMA

Defining Characteristics: Headache, dizziness, and hot flashes may occur. Vasodilation most common, with 67.9% incidence. Sweating may affect 5% of patients. Tumor flare may also occur initially (bone and tumor pain, transient increase in tumor size due to transient increase in testosterone levels). Breast tenderness has been reported. Peripheral edema may occur in 8% of patients.

Nursing Implications: Inform patient that symptoms may occur, that flare reaction will subside after the initial 2 weeks of therapy. Encourage patient to report symptoms early. Develop symptom management plan with patient and physician.

II.   POTENTIAL SEXUAL DYSFUNCTION related to LIBIDO, IMPOTENCE

Defining Characteristics: Frequently causes decreased libido and erectile impotence in men. Gynecomastia occurs in 3–6.9% of patients. In women, amenorrhea occurs after 10 weeks of therapy.

Nursing Implications: As appropriate, explore with patient and significant other the issues of reproductive and sexual patterns and the impact chemotherapy may have on them. Discuss strategies to preserve sexuality and reproductive health.

III.   DEPRESSION, POTENTIAL, related to DRUG EFFECT

Defining Characteristics: Depression may affect up to 5.3% of patients, and less commonly, patients may develop emotional lability, insomnia, nervousness, anxiety.

Nursing Implications: Assess baseline affect and usual coping strategies. Teach patient to report change in affect. Assess effectiveness of coping strategies, encourage patient to verbalize feelings, and provide emotional support. Assess need for referral to psychiatric nurse specialist or social worker if supportive efforts ineffective.

IV.   ALTERED NUTRITION, LESS THAN BODY REQUIREMENTS, related to GI SIDE EFFECTS

Defining Characteristics: Anorexia, nausea, and vomiting may occur rarely, with an incidence of < 5%.

Nursing Implications: If patients experience symptoms, encourage small, frequent feedings of favorite foods, especially high-calorie, high-protein foods. Monitor weight weekly. Assess incidence and pattern of nausea, vomiting, or anorexia if they occur. Discuss need for antiemetic with physician and patient.

V.   ALTERATION IN SKIN INTEGRITY, POTENTIAL, related to INSERTION AND REMOVAL OF 12-MONTH IMPLANT

Defining Characteristics: Insertion and removal of implant caused local site bruising (34.8%) and burning (5.6%). In general, the reactions lasted 2 weeks, and then resolved completely. In about 10% of patients, reactions lasted longer than 2 weeks, or reactions did not develop until after 2 weeks.

Nursing Implications: Assess baseline skin integrity after implant insertion or removal. Teach patient that these reactions may occur, and will resolve, usually within 2 weeks. Teach patients to use local measures to minimize feeling of burning.

Drug: lomustine (CCNU, CeeNU)

Class: Alkylating agent (nitrosourea).

Mechanism of Action: Nitrosourea alkylates DNA with a reactive chloroethyl carbonium ion, producing strand breaks and crosslinks that inhibit RNA and DNA synthesis. Interferes with enzymes and histidine utilization. Is cell cycle phase nonspecific.

Metabolism: Completely absorbed from GI tract. Metabolized rapidly, partly protein bound. Undergoes hepatic recirculation. Lipid soluble: crosses BBB; 75% excreted in urine within 4 days.

Indication: Shown to be useful as a single agent in addition to other treatment modalities, or in established combination therapy with other approved chemotherapeutic agents in (1) brain tumors both primary and metastatic, in patients who have already received appropriate surgical and/or radiotherapeutic procedures; (2) Hodgkin's disease, as secondary therapy in combination with other approved drugs in patients who relapse while being treated with primary therapy, or who fail to respond to primary therapy.

Dosage/Range:
- 130 mg/m² PO every 6 weeks.
- 100 mg/m² if given with other myelosuppressive drugs.

Drug Preparation:
- Oral. Available in 10-mg, 30-mg, and 100-mg capsules.

Drug Administration:
- Administer on an empty stomach at bedtime.
- Patient teaching (FDA, 2009):
  - Patients should be told that lomustine is an anticancer drug and belongs to the group of medicines known as alkylating agents.
  - In order to provide the proper dose of lomustine (CeeNU), patients should be aware that there may be two or more different types and colors of capsules in the container dispensed by the pharmacist.
  - Patients should be told that lomustine (CeeNU) is given as a single oral dose and will not be repeated for at least 6 weeks.
  - Patients should be told that nausea and vomiting may occur, to take anti-nausea medicine to prevent this; if it occurs, it usually lasts less than 24 hours, although loss of appetite may last for several days.
  - If any of the following reactions occur, notify the physician: fever, chills, sore throat, unusual bleeding or bruising, shortness of breath, dry cough, swelling of feet or lower legs, mental confusion, or yellowing of eyes and skin.
  - Patients should be told to wear gloves when handling lomustine (CeeNU) capsules.

Drug Interactions:
- Myelosuppressive drugs increase hematologic toxicity; reduce dose.

Lab Effects/Interference:
- Decreased CBC.
- Increased LFTs, RFTs.

Special Considerations:
- Give orally on an empty stomach.
- Consumption of alcohol should be avoided for a short period after taking lomustine.
- Absorbed 30–60 minutes after administration; consequently, vomiting does not usually affect efficacy.

Potential Toxicities/Side Effects and the Nursing Process

I.   INFECTION AND BLEEDING related to MYELOSUPPRESSION

Defining Characteristics: Nadir of platelets: 26–34 days, lasting 6–10 days; nadir of WBC: 41–46 days, lasting 9–14 days. Delayed and cumulative bone marrow depression with successive dosing: recovery takes 6–8 weeks. Bone marrow depression is dose-limiting toxicity.

Nursing Implications: Drug should be administered every 6–8 weeks due to delayed nadir and recovery. Monitor CBC, platelets prior to drug administration (WBC > 4,000/mm^3 and platelets > 100,000/mm^3). Dispense only one dose at a time.

II.   ALTERATION IN NUTRITION, LESS THAN BODY REQUIREMENTS, related to NAUSEA/VOMITING, ANOREXIA, DIARRHEA

Defining Characteristics: Onset of nausea/vomiting occurs 2–6 hours after taking dose; may be severe. Anorexia may last for several days. Diarrhea is uncommon.

Nursing Implications: Administer drug on an empty stomach at bedtime. Premedicate with antiemetic and sedative or hypnotic to promote sleep. Discourage food or fluid intake for 2 hours after drug administration. Encourage small, frequent feedings of favorite foods. Encourage high-calorie, high-protein foods; monitor weekly weights. Encourage patient to report onset of diarrhea. Administer or teach patient to self-administer antidiarrheal medication.

III.   ALTERATION IN URINARY ELIMINATION related to RENAL COMPROMISE

Defining Characteristics: After prolonged therapy with high cumulative doses, tubular atrophy, glomerular sclerosis, and interstitial nephritis have occurred, leading to renal failure.

Nursing Implications: Monitor BUN, creatinine prior to dosing, especially in patients receiving prolonged or high cumulative dose therapy. If abnormalities are noted, a creatinine clearance should be determined.

IV.   POTENTIAL FOR SEXUAL DYSFUNCTION related to MUTAGENIC AND TERATOGENIC QUALITIES OF LOMUSTINE

Defining Characteristics: Drug is teratogenic, mutagenic, and carcinogenic.

Nursing Implications: As appropriate, discuss birth control measures.

V.   ACTIVITY INTOLERANCE related to LETHARGY, CONFUSION

Defining Characteristics: Neurologic dysfunction may occur rarely: confusion, lethargy, disorientation, ataxia.

Nursing Implications: Perform neurologic assessment as part of prechemotherapy assessment. Assess orientation and level of consciousness, gait, activity tolerance.

VI. POTENTIAL SENSORY/PERCEPTUAL ALTERATIONS (VISUAL) related to OCULAR DAMAGE

Defining Characteristics: Ocular damage may occur rarely: optic neuritis, retinopathy, blurred vision.

Nursing Implications: Assess vision during prechemotherapy assessment. Encourage patient to report any visual changes.

Drug: mechlorethamine hydrochloride (Mustargen, nitrogen mustard, HN₂)

Class: Alkylating agent.

Mechanism of Action: Produces interstrand and intrastrand crosslinkages in DNA, causing miscoding, breakage, and failures of replication. Cell cycle phase nonspecific.

Metabolism: Undergoes chemical transformation after injection with less than 0.01% excreted unchanged in urine. Drug is rapidly inactivated by body fluids. 50% of the inactive metabolites are excreted in the urine within 24 hours.

Indication: (1) IV for the palliative treatment of Hodgkin's disease (Stages III, IV), lymphosarcoma, chronic myelocytic or chronic lymphocytic leukemia, polycythemia vera, mycosis fungoides, and bronchogenic carcinoma; (2) intrapleurally, intraperitoneally, or intrapericardially for the palliative treatment of metastatic carcinoma resulting in effusion.

Contraindication: In patients with known infectious disease and in patients who have previously had anaphlyactic reactions to nitrogen mustard.

Dosage/Range:
- IV: 0.4 mg/kg, or 12–16 mg/m² IV as single agent; 6 mg/m² IV days 1 and 8 of 28-day cycle with MOPP regimen.
- Topical: Dilute 10 mg in 60 mL sterile water; apply with rubber gloves.
- Intracavitary: Pleural, peritoneal, pericardial: 0.2–0.4 mg/kg.

Drug Preparation:
- Add sterile water or 0.9% sodium chloride to each vial. Wear eye and hand protection when mixing.
- Administer via sidearm or rapidly running IV.
- Drug must be used within 15 minutes of reconstitution.

Drug Administration:
- Intravenous: This drug is a potent vesicant. Give through a freely running IV to avoid extravasation, which can lead to ulceration, pain, and necrosis. Check hospital's policy and procedure for administration of a vesicant.

Drug Interactions:
- Myelosuppressive drugs: Additive hematologic toxicity; dose-reduce or monitor patient closely.
- Sodium thiosulfate: inactivates drug.

Lab Effects/Interference:
- Decreased CBC.
- Increased uric acid, RFTs.

Special Considerations:
- Drug is a vesicant. Give through a running IV to avoid extravasation. Antidote is sodium thiosulfate: dilute 4 mL sodium thiosulfate injection USP (10%) with 6 mL sterile water for injection, USP, and inject subcutaneously in area of infiltration.
- Nadir is 6–8 days after treatment.
- Side effects occur in the reproductive system, such as amenorrhea and azoospermia.
- Severe nausea and vomiting.
- Systemic toxic effects may occur with intracavitary drug administration.

Potential Toxicities/Side Effects and the Nursing Process

I.   ALTERATION IN NUTRITION, LESS THAN BODY REQUIREMENTS, related to NAUSEA AND VOMITING, ANOREXIA, DIARRHEA

Defining Characteristics: Nausea and vomiting occur in ~100% of patients, within 30 minutes to 2 hours of drug administration, and up to 8 hours afterward. Nausea and vomiting can be severe, but can be prevented by the use of combination antiemetics such as serotonin antagonist (granisetron or ondansetron) and dexamethasone. Anorexia and taste distortion (metallic taste) occur commonly. Diarrhea may occur up to several days after drug administration.

Nursing Implications: Premedicate with combination antiemetics such as serotonin antagonist (granisetron or ondansetron) and dexamethasone. Continue prophylactically. Antiemetic and sedative may need to be started the evening before if patient develops anticipatory nausea and vomiting. Encourage small, frequent feedings of cool, bland foods, dry toast, crackers. Monitor I/O to detect fluid volume deficit. Notify physician of the need for more aggressive antiemetic if vomitus > 750 mL. Encourage small, frequent feedings of high-calorie, high-protein foods. Encourage use of spices for anorexia and obtain weekly weights. Encourage patient to report onset of diarrhea. Administer or teach patient to self-administer antidiarrheal medication and teach diet modifications (low residue) as appropriate.

II.   INFECTION AND BLEEDING related to BONE MARROW DEPRESSION

Defining Characteristics: Potent myelosuppressant with nadir 6–8 days, recovery in 4 weeks. Patients at risk for profound bone marrow depression are those with previous extensive XRT, previous chemotherapy, or compromised bone marrow function. Lymphocyte depression occurs within 24 hours of drug dose.

Nursing Implications: Evaluate WBC, with neutrophil, and platelet count, and discuss any abnormalities with physician prior to drug administration. Assess for signs/symptoms of infection or bleeding; instruct patient in signs/symptoms of infection and bleeding, and to notify nurse or physician if they arise. Teach patient self-care measures to minimize risk of infection and bleeding, including avoidance of OTC aspirin-containing medications. Assess patient's Hgb/HCT and signs/symptoms of fatigue; teach patient self-assessment and to alternate rest and activity as needed. Transfuse red blood cells and platelets per physician order.

III. IMPAIRED SKIN INTEGRITY related to ALOPECIA, DRUG EXTRAVASATION

Defining Characteristics: Alopecia usually occurs as diffuse thinning. Drug is a potent vesicant, causing tissue necrosis and sloughing if extravasation occurs. Thrombosis or thrombophlebitis may occur despite all precautions, and venous access device may be required. Delayed cutaneous hypersensitivity is seen with topical application.

Nursing Implications: Discuss with patient hair loss, anticipated impact, and strategies to decrease distress, e.g., obtaining wig prior to hair loss. Assess body disturbance from hyperpigmentation and discuss strategies to minimize this, e.g., nail polish. Drug must be administered via patent IV. Assess need for venous access device early. Delayed cutaneous hypersensitivity (topical application) is not an indication to stop the drug. Discuss symptomatic management with physician. If extravasation is suspected, stop drug; aspirate any residual drug and blood from IV tubing, IV catheter/needle, and IV site if possible; instill antidote, sodium thiosulfate (1/6 molar), into area of apparent infiltration as per physician orders and institutional policy and procedure; apply cold or topical medication as per physician orders and institutional policy and procedure. Assess site regularly for pain, progression of erythema, induration, and for evidence of necrosis. When in doubt about whether drug is infiltrating, TREAT AS AN INFILTRATION. Teach patient to assess site, and instruct to notify physician if condition worsens. Arrange next clinic visit for assessment of site depending on drug, amount infiltrated, extent of potential injury, and patient variables. Document in patient's record as per institutional policy. Warm packs may decrease discomfort of phlebitis. Have standing orders and sodium thiosulfate injection USP (10%) close by in the event of actual infiltration of drug; dilute sodium thiosulfate with sterile water for injection and inject subcutaneously in area of infiltration.

IV. ALTERATION IN COMFORT related to CHILLS, FEVER, DIARRHEA

Defining Characteristics: Chills, fever, diarrhea may occur after drug administration. Also weakness, drowsiness, headache may occur.

Nursing Implications: Assess patient for these symptoms during hour following treatment. Instruct patient to report these symptoms and teach self-management at home if outpatient. Provide symptomatic management per physician with acetaminophen, antidiarrheal medication.

V.   POTENTIAL SEXUAL DYSFUNCTION related to DRUG EFFECTS

Defining Characteristics: Drug is teratogenic, carcinogenic. Amenorrhea occurs in females. Impaired spermatogenesis occurs in males. If administered to pregnant patients, spontaneous abortion or fetal abnormalities may occur.

Nursing Implications: As appropriate, explore with patient and partner issues of reproductive and sexual patterns, and anticipated impact chemotherapy will have. Discuss strategies to preserve sexuality and reproductive health (sperm banking, contraception).

VI.   POTENTIAL FOR SENSORY/PERCEPTUAL ALTERATIONS related to CRANIAL NERVE INJURY

Defining Characteristics: Tinnitus, deafness, and other signs of eighth cranial nerve damage occur rarely, with high drug doses or regional perfusion techniques. Temporary aphasia and paresis occur very rarely.

Nursing Implications: Assess hearing ability, presence of tinnitus prior to drug doses. If high doses of drug are given, or regional perfusion used, schedule patient for periodic audiometry. Instruct patient to report signs/symptoms of hearing loss.

Drug: melphalan hydrochloride (Alkeran, L-phenylalanine mustard, L-PAM, L-sarcolysin)

Class: Alkylating agent.

Mechanism of Action: Prevents cell replication by causing breaks and crosslinkages in DNA strands with subsequent miscoding and breakage. Cell cycle phase nonspecific. Drug is derivative of nitrogen mustard.

Metabolism: Variable bioavailability after oral administration, especially if taken with food. Therefore, dose is titrated to WBC count; 20–50% of drug is excreted in feces over 6 days, 50% excreted in urine within 24 hours. After IV administration, parent compound disappears from plasma, with a half-life of about 2 hours.

Indications: (1) PO: for the palliative treatment of multiple myeloma, and for the palliation of nonresectable epithelial carcinoma of the ovary; (2) IV: palliative treatment of patients with multiple myeloma for whom oral therapy is not appropriate.

Contraindications: Patients whose disease has shown prior resistance to melphalan, and patients with demonstrated hypersensitivity to the drug.

Dosage/Range:
- **Multiple myeloma:** PO: Several regimens, including 0.25 mg/kg/day × 4 days, in combination with prednisone 2 mg/kg/day, repeated every 6 weeks; OR 6 mg/m^2 orally

daily × 5 days every 6 weeks for myeloma; OR 0.1 mg/kg PO × 2–3 weeks, then maintenance of 2–4 mg daily when bone marrow has recovered.
* **Bone marrow transplantation:** 50–60 mg/m² IV, but may be as high as 140–200 mg/m² (investigational).

Drug Preparation:
* Oral: Available in 2-mg tablets. Take on empty stomach.
* IV: Reconstitute 50-mg vial with 10 mL of provided diluent resulting in concentration of 5 mg/mL. Further dilute in 100–150 mL to produce a final concentration ≤ 2 mg/mL in 0.9% sodium chloride. Use provided 0.45-mm filter. Administer over 30–45 minutes. Stable for 1 hour at room temperature.

Drug Administration:
* Serious hypersensitivity reactions reported with IV administration.
* IV drug can cause anaphylaxis.
* IV drug is an irritant—avoid extravasation.

Drug Interactions:
* Myelosuppressive chemotherapy: Increases hematologic toxicity; dose-reduce or monitor patient very carefully.
* Cyclosporine: Increases nephrotoxicity.
* H₂ blockers: may decrease oral melphalan bioavailability.

Lab Effects/Interference:
* Decreased CBC.

Special Considerations:
* Nadir is 14–21 days after treatment.
* Increased risk of nephrotoxicity when given with cyclosporine.
* Drug dose reductions are recommended in patients with renal compromise.
* Drug is used in regional perfusion.

Potential Toxicities/Side Effects and the Nursing Process

I. INFECTION AND BLEEDING related to BONE MARROW DEPRESSION

Defining Characteristics: Bone marrow depression may be pronounced; leukopenia and thrombocytopenia occur 14–21 days after intermittent dosing schedules. May be delayed in onset, and cumulative with nadir extended to 5–6 weeks. Combined immunosuppression from disease (e.g., multiple myeloma) and drug may prolong vulnerability to infection. Thrombocytopenia may be persistent.

Nursing Implications: Evaluate WBC, with neutrophil, and platelet count and discuss any abnormalities with physician prior to drug administration. Assess for signs/symptoms of infection or bleeding; instruct patient in signs/symptoms of infection and bleeding, and to notify nurse or physician if they arise. Teach patient self-care measures to minimize risk of infection and bleeding, including avoidance of OTC aspirin-containing medications.

Assess patient for Hgb/HCT and signs/symptoms of fatigue; teach patient self-assessment and to alternate rest and activity as needed. Transfuse packed red blood cells and platelets per physician order.

II.   ALTERATION IN NUTRITION, LESS THAN BODY REQUIREMENTS, related to NAUSEA AND VOMITING, ANOREXIA

Defining Characteristics: Nausea and vomiting are mild at low, continuous dosing; severe following high doses. Anorexia occurs rarely.

Nursing Implications: Administer drug (oral) on empty stomach. Premedicate with antiemetic (oral) 1 hour before oral dose. Use aggressive antiemetic regimen for IV Alkeran. Encourage small, frequent feedings of favorite foods, especially high-calorie, high-protein foods. Encourage use of spices and obtain weekly weights.

III.   ALTERATION IN CARDIAC OUTPUT, PERFUSION related to ANAPHYLAXIS

Defining Characteristics: Severe hypersensitivity reactions can occur with IV administration, including diaphoresis, hypotension, and cardiac arrest.

Nursing Implications: Review standing orders for management of patient in anaphylaxis and identify location of anaphylaxis kit containing epinephrine 1:1,000, hydrocortisone sodium succinate (Solu-Cortef), diphenhydramine HCl (Benadryl), aminophylline, and others. Prior to drug administration, obtain baseline vital signs and record mental status. Administer drug slowly, diluted as per physician's order. Observe for following signs/symptoms, usually occurring within first 15 minutes of infusion. Subjective signs are generalized itching, nausea, chest tightness, crampy abdominal pain, difficulty speaking, anxiety, agitation, sense of impending doom, uneasiness, desire to urinate/defecate, dizziness, chills. Objective signs are flushed appearance (angioedema of face, neck, eyelids, hands, feet), localized or generalized urticaria, respiratory distress ± wheezing, hypotension, cyanosis. For generalized allergic reaction, stop infusion and notify physician. Place patient in supine position to promote perfusion of visceral organs. Monitor VS. Provide emotional reassurance to patient and family. Maintain patent airway and have CPR equipment ready if needed. Document incident. Discuss with physician desensitization for further dosing versus drug discontinuance.

IV.   POTENTIAL SEXUAL DYSFUNCTION related to DRUG EFFECTS

Defining Characteristics: Potentially mutagenic and teratogenic.

Nursing Implications: Encourage patient to verbalize goals about family; discuss options, such as sperm banking. As appropriate, discuss or refer for counseling about birth control measures during therapy.

V. POTENTIAL FOR INJURY related to SECOND MALIGNANCY

Defining Characteristics: Acute myelogenous and myelomonocytic leukemias may occur after continuous long-term dosing, especially in patients with ovarian cancer and multiple myeloma. Heralded by preleukemic pancytopenia of several weeks' duration. Chromosomal abnormalities characteristic of acute leukemia.

Nursing Implications: Patients receiving prolonged continuous therapy should be closely followed during and after treatment.

VI. POTENTIAL FOR IMPAIRED GAS EXCHANGE related to PULMONARY TOXICITY

Defining Characteristics: Rare, but may occur, especially with continued chronic dosing. Bronchopulmonary dysplasia and pulmonary fibrosis.

Nursing Implications: Assess pulmonary status for signs/symptoms of pulmonary dysfunction. Assess lung sounds prior to dosing. Instruct patient to report cough or dyspnea. Discuss PFTs to be performed periodically with physician. Long-term follow-up is important.

VII. IMPAIRED SKIN INTEGRITY related to ALOPECIA, MACULOPAPULAR RASH, URTICARIA

Defining Characteristics: Alopecia is minimal if it occurs at all. Maculopapular rash and urticaria are infrequent.

Nursing Implications: Assess skin integrity and presence of rash, urticaria, alopecia prior to dosing. Assess impact of these alterations on patient and develop plan to manage symptom distress.

Drug: mercaptopurine (PURIXAN oral suspension, Purinethol, 6-MP)

Class: Nucleoside metabolic inhibitor (antimetabolite).

Mechanism of Action: Nucleoside metabolic inhibitor that is activated to form 6-thioguanine nucleotides (6-TGNs). When the cell uses 6-TGN (a false metabolite) to make nucleic acids instead of purine bases, it causes the cell's cell cycle to stop and the cell to die. The drug also has other actions. Cell cycle phase specific for S phase.

Metabolism: Absorption of oral dose is incomplete with approximately 50% bioavailability. There is bioequivalence between tablet and suspension in bioavailability, although the mean Cmax following oral suspension was 34% higher than the tablet. Does not cross BBB. Metabolized by two major pathways: (1) thiol methylation catalyzed by the enzyme thiopurine S-methyltransferase (TPMT) to form an inactive metabolite, and (2) oxidation catalyzed by the enzyme xanthine oxidase into another inactive metabolite. Elimination half-life is about 2 hrs. About 46% of the dose is excreted in the urine in the first 24 hrs. There is genetic polymorphism in the TPMT gene. About 0.3% of Caucasians and African Americans have 2 non-functional alleles (copies of the genes, called homozygous-deficient), so this metabolic pathway is inactive. Ten percent of patients have one TPMT non-functional allele (heterozygous) leading to low or intermediate TPMT activity, and 90% of patients have normal TPMT activity with two functional alleles. If TPMT is inactive (homozygous-deficient patients) or reduced (low or intermediate TPMT activity), mercaptopurine is incompletely metabolized by one pathway; if normal mercaptopurine doses are administered, there is higher risk of severe mercaptopurine toxicity. TPMT genotyping or phenotyping (red blood cell TPMT activity) helps to identify patients who are homozygous-deficient or who have low/intermediate TPMT activity. See package insert for TPMT testing details.

Indication: Mercaptopurine is indicated for the treatment of patients with ALL as a component of a combination maintenance therapy regimen; drug is not indicated for but is used to treat some patients with other cancers, Chrohn's disease, and ulcerative colitis.

Dosage/Range:
Maintenance:
- Starting dose in multi-agent combination chemotherapy 1.5–2.5 mg/kg (50–75 mg/m^2) for acute lymphoblastic leukemia (ALL), oral.
  - After beginning mercaptopurine, dose should be determined by periodic ANC and platelet counts.
  - Monitor serum transaminase levels, alkaline phosphatase, and bilirubin levels weekly at the beginning of therapy, then monthly. Monitor LFTs daily, more frequently in patients who are receiving other potentially hepatotoxic drugs or with preexisting liver disease.
  - Reduce dose in cases of hepatic or renal dysfunction.
  - Interrupt mercaptopurine when clinical or laboratory evidence suggests hepatotoxicity.
  - Start at low end of dosing range, patients with:
    - Elderly: greater frequency of decreased hepatic, renal, or cardiac function; other concommitant disease; other drug therapy.
    - Renal impairment: increase the dosing interval to 36–48 hr; adjust subsequent doses on efficacy and toxicity.
    - Hepatic impairment: monitor transaminases and bilirubin; monitor closely for toxity; hold or adjust the dose of mercaptopurine.
- TPMT-deficient patients: perform TPMT testing; should be considered in patients who experience severe bone marrow toxicities.
  - Homozygous-deficient patients may require a 90% dose reduction (patient receives only 10% of standard dose).
  - Heterozygous TPMT-deficiency patients usally tolerate recommended mercaptopurine dose, but some patients do require a dose reduction.
  Avoid coadministration with allopurinol, as allopurinol inhibits xanthine oxidase; if they must be coadministered, mercaptopurine dose must be reduced by at least 25% of the normal dose.

Drug Preparation:
- Oral: tablet, none; available in 50-mg tablets.
- Oral suspension (PURIXAN, 2,000 mg/100 mL or 20 mg/mL): Shake bottle vigorously for at least 30 seconds to ensure it is well mixed; color will be pink to brown viscous oral

suspension. Once opened, drug should be used within 6 weeks. Ask pharmacist to give patient oral syringe and suitable adaptor, based on patient's dosing requirement.
- Tablet has been available since 1953, but precise BSA dosing and dose adjustments are difficult with the tablet; oral suspension provides more accurate and consistent dosing.

Drug Administration:
Oral.
- Teach patient how to administer mercaptopurine using gloves. If oral suspension, demonstrate how to draw up prescribed dose in a syringe.
- If the syringe will be used for multiple use, teach patient and caregivers to (1) wash the syringe with warm, soapy water and rinse well; (2) hold the syringe under water and move the plunger up and down several times to make sure the inside of the syringe is clean; (3) ensure the syringe is completely dry before using the syringe again for dosing; (4) store the syringe in a hygienic place, along with the medicine.
- Lab tests:
  - CBS/differential, transaminases, bilirubin.
  - Bone marrow should be evaluated in patients with prolonged or repeated marrow suppression to assess leukemia status and marrow cellularity.
  - Evaluate TPMT status in patients with severe bone marrow toxicity (clinical and/or laboratory), or repeated episodes of myelosuppression.
- Drug is cytotoxic; teach patient and caregiver to use special handling and how to dispose of hazardous waste.

Drug Interactions:
Drugs that decrease the clearance of mercaptopurine and increase drug serum levels do so by (1) inhibiting first-pass oxidative metabolism by xanthine oxidase; or by (2) inhibiting TPMT enzyme. Avoid coadministration; if drugs must be coadministered, mercaptopurine dose must be reduced.
- Allopurinol: increased bone marrow suppression, nausea, vomiting; reduce dose to 25–35% of normal.
- Myelosuppressants (e.g., chemotherapy, trimethoprim-sulfamethoxazole): increased BMD; monitor patient closely.
- Warfarin: may decrease anticoagulant effect; monitor closely and dose based on PT or INR.
- Aminosalicylate derivatives (e.g., olsalazine, mesalamine, sulfasalazine): may inhibit TPMT. If coadministered, use the lowest dose of each drug and monitor the patient closely for BMD.
Vaccines: mercaptopurine is immunosuppressive and may impair the immune response to vaccines; there may be risk of infection with live virus vaccines.

Lab Effects/Interference:
- Decreased CBC.
- Increased LFTs.
- Increased RFTs: tumor lysis.

Special Considerations:
- Drug is hepatotoxic; reports of death associated with hepatic necrosis have been reported. Risk for hepatic injury is increased when recommended dose is exceeded. Clinical

jaundice appears in the first 1–2 months of treatment, but it has been reported as early as 1 week and as late as 8 years. Anorexia, diarrhea, jaundice, and ascites may appear. Reports of jaundice resolving after drug interruption, and reappearance with rechallenge have been documented. Monitor LFTs weekly when beginning mercaptopurine, then at least monthly.

- Teach women of reproductive potential to avoid pregnancy. Drug can cause embryo-fetal toxicity. If drug is used in pregnancy or if the woman becomes pregnant while taking drug, apprise patient of potential hazard to the fetus. Drug increases risk of abortions in first trimester as well as later in the pregnancy; stillbirth was seen after the first trimester as well.
- Nursing mothers should decide whether to discontinue nursing or the drug.
- Most common (>20%) adverse reactions in clinical trials were myelosuppression (anemia, neutropenia, lymphopenia, thrombocytopenia). Adverse reactions occurring 5–20% were anorexia, nausea, vomiting, diarrhea, malaise, rash. Rare reactions (<5%) were urticaria, hyperuricemia, oral lesions (thrush), elevated transaminases, hyperbilirubinemia, hyperpigmentation. Delayed or late toxicities include hepatic fibrosis, hyperbilirubinemia, alopecia, pulmonary fibrosis, oligospermia, secondary malignancies.
- Drug is mutagenic in animals and humans, carcinogenic in animals, and may increase risk of secondary malignancies.
  - Rarely, hepatosplenic T-cell lymphoma has been described in adolescents and young adults receiving tumor necrosis factor (TNF) blockers and azathioprine and/ or mercaptopurine, as well as those receiving mercaptopurine alone, for treatment of Crohn's disease or ulcerative colitis (FDA, 2011). Drug is NOT approved for this use.
  - Patients with RA, Crohn's disease, ankylosing spondylitis, psoriatic arthritis, and plaque psoriasis may be more likely to develop lymphoma than the general population. If patient develops splenomegaly, hepatomegaly, abdominal pain, persistent fever, night sweats, and weight loss, discuss with physician, NP/PA further evaluation.

Potential Toxicities/Side Effects and the Nursing Process

I.   POTENTIAL FOR INFECTION AND BLEEDING related to BONE MARROW DEPRESSION

Defining Characteristics: Nadir varies from 5 days to 6 weeks after treatment. Leukopenia more prominent than thrombocytopenia. Blood counts may continue to fall after therapy is stopped. Drug fever may occur rarely, but other causes, such as sepsis in the setting of ALL, must be ruled out first.

Nursing Implications: Evaluate WBC, with neutrophil, and platelet count, which should be monitored closely, and discuss any abnormalities with physician prior to drug administration. Assess for signs/symptoms of infection or bleeding; instruct patient to notify nurse or physician if they arise. Teach patient self-care measures to minimize risk of infection and bleeding, including avoidance of OTC aspirin-containing medications. Assess patient's Hgb/HCT and signs/symptoms of fatigue; teach patient self-assessment and to alternate rest and activity as needed. Discuss dose modifications based on CBC/differential for severe neutropenia and thrombocytopenia.

II. ALTERATION IN NUTRITION, LESS THAN BODY REQUIREMENTS, related to HEPATOTOXICITY, GI SYMPTOMS

Defining Characteristics: Reversible cholestatic jaundice may develop after 2–5 months of treatment. Hepatic necrosis may develop. Nausea, vomiting, anorexia, diarrhea are infrequent. Stomatitis uncommon, but appears as white patchy areas similar to thrush.

Nursing Implications: Monitor transaminases, alkaline phosphatase, and bilirubin weekly at drug initiation, then monthly during treatment. Notify physician of any elevations. Assess for signs/symptoms of hepatotoxicity, which is an indication for discontinuing treatment. Instruct patient to report GI side effects and to perform self-care measures as appropriate.

III. POTENTIAL FOR IMPAIRED SKIN INTEGRITY related to RASH

Defining Characteristics: Skin eruptions; rash may occur.

Nursing Implications: Advise patient these changes may occur. Instruct patient in symptomatic care if distress related to skin reactions occurs.

Drug: methotrexate (Amethopterin, Mexate, Folex)

Class: Antimetabolite, folic acid antagonist.

Mechanism of Action: Blocks the enzyme dihydrofolate reductase (DHFR), which inhibits the conversion of folic acid to tetrahydrofolic acid, resulting in an inhibition of the key precursors of DNA, RNA, and cellular proteins. May synchronize malignant cells in the S phase: at high plasma levels, passive entry of the drug into tumor cells can potentially overcome drug resistance.

Metabolism: Following parenteral administration, drug is completely absorbed. Oral drug is absorbed from GI tract in a dose-dependent manner: 60% bioavailability at 30 mg/m^2 or lower doses; but at doses > 80 mg/m^2, bioavailability is significantly less (possibly due to saturation effect). Peak plasma levels are reached in 1–2 hours. Drug is 50% protein-bound; concurrent use of drugs that displace methotrexate from serum albumin should be avoided. Salicylates, sulfonamides, Dilantin, some antibacterials—including tetracycline, chloramphenicol, para-aminobenzoic acid—and alcohol should be avoided, as they will delay excretion. Plasma half-life is 2 hours; 50–100% of dose is excreted into the systemic circulation, with peak concentration 3–12 hours after administration. At high doses, drug crosses blood–brain barrier (BBB), but high CSF concentrations of drug require IT administration. After absorption, drug is metabolized via hepatic and intracellular processes; some active metabolites may be retained in tissue with prolonged drug release, so effusions should be tapped prior to administration of high doses. After oral administration, some drug is partially metabolized by intestinal flora. The drug half-life is 3–10 hr for doses < 30 mg/m^2 while the terminal half-life for high doses is 8–15 hrs. Drug is principally excreted via the kidneys, and it is dose- and route-dependent. After IV drug administration, most (80–90%) of unchanged drug is excreted via the kidneys (glomerular filtration and active tubular secretion) in the urine within 24 hr. Less than 10% of drug is excreted in the bile. Toxicity is believed to be the result of high methotrexate serum levels due to delayed drug excretion (with subsequent longer time of drug exposure), caused by renal impairment, third space effusion, or other factors.

Indication:

- Cancer: (1) gestational choriocarcinoma, chorioadenoam destruens and hydatidiform mole; (2) ALL for prophylaxis of meningeal leukemia and used as maintenance therapy in combination with other chemotherapy agents; (3) meningeal leukemia; (4) alone or in combination with other anticancer agents in the treatment of breast cancer, epidermoid cancers of head and neck, advanced mycosis fungoides (cutaneous T cell lymphoma, lung cancer, particularly squamous cell and small cell types, and advanced stage NHL); (5) high doses with leucovorin rescue in combination with other chemotherapy agents in nonmetastatic osteosarcoma after surgical resection or amputation of the primary tumor.
- Rheumatoid Arthritis.
- Psoriasis.

Dosage/Range:

- Cancer.
- Oral: preferred for low doses.
- IV: Low: 10–50 mg/m^2; med: 100–500 mg/m^2; high: 500 mg/m^2 and above with leucovorin rescue.
- IM: 25 mg/m^2.
- IT: 10–15 mg/m^2 with preservative-free diluent ONLY.
- Rheumatoid Arthritis (RA), juvenile RA, psoriasis: single oral dose 7.5 mg once weekly, or divided oral doses of 2.5 mg at 12-hour intervals for 3 doses, given as a course once a week.

Drug Preparation:

- 5-, 50-, 100-, and 200-mg vials are available already reconstituted.
- Powder is available in vials without preservative for IT and high-dose administration (reconstitute with preservative-free 0.9% sodium chloride).

Drug Administration:

- 5–149 mg: slow IVP.
- 150–499 mg: IV drip over 20 minutes.
- **Higher Doses:** 500–1,500 mg or higher per m^2: infusion with leucovorin rescue.
- High Dose: 12–15 gm/m^2: Minimum dose must produce a peak serum methotrexate concentration of 1,000 micromolar (10^{-3} mol/L). Usually administered as a 4-hour infusion. Leucovorin (15 mg PO or IV) every 6 hours, beginning 24 hours after the start of the methotrexate infusion.
- Assess labs: proceed only if WBC > 1,500/mL, ANC > 200/mL, platelets > 75,000/mL, serum bilirubin < 1.2 mg/dL, SGPT < 450U; serum creatinine WNL, creatinine clearance > 60 mL/min.
- Assess patient and proceed only if: absence of mucositis, or healing of existing mucositis; any effusion, e.g., pleural, has been drained dry prior to methotrexate; well hydrated (e.g., 1 L/m^2 IV fluid over 6 hr) prior to methotrexate with bicarbonate to alkalinize urine and maintain pH > 7.0 during methotrexate and leucovorin therapy. After initial prechemotherapy hydration, continue hydration at 3 L/m^2/day during methotrexate infusion,

and for 2 days after the infusion has been completed. Assess serum creatinine prior to each subsequent treatment course. If creatinine has increased by 50% or more compared to prior value, reassess and document creatine clearance > 60 mL/min (even if serum creatinine is still WNL).

- Adjust leucovorin dose based on serum methotrexate levels:
  - Normal Methotrexate elimination: serum level 10 micromolar at 24 hr after administration, 1 micromolar at 48 hr, and < 0.2 micromolar at 72 hr: leucovorin dose 15 mg (PO, IM, IV) q 6 hr × 60 hr (10 doses starting 24 hr after start of methotrexate infusion).
  - Delayed Late Methotrexate elimination: serum methotrexate level remaining > 0.2 micromolar at 72 hr, and > 0.05 micromolar at 96 hr after administration: continue 15 mg leucovorin (PO, IM, IV) q 6 hr until methotrexate level is < 0.05 micromolar.
  - Delayed Early Methotrexate elimination and/or evidence of acute renal injury: serum methotrexate level of ≥ 50 micromolar at 24 hr, or ≥ 5 micromolar at 48 hr after administration; OR ≥ 100% increase in serum creatinine at 24 hr after methotrexate administration (e.g., increase from 0.5 mg/dL to 1 mg/dL or more); leucovorin 150 mg IV q 3 hr until methotrexate level is < 1 micromolar; then 15 mg IV q 3 hr until methotrexate level is < 0.05 micromolar.

Drug Interactions:

- Protein-bound drugs (aspirin, sulfonamides, sulfonylureas, phenytoin, tetracycline, chloramphenicol) increase toxicity; give together cautiously and monitor patient closely.
- NSAIDs (nonsteroidal anti-inflammatory drugs, e.g., indomethacin, ketoprofen) increased and prolonged methotrexate levels; DO NOT administer concurrently with high doses of methotrexate; monitor patients closely who are receiving moderate or low-dose methotrexate, if given concurrently. Patients with RA appear to tolerate concomitant NSAIDs and methotrexate at 7.5 mg dose.
- Cotrimoxazole increased methotrexate serum level; DO NOT use concurrently.
- Proton pump inhibitors (PPIs, omeprazole, esomeprazole, pantoprazole): elevated and prolonged methotrexate serum levels; DO NOT use concurrently with high-dose methotrexate. Ranitidine did not cause changes in methotrexate levels.
- Warfarin: anticoagulant effect may increase; monitor INR closely.
- 5-FU: enhanced antitumor effect of 5-FU when methotrexate is given 24 hours before 5-FU.
- Folic acid: may reduce antitumor effect of methotrexate; do not coadminister.
- Thymidine, leucovorin: rescues normal cells from methotrexate effect; may nullify antitumor effect if given close to the time of methotrexate; usually given 24 hours after methotrexate. High-dose leucovorin may reduce the efficacy of IT methotrexate.
- L-asparaginase: reduces methotrexate antitumor effects.
- 6-mercaptopurine (6-MP): methotrexate increases 6-MP plasma levels; if given together, adjust 6-MP dose.
- Oral antibiotics (tetracycline, non-absorbable broad spectrum) may decrease intestinal absorption of methotrexate or interfere with drug metabolism; do not coadminister when methotrexate is given orally.
- Penicillins: may increase methotrexate serum levels at any methotrexate dose; use together cautiously if at all, and monitor patient closely for toxicity.

- Theophylline: methotrexate may decrease theophylline clearance; monitor theophylline levels and adjust dose.
- Folate deficiencies (e.g., trimethoprim/sulfamethoxazole) may increase risk of bone marrow suppression; do not coadminister.

Lab Effects/Interference:
- Decreased CBC.
- Increased LFTs, RFTs.

Special Considerations:
- High doses cross the BBB; reconstitute with preservative-free 0.9% sodium chloride.
- With high doses (12–15 g/m²), urine should be alkalinized both before and after administration, as the drug is a weak acid and can crystallize in the kidneys at an acid pH. Alkalinize with bicarbonate; add to pre- and posthydration fluids. High doses should only be given under the direction of a qualified oncologist at an institution that can provide rapid serum methotrexate level readings and has adequate leucovorin stores if needed.
- Leucovorin rescue must be given on time per orders to prevent excessive toxicity and to achieve maximum therapeutic response (see leucovorin calcium).
- Avoid folic acid and its derivatives during methotrexate therapy. Kidney function must be adequate to excrete drug and avoid excessive toxicity. Check BUN and creatinine before each dose.

Potential Toxicities/Side Effects and the Nursing Process

I. ALTERATION IN NUTRITION, LESS THAN BODY REQUIREMENTS, related to GI SIDE EFFECTS

Defining Characteristics: Nausea and vomiting are uncommon with low dose; more common (39%) with higher and high dose; may occur during drug administration and last 24–72 hours. Anorexia is mild. Stomatitis is a common indication for interruption of therapy: occurs in 3–5 days with high dose, 3–4 weeks with low dose; appears initially at corners of mouth. Stomatitis precedes bone marrow depression. Diarrhea is common and is an indication for interruption of therapy, as enteritis and intestinal perforation may occur; melena, hematemesis may occur. Hepatotoxicity is usually subclinical and reversible, but can lead to cirrhosis; increased risk of hepatotoxicity when given with other agents, like alcohol; transient increase in LFTs with high dose 1–10 days after treatment—may cause jaundice.

Nursing Implications: Premedicate with antiemetics if giving high-dose methotrexate; continue prophylactically for 24 hours (at least) to prevent nausea and vomiting. Encourage small, frequent feedings of cool, bland foods and liquids. Assess for symptoms of fluid and electrolyte imbalance: monitor I/O, daily weights if administered to inpatient. Assess oral cavity every day. Teach patient oral assessment and mouth care regimens. Encourage patient to report early stomatitis. Provide pain relief measures, if indicated. Explore patient compliance to rescue; discuss increase in rescue dose if moderate GI toxicity. Assess patient for diarrhea: guaiac all stools; encourage patient to report onset of diarrhea. Administer or teach patient to self-administer antidiarrheal medications. Monitor LFTs prior to drug dose, especially with high-dose methotrexate. Assess patient prior to and during treatment for signs/symptoms of hepatotoxicity.

II. POTENTIAL FOR INFECTION AND BLEEDING related to BONE MARROW DEPRESSION

Defining Characteristics: Nadir is seen 4–7 days after drug administration, with recovery by day 14. Bone marrow depression occurs in about 10% of patients.

Nursing Implications: Monitor CBC and platelet count prior to drug administration, as well as signs/symptoms of infection or bleeding. Instruct patient in self-assessment of signs/symptoms of infection or bleeding measures to decrease risk. Administer leucovorin calcium as ordered.

III. POTENTIAL FOR ALTERATION IN URINARY ELIMINATION related to RENAL TOXICITY

Defining Characteristics: As an organic acid, methotrexate is insoluble in acid urine. At doses greater than 1 g/m² (i.e., high dose), drug may precipitate in renal tubules, causing acute renal tubular necrosis (ATN).

Nursing Implications: Prehydrate patient with alkaline solution for several hours prior to drug administration. Maintain high urine output with a urine pH greater than 7.0 (hydration fluid may need further alkalinization); dipstick each void. Record I/O. Monitor BUN and serum creatinine before, during, and after drug administration. Increases in these values may require methotrexate dose reductions or leucovorin dose increases.

IV. POTENTIAL FOR IMPAIRED GAS EXCHANGE related to PULMONARY TOXICITY

Defining Characteristics: Pneumothorax (high dose): rare, occurs within first 48 hours after drug administration in patients with pulmonary metastasis. Allergic pneumonitis (high dose): rare but accompanied by eosinophilia, patchy pulmonary infiltrates, fever, cough, shortness of breath. Occurs 1–5 months after initiation of treatment. Pneumonitis (low-dose) symptoms usually disappear within a week, with or without use of steroids; interstitial pneumonitis may be a fatal complication.

Nursing Implications: Assess for signs/symptoms of pulmonary dysfunction before each dose and between doses (see Defining Characteristics section). Discuss PFTs to be performed periodically with physician. Assess lung sounds prior to drug administration. Instruct patient to report cough or dyspnea.

V.   POTENTIAL FOR ALTERATION IN SKIN INTEGRITY related to ALOPECIA, DERMATITIS

Defining Characteristics: Alopecia and dermatitis are uncommon. Pruritus, urticaria may occur. Photosensitivity, sunburnlike rash 1–5 days after treatment; also, patient can develop radiation recall reaction.

Nursing Implications: Assess patient for signs/symptoms of hair loss. Discuss with patient impact of hair loss and strategies to minimize distress. Instruct patient to avoid sun if possible and to stay covered or wear sunblock if sun exposure is unavoidable.

VI.   POTENTIAL FOR SENSORY AND PERCEPTUAL ALTERATIONS related to CNS CHANGES

Defining Characteristics: CNS effects: dizziness, malaise, blurred vision. IT administration may increase CSF pressure. Brain XRT followed by IV methotrexate may also cause neurologic changes.

Nursing Implications: Monitor for CNS effects of drug: dizziness, blurred vision, malaise. Monitor for symptoms of increased CSF pressure: seizures, paresis, headache, nausea and vomiting, brain atrophy, fever. If IV methotrexate follows brain XRT, monitor for symptoms of increased CSF pressure.

VII.   POTENTIAL FOR ALTERATIONS IN COMFORT related to PAIN

Defining Characteristics: Sometimes causes back pain during administration.

Nursing Implications: Monitor patient for back and flank pain. Slow down infusion rate if it occurs. Administer analgesics if pain occurs (must avoid aspirin-containing products, as they displace methotrexate from serum albumin).

Drug: mitomycin (mitomycin C, Mutamycin, 3 Mitozytrex)

Class: Antitumor antibiotic.

Mechanism of Action: Drug acts as alkylating agent and inhibits DNA synthesis by crosslinking of DNA. Alkylating and crosslinking mitomycin metabolites interfere with structure and function of DNA.

Metabolism: Drug is rapidly cleared by the liver. May need to modify dose in presence of liver abnormalities; 10% of drug is excreted unchanged.

Indication: In combination therapy for the treatment of disseminated adenocarcinoma of the stomach or pancreas, and as palliative treatment when other modalities have failed. Not to be used as a single-agent primary therapy.

Contraindications: Patients with thrombocytopenia, coagulation disorder, or increase in bleeding tendency due to other causes; patients hypersensitive to the drug or who have had an idiosyncratic reaction in the past.

Dosage/Range:
- 10 mg/m² IV every 8 weeks, with 5-FU and doxorubicin (FAM regimen).
- Bladder instillations 20–40 mg in 20–40 mL of water.
- May be used at different dosages for autologous bone marrow transplant.

Drug Preparation:
- Depending on vial size, dilute with sterile water to obtain concentration of 0.5 mg/mL.

Drug Administration:
- IV: Drug is potent vesicant.
- Give through the sidearm of a patent, running IV to avoid extravasation, which can lead to ulceration, pain, and necrosis. Check individual hospital policy for administration of a vesicant.

Drug Interactions:
- Myelosuppressive agents: Additive toxicity if overlapping nadirs, use cautiously.

Lab Effects/Interference:
- Decreased CBC, especially WBC and platelets.
- Hemolytic uremic syndrome (rare): Decreased hemoglobin, platelets, and increased creatinine.

Special Considerations:
- Indicated for treatment of disseminated adenocarcinoma of the stomach or pancreas in proven combinations with other approved chemotherapeutic agents and as palliative treatment when other modalities have failed.
- May cause interstitial pneumonitis; monitor patient for acute dyspnea and bronchospasm. Risk increases after a cumulative dose of > 60 mg.
- If patient requires surgery and has received mitomycin C together with other antineoplastics, the patient is at risk for ARDS. fiO₂ should be < 50%, and fluid status should be monitored closely.
- Rarely, hemolytic uremic syndrome can occur (characterized by rapid fall in hemoglobin, renal failure, severe thrombocytopenia) and progress to pulmonary edema and hypotension. The risk increases as the cumulative dose exceeds 60 mg.
- Drug may be given intra-arterially.
- Manufacturer's recommendations on dosage modification based on hematologic toxicity (NADIR AFTER PRIOR DOSE).

Potential Toxicities/Side Effects and the Nursing Process

I.   POTENTIAL FOR INFECTION related to MYELOSUPPRESSION

Defining Characteristics: Myelosuppression is the dose-limiting toxicity. Toxicity is delayed and cumulative. Initial nadir occurs at approximately 4–6 weeks. Usually by the third course, 50% drug modifications are necessary.

Nursing Implications: Monitor WBC, HCT, platelets prior to drug administration. Monitor patients for signs/symptoms of infection. Teach patient self-assessment. Drug dosage should be reduced or held for lower-than-normal blood values.

II.   ALTERATION IN NUTRITION, LESS THAN BODY REQUIREMENTS, related to NAUSEA, VOMITING, ANOREXIA, STOMATITIS

Defining Characteristics: Mild-to-moderate nausea and vomiting occur within 1–2 hours, lasting up to 3 days, but may be prevented by adequate premedication. Anorexia occurs commonly, and stomatitis may occur.

Nursing Implications: Premedicate with aggressive antiemetics, i.e., serotonin antagonist to prevent nausea and vomiting at least for the first treatment. Encourage small, frequent feedings of cool, bland foods and liquids. Teach patient and family member preparation of meals in advance, and encourage the use of spices when patient has little appetite. Teach patient oral assessment and oral hygiene regimen, and encourage patient to report early stomatitis.

III.   POTENTIAL FOR ACTIVITY INTOLERANCE related to FATIGUE

Defining Characteristics: Fatigue is common.

Nursing Implications: Assess baseline activity level. Teach patient to report fatigue and activity intolerance. Teach self-management strategies, including alternating rest and activity periods, as well as stress reduction.

IV.   POTENTIAL FOR IMPAIRED SKIN INTEGRITY related to DRUG EXTRAVASATION, ALOPECIA

Defining Characteristics: Extravasation of drug can cause severe tissue necrosis, erythema, burning, tissue sloughing. Delayed erythema or ulceration has been reported weeks to months after drug dose, at the injection site or distant from it, and despite the fact that there was no evidence of extravasation. Alopecia occurs frequently.

Nursing Implications: Use scrupulous IV technique to prevent extravasation of the drug. If there is doubt as to whether drug has infiltrated, treat as an infiltration, aspirate any drug in the tubing, and discontinue IV. IV line must be patent. Assess for need of venous access device early. Refer to hospital policy for management of extravasation, and see beginning of this chapter. Assess site regularly for pain, progression of erythema, induration, and evidence of necrosis. Discuss with patient hair loss, anticipated impact, and strategies to decrease distress, e.g., obtaining wig prior to hair loss.

V. POTENTIAL FOR INJURY related to HEMOLYTIC UREMIC SYNDROME

Defining Characteristics: 2% of patients may experience significant increase in creatinine unrelated to total dose or duration of therapy. Thrombotic microangiopathy may occur with anemia, thrombocytopenia. Blood transfusions may exacerbate condition. Can often be fatal.

Nursing Implications: Monitor renal function, HCT, and platelets prior to each drug dose; hold dose if serum creatinine is > 1.7 mg/dL. If renal failure occurs, hemofiltration or dialysis may be necessary. Discuss risks and benefits with physician and patient if renal insufficiency is present and blood transfusion(s) is required.

VI. POTENTIAL ALTERATION IN OXYGENATION related to INTERSTITIAL PNEUMONITIS

Defining Characteristics: Rarely, interstitial pneumonitis occurs and can be quite severe (ARDS). Signs/symptoms include nonproductive cough, dyspnea, hemoptysis, pneumonia, pulmonary infiltrates on X-ray. Incidence may be reduced by dexamethasone 20 mg IV prior to dose (Chang et al., 1986).

Nursing Implications: Assess baseline pulmonary status, and monitor prior to each drug dose. Teach patient to report dyspnea, new-onset cough, or any respiratory symptoms. Discuss abnormalities with physician, and plan for further diagnostic workup.

VII. POTENTIAL FOR INJURY related to VENO-OCCLUSIVE DISEASE OF THE LIVER AFTER BONE MARROW TRANSPLANT

Defining Characteristics: Hepatic veno-occlusive disease has been reported in patients who have received mitomycin C and autologous bone marrow transplant. Signs/symptoms are abdominal pain, hepatomegaly, and liver failure.

Nursing Implications: Assess baseline LFTs, and monitor periodically during therapy. Notify physician of any abnormalities, and discuss further diagnostic workup and management. Refer to autologous bone marrow transplant protocol.

Drug: mitotane (Lysodren)

Class: Antihormone.

Mechanism of Action: Adrenocortical suppressant with direct cytotoxic effect on mitochondria of adrenal cortical cells. Forces a drop in steroid secretion and alters the peripheral metabolism of steroids.

Metabolism: 34–45% of oral dose is absorbed from the GI tract. Metabolized partly in the liver and kidneys to a water-soluble metabolite that is then excreted in the bile and urine. Small amount of drug passes into the CSF.

Indication: In the treatment of inoperable adrenal corticoid carcinoma of both functional and nonfunctional types.

Dosage/Range:
- Dose ranges from 2–16 g/day PO.
- Usual doses 2–10 g/day.
- Treatment usually begins with low doses (2 g/day) and gradually increases.
- Daily dose is divided into 3–4 doses.
- Reduce dose in patients with hepatic dysfunction.

Drug Preparation:
- None.

Drug Administration:
- Oral. Available as a 500-mg tablet.

Drug Interactions:
- Neurotoxic drugs may have additive toxicity; use cautiously.
- Warfarin: may decrease anticoagulant effect; monitor INR and increase dose as needed.
- Spirolactone: may decrease mitotane effectiveness; do not use together.
- Steroids: decreased steroid effect requiring increased steroid dose.
- Phenytoin, cyclophosphamide, barbiturates: assess effect and need for dose adjustment.

Lab Effects/Interference:
- None.

Special Considerations:
- Hypersensitivity reactions are rare but have occurred.
- Use cautiously in patients with hepatic dysfunction.
- If patient undergoes stress (infection, trauma, shock), requires IV steroids.
- Drug may cause lethargy and somnolence; teach patient not to operate heavy equipment or drive until the effect of the drug is known.

Potential Toxicities/Side Effects and the Nursing Process

I.   ALTERATION IN NUTRITION, LESS THAN BODY REQUIREMENTS, related to GI SIDE EFFECTS

Defining Characteristics: Nausea and vomiting occur in 75% of patients and may be dose-limiting toxicity. Anorexia may also occur. Diarrhea occurs in 20% of patients.

Nursing Implications: Nausea and vomiting may be reduced by beginning therapy with a low dose and increasing it as tolerated. Premedicate with antiemetics to prevent nausea and vomiting; continue as needed. Encourage small, frequent meals of cool, bland foods and liquids. Inform patient that nausea and vomiting can occur; encourage patient to report onset. Encourage patient to report onset of diarrhea. Administer or teach administration of antidiarrheal medication. If diarrhea is protracted, ensure adequate hydration, monitor I/O and electrolytes, teach perineal hygiene.

II. POTENTIAL FOR INJURY related to NEUROLOGIC TOXICITY

Defining Characteristics: Lethargy and somnolence are most common; resolve with discontinuation of therapy. Dizziness, vertigo occur in about 15% of patients. Other CNS manifestations are depression, muscle tremors, confusion, headache.

Nursing Implications: Teach the patient and family about possible neurologic toxicity; assess safety of planned activities (e.g., patient should avoid activities that require alertness). Encourage patient and family to report onset of symptoms, as they may necessitate discontinuing therapy.

III. POTENTIAL FOR IMPAIRED SKIN INTEGRITY related to RASH

Defining Characteristics: Skin irritation or rash occurs in about 15% of patients. Sometimes resolves during treatment.

Nursing Implications: Inform patient that rash is expected and will resolve when treatment is finished. Assess skin for integrity; recommend measures to decrease irritation, if indicated.

Drug: mitoxantrone (Novantrone)

Class: New class of antineoplastics—anthracenediones. Antitumor antibiotic.

Mechanism of Action: Inhibits both DNA and RNA synthesis regardless of the phase of cell division. Intercalates between base pairs, thus distorting DNA structure. DNA-dependent RNA synthesis and protein synthesis are also inhibited.

Metabolism: Excreted in both the bile and urine for 24–36 hours as virtually unchanged drug. Mean half-life is 5.8 hours. Peak levels achieved immediately. FDA-approved for acute nonlymphocytic leukemia in adults.

Indication: (1) For reducing neurologic disability and/or frequency of clinical relapses in patients with secondary (chronic) progressive, progressive relapsing, or worsening relapsing-remitting multiple sclerosis (MS); it is NOT indicated for treatment of patients with primary progressive MS; (2) in combination with corticosteroids as initial chemotherapy for the treatment of patients with pain related to advanced hormone-refractory prostate cancer; (3) in combination with other approved drug(s) for the initial therapy of acute nonlymphocytic leukemia (ANLL) in adults (includes myelogenous, promyelocytic, monocytic, and erythroid acute leukemias).

Dosage/Range:
- 12 mg/m^2 IV daily for 3 days, in combination with cytosine arabinoside 100 mg/m^2/ day × 7 days continuous infusion for induction therapy of ANLL.
- 12 mg/m^2 IV day 1 every 21 days for prostate cancer, in combination with prednisone 5 mg PO twice a day.
- **Multiple sclerosis:** 12 mg/m^2 IV every 3 months, maximum lifetime dose 140 mg/m^2.

Drug Preparation:
- Available as dark-blue solution in 2-mg/mL vials: 10-mL (20-mg), 12.5-mL (25-mg), and 15-mL (30-mg) multidose vials.
- May be diluted in 5% dextrose, 0.9% sodium chloride, or 5% dextrose in 0.9% sodium chloride.
- Solution is chemically stable at room temperature for at least 48 hours.
- Intact vials should be stored at room temperature. If refrigerated, a precipitate may form. This precipitate can be redissolved when vial is warmed to room temperature.

Drug Administration:
- IV push over 3 minutes through the sidearm of a patent, freely running infusion.
- IV bolus over 5–30 minutes.

Drug Interactions:
Myelosuppressive agents: Increased hematologic toxicity if nadir overlaps; use together cautiously.

Lab Effects/Interference:
- Decreased CBC.
- Decreased electrolytes.
- Increased LFTs, uric acid.
- Decreased LVEF.

Special Considerations:
- Nonvesicant. There have been rare reports of tissue necrosis after drug infiltration.
- Incompatible with admixtures containing heparin.
- Patient may experience blue-green urine for 24 hours after drug administration.
- Cardiotoxicity is less than that of doxorubicin or daunorubicin, but risk increases with a cumulative dose of 140 mg/m^2 in patients without a history of prior anthracycline use, and 120 mg/m^2 if prior anthracycline treatment. Monitor LVEF, and discontinue drug if there is a 15–20% decrease in LVEF.

Potential Toxicities/Side Effects and the Nursing Process

I.   POTENTIAL FOR INJURY related to BONE MARROW DEPRESSION

Defining Characteristics: Potent bone marrow depression; nadir 9–10 days. Granulocytopenia is usually the dose-limiting toxicity, and toxicity may be cumulative. Thrombocytopenia uncommon, but can be severe when it occurs. Hypersensitivity has been reported occasionally with hypotension, urticaria, dyspnea, rashes.

Nursing Implications: Monitor WBC, HCT, platelets prior to drug administration. Instruct patient in self-assessment for signs/symptoms of infection. Drug dosage should be reduced or held for lower-than-normal blood values. Instruct patient in self-assessment of signs/ symptoms of bleeding. Prior to drug administration, obtain baseline vital signs. Observe for signs/symptoms of allergic reaction. Subjective signs/symptoms: generalized itching, dizziness. Objective signs/symptoms: flushed appearance (angioedema of face, neck, eyelids, hands, feet), localized or generalized urticaria. Document incident. Discuss with physician desensitization for future dose versus drug discontinuance.

II. POTENTIAL FOR ALTERATION IN CARDIAC OUTPUT related to CARDIOTOXICITY

Defining Characteristics: CHF with decreased LVEF occurs in about 3% of patients. Increased cardiotoxicity with cumulative dose greater than 180 mg/m^2; cumulative lifetime dose must be reduced if patient has had previous anthracycline therapy.

Nursing Implications: Assess for signs/symptoms of cardiomyopathy. Assess quality and regularity of heartbeat. Baseline EKG. Instruct patient to report dyspnea, shortness of breath, swelling of extremities, orthopnea. Discuss frequency of GBPS with physician.

III. ALTERATION IN NUTRITION, LESS THAN BODY REQUIREMENTS, related to NAUSEA/VOMITING AND MUCOSITIS

Defining Characteristics: Nausea and vomiting are typically not severe and occur in 30% of patients. Mucositis is more common with prolonged dosing; occurs in 5% of patients, usually within 1 week of therapy.

Nursing Implications: Premedicate with antiemetic and continue prophylactically for 24 hours to prevent nausea and vomiting, at least for the first treatment. Encourage small, frequent feedings of cool, bland foods and liquids. Teach patient oral assessment and oral hygiene regimen. Encourage patient to report early stomatitis.

IV. POTENTIAL FOR IMPAIRED SKIN INTEGRITY related to ALOPECIA AND EXTRAVASATION

Defining Characteristics: Alopecia is mild to moderate; occurs in 20% of patients. Drug is not a vesicant. Stains skin blue without ulcers. There have been rare reports of tissue necrosis following extravasation.

Nursing Implications: Discuss with patient impact of hair loss. Suggest wig as appropriate prior to actual hair loss. Explore with patient response to actual hair loss and plan strategies to minimize distress, e.g., wig, scarf, cap. Use careful technique during venipuncture and IV administration. Administer drug through freely flowing IV, constantly monitoring IV site and patient response.

V.   POTENTIAL FOR ANXIETY related to ABNORMAL COLOR OF URINE SCLERA

Defining Characteristics: Urine will be green-blue for 24 hours. Sclera may become discolored blue.

Nursing Implications: Explain to patient changes that may occur with therapy and that they are only temporary.

VI.   POTENTIAL SEXUAL DYSFUNCTION related to DRUG EFFECT

Defining Characteristics: Drug is mutagenic and teratogenic.

Nursing Implications: As appropriate, explore with patient and partner issues of reproductive and sexuality patterns and impact chemotherapy may have. Discuss strategies to preserve sexual and reproductive health (e.g., sperm banking, contraception).

Drug: nelarabine (Arranon)

Class: Nucleoside metabolic inhibitor (Antimetabolite).

Mechanism of Action: Drug is a pro-drug of deoxyguanosine analogue of ara-G (9-β-arabinofuranosylguanine), a cytotoxic agent. It is demethylated and converted into the active 5'-triphosphate ara-GTP. Ara-GTP accumulates in leukemic blasts and enters DNA where it causes inhibition of DNA synthesis and cell death. It may have other mechanisms as well.

Metabolism: Nelarabine and ara-G are rapidly eliminated from the plasma with a half-life of about 30 minutes and 3 hours, respectively. Both are extensively distributed throughout the body, and are not substantially bound to plasma proteins. Nelarabine and ara-G are partially excreted via the kidneys, 5–10% and 20–30%, respectively.

Indication: Treatment of patients with T-cell acute lymphoblastic leukemia and T-cell lymphoblastic lymphoma whose disease has not responded to or has relapsed following treatment with at least 2 chemotherapy regimens. This use is based on induction of CRs; randomized clinical trials demostrating increased survival or other clinical benefit have not been done.

Dosage/Range:
- *Adult:* 1,500 mg/m^2 IV over 2 hours on days 1, 3, 5, repeated every 3 weeks.
- *Pediatric:* 650 mg/m^2 IV over 1 hour on days 1, 2, 3, 4, 5, repeated every 3 weeks.
- Duration of treatment has not been determined; in clinical trials, treatment continued until disease progression, unacceptable toxicity, or patient became a candidate for a bone marrow transplant.

Drug Preparation:
- Drug available in 250-mg vials, 5 mg/mL.
- Appropriate (undiluted) dose of nelarabine should be transferred into polyvinyl chloride (PVC) infusion bags or glass containers, and administered as a 2-hour infusion in adults and a 1-hour infusion in pediatric patients. Drug is stable for 8 hours at up to 30°C in PVC infusion bags. Drug should not be used in patients with creatinine clearance of < 50 mL/minute. Drug should be discontinued for grade 2 or higher neurotoxicity (CTCAE), and dosage should be delayed for other toxicity, including hematologic toxicity.

Drug Interactions:
- None known.

Lab Effects/Interference:
- *Pediatric patients*: serum transaminases, bilirubin, creatinine; ↓ serum potassium, albumin, calcium, glucose, magnesium.
- *Adults*: glucose, AST.
- *Both*: anemia, neutropenia, thrombocytopenia.

Special Considerations:
- Drug is a potent antineoplastic with potentially significant neurotoxicity, which is dose limiting, characterized by somnolence, confusion, convulsions, ataxia, paresthesias, and hypoesthesia. Severe neurotoxicity includes coma, status epilepticus, craniospinal demyelination, or ascending neuropathy (like Guillain-Barré syndrome).
- Drug is a potent teratogen. Women of childbearing potential should avoid pregnancy. If drug is used during pregnancy or if patient becomes pregnant while taking the drug, the patient should be warned of potential hazard to the fetus. Nursing mothers should not breastfeed while receiving the drug.
- The risk of adverse events may be increased in patients with severe hepatic impairment (bilirubin > 3.0 mg/dL); closely monitor these patients for toxicities.
- The most common side effects in pediatric patients were bone marrow depression, headache, and vomiting; most common in adult patients were fatigue, nausea, vomiting, constipation, bone marrow depression, cough and dyspnea, somnolence and dizziness, and fever.

Potential Toxicities/Side Effects and the Nursing Process

I.   POTENTIAL FOR INJURY related to TUMOR LYSIS SYNDROME (TLS)

Defining Characteristics: May develop with initial therapy if patient has a large tumor burden; results from rapid lysis of tumor cells. This usually begins 1–5 days after initiation of therapy, and causes elevations in serum uric acid, potassium, phosphorus, BUN, creatinine.

Nursing Implications: If this is induction therapy for a patient with acute leukemia or high tumor burden, expect medical orders to include IV hydration at 150 mL/hour with urine alkalinization, allopurinol prophylaxis, strict monitoring of I/O, daily weight, and total body fluid balance determination. Monitor baseline and daily serum BUN, creatinine, potassium, phosphorus, uric acid, and calcium. Monitor for renal, cardiac, neuromuscular signs/symptoms of TLS.

II.   INFECTION AND BLEEDING related to BONE MARROW DEPRESSION

Defining Characteristics: In pediatric patients, bone marrow depression is very common anemia 95% (45% grade 3), neutropenia 94% (17% grade 3), and thrombocytopenia 88% (27% grade 3). In adults, anemia affects 99% of patients (20% grade 3), thrombocytopenia 86% (37% grade 3), and neutropenia 81% (14% grade 3), and 12% had febrile neutropenia.

Nursing Implications: Assess WBC, neutrophil, and platelet count, and discuss any abnormalities with physician prior to drug administration; assess for signs/symptoms of skin infections (all mucosal surfaces, body orifices) and bleeding; instruct patient in signs/symptoms of infection and bleeding, as well as to report them or come to the emergency room. Teach patient self-care measures to minimize risk of infection and bleeding, including avoidance of OTC aspirin-containing medications. Assess patient's Hgb/HCT and signs/symptoms of fatigue; teach patient self-assessment and to alternate rest and activity as needed.

III.   POTENTIAL FOR INJURY related to NEUROTOXICITY

Defining Characteristics: Neurologic events occurred in 64% of patients. In pediatric studies, most common events were headache (17%), peripheral neuropathy (12%, sensory and/or motor), somnolence (7%), hypoesthesia (6%), seizures (6%, including grand mal and status epilepticus), paresthesia (4%), tremor (4%). Rare grade 3–4 events were status epilepticus (1 fatal), hypertonia, and 3rd nerve paralysis. In adults, somnolence was most common (23%), followed by dizziness (21%), peripheral neuropathy (21%, including motor and/or sensory), hypoesthesia (17%), headache (15%), paresthesia (15%), ataxia (9%), depressed level of consciousness (6%), tremor (5%), blurred vision (4%), amnesia (3%). Grade 3 events in adults were rare and included aphasia, convulsion, hemiparesis, loss of consciousness, while grade 4 events included cerebral hemorrhage, coma, intracranial hemorrhage, leukoencephalopathy.

Nursing Implications: Assess baseline neurologic status, including sedation level, blurred vision, presence of numbness or tingling, difficulty with fine motor movement, such as buttoning clothes, unsteadiness when walking, or tripping. Teach patient that serious neurologic side effects may occur. Pediatric: extreme sleepiness, seizures, coma, peripheral neuropathy, weakness, and paralysis. Adult: sleepiness, dizziness, peripheral neuropathy, rarely seizure, aphasia, hemiparesis, loss of consciousness. Teach patient to notify the provider/go to ED immediately if they occur. Teach adult patient not to drive or operate heavy machinery if sleepiness occurs.

IV. ALTERED NUTRITION, LESS THAN BODY REQUIREMENTS, related to NAUSEA AND VOMITING, STOMATITIS, DIARRHEA, CONSTIPATION, HEPATOTOXICITY

Defining Characteristics: Nausea and vomiting are common in adults, but less common in children (10%). In adults, nausea affects 41%, vomiting 22%, diarrhea 22%, and constipation 21%. In adults, 8% of patients developed stomatitis. Nausea and vomiting can be successfully prevented with combination antiemetics. Rarely dysgeusia can occur. Drug should be used cautiously in patients with impaired hepatic function, and the patient monitored closely for toxicity.

Nursing Implications: Premedicate with antiemetics and revise regimen based on prior response to treatment. If patient develops nausea/vomiting, assess fluid and electrolyte balance and the need for replacements. Assess oral mucosa prior to chemotherapy, and teach patient oral hygiene regimen and self-assessment; encourage patient to report diarrhea, discuss use of antidiarrheals with physician, and teach self-care PRN. Since patients become neutropenic, all mucosal surfaces need to be assessed for infection, and patients must be taught scrupulous perineal hygiene. Monitor LFTs prior to, during, and after therapy.

V. ALTERATION IN COMFORT related to FATIGUE, FEVER, ASTHENIA, EDEMA, PAIN, RIGORS, MYALGIAS

Defining Characteristics: Fatigue affects 50% of adults, and can be severe in 10%. Pyrexia affects 23% and asthenia 17%. Peripheral edema affects 15%, pain 11%, rigors 8%, myalgias 13%, arthralgias 9%, muscular weakness 8%.

Nursing Implications: Assess comfort level/symptoms experienced at baseline and prior to each dose, then prior to each cycle. Teach patient to alternate rest and activity periods to manage or prevent fatigue. Teach patient to report fevers (> 100.5°F) and rigors right away, and to come to the clinic or ED. Teach patient symptomatic management of myalgias, arthralgias (e.g., local application of heat, acetaminophen if permitted).

Drug: nilutamide (Nilandron)

Class: Antiandrogen.

Mechanism of Action: Irreversibly binds to androgen receptors and inhibits androgen binding. Unlike steroidal antiandrogens, nilutamide binds specifically to adrenal androgen receptor in the nucleus of androgen-sensitive prostate cancer cells. It does not interact with progestin or glucocorticoid receptors.

Metabolism: Following oral administration, nilutamide is rapidly and completely absorbed, with 80% plasma protein binding. Steady-state levels are achieved after about 2 weeks. Though the drug is extensively metabolized in the liver, it appears that the parent drug is the active compound. The drug is excreted in the urine as metabolites. Renal impairment does not alter the properties of the drug.

Indication: In combination with surgical castration for the treatment of metastatic prostate cancer, Stage D2.

Contraindications: Patients with
- Severe hepatic impairment (baseline hepatic enzymes should be evaluated prior to treatment).
- Severe respiratory insufficiency.
- Hypersensitivity to nilutamide or any component of this preparation.

Dosage/Range:
- 300 mg/day orally for 30 days and then 150 mg/day.

Drug Preparation/Administration:
- Oral. Start the day of or day after surgical castration for maximal benefit.

Drug Interactions:
- Has been shown to inhibit the liver cytochrome P450 isoenzymes and may decrease the metabolism of compounds requiring these systems. Monitor patients closely for toxicity if the patient is also taking phenytoin or theophylline.
- Warfarin: nilutamide may decrease warfarin metabolism, resulting in increased anticoagulation; monitor INR closely and the dose accordingly.
- Alcohol: rare disulfiram reaction (flushing, throbbing in head and neck, headache, dyspnea, nausea/vomiting, sweating, chest pain, palpitation, hypotension, vertigo, uneasiness, and confusion).

Lab Effects/Interference:
- Causes increased liver enzymes (see below); may cause increased serum glucose.

Special Considerations:
- Hepatitis has been described, with rare cases of death or hospitalization related to severe liver injury reported. Monitor LFTs baseline and during therapy. If transaminases rise to greater than 2–3 times the upper limit of normal, therapy should be discontinued.
- Interstitial pneumonitis has been reported in 2% of patients. Monitor PFTs and CXR baseline and during therapy. If symptoms occur, or if interstitial pneumonitis suspected (CXR or 20–25% decrease in DLCO and FVC), nilutamide should be discontinued. Teach patient to report any new or worsening SOB. Post-marketing reports have described patients with pulmonary fibrosis, which led to hospitalization and death.
- Rarely, aplastic anemia may occur.

Potential Toxicities/Side Effects and the Nursing Process

I.   ALTERATION IN NUTRITION, LESS THAN BODY REQUIREMENTS, related to NAUSEA, ANOREXIA, CONSTIPATION, CHANGES IN LFTs

Defining Characteristics: Nausea, anorexia occur infrequently. Constipation and increased LFTs are common, affecting 10–50% of patients.

Nursing Implications: Teach patient to report occurrence of loss of appetite or nausea. Encourage small, frequent feedings and consider antiemetic if necessary. Teach the patient to monitor bowel status and to eat foods high in roughage and prunes, to hydrate well, and to take stool softeners as needed to prevent constipation. Monitor baseline and during treatment. Discuss change in treatment if AST, ALT increase by 2–3 times ULN.

II. ALTERATION IN CARDIAC OUTPUT related to HYPERTENSION, ANGINA

Defining Characteristics: Angina occurs in 2% of patients; unclear whether increased incidence of hypertension (9%) due to drug alone.

Nursing Implications: Instruct patient in signs and symptoms of angina, and to report to physician if they occur. Monitor BP on follow-up visits.

III. ALTERATION IN COMFORT related to DIZZINESS, HOT FLASHES, DYSPNEA, VISUAL CHANGES

Defining Characteristics: Hot flashes occur in 28% of patients and are the most common side effect. Dyspnea is rare but is related to interstitial pneumonitis, a serious side effect of the drug; if it occurs, it is usually during the first 3 months of treatment. Patients of Asian heritage are at risk. Many patients experience impaired adaptation to light and, less commonly, changes in color vision.

Nursing Implications: Inform patient that side effects may occur and to report dyspnea immediately to physician, as therapy must be discontinued if it occurs. Baseline chest X-ray and PFTs should be done prior to treatment; if interstitial pneumonitis is suspected, the drug should be discontinued. Patients should be discouraged from driving at night because of visual changes and may find it helpful to wear tinted glasses during the day.

Drug: omacetaxine mepesuccinate for injection (Synribo)

Class: Protein synthesis inhibitor.

Mechanism of Action: Not fully understood, but protein synthesis inhibition is independent of Bcr-Abl binding. The drug is a semisynthetic derivative from cephalotaxine, an extract from the *Cephalotaxus* leaf. Drug reduces the oncoprotein levels of Bcr-Abl, as well as Mcl-1, a member of the anti-apoptosis Bcl-2 family.

Metabolism: After subcutaneous injection, peak serum level is reached in 30 minutes, and mean half-life is about 6 hours. Drug plasma protein binding is ≤ 50%. Drug metabolism is primarily hydrolysis into 4'-DMHHT without microsomal activity, and while elimination route is unknown, < 15% of drug is excreted unchanged in the urine.

Indication: Treatment of adult patients with chronic or accelerated phase chronic myelogenous leukemia (CML) with resistance and/or intolerance to two or more tyrosine kinase inhibitors.

Dosage/Range:
- **Induction dose:** 1.25 mg/m^2 administered by subcutaneous injection twice daily × 14 consecutive days in a 28-day cycle; assess weekly CBC/differential.
- **Maintenance dose:** 1.25 mg/m^2 administered by subcutaneous injection twice daily × 7 consecutive days in a 28-day cycle; assess weekly CBC/differential during initial maintenance, then every 2 weeks or as clinically indicated.
- **Dose Modifications**
  - **Hematologic:** Grade 4 neutropenia (ANC < 500 cells/mm^3) or grade 3 thrombocytopenia (platelets < 50,000 cells/mm^3) during a cycle, delay the next cycle until ANC ≥ 1,000 cells/mm^3 and platelet count is ≥ 50,000 cells/mm^3. Also, reduce the number of treatment days by 2 the next cycle, e.g., to 5 days.
  - **Other toxicity:** Interrupt or delay drug until toxicity is resolved, and manage symptomatically.

Drug Preparation:
- Drug is available in a single-use vial containing 3.5 mg of omacetaxine mepesuccinate as a preservative-free, lypholized powder.
- Reconstitute with 1 mL of 0.9% Soduim Chloride Injection USP; gently swirl until solution is clear (should take < 1 minute). The final concentration is 3.5 mg/mL omacetaxine mepesuccinate.
- Inspect for particulate matter and discoloration, and do not use if found.
- Use within 12 hours of reconstitution when stored at room temperature, and 24 hours if refrigerated at 2°C–8°C (36°F–46°F). Protect from light.

Drug Administration: Teach patient to
- Self-administer drug subcutaneously and to rotate sites, or teach caregiver.
- Have weekly CBC/differential as above.
- Prepare drug, handle and store drug properly, and how to clean up accidental spillage of hazardous drug.
- Hazardous waste disposal and spill management. (Discard used needle, syringe, vials in biohazard container; do not recap or clip used needle, do not place used equipment in household trash or recycling bin; if drug accidentally spills, keep using protective eye wear and gloves, wipe spilled liquid with absorbent pad, and wash the area with soap and water. Then place pad and gloves in biohazard container and wash hands thoroughly. Return the biohazard container to the clinic or pharmacy for final disposal.)
- Ensure patient has necessary supplies for home administration: reconstituted omacetaxine mepesuccinate for injection in prefilled syringes with capped needle for subcutaneous injection (filled with patient-specific dose), protective eyewear, gloves, appropriate biohazard container, absorbent pad(s) for placement of administrative materials and for accidental spillage, alcohol swabs, gauze pads, ice packs or cooler for transportation of reconstituted omacetaxine mepesuccinate for injection syringes.
- If a patient or caregiver cannot be trained for some reason, the drug should be administered by a healthcare professional.

Drug Interactions: Drug is a P-glycoprotein (P-gp) substrate in vitro, but does not inhibit P-gp mediated efflux of loperamide, e.g., clinically.

Lab Effects/Interference:
- Decreased WBC, neutrophil, lymphocyte, platelet, red blood cell counts.
- Increased blood glucose.
- Increased ALT, bilirubin, creatinine, and uric acid.

Special Considerations:
Most common adverse reactions in patients with CML-chronic and accelerated phases (frequency ≥ 20%): thrombocytopenia, anemia, neutropenia, diarrhea, nausea, fatigue, asthenia, injection-site reaction, pyrexia, infection, and lymphopenia.

Warnings and Precautions:
- Myelosuppression: Severe and fatal thrombocytopenia, neutropenia, and anemia. Monitor hematologic parameters frequently.
- Bleeding: Severe thrombocytopenia and increased risk of hemorrhage may occur; fatal cerebral hemorrhage, and severe, nonfatal GI hemorrhage has occurred.
- Hyperglycemia: Drug can induce glucose intolerance with grades 3 or 4 hyperglycemia in 11% of patients. Hyperosmolar, nonketotic hyperglycemia may rarely occur. Monitor blood glucose levels frequently, especially in patients with diabetes or risk factors for diabetes. Avoid using drug in patients with poorly controlled diabetes mellitus, waiting until diabetes is well controlled.
- Embryo-fetal toxicity: Counsel women of reproductive potential to use effective contraceptives to avoid becoming pregnant, as drug is fetotoxic.

Potential Toxicities/Side Effects and the Nursing Process

I. POTENTIAL FOR INFECTION, BLEEDING AND FATIGUE related to BONE MARROW SUPPRESSION

Defining Characteristics: Grades 3–4 thrombocytopenia occurred in 85% and 88% of patients respectively, while neutropenia occurred in 81% and 71%. Grades 3–4 anemia occurred in 62% and 80% respectively. 3% of patients died from myelosuppression. Fatalities from cerebrovascular hemorrhage occurred in 2% of patients.

Nursing Implications: Monitor CBC/differential and platelet count weekly during induction and initial maintenance, then every 2 weeks during later maintenance, or as clinically indicated. Teach patients to report right away signs/symptoms of infection (e.g., fever ≥ 100.4°F, sore throat, sputum production, difficulty breathing, painful urination) or bleeding. Teach patient to avoid OTC preparations containing aspirin, NSAIDs, or other drugs that increase the potential for bleeding.

II. ALTERATION IN NUTRITION, POTENTIAL related to DIARRHEA, NAUSEA, CONSTIPATION, VOMITING, HYPERGLYCEMIA

Defining Characteristics: Diarrhea occurred in 41% of patients, nausea 35%, constipation 14%, vomiting 12%, while hyperglycemia occurred in 10–15% and hypoglycemia 6–8%. Hyperosmolar nonketotic hyperglycemia may rarely occur.

Nursing Implications: Monitor blood glucose levels baseline and frequently during therapy, especially in patients with diabetes or risk factors for diabetes. Teach patient dietary as well as pharmacologic control of diarrhea, nausea, vomiting, or constipation.

III.   ALTERATION IN COMFORT, POTENTIAL related to INJECTION-SITE REACTIONS, ARTHRALGIA, FEVER, FATIGUE, ASTHENIA, PERIPHERAL EDEMA

Defining Characteristics: Injection-site reactions occurred in 35%, fatigue in 29% (5% grades 3–4), pyrexia 25%, asthenia 23%, peripheral edema 16%, arthralgia 19%, and headache 20%.

Nursing Implications: Teach patient that these reactions may occur, and to manage them symptomatically. Assess prior injection site at each visit and rotate sites. Discuss more aggressive symptom management strategies as needed with physician or NP/PA.

Drug: oxaliplatin (Eloxatin)

Class: Alkylating agent (third-generation platinum analogue).

Mechanism of Action: Blocks DNA replication and transcription into RNA by causing intrastrand and interstrand crosslinks in DNA strands. It is cell cycle nonspecific. DNA mismatch repair enzymes are unable to repair these errors, and the cell dies. Drug may also bind to proteins in the cell nucleus and cytoplasm to further injure the cell.

Metabolism: Heavily bound (98%) to plasma proteins; following 2-hour drug infusion, 15% of drug is found in plasma and 85% in tissue or excreted in the urine; 40% of the drug binds irreversibly in red blood cells within 2–5 hours of administration. The drug concentrates in the kidney and spleen, and is excreted as platinum-containing metabolites.

Indication: In combination with infusional 5-fluorouracil (5-FU)/leucovorin for
- Adjuvant treatment of stage III colon cancer in patients who have undergone complete resection of the primary tumor.
- Treatment of advanced colorectal cancer (CRC).

Dosage/Range:
- FOLFOX4 every 2 weeks:
- *Day 1*: Oxaliplatin 85 mg/m² IV infusion in 250–500 mL D₅W and leucovorin 200 mg/m² IV infusion in D₅W, each over 2 hours simultaneously in separate bags using a Y-line, followed by 5-FU 400 mg/m² IVB over 2–4 minutes, followed by 5-FU 600 mg/m² in 500 mL D₅W as a 22-hour continuous infusion.
- *Day 2*: Leucovorin 200 mg/m² IV infusion over 2 hours, followed by 5-FU 400 mg/m² IVB over 2–4 minutes, followed by 5-FU 600 mg/m² in 500 mL D₅W as a 22-hour continuous infusion.

Dose Reduction:

Reduce the dose of oxaliplatin to 75 mg/m^2 in patients receiving **adjuvant therapy** or 65 mg/m^2 in patients with advanced CRC:

- Persistent grade 2 neurotoxicity that does not resolve.
- After recovery from grade 3–4 GI toxicities (despite prophylactic treatment) or grade 4 neutropenia or grade 3–4 thrombocytopenia. Delay next dose until neutrophils ≥ 1.5×10^9/L and platelets ≥ 75 × 10^9/L.

For patients with severe renal impairment (CrCl < 30 mL/min), initial recommended dose is 65 mg/m^2. Discontinue oxaliplatin if there are persistent grade 3 neurosensory events.

Drug Preparation:

- Further dilute in 250–500 mL of 5% dextrose injection.
- DO NOT use chloride-containing solutions or sodium chloride.
- DO NOT use aluminum needles or infusion sets containing aluminum.

Drug Administration:

- Administer IV infusion over 2 or more hours through central line, preferably.

Drug Interactions:

- Incompatible with 5-FU and other highly alkaline solutions.
- Incompatible with chloride-containing solutions (forms precipitate).
- Physically incompatible with diazepam (forms precipitate).
- Incompatible with cefepime, cefoperazone, dantrolene.
- Nephrotoxic drugs: renal excretion of oxaliplatin could be reduced with increased serum levels of oxaliplatin.
- 5-FU: At high doses (130 mg/m^2), increases plasma levels of 5-FU by 20%.
- Bevacizumab: increased response rate and survival in metastatic CRC when combined with FOLFOX.

Lab Effects/Interference:

- Decreased CBC, especially WBC and platelets.
- Elevated LFTs.

Special Considerations:

- In the MOSAIC study of 2246 patients receiving adjuvant chemotherapy for colon cancer, stage III patients receiving FOLFOX4 had a superior survival compared with patients receiving 5-FU/LV alone (24% risk reduction for recurrence) 4 years out (de Gramont, 2007). In addition, 99% of patients with grade 3 neurotoxicity had resolved or decreased by 1 year posttreatment (de Gramont et al., 2003).
- Peripheral neuropathy (sensory) is dose-limiting toxicity (DLT). Two distinct neurotoxicity syndromes: acute, lasting less than 14 days, and chronic persistent peripheral neuropathy (PN) similar to cisplatin, which is the DLT.
- Rare pulmonary fibrosis and veno-occlusive disease of the liver occur.

Potential Toxicities/Side Effects and the Nursing Process

I.   SENSORY/PERCEPTUAL ALTERATIONS related to ACUTE SENSORY NEUROPATHY

Defining Characteristics: Acute neurotoxicity appears related to ion channelopathy. It is common, affecting many patients. It is temporary, and occurs during, within hours of, or up to 14 days following oxaliplatin administration. Often precipitated by exposure to cold and characterized by dysesthesias, transient paresthesias, or hypesthesias of the hands, feet, perioral area, and throat. Acute events can be minimized by slower infusion of oxaliplatin, increasing the infusion time from 2 to 6 hours, as this lowers peak serum levels. Studies are ongoing to determine whether glutamine can prevent these, and also studies exploring 1 g calcium/1 g magnesium IVB prior to and after the oxaliplatin infusion. Most frightening for patients is pharyngolaryngeal dysesthesia characterized by a sensation of discomfort or tightness in the back of the throat and inability to breathe. It may be accompanied by jaw pain, and is often precipitated by exposure to cold. Cramping of muscles, such as fisted hand, occurs due to prolonged action potential. Rarely, dysarthria (difficulty articulating words), eye pain, and a feeling of chest pressure can occur.

Nursing Implications: Teach patient that acute neurotoxicity can occur but is not dangerous. Teach patient to minimize occurrence by avoiding exposure to cold during and for 3–5 days after drug administration, such as wearing scarves over the face in the winter, warm gloves if going outside or reaching into the refrigerator or freezer. Teach patient to avoid exposure to cold and cold liquids, if lip paresthesias present. Teach patient to use straw if drinking cool liquids. Teach patient to avoid cold air conditioning in the car or home during the summer. Teach patient how to reassure themselves they are breathing if pharyngolaryngeal dysesthesia occurs (cup hands in front of mouth or hold mirror so that breath can be felt or seen on the mirror). Teach patient to warm area, such as fingers or toes, if they become cold; for example, running warm water over affected area may help resolve the feeling. Do not use ice chips before and during 5-FU infusions to prevent stomatitis.

II.   SENSORY/PERCEPTUAL ALTERATIONS related to PERSISTENT, CHRONIC SENSORY NEUROPATHY

Defining Characteristics: Peripheral neurotoxicity affects some patients, and risk increases as cumulative doses > 800 mg/m^2. Symptoms include paresthesias, dysesthesias, hypoesthesias, in a stocking-and-glove distribution, and altered proprioception (knowing where body parts are in relation to the whole). This can become manifested as difficulty writing, walking, swallowing, and buttoning buttons. IF allowed to progress, motor pathways will become involved. When drug is stopped, symptoms may get worse, but in general, symptoms resolve in 4–6 months in many patients. Ongoing studies in patients with advanced CRC are looking at temporarily stopping the drug when grade 2 or 3 neurotoxicity occurs, continuing the 5-FU/LV as maintenance, or stopping chemotherapy drugs and resuming after 12 cycles of maintenance or when disease progression occurs. This has shown to reduce the incidence and intensity of PN (OPTIMOX trial). In the MOSAIC trial, an adjuvant trial, although some patients developed grade 3 neurotoxicity after 6 months, most patients had complete resolution of grade 3 toxicity (de Gramont et al., 2003).

Nursing Implications: Assess baseline neurologic status (sensory and motor); instruct patient to report signs/symptoms. Identify patients at risk: those with preexisting neuropathies (e.g., ethanol- and diabetes mellitus-related). Assess sensory and motor function, and monitor over time prior to each treatment, such as picking up a dime from a smooth/flat surface, buttoning shirt, and writing name. Specifically, assess whether function is impaired, as this necessitates a dose reduction. If the patient is unable to perform activities of daily living, this necessitates drug cessation. In either case, discuss with physician, as complete neurologic exam should be performed before treatment decision as to drug holiday or discontinuance based on grade of neurotoxicity. Assess impact on patient and quality of life.

III. POTENTIAL FOR INFECTION, BLEEDING, AND FATIGUE related to BONE MARROW DEPRESSION

Defining Characteristics: Mild leukopenia, and mild to moderate thrombocytopenia occur. Febrile neutropenia is very uncommon. Anemia is common.

Nursing Implications: Assess baseline CBC, WBC, differential, and platelet count prior to chemotherapy, as well as signs/symptoms of infection, bleeding, or fatigue. Teach patient signs/symptoms of infection or bleeding, and to report these immediately. Teach patient self-care measures to minimize risk of infection and bleeding. This includes avoidance of crowds, proximity to people with infections, and OTC aspirin-containing medications. Teach energy-conserving techniques and ways to minimize fatigue, such as gentle exercise as tolerated.

IV. ALTERATION IN NUTRITION, LESS THAN BODY REQUIREMENTS, related to NAUSEA AND VOMITING, DIARRHEA, HEPATOTOXICITY

Defining Characteristics: Nausea and vomiting occur commonly and are severe if patient does not receive aggressive antiemesis. Diarrhea commonly occurs in combination with 5-FU/LV. Hepatotoxicity may occur manifested by increases in transaminases and alkaline phosphatase, whereas increases in bilirubin may be related to the concomitant 5-FU/LV, as the incidence was similar in the group receiving FOLFOX compared with patients receiving only 5-FU/LV. Liver biopsies showed peliosis, nodular regenerative hyperplasia, or sinusoidal alterations, perisinusoidal fibrosis, and veno-occlusive lesions.

Nursing Implications: Premedicate patient with aggressive combination antiemetics: serotonin antagonist (granisetron or ondansetron) and dexamethasone. Encourage small, frequent feedings of cool, bland foods. Instruct patient to report nausea, and teach self-administration of antiemetics if patient is receiving drug as an outpatient. Teach the patient to report diarrhea that does not respond to usual antidiarrheal medicine and diet modification so that more aggressive management can be instituted and prevent dehydration and electrolyte imbalance. If LFTs are significantly elevated, the drug should be stopped, and hepatic dysfunction, unexplainable by liver metastases, should be evaluated.

V.   POTENTIAL FOR INJURY related to DELAYED HYPERSENSITIVITY OR ANAPHYLAXIS REACTIONS (often after 8–12 cycles of therapy)

Defining Characteristics: Delayed hypersensitivity may occur after 10–12 cycles of therapy with symptoms ranging from local rash or vague symptoms such as new onset of vomiting, to anaphylaxis and severe hypersensitivity (characterized by dyspnea, hypotension requiring treatment, angioedema, and generalized urticaria). Anecdotal reports show successful desensitization using carboplatin desensitization regimens.

Nursing Implications: Assess baseline VS and mental status prior to drug administration. If patient has symptoms, discuss premedication using corticosteroid, antihistamine, and H_2 antagonist as ordered. Monitor VS every 15 minutes, and remain with patient during first 15 minutes of drug infusion. Stop drug if signs/symptoms of hypersensitivity or anaphylaxis occur, and notify physician. *Subjective symptoms:* generalized itching, nausea, chest tightness, crampy abdominal pain, difficulty speaking, anxiety, agitation, sense of impending doom, uneasiness, desire to urinate/defecate, dizziness, chills. *Objective signs:* flushed appearance; angioedema of face, neck, eyelids, hands, feet; localized or generalized urticaria; respiratory distress with or without wheezing; hypotension; cyanosis. Provide fluid resuscitation for hypotension per MD order, and maintain a patent airway.

Drug: paclitaxel (Taxol)

Class: Taxoid, mitotic inhibitor.

Mechanism of Action: Promotes early microtubule assembly and prevents depolymerization necessary for normal mitosis and cell division, resulting in cell death in G_2 and M phases of the cell cycle.

Metabolism: Extensively protein-bound, resulting in an initial sharp decline in serum level. Metabolized primarily by hepatic hydroxylation using the P450 enzyme system. Metabolites are excreted in the bile. Less than 10% of the intact drug is excreted in the urine.

Indication: (1) First-line and subsequent treatment of patients with advanced ovarian cancer; as first line, in combination with cisplating; (2) adjuvant treatment of node-positive breast cancer patients, administered sequentially to standard doxorubicin-containing combination chemotherapy; (3) treatment of patients with metastatic breast cancer after failure of combination chemotherapy, or relapse within 6 months of adjuvant chemotherapy (which included an anthracycline unless clinically contraindicated); (4) in combination with cisplatin, for the first-line treatment of NSCLC in patients who are not candidates for potentially curative surgery and/or RT; (5) second-line treatment of patients with AIDS-related Kaposi's sarcoma (KS).

Contraindication: (1) Patients with a history of hypersensitvity reactions to paclitaxel injection or other drugs formulated in plyoxy 35 castor oil, NF; (2) patients with solid tumors having a baseline ANC <1,500 cells/mm³ or in patients with AIDS-related KS with a baseline ANC < 1,000 cells/mm³.

Dosage/Range:

- Dose-reduce if hepatic dysfunction.
- Breast cancer:
- **Adjuvant treatment** of patients with LN-positive breast cancer, administered sequentially to standard doxorubicin containing combination chemotherapy (benefit at 30 months for ER/PR negative tumors): Adjuvant node-positive breast cancer: 175 mg/m² IV over 3 hours, every 3 weeks, for 4 courses, administered sequentially to doxorubicin-containing combination chemotherapy.
- **Advanced breast** cancer after failure of combination therapy for metastatic disease or relapse within 6 months of adjuvant therapy (containing an anthracycline except if not tolerated): 175 mg/m² IV over 3 hours, every 3 weeks; if tumor overexpresses HER2 protein, given in combination with trastuzumab.
- **Ovarian cancer:** First-line (in combination with cisplatin) and subsequent therapy for patients with advanced ovarian cancer.
- Previously *untreated* ovarian cancer: 135 mg/m² IV over 24 hours, followed by cisplatin 75 mg/m² every 3 weeks or paclitaxel 175 mg IV over 3 hours followed by cisplatin 75 mg/m² q 3 weeks.
- Previously treated ovarian cancer: 135 mg or 175 mg/m² IV over 3 hours every 3 weeks.
- **Non-small-cell lung cancer:** First-line treatment (in combination with cisplatin) in patients who are not candidates for surgical or radiation curative therapy: non–small-cell lung cancer (NSCLC): 135 mg/m² IV over 24 hours, followed by cisplatin 75 mg/m² repeated every 3 weeks.
- **AIDS-related Kaposi's sarcoma:** Second-line treatment: 135 mg/m² IV over 3 hours, repeated every 3 weeks, or 100 mg/m² IV over 3 hours, repeated every 2 weeks (dose intensity of 45–50 mg/m² per week).

Other doses:

- Metastatic breast cancer, weekly paclitaxel 80 mg/m² IV over 1 hour q wk.
- Advanced or metastatic NSCLC: weekly paclitaxel 50 mg/m² IV over 1 hour in combination with carboplatin AUC 2 with concurrent XRT and after completion of XRT, paclitaxel 200 mg/m² and carboplatin AUC 6 q 3 weeks × 2 cycles.
- Ovarian, intraperitoneal: 60–65 mg/m².
- Less myelosuppression with 3-hour vs 24-hour infusion.

Drug Preparation:

- Drug is poorly soluble in water, so is formulated using polyoxyethylated castor oil (Cremophor EL) and dehydrated alcohol.
- Further dilute in 5% dextrose or 0.9% sodium chloride.

Drug Administration:

- Glass or polyolefin containers MUST BE USED, and polyethylene-lined administration sets must be used. DO NOT USE polyvinylchloride containers or tubing

since the polyoxyethylated castor oil (Cremophor EL) causes leaching of plasticizer diethylhexylphthalate (DEHP) from polyvinylchloride plastic into the infusion fluid. Do not use Chemo Dispensing Pin device or similar devices since the device may cause the stopper to collapse, sacrificing sterility of the paclitaxel solution.
- Inline filter of < 0.22 microns MUST be used.
- Assess vital signs baseline, and remain with patient during first 15 minutes of infusion. Monitor vital signs every 15 minutes or per hospital policy.
- **Assess CBC:** Patients with solid tumors: absolute neutrophil count (ANC) must be at least 1,500 cells/mm^3 and platelet count at least 100,000/mm^3; patients with AIDS-related Kaposi's sarcoma: ANC at least 1,000 cells/mm^3.

Premedication with corticosteroids:
- Solid tumors: Dexamethasone 20 mg PO 12 and 6 hours prior to treatment. Administer diphenhydramine 50 mg and H$_2$ antagonist (cimetidine 300 mg, famotidine 20 mg, or ranitidine 50 mg) IV 30–60 minutes prior to treatment.
- AIDS-related Kaposi's sarcoma: Dexamethasone 10 mg PO 12 and 6 hours prior to treatment; administer diphenhydramine 50 mg and H$_2$ antagonist (cimetidine 300 mg, famotidine 20 mg, or ranitidine 50 mg) IV 30–60 minutes prior to treatment.
- Administer paclitaxel IV over 3 hours via infusion controller.
- DO NOT give drug as a bolus, as this may cause bronchospasm and hypotension.
- Assess for hypersensitivity reaction (most often occurs during first 10 minutes of infusion) and for cardiovascular effects (arrhythmia, hypotension).
- Keep resuscitation equipment nearby.
- Administer paclitaxel first when given in combination with cisplatin or carboplatin. There is increased cytotoxic activity when given in this sequence.
- Paclitaxel is being studied as a radiosensitizer, given weekly doses 80–100 mg/m^2 as a 1-hour infusion.
- Intraperitoneal infusion (investigational): Dilute dose into 1–2 liters of 0.9% NS, or as ordered; warm to 37°C and infuse as rapidly as tolerated into peritoneal cavity; assist patient to change position every 15 minutes per protocol × 2 hours to maximize distribution in peritoneal cavity.

Drug Interactions:
- Cisplatin: Myelosuppression is more severe when cisplatin is administered prior to paclitaxel (due to 33% reduction in paclitaxel clearance from the plasma). Therefore, paclitaxel must be given prior to cisplatin when drugs are administered sequentially.
- Carboplatin: Possible increased cytotoxicity when given *after* taxol. Also, combination of paclitaxel and carboplatin results in less thrombocytopenia than would be expected from dose of carboplatin alone (etiology of platelet-sparing effect unknown).
- Paclitaxel is metabolized by P450 cytochrome isoenzymes CYP2C8 and CYP3A4. Potential interactions may occur, including antiretroviral protease inhibitors. Use together cautiously with other drugs metabolized by this system (CYP2C8 and CYP3A4 inducers: carbamazine, phenytoin, phenobarbital, rifampin: may decrease serum level of paclitaxel and decrease effect; CYP2C8 and CYP3A4 inhibitors: ethinyl estradiol, fluconazole, ketoconazole, sulfonamides, testosterone, tretinoin, ciprofloxacin, clarithromycin,

doxycycline, erythromycin, grapefruit juice, isoniazid, protease inhibitors, verapamil: may increase serum level of paclitaxel with increased risk of toxicity). Use together cautiously, if at all.

- Doxorubicin and liposomal doxorubicin: Increased incidence of neutropenia and stomatitis when paclitaxel is administered prior to doxorubicin (due to 30–35% decrease in doxorubicin clearance, possibly due to competition for biliary excretion of both agents). Therefore, doxorubicin should be given prior to paclitaxel or sequentially rather than concomitantly.
- Doxorubicin: Increased risk of cardiotoxicity when given in combination with paclitaxel, with sharp increase in risk of congestive heart failure once cumulative dose of doxorubicin is > 380 mg/m^2 (Minotti et al., 2001). Give sequentially rather than concomitantly.
- Cyclophosphamide: Increased myelosuppression when cyclophosphamide given before paclitaxel; give sequentially rather than concomitantly.
- Beta-blockers, calcium channel blockers, digoxin: Additive bradycardia may occur; assess/monitor patients closely.
- Immunosuppressive agents, other antineoplastic agents: Additive immunosuppression may occur; assess toxicity and patient response closely.
- Trastuzumab: Increased risk of cardiotoxicity, but studies have shown no increased cardiac events when used together (Dang et al., 2006).
- St. John's wort: May increase paclitaxel serum level; do not use together.

Lab Effects/Interference:
- Decreased CBC.
- Increased LFTs.

Special Considerations:
- Drug has radiosensitizing effects.
- Drug is embryotoxic; avoid use in pregnancy. Women of childbearing age should use effective contraception.
- Drug may be excreted in breastmilk, so breastfeeding should be avoided during drug therapy.
- ANC should be ≥ 1,500/mm^3 prior to initial or subsequent doses of paclitaxel.
- Dose reductions: 20% dose reduction if severe neuropathy or severe neutropenia (ANC < 500/mm^3 for 7 or more days) develop and/or consider addition of colony-stimulating factor support with next cycle; 25–50% dose reduction if hepatic dysfunction (hepatic metastasis > 2 cm) occurs (Chabner and Longo, 2001); 50% or more dose reduction for moderate or severe hyperbilirubinemia or significantly increased serum transferase levels, with dose of paclitaxel not exceeding 50–75 mg/m^2 IV over 24 hours, or 75–100 mg/m^2 IV over 3 hours; if AST > 2 times upper limit of normal, patient dose should not exceed 50 mg/m^2 IV over 24 hours.
- One-hour infusion of paclitaxel as well as weekly dosing regimens are being studied/ used. Lower doses, e.g., 80–100 mg/m^2 IV over 1 hour weekly × 3 with 1 week off per cycle, weekly × 6 with 2 weeks off per cycle, or weekly × 12 weeks, appear to inhibit angiogenesis, and allow for increased dose density.

Potential Toxicities/Side Effects and the Nursing Process

I.   POTENTIAL FOR INJURY related to HYPERSENSITIVITY OR ANAPHYLAXIS REACTIONS

Defining Characteristics: Hypersensitivity occurs in 10% of patients, with anaphylaxis and severe hypersensitivity reactions in 2–4% (characterized by dyspnea, hypotension requiring treatment, angioedema, and generalized urticaria). Reaction is to Cremophor in paclitaxel preparation. Signs/symptoms include tachycardia, wheezing, hypotension, facial edema; incidence of supraventricular tachycardia with hypotension and chest pain occurs in 1–2%. Patients who have severe hypersensitivity reaction should not be rechallenged with drug. Those who have less severe reactions have received 24 hours of corticosteroid prophylaxis, and have been successfully rechallenged with drug infused at a slower rate.

Nursing Implications: Assess baseline VS and mental status prior to drug administration. Ensure that patient has taken dexamethasone premedication, and administer diphenhydramine and H_2 antagonist as ordered. Monitor VS every 15 minutes, and remain with patient during first 15 minutes of drug infusion as most reactions occur during the first 10 minutes. Stop drug if cardiac arrhythmia (irregular apical pulse), hypotension, or hypertension occur, and discuss continuance of infusion with physician. Recall signs/symptoms of anaphylaxis, and if these occur, stop drug immediately and notify physician. *Subjective symptoms:* generalized itching, nausea, chest tightness, crampy abdominal pain, difficulty speaking, anxiety, agitation, sense of impending doom, uneasiness, desire to urinate/defecate, dizziness, chills. *Objective signs:* flushed appearance; angioedema of face, neck, eyelids, hands, feet; localized or generalized urticaria; respiratory distress with or without wheezing; hypotension; cyanosis. Review standing orders or nursing procedure for patient management of anaphylaxis, and be prepared to stop drug immediately if signs/symptoms occur, keep IV line open with 0.9% sodium chloride, notify physician, monitor VS, and administer ordered medications, which may include epinephrine 1:1,000, hydrocortisone sodium succinate, and diphenhydramine. Teach patient the potential of a hypersensitivity or anaphylactic reaction and to immediately report any unusual symptoms.

II.   POTENTIAL FOR INFECTION AND BLEEDING related to BONE MARROW DEPRESSION

Defining Characteristics: Neutropenia may be severe, especially when drug is administered via 24-hour infusion. Neutropenia is also more severe when cisplatin precedes paclitaxel in sequential administration, as it reduces paclitaxel clearance by 33%. Neutropenia is also more pronounced in patients who have received prior radiotherapy. Nadir is 7–11 days after dose with recovery in 1 week. Neutropenia is dose-dependent, with severe neutropenia (ANC < 500/mm³) occurring in 47–67% of patients. Anemia occurs frequently, but thrombocytopenia is uncommon.

Nursing Implications: Assess baseline CBC, WBC, differential, and platelet count prior to chemotherapy, as well as signs/symptoms of infection or bleeding. Teach patient the signs/symptoms of infection or bleeding, and to report these immediately, and teach patient self-care measures to minimize risk of infection and bleeding. This includes avoidance of crowds, proximity to people with infections, and OTC aspirin-containing medications. Administer paclitaxel PRIOR to cisplatin or carboplatin when either is given in combination with paclitaxel. Teach patient self-administration of G-CSF as ordered to prevent severe neutropenia. Transfuse red blood cells and platelets per physician order.

III. SENSORY/PERCEPTUAL ALTERATIONS related to SENSORY NEUROPATHY

Defining Characteristics: Frequency and incidence is dose-dependent but appears not to be influenced by infusion duration. Overall incidence is 60%, with 3% severe neuropathy in women with breast or ovarian cancer treated with single-agent paclitaxel, but severe neuropathy occurred in 8–13% of patients with NSCLC who also received cisplatin. Onset related to cumulative dose, with incidence after first course 27% and remainder occurring after 2–10 courses. Sensory symptoms usually resolve after 2 or more months following paclitaxel discontinuance. Sensory alterations are paresthesias in a glove-and-stocking distribution, and numbness. There may be a symmetrical loss of sensation, vibration, proprioception, temperature, and pinprick. Sensory and motor neuropathy may occur in patients receiving both paclitaxel and cisplatin. There is an increased risk for motor and autonomic dysfunction in patients with neuropathy from diabetes mellitus or alcohol ingestion prior to treatment with paclitaxel. Arthralgias and myalgias affect 60% of patients, and begin 2–3 days after treatment; they resolve in a few days; may be ameliorated by low-dose dexamethasone.

Nursing Implications: Assess baseline neurologic status. Instruct patient to report signs/symptoms of pins-and-needles sensation, numbness, pain, increased discomfort with certain sensations, especially in the extremities, or motor weakness. Identify patients at risk: those with history of cisplatin use or with preexisting neuropathies (ethanol- and diabetes mellitus-related). Assess sensory and motor function prior to each treatment, and if abnormality found, assess impact on patient function, safety, independence, and quality of life. Test patient's ability to button a shirt or pick up a dime from a flat surface. If severely impacting safety or quality of life, discuss with patient and physician drug reduction (20%) or discontinuance or use of cytoprotective agent. Teach self-care strategies, including maintaining safety when walking, getting up, taking bath, or washing dishes, and discuss inability to sense temperature and the need to keep extremities warm in cold weather. See NCI Common Toxicity Criteria Adverse Effects, *Appendix II:* grade 3 motor = objective weakness, interfering with ADLs; grade 3 sensory = sensory loss or paresthesia interfering with ADLs; grade 4 motor = paralysis; grade 4 sensory = permanent sensory loss that interferes with function.

IV.   ALTERATION IN SKIN INTEGRITY related to ALOPECIA, ONYCHOLYSIS

Defining Characteristics: Complete alopecia occurs in most patients and is reversible. Onycholysis may occur in patients receiving weekly paclitaxel, and risk increases after the sixth course.

Nursing Implications: Discuss potential impact of hair loss prior to drug administration. Discuss coping strategies and plan to minimize body image distortion (e.g., wig, scarf, cap). Assess patient for signs/symptoms of hair loss. Assess patient's response and use of coping strategies, and help patient to build on effective strategies. If the patient is receiving weekly paclitaxel, teach fingernail care (keep clean and well manicured).

V.   ALTERATION IN NUTRITION, LESS THAN BODY REQUIREMENTS, related to NAUSEA AND VOMITING, DIARRHEA, STOMATITIS, HEPATOTOXICITY

Defining Characteristics: Nausea and vomiting occur commonly in 52% of patients and are mild and preventable with antiemetics. Diarrhea occurs in 38% of patients and is mild. Stomatitis occurs in 31% and is mild, appears to be dose- and schedule-dependent, and is more common with 24-hour infusions than 3-hour infusions. Mild increase in LFTs may occur (7% bilirubin, 22% alk phos, 19% AST). Rarely, hepatic necrosis and hepatic encephalopathy leading to death have been reported. If severe hepatic dysfunction occurs, paclitaxel dose should be reduced (see Special Considerations section).

Nursing Implications: Premedicate patient with antiemetic (either serotonin antagonist or dopamine antagonist). Encourage small, frequent meals of cool, bland foods. Instruct patient to report nausea, and teach self-administration of antiemetics if receiving drug as an outpatient. If nausea/vomiting occur and is severe, assess for signs/symptoms of fluid/ electrolyte imbalance. Encourage patient to report onset of diarrhea and to self-administer antidiarrheal medications. Assess baseline oral mucous membranes. Teach patient oral assessment and to report any alterations. Assess LFTs prior to drug administration and periodically during treatment.

VI.   POTENTIAL ALTERATION IN CIRCULATION related to HYPOTENSION, ARRHYTHMIA

Defining Characteristics: Hypotension during first 3 hours of infusion in 12% of patients, and transient, asymptomatic bradycardia in 30% of patients have been reported; most often patients did not require intervention. Significant cardiovascular events (syncope, rhythm abnormalities, hypertension, and venous thrombosis) occurred in 1% of patients receiving single-agent paclitaxel, but the incidence was 12–13% in patients with NSCLC receiving cisplatin as well. Of those patients with normal baseline EKGs at the beginning of pacli-taxel therapy, 14% of patients developed an abnormal EKG tracing (nonspecific repolar-ization abnormalities, sinus bradycardia, sinus tachycardia, premature beats). Whether or not the patient received prior anthracycline therapy did not influence these events. Prior anthracycline therapy did influence the rare incidence of CHF. Rarely, patients developed myocardial infarction, atrial fibrillation, and supraventricular tachycardia. For patients receiving doxorubicin in combination with paclitaxel, there is increased risk of CHF once the cumulative dose of doxorubicin is > 380 mg/m^2 (Gianni et al, 1998). Severe conduction abnormalities have been described in < 1% of patients, and required pacemaker insertion in some patients. The drug should be used cautiously in patients with coronary artery disease or prior myocardial infarction within past 6 months, as well as in patients with a history of arrhythmia who are being treated with beta-blockers, calcium channel blockers, or digoxin.

Nursing Implications: Assess baseline cardiac status, history, and risk for development of CHF. Closely monitor patient during paclitaxel infusion, especially if patient has history of hypertension, or is on cardiac medications (see Drug Interactions section). Teach patient to report any dyspnea, SOB, chest pain, or heart palpitations, or any unusual feeling. If any abnormalities occur, stop infusion as appropriate and discuss further management with physician. If patient is receiving doxorubicin and paclitaxel, discuss with physician stopping combination therapy when cumulative doxorubicin dose is 340–380 mg/m^2, and continuing paclitaxel as a single agent, as this does not increase risk of CHF (Gianni et al., 1998). If the patient develops significant conduction abnormalities, discuss medical management with physician, and expect that patient will have cardiac monitoring during subsequent paclitaxel therapy.

VII.   ALTERATION IN COMFORT related to FATIGUE, ARTHRALGIAS AND MYALGIAS

Defining Characteristics: Fatigue occurs commonly, and arthralgias and myalgias affect about 44% of all patients, with 8% experiencing severe symptoms. Arthralgias and myalgias commonly occurred 2–3 days after the drug was given, and resolved within a few days.

Nursing Implications: Teach patient that fatigue may occur, and ways to minimize exertion and energy expenditure by alternating rest and activity, and organizing chores so that they are done as efficiently as possible. Arthralgias and myalgias may be troublesome, and can be managed with NSAIDs, application of warmth, and other comfort measures. Some patients report that swimming is helpful in minimizing discomfort. Studies of gabapentin, glutamine, and steroids have been disappointing. Opioids may be needed if severe.

Drug: paclitaxel protein-bound particles for injectable suspension (albumin-bound), [Abraxane]

Class: Microtubule inhibitor. Drug (Abraxane) is paclitaxel that is formulated so that paclitaxel is bound in albumin (protein) nanoparticles; it is a mitotic inhibitor, like generic paclitaxel.

Metabolism: Paclitaxel protein-bound particles for injectable suspension (Abraxane) are highly protein bound (89–99%). The half-life is approximately 27 hours. Paclitaxel protein-bound particles for injectable suspension (Abraxane) is metabolized in the liver, primarily by CYP2C8 into 6-alpha-hydroxypaclitaxel, and by CYP3A4 into two minor metabolites. Fecal excretion was approximately 20% of the administered drug, and little drug was excreted in the urine (<1%) in clinical trials.

Indications: Indicated for the treatment of patients with
- (1) Metastatic Breast Cancer (MBC) after failure of combination chemotherapy for MBC or relapse within 6 months of adjuvant chemotherapy. Prior therapy should have included an anthracycline unless clinically contraindicated;
- (2) NSCLC, locally advanced or metastatic, as first line therapy, in combination with carboplatin, in patients who are not candidates for curative surgery or radiation therapy;
- (3) Metastatic adenocarcinoma of the pancreas as first-line treatment in combination with gemcitabine.

Contraindications: (1) ANC < 1,500 cells/mm^3; (2) severe hypersensitivity reaction to Abraxane.

Dosage/Range:
- Paclitaxel protein-bound particles for injectable suspension (albumin-bound) is different from generic paclitaxel and cannot be substituted for it.
- Metastatic Breast Cancer (MBC) after failure of combination chemotherapy, or relapse within 6 months of adjuvant chemotherapy: 260 mg/m^2 IV infusion over 30 minutes every 3 weeks.
- NSCLC: 100 mg/m^2 IV infusion over 30 min on days 1, 8, 15 of each 21-day cycle, together with carboplatin given IV on day 1 of each 21-day cycle immediately after paclitaxel protein-bound particles for injectable suspension is given.
- Adenocarcinoma of the pancreas: 125 mg/m2 IV infusion over 30–40 minutes on days 1, 8, and 15 of each 28-day cycle. Administer gemcitabine immediately after paclitaxel protein-bound particles for injectable suspension (Abraxane) is given on days 1, 8, and 15 of each 28-day cycle.
- Do not administer drug to patients with baseline ANC < 1,500 cells/mm^3. Assess CBC/ differential frequently, including prior to day 1 for MBC patients, and days 1, 8, 15 for NSCLC and pancreatic cancer patients.
- Dose reductions or discontinuation may be needed for severe hematologic, neurologic, cutaneous, or GI toxicities (see package insert).
- Reduce starting dose in patients with moderate to severe hepatic impairment (see package insert).
- No dose adjustment needed for patients with mild hepatic impairment. Hold drug if AST > 10X ULN or bilirubin > 5X ULN.
- Dose reduction or interruption may be needed based on severe hematologic, neurologic, cutaneous, or gastrointestinal toxicities (see package insert).

Drug Preparation/Administration:
- This drug is protein (albumin)-bound paclitaxel, and it must be distinguished from other, nonprotein-bound paclitaxel formulations, such as generic paclitaxel. Do not substitute for or with other paclitaxel formulations.
- Drug is contraindicated in patients with ANC < 1,500 cells/mm^3, or prior severe hypersensitivity reaction to paclitaxel protein-bound particles for injectable suspension (Abraxane).

- Available in single-use 100-mg lyophilized powder vials. The vial should be reconstituted with 20 mL of 0.9% Sodium Chloride, USP prior to IV infusion (see package insert for specific instructions). If not used immediately after mixing, the reconstituted vial may be stored in refrigerator for up to 8 hours; it should be protected from bright light by placing it in the original carton (see package insert). See package insert for preparation instructions and stability information. Solution will be milky white.
- Administer only if baseline ANC is $\geq$ 1,500 cells/mm^3.
- Dose-reduce for neutropenia or neuropathy.
- The use of specialized DEHP-free solution containers and administration sets is not necessary; do not use an in-line filter.
- DO NOT substitute for other paclitaxel formulations.
- No premedication is generally required, as with generic paclitaxel.
- Administer by IV infusion over 30 minutes.
- Drug is an irritant; monitor for injection-site reactions.

Drug Interactions:
- These are the same as generic, nonprotein-bound paclitaxel.
- Paclitaxel is metabolized by P450 cytochrome isoenzymes CYP2C8 and CYP3A4. Potential interactions may occur. Use cautiously with other drugs metabolized by this system (CYP2C8 and CYP3A4):
  Inducers: e.g., carbamazepine, efavirenz, nevirapine, phenytoin, rifampicin
  Inhibitors: e.g., cimetidine, erythromycin, fluoxetine, gemfibrozil, indinivir, ketoconazole and other imidazole antifungals, nelfinavir, ritonavir, saquinivir
- Use caution when administering paclitaxel protein-bound particles for injectable suspension (Abraxane) together with inhibitors or inducers of either CYP2C8 or CYP3A4; avoid coadministration if possible.

Lab Effects/Interference:
- Decreased white and red cell counts, neutrophil count, platelet count.
- Increased alkaline phosphatase, AST, ALT, bilirubin.

Special Considerations:
- Drug is a Cremophor-free, protein-engineered nanotransporter of paclitaxel. No premedication for hypersensitivity is generally required prior to administration of paclitaxel protein-bound particles for injectable suspension (Abraxane).
- Drug needs no special tubing or filter.
- Most common adverse reactions for patients are (1) *metastatic breast cancer:* alopecia, neutropenia, sensory neuropathy, abnormal ECG, fatigue/asthenia, myalgia/arthralgia, AST elevation, alkaline phosphatase elevation, anemia, nausea, infections, diarrhea; (2) *NSCLC:* anemia, neutropenia, thrombocytopenia, alopecia, peripheral neuropathy, nausea, fatigue; and (3) *adenocarcinoma of the pancreas:* neutropenia, fatigue, peripheral neuropathy, nausea, alopecia, peripheral edema, diarrhea, pyrexia, vomiting, decreased appetite, rash, dehydration.

Paclitaxel protein-bound particles for injectable suspension (Abraxane) has the following special warnings and precautions:

- Drug causes myelosuppression (primarily neutropenia), which is dose-dependent and a dose-limiting toxicity; monitor CBC and hold/reduce dose as needed; dose modify per package insert.
- Sensory neuropathy occurs frequently and may require dose reduction or treatment interruption.
- Sepsis has occurred in 5% of patients with or without neutropenia who received drug in combination with gemcitabine. Risk factors for severe or fatal sepsis included biliary obstruction or presence of biliary stent. If a patient becomes febrile, regardless of ANC, broad spectrum antibiotics should be initiated. For febrile neutropenia, interrupt Abraxane and gemcitabine until fever resolves and ANC ≥ 1,500, then resume at a reduced dose; see package insert.
- Pneumonitis has occurred in 4% of patients receiving the drug with gemcitabine. Monitor patients for signs/symptoms and interrupt drugs during evaluation of pneumonitis; if pneumonitis diagnosed, permanently discontinue treatment with both drugs.
- Severe hypersensitivity reactions with sometimes fatal outcomes have been reported. Do not re-challenge the patient with this drug.
- Increased serum LFT levels and toxicity can occur in patients with hepatic impairment. The starting dose for patients with moderate to severe hepatic impairment should be reduced (see package insert). Monitor LFTs and administer with caution.
- Drug contains albumin derived from human blood, which has a theoretical risk of viral transmission.
- Drug can harm the fetus. Counsel women of reproductive potential, as well as men, to use effective contraception to avoid pregnancy.

Potential Toxicities/Side Effects and the Nursing Process

I.   POTENTIAL FOR INFECTION AND BLEEDING related to BONE MARROW DEPRESSION

Defining Characteristics: Neutropenia is dose-dependent and reversible, and is a dose-limiting toxicity of paclitaxel protein-bound particles for injectable suspension. Grade 3–4 neutropenia occurred in 34% of patients with MBC, 47% in patients with NSCLC, and 38% in patients with pancreatic cancer. Infectious complications occurred in 24% of patients, with oral candidiasis, respiratory tract infection, and pneumonia the most commonly reported. Thrombocytopenia is uncommon, with bleeding reported in 2% of patients. Anemia occurred in 33% of patients and was severe in 1% of patients (Hgb < 8 g/dL). Sepsis occurred in 5% of patients with or without neutropenia, and risk of severe/fatal sepsis was increased in patients with biliary obstruction or presence of biliary stent.

Nursing Implications: Assess baseline CBC, WBC, differential, and platelet count prior to chemotherapy, as well as signs/symptoms of infection or bleeding. Teach patient the signs/symptoms of infection or bleeding, and to report these immediately, and teach patient self-care measures to minimize risk of infection and bleeding. This includes avoidance of crowds, proximity to people with infections, and OTC aspirin-containing medications. Do not administer paclitaxel protein-bound particles for injectable suspension to patients with a baseline ANC < 1,500 cells/mm^3. Assess the patient with biliary obstruction or presence of biliary stents closely for fever. If a patient becomes febrile, broad spectrum antibiotics should be started immediately regardless of ANC. If the patient develops febrile neutropenia, interrupt paclitaxel protein-bound particles for injectable suspension (Abraxane) and gemcitabine until fever resolves and ANC ≥ 1,500, then resume treatment at a reduced dose level (see package insert). Drug dose should be reduced for neutropenia or thrombocytopenia per package insert. Administer paclitaxel protein-bound particles for injectable suspension PRIOR to cisplatin or carboplatin when either is given in combination with paclitaxel.

II. SENSORY/PERCEPTUAL ALTERATIONS related to SENSORY NEUROPATHY, OCULAR AND VISUAL DISTURBANCES

Defining Characteristics: Sensory neuropathy is dose-related, schedule-dependent, and common in patients receiving paclitaxel protein-bound particles for injectable suspension. Incidence in patients with MBC receiving 260 mg/m2 every 3 weeks was 71%, compared to 56% in patients receiving paclitaxel in metastatic breast cancer studies. Grade 3 neuropathy occurred in 10%, and 14/24 patients had documented improvement after a median of 22 days. No grade 4 severity has been reported in clinical trials. Incidence of peripheral neuropathy in patients with NSCLC was 48% (compared to 64% for patients receiving paclitaxel every 3 weeks) and 54% in patients with adenocarcinoma of the pancreas. Motor or autonomic neuropathy (e.g., ileus) occurs rarely. Ocular/visual disturbances may occur in 13% of the patients, especially at doses higher than recommended; in the literature, persistent optic nerve damage related to generic paclitaxel has been reported.

Nursing Implications: Assess baseline neurologic status. Instruct patient to report signs/ symptoms of pins-and-needles sensation (paresthesias), numbness, pain, increased discomfort with certain sensations (dysesthesias), especially in the extremities, or motor weakness. Identify patients at risk: those with history of cisplatin use or with preexisting neuropathies (ethanol- and diabetes mellitus-related). Assess sensory and motor function prior to each treatment, and if abnormality found, assess impact on patient function, safety, independence, and quality of life. Test patient's ability to button a shirt or pick up a dime from a flat surface. Teach self-care strategies as needed, including maintaining safety when walking, getting up, taking bath, or washing dishes; explain inability to sense temperature and the need to keep extremities warm in cold weather (see NCI Common Toxicity Criteria). Teach the patient to report any ocular or visual disturbance, and discuss management or need for ophthalmologic consultation with physician. Grades 1 or 2 peripheral neuropathy generally do not require dose adjustment. If grades 3 or higher, hold paclitaxel protein-bound particles for injectable suspension (Abraxane) until signs/symptoms resolve/improve to ≤ grade 1 or 2 for patients with MBC or until resolution to ≤ grade 1 for patients with either NSCLC or pancreatic cancer, followed by a dose reduction for all subsequent courses of paclitaxel protein-bound particles for injectable suspension (Abraxane) [see package insert].

III.   ALTERATION IN SKIN INTEGRITY related to ALOPECIA

Defining Characteristics: Alopecia occurs commonly (90% in patients with MBC studied, 56% in patients with NSCLC, and 50% in patients with adenocarcinoma of the pancreas).

Nursing Implications: Discuss potential impact of hair loss prior to drug administration. Discuss coping strategies and plan to minimize body image distortion (e.g., wig, scarf, cap). Assess patient for signs/symptoms of hair loss. Assess patient's response and use of coping strategies, and help patient to build on effective strategies.

IV.   ALTERATION IN NUTRITION, LESS THAN BODY REQUIREMENTS, related to NAUSEA/VOMITING AND DIARRHEA

Defining Characteristics: Side effects that may affect nutrition are the following, with incidences for patients with MBC, NSCLC, and adenocarcinoma of the pancreas indicated for each: nausea occurred in 30% of patients with MBC, 27% in patients with NSCLC, and 54% in patients with adenocarcinoma of pancreas; vomiting in 18%, 12%, and 36% of patients respectively; and diarrhea in 27%, 15%, and 44% of patients respectively.

Nursing Implications: Premedicate patient with antiemetic if needed. Encourage small, frequent meals of cool, bland foods. Instruct patient to report nausea, and teach self-administration of antiemetics. If nausea/vomiting occurs and is severe, assess for signs/symptoms of fluid/electrolyte imbalance. Assess bowel elimination pattern and oral mucosa baseline prior to each treatment. Teach patient to report diarrhea unrelieved with self-administered anti-diarrheal medications and adequate fluid replacement.

V.   ALTERATION IN COMFORT related to FATIGUE, ARTHRALGIAS, AND MYALGIAS

Defining Characteristics: Fatigue is common, with fatigue/asthenia affecting 47% of patients with MBC, 25% of patients with NSCLC, and 59% of patients with adenocarcinoma of the pancreas. Arthralgias and myalgias affect about 44% of MBC patients, with 8% experiencing severe symptoms. Arthralgias occurred in 13% and myalgias 10% in patients with NSCLC, and 11% and 10% respectively in patients with adenocarcinoma of the pancreas. Arthralgias and myalgias commonly occurred 2–3 days after the drug was given, and resolved within a few days.

Nursing Implications: Teach patient that fatigue may occur, and ways to minimize exertion and energy expenditure by alternating rest and activity, and organizing chores so that they are done as efficiently as possible. Teach patient that arthralgias and myalgias may occur, teach self-care measures to reduce discomfort, and advise patient to report discomfort that does not resolve.

Drug: pegasparaginase (Oncaspar)

Class: Miscellaneous agent (enzyme).

Mechanism of Action: Pegasparaginase is a modified form of L-asparaginase, wherein units of monomethoxypolyethylene glycol (PEG) are covalently conjugated to L-asparaginase, forming the active ingredient PEG-L-asparaginase. The enzyme hydrolyzes serum asparagine, a nonessential amino acid for both normal and leukemic cells. Unlike normal cells, leukemic cells are unable to synthesize their own asparagine (lack the enzyme asparagine synthetase and thus require exogenous L-asparagine), resulting in cell death.

Metabolism: Unclear. Elimination half-life is significantly prolonged with pegylated formulation of 5.5–7 days, compared to Erwinia asparaginase, of 16 hours, and native E.coli L-asparaginase of 26–30 hours. One dose of pegylated L-asparaginase of 2,500 IU/m^2 achieves similar levels of asparagine depletion as 9 doses of native E.coli L-asparaginase during induction, and 6 doses during each delayed intensification phase (Oncaspar package insert, 2006).

Indication: For the treatment of patients with (1) acute lymphoblastic leukemia (ALL, as first-line treatment as part of a multi-agent chemotherapeutic regimen; (2) acute lymphoblastic leukemia in patients hypersenisitive to asparaginase, as a component of a multi-agent chemotherapeutic regimen.

Contraindication: Patients with a history of (1) serious allergic reactions to Oncaspar; (2) serious thrombosis with prior L-asparaginase therapy; (3) pancreatitis with prior L-asparaginase therapy; (4) serous hemorrhagic events with prior L-asparaginase therapy.

Dosage/Range:
- Recommended dose is 2,500 international units/m^2 IM or IV every 14 days.

Drug Preparation:
- Available as a 3750 international units/5 mL single-use vial.
- For intravenous use, reconstitute with sterile water for injection, and dilute further in 100 cc NS or D5W. If giving IM, reconstitute in no more than 2 cc NS for injection. If more than 2 cc of NS is used, more than one injection site must be used.
- Do not administer Oncaspar if the drug has been frozen, stored at room temperature (+15°C–25°C; 59°F–77°F) for >48 hours, or if the drug has been shaken or vigorously agitated.
- Inspect solution for particulate matter and/or discoloration prior to administration; if present, do not use.

Drug Administration:
- IM is the preferred route of administration because of the lower incidence of hepatotoxicity, coagulopathy, and gastrointestinal and renal disorders, as compared with the intravenous route.
- When administered IM, the volume at the injection site should be less than or equal to 2 mL; if volume to administer is larger than 2mL, use multiple injection sites.

- When administered IV: mix in 100 mL of sodium chloride or dextrose injection 5%, infuse over a period of 1–2 hours; piggyback into a plain infusion that is already infusing.
- Observe patient during and for 1 hour after drug administration, as anaphylaxis may occur.

Drug Interactions:

- Nonsteroidal anti-inflammatory drugs (NSAIDs), aspirin, dipyridamole, heparin, warfarin, and blood-dyscrasia-causing medications: Pegasparaginase causes imbalances in coagulation factors, predisposing patients to bleeding and/or thrombosis.
- Hepatotoxic medications (increased risk of toxicity).
- **Methotrexate:** Drug antagonizes antifolate effects of MTX if given before MTX administration. If given 24 hours after MTX, its antifolate activity will be terminated at that point.
- Vaccines, both live and killed virus: Patient's antibody response to the killed vaccine may be reduced for up to 1 year by the immunosuppression brought on by pegasparaginase. Such immunosuppression may also potentiate the replication of live-virus vaccines, increase the side effects of the vaccine virus, and/or may decrease the patient's antibody response to the vaccine.

Lab Effects/Interference:

- Increased LFTs, serum glucose, BUN, and uric acid.
- Prolonged PT.

Special Considerations:

- Drug should NOT be given in patients with:
  - Pegasparaginase allergy,
- Bleeding disorders associated with prior asparaginase therapy,
- Pancreatitis, or history of.
- Hypersensitivity reactions occur more frequently with pegasparaginase than with the vast majority of chemotherapeutic agents. Patients must be closely monitored for signs of allergic/anaphylactic reactions. Ensure immediate access to adverse-reaction kit.

Potential Toxicities/Side Effects and the Nursing Process

I.   POTENTIAL FOR INJURY related to HYPERSENSITIVITY OR ANAPHYLACTIC REACTIONS

Defining Characteristics: Occurs less often with IM route of administration. May be life-threatening reaction, but is usually mild.

Nursing Implications: Discuss with physician use of test dose prior to drug administration. Assess baseline VS and mental status prior to drug administration. Review standing orders or nursing procedure for management of anaphylaxis and be prepared to stop drug immediately if signs/symptoms occur; keep IV line open with 0.9% sodium chloride, notify physician, monitor vital signs, and administer ordered medications, which may include epinephrine 1:1,000, hydrocortisone sodium succinate, and diphenhydramine. Teach patient the potential of a hypersensitivity or anaphylactic reaction and to report any unusual symptoms immediately. *Escherichia coli* preparation of L-asparaginase and *Erwinia carotovora* preparation are non-cross-resistant, so if an anaphylactic reaction occurs with one, the other preparation may be used.

II.   POTENTIAL FOR INJURY related to HEPATIC DYSFUNCTION OR THROMBOEMBOLISM

Defining Characteristics: Most patients have elevated LFTs starting within first 2 weeks of treatment, e.g., SGOT, bili, and alk phos. Hepatically derived clotting factors may be depressed, resulting in excessive bleeding or blood clotting. Relatively uncommon.

Nursing Implications: Monitor SGOT, bili, alk phos, albumin, and clotting factors CPT, PTT, fibrinogen. Teach patient of the potential for excessive bleeding or blood clotting, and instruct to report any unusual symptoms. Assess patient for signs/symptoms of bleeding.

III.   ALTERED NUTRITION, LESS THAN BODY REQUIREMENTS, related to NAUSEA/VOMITING, ANOREXIA, HYPERGLYCEMIA

Defining Characteristics: Many patients experience mild-to-moderate nausea and vomiting. Anorexia commonly occurs. Hyperglycemia is a transient reaction caused by effects on the pancreas with decreased insulin synthesis. Pancreatitis occurs in some patients.

Nursing Implications: Premedicate with antiemetics and continue prophylactically for 24 hours to prevent nausea and vomiting. Encourage small, frequent meals of cool, bland foods and liquids, as well as favorite foods, especially high-calorie, high-protein foods. Encourage use of spices and do weekly weights. Teach patient about the potential of hyperglycemia and pancreatitis, and instruct to report any unusual symptoms: e.g., increased thirst, urination, and appetite (hyperglycemia) and abdominal or stomach pain, constipation, or nausea and vomiting (pancreatitis). Monitor serum glucose, amylase, and lipase levels periodically during treatment. Report any laboratory elevations to physician. Treat hyperglycemia issues with diet or insulin as ordered by physician. Treat pancreatitis per physician orders.

IV.   SENSORY/PERCEPTUAL ALTERATIONS related to NEUROTOXICITY

Defining Characteristics: Neurotoxicity may occur in some patients—commonly, lethargy, drowsiness, and somnolence; rarely coma. Seen more frequently in adults.

Nursing Implications: Teach patient about the potential of CNS toxicity, and instruct to report any unusual symptoms. Obtain baseline neurologic and mental function. Assess patient for any neurologic abnormalities and report changes to physician. Discuss with patient the impact of malaise on his/her general sense of well-being and strategies to minimize the distress.

V. INFECTION, BLEEDING, AND FATIGUE related to BONE MARROW DEPRESSION

Defining Characteristics: Bone marrow depression is not common. Mild anemia may occur. Serious leukopenia and thrombocytopenia are rare.

Nursing Implications: Monitor CBC, platelet count prior to drug administration, as well as signs/symptoms of infection, bleeding, or anemia. Instruct patient in self-assessment of signs/symptoms of infection, bleeding, or anemia and to report immediately.

Drug: pemetrexed (Alimta)

Class: Folate analog metabolic inhibitor [multitargeted antifolate (antimetabolite)].

Mechanism of Action: Inhibits key metabolic enzymatic steps (thymidylate synthase [TS], dihydrofolate reductase [DHFR], and glycinamide ribonucleotide formyltransferase [GARFT]) critical to pyrimidine and purine synthesis, thus preventing DNA synthesis and cell division. Drug is carried into tumor cells via reduced folate carriers, metabolized intracellularly to polyglutamated form of pemetrexed that potently inhibits purine and pyrimidine synthesis. Antitumor effect dependent upon size of cellular folate pools, so folic acid must be coadministered to increase drug efficacy and minimize toxicity. Polyglutamates accumulate in the cell, with a long cellular half-life, and increased cytotoxicity. It is active in the S phase of the cell cycle.

Metabolism: Following IV administration, peak plasma levels are achieved within 30 minutes. Drug is widely distributed in body tissues, especially liver, kidneys, small intestines, and colon. Excreted by kidneys (glomerular and tubular) into the urine, with up to 90% of the drug excreted unchanged during the first 24 hours after administration. Plasma half-life is about 3 hours, with prolonged terminal half-life of 20 hours.

Indications:
- (1) Locally advanced or metastatic nonsquamous NSCL (a) initial treatment in combination with cisplatin; (b) as maintenance treatment of patients whose disease has not progressed after 4 cycles of platinum-based first-line chemotherapy; (c) after prior chemotherapy as a single-agent;
- (2) Mesothelioma: in combination with cisplatin.
- Pemetrexate is not indicated for the treatment of patients with squamous cell NSCLC.

Dosage/Range:
- Combination use in nonsquamous NSCLC and mesothelioma: 500 mg/m^2 IV on day 1 of each 21-day cycle, in combination with cisplatin 75 mg/m^2 IV over 2 hours, beginning 30 minutes after the end of the pemetrexed dose.
- Single-agent use in NSCLC, 500 mg/m^2 IV day 1 of each 21-day cycle.

Dose reduction: Dose reductions or discontinuation may be needed based on toxicities from the preceding cycle of therapy. These reductions are based on NCI's CTCAE:

- Pemetrexed plus cisplatin:
  - Hematologic: Nadir ANC < 500 cells/mm³, and platelet count ≥ 50,000 cells/mm³. DOSE-REDUCE both drugs to 75% of previous doses.
  - Hematologic: Nadir platelets < 50,000 cells/mm³ without bleeding regardless of ANC nadir. DOSE-REDUCE both drugs to 75% of previous doses; if bleeding present, dose-reduce both drugs to 50% of previous doses.
- For nonhematologic grade 3 or higher toxicities, pemetrexed should be withheld until resolution to less than or equal to patient's pre-therapy value, then resume at:
  - Any grade 3 or 4 toxicity (except mucositis): 75% of previous dose of both drugs.
  - Any diarrhea requiring hospitalization, or grade 3 or 4 diarrhea: 75% of previous dose of both drugs.
  - Grade 3 or 4 mucositis: 50% of previous dose of pemetrexed, and 100% of cisplatin dose.
- Neurotoxicity:
  - If grade 1 neurotoxicity, no dose modifications of either drug.
  - If grade 2 neurotoxicity, 100% pemetrexed dose, and dose-reduce cisplatin to 50% of previous dose.
  - If grade 3 or 4 neurotoxicity, discontinue therapy.
- Permanently discontinue pemetrexate if a patient experiences grade 3 or 4 hematologic or nonhematologic toxicity after 2 dose reductions, or immediately for grade 3 or 4 neurotoxicity.

Drug Preparation.
- Drug available in 100-mg and 500-mg vials for injection.
- Reconstitute pemetrexed 100-mg vial by adding 4.2 mL and 500-mg vial by adding 20 mL 0.9% sodium chloride for injection, resulting in a concentration of 25 mg/mL.
- Aseptically remove dose and add to 100 mL 0.9% sodium chloride for injection infusion bag.

Administration:
- Assess labs prior to each cycle, which must be: ANC ≥ 1,500 cells/mm³, platelet count ≥ 100,000 cells/mm³, and CrCl ≥ 45 mL/min. Patients should also be monitored for nadir and recovery, e.g., days 8 and 15 of each cycle.
- Do not administer pemetrexate if CrCl < 45 mL/min.
- Ensure patient has taken premedication prior to initial dose of pemetrexed and continuing through treatment:
  - Folic acid supplement (400 to 1,000 micrograms) PO once daily beginning 1 week prior to initial treatment, and continuing throughout treatment and 21 days posttreatment.
  - Vitamin B_{12} (1,000 micrograms) IM injections every 3 cycles, beginning 1 week prior to first treatment, and continuing throughout treatment every 3 cycles thereafter. Subsequent vitamin B_{12} injections (after the initial dose) can be given the same day as pemetexed administration.
  - Dexamethasone 4 mg PO twice daily on the day before, day of, and day after treatment to help prevent skin rash.

- Ensure that patients with mild to moderate renal insufficiency (Cr Cl 45–79 mL/min) have stopped NSAIDs with short elimination half-lives (e.g., diclofenac, indomethacin) at least 2 days prior to receiving pemetrexed: the day of administration and for two days following. Patients with normal renal function (CrCl ≥ 80 mL/min) can take NSAIDs (e.g., ibuprofen 400 mg qid), without significantly reducing pemetrexed clearance.
- Administer as a 10-minute IV infusion.

Drug Interactions:
- Nephrotoxic drugs: potentially delayed pemetrexed excretion.
- Drugs secreted by renal tubules (e.g., probenecid): potential delayed pemetrexed excretion.
- Thymidine: rescues normal cells.
- Leucovorin: decreases antitumor effect of pemetrexed; do not coadminister.
- 5-FU: may increase antitumor effect of pemetrexed.
- Ibuprofen and other NSAIDs, in people with normal renal function: 20% increase in AUC of pemetrexed, due to 20% reduction in pemetrexed clearance.
- NSAIDs (short half-lives, e.g., ibuprofen): AVOID if renal compromise (creatinine clearance < 80 mL/min), stop NSAIDs 2 days prior to pemetrexed administration, the day of administration, and for 2 days following pemetrexed administration.
- NSAIDs (long half-lives): stop NSAID 5 days before, the day of, and for 2 days following pemetrexed administration.
- If patient must continue NSAIDs, 24-hour creatinine clearance should be > 80 mL/min.
- Lactated Ringer's or Ringer's Injection USP: physical incompatibility with pemetrexed; do not use together.

Lab Effects/Interference:
- Transient increase in serum transaminases and bilirubin.

Special Considerations:
- Do not administer drug if creatinine clearance is < 45 mL/min using Cockcroft and Gault formula (estimated creatinine clearance): (140 - age in years) × actual body weight (kg); males: 72 × serum creatinine (mg/dL) = mL/min; females: estimated creatinine clearance for males × 0.85.
- Pemetrexed is fetotoxic and teratogenic. Women of childbearing age should use effective birth control measures. Women should not breastfeed an infant while receiving pemetrexed.
- Patients with Stage IIIB or IV NSCLC who receive platinum-based induction therapy for 4 cycles followed by maintenance therapy with pemetrexate (500 mg/m^2), had significantly longer time to progression compared with patients who received placebo (4 months vs 2 months, $p < .0001$), and longer OS when patients with squamous cell NSCLC were removed (15.5 months vs 10.3 months, $p < .0001$). In subset analysis, there was no survival advantage for patients with squamous cell histology NSCLC (Ciuleanu et al., 2008).
- Premedication regimen is necessary to reduce severity of hematologic and GI toxicity: supplementation with oral folic acid, IM Vitamin B$_{12}$.
- Use caution in patients with mild to moderate renal insufficiency (cr cl 45–79 mL/min) who are also taking NSAIDs. Stop NSAIDs at least 2 days prior to administering pemetrexed: the day of administration and for two days following.

Potential Toxicities/Side Effects and the Nursing Process

I. POTENTIAL INFECTION, BLEEDING, AND FATIGUE related to BONE MARROW DEPRESSION

Defining Characteristics: Bone marrow depression is dose-limiting toxicity. Nadir is day 8 with recovery by day 15 of each cycle. Neutropenia occurred in 58% of patients, with grade 3 (19%), and grade 4 (5%). For grades 3 and 4 neutropenia, the incidence in between patients who were fully supplemented was 24%, in contrast to patients who were never supplemented (38%). The overall incidence of thrombocytopenia is 27%, with grades 3 and 4 (4% and 1%, respectively). Anemia occurred in 33% of patients overall.

Nursing Implications: Assess baseline CBC, WBC, differential and ANC, and platelet count prior to chemotherapy as well as for signs and symptoms of infection, bleeding, or anemia. Ensure labs ANC > 1,500 cells/mm³, platelets > 100,000 cells/mm³, AND creatinine clearance > 45 mL/min prior to drug administration. Ensure that patient has taken vitamin supplements prior to drug administration: low-dose oral folic acid or multivitamin with folic acid daily (at least 5 daily doses of folic acid must be taken during the 7-day period prior to the first dose of pemetrexed, and dosing should continue during the full course of therapy, and for 21 days after the last drug dose; vitamin B₁₂ 100 micrograms IM during the week prior to cycle 1, then every 3 cycles; subsequent doses can be given on same day as pemetrexed treatment). Discuss dose reductions based on nadir counts with physician as needed. Teach patient signs/symptoms of infection, and bleeding, and instruct to report them right away. Teach measures to minimize infection and bleeding, such as avoidance of crowds and proximity to people with infection, and to avoid aspirin or NSAID-containing medications. Teach patient strategies to minimize fatigue, such as alternating rest with activity, and ways to organize shopping to minimize energy expenditure.

II. POTENTIAL ALTERATION IN NUTRITION, LESS THAN BODY REQUIREMENTS, related to NAUSEA, CONSTIPATION, ANOREXIA, DIARRHEA, STOMATITIS

Defining Characteristics: Nausea occurs in 84% of patients, vomiting 58%, constipation 44%, anorexia 35%, stomatitis/pharyngitis 28%, and diarrhea 26%, in combination with cisplatin.

Nursing Implications: Premedicate with antiemetics, and ensure patient has antiemetics to take to prevent delayed emesis from cisplatin. Teach patient and family delayed emesis regimen. Encourage small, frequent meals of cool, bland foods, and to increase fluid intake. Assess oral mucosa prior to drug administration and instruct patient to report changes. Teach patient oral hygiene measures and self-assessment. Instruct patient to report diarrhea, to self-administer prescribed antidiarrheal medications and to drink adequate fluids. Monitor LFTs baseline and periodically during therapy. Notify physician of any abnormalities and discuss implications as drug studied only in patients with elevated LFTs related to liver metastases.

III.   ALTERATION IN SKIN INTEGRITY related to RASH

Defining Characteristics: Incidence of rash with or without desquamation was 22%.

Nursing Implications: Assess baseline skin integrity. Teach patient that this may occur, and to take recommended dexamethasone premedication 4 mg po bid the day before, the day of, and the day after pemetrexed administration. Teach patient potential side effects of corticosteroid administration, including difficulty sleeping, mood alterations, and depression.

IV.   POTENTIAL FOR IMPAIRED GAS EXCHANGE related to DYSPNEA

Defining Characteristics: Dyspnea was reported in 66% of patients receiving pemetrexed and cisplatin therapy; 10% had grade 3 dyspnea, and 1% had grade 4 toxicity.

Nursing Implications: Teach patient that this may occur, and to report it right away if severe or worsening. Assess baseline pulmonary status, at rest, and with activity. Assess oxygen saturation with vital signs. Discuss severe or worsening dyspnea with physician.

Drug: pentostatin (Nipent, 2-deoxycoformycin)

Class: Antimetabolite.

Mechanism of Action: Isolated from fermentation cultures of *Streptomyces antibioticus*. Drug is a potent inhibitor of adenosine deaminase (ADA), which is found in lymphocytes, with T cells (and T-cell malignancies) having higher levels of ADA than B cells (and B-cell malignancies). By blocking ADA, pentostatin is believed to block DNA and RNA synthesis, resulting in cell death. It causes cells to arrest in G_1–S phases of the cell cycle, but also appears to act in a non–cell cycle specific way.

Metabolism: Is not absorbed orally. After IV administration drug distributes widely in body tissue and water, low protein binding, and crosses blood–brain barrier with up to 12% identified in the CSF within 24 hours of administration. Liver metabolizes minimal amount of drug. More than 90% of drug and metabolites are excreted unchanged in the urine, with half-life of drug about 6 hours unless impaired renal function.

Indications: As a single-agent in the treatment of hairy cell leukemia (both untreated and alpha-interferon refactory) in patients with active disease (e.g., clinically significant anemia, neutropenia, thrombocytopenia, or disease-related symptoms).

Dosage/Range:
Hairy cell leukemia:
- 4 mg/m² IV every other week until complete response if tolerated well and then two additional doses. Discontinue after 6 months of treatment if no response or if only partial response after 12 months.
- Check baseline serum creatinine and 24-hour creatinine clearance, and repeat serum creatinine before each dose.

- Dose-reduce to 2–3 mg/m^2 IV if creatinine clearance 50–60 mL/min and benefit justifies risk of toxicity.
- Hydration: 500 mL to 1 L of fluid before drug, followed by 1,000 mL after drug administration to ensure adequate urine output (and drug excretion).

Drug Preparation:
- Available in single-use 10-mg vials, which are reconstituted with 5-mL sterile water (2 mg/mL).
- Stable at room temperature for 8 hours.

Drug Administration:
- IV push over 5 minutes or IV infusion over 20–30 minutes in a 50-mL bag of D$_5$W or 0.9% NS after prehydration and followed by posthydration.
- Hold drug if patient has ANC < 200/mm^3 (when baseline count was > 500/mm^3), active infection, severe reactions to drug, CNS toxicity, or increased serum creatinine.
- Assess renal function prior to initial treatment, including a serum creatinine or creatinine clearance assay; CBC/differential and serum creatinine should be assessed prior to each dose, and more frequently if needed.

Drug Interactions:
- Fludarabine: fatal pulmonary toxicity; do not coadminister.
- Bone marrow-suppressing agents: increased bone marrow depression.
- High-dose cyclophosphamide (BMT): possible fatal cardiotoxicity.
- Vidarabine: decreased metabolism, with increased activity and toxicity of vidarabine.
- CNS depressants (sedative, hypnotics): increased CNS toxicity possible.

Lab Effects/Interference:
- Increased AST, ALT, alkaline phosphatase, LDH, uric acid, serum creatinine.
- Decreased WBC (lymphocytes and granulocytes).

Special Considerations:
Warnings:
- Myelosuppression during the first few courses may occur. Ensure that patient does not have an infection, as this may worsen and be fatal.
  - Patients with infection prior to starting pentostatin should be treated only if potential benefit justifies the potential risk
  - Patients with progressive hairy cell leukemia may have worsening of neutropenia during initial courses; monitor CBC/differential more frequently in these patients. If severe neutropenia continues beyond the initial cycles, patient's disease status should be evaluated, including a bone marrow biopsy.
- Elevations in LFTs occur and are generally reversible.
- Renal toxicity may occur, and elevated serum creatinine is usually reversible.
- Rashes are common and may occasionally be severe. Rash may worsen with continued treatment.
- Acute pulmonary edema and hypotension have been reported when pentostatin is combined with carmustine, etoposide, and high-dose cyclophosphamide as part of the ablative regimen for BMT.

• Drug can cause fetal harm. Teach women of reproductive potential to use effective contraception to avoid pregnancy. If the patient is treated or becomes pregnant while receiving the drug, the patient should be apprised of the potential hazard to the fetus.

• Use cautiously with reduced dose, or not at all, in patients with abnormal renal function, as > 90% of drug and metabolites excreted intact in urine.

• Rarely, angina, myocardial infarction, CHF, acute arrhythmias, and pulmonary toxicity may occur. Risk highest in patients with prior cardiac dysfunction.

Potential Toxicities/Side Effects and the Nursing Process

I.   POTENTIAL FOR INFECTION AND BLEEDING related to BONE MARROW DEPRESSION

Defining Characteristics: Dose-limiting leukopenia, with nadir occurring on days 10–14 and recovery by days 21–27. Profound immunosuppression, with both B and T cells reduced, and increasing risk of viral, bacterial, fungal, and parasitic infections. Less frequent thrombocytopenia. Potent immunosuppressant, with suppressed B and T lymphocytes, and helper T cells during and after treatment for months to years. Immunosuppression increases risk of infection by virus, encapsulated bacteria, fungi, and parasites. In patients with advanced hairy cell leukemia, neutropenia may worsen.

Nursing Implications: Assess 24-hour urine for creatinine clearance to determine whether treatment can be given. Assess CBC with differential, platelet count, and serum creatinine before each drug administration, as well as signs/symptoms of infection or bleeding. Instruct patient in self-assessment of signs/symptoms of infection or bleeding and risk reduction. Teach the patient to call provider immediately for signs/symptoms of infection. Discuss with physician whether prophylactic antimicrobials are indicated. Before each treatment, assess patient tolerance of preceding treatment, especially CNS, gingival bleeding or infection, or other potential sources of infection.

II.   ALTERATION IN NUTRITION, LESS THAN BODY REQUIREMENTS, related to NAUSEA/VOMITING, ANOREXIA, AND DIARRHEA

Defining Characteristics: Nausea and vomiting occur commonly but are mild. Diarrhea and anorexia may affect 10–50% of patients.

Nursing Implications: Premedicate with antiemetics, and ensure patient has antiemetics to take at home if needed. Teach patient and family self-administration of antiemetics if needed at home. Encourage small, frequent meals of cool, bland foods and increase in fluid intake. Assess oral mucosa and gums before drug administration and instruct patient to report changes. Teach patient oral hygiene measures and self-assessment. Instruct patient to report diarrhea, to self-administer prescribed antidiarrheal medications, and to drink adequate fluids.

III. SENSORY/PERCEPTUAL ALTERATIONS related to CONFUSION, ACTIVITY INTOLERANCE, FATIGUE

Defining Characteristics: Drug passes through blood–brain barrier into CNS with resulting dose-related headache, lethargy, and fatigue. Less commonly, blurred vision, confusion, depression, dizziness, coma may occur. Conjunctivitis, photophobia, and diplopia, as well as ototoxicity may occur.

Nursing Implications: Assess neurologic, mental status, and intactness of vision and hearing baseline before each treatment. Instruct patient to report any alterations in thinking, behavior, sensation, perception. Develop a plan of care with patient and family if side effects develop to manage distress and promote safety. Drug should be stopped if confusion, hallucinations, and coma occur.

IV. ALTERATION IN COMFORT related to FEVER, CHILLS, MYALGIAS, ARTHRALGIAS

Defining Characteristics: Fever and chills affect 10–50% of patients, whereas myalgias and arthralgias are less common.

Nursing Implications: Assess baseline comfort status. Teach patient these symptoms may occur and self-management techniques, including increased oral fluid intake to at least 1,500 mL/24 hours, calling provider if temperature ≥ 100.4°F, and warm soaks for arthralgias and myalgias.

Drug: polifeprosan 20 with carmustine (BCNU) implant (Gliadel®)

Class: Alkylating agent.

Mechanism of Action: Wafer (copolymer) containing carmustine is implanted in the surgical cavity created when brain tumor is resected. In water, the anhydride bonds of the wafer are hydrolyzed, releasing the carmustine into the surgical cavity. The carmustine diffuses into the surrounding brain tissue, reaching any residual tumor cells, and causing cell death by alkylating DNA and RNA.

Metabolism: Unknown. Dime-sized wafer is biodegradable in brain tissue, with a variable rate. More than 70% of the copolymer degrades by 3 weeks, slowly releasing 7.7 mg of carmustine in concentrations. In some patients, wafer fragments remained up to 232 days after implantation, with almost all drug gone.

Indication: For the treatment of patients with:
• Newly diagnosed high-grade malignant glioma, as an adjunct to surgery and radiation.
• Recurrent glioblastoma multiforme as an adjunct to surgery.

Dosage/Range:
- Each wafer contains 7.7 mg of carmustine, and the recommended dose is eight wafers, or a total dose of 61.6 mg of carmustine.

Drug Preparation:
- Drug must be stored at or below 20°C (−4°F) until time of use.
- Unopened foil packages can stay at room temperature for a maximum of 6 hours at a time. The manufacturer recommends that the treatment box be removed from the freezer and taken to the operating room just prior to surgery.
- The box and pouches should be opened just before the surgeon is ready to implant the wafers. Open the sealed treatment box and remove double foil packages, handling the unsterile outer foil packet by the crimped edge VERY CAREFULLY to prevent damage to the wafers. See product information for opening the inner foil pouch and removing the wafer with sterile technique.
- Chemotherapy precautions should be used to limit exposure to the chemotherapy: surgical instruments used to remove and implant the wafers should be kept separate from other instruments and sterile fields, and should be cleaned after the procedure according to hospital chemotherapy procedure; all personnel handling the wafers or the inner foil pouches containing the wafers should wear double gloves, which, along with unused wafers or fragments, inner foil packages, and opened outer foil package, should be disposed of as chemotherapeutic waste.

Drug Administration:
- Neurosurgeon places eight wafers into surgical resection cavity if size and shape appropriate; wafers are placed contiguously or with slight overlapping.
- Wafer may be broken into two pieces *only* if needed.

Drug Interactions:
- Unknown but unlikely, as drug is probably not systemically absorbed.

Lab Effects/Interference:
- Unknown, but unlikely.

Special Considerations:
- Manufacturer reports that in a study of 222 patients with recurrent glioma who failed initial surgery and radiotherapy, the 6-month survival rate after surgery increased from 47% (placebo) to 60%, and in patients with glioblastoma multiforme, the 6-month survival for patients receiving placebo was 36% versus 56% for patients receiving polifeprosan 20 with carmustine implant.
- Patients require close monitoring for complications of craniotomy, as intracerebral mass effect has occurred that does not respond to corticosteroid treatment; in one case, this resulted in brain herniation.
- Studies have not been conducted during pregnancy or in nursing mothers. Carmustine is a known teratogen, and is embryotoxic. Use during pregnancy should be avoided, and mothers should stop nursing during use of the drug.

Potential Toxicities/Side Effects and the Nursing Process

I. POTENTIAL SENSORY/PERCEPTUAL ALTERATIONS related to SEIZURES, BRAIN EDEMA, MENTAL STATUS CHANGES

Defining Characteristics: In clinical testing, the incidence of new or worsened seizures was 19% in both the group receiving the implant and those receiving the placebo. Seizures were mild to moderate in severity. In patients with new or worsened seizures postoperatively, the group receiving the implant had a 56% incidence, with median time to first new or worsened seizure of 3.5 days, versus placebo incidence of 9%, and median time to first new or worsened seizure of 61 days. Incidence of brain edema was 4%, and there were cases of intracerebral mass effect that did not respond to corticosteroids. Other nervous system effects were hydrocephalus (3%), depression (3%), abnormal thinking (2%), ataxia (2%), dizziness (2%), insomnia (2%), visual field defect (2%), monoplegia (2%), eye pain (1%), coma (1%), amnesia (1%), diplopia (1%), and paranoid reaction (1%). Rarely (< 1%), cerebral infarct or hemorrhage may occur.

Nursing Implications: Monitor neurovital signs closely postoperatively, and notify physician of any abnormalities. If intracranial pressure increases, a mass effect is suspected, and if it is nonresponsive to corticosteroids, expect the patient to be taken to surgery, with possible removal of wafer or remnants. Assess baseline mental status and regularly during postoperative care. Validate changes with family members. Discuss abnormalities with physician immediately and continue to monitor closely.

II. POTENTIAL FOR INFECTION related to HEALING ABNORMALITIES

Defining Characteristics: Most abnormalities were mild to moderate, occurred in 14% of patients, and included cerebrospinal leaks, subdural fluid collections, subgaleal or wound effusions, and breakdown. The incidence of intracranial infection (e.g., meningitis or abscess) was 4%. Incidence of deep wound infection was 6% (same as placebo) and included infection of subgaleal space, bone, meninges, and brain tissue.

Nursing Implications: Using aseptic technique, assess postoperative wound/dressing immediately postoperatively, and regularly thereafter. Assess systematically for signs/symptoms of infection or wound breakdown. Notify physician immediately and discuss antimicrobial therapy.

III. ALTERATION IN NUTRITION, LESS THAN BODY REQUIREMENTS, related to GI SIDE EFFECTS, ELECTROLYTE ABNORMALITIES

Defining Characteristics: Rarely, GI disturbances occurred: diarrhea (2%), constipation (2%), dysphagia (1%), gastrointestinal hemorrhage (1%), fecal incontinence (1%). Hyponatremia (3%), hyperglycemia (3%), and hypokalemia (1%) also occurred.

Nursing Implications: Assess baseline nutritional status, including electrolytes. Assess bowel elimination status and monitor nutritional and bowel elimination status closely during postoperative time. Discuss interventions for abnormalities with physician.

IV. ALTERATION IN CIRCULATION, POTENTIAL, related to CHANGES IN BLOOD PRESSURE

Defining Characteristics: Hypertension occurred in 3% of patients, and hypotension in 1%.

Nursing Implications: Assess baseline VS and monitor closely during postoperative phase. Discuss abnormalities with physician.

V. ALTERATION IN COMFORT related to EDEMA, PAIN, ASTHENIA

Defining Characteristics: The following occur rarely: peripheral edema (2%), neck pain (2%), rash (2%), back pain (1%), asthenia (1%), chest pain (1%).

Nursing Implications: Assess baseline comfort level and monitor closely during postoperative phase. Provide comfort measures. If ineffective, discuss symptom-management strategies with physician.

Drug: pralatrexate injection (Folotyn)

Class: Folate analog metabolic inhibitor (antimetabolite).

Mechanism of Action: Drug is a folate analog metabolic inhibitor. It competively inhibits the enzyme dihydrofolate reductase; it also competitively inhibits polyglutamylation by the enzyme folylpolyglutamyl synthetase, resulting in the depletion of thymidine, and other essential biologic molecules. Thus, the cell, as it goes to divide, lacks the essential DNA building blocks, is unable to complete the synthesis phase, and dies.

Metabolism: Following IV administration of pralatrexate, the terminal half-life of the drug is 12–18 hours; the pharmokinetics do not change significantly over multiple treatment cycles, and the drug does not accumulate. The drug is 67% bound to plasma proteins and is not a substrate for P-glycoprotein-mediated transport; nor does it inhibit it. Drug does not appear to inhibit or induce the hepatic CYP450 microenzyme system. 34% of IV pralatrexate is excreted unchanged in the urine. Patients with moderate to severe renal impairment should be monitored closely, as the drug has not been studied in these patients.

Indication: For the treatment of patients with relapsed or refractory peripheral T-cell lymphoma. Indication is based on overall response rate; clinical benefit (e,g., improvement in PFS or OS has not been demonstrated).

Dose Modifications for Mucositis (NCI CTCAE version 3.0 grading) [Folotyn PI 5.2012]

Mucositis Grade Day of Treatment	Action	Dose Upon Recovery to ≤ Grade 1
1: Grade 2	Omit dose	Continue prior dose
2: Grade 2 recurrence	Omit dose	20 mg/m²
3. Grade 3	Omit dose	20 mg/m²
4: Grade 4	STOP THERAPY	

Dose Modifications for Hematologic Toxicities [Folotyn PI 5.2012]

Blood Count Day of Treatment	Duration of Toxicity	Action	Dose Upon Restart
Platelet < 50,000/µL	1 week	Omit dose	Continue prior dose
Platelet < 50,000/µL	2 weeks	Omit dose	20 mg/m²
Platelet < 50,000/µL	3 weeks	STOP THERAPY	None
ANC 500–1,000/µL without fever	1 week	Omit dose	Continue prior dose
ANC 500–1,000/µL with fever or ANC < 500/µL	1 week	Omit dose, give G-CSF or GM-CSF support	Continue prior dose with G-CSF or GM-CSF support
ANC 500–1,000/µL with fever or ANC < 500/µL	2 weeks or recurrence	Omit dose, give G-CSF or GM-CSF support	20 mg/m² with G-CSF or GM-CSF support
ANC 500–1,000/µL with fever or ANC < 500/µL	3 weeks or 2nd recurrence	STOP THERAPY	None

Dose Modification for All Other Treatment-Related Toxicities (NCI CTCAE version 3.0 grading) [Folotyn PI 5.2012]

Toxicity Grade Day of Treatment	Action	Dose Upon Recovery ≤ Grade 2
Grade 3	Omit dose	20 mg/m²
Grade 4	STOP THERAPY	

Dosage/Range:

- 30 mg/m² IV push over 3–5 minutes once weekly for 6 weeks in a 7-week cycle.
- Patients must also take vitamin B₁₂ 1 mg IM every 8–10 weeks and folic acid 1.0–1.25 mg PO daily.
- Treatment interruption or dose reduction to 20 mg/m² IV may be needed to manage toxicity. DO NOT make up any omitted doses, and do not reescalate dose once reduced.

• Use caution and monitor closely for drug side effects in patients with decreased renal function, as drug has not been studied in this population.
• Persistent elevation of LFTs may indicate liver toxicity and require dose modification. Monitor patients' LFTs closely.
• See Folotyn package insert for dose modifications.

Drug Preparation:
• Pralatrexate is available as sterile, single-use vials at a concentration of 20 mg/mL: 20 mg pralatrexate in a 1-mL solution, or 40-mg vial in 2 mL.
• Drug should be refrigerated at 2–8°C (36–46°F) and stored in its original carton to protect from light.
• Verify that solution is a clear yellow solution without particulate matter prior to drawing up the calculated dose of pralatrexate injection. Discard any drug remaining in the vial, as the drug contains no preservatives.
• Unopened vials in the original carton are stable at room temperature for 72 hours only.

Drug Administration:
• Administer if patient assessment adequate: mucositis is grade 0 or 1; platelet count ≥ 100,000/microL for first dose, and ≥ 50,000/microL for all subsequent doses; ANC ≥ 1,000/microL. Otherwise, see dose modification tables in Folotyn package insert.
• Administer IV push over 3–5 minutes via the side port of a patent, freely flowing IV of 0.9% sodium chloride injection, USP, once weekly for 6 weeks in a 7-week cycle.
• Folic acid supplementation should begin 10 days prior to first dose of pralatrexate and continue through treatment and for 30 days after the last dose of pralatrexate.
• Vitamin B_{12} 1 mg IM should be given no more than 10 weeks before the first dose of pralatrexate and continue every 8–10 weeks. Injections during pralatrexate therapy can be given on the same day as the pralatrexate.
• Assess blood counts and oral mucosa prior to administration of each dose: omit or modify dose per MD for grade 2 or higher stomatitis, DO NOT make up any omitted doses. Once a dose reduction occurs, do not reescalate.
• Assess renal and hepatic function, along with other serum chemistries, prior to the first and fourth doses of each cycle. Patients with moderate to severe renal impairment should be monitored closely both for systemic toxicity (due to increased drug exposure) and with renal function testing prior to each dose. Pralatrexate can cause LFT abnormalities. If LFTs are persistently increased, this may indicate liver toxicity and require dose modification.

Drug Interactions:
• Drugs that are renally cleared (e.g., probenecid, NSAIDs, trimethoprim/sulfamethoxazole) may decrease pralatrexate clearance with risk of increased pralatrexate toxicity.

Lab Effects/Interference:
• Hypokalemia in 15% of patients; 13% elevated liver function tests (ALT, AST).

Special Considerations:
- Patients must receive supplements in folic acid and vitamin B_{12} during pralatrexate therapy to minimize bone marrow suppression and mucositis. Blood counts should be monitored closely.
- Women of childbearing age should use effective contraception, as drug can cause fetal harm. If the patient becomes pregnant, she should be informed of potential harm to the fetus. Nursing mothers should choose between receiving the drug and not nursing or discontinuing the drug to nurse.
- Drug is dose-modified or interrupted for bone marrow suppression and mucositis, as well as grade 3 or higher liver test abnormalities. If the patient has moderate to severe renal impairment, use drug cautiously and monitor closely.
- Patients with renal impairment are at higher risk for toxicity due to increased serum drug concentrations. Monitor patient's renal function and systemic toxicity, and discuss dose adjustment with physician or NP/PA. Drug should not be given to patients with end-stage renal disease, including those undergoing dialysis unless potential benefit exceeds potential risk.
- The most common adverse effects are mucositis (70%), thrombocytopenia (41%), nausea (40%), fatigue (26%). Common serious adverse events are pyrexia, mucositis, sepsis, febrile neutropenia, dehydration, and thrombocytopenia.
- Dermatologic reactions can occur, including skin exfoliation, ulceration, and toxic epidermal necrolysis (TEN), as well as tymor lysis syndrome. These reactions may be progressive and rarely fatal. If patient develops a skin reaction, monitor the patient closely. If the skin reaction is severe, hold or discontinue pralatrexate.
- If patient has high tumor burden prior to first dose, prophylax against tumor lysis syndrome per physician (e.g., allopurinol, hydration, urine alkalinization).

Potential Toxicities/Side Effects and the Nursing Process

I. POTENTIAL FOR INFECTION, BLEEDING, AND FATIGUE related to BONE MARROW DEPRESSION

Defining Characteristics: Major dose-limiting toxicity. Thrombocytopenia occurs in 41% of patients overall, with 14% grade 3 and 19% grade 4. Anemia occurs in 34% of patients, with 17% grade 3 and 2% grade 4. Neutropenia occurs in 24% of patients, with 13% grade 3 and 7% grade 4. Pyrexia occurs in 14% of patients, fatigue in 36% of patients, and epistaxis in 26% of patients. Upper respiratory infections occur in 10% of patients.

Nursing Implications: Monitor CBC and platelet count prior to drug administration, as well as signs/symptoms of infection, bleeding, and anemia. Instruct patient in self-assessment of signs/symptoms of infection (e.g., fever, chills, cough, SOB, pain or burning on urination), bleeding (e.g., epistaxis), and anemia (e.g., fatigue and tiredness) and to report this immediately. Ensure that patient is taking folic acid and receiving vitamin B_{12}. Teach patient self-care measures to minimize risk of infection and bleeding. This includes avoidance of crowds and proximity to people with infections, and avoidance of OTC aspirin-containing medications. Administer platelet and red cell transfusions per physician order.

II.   ALTERATION IN NUTRITION, LESS THAN BODY REQUIREMENTS, related to MUCOSITIS, NAUSEA, VOMITING, DIARRHEA, CONSTIPATION

Defining Characteristics: Mucositis is dose limiting and occurs in 70% of patients (17% gr 3, 4% gr 4). Nausea occurs in 40% and vomiting in 25%. Diarrhea occurs in 21%, constipation in 33%, anorexia in 15%.

Nursing Implications: Teach patient to take oral folic acid supplement as directed and emphasize that nonadherence can result in severe toxicity. Assess mucositis prior to each dose administration, and dose-reduce as directed by physician based on past grade of mucositis. Premedicate with antiemetics 30 minutes before taking procarbazine to prevent nausea and vomiting prior to drug administration and teach patient self-administration of antiemetics at home. Encourage small, frequent meals of cool, bland foods and liquids. Encourage patients to report onset of mucositis, diarrhea, constipation, and anorexia and to report if symptoms persist despite intervention for 24 hours. Teach patient to self-administer antidiarrheal medications or anticonstipation medications as appropriate, along with dietary modification.

III.   POTENTIAL FOR IMPAIRED SKIN INTEGRITY related to RARE DERMATITIS REACTIONS

Defining Characteristics: Rash occurs in 15% of patients. Rarely, severe dermatologic reactions occur and can be fatal (e.g., skin exfoliation, ulceration, and toxic epidermal necrolysis [TEN]). Pruritus occurs in 14% of patients. Edema occurs in 30% of patients.

Nursing Implications: Assess patient for changes in skin, and teach patient to report them right away (e.g., rash, peeling or loss of skin, sores, or blisters). Discuss management and impact on drug administration with physician prior to administration.

Drug: procarbazine hydrochloride (Matulane)

Class: Miscellaneous agent.

Mechanism of Action: Uncertain but appears to affect preformed DNA, RNA, and protein. It is a methylhydrazine derivative and acts as an alkylating agent. Cell cycle nonspecific.

Metabolism: Metabolized to active metabolites in the liver by the P450 microenzyme system. Rapidly and completely absorbed from the GI tract with peak plasma levels within 1 hour. Procarbazine metabolites taken up by lymph nodes and bone marrow, and cross the BBB, with peak CSF levels occurring in 30–90 minutes. Also metabolized in red blood cells and kidney. Most of the drug (5%) and metabolites (70%) are excreted in the urine. Elimination half-life is 1 hour.

Indication: In combination with other anticancer drugs for the treatment of stage III and IV Hodgkin's disease, e.g., MOPP regimen (nitrogen mustard, vincristine, procarbazine, prednisone).

Dosage/Range:
- 100 mg/m^2 orally, daily from 7–14 days every 4 weeks as part of the MOPP regimen.
- Brain tumors: 60 mg/m^2 orally every day × 14 days as part of the PCV regimen.

Drug Preparation:
- None.

Drug Administration:
- Oral.
- Available in 50-mg capsules.

Drug Interactions:
- Procarbazine is synergistic with CNS depressants. Barbiturate, antihistamine, narcotic, and hypotensive agents or phenothiazine antiemetics should be used with caution.
- Disulfiram (Antabuse)-like reaction may result if the patient consumes alcohol. Symptoms include headache, respiratory difficulties, nausea and vomiting, chest pain, hypotension, and mental status changes.
- Exhibits weak MAO (monoamine oxidase) inhibitor activity. Foods containing high amounts of tyramine should be avoided: substances such as beer, wine, cheese, brewer's yeast, chicken livers, and bananas. Consumption of foods high in tyramine in combination with procarbazine may lead to intracranial hemorrhage or hypertensive crisis.
- Levodopa, meperidine: hypertension when either is taken with procarbazine. Avoid coadministration.
- Sympathomimetics, tricyclic antidepressants: CNS excitation, hypertension, palpitations, angina, hypertensive crisis; avoid coadministration.
- Antidiabetic (sulfonylurea, insulin): potentiation of hypoglycemic effect. Monitor blood sugar closely and adjust dose as needed.
- When taken in combination with digoxin, there is a decreased bioavailability of digoxin.

Lab Effects/Interference:
- Decreased CBC.
- Increased LFTs, RFTs.

Special Considerations:
- Discontinue if CNS signs/symptoms (paresthesia, neuropathy, confusion), stomatitis, diarrhea, or hypersensitivity reaction occur.
- Patients with G$_6$PD should be monitored closely for hemolytic anemia.
- Patients may develop hypersensitivity reaction (pruritus, urticaria, maculopapular rash, flushing) responding to steroid therapy and continuation of drug. If pulmonary infiltrates develop, procarbazine should be discontinued.

Potential Toxicities/Side Effects and the Nursing Process

I.   POTENTIAL FOR INFECTION AND BLEEDING related to BONE MARROW DEPRESSION

Defining Characteristics: Major dose-limiting toxicity. Thrombocytopenia occurs in 50% of patients, evidenced by a delayed onset (28 days after treatment) and lasting 2–3 weeks. Leukopenia seen in two-thirds of patients, with nadirs occurring after initial thrombocytopenia. Anemias may be due to bone marrow depression or hemolysis.

Nursing Implications: Monitor CBC, platelet count prior to drug administration, as well as signs/symptoms of infection, bleeding, and anemia. Instruct patient in self-assessment of signs/symptoms of infection, bleeding, and anemia and to report this immediately. Dose reduction often necessary (35–50%) if compromised bone marrow function. Platelet and red cell transfusions per physician order.

II.   ALTERATION IN NUTRITION, LESS THAN BODY REQUIREMENTS, related to NAUSEA, VOMITING, DIARRHEA

Defining Characteristics: Nausea and vomiting occur in 70% of patients and may be a dose-limiting toxicity. Diarrhea is uncommon, but rarely may be protracted and thus would be an indication for dose reduction.

Nursing Implications: Teach patient to premedicate with antiemetics 30 minutes before taking procarbazine to prevent nausea and vomiting. Encourage small, frequent meals of cool, bland foods and liquids. Minimize nausea and vomiting by dividing the total daily dosage into 3–4 doses. Also, taking the pills at bedtime may decrease the sense of nausea. May administer nonphenothiazine antiemetics. Encourage patients to report onset of diarrhea. Administer, or teach patient to self-administer, antidiarrheal medications.

III.   POTENTIAL FOR SENSORY/PERCEPTUAL ALTERATIONS

Defining Characteristics: Symptoms occur in 10–30% of patients and are seen as lethargy, depression, frequent nightmares, insomnia, nervousness, or hallucinations. Tremors, coma, convulsions are less common. Symptoms usually disappear when drug is discontinued. Crosses into CSF.

Nursing Implications: Teach patient the potential for neurotoxicity and provide early counseling about these effects. Assess patients for any symptoms of neurotoxicity. Discuss strategies with patient to preserve general sense of well-being. Obtain baseline neurologic and motor function. CNS toxicity may be manifested as reactions to other drugs, e.g., barbiturates, narcotics, and phenothiazine antiemetics.

IV. ACTIVITY INTOLERANCE related to PERIPHERAL NEUROPATHY

Defining Characteristics: 10% of patients exhibit paresthesias, decrease in deep tendon reflexes. Foot drop and ataxia occasionally reported. Reversible when drug is discontinued.

Nursing Implications: Obtain baseline neurologic and motor function. Assess patient for any changes in motor function, e.g., ability to pick up pencils or buttons.

V. ALTERATION IN COMFORT related to FLU-LIKE SYNDROME

Defining Characteristics: Fever, chills, sweating, lethargy, myalgias, and arthralgias commonly occur at the beginning of therapy.

Nursing Implications: Teach patient the potential for flu-like syndrome and how to distinguish from actual infection. Instruct patient to report any changes in condition.

VI. POTENTIAL FOR IMPAIRED SKIN INTEGRITY related to RARE DERMATITIS REACTIONS

Defining Characteristics: Rarely occurs as alopecia, pruritus, rash, hyperpigmentation.

Nursing Implications: Assess patient for changes in skin, nails, and hair loss. Discuss with patient impact of changes and strategies to minimize distress, e.g., wearing nail polish, long-sleeved tops, wigs, scarves, caps.

VII. POTENTIAL SEXUAL DYSFUNCTION related to DRUG EFFECTS

Defining Characteristics: Drug is teratogenic. Causes azoospermia. Causes cessation of menses, although may be reversible.

Nursing Implications: As appropriate, explore with patient and partner issues of reproductive and sexuality patterns and the impact chemotherapy may have. Discuss strategies to preserve sexual and reproductive health (e.g., sperm banking, contraception).

Drug: progestational agents: medroxyprogesterone acetate (Provera, Depo-Provera), megestrol acetate (Megace)

Class: Hormone.

Mechanism of Action: Unclear, but progestational agents compete for androgen and progestational receptor sites on the cell. Has potent antiestrogenic properties that disturb estrogen receptor cycle. Also increases synthesis of RNA by interacting with DNA.

Metabolism: Rapidly absorbed from GI tract. Metabolized in the liver. Excreted in the urine. Peak plasma levels reached in 1–3 hours; biologic half-life, 3.5 days.

Dosage/Range:
Medroxyprogesterone acetate:
• Provera: 20–80 mg PO daily.
• Depo-Provera:
  • 400–800 mg IM every month
  • 100 mg IM three times weekly
  • 1,000–1,500 mg daily (high dose)
• *Megestrol acetate:*
  • Megace, mg PO qid (breast cancer): 80 mg PO qid (endometrial cancer).

Drug Preparation:
• IM preparation is ready to use; shake vial well before drawing up medication.

Drug Administration:
• Give via deep IM injection.

Drug Interactions:
• None.

Lab Effects/Interference:
• Increased LFTs.
• Changes in TFTs.

Special Considerations:
• Patients may become sensitive to oil carrier (oil in which drug is mixed).
• Small risk of hypersensitivity reaction.

Potential Toxicities/Side Effects and the Nursing Process

I.   POTENTIAL FOR INJURY related to FLUID RETENTION, THROMBOEMBOLISM

Defining Characteristics: Fluid retention. Thromboembolic complications may occur. Sterile abscess may occur with IM injection.

Nursing Implications: Inform patient of potential for fluid retention and of signs/symptoms to watch for and to report to nurse or physician. Assess for signs/symptoms of fluid overload. Teach patient and family signs/symptoms of thromboembolic events: positive Homan's sign, localized pain, tenderness, erythema, sudden CNS changes, shortness of breath. Instruct patient to notify nurse or physician if any of the above occur. Give drug via deep IM injection: apply pressure to injection site after administering. Inspect used sites; rotate sites systematically.

II. ALTERED NUTRITION, LESS THAN BODY REQUIREMENTS, related to NAUSEA

Defining Characteristics: Nausea is rare.

Nursing Implications: Inform patient that nausea can occur; encourage patient to report nausea. Encourage small, frequent meals of cool, bland foods and liquids.

Drug: streptozocin (Zanosar)

Class: Alkylating agent (nitrosourea).

Mechanism of Action: A weak alkylating agent (nitrosourea) that causes interstrand crosslinking in DNA and is cell cycle phase nonspecific. Appears to have some specificity for neoplastic pancreatic endocrine cells. Glucose attached to nitrosourea appears to diminish myelotoxicity.

Metabolism: 60–70% of total dose and 10–20% of parent drug appear in urine. Drug is rapidly eliminated from serum in 4 hours, with major concentrations occurring in liver and kidneys. Drug half-life is 35 minutes. Drug metabolized in the liver, and metabolites excreted in the urine.

Indication: For the treatment of patients with metastatic islet cell carcinoma of the pancreas (functional and nonfunctional).

Dosage/Range:
- 500 mg/m^2 IV daily × 5 days. Repeat every 3–4 weeks; OR
- 1,000–1,500 mg/m^2 IV every week × 6 followed by observation.
- Dose-reduce (DR) based on 24-hour creatinine clearance (10–50 mL/min = 25% reduction; < 10 mL/min = 50% reduction).

Drug Preparation:
- Add sterile water or 0.9% sodium chloride to vial.
- If powder or solution contacts skin, wash immediately with soap and water.
- Solution is stable 48 hours at room temperature, 96 hours if refrigerated.

Drug Administration:
- Assess renal function before each cycle.
- Administer via pump over 1 hour.
- Has also been given as continuous infusion or continuous arterial infusion into the hepatic artery.
- If local pain or burning occurs, slow infusion and apply cool packs above injection site.
- Irritant; avoid extravasation.
- Administer with 1–2 L of hydration to prevent nephrotoxicity.

Drug Interactions:
- Nephrotoxic drugs (cisplatin, aminoglycosides, amphotericin B): additive nephrotoxicity; avoid concurrent use if possible.

- Steroids: increase risk of severe hyperglycemia.
- Phenytoin: antagonism of antitumor effect; do not coadminister.
- Doxorubicin: increased half-life of doxorubicin, resulting in increased myelosuppression.

Lab Effects/Interference:
- Decreased CBC.
- Increased RFTs (especially BUN).
- Increased LFTDH.
- Changes in glucose, phosphorus, albumin serum levels.

Special Considerations:
- Renal function must be monitored closely.
- Drug is an irritant; give IV short infusion over 15–30 minutes or as a 6-hour infusion.

Potential Toxicities/Side Effects and the Nursing Process

I.   POTENTIAL FOR ALTERATION IN URINARY ELIMINATION related to RENAL DYSFUNCTION

Defining Characteristics: 60% of patients experience renal dysfunction. Usually transient proteinuria and azotemia, but this may progress to permanent renal failure, especially if other nephrotoxic drugs are given concurrently. Signs/symptoms include proteinuria, increased BUN, hypophosphatemia, glycosuria, renal tubular acidosis, decreased creatinine clearance. Hypophosphatemia is probably earliest sign of renal dysfunction.

Nursing Implications: Closely monitor BUN, creatinine, phosphorus, urine protein, and 24-hour creatinine clearance prior to each treatment. Monitor BUN, creatinine, pH of urine, glucose/protein of urine every shift during therapy. Discuss dose reduction with physician based on creatinine clearance. Strictly monitor I/O during therapy. Hydration per physician, but usually 2–3 L/day. Rarely, renal toxicity may present as glucosuria, hypophosphatemia, and diabetes insipidus.

II.   ALTERATION IN NUTRITION, LESS THAN BODY REQUIREMENTS, related to GI SIDE EFFECTS

Defining Characteristics: Nausea and vomiting occur in up to 90% of patients, beginning 1–4 hours after drug dose, and can be significantly reduced when drug is given as continuous infusion. Nausea and vomiting may worsen during 5-consecutive-day therapy; increased severity with doses > 500 mg/m^2. 10% of patients experience diarrhea with abdominal cramping. LFTs may be elevated but normalize with time. Hepatotoxicity occurs in approximately 50% of patients. Liver enzymes increase 2–3 weeks after therapy; albumin decreases, but symptoms rarely occur. May also develop painless jaundice.

Nursing Implications: Premedicate with antiemetics and continue prophylactically for 24 hours; use aggressive antiemetics when drug is given IV over 1 hour (serotonin antagonists effective). Encourage small, frequent feedings of cool, bland foods and liquids. If patient has nausea or vomiting, discuss with physician more aggressive antiemetics.

TREATMENT

Monitor I/O closely and replace fluids. Encourage patient to report onset of diarrhea. Administer or teach patient to self-administer antidiarrheal medications. Teach patient diet modifications. Monitor LFTs prior to each treatment (alk phos, SGOT, SGPT, albumin). Assess for signs/symptoms of hepatic dysfunction: jaundice, yellowing of skin, sclera; orange-colored urine; white or clay-colored stools; itchy skin.

III. ALTERATIONS IN GLUCOSE METABOLISM related to HYPOGLYCEMIA

Defining Characteristics: Appears that damage to pancreatic beta cells causes sudden release of insulin, with resulting hypoglycemia in about 20% of patients. Hyperglycemia may occur in patients with insulinomas and decreased glucose tolerance. Increased fasting or postprandial blood levels may occur.

Nursing Implications: Monitor serum glucose levels every day or more frequently as needed; check urine glucose. Assess for, and instruct patient to report, the following signs/symptoms of hypoglycemia: muscle weakness and lethargy, perspiration, flushed feeling, restlessness, headache, confusion, trembling, epigastric hunger pains. If signs/symptoms are found, encourage patient to eat or drink high-glucose food and juice and notify physician. Hypoglycemia can be prevented with nicotinamide. Assess for signs/symptoms of hyperglycemia in patient with insulinomas and instruct patient in self-assessment.

IV. POTENTIAL FOR INFECTION AND BLEEDING related to BONE MARROW DEPRESSION

Defining Characteristics: Bone marrow depression occurs in about 9–20% of patients. Nadir 1–2 weeks after administration. Occasionally, severe leukopenia and thrombocytopenia occur. Mild anemia may occur.

Nursing Implications: Monitor CBC, platelets prior to drug administration, as well as assess for signs/symptoms of infection or bleeding. Instruct patient in self-assessment of signs/symptoms of infection or bleeding.

V. POTENTIAL FOR INJURY related to SECONDARY MALIGNANCIES

Defining Characteristics: Drug is carcinogenic; secondary malignancies are well described.

Nursing Implications: Patients receiving prolonged therapy should be screened periodically.

Drug: tamoxifen citrate (Nolvadex, Soltamox oral solution)

Class: Antiestrogen.

Mechanism of Action: Nonsteroidal antiestrogen that competitively binds to estrogen receptors, forming an abnormal complex that migrates to the cell nucleus and inhibits DNA synthesis. Also, appears to stimulate secretion of transforming growth factor beta, which proceeds to inhibit genes that stimulate cell proliferation. Activity is cell cycle specific in mid-G1 phase.

Metabolism: Drug is a prodrug, and active metabolite is produced after metabolism by CYP2D6 pathway. Well absorbed from GI tract with a high degree of protein binding and peak plasma levels in 4–6 hours. Widely distributed in body tissue, especially areas where estrogen receptors are expressed. Metabolized by P450 microenzyme system in liver (CYP3A4, CYP2D6). Undergoes enterohepatic circulation, prolonging blood levels. Excreted in feces. Elimination half-life is 7–14 days.

Indications: (1) Metastatic breast cancer (MBC) in women and men; in premenopausal women, with MBC, tamoxifen is an alternative to oophorectomy or radiation of the ovaries (estrogen positive most likely to benefit); (2) adjuvant treatment of node-positive breast cancer in women after total mastectomy or segmental mastectomy, axillary dissection, and breast irradiation (most benefit in subgroup with 4+ positive axillary lymph nodes); (3) treatment of axcillary node-negative breast cancer after total mastectomy or segmental mastectomy, axillary dissection, and breast irradiation; (4) women with ductal carcinoma in situ (DCIS) to reduce risk of invasive breast cancer.
- Tamoxifen reduces the occurrence of contralateral breast cancer in patients receiving adjuvant tamoxifen for breast cancer.
- While past data support 5 years of adjuvant tamoxifen therapy, in women with early-stage breast cancer, 10 years of tamoxifen threapy further reduces the risk of recurrence and breast cancer mortality (Davies et al., 2013).

Dosage/Range:
- 20 mg PO daily (most often, 10 mg bid).
- Recommended testing for CYP2D6 gene function, as poor metabolizers do not achieve same drug benefit as patients who are normal metabolizers.

Drug Preparation:
- Available in 10-mg tablets or oral liquid solution (10 mg/5 mL).

Drug Administration:
- Oral.

Drug Interactions:
- Anticoagulants: increased PT; monitor PT closely and reduce anticoagulant dose as needed.
- CYP3A4, -2D6 inducers (carbamazepine, glucocorticoids, phenobarbital, phenytoin, rifamycin, nevirapine): may decrease serum level of tamoxifen.
- CYP3A4, -2D6 inhibitors (ciprofloxacin, clarithromycin, doxycycline, erythromycin, imatinib, diclofenac, nicardipine, nefazodone, protease inhibitors, verapamil, quinidine, cimetidine, codeine, fluoxetine, haloperidol, paroxetine, fluoxetine, sertraline): may block the activation of tamoxifen as tamoxifen, is a prodrug, and must be activated into the therapeutic metabolite.
- Drugs activated by P450 system: may inhibit metabolic activation of cyclophosphamide.
- Letrozole: decreased letrozole serum levels by 37%; do not give concurrently.
- St. John's wort: decreased tamoxifen serum level; do not give concurrently.

Lab Effects/Interference:
- Decreased CBC.
- Increased LFTs.
- Increased Ca.
- Interference in lab tests such as TFTs and hyperlipidemia.

Special Considerations:
- Measurements of estrogen receptors in tumor are important in predicting tumor response and should be performed at same time as biopsy and before antiestrogen treatment is started.
- Avoid antacids within 2 hours of taking enteric-coated tablets.
- A flare reaction with bone pain and hypercalcemia may occur. Such reactions are short-lived and usually result in a tumor response if therapy is continued.
- No evidence exists that doses > 20 mg/day are more efficacious.
- Tamoxifen resulted in a significant decrease in development of invasive breast cancer in women with atypical hyperplasia (88%). ATLAS study confirmed that 10 years of adjuvant tamoxifen superior to 5 years in preventing breast cancer recurrence (16.7% vs 19.2%) [Davies et al., 2013].
- Rare side effects include uterine sarcoma, stroke, uterine cancer, blood clot formation.
- Tamoxifen is being studied as an adjunct to in vitro fertilization (IVF) for women with breast cancer who wish to have a child, given with FSH. The addition of either tamoxifen or letrozole with FSH increased the number of ovarian follicles, more mature eggs, and more embryos (Oktay et al., 2005).
- Use cautiously in patients with abnormal liver function or history of thromboembolic disease.
- Patients should be taught to notify physician immediately if patient develops abnormal uterine bleeding, pelvic pain, pain in the legs, or breathing problems.
- One study showed that women taking tamoxifen plus an SSRI that was a moderate-to-potent inhibitor of CYP2D6 (e.g., fluoxeine [Prozac], paroxetine [Paxil], sertraline [Zoloft]) had more than double the risk of breast cancer recurrence compared to those not taking them. The following SSRIs had NO effect on breast cancer recurrence: citalopram (Celexa), escitalopram (Lexapro), and fluvoxamine (Luvox) (Aubert et al., 2009).

Potential Toxicities/Side Effects and the Nursing Process

I.   POTENTIAL FOR SEXUAL DYSFUNCTION related to CHANGES IN MENSES, HOT FLASHES

Defining Characteristics: May cause menstrual irregularity, hot flashes, milk production in breasts, vaginal discharge, and bleeding. Symptoms occur in about 10% of patients and are usually not severe enough to discontinue therapy. Drug may cause endometrial hyperplasia, polyps, and endometrial cancer.

Nursing Implications: As appropriate, explore with patient and partner issues of reproductive and sexuality patterns and the impact drug may have on them. Discuss strategies to preserve sexual and reproductive health. Teach patient that she should be closely followed by a gynecologist for annual endometrial biopsies and to report immediately abnormal uterine bleeding, or pelvic pain.

II.   POTENTIAL FOR ALTERATION IN CIRCULATION related to THROMBOEMBOLISM

Defining Characteristics: Tamoxifen has been associated with thromboembolic events and is associated with antithrombin III deficiency.

Nursing Implications: Teach patient to minimize likelihood of developing DVT, such as to avoid sitting in the same position for long periods, especially on airplanes, and to get up and walk regularly to increase venous return from the lower extremities. Teach patient to report immediately or go to the emergency department if pain in the lower extremities develops or the patient develops abrupt onset of dyspnea, shortness of breath, or any pulmonary symptom.

III.   POTENTIAL FOR ALTERATION IN COMFORT related to FLARE REACTION

Defining Characteristics: May cause flare reaction initially (bone and tumor pain, transient increase in tumor size). Nausea, vomiting, and anorexia may occur.

Nursing Implications: Inform patient of possibility of flare reaction, signs/symptoms to be aware of, and encourage patient to report any signs/symptoms. Inform patient of possibility of nausea, vomiting, and anorexia. Encourage small, frequent meals of high-calorie, high-protein foods.

IV.   POTENTIAL FOR SENSORY/PERCEPTUAL ALTERATION related to VISUAL CHANGES

Defining Characteristics: Retinopathy has been reported with high doses. Corneal changes, cataracts, decreased visual acuity, and blurred vision have occurred. Headache, dizziness, and light-headedness are rare.

Nursing Implications: Obtain visual assessment prior to starting therapy. Encourage patient to report any visual changes and discuss evaluation by ophthalmologist depending upon symptom(s). Instruct patient to report headache, dizziness, light-headedness.

V.   POTENTIAL FOR INFECTION AND BLEEDING related to BONE MARROW DEPRESSION

Defining Characteristics: Mild, transient leukopenia and thrombocytopenia occur rarely.

Nursing Implications: Monitor CBC, platelets prior to drug administration and after therapy has begun. Instruct patient in self-assessment of signs/symptoms of infection or bleeding.

VI. POTENTIAL FOR SKIN INTEGRITY IMPAIRMENT related to RASH, ALOPECIA

Defining Characteristics: Skin rash, alopecia, peripheral edema are rare.

Nursing Implications: Assess patient for signs/symptoms of hair loss, edema, and skin rash. Instruct patient to report any of these symptoms. Discuss with patient the impact of skin changes.

VII. POTENTIAL FOR INJURY related to HYPERCALCEMIA

Defining Characteristics: Hypercalcemia uncommon.

Nursing Implications: Obtain serum calcium levels prior to therapy and at regular intervals during therapy. Instruct patient in signs/symptoms of hypercalcemia: nausea, vomiting, weakness, constipation, loss of muscle tone, malaise, decreased urine output.

Drug: temozolomide (Temodar)

Class: Alkylating agent.

Mechanism of Action: Drug is a member of the imidazotetrazine class and is the active metabolite of dacarbazine in an oral form. Drug is a prodrug, forming the metabolite monomethyl triazenoimidazole carboxamide (MTIC) when chemically degraded, and is further metabolized to 5-aminoimidazole-4-carboxamide (AIC), the active cytotoxic metabolite. Drug is lipophilic and can pass through the BBB, where it has been shown to be effective against some brain tumors, possibly because of the alkaline pH. MTIC causes alkylation of DNA and RNA strands, and DNA, RNA, and protein synthesis is inhibited.

Metabolism: Well absorbed from the GI tract following oral dose (100% bioavailability), with peak concentrations in 1 hour when taken on empty stomach. The elimination half-life is 1.8 hours. The drug is degraded into MTIC in plasma and tissues. 15% of drug is excreted unchanged in the urine. Differs from dacarbazine in that formation of MTIC does not require liver metabolism. Food decreases the rate and extent of drug absorption. IV formulation.

Indication: For the treatment of adult patients with (1) newly diagnosed glioblastoma multiforme (GBM) concomitantly with RT and then as maintenance treatment; (2) refractory anaplastic astrocytoma in patients who have experienced disease progression on a drug regimen containing nitrosurea and procarbazine.

Dosage/Range:
Refractory anaplastic astrocytoma that has failed prior chemotherapy:
- 150 mg/m^2/day orally × 5 days if patient has received prior chemotherapy, repeated every 28 days.
- Dose should be adjusted to keep ANC 1,000–1,500/mm^3 and platelet count 50,000–100,000/mm^3.

Newly diagnosed glioblastoma multiforme (GBM) concomitantly with (at the same time as) radiotherapy and then as maintenance treatment:

- 75 mg/m² orally, daily starting the first day of RT through the last day of RT, for 42 days (maximum 49 days) as long as ANC > 1,500 cells/mm³, platelet count > 100,000 cells/mm³, and other toxicity (except alopecia, nausea, vomiting) are less than grade 1 (CTCAE).
- Prophylaxis for *Pneumocystis carinii* pneumonia while receiving concomitant RT and temozolomide, continuing to 4 weeks after completion of RT.
- Maintenance dose (temozolomide orally daily × 5, then 23 days without treatment, repeated × 6):
  - Cycle 1: Temozolomide 150 mg/m² orally daily × 5, then 23 days without treatment (as long as ANC > 1,500 cells/mm³, platelet count > 100,000 cells/mm³, and other toxicity [except alopecia, nausea, vomiting] are less than grade 1 [CTCAE]).
  - Cycle 2–6: Temozolomide 200 mg/m² orally daily × 5 then 23 days without treatment, repeated for 5 more cycles (as long as ANC > 1,500 cells/mm³, platelet count > 100,000 cells/mm³, and other toxicity [except alopecia, nausea, vomiting] are < grade 1 [CTCAE]).
  - Monitor CBC on day 22 then weekly until ANC > 1,500 cells/mm³, and platelets > 100,000 cells/mm³.
  - See package insert for dose reductions based on nadir counts and worst CTCAE toxicity.

Drug Preparation:
- None.
- Available in 180-mg, 140-mg, 20-mg, and 5-mg strengths.
- Drug is stored at room temperature, protected from light and moisture.
- IV: Available as 100-mg powder for injection. Dose is the same dose as the oral dose. Add 41 mL sterile water for injection resulting in a concentration of 2.5 mg/mL. Bring vial to room temperature prior to mixing. Gently swirl to mix, and use within 14 hours of reconstitution. Leave vial at room temperature once mixed. Aseptically withdraw ordered dose, where 40 mL per vial is 100 mg (2.5 mg/mL). Discard any remaining solution. Transfer ordered dose into an empty 250-mL PVC infusion bag, and administer via pump over 90 min.
- Dose based on nadir WBC, platelet count, as well as the counts on day of treatment.

Drug Administration:
- Give orally with full glass of water on an empty stomach. Patient should take medicine at around the same time of day each day, e.g., bedtime.
- Do not crush or dissolve capsule.
- Administer IV over 90 minutes. Shorter dosing times may result in suboptimal dosing. Flush line before and after temozolomide infusion. Do not infuse with any other medication.

Drug Interactions:
- Valproic acid: reduces temozolomide clearance by 5% but may not be clinically significant; monitor drug effect closely if used together.

Lab Effects/Interference:
• Elevated liver function tests (e.g., ALT, AST; occur in up to 40% of patients), increase in alk phos.
• Decreased WBC, Hgb, and platelet count.
• Hyperglycemia.
• Elevated renal function tests.

Special Considerations:
• Drug has been used for treatment of glioma after first relapse and advanced metastatic malignant melanoma, high-grade malignant glioma (glioblastoma multiforme, anaplastic astrocytoma) and is being studied in a variety of solid tumors.
• Drug causes severe myelosuppression, and thrombocytopenia is the dose-limiting factor.
• Use with caution, if at all, in the following patients: hypersensitive to dacarbazine; myelosuppressed; have bacterial or viral infection; have renal dysfunction; have received prior chemotherapy or radiation; and women who are pregnant or who are breastfeeding.
• Rarely (1% of patients), hypercalcemia may occur with the 5-day regimen.
• PET (positive emission tomography) scanning showed reduced uptake of fluorodeoxyglucose (FDG) in patients who responded in 7–14 days following a 5-day course of treatment, as opposed to those patients who did not respond, and who showed increased FDG uptake (Newlands et al., 1997).
• Overall response rate in some studies of patients with malignant glioma that had recurred or progressed after surgery and radiation therapy was 15–25% and 30% in newly diagnosed patients prior to XRT (Bower et al., 1997).
• Laboratory monitoring: With concurrent RT, monitor CBC baseline then weekly during treatment; for 28-day treatment cycles, baseline CBC on day 1 then 21 days after the first dose.

Warnings and Precautions:
• Myelosuppression, including prolonged pancytopenia, which may result in aplastic anemia.
  • Patient must have ANC > 1,500 cells /mm^3 and platelets at least 100,000/mm^3 prior to dosing.
  • Assess CBC/differential on day 22 (21 days after first dose) or within 48 hrs of that day, and weekly until the ANC is >1,500 cells/mm^3, and platelet count is >100,000/mm^3.
  • Geriatric patients have a higher risk to develop myelosuppression.
• Cases of myelodysplastic syndrome and secondary malignancies have been described.
• For patients with newly diagnosed GBM receiving concomitant RT for 42 days, concurrent oral prophylaxis with co-trimoxazole (Bactrim) is required, as patients may develop opportunistic *Pneumocystis* pneumonia (PCP). In addition, all patients receiving steroids on temozolomide should be monitored closely for the occurrence of PCP.
• Laboratory tests: for concomitant treatment phase with RT, assess CBC prior to treatment initiation and weekly during treatment. For 28-day cycles, assess CBC prior to treatment on day 1 and day 22 of each cycle. As needed, assess CBC weekly until recovery of ANC to >1,500 cells/mm^3 and platelet count is > 100,000/mm^3.

- Fatal and severe hepatotoxicity have been reported. Assess LFTs baseline, and midway through first cycle, prior to each subsequent cycle, and 2–4 weeks after last dose of temozolomide.
- Drug causes fetal harm. Teach women of reproductive potential to use effective contraception to avoid pregnancy. Nursing mothers should make a decision to stop nursing or to discontinue the drug, taking into account the importance of the drug to the mother's health.
- Infusion time: study showed bioequivalence when infusion time was 90 minutes, so drug must be infused over this time.

Potential Toxicities/Side Effects and the Nursing Process

I. POTENTIAL FOR INFECTION, BLEEDING, AND FATIGUE related to BONE MARROW DEPRESSION

Defining Characteristics: Thrombocytopenia and leukopenia are dose-limiting factors and occur in grade 2 or higher 40% of the time. This does not usually require administration of G-CSF. Nadir at 21–22 days, unless using 5-day treatment schedule, where nadir is day 28–29. Recovery for platelets is 7–42 days and in shorter time for WBC. Anemia may also occur, but is infrequent and less severe. Severity of bone marrow depression depends on dose and schedule, as well as disease process. In one trial, patients with malignant glioma had severe lymphopenia (41% grade 3 and 15% grade 4).

Nursing Implications: Assess baseline WBC, differential, platelet, and Hgb/HCT prior to chemotherapy, as well as for signs/symptoms of infection or bleeding. Teach patient signs/symptoms of infection and bleeding and to report these immediately; teach patient self-care measures to minimize risk of infection and bleeding. This includes avoidance of crowds, proximity to people with infections, and OTC aspirin-containing medications. Teach patient to report fatigue and teach measures to conserve energy, such as alternating rest and activity periods. Discuss transfusion of red blood cells as needed.

II. ALTERED NUTRITION, LESS THAN BODY REQUIREMENTS, related to NAUSEA AND VOMITING, STOMATITIS, AND DIARRHEA

Defining Characteristics: Nausea and vomiting occur in 75% of patients, usually grade 1 or 2, and usually occurring on day 1. In one trial, using a 5-day treatment regimen, 21% had grade 3 nausea, and 23% had grade 4. Stomatitis may occur in up to 20% of patients. Diarrhea, constipation, and/or anorexia may affect up to 40% of patients.

Nursing Implications: Teach patient to self-medicate with antiemetics (serotonin antagonist effective) 1 hour prior to dose and suggest evening dosing to minimize nausea/vomiting. Encourage small, frequent feedings of cool, bland foods. Teach patient to notify provider right away if nausea/vomiting persists. Assess oral mucosa prior to drug administration and teach patient to report changes. Teach patient oral hygiene measures and self-assessment.

Teach patient to report diarrhea, to self-administer prescribed antidiarrheal medications, and to drink adequate fluids. Teach patient to report constipation, and manage with stool softeners or laxatives. If patient has anorexia, teach patient to select acceptable foods and to eat small portions q 2 hours and at bedtime. Teach patient to keep a diary documenting when medications are taken and side effects and to bring in medication bottle for a pill count to evaluate ability to adhere to regimen.

III.   ALTERATION IN SKIN INTEGRITY/COMFORT related to RASH, PRURITUS, ALOPECIA

Defining Characteristics: Skin rash, itching, and mild alopecia may occur, and are mild.

Nursing Implications: Teach patient about the possibility of these side effects and to notify the nurse if any develop. Discuss rash with physician if moderate or severe. Teach patient local symptom-management strategies for itch. Reassure patient that hair loss is usually thinning with mild hair loss and will grow back.

IV.   ACTIVITY INTOLERANCE, POTENTIAL, related to CENTRAL NERVOUS SYSTEM EFFECTS

Defining Characteristics: Lethargy (up to 40% in patients with malignant glioma), fatigue, headache, ataxia, and dizziness may occur; in clinical testing, it was unclear whether this was due to neurologic disease (i.e., malignant glioma), concurrent other drug therapy, or temozolomide.

Nursing Implications: Assess baseline energy and activity level. Teach patients that these side effects may occur, especially if the primary diagnosis is malignant glioma. Teach patient to report them. Teach patient to alternate rest and activity periods, to use supportive device such as a cane if ataxia or dizziness occurs, and other measures to maximize activity tolerance and to prevent injury.

Drug: thioguanine (Tabloid, 6-thioguanine, 6-TG)

Class: Thiopurine antimetabolite.

Mechanism of Action: Converts to monophosphate nucleotides and inhibits *de novo* purine synthesis. The nucleotides are also incorporated into DNA. Cell cycle specific for S phase. Thioguanine interferes with nucleic acid biosynthesis, resulting in sequential blockage of the synthesis and utilization of the purine nucleotides.

Metabolism: Oral absorption is incomplete (30%) and variable, with a plasma half-life of 11 hours. Food may affect absorption. Drug is metabolized in the liver by deamination and methylation. Metabolites are excreted in the urine and feces.

Indication: For remission induction and remission consolidation treatment of patients with acute nonlymphocytic leukemias (not recommended during maintenance due to high risk of liver toxicity).

Dosage/Range:
- **Children and adults:** 100 mg/m^2 orally every 12 hours for 5–10 days, usually in combination with cytarabine and then 100 mg/m^2 orally every 12 hours for 5 days repeated every 4 weeks for maintenance.
- 1–3 mg/kg orally daily OR 75–200 mg/m^2/day orally in one to two divided doses × 5–7 days or until remission.

Drug Preparation:
- Available in 40-mg tablets.

Drug Administration:
- Given orally between meals; can be given as a single dose.

Drug Interactions:
- Busulfan: increased hepatotoxicity; use caution when used together; monitor patient closely during long-term therapy.
- Other hepatotoxic drugs: increased risk of hepatotoxicity.

Lab Effects/Interference:
- Decreased CBC.
- Increased LFTs.
- Increased uric acid.

Special Considerations:
- Oral dose is to be given on empty stomach to facilitate absorption.
- Dose is titrated to avoid excessive stomatitis and diarrhea.
- Thioguanine can be used in full doses with allopurinol.
- Veno-occlusive disease of the liver can rarely occur; monitor LFTs baseline and during treatment.

Potential Toxicities/Side Effects and the Nursing Process

I.   ALTERATION IN NUTRITION, LESS THAN BODY REQUIREMENTS, related to GI SIDE EFFECTS

Defining Characteristics: Nausea and vomiting occur commonly, especially in children, but are dose-related; anorexia is rare; stomatitis is rare, but most common with high doses; hepatotoxicity is rare, but may be associated with hepatic veno-occlusive disease or jaundice.

Nursing Implications: Treat symptomatically with antiemetics. Encourage small, frequent feedings of cool, bland foods and liquids. If vomiting occurs, assess for fluid and electrolyte imbalance. Monitor I/O and daily weights if patient is hospitalized. Encourage small, frequent meals of favorite foods, especially high-calorie, high-protein foods. Encourage use of spices and obtain weekly weights. Teach oral assessment and oral hygiene regimen. Encourage patient to report early stomatitis. Provide pain relief measures, if indicated. Monitor LFTs prior to drug dose. Assess patient prior to and during treatment for signs/ symptoms of hepatotoxicity. Discuss drug dose reduction if mucositis or diarrhea occurs and is severe.

II. POTENTIAL FOR INFECTION AND BLEEDING related to BONE MARROW DEPRESSION

Defining Characteristics: Bone marrow depression occurs 1–4 weeks after treatment, with nadir 10–14 days and recovery by day 21. Leukopenia and thrombocytopenia are most common. Immunosuppression may occur, with increased risk of bacterial, fungal, and parasitic infections.

Nursing Implications: Monitor CBC, platelet count prior to drug administration as well as for signs/symptoms of infection or bleeding. Instruct patient in self-assessment of signs/ symptoms of infection or bleeding. Administer platelet, red cell transfusions per physician's order.

III. POTENTIAL FOR SENSORY/PERCEPTUAL ALTERATION related to LOSS OF VIBRATORY SENSE

Defining Characteristics: Loss of vibratory sensation; unsteady gait may occur.

Nursing Implications: Assess vibratory sensation, gait before each dose and between treatments. Report changes to physician. Encourage patient to report any changes.

Drug: thiotepa (Thioplex, Tepadina, triethylenethiophosphoramide)

Class: Alkylating agent.

Mechanism of Action: Selectively reacts with DNA phosphate groups to produce chromosome crosslinkage with blocking of nucleoprotein synthesis. Acts as a polyfunctional alkylating agent. Cell cycle phase-nonspecific agent. Mimics radiation-induced injury.

Metabolism: Rapidly cleared following IV administration and 40% bound to plasma proteins. Slow onset of action, slowly bound to tissues, extensively metabolized. Metabolized by the P450 microenzyme system in the liver with 63% of dose eliminated in urine within 24–72 hours. When high doses are given in the transplant setting, some of the drug is excreted as perspiration.

Indication: (1) Treatment of adenocarcinoma of the breast and ovarian cancer; (2) controlling intracavitary effusions secondary to diffuse or localized neoplastic diseases; (3) treatment of superficial papillary carcinoma of the urinary bladder; and (4) lymphomas, such as lymphosarcoma and Hodgkin's disease.

Dosage/Range:

Intravenous:

- 8 mg/m^2 (0.2 mg/kg) IV every day × 5 days, repeated every 3–4 weeks, OR
- 0.3–0.4 mg/kg IV, every 1–4 weeks.
- High dose (transplant): 180–1100 mg/m^2 IV.

Intracavitary:

- Bladder: 60 mg in 30–60 mL sterile water once a week for 3–4 weeks.

Intracavitary (effusions):

- 0.6–0.8 mg/kg every 1–4 weeks.

Drug Preparation:

- Add sterile water to vial of lyophilized powder.
- Further dilute with 0.9% sodium chloride or 5% dextrose.
- Do not use solution unless it is clear.
- Refrigerate vial until use (reconstituted solution is stable for 5 days).

Drug Administration:

- IV, IM; intracavitary, intratumor, intra-arterial.

Drug Interactions:

- Myelosuppressive drugs: additive hematologic toxicity.

Lab Effects/Interference:

- Decreased CBC (especially WBC and platelets).
- Increased LFTs and RFTs.

Special Considerations:

- Hypersensitivity reactions have occurred with this drug.
- Is an irritant; should be given IVP via a sidearm of a running IV.
- Increased neuromuscular blockage when given with nondepolarizing muscle relaxants.
- Monitor CBC in patients receiving intravesicular administration of drug, as systemic absorption may occur.
- Second malignancies may occur (e.g., AML, breast and lung cancers).
- High-dose therapy: mucositis, nausea and vomiting, skin changes (skin bronzing, rash, flaking/desquamation of skin).

Potential Toxicities/Side Effects and the Nursing Process

I.   POTENTIAL FOR INFECTION AND BLEEDING related to BONE MARROW DEPRESSION

Defining Characteristics: Nadir is 5–30 days after drug administration (WBC 7–10 days, platelets day 21), with recovery of WBC by day 21 and platelets by day 28–35. Thrombocytopenia and leukopenia may occur. Anemia may occur with prolonged use. May be cumulative toxicity with recovery of bone marrow in 40–50 days. Thrombocytopenia is dose-limiting.

Nursing Implications: Monitor CBC, platelet count prior to drug administration; monitor for signs/symptoms of infection or bleeding. Instruct patient in self-assessment of signs/symptoms of infection (e.g., temperature > 100.4°F, chills, rigors, colored sputum, burning when urinating, difficulty breathing) or bleeding and to report them immediately. Teach self-care strategies to protect patient from infection (e.g., avoiding crowds, people with colds, handwashing) and bleeding (e.g., wearing gloves when gardening, using electric shaver rather than razor). Administer red cells and platelet transfusions per physician's orders.

II. ALTERATION IN NUTRITION, LESS THAN BODY REQUIREMENTS, related to GI SIDE EFFECTS

Defining Characteristics: Nausea and vomiting occur in 10–15% of patients; dose-dependent; occurs 6–12 hours after drug dose; anorexia occurs occasionally.

Nursing Implications: Premedicate with antiemetics especially with parenteral dosing of high dose. Continue antiemetics at least 12 hours after drug is given. Encourage small, frequent meals of cool, bland, dry foods, and favorite foods, especially high-calorie, high-protein foods. Encourage use of spices; assess weight weekly. Teach patient to report diarrhea that does not resolve in 24 hours and self-administration of antidiarrheals if at home and to increase oral fluids to 2–3 liters a day.

III. POTENTIAL SEXUAL DYSFUNCTION related to DRUG EFFECT

Defining Characteristics: Drug is mutagenic. Sterility may be reversible and incomplete. Amenorrhea often reverses in 6–8 months.

Nursing Implications: As appropriate, explore with patient and partner issues of reproductive and sexuality patterns and the anticipated impact chemotherapy may have. Discuss strategies to preserve sexuality and reproductive health (e.g., sperm banking).

IV. POTENTIAL FOR INJURY related to ALLERGIC REACTION

Defining Characteristics: Allergic responses occur rarely: hives, bronchospasm, skin rash (dermatitis). Secondary malignancies may occur with prolonged therapy.

Nursing Implications: Assess for signs/symptoms of allergic response during drug administration. Stop drug if bronchospasm occurs and notify physician. If symptomatic, institute emergency measures such as bronchodilator, and support other vital signs as needed. Discuss symptomatic treatment with physician. Instruct patient receiving prolonged therapy about importance of regular health maintenance examinations during and after therapy by primary care provider and oncologist.

V.   ALTERATION IN COMFORT related to DIZZINESS, FEVER, PAIN

Defining Characteristics: Dizziness, headache, fever, and local pain may occur.

Nursing Implications: Assess for alterations in comfort. Treat symptomatically.

Drug: topotecan hydrochloride for injection (Hycamtin)

Class: Topoisomerase I inhibitor.

Mechanism of Action: Topoisomerase I causes reversible single-strand breaks in DNA, which permits relaxation of DNA helix prior to DNA replication. Topotecan binds to the topoisomerase I-DNA complex, thus preventing repair (religation) of the strand breaks. When the cell tries to synthesize DNA, replication enzymes interact with the complex, and this leads to double-strand DNA breaks that cannot be repaired; thus, drug prevents DNA synthesis and replication and leads to cell death.

Metabolism: After IV administration, extensively tissue-bound, with about 35% of drug bound to plasma proteins. Crosses BBB. 30% of dose is excreted in the urine. Patients with moderate renal impairment have a 33% decrease in plasma clearance; patients with moderate impairment require a dosage adjustment. Minor metabolism by the liver, so patients with liver dysfunction do not require dose modification. The oral formulation is rapidly absorbed with peak plasma concentration occurring between 1 to 2 hours and 40% bioavailability. Drug demonstrates biexponential pharmacokinetics, and the mean terminal half-life is 3–6 hours. Drug binds to plasma proteins 35%. 57% of the oral dose (five daily doses) was recovered; 20% was excreted in the urine and 33% in the feces.

Indication: For (1) metastatic carcinoma of the ovary after failure of initial or subsequent chemotherapy; (2) small cell lung cancer (SCLC) extensive disease after failure of first-line chemotherapy; (3) combination therapy with cisplatin for Stage IVB recurrent, or persistent carcinoma of the cervix that is not amenable to curative treatment with surgery and/or RT; (4) as an oral capsule for the treatment of relapsed SCLC in patients with a prior complete or partial response and who are at least 45 days from the end of first-line therapy.

Dosage/Range:

- IV: Metastatic carcinoma of the ovary after failure of initial or subsequent chemo: 1.5 mg/m^2 IV infusion over 30 minutes for 5 consecutive days (days 1–5) every 21 days. (Some oncologists use dose of 1.25 mg/m^2, which the manufacturer says has equal efficacy.) Minimum of 4 courses as tumor response may be delayed. Median time to response is 9–12 weeks.
- IV: Small-cell lung cancer (SCLC) after failure of first-line chemotherapy: same as ovarian cancer dose, cycle length, and recommended minimum of 4 courses in the absence of disease progression. Median time to response was 5–7 weeks.

- IV: Cervical cancer: 0.75 mg/m² IV over 30 minutes, on days 1, 2, 3 followed by cisplatin 50 mg/m² IV infusion on day 1 repeated every 21 days.
- Verify BSA area prior to drug preparation and dispensing; recommended dosage should generally NOT exceed 4 mg IV.
- PO: relapsed small cell lung cancer: 2.3 mg/m²/day orally once daily for 5 consecutive days repeated every 21 days.

Dose Reduction:
- **IV: Ovarian and SCLC:**
  - Neutropenia ANC < 1,500 cells/mm³ or platelet count falls to < 25,000 cells/mm³ during treatment, decrease next dose by 0.25 mg/m² or add G-CSF beginning on day 6 (24 hours after the last dose of topotecan).
  - Counts must be ANC > 1,000 cells/mm³, platelet count > 100,000 cells/mm³, and Hgb 9.0 g/dL before resuming next cycle.
- **IV: Cervical cancer:**
  - Severe, febrile neutropenia (ANC < 1,000 cells/mm³ with temperature of 38°C or 100.4°F), reduce dose to 0.60 mg/m² for subsequent courses or add G-CSF beginning on day 4 to avoid dose reduction (24 hours after the last dose of topotecan). If febrile neutropenia again develops despite G-CSF, reduce dose to 0.45 mg/m² for subsequent courses.
  - If platelet count falls < 25,000cells/mm³, reduce doses to 0.60 mg/m² for subsequent cycles.
  - Serum creatinine must be ≤ 1.5 g/dL to administer topotecan with cisplatin.
- **Moderate renal impairment** (creatinine clearance 20–39 mL/min): 0.75 mg/m² should be the starting dose.
- **PO:** relapsed SCLC: (1) moderate renal impairment (CrCl 30–49 mL/min): reduce dose to 1.8 mg/m²; (2) ANC must recover to > 1,000 cells/mm³, platelets to >100,000cells/mm³, and hemoglobin to ≥ 9g/dL with transfusion if necessary; (3) severe neutropenia (neutrophils < 500 cells/mm³ with fever or infection or lasting for 7 or more days) or neutropenia (ANC 500–1,000 cells/mm³) lasting beyond day 21 of the treatment course: reduce dose by 0.4 mg/m²/day for subsequent courses; similarly reduce dose if the platelet count falls < 25,000 cells/mm³; (4) grade 3 or 4 diarrhea: reduce dose by 0.4 mg/m² for subsequent courses.

See package insert for all dose modifications.

Drug Preparation:
- IV formulation available as a 4-mg vial.
- Reconstitute vial with 4 mL sterile water for injection.
- Further dilute in 0.9% sodium chloride or 5% dextrose.
- Use immediately.
- PO formulation: Available as 0.25-mg capsules (opaque white to yellowish white) and 1.0-mg capsules (opaque pink).

Drug Administration:
- Baseline ANC for initial course must be > 1,500/mm³ and platelets > 100,000/mm³, and for subsequent courses, ANC > 1,000/mm³, platelets > 100,000/mm³, and hemoglobin ≥ 9 mg/dL.

* Ovarian and SCLC: Administer 1.5 mg/m^2 IV over 30 minutes, days 1-5, with cycle repeated q 21 days.
* G-CSF may be required if neutropenia develops.
* Cervical cancer: 0.75 mg/m^2 IV days 1, 2, 3 followed by cisplatin 50 mg/m^2 IV over 1 hour on day 1 of the cycle, and the cycle repeated every 21 days.
* Avoid extravasation of drug, as severe reactions have been reported.
* Oral: teach patient to take with or without food; capsule must be swallowed whole and must not be chewed, crushed, or divided. If patient vomits after taking the dose, the patient should not take a replacement dose.

Drug Interactions:
* PO: P = glycoprotein inhibitors (e.g., cyclosporine A, elacridar, ketoconazole, ritonavir, and saquinavir): increase topotecan exposure; avoid concurrent use.
* G-CSF: can prolong duration of neutropenia, so do not initiate until day 6 of a 5-day course of therapy, or day 4 of a 3-day course (24 hours after the last dose of topotecan).
* Platinum, other cytotoxic agents: increased severity of myelosuppression. Administering cisplatin on day 1 of a 5-day course of topotecan required lower doses of each agent, compared to coadministration on day 5 of the dosing schedule of topotecan.

Lab Effects/Interference:
* Decreased CBC.
* Increased LFTs, RFTs.

Special Considerations:
* IV: Minimum of 4 courses needed, as clinical responses delayed.
* Neutropenic colitis may occur, and fatalities have been reported. Consider this in the differential if patient presents with fever, neutropenia, abdominal pain.
* Interstitial lung disease (ILD) has been reported and may be fatal. Underlying risk factors include history of ILD, pumonary fibrosis, lung cancer, thoracic exposure to radiation, use of pneumotoxic drugs, and colony-stimulating factors. Monitor patients for pulmonary symptoms (e.g., cough, fever, dyspnea, and/or hypoxia). Discontinue topotecan if ILD confirmed.
* Contraindicated in patients with history of severe hypersensitivity reactions to topotecan or any of the components; pregnant or breastfeeding mothers; patients with severe bone marrow depression.
* Drug is fetotoxic. Teach women of reproductive potential to use effective contraception to avoid pregnancy. If the drug is used during pregnancy or if the patient becomes pregnant while receiving the drug, apprise the patient of the potential hazard to the fetus.
* Nursing mothers should make a decision whether to discontinue nursing or to discontinue the drug, taking into account the importance of the drug to the mother's health.
* Oral formulation: Teach patient to store pills out of reach of children and pets, at controlled room temperature, and protected from light.

Potential Toxicities/Side Effects and the Nursing Process

I.   INFECTION AND BLEEDING related to BONE MARROW DEPRESSION

Defining Characteristics: IV formulation: Myelosuppression is the dose-limiting toxicity. Severe grade 4 neutropenia is seen during the first course of therapy in 60% of patients.

Febrile neutropenia or sepsis may occur in up to 26% of patients. Nadir occurs on day 11. Prophylactic G-CSF is needed in 27% of courses after the first cycle. Thrombocytopenia (grade 4 with platelet count < 25,000/mm³) occurs in 26% of patients. Platelet nadir occurs on day 15. Severe anemia (Hgb < 8 g/dL) occurs in 40% of patients, and transfusions were needed for 56% of patients. Oral formulation: Grades 3–4 neutropenia occurred in 61% of patients, anemia in 25%, and thrombocytopenia in 37%.

Nursing Implications: Monitor CBC and platelet count prior to drug administration as well as signs/symptoms of infection or bleeding. Assess renal function baseline and prior to each treatment. Discuss dose reductions with physician (see Special Considerations section). Instruct patient in self-assessment of signs/symptoms of infection or bleeding. Administer RBCs and platelet transfusions per physician's orders. Teach patient self-administration of G-CSF as ordered. Discuss dose modification with physician depending on severity of bone marrow depression.

II.   ALTERATION IN NUTRITION, LESS THAN BODY REQUIREMENTS, related to NAUSEA AND VOMITING, DIARRHEA, ELEVATED LFTS

Defining Characteristics: IV formulation: Nausea occurs in 77% of patients, and vomiting in 58% without premedication with antiemetics. Diarrhea occurs in 42% of patients, while constipation occurs in 39%. Abdominal pain may occur in 33% of patients. Aspirate aminotransferase (AST, previously SGOT) and alanine aminotransferase (ALT, previously SGPT) elevations occur in 5% of patients. Oral formulation: Grades 3–4 nausea occurred in 27% of patients and vomiting in 19%. Diarrhea occurred in 14%.

Nursing Implications: Premedicate with a serotonin antagonist or dopamine antagonist antiemetic, and continue prophylactically for 24 hours to prevent nausea and vomiting, at least for the first treatment. Teach patient to take oral antiemetics 1 hour before taking oral topotecan. Encourage small, frequent feedings of cool, bland, dry foods. Assess for symptoms of fluid and electrolyte imbalance: monitor I/O and daily weights if administered to an inpatient. Teach patient oral assessment and oral hygiene regimen. Encourage patient to report early stomatitis. Provide pain relief measures if indicated (e.g., topical anesthetics). Encourage patient to report onset of diarrhea. Administer or teach patient to self-administer antidiarrheal medication. Ensure adequate hydration, monitor I/O. Monitor LFTs baseline and periodically during treatment. Discuss dose modification with physician depending on severity of diarrhea in patients receiving oral topotecan.

III.   POTENTIAL FOR HEPATOTOXICITY related to HYPOALBUMINEMIA, PREEXISTING HEPATIC INSUFFICIENCY (IV formulation)

Defining Characteristics: Evidence of increased drug toxicity in patients with low protein and hepatic dysfunction. Dose reductions may be necessary.

Nursing Implications: Monitor LFTs prior to drug dose. Assess patient prior to administering drug and during treatment for signs/symptoms of hepatotoxicity.

IV.   POTENTIAL FOR SKIN INTEGRITY IMPAIRMENT related to ALOPECIA (oral formulation)

Defining Characteristics: Alopecia occurs in 10–20% of patients.

Nursing Implications: Assess patient for signs/symptoms of hair loss. Instruct patient to report any of these symptoms. Discuss with patient the impact of skin changes.

Drug: toremifene citrate (Fareston)

Class: Estrogen agonist/antagonist; selective estrogen receptor modulator (SERM).

Mechanism of Action: Nonsteroidal estrogen antagonist: competitively binds directly to estrogen receptors in breast cancer cells, preventing estrogen from binding. Has four to five times more affinity for estrogen receptor than tamoxifen.

Metabolism: Well absorbed following oral dose. Highly protein-bound (99%). Peak serum level after single dose is 3 hours, with terminal half-life of 5–6.2 days. Extensively metabolized in the liver by the P450 enzyme system. Increased terminal half-life (decreased clearance) in patients with hepatic dysfunction to 10.9 days and 21 days for the principal metabolite. Clearance not significantly changed with renal impairment. Excreted in feces and, to a lesser extent, urine.

Indication: Treatment of women with estrogen-receptor positive or unknown, metastatic breast cancer.

Contraindication: Patients with known hypersensitivity to drug. Toremifene citrate should not be prescribed to patients with congenital/acquired QT prolongation (long QT syndrome), uncorrected hypokalemia, or uncorrected hypomagnesemia.

Dosage/Range:
- 60 mg orally, daily; generally continued until disease progression.
- Assess baseline CBC/ LFTs; electrolytes including serum potassium, magnesemium, and calcium, and these should be reassessed periodically. Patents at risk for prolonged QTc should have an ECG baseline, which should be reassessed periodically during therapy.

Drug Preparation/Administration:
- None.

Drug Interactions:
- Warfarin: increased anticoagulation effect; monitor INR and dose accordingly.
- Thiazide diuretics: increases risk of hypercalcemia (decreased calcium excretion).
- CYP3A4 inducers (carbamazepine, phenobarbital, phenytoin, ranitidine, rifampin), and St. John's wort: may decrease toremifene serum level and effect; assess for inadequate dose, and discontinue St. John's wort.
- CYP3A4 inhibitors (ciprofloxacin, clarithromycin, doxycycline, erythromycin, isoniazid, itraconazole, propofol, verapamil, others): may increase toremifene serum level and toxicity; assess for adverse effects.

- Metabolism is inhibited by testosterone and cyclosporin.
- Appears to enhance inhibition of multidrug-resistant cell lines by vinblastine.
- Appears to be cross-resistant with tamoxifen.

Lab Effects/Interference:
- Decreased WBC and platelets (mild).
- Hypercalcemia.
- Increased alkaline phosphatase, bilirubin, calcium, AST.
- Prolonged QTc interval.

Special Considerations:
- Monitor CBC and LFTs baseline and periodically during treatment.
- Cataracts may develop, so patient should be taught to have eye exams by an ophthalmologist baseline and then twice yearly.
- Activity, side effects, toxicity in postmenopausal women or women with unknown receptor status appear similar.
- In general, do not use drug in patients with history of thromboembolic events or as long-term therapy in women with endometrial hyperplasia.

Warnings and Precautions:
- Prolongation of QTc interval, which can result in torsades de pointes, a type of ventricular tachycardia, causing syncope, seizure, and/or sudden death.
  - Avoid use in patients with long QT syndrome, and/or uncorrected hypokalemia and hypomagnesemia. Use cautiously in patients with CHF, hepatic impairment, and electrolyte abnormalities.
  - Correct hypokalemia and hypomagnesemia if they exist, prior to starting toremifene citrate, and monitor these electrolytes throughout treatment.
  - Patients at increased risk should have an ECG baseline, including QTc interval, and as clinically indicated.
  - Patient should avoid taking drugs that prolong QTc with toremifene citrate (e.g., certain anti-arrhythmics, potent CYP3A4 inhibitors), and should discuss alternatives with their physician or NP/PA.
- Hypercalcemia and tumor flare: patients with bone metastases are at increased risk for this, which happens during the first few weeks of treatment.
  - Tumor flare is characterized by diffuse musculoskeletal pain and erythema, together with increased size of tumor lesions that later regress; hypercalcemia may also occur.
  - If hypercalcemia occurs, discuss management with physician or NP/PA; if severe, toremifene citrate should be discontinued.
  - Monitor patients with bony metastases closely for hypercalcemia during the first weeks of therapy.
- Drug is approved for use in post-menopausal women. If used by premenopausal women, the patient should be taught to use effective (nonhormonal) contraception to avoid pregnancy.

- Use in pregnancy: drug can cause fetal harm; if the drug is used during pregnancy, or if the patient becomes pregnant while taking the drug, the patient should be apprised of the potential hazard to the fetus.
- Nursing mothers should decide whether to discontinue nursing or to discontinue the drug, taking into account the importance of the drug to the mother's health.
- Patients are at risk for endometrial cancer. Teach patient to have a baseline then annual gynecology exam with endometrial biopsy. Teach patient to call provider for a gynecologic exam right away if vaginal bleeding occurs.

Potential Toxicities/Side Effects and the Nursing Process

I. POTENTIAL FOR SEXUAL DYSFUNCTION related to MENSTRUAL IRREGULARITIES, HOT FLASHES

Defining Characteristics: Similar to tamoxifen toxicity profile. May cause menstrual irregularity, hot flashes (most common), milk production in breasts, and vaginal discharge and bleeding.

Nursing Implications: As appropriate, explore with patient and partner issues of reproductive and sexuality patterns and the impact drug may have on them. Discuss strategies to preserve sexual and reproductive health.

II. POTENTIAL FOR ALTERATION IN COMFORT related to FLARE REACTION

Defining Characteristics: May cause flare reaction initially (bone and tumor pain, transient increase in tumor size). Nausea, vomiting, and anorexia may occur. Tremor may occur and be significant in some patients.

Nursing Implications: Inform patient of flare reaction, signs/symptoms to be aware of, and encourage patient to report any signs/symptoms. Inform patient of possibility of nausea, vomiting, and anorexia. Encourage small, frequent feedings of high-calorie, high-protein foods. Teach patients to report tremor, and discuss impact on self-care ability and comfort. If patient has brain or vertebral metastases, observe closely; any transient increase in tumor size may cause severe neurologic symptoms.

III. POTENTIAL FOR INFECTION AND BLEEDING related to BONE MARROW DEPRESSION

Defining Characteristics: Mild, transient leukopenia and thrombocytopenia occur rarely. Lowest WBC count in clinical trials was $2,500/mm^3$.

Nursing Implications: Monitor CBC and platelet count prior to drug administration and after therapy has begun. Instruct patient in self-assessment of signs/symptoms of infection or bleeding.

IV. POTENTIAL FOR SKIN INTEGRITY IMPAIRMENT related to RASH, ALOPECIA

Defining Characteristics: Skin rash, alopecia, and peripheral edema are rare.

Nursing Implications: Assess patient for signs/symptoms of hair loss, edema, and skin rash. Instruct patient to report any of these symptoms. Discuss with patient the impact of skin changes.

Drug: trimetrexate (Neutrexin)

Class: Antimetabolite.

Mechanism of Action: Nonclassical folate antagonist; potent inhibitor of dihydrofolate reductase. May be able to overcome mechanism(s) of methotrexate resistance as drug reaches higher concentration within tumor cells. Also, inhibits growth of parasitic infective agents (causing *Pneumocystis carinii* pneumonia [PCP], toxoplasmosis) in patients with immunodeficiency or myelodysplastic disorders.

Metabolism: Significant percentage of drug is protein-bound. Metabolized by liver; 10–20% of dose is excreted by kidneys in 24 hours.

Indication: With concurrent leucovorin administration, as an alternative therapy for the treatment of moderate to severe *Pneumocystis carinii* pneumonia (PCP) in immunocompromised patients, including patients with acquired immune deficiency syndrome (AIDS) who are intolerant of, or are refractory to, trimethoprim-sulfamethoxazole therapy, or for whom trimethoprim-sulfamethoxazole is contraindicated.

Dosage/Range:
For PCP indication:
- 45 mg/m^2 daily IV infusion over 60–90 minutes × 21 days.
- Leucovorin 20 mg/m^2 IV over 5–10 minutes q 6 hours (80 mg/m^2 24-hour total dose), or 20 mg/m^2 PO qid for days of trimetrexate treatment, extending 72 hours past the last dose of trimetrexate, for a total of 24 days.

Drug Preparation:
- Reconstitute with 2 mL 5% dextrose USP or sterile water for injection (12.5 mg of trimetrexate/mL).
- Filter with 0.22-μm filter prior to further dilution; observe for cloudiness or precipitate.
- Further dilute in 5% dextrose to a final concentration of 0.25–2.00 mg/mL.
- Stable 24 hours at room temperature or refrigerated.

Drug Administration:
- IV infusion over 60 minutes.
- Incompatible with chloride solutions, as precipitate forms immediately, and leucovorin.
- Leucovorin can be started either before or after first trimetrexate dose, but ensure that IV line is flushed with at least 10 mL of 5% dextrose between drugs.

Drug Interactions:
- Drug is metabolized by P450 enzyme system, so interactions are possible with erythromycin, fluconazole, ketoconazole, rifabutin, rifampin, protease inhibitors.

Lab Effects/Interference:
- Decreased CBC.
- Increased LFTs, RFTs (especially creatinine).
- Decreased Ca, Na.

Special Considerations:
- Increased toxicity is seen in patients with low protein (drug is highly protein-bound) and hepatic dysfunction. Dose reduction is indicated.
- Leukopenia is dose-limiting toxicity.
- Other side effects are nausea and vomiting, rash, mucositis, AST elevations, thrombocytopenia.
- Drug is fetotoxic and embryotoxic. Women of childbearing age should use contraceptive measures to prevent pregnancy while receiving the drug.
- Zidovudine (AZT) therapy should be interrupted while receiving trimetrexate.
- Use cautiously in patients with renal, hepatic, or hematologic impairment.
- Transaminase levels or alk phos > 5 times upper limit of normal: HOLD DOSE.
- Serum creatinine ≥ 2.5 mg/dL due to trimetrexate: HOLD DOSE.
- Severe mucosal toxicity (unable to eat): HOLD DOSE, and continue leucovorin.
- Temperature ≥ 40.5°C (105°F) uncontrolled by antipyretics: HOLD DOSE.
- Hematologic toxicity: HOLD DOSE and consult package insert.

Potential Toxicities/Side Effects and the Nursing Process

I.   INFECTION AND BLEEDING related to BONE MARROW DEPRESSION

Defining Characteristics: Leukopenia is a dose-limiting toxicity. Thrombocytopenia also occurs commonly.

Nursing Implications: Monitor CBC, platelet count prior to drug administration, as well as for signs/symptoms of infection or bleeding. Instruct patient in self-assessment of signs/symptoms of infection or bleeding. Administer red cells and platelet transfusions per physician's orders.

II.   ALTERATION IN NUTRITION, LESS THAN BODY REQUIREMENTS, related to GI SIDE EFFECTS

Defining Characteristics: Nausea and vomiting have been reported in clinical trials; drug has been reported to cause stomatitis; diarrhea may occur also.

Nursing Implications: Premedicate with antiemetics and continue prophylactically for 24 hours to prevent nausea and vomiting, at least for the first treatment. Encourage small, frequent feedings of cool, bland, dry foods. Assess for symptoms of fluid and electrolyte imbalance: monitor I/O, daily weights if administered to an inpatient. Teach patient oral assessment and oral hygiene regimen. Encourage patient to report early stomatitis. Provide pain relief measures if indicated (e.g., topical anesthetics). Encourage patient to report onset of diarrhea. Administer or teach patient to self-administer antidiarrheal medication. Guaiac all stools. Ensure adequate hydration; monitor I/O.

III. POTENTIAL FOR IMPAIRED SKIN INTEGRITY related to ALOPECIA

Defining Characteristics: Alopecia is total in 42% of patients.

Nursing Implications: Discuss with patient the impact of hair loss. As appropriate, suggest wig prior to actual hair loss. Explore patient's response to actual hair loss and plan strategies to minimize distress (e.g., wig, scarf, cap).

IV. ALTERATION IN COMFORT related to HEADACHE

Defining Characteristics: Headache occurs in 21% of patients. Paresthesias may affect 9% of patients.

Nursing Implications: Teach patient that headache may occur and is usually relieved by acetaminophen. Instruct patient to report headache that is not relieved by usual methods.

V. ALTERATION IN OXYGEN, POTENTIAL, related to DYSPNEA

Defining Characteristics: Dyspnea may occur in 20% of patients, and is severe in 4% of patients.

Nursing Implications: Assess baseline pulmonary status, including presence of dyspnea, and history since last treatment prior to successive drug administrations. Instruct patient to report new onset or worsening of dyspnea. Discuss occurrences with physician to determine further diagnostic evaluation.

Drug: triptorelin pamoate (Trelstar LA, Trelstar Depot)

Class: Gonadotropin-releasing hormone (GnRH) agonist.

Mechanism of Action: Potently inhibits gonadotropin secretion, resulting in an initial surge in circulating levels of luteinizing hormone (LH), follicle-stimulating hormone (FSH), testosterone, and estradiol, and then after 2 to 4 weeks of continued drug administration, sustained decreases in LH and FSH secretion, resulting in a reduction of testosterone similar to surgical castration serum levels. This removes the hormonal stimulation from prostate cancer cells and stops the growth and proliferation of prostate cells. The drug effect is reversible following discontinuance of the drug.

Metabolism: After IM administration, the drug probably undergoes metabolism by the liver, with excretion by liver and kidneys.

Indication: For the palliative treatment of patients with advanced prostate cancer.

Contraindication: (1) Known hypersensitvity to drug or its components or other GnRH agonists, or GnRH; (2) pregnancy.

Dosage/Range:
- Trelstar depot: 3.75 mg IM once every 4 weeks.
- Trelstar LA: 11.25 mg IM once every 12 weeks.
- Trelstar LA: 22.5 mg IM every 24 weeks (6 months).

Drug Preparation:
- Using the manufacturer's Clip'n'Ject system, reconstitute drug vial with 2 mL sterile water, shake well, inspect milky solution that results.
- Draw up and administer using the Clip'n'Ject (see package insert).

Drug Administration:
- Administer in large muscle and rotate sites.
- Administer Trelstar LA in buttock.
- Monitor patients closely after first two treatments, as anaphylaxis with or without angioedema may rarely occur.
- Monitor serum testosterone levels baseline and periodically.
- Monitor patients with bony metastases or disease that could cause ureteral obstruction closely after initial treatment, as flare may cause ureteral obstruction or spinal cord compression, depending on location of metastases. In extreme cases, orchiectomy may be required to relieve obstruction of ureters.

Lab Effects/Interference:
- Decreased serum testosterone levels.
- Chronic or continuous administration of triptorelin results in suppression of pituitary-gonadal axis; diagnostic tests of pituitary-gonadal function during treatment and after therapy ends may be misleading.

Special Considerations:
- 6-month formulation maintains > 98% of patients below castrate level at 6 and 12 months.
- Monitor drug effectiveness (serum testosterone level, PSA).
- Drug is used off-label for the treatment of patients with endometriosis, in vitro fertilization, and ovarian cancer.
- Rarely can cause pituitary apoplexy (pituitary infarction) in patients who have anadenoma, characterized by sudden headache, vomiting, visual changes, ophthalmoplegia (paralysis or weakness of the muscles that control eye movement), altered mental status, and sometimes cardiovascular collapse after the first dose (within hours to 2 weeks). Emergency medical care is required.

Warnings and Precautions:

- Hypersensitivity reactions (HSRs) including anaphylactic shock, hypersensitivity, and angioedema have been reported. If HSRs occur, discontinue drug immediately and provide supportive and symptomatic care in concert with physican and/or NP/PA.
- Transient increase in serum testosterone may occur, resulting in worsening of signs and symptoms or new onset of symptoms of prostate cancer during first few weeks of treatment. These include bone pain, neuropathy, hematuria, or ureteral or bladder outlet obstruction.
- Spinal cord compression and renal impairment have been reported. If spinal cord compression or renal impairment develop and cannot be managed with standard treatment, an orchiectomy should be considered.
- Hyperglycemia and diabetes have been reported in men receiving GnRH agoinsts. Monitor blood glucose or HbA1c baseline and periodically, and manage appropriately.
- Cardiovascular diseases, including increased risk of developing MI, sudden cardiac death, and stroke have been reported. Monitor patients for signs suggestive of cardiovascular disease, and discuss management with physician or NP/PA.

Potential Toxicities/Side Effects and the Nursing Process

I. ALTERATION IN COMFORT related to HOT FLASHES, TUMOR FLARE, LEG PAIN, EYE PAIN, HEADACHE, EDEMA

Defining Characteristics: Initially, drug causes increased LH secretion, resulting in increased testosterone secretion and tumor flare. Usually disappears after 2 weeks. Headache, dizziness, and hot flashes may occur. Vasodilation most common. Tumor flare may also occur initially (bone and tumor pain, transient increase in tumor size due to transient increase in testosterone levels). Breast tenderness has been reported. Peripheral edema, leg and eye pain, headache may occur.

Nursing Implications: Inform patient that symptoms may occur and that flare reaction will subside after the initial 2 weeks of therapy. Assess and document pain score baseline, and teach patient to report pain, especially if it is new onset of back pain that may be radicular, or pelvic pain, hematuria, or urinary retention. Encourage patient to report symptoms early. Triage symptoms, and discuss emergency management if severe symptoms develop. Develop symptom management plan with patient and physician. Monitor patients with disease near ureters or bony metastases closely after initial treatment, as ureteral obstruction and spinal cord compression have occurred.

II. POTENTIAL SEXUAL DYSFUNCTION related to LIBIDO, IMPOTENCE

Defining Characteristics: Frequently causes decreased libido and erectile impotence in men. Gynecomastia occurs in 1–10% of patients. In women, amenorrhea occurs after 10 weeks of therapy.

Nursing Implications: As appropriate, explore with patient and significant other issues of reproductive and sexual patterns and the impact chemotherapy may have on them. Discuss strategies to preserve sexuality and reproductive health.

III.   DEPRESSION, POTENTIAL, related to DRUG EFFECT

Defining Characteristics: Depression may affect up to 5.3% of patients and, less commonly, patients may develop emotional lability, insomnia, nervousness, and anxiety.

Nursing Implications: Assess baseline affect and usual coping strategies. Teach patient to report change in affect. Assess effectiveness of coping strategies. Encourage patient to verbalize feelings, and provide emotional support. Assess need for referral to psychiatric nurse specialist or social worker if supportive efforts ineffective.

IV.   ALTERED NUTRITION, LESS THAN BODY REQUIREMENTS, related to GI SIDE EFFECTS

Defining Characteristics: Anorexia, nausea, and vomiting may occur rarely.

Nursing Implications: If patients experience symptoms, encourage small, frequent feedings of favorite foods, especially high-calorie, high-protein foods. Monitor weight weekly. Assess incidence and pattern of nausea, vomiting, or anorexia if they occur. Discuss need for antiemetic with physician and patient.

Drug: valrubicin (Valstar)

Class: Anthracycline antitumor antibiotic.

Mechanism of Action: Semisynthetic analogue of doxorubicin; drug is highly lipophilic and is made soluble in Cremophor EL. Apparently, the drug does not interact with negatively charged molecules, and thus is less irritating to bladder mucosa. Drug metabolites appear to inhibit topoisomerase II so that cellular DNA cannot replicate, thus inhibiting DNA synthesis and causing chromosomal damage and cell death.

Metabolism: Drug is well absorbed by bladder mucosa with little, if any, systemic absorption unless bladder is injured/perforated. Used for bladder instillation, and excreted unchanged in the urine (98.6%).

Indication: For intravesical therapy of BCG-refractory carcinoma *in situ* of the urinary bladder in patients for whom immediate cystectomy would be associated with unacceptable morbidity or mortality.

Contraindication: Patients with (1) known hypersensitivity to anthracyclines or polyoxy castor oil; (2) concurrent UTIs; (3) a small bladder capacity (e.g., unable to tolerate a 75 mL instillation).

Dosage/Range:
- Intravesicular therapy of BCG-refractory carcinoma in situ of the urinary bladder: 800 mg q week × 6 weeks.
- High incidence of metastases in patients receiving drug in clinical trials, probably due to delayed cystectomy. Therefore, therapy should be discontinued in patients not responding to treatment after 3 months.

Drug Preparation:
- Available as injection form, 200 mg in 5-mL vial, which should be stored in the refrigerator 2–8°C (36–46°F).
- Remove vials from refrigerator and allow to warm to room temperature without heating; dilute by adding 800 mg (20 mL) to 55 mL of 0.9% normal saline injection, USP.

Drug Administration:
- Bladder lavage by intravesicular administration of drug (total volume of 75 mL when diluted as above), allowed to dwell for 2 hours, and then voided out.
- Non-PVC tubing and non-DEHP containers and administration sets should be used to prevent leaching of PVC into drug volume (due to Cremophor EL).

Drug Interactions:
- None known due to limited, if any, systemic absorption.

Lab Effects/Interference:
- Hyperglycemia.

Special Considerations:
- Contraindicated in patients with hypersensitivity to anthracycline antibiotic Cremophor EL, or any drug components, during pregnancy, in breastfeeding mothers, or in patients with urinary tract infection at time treatment is planned or with small bladder unable to hold 75 mL.
- Drug should NOT be given if bladder is injured, inflamed, or perforated, as systemic absorption will occur via loss of mucosal integrity.
- Use with caution in patients with severe irritable bladder symptoms, as drug may cause symptoms of irritable bladder (during instillation and dwell time).
- Teach patients that urine will be red- or pink-tinged for 24 hours.
- Patients with diabetes need to check blood glucose levels, as hyperglycemia may occur with treatment (1% incidence).

Potential Toxicities/Side Effects and the Nursing Process

I. ALTERATION IN URINE ELIMINATION related to DRUG EFFECTS

Defining Characteristics: Intravesicular administration of drug is associated with signs/symptoms of bladder irritation: frequency (61% of patients), dysuria (56%), urgency (57%), bladder spasm (31%), hematuria (29%), pain in bladder (28%), incontinence (22%), cystitis (15%), and urinary tract infection (15%). Less commonly, nocturia (7%), burning on urination (5%), urinary retention (4%), pain in the urethra (3%), pelvic pain (1%).

Nursing Implications: Assess baseline urinary elimination pattern, history of signs/symptoms of bladder irritation. Teach patient that these side effects may occur and to report them. Teach patient to drink 3 L of fluid for at least 2–3 days beginning day of treatment to flush bladder. Reassure patient that signs/symptoms will resolve and to report any persistent symptoms.

II.   ALTERATION IN OXYGENATION, POTENTIAL, related to RARE CARDIAC EFFECTS

Defining Characteristics: Rarely, chest pain may occur (2%), as may vasodilation (2%) or peripheral edema (1%).

Nursing Implications: Assess patient's baseline cardiac status, and history of chest pain, peripheral edema. Teach patient to report any pain, or swelling in hands or feet. If this occurs, discuss management with physician. If possible, do EKG while patient is having chest pain to see if ischemia exists. Systemic absorption is possible only if bladder mucosal surfaces are injured, so this should be considered.

III.   ALTERATION IN COMFORT, POTENTIAL, related to PAIN, RASH, WEAKNESS, MYALGIA

Defining Characteristics: The following discomfort may occur: headache (4%), malaise (4%), dizziness (3%), fever (2%), rash (3%), abdominal pain (5%), weakness (4%), back pain (3%), myalgia (1%).

Nursing Implications: Assess baseline comfort level, and any pain and the usual pain relief plan. Teach patient that these problems may occur rarely and to report them if they do. Teach patient these symptoms should resolve, and to use local measures to minimize discomfort. Teach patient to report any symptoms that do not resolve or that become worse.

IV.   ALTERATION IN NUTRITION, POTENTIAL, related to NAUSEA, DIARRHEA, VOMITING

Defining Characteristics: Rarely, gastrointestinal symptoms may occur: nausea affects approximately 5% of patients, diarrhea 3% of patients, and vomiting 2% of patients.

Nursing Implications: Assess baseline nutritional status, history of nausea, vomiting, or diarrhea. Teach patient that these may occur rarely and to report them if they do. If patient does develop symptoms, teach patient to take antiemetic medication as ordered, and OTC antidiarrheal medicine. Teach patient to call right away if symptoms do not resolve.

Drug: vinblastine (Velban)

Class: Plant alkaloid extracted from the periwinkle plant (*Vinca rosea*).

Mechanism of Action: Drug binds to microtubular proteins, thus arresting mitosis during metaphase; may inhibit RNA, DNA, and protein synthesis. Cell cycle-specific for M phase and active in S phase.

Metabolism: About 10% of drug is excreted in feces. Vinblastine is partially metabolized by the liver (P450 microenzyme system). Minimal amount of the drug is excreted in urine and bile. Dose modification may be necessary in the presence of hepatic failure.

Indication: For the palliative treatment of generalized Hodgkin's Disease (Stages III, IV), lymphocytic lymphoma (nodular and diffuse, poorly and well differentiated), histiocytic lymphoma, mycosis fungoides (advanced stages), advanced carcinoma of the testis, Kaposi's sarcoma, Letterer-Siwe disease (histiocytosis X).

Contraindication: Patients with (1) significant granulocytopenia unless resulting from disease being treated; (2) bacterial infection must be brought under control prior to initiation of vinblastine.

Dosage/Range:
- 0.1 mg/kg; 6 mg/m² IV weekly: continuous infusion 1.5–2.0 mg/m²/d in 1 L D₅W or NS × 5 days.
- Dose-reduce (50%) for bilirubin 1.5–3 mg/dL or AST 60–180 units/L; dose-reduce 75% if bilirubin 3–5 mg/dL and hold for bilirubin > 5 mg/dL or AST > 180 units/L.

Drug Preparation:
- Available in 10-mg vials. Store in refrigerator until use. Prepared syringes containing the drug must be packaged in an overwrap that is labeled "DO NOT REMOVE COVERING UNTIL MOMENT OF INJECTION. FATAL IF GIVEN INTRATHECALLY. FOR INTRAVENOUS USE ONLY."

Drug Administration:
- IV: This drug is a vesicant. Give slow IVP over 1–2 min through the sidearm of a running IV so as to avoid extravasation, which can lead to ulceration, pain, and necrosis. Refer to individual hospital policy and procedure for administration of a vesicant. Ensure there is no confusion, as drug is fatal if given intrathecally (IT).

Drug Interactions:
- CYP3A4 inhibitors (itraconazole, erythromycin, others): increased serum drug level of vinblastine; do not use together or assess possible toxicity and dose-reduce vinblastine.
- CYP3A4 inducers (carbamazepine, dexamethasone, phenytoin, others): decreased serum levels of vinblastine; do not use together or assess need to increase dose of vinblastine.
- St. John's wort: may increase vinblastine toxicity; do not administer concomitantly.
- Grapefruit juice: may increase vinblastine toxicity; do not administer concomitantly.
- Decreased pharmacologic effects of phenytoin when given with this drug; check phenytoin levels and dose-modify based on levels.
- Increases cellular uptake of methotrexate by certain malignant cells when administered sequentially, but less so than vincristine.
- Antigout medicines: may decrease effect of vinblastine. Do not use together if possible.

Lab Effects/Interference:
- Decreased WBC.

Special Considerations:
- Drug is a vesicant; give through a running IV to avoid extravasation.
- Dose modification may be necessary in the presence of hepatic failure.
- Teach women of childbearing potential to use effective contraception to avoid pregnancy. If drug is used in pregnancy or if the patient becomes pregnant while receiving the drug,

the patient should be apprised of the potential hazard to the fetus. Nurisng mothers should make a decision whether to discontinue nursing or discontinue the drug, taking into account the importance of the drug to the mother's health.

* Aspermia has been reported in men.
* Leukopenia is dose-limiting, with nadir day 5–10 days after a dose, and recovery to pretreatment levels 7–14 days after treatment.
* IV administration only; drug is fatal if administered intrathecally. Prepared syringes containing the drug must be packaged in an overwrap that is labeled "DO NOT REMOVE COVERING UNTIL MOMENT OF INJECTION. FATAL IF GIVEN INTRATHECALLY. FOR INTRAVENOUS USE ONLY."
* If inadvertent IT administration of vinca alkaloids occurs, **immediate** neurosurgical intervention is necessary to prevent ascending paralysis leading to death. The competent physician should (Bedford Labs, 2014):
  * Remove as much CSF as is safely possible through lumbar access.
  * Insert epidural catheter into subarachnoid space via the intervertebral space above initial lumbar access and irrigate the CSF with lactated Ringer's solution. Fresh frozen plasma should be requested and, when available, 25 mL should be added to every 1 liter of lactated Ringer's solution.
  * Neurosurgeon should insert an intraventricular drain or catheter and continue CSF irrigation with fluid removed through the lumbar access, connected to a closed drainage system. Lactated Ringer's solution should be given by continuous infusion at 150 mL/hour or a rate of 75 mL/hr when fresh frozen plasma has been added as above.
  * Rate of infusion should be adjusted to maintain a spinal fluid protein level of 150 mg/dL.
  * The following measures have also been used, but may not be essential: gluamic acid, 10 gm, IV over 24 hours, followed by 500 mg 3 × daily by mouth for 1 month. Folinic acid has been administered IV as a 100 mg bolus and then infused at a rate of 25 mg/hr × 24 hours, then bolus doses of 25 mg every 6 hours for 1 week. Pyridoxine has been given at a dose of 50 mg every 8 hours by IV infusion over 30 min.

Potential Toxicities/Side Effects and the Nursing Process

I.   POTENTIAL FOR INFECTION AND BLEEDING related to BONE MARROW DEPRESSION

Defining Characteristics: May cause severe bone marrow depression; nadir 4–10 days. Neutrophils greatly affected. In patients with prior XRT or chemotherapy, thrombocytopenia may be severe.

Nursing Implications: Monitor CBC, platelet count prior to drug administration. Assess for signs/symptoms of infection or bleeding. Instruct patient in self-assessment of signs/ symptoms of infection or bleeding. Dose reduction if hepatic dysfunction: 50% if bili > 1.5 mg/dL; 75% if bili > 3.0 mg/dL. Administer red blood cell and platelet transfusions per physician's orders.

II. POTENTIAL FOR SENSORY/PERCEPTUAL ALTERATIONS related to PERIPHERAL OR CENTRAL NEUROPATHY

Defining Characteristics: Occur less frequently than with vincristine. Occur in patients receiving prolonged or high-dose therapy. Symptoms: paresthesias, peripheral neuropathy, depression, headache, malaise, jaw pain, urinary retention, tachycardia, orthostatic hypotension, seizures. Rare ocular changes: diplopia, ptosis, photophobia, oculomotor dysfunction, optic neuropathy.

Nursing Implications: Assess sensory/perceptual changes prior to each drug dose, especially if dose is high (> 10 mg) or patient is receiving prolonged therapy. Notify physician of alterations. Discuss with patient the impact changes have had, as well as strategies to minimize dysfunction and decrease distress.

III. ALTERATION IN BOWEL ELIMINATION related to CONSTIPATION

Defining Characteristics: Constipation results from neurotoxicity (central) and is less common than with vincristine. Risk factor: high dose (> 20 mg). May lead to adynamic ileus, abdominal pain.

Nursing Implications: Assess bowel elimination pattern with each drug dose, especially if dose > 20 mg. Teach patient to promote bowel elimination with fluids (3 L/day), high-fiber, bulky foods, exercise, stool softeners. Suggest laxative if unable to move bowels at least once a day. Instruct patient to report abdominal pain.

IV. ALTERATION IN NUTRITION, LESS THAN BODY REQUIREMENTS, related to GI SIDE EFFECTS

Defining Characteristics: Nausea and vomiting rarely occur. Stomatitis is uncommon but can be severe.

Nursing Implications: Premedicate with antiemetics and continue prophylactically for 24 hours to prevent nausea and vomiting, at least for the first treatment. Encourage small, frequent feedings of cool, bland foods and liquids. Assess for symptoms of fluid and electrolyte imbalance: monitor I/O, daily weights if administered to an inpatient. Teach patient oral assessment. Teach, reinforce teaching, regarding oral hygiene regimen. Encourage patient to report early stomatitis. Provide pain relief measures if indicated (e.g., topical anesthetics).

V. POTENTIAL FOR IMPAIRED SKIN INTEGRITY related to ALOPECIA

Defining Characteristics: Alopecia is reversible and mild and occurs in 45–50% of patients receiving drug. Drug is a potent vesicant and can cause irritation and necrosis if infiltrated.

Nursing Implications: Discuss with patient the impact of hair loss. Suggest wig as appropriate prior to actual hair loss. Explore with patient response to actual hair loss and plan strategies to minimize distress (e.g., wig, scarf, cap). Careful technique is used during venipuncture and intravenous administration. Administer vesicant through freely flowing IV, constantly monitoring IV site and patient response. Nurse should be THOROUGHLY familiar with institutional policy and procedure for administration of a vesicant agent. If vesicant drug is administered as a continuous infusion, drug must be given through a PATENT CENTRAL LINE. If extravasation is suspected, stop drug administration and aspirate any residual drug and blood from IV tubing, IV catheter/needle, and IV site if possible. If drug infiltration is suspected, manufacturer suggests the following after withdrawing any remaining drug from IV: local installation of hyaluronidase; application of moderate heat. Assess site regularly for pain, progression of erythema, induration, and evidence of necrosis. When in doubt about whether drug is infiltrating, TREAT AS AN INFILTRATION. Teach patient to assess site, and instruct to notify physician if condition worsens. Arrange next clinic visit for assessment of site depending on drug, amount infiltrated, extent of potential injury, and patient variables. Document in patient's record as per institutional policy and procedure.

VI.   POTENTIAL FOR SEXUAL DYSFUNCTION related to REPRODUCTIVE HAZARD

Defining Characteristics: Drug is possibly teratogenic. Likely to cause azoospermia in men.

Nursing Implications: As appropriate, explore with patient and partner issues of reproductive and sexuality patterns and the anticipated impact chemotherapy may have. Discuss strategies to preserve sexual health (e.g., sperm banking).

Drug: vincristine (Oncovin)

Class: Plant alkaloid extracted from the periwinkle plant (*Vinca rosea*).

Mechanism of Action: Drug binds to microtubular proteins, thus arresting mitosis during metaphase. Cell cycle-specific for M phase and active in S phase.

Metabolism: The primary route for excretion is via the liver (P450 microenzyme system) with about 70% of the drug being excreted in feces and bile. These metabolites are a result of hepatic metabolism and biliary excretion. A small amount is excreted in the urine. Dose modification may be necessary in the presence of hepatic failure.

Indication: For the treatment of patients with acute leukemia. In addition, in combination with other oncolytic agents in the treatment of patients with Hodgkin's disease, NHL, rhabdomyosarcoma, neuroblastoma, and Wilms' tumor.

Contraindication: Patients with the demyelinating form of Charcot-Marie-Tooth syndrome.

Dosage/Range:
- 0.4–1.4 mg/m^2 weekly (initially limited to 2 mg per dose).

Drug Preparation:
- Supplied in 1-mg, 2-mg, and 5-mg vials. Refrigerate vials until use. Prepared syringes containing the drug must be packaged in an overwrap that is labeled "DO NOT REMOVE COVERING UNTIL MOMENT OF INJECTION. FATAL IF GIVEN INTRATHECALLY. FOR INTRAVENOUS USE ONLY."
- To reduce potential for fatal medication errors due to incorrect route of administration, vincristine sulphate injection should be diluted in a flexible plastic container and prominently labeled as indicated for IV use only.

Drug Administration:
- IV: This drug is a vesicant. Give IVP through sidearm of a running IV to avoid extravasation, which can lead to ulceration, pain, and necrosis. Refer to hospital's policy and procedure for administration of a vesicant.

Drug Interactions:
- Neurotoxic drugs: additive neurotoxicity can occur; use cautiously.
- CYP3A4 inhibitors (itraconazole, erythromycin, others): increased serum drug level of vincristine; do not use together, or assess possible toxicity and dose-reduce vincristine.
- CYP3A4 inducers (carbamazepine, dexamethasone, phenytoin, others): decreased serum levels of vincristine; do not use together, or assess need to increase dose of vincristine.
- St. John's wort: may increase vincristine toxicity; do not administer concomitantly.
- Grapefruit juice: may increase vincristine toxicity; do not administer concomitantly.
- Asparaginase: when given prior to vincristine, will decrease vincristine excretion, with resulting increased neurotoxicity; give vincristine 12–24 hours before asparaginase.
- Decreased bioavailability of digoxin when given with this drug.
- Increased cellular uptake of methotrexate by some malignant cells when given sequentially.

Lab Effects/Interference:
- Decreased WBC, platelets.
- Increased uric acid.

Special Considerations:
- Dose is a vesicant; give through a running IV to avoid extravasation.
- Dose modifications may be necessary in the presence of hepatic failure.
- Drug has been given INTRATHECALLY by error, resulting in death. Ensure that vincristine is labeled "For IV use only." In some institutions, vincristine is mixed in a bag to prevent this error; however, this requires very careful administration, as drug is a vesicant.
- IV administration only; drug is fatal if administered intrathecally. Prepared syringes containing the drug must be packaged in an overwrap that is labeled "DO NOT REMOVE COVERING UNTIL MOMENT OF INJECTION. FATAL IF GIVEN INTRATHECALLY. FOR INTRAVENOUS USE ONLY."

- If inadvertent IT administration of vinca alkaloids occurs, **immediate** neurosurgical intervention is necessary to prevent ascending paralysis leading to death. The competent physician should (Bedford Labs, 2014):
  - Remove as much CSF as is safely possible through lumbar access.
  - Insert epidural catheter into subarachnoid space via the intervertebral space above initial lumbar access and irrigate the CSF with lactated Ringer's solution. Fresh frozen plasma should be requested and, when available, 25 mL should be added to every 1 liter of lactated Ringer's solution.
  - Neurosurgeon should insert an intraventricular drain or catheter and continue CSF irrigation with fluid removed through the lumbar access, connected to a closed drainage system. Lactated Ringer's solution should be given by continuous infusion at 150 mL/hour or a rate of 75 mL/hr when fresh frozen plasma has been added as above.
  - Rate of infusion should be adjusted to maintain a spinal fluid protein level of 150 mg/dL.
- The following measures have also been used, but may not be essential: gluamic acid, 10 gm, IV over 24 hours, followed by 500-mg 3 times daily by mouth for 1 month. Folinic acid has been administered IV as a 100 mg bolus and then infused at a rate of 25 mg/hr x 24 hours, then bolus doses of 25 mg every 6 hours for 1 week. Pyridoxine has been given at a dose of 50 mg every 8 hrs by IV infusion over 30 min.
- Liposomal vincristine (Marqibo) is FDA-approved for treatment of patients with Philadelphia chromosome-negative acute lymphoblastic leukemia (ALL), who have relapsed at least twice or whose ALL has progressed after two or more anti-leukemia regimens. This drug is different from vincristine (Oncovin). Drug dose is different from vincristine sulfate injection—verify drug name and dose prior to preparation and administration to avoid overdosage.

Potential Toxicities/Side Effects and the Nursing Process

I.   POTENTIAL FOR SENSORY/PERCEPTUAL ALTERATIONS related to PERIPHERAL CENTRAL NEUROPATHY

Defining Characteristics: Peripheral neuropathies occur as a result of toxicity to nerve fibers: absent deep tendon reflexes, numbness, weakness, myalgias, cramping, and late severe motor difficulties. Reversal or discontinuance of therapy is necessary. Increased risk exists in elderly. Cranial nerve dysfunction may occur (rare), as well as jaw pain (trigeminal neuralgia), diplopia, vocal cord paresis, mental depression, and metallic taste.

Nursing Implications: Assess sensory/perceptual changes prior to each drug dose, e.g., presence of numbness or tingling of fingertips or toes. Assess for loss of tendon reflexes: foot drop, slapping gait. Assess for motor difficulties: clumsiness of hands, difficulty climbing stairs, buttoning shirt, walking on heels. Notify physician of alterations; discuss holding drug if loss of deep tendon reflexes occurs. Discuss with patient the impact alterations have had, and strategies to minimize dysfunction and decrease distress. Discuss with patient type of alteration: memory and sensory/perceptual changes are temporary and reversible when drug is stopped. Assess patient for signs/symptoms of nerve dysfunction before each dose. Notify physician of any changes.

II.   ALTERATION IN BOWEL ELIMINATION related to CONSTIPATION

Defining Characteristics: Autonomic neuropathy may lead to constipation and paralytic ileus. A concurrent use of vincristine, narcotic analgesics, or cholinergic medication may increase risk of constipation.

Nursing Implications: Assess bowel elimination pattern prior to each chemotherapy administration. Teach patient to include bulky and high-fiber foods in diet, increase fluids to 3 L/day, and exercise moderately to promote elimination. Suggest stool softeners if needed. Teach patient to use laxative if unable to move bowels at least once every 2 days. Instruct patient to report abdominal pain.

III.   POTENTIAL FOR IMPAIRED SKIN INTEGRITY related to ALOPECIA

Defining Characteristics: Complete hair loss occurs in 12–45% of patients. Both men and women are at risk for body image disturbance. Hair will grow back. Dermatitis is uncommon. Drug is potent vesicant causing irritation and necrosis if infiltrated.

Nursing Implications: Discuss with patient anticipated impact of hair loss. Suggest wig or toupee as appropriate prior to actual hair loss. Explore with patient response to actual hair loss and plan strategies to minimize distress (e g , wig, scarf, cap). Assess impact on patient body image, comfort. Careful technique is used during venipuncture and intravenous administration. Administer vesicant through freely flowing IV, constantly monitoring IV site and patient response. Nurse should be THOROUGHLY familiar with institutional policy and procedure for administration of a vesicant agent. If vesicant drug is administered as a continuous infusion, drug must be given THROUGH A PATENT CENTRAL LINE. When administering the drug, if extravasation is suspected, TREAT IT AS AN INFILTRATION. Stop drug administration and aspirate any residual drug and blood from IV tubing, IV catheter/needle, and IV site if possible. Manufacturer suggests the following after withdrawing any remaining drug from IV: local installation of hyaluronidase, application of moderate heat. Assess site regularly for pain, progression of erythema, induration, and evidence of necrosis. Teach patient to assess site and notify physician if condition worsens. Arrange next clinic visit for assessment of site depending on drug, amount infiltrated, extent of potential injury, and patient variables. Document in patient's record as per institutional policy and procedure.

IV.   POTENTIAL FOR INFECTION AND BLEEDING related to BONE MARROW DEPRESSION

Defining Characteristics: Rare myelosuppression, mild when it occurs. Nadir 10–14 days after treatment begins.

Nursing Implications: Monitor CBC, HCT, platelet count prior to drug administration. Dose reduction if hepatic dysfunction: 50% reduction if bili > 1.5 mg/dL; 75% reduction if bili > 3.0 mg/dL.

V.   POTENTIAL SEXUAL DYSFUNCTION related to IMPOTENCE

Defining Characteristics: Impotence may occur related to neurotoxicity.

Nursing Implications: As appropriate, explore with patient and partner issues of reproductive and sexuality patterns, and impact chemotherapy may have. Discuss strategies to preserve sexual health, e.g., alternative expressions of sexuality. Reassure patient that impotency, if it occurs, is usually temporary, and reversible after drug discontinuance.

Drug: vinorelbine tartrate (Navelbine)

Class: Semisynthetic vinca alkaloid derived from vinblastine.

Mechanism of Action: Inhibits mitosis at metaphase by interfering with microtubule assembly. Specifically, it inhibits tubulin polymerization and binds preferentially to microtubules during mitosis so that mitosis is blocked at G_2–M phase, causing cell death. Also appears to interfere with some aspects of cellular metabolism, including cellular respiration and nucleic acid biosynthesis. Cell cycle-specific.

Metabolism: Slow elimination; extensive tissue binding (80% bound to plasma proteins); metabolized by the liver (P450 microenzyme system). Terminal half-life is 27–43 hours. Excreted in feces (46%) and urine (18%). The investigational oral form 60–80 mg/m^2 results in comparable serum levels to that of 25- to 30-mg/m^2 IV formulation. The drug is well absorbed following oral administration, T_{max} reached in 1.5 to 3 hours. The drug is significantly taken up by lung tissue, and has an elimination half-life of 35 to 40 hours. Bioavailability of the oral capsules is 33–43%, probably because of incomplete absorption and a first-pass effect in the liver. Vomiting 3 hours after swallowing the dose does not reduce the absorption of the drug.

Indication: Drug indicated as single agent or in combination with cisplatin for the first-line treatment of ambulatory patients with advanced, unresectable, non–small-cell lung cancer (NSCLC).
- Patients with stage IV NSCLC:, vinorelbine as a single agent.
- Patients with stage III, in combination with cisplatin.

Contraindications: Patients with a pretreatment ANC < 1,000 cells/mm^3.

Dosage/Range:
- IV:
  - Single agent, initial dose: 30 mg/m^2 IV over 6–10 minutes weekly until progression or dose-limiting toxicity.
  - In combination with cisplatin: 25 mg/m^2 IV every week in combination with cisplatin 100 mg/m^2 given every 4 weeks. Assess CBC/differential weekly and dose-reduce as necessary. In SWOG study, most patients required a 50% dose reduction at day 15 of each cycle, and a 50% dose reduction of cisplatin by cycle 3.
  - In combination with cisplatin: 30 mg/m^2 IV as a weekly dose, and cisplatin 120 mg/m^2 given on days 1 and 29 then every 6 weeks.

- Dose modifications
  - **Hematologic toxicity:** See package insert. If ANC on day of treatment is 1,000–1,499/ mm³, use 50% dose (i.e., 15 mg/m²); drug should be held if ANC < 1,000/mm³. If drug is held for 3 consecutive weeks because ANC < 1,000/mm³, discontinue drug.
  - If patient develops neutropenic fever or sepsis or drug is held for neutropenia for 2 consecutive doses due to granulocytopenia, dose should be:
    - ANC on day of treatment: ≥ 1,500, give 75% of starting dose.
    - ANC on day of treatment: 1,000–1,499: give 37.5% of starting dose.
  - Hepatic dysfunction: if total bili is 2.1–3.0 mg/dL, give 50% of initial dose (i.e., 15 mg/m²); if total bili is > 3.0 mg/dL, give 25% of starting dose (i.e., 7.5 mg/m²).
  - If patient requires dose adjustment for both hematologic toxicity and hepatic insufficiency: use the lower of the doses.
  - If grade 2 or higher neurotoxicity occurs, discontinue vinorelbine.

Drug Preparation:
- Drug is available as 10 mg/mL in 1- or 5-mL vials.
- Further dilute drug in syringe or IV bag in 0.9% sodium chloride or 5% dextrose to a final concentration of 1.5–3.0 mg/mL in a syringe, or 0.5–2.0 mg/mL in an IV bag.
- Prepared syringes containing the drug must be packaged in an overwrap that is labeled "DO NOT REMOVE COVERING UNTIL MOMENT OF INJECTION. FATAL IF GIVEN INTRATHECALLY. FOR INTRAVENOUS USE ONLY."
- Stable for 24 hours if refrigerated.
- Also available as a 40-mg gelatin capsule.

Drug Administration:
- Assess CBC/differential, as ANC must be 1,000 cells/mm³ or higher prior to drug administration.
- Infuse diluted drug IV over 6–10 minutes into sidearm port of freely flowing IV infusion, either peripherally or via central line. Use port CLOSEST TO THE IV BAG, not the patient.
- Flush vein with at least 75–125 mL of IV fluid after drug infusion.
- Drug is a vesicant; use vesicant precautions.
- Oral capsule should be taken on an empty stomach at bedtime.

Drug Interactions:
- Increased granulocytopenia occurs when given in combination with cisplatin.
- Possible pulmonary reactions occur when given in combination with mitomycin C, characterized by dyspnea and severe bronchospasm. May require management with bronchodilators, corticosteroids, and/or supplemental oxygen.
- CYP3A4 inhibitors (itraconazole, erythromycin, omeprazole, fluoxetine, others): increased serum drug level of vinorelbine; do not use together or assess possible toxicity and dose-reduce vinorelbine.
- CYP3A4 inducers (carbamazepine, dexamethasone, phenytoin, others): decreased serum levels of vinorelbine; do not use together or assess need to increase dose of vinorelbine. Monitor phenytoin levels and dose-modify depending upon levels, as levels may be low.

- Paclitaxel, docetaxel: give paclitaxel or docetaxel before vinorelbine to reduce myelosuppression (reverse sequence increases toxicity of paclitaxel or docetaxel).
- St. John's wort: may decrease vinorelbine effectiveness; do not give together.
- Grapefruit juice: inhibits CYP3A4 enzymes, which may increase toxicity of vinorelbine; do not use together.

Lab Effects/Interference:
- Decreased CBC (especially WBC).
- Increased LFTs.

Special Considerations:
- Drug is embryotoxic and mutagenic, so female patients of childbearing age should use effective contraception. If a patient becomes pregnant while receiving the drug, the patient should be apprised of the potential hazard to the fetus.
- Administer cautiously to patients with hepatic insufficiency. Contraindicated in patients with ANC < 1,000/mm^3.
- Use drug cautiously in patients with reduced bone marrow reserve (e.g., prior irradiation or chemotherapy).
- Drug may cause a radiation recall reaction in patients who have had prior RT.
- Avoid contamination of the eye when administering the drug. Severe eye irritation may occur; if it does, the eye should immediately be flushed with water.
- Monitor patients with history of or preexisting neuropathy for new or worsening signs and symptoms of neuropathy while receiving the drug.
- Patients should be taught to contact their physician or NP/PA if they experience increased SOB, cough, or new pulmonary symptoms, or if they experience abdominal pain or constipation.

Potential Toxicities/Side Effects and the Nursing Process

I.   INFECTION AND BLEEDING related to BONE MARROW DEPRESSION

Defining Characteristics: Leukopenia is dose-limiting toxicity; bone marrow depression noncumulative and short-lived (< 7 days), with nadir at 7–10 days. Use with caution in patients with history of prior radiotherapy or chemotherapy. Severe thrombocytopenia and anemia are uncommon.

Nursing Implications: Monitor CBC, ANC, HCT, and platelet count prior to drug administration, as well as for signs/symptoms of infection or bleeding. Instruct patient in self-assessment of signs/symptoms of infection or bleeding. Teach patient self-care measures, including avoidance of OTC aspirin-containing medications. Dose reduction necessary for hematologic toxicity (see Special Considerations section).

II.   POTENTIAL FOR SENSORY/PERCEPTUAL ALTERATIONS related to NEUROLOGIC TOXICITY

Defining Characteristics: Incidence of mild-to-moderate neuropathy is 25%. Paresthesias occur in 2–10% of patients, but incidence is increased if patient has received prior chemotherapy with vinca alkaloids or abdominal XRT. Decreased deep tendon reflexes occur in 6–29% of patients. Constipation may occur in 29% of patients. Neuropathy is reversible.

Nursing Implications: Assess baseline neuromuscular function, and reassess prior to drug infusion, especially in the presence of paresthesias; risk is increased if drug is given concurrently with cisplatin. Teach patient to report any changes in sensation or function. Identify strategies to promote comfort and safety.

III. ALTERATION IN NUTRITION, LESS THAN BODY REQUIREMENTS, related to NAUSEA/VOMITING, DIARRHEA, STOMATITIS, HEPATOTOXICITY

Defining Characteristics: Incidence of nausea/vomiting increases with oral dosing; mild in IV dosing, with an incidence of 44%. Vomiting occurs in 20% of patients. Diarrhea increases with oral dosing (17% incidence). Stomatitis is mild to moderate with < 20% incidence. Transient increases in LFTs (AST) occur in 67% of patients, and are without clinical significance.

Nursing Implications: Premedicate with antiemetic, such as a serotonin antagonist, prior to drug administration. Encourage small, frequent meals of cool, bland foods and liquids. Assess for symptoms of fluid/electrolyte imbalance if patient has severe nausea and vomiting. Monitor I/O, daily weights, and lab electrolyte values. Encourage patient to report onset of diarrhea. Administer, or teach patient to self-administer, antidiarrheal medications. Teach patient oral assessment. Teach and reinforce teaching of systemic oral hygiene regimen. Instruct patient to report early stomatitis, and provide pain relief measures as needed. Assess LFTs prior to drug administration baseline and periodically during treatment. Dose modifications may be necessary for hepatic dysfunction (see Special Considerations section).

IV. POTENTIAL FOR ALTERATION IN SKIN INTEGRITY related to ALOPECIA, EXTRAVASATION

Defining Characteristics: Gradual alopecia occurs in 10% of patients, rarely progressing to complete hair loss or requiring a wig. Severity is related to treatment duration. Drug is a moderate vesicant, primarily causing venous irritation and phlebitis; 30% of patients experience injection-site reactions commonly characterized by erythema, vein discoloration, tenderness; rarely, pain and venous irritation at sites proximal to injection site.

Nursing Implications: Discuss potential impact of hair loss prior to drug administration; also assess coping strategies, and plans to minimize body-image distortion (e.g., wig, scarf, cap). Assess patient for signs/symptoms of hair loss. Assess patient's response and use of coping strategies. Scrupulous venipuncture technique is used during venipuncture. Administer vesicant through freely flowing IV via IV port closest to IV fluid bag, not patient, and administer maximally diluted drug over 6–10 minutes (not longer). If extravasation is suspected, TREAT AS AN INFILTRATION and aspirate any remaining drug from IV tubing, locally instill hyaluronidase in area of suspected infiltration, and apply moderate heat. Assess site regularly for pain, progression of erythema, and evidence of necrosis. Document in patient's record. Schedule next clinic visit for assessment of site depending on drug, amount infiltrated, extent of potential injury, and other patient variables.

V. POTENTIAL FOR SEXUAL/REPRODUCTIVE DYSFUNCTION related to TERATOGENICITY

Defining Characteristics: Drug is teratogenic and fetotoxic.

Nursing Implications: As appropriate, explore with patient and partner issues of reproductive and sexuality patterns and the anticipated impact chemotherapy may have. Counsel female patients of childbearing age in contraceptive options.

Chapter 2
Biologic Response Modifier Therapy

Surgery, chemotherapy, and radiation therapy are the three most commonly used treatments against cancer. Biotherapy, or the use of biologic response modifiers (BRMs), comprises the fourth traditional treatment modality for cancer management. BRMs work in a variety of ways to modify the immune response so that cancer cells are injured, killed, or prevented from dividing. This category includes antibodies, cytokines, and other substances that stimulate the immune system (hemopoietic growth factors). Biologic/immune targeted therapy has recently been greatly expanded to include gene therapy and immunotherapeutic agents, such as vaccines and immune checkpoint inhibitors. In this book, *Chapter 4* addresses new agents that target specific abnormal molecular and immune events that promote malignant transformation, such as overexpression of cell surface growth factor receptors like epidermal growth factor receptor (EGFR). Inhibitors that target abnormal signal transduction and transcription factors are also included in *Chapter 4*. Monoclonal antibodies are classically targeted against molecular flaws, such as the monoclonal antibody targeting vascular endothelial growth factor (VEGF), bevacizumab (Avastin), an angiogenesis inhibitor, and epidermal growth factor receptor inhibitor cetuximab (Erbitux). Even though they are technically biologic agents, for this publication, they appear in *Chapter 4, Molecularly Targeted Therapies*.

Biologic response modifiers can:

- Have direct antitumor activity or help cancer cells become recognizable as foreign so that the host immune system can kill the cancer cells.
- Restore, augment, or modulate the host's immune system, such as inhibiting viral infection and activating natural killer (NK) and lymphocyte-activated killer (LAK) cells.
- Help the host's normal ability to repair or replace damaged cells (e.g., damaged by chemotherapy or radiotherapy).
- Interfere with tumor cell differentiation, transformation, or metastasis.

Cytokines are substances released from activated lymphocytes and include the interferons (IFNs), interleukins (ILs), tumor necrosis factor (TNF), and colony-stimulating factors (CSFs). Other BRMs are the monoclonal antibodies (MoAbs or MAbs) and vaccines.

Interferons occur naturally in the body and were the first cytokine to be studied. The interferons can be divided into two types: Type I IFNs bind to cell surface receptors on effector cells. Type I IFNs include IFN-α and IFN-β, which bind to α and β cell surface receptors on effector cells, respectively. Type II IFNs, such as IFN-γ, bind to different cell surface receptors. Interferons of both groups help to regulate the immune system, improve resistance to invading microorganisms, and halt cell proliferation, but each interferon subgroup has specific functions as well (as discussed in this chapter).

IFN-α is stimulated by viruses and tumor cells; its antiviral activity is greater than its antiproliferative activity, which is greater than its immunomodulatory effects. There are 20 subtypes of IFN-α. IFN-β is also stimulated by viruses; it has equal antiviral, antiproliferative, and immunomodulatory effects. There are two subtypes of IFN-β. IFN-γ is stimulated by cell-mediated immune response and IL-2; it is released by activated T lymphocytes and NK cells. Its immunomodulatory action is greater than its antiproliferative effect, which is greater than its antiviral effect. There are two types of this interferon. IFN-α-2a is used in the treatment of hairy-cell leukemia, acquired immunodeficiency syndrome (AIDS)-related Kaposi's sarcoma, chronic myelogenous leukemia (CML), chronic hepatitis C, and adjuvant therapy of malignant melanoma. IFN-α-2b is used for condyloma acuminata, hepatitis B and C, hairy-cell leukemia, high-risk malignant melanoma, and AIDS-related Kaposi's sarcoma. A new formulation, peginterferon alfa-2b (Sylatron), is now FDA-approved for treatment of patients with melanoma with microscopic or gross nodal involvement within 84 days of definitive surgical resection, including complete lymphadenectomy. IFN-β-1a is being studied as to its usefulness in treating AIDS-related Kaposi's sarcoma, metastatic renal cell cancer, malignant melanoma, and cutaneous T-cell lymphoma. IFN-γ is used for B-cell malignancies, chronic myelogenous leukemia, and renal cell cancer, and is being studied in ovarian cancer. Common side effects of interferons include flulike symptoms, anorexia, and fatigue.

Colony-stimulating factors include hematopoietic growth factors. They too occur naturally in the body and help immature blood cell elements develop into mature, effective white blood cells, red blood cells, and platelets. Recombinant DNA techniques have permitted the manufacture of large quantities of these substances. An "r" prefix (e.g., r-IL-2) indicates that it was produced using recombinant technology.

The use of colony-stimulating growth factors has permitted increased doses of chemotherapy to be given safely. Filgrastim (Neupogen) and tbo-filgrastim (Neutroval, Granix) are granulocyte-colony-stimulating factors (G-CSF) approved to prevent infection related to febrile neutropenia following bone marrow suppressive chemotherapy, as well as for other uses, and a sustained-duration pegylated formulation requiring less frequent dosing is available (pegfilgrastim or Neulasta). This is called primary prophylaxis and begins after the first cycle of chemotherapy. Primary prophylaxis is used to prevent febrile neutropenia in high-risk patients (e.g., age, medical history, disease characteristics, expected chemotherapy myelotoxicity) (Smith et al., 2015). Secondary prophylaxis is when the growth factor is used to prevent the recurrence of febrile neutropenia in a patient who has not used growth factor in the past, and therapeutic use is when the growth factor is used at the time of neutropenia or neutropenic fever in high-risk individuals, such as those with sepsis syndrome, pneumonia, or fungal infection (Barbour and Crawford, 2007).

In order to provide guidance and recommendations for evidence-based practice, the American Society of Clinical Oncology (ASCO) published guidelines for the use of colony-stimulating factors. In 2015, ASCO updated recommendations for the use of white blood cell growth factors, creating an evidence-based practice guideline. The guideline emphasizes that the reduction of febrile neutropenia is an important clinical outcome justifying the use of CSFs, regardless of the impact on other factors, when the risk of febrile neutropenia is 20% or more and there is no other equally effective anticancer regimen that does not require CSFs available. An example of a common breast cancer regimen with a 20% or greater incidence of febrile neutropenia is Adriamycin and Cytoxan followed by Taxol (AC T). Additional regimens can be found in the 2014 Myeloid Growth Factor NCCN Guideline, found at http://www.nccn.org. Patient factors and comorbidities can also increase the risk for febrile neutropenia; these include a history of severe neutropenia with similar chemotherapy, extensive prior chemotherapy, poor performance or nutritional status, age older than 65 years, bone marrow involvement with tumor, open wounds, and liver disease (NCCN, 2014). In addition, CSFs permit the administration of dose-dense chemotherapy regimens as part of a clinical trial or as supported by efficacy data. Dose dense regimens that require CSFs should only be used in a clinical trial or if supported by strong evidence to support efficacy (Smith et al., 2015). For example, prophylactic G-CSF permits patients with diffuse aggressive lymphoma, aged 65 or older who are being treated with curative intent, to have reduced risk of febrile neutropenia and infections (Smith et al., 2006). NCCN guidelines (2014) suggest that patients with solid tumors or nonmyeloid malignancies should be evaluated for risk of febrile neutropenia prior to the first cycle of chemotherapy in terms of disease, chemotherapy regimen (high dose, dose dense, or standard dose), patient risk factors (e.g., age 65 or older, prior history of neutropenia), and treatment intent (e.g., cure vs. control vs. palliation). If the risk of febrile neutropenia is high (> 20%), CSF as primary prophylaxis should be used. If the risk is intermediate (10–20%), consider CSF. If it is low, < 10%, CSF should not be prescribed. Following the first cycle of chemotherapy, and with subsequent cycles, if the patient develops febrile neutropenia or a dose-limiting neutropenic event, and G-CSF was used with cycle 1, consider dose reduction or change in treatment regimen. If G-CSF was not used before, consider secondary prophylaxis with CSF. If no febrile or other dose-limiting neutropenic event occurred, reassess after each subsequent treatment cycle. Febrile neutropenia is defined as a single temperature $\geq 38.3°C$ ($101°F$) orally or $\geq 38°C$ ($100.4°F$) over 1 hour; neutropenia is defined as < 500 neutrophils/mm^3 or < 1,000 neutrophils/mm^3 with an anticipated decline to ≤ 500 cells/mm^3 over the next 48 hours. NCCN (2014) recommendations for use of CSF to treat patients who present with febrile neutropenia are as follows: if the patient is currently receiving prophylactic G-CSF (e.g., filgrastim or sargramostim), continue it. If the patient has received prophylactic pegfilgrastim, do not give additional G-CSF. If the patient did not receive prophylactic CSF and has risk factors for an infection-associated complication (e.g., sepsis syndrome, age > 65 years, severe neutropenia with ANC < 100/mm^3, neutropenia expected to last more than 10 days in duration, pneumonia, invasive fungal infection, hospitalized at the time of fever, prior episode of febrile neutropenia, and other clinically documented infections), consider giving G-CSF.

Sargramostim, or granulocyte-macrophage colony-stimulating factor (GM-CSF), is approved for myeloid reconstitution after autologous bone marrow transplantation and for other uses. It is now being studied in use with dendritic cell vaccines. Both G-CSF and GM-CSF can be used to mobilize stem cells that will be used to rescue the bone marrow after high-dose chemotherapy.

EPO or rHuEPO (erythropoietin) has become standard therapy as an adjunct to chemotherapy in certain regimens. Together with the American Society of Hematology Colleagues, ASCO guidelines assert that there is strong evidence to use epoetin as a treatment option for patients with chemotherapy-associated anemia with a hemoglobin concentration below 10 g/dL (Rizzo et al., 2002). However, despite beliefs that increasing the hemoglobin beyond 12 g/dL would improve patient response and quality of life, studies showed the converse; in fact, using erythropoiesis-stimulating agents (ESAs) to target a hemoglobin of 12 g/dL or higher in cancer patients resulted in shortened time to tumor progression in patients with advanced head and neck cancer receiving radiation therapy, shortened overall survival, increased deaths related to disease progression in patients with metastatic breast cancer receiving chemotherapy, and increased risk of death in cancer patients not receiving chemotherapy or radiation therapy (FDA, 2007). Three meta-analyses confirmed these findings in patients with breast, NSCLC, head and neck, lymphoid, and cervical cancers, while two did not (NCCN, 2014). As a result, the FDA issued an alert (on March 9, 2008) that required all ESA package inserts to add to the black-box warning that ESAs be used only on label (e.g., while patients are receiving myelosuppressive chemotherapy). ESAs are *not* indicated when the anticipated outcome is cure. In addition, Medicare (CMS) revised their guidelines to tighten reimbursement for ESAs. The target hemoglobin has now been changed to 10 g/dL, with initiation tied to Hgb < 10 g/dL (HCT < 30%) for a maximum of 8 weeks, and the threshold for holding ESAs is the lowest dose necessary to avoid RBC transfusion (NCCN, 2014). In addition, it is imperative to analyze the patient's iron status and replete as necessary. IV iron appears to be superior to oral iron (NCCN, 2014). The NCCN Cancer and Chemotherapy-Induced Anemia Guidelines specify recommendations for administering parenteral iron products (e.g., iron dextran, ferric gluconate, iron sucrose) (NCCN, v.1, 2014).

In February 2010, the FDA required that oncologists/hematologists comply with their Risk Evaluation and Mitigation Strategy (REMS), which was developed by Amgen at the FDA's direction. This requires that within 1 year, physicians and hospitals must register, undergo training, and be certified through the ESA APPRISE Oncology Program in order to continue to prescribe and dispense ESAs. In addition, healthcare professionals must give all patients receiving ESAs the FDA-approved Medication Guide containing information about the drugs' risks and benefits. An example of the patient guide is found at http://www.fda.gov/downloads/Drugs/DrugSafety/UCM085918.pdf. Patients are required to sign the ESA APPRISE Oncology Patient and Healthcare Professional (HCP) Acknowledgment Form, which documents that the HCP has discussed the risks of ESAs with the patient. Specifically, the guide informs the patient that the prescribed ESA may make the tumor grow faster, the patient may die sooner, and the patient may develop blood clots and serious heart problems (e.g., MI, CHF, or stroke) if the drug is used to increase the hemoglobin beyond "the amount needed to avoid red blood cell transfusions." In addition, the guide suggests questions to ask the physician.

In summary, when ESAs are prescribed, based on FDA and NCCN Guidelines (v.3; 2014):

- First, evaluate cause of anemia if Hgb < 10 g/dL or ≥ 2 g/dL below baseline, and if no cause found, consider anemia related to inflammation or myelosuppressive chemotherapy.
- Use the lowest dose to prevent red blood cell transfusion.
- Use only for treatment of anemia due to concomitant myelosuppressive chemotherapy (noncurative).
- Use fixed titration.
- ESAs are not indicated for patients receiving myelosuppressive therapy when the anticipated outcome is cure.
- Discontinue ESA therapy following the completion of a chemotherapy course.

Platelet growth factor, oprelvekin (Neumega), or IL-11 can be used to prevent and treat thrombocytopenia after myelosuppressive chemotherapy and results in a modest increase in platelets; however, it has side effects that have limited its utility. A new agent, romiplostim (Nplate), is a "peptibody" or peptide antibody that mimics the activity of thrombopoietin to stimulate platelet production. Clinical trials in patients with immune thrombocytopenia purpura (ITP) have shown significant benefit (Kuter et al., 2008). The drug has recently been FDA-approved for the treatment of thrombocytopenia in patients with chronic immune (idiopathic) thrombocytopenia purpura (ITP). An oral agent, eltrombopag (Promacta), works similarly and is also FDA-approved for treatment of ITP. Research continues on thrombopoietin (TPO), which has a peak effect in 12 days, which often is when the nadir effect of chemotherapy occurs. Common side effects of colony-stimulating factors may include bone pain, fatigue, anorexia, and fever.

IL-2 is another naturally occurring cytokine that is made using recombinant technology. It is indicated for the treatment of adults with metastatic renal cell carcinoma and adults with metastatic malignant melanoma; recently, an inhaled high-dose form given together with dacarbazine has been shown to reduce lung metastases from malignant melanoma (Enk et al., 2000). IL-12 is gaining much attention due to its ability to stimulate NK activity and antitumor potential, as well as its synergistic action with IL-2, GM-CSF, and calcium ionophore to enhance dendritic cell function (Bedrosian et al., 2000). IL-12 is being studied in gene therapy (Divino et al., 2000). Side effects of interleukins include flulike symptoms, fatigue, and anorexia, as well as substance-specific side effects; for example, IL-2 can cause serious side effects, depending upon dose, such as capillary leak syndrome. Research exploring the cytokine IL-7 shows that in the recombinant form given SQ every other day for 2 weeks, patients' immune systems are stimulated to make large numbers of T-helper lymphocytes (CD4+ increased by 300%), and cytotoxic CD8 + cells increased by over 400%; the elevated T cells remained elevated for 6 weeks after the end of therapy (Sportes et al., 2008).

While many BRMs are still investigational (i.e., being studied in clinical research trials to determine their effectiveness, optimal dose, and method of administration), many are quickly being approved for use. Expected side effects vary according to agent, dose, and patient characteristics. In general, flulike symptoms (fever, chills, rigor, malaise, arthralgias, headache, myalgias, and anorexia) may occur. Routes of administration include intravenous (IV), intramuscular (IM), intraperitoneal (IP), subcutaneous (SQ), intralesional, inhaled, and topical.

Currently, palifermin or recombinant human keratinocyte growth factor has shown remarkable success in decreasing the oral mucositis associated with bone marrow transplant, and it has been approved by the FDA for use in patients undergoing bone marrow transplantation.

While G-CSF is often used in stem cell mobilization for patients undergoing high-dose chemotherapy with stem cell transplant, a new agent, plerixafor (Mozobil), has recently been FDA-approved for mobilization of peripheral blood hematopoietic stem cells.

Finally, monoclonal antibodies are produced to target a single foreign antigen, and they are designed to attach to specific cancer antigens. Monoclonal antibodies can become targeted therapies and have demonstrated an active role in molecularly targeted therapies. Therefore, further discussion of monoclonal antibodies and specific agents can be found in *Chapter 4,* Molecularly Targeted Therapies.

References

Amgen Inc. Neupogen (filgrastim) [package insert]. Thousand Oaks, CA, February 2014.

Barbour SY, Crawford J. Hematopoietic Growth Factors. Pazdur R, Coia LR, Hoskins WJ, Wagman LD (eds). *Cancer Management: A Multidisciplinary Approach,* 10th ed. Lawrence, KS: CMP Healthcare Media LLC; 2007.

Battiato LA. Biologic and Targeted Therapy. Yarbro CH, Frogge MH, Goodman M, eds. *Cancer Nursing: Principles and Practice,* 6th ed. Sudbury, MA: Jones & Bartlett Learning, 2005; 510–559.

Bedrosian L, Roras JG, Xu S. Granulocyte-Macrophage Colony-Stimulating Factor, Interleukin-2a and Interleukin-12 Synergize with Calcium Ionophore to Enhance Dendritic Cell Function. *J Immunother* 2000; 23(3) 311–320.

Bernstein SH. Future of Basic/Clinical Hematopoiesis: Research in the Era of Hematopoietic Growth Factor Availability. *Semin Oncol* 1992; 19(4) 441–448.

Bronchud MH, Scarffe JH, Thatcher N, et al. Phase I/II Study of Recombinant Human Granulocyte Colony-Stimulating Factor in Patients Receiving Intensive Chemotherapy for SCLC. *Br J Cancer* 1987; 56809–56813.

Eggermont AM, Suciu S, Santinami M, et al. Adjuvant Therapy with Pegylated Interferon Alfa-2b Versus Observation Alone in Resected Stage III Melanoma; Final Results of EORTC 18991, a Randomised Phase III Trial. *Lancet* 2008; 372(9633) 117–126.

Egrie JC, Dwyer E, Lykos M, et al. Novel Erythropoiesis Stimulating Protein (NESP) Has a Longer Serum Half-Life and Greater in Vivo Biological Activity than Recombinant Human Erythropoietin (rHuEPO). *Blood* 1997; 90(10) abstract 243 (Suppl 1).

Enk AH, Nashan D, Rubben A, Knop J. High-Dose Inhalation Interleukin-2 Therapy for Lung Metastases in Patients with Malignant Melanoma. *Cancer* 2000; 88(9) 2042–2046.

Federal Drug Administration. Erythropoiesis Stimulating Agent Warning. March 9, 2008. http://www .fda.gov/cder/drug/infopage/RHE/default.htm. Accessed July 9, 2008.

Gabrilove JL, Cleeland CS, Livingston RB. Clinical Evaluation of Once Weekly Dosing of Epoetin Alfa in Chemotherapy Patients: Improvements in Hemoglobin and Quality of Life Are Similar to Three Times Weekly Dosing. *J Clin Oncol* 2001;19(11) 2875–2882.

Genzyme Corporation. Thyrogen (package insert). Cambridge, MA: Genzyme Corp. March 2014.

GlaxoSmithKline. Promacta (eltrombopag) [Package insert]. Research Triangle Park, NC, February 2014.

Kammula US, White D, Rosenberg SA. Trends in the Safety of High-Dose Bolus Interleukin-2 Administration in Patients with Metastatic Cancer. *Cancer* 1998; 83(4) 797–805.

Kuter DJ, Bussel JB, Lyons RM, et al. Efficacy of Romiplostim in Patients with Chronic Immune Thrombocytopenic Purpura: A Double-Blind Randomised Controlled Trial. *Lancet* 2008; 371(9610) 395–403.

Merck and Co, Inc. Intron A [Package insert]. Whitehouse Station, NJ, April 2014.

Merck and Co, Inc. Zostavax [package insert]. Whitehouse Station, NJ, February 2014.

National Comprehensive Cancer Network (NCCN). *Clinical Practice Guidelines Cancer and Treatment Related Anemia* v3.2014. http://www.nccn.org. Accessed June 7, 2014.

National Comprehensive Cancer Network (NCCN). *Clinical Practice Guidelines Myeloid Growth Factors* v2. 2014, http://www.nccn.org. Accessed August 13, 2014.

Pacini F, Molinaro E, Castagna MG, Lippi F, Ceccarelli C, Agate L, Elisei R, Pinchera A. Ablation of Thyroid Residues with 30 mCi 131I: A Comparison in Thyroid Cancer Patients Prepared with Recombinant Human TSH or Thyroid Hormone Withdrawal. *J Clin Endocrinol Metab* 2002; 87 4063–4068.

Rizzo JD, Lichtin AE, Woolf SH, et al. Use of Epoetin in Patients with Cancer: Evidence-Based Clinical Practice Guidelines of the American Society of Clinical Oncology and the American Society of Hematology. *Blood* 2002; 100(7) 2303–2320.

Simpson C, Seipp CA, Rosenbery SA. The Current Status and Future Applications of Interleukin-2 and Adoptive Immunotherapy in Cancer Treatment. *Semin Oncol Nurs* 1988; 4132–4141.

Smith TJ, Bohike L, Lyman GH, et al. Recommendations for the use of WBC growth factors: American Society of Clinical Oncology Clinical practice guideline update. [Published ahead of print July 13, 2015]. *J Clin Oncol*. doi: 10.1200/JCO.2015.62.3488.

Spielberger R, Emmanouilides C, Stiff P, et al. Use of Recombinant Human Keratinocyte Growth Factor (rHuKGF) Can Reduce Severe Oral Mucositis in Patients with Hematologic Malignancies Undergoing Autologous Peripheral Blood Progenitor Cell Transplantation (Auto-PBPCT) after Radiation-Based Conditioning–Results of a Phase 3 Trial. *Proc Am Soc Clin Oncol* 2003; 2(2) 122, abstract 3642.

Sportes C, Hakim FT, Memon SA, et al. Administration of rhIL-7 in Humans Increases in Vivo TCR Repertoire Diversity by Preferential Expansion of Naïve T Cell Subsets. *J Exp Med* 2008. Accessed June 23, 2008.

Swanson G, Bergstrom K, Stump E, et al. Growth Factor Usage Patterns and Outcomes in the Community Setting: Collection Through a Practice-Based Computerized Clinical Information System. *J Clin Oncol* 2000; 18(8) 1764–1770.

Teva Pharmaceuticals USA. Tbo-filgrastim (Granix) [package insert]. North Wales, PA, August 2012.

Timar J, Ladanyi A, Forster-Horvath C, et al. Neoadjuvant Immunotherapy of Oral Squamous Cell Carcinoma Modulates Intratumoral CD4/CD8 Ratio and Tumor Microenvironment: A Multicenter Phase II Clinical Trial. *J Clin Oncol* 2005; 23(15) 3421–3432.

Drug: aldesleukin (interleukin-2, Proleukin)

Class: Cytokine.

Mechanism of Action: Interleukin-2 (IL-2), previously called T-cell growth factor, is produced by helper T cells following antibody-antigen reaction (processed antigen is mounted on macrophage) and IL-1. IL-2 amplifies the immune response to an antigen by immunomodulation and immunorestoration. IL-2 stimulates T-lymphocyte proliferation, enhances killer T-cell activity, increases antibody production (secondary to increased B-cell proliferation), helps to increase synthesis of other cytokines (IFNs, IL-1, -3, -4, -5, -6, CSFs), and stimulates production and activation of natural killer (NK) cells and other cytotoxic cells (LAK and TIL).

Metabolism: The half-life of distribution is 13 minutes, whereas the elimination half-life is 85 minutes.

Indication: For the treatment of adults with (1) metastatic renal cell carcinoma; (2) metastatic melanoma. Patient selection must be careful and exclude patients with significant cardiac, pulmonary, renal, hepatic, or CNS impairment.

Contraindications: In (1) patients with a known history of hypersensitvity to IL-2 or any component of Proleukin; (2) patients with an abnormal thallium stress test or abnormal pulmonary function tests, and those with organ allografts. Retreatment with (3) Proleukin is contraindicated in patients who have experienced the following drug-related toxicities while receiving an earlier course of therapy:

- Sustained ventricular tachycardia (≥ 5 beats), uncontrolled cardiac rhythm disturbances, EKG changes showing angina or MI, cardiac tamponade.
- Intubation > 72 hours.
- Renal failure requiring dialysis > 72 hours.
- Coma or toxic psychosis lasting > 48 hours; difficult to control seizures.
- Bowel ischemia or perforation, GI bleeding requiring surgery.

Delay with resumption of dose after resolution of symptoms and condition resolved or ruled out:
- Persistent atrial fibrillation, supraventricular tachycardia, or bradycardia.
- Hypotension (SBP < 90 mm Hg with need for pressors).
- EKG change showing MI, ischemia, myocarditis.
- O_2 saturation < 90%.
- Mental status changes (confusion, agitation).
- Sepsis.
- Serum creatinine > 4.5 mg/dL or ≥ 4 mg/dL with severe volume overload, acidosis, or hyperkalemia; persistent oliguria, urine output < 10 mL/hr for 16–24 hours with increasing serum creatinine.
- Signs of hepatic failure (encephalopathy, increasing ascites, liver pain, hypoglycemia): stop this course of treatment and reinitiate new course after at least 7 weeks of rest.
- Stool guaiac repeatedly > 3–4+.
- Bullous dermatitis or marked worsening of preexisting skin condition (do not use topical steroid therapy).

Dosage/Range:
Metastatic renal cell carcinoma and metastatic malignant melanoma:
- 600,000 IU/kg (0.037 mg/kg) IVB over 15 minutes every 8 hours for a maximum of 14 doses over 5 days and then a 9-day rest, followed by 14 additional doses every 8 hours, for a maximum of 28 doses per course as tolerated. Evaluate for response 4 weeks after completion of a course and before the next treatment course. Tumor shrinkage should be seen before retreatment. Seven-week rest period should separate discharge from the hospital and retreatment. Delay and drug holiday should be used rather than drug dose reduction to manage toxicity.

Drug Preparation:
- Vial containing 22 million international units (1.3 mg) should be reconstituted with 1.2 mL of sterile water for injection, USP so each mL contains 18 million international units of drug. DO NOT SHAKE. Further dilute in 50 mL of 5% dextrose injection, USP. If dose is < 1.5 mg, use a smaller volume. Refrigerate and use within 48 hours of preparation. Bring to room temperature before administration.

Drug Administration:
- Final concentration should be between 30–70 μg/mL.
- Use plastic IV bags instead of glass bottles, and do not use in-line filters.
- Administer IV over 15 minutes.

Drug Interactions:
- Potentiation of CNS effects when given in combination with psychotropic drugs.
- The combination with nephrotoxic, myelotoxic, cardiotoxic, or hepatotoxic drugs will increase toxicity of aldesleukin in these organ systems.
- Increased risk of hypersensitivity reactions when sequential high-dose aldesleukin combined with dacarbazine, cisplatin, tamoxifen, and IFN-α.
- IFN-α and aldesleukin concurrently: increased risk of myocardial injury (MI, myocarditis, severe rhabdomyolysis).
- Glucocorticoid steroids: decreased antitumor effectiveness. Do not use together.
- β-Blockers, antihypertensives: potentiate hypotension of aldesleukin.
- Iodinated contrast medium: increased risk of atypical adverse reaction (12.6% incidence) characterized by fever, chills, nausea, vomiting, pruritus, rash, diarrhea, hypotension, edema, and oliguria and typically happens when contrast is given within 4 weeks of aldesleukin dosing.

Lab Effects/Interference:
- Anemia, leukopenia, thrombocytopenia.
- Elevated LFTs.
- Increased serum creatinine.
- Acidosis.

Special Considerations:
- Patient must have NORMAL cardiac, pulmonary, hepatic, renal (serum creatinine ≤ 1.5 mg/dL), and CNS function before treatment and be free of any known infection.
- Baseline testing includes the following, which should be repeated daily during drug administration:
  - Standard CBC, differential, and platelet counts.
  - Blood chemistries (including electrolytes, renal, and hepatic function tests).
  - Chest X-ray.
  - Baseline PFTs with arterial blood gases (ABGs) with FEV_1 > 2 liters or ≥ 75% predicted for height and age prior to starting therapy.
  - Baseline stress thallium study with normal ejection fraction and unimpaired wall motion.
  - Daily monitoring during therapy of VS including pulse oximetry, cardiopulmonary exam, weight, and fluid I/O. If the patient has a systolic BP < 90 mm Hg, patient should receive continuous telemetry, EKG documentation of any abnormal rhythm, and hourly VS monitoring. If patient develops dyspnea, assess ABGs. If angina develops, patient should have cardiac enzyme evaluation and further cardiac workup.
- Drug may worsen symptoms of patients with unknown/untreated CNS metastases. Thorough evaluation and treatment of CNS metastases should precede the treatment so that the patient has a negative scan before starting aldesleukin.

- Aldesleukin is associated with capillary leak syndrome (CLS), characterized by loss of vascular tone and extravasation of plasma proteins and fluid into the extravascular space; this results in hypotension and reduced organ perfusion, which can be severe and fatal. CLS may be associated with cardiac arrhythmias, angina, myocardial infarction, respiratory insufficiency requiring intubation, GI bleeding or infarction, renal insufficiency, edema, and mental status changes.
- Aldesleukin is associated with impaired neutrophil function (reduced chemotaxis), with increased risk of disseminated infection (e.g., sepsis, bacterial endocarditis). Preexisting bacterial infections should be fully treated before starting aldesleukin therapy. Patients with indwelling central lines are at high risk for infection with gram-positive microorganisms; antibiotic prophylaxis with oxacillin, nafcillin, ciprofloxacin, or vancomycin has been shown to reduce the incidence of staphylococcal infections.
- Drug should be withheld in patients with moderate to severe lethargy or somnolence, because aldesleukin administration can result in coma.
- Use caution when patient is receiving other drugs that are hepatic or renally toxic.
- Drug may increase rejection in allogeneic transplant patients, exacerbation of autoimmune disease, and inflammatory disorders.
- Drug should be used during pregnancy only if the potential benefit justifies the potential risk to the fetus.
- Nursing mothers should make a decision to discontinue nursing or to discontinue the drug, taking into consideration the importance of the drug to the mother's health.

Potential Toxicities/Side Effects (Dose-1 and Schedule-Dependent) and the Nursing Process

I.   ALTERATION IN COMFORT related to FLULIKE SYNDROME

Defining Characteristics: Chills may occur 2–4 hours after dose; rigors are possible; fever to 39–40°C (102–104°F), and headache. Myalgia and arthralgias may occur at high doses because of accumulation of cytokine deposits/lymphocytes in joint spaces. The incidence of chills is 52%, fever 29%, malaise 27%, asthenia 23%, anorexia 20%.

Nursing Implications: Assess baseline T, VS, neurologic status, and comfort level, and monitor every 4–6 hours if patient is in hospital. Discuss with physician premedication and regular dosing of antipyretic (e.g., acetaminophen ± diphenhydramine, NSAID). If patient is in hospital and experiences rigor, discuss with physician IV meperidine and monitor BP for hypotension.

II.   SENSORY/PERCEPTUAL ALTERATION related to CNS EFFECTS

Defining Characteristics: Confusion, irritability, disorientation, impaired memory, expressive aphasia, sleep disturbances, depression, hallucinations, and psychoses may occur, resolving within 24–48 hours after last drug dose. Mental status abnormalities exaggerated by anxiety and sleep deprivation.

Nursing Implications: Assess baseline mental status and neurologic status before drug administration. Assess patient for changes (impaired memory/attention, disorientation, slow/vague responses to questions, increased lethargy) during treatment. Teach patient to report signs/symptoms. Provide information, emotional support, and interventions to ensure safety if signs/symptoms occur.

III. ALTERATION IN CARDIAC OUTPUT related to HYPOTENSION (HIGH-DOSE THERAPY)

Defining Characteristics: Increased risk with dose > 100,000 IU/kg. Capillary leak syndrome (peripheral edema, CHF, pleural effusions, and pericardial effusions) may occur and is reversible once treatment is stopped. Atrial arrhythmias may occur; occasionally, supraventricular tachycardia, myocarditis, chest pain; and rarely, myocardial infarction. IL-2 causes peripheral vasodilation, decreased systemic vascular resistance, and hypotension that may lead to decreased renal perfusion. A decrease in SBP occurs 2–12 hours after start of therapy and typically will progress to significant hypotension (SBP < 90 mm Hg or a 20-mm Hg drop from baseline SBP) with hypoperfusion. In addition, protein and fluids will extravasate into the extravascular space, forming edema and new effusions.

Nursing Implications: Assess baseline cardiopulmonary status and patients at risk (the older population, those with preexisting cardiac dysfunction). Monitor VS and pulse oximetry frequently, at least q 4 hour (if hypotensive, q 1 hr), noting rate, rhythm of heartbeat, blood pressure, urinary output, fluid status. I/O q 4 hours or more frequently, and daily weights during therapy. Discuss any abnormalities with physician, and revise plan as needed (e.g., diuretics, plasma expanders). Instruct patient to report signs or symptoms of dyspnea, chest pain, edema, or other abnormalities immediately. Hypotension requires fluid replacement, and patient should be monitored with continuous cardiac monitoring if SBP < 90 mm Hg. Any ectopy should be documented on ECG. Manufacturer states that early administration of dopamine (1–5 mcg/kg/min) to patients with capillary leak syndrome before the onset of hypotension can improve organ perfusion and preserve urinary output. Increased dopamine doses (6–10 mcg/kg/min) or the addition of phenylephrine hydrochloride (1–5 mcg/kg/min) to low-dose dopamine has been described. After blood pressure is stabilized, the use of diuretics is often effective in relieving edema and pulmonary congestion.

IV. POTENTIAL ALTERATION IN OXYGENATION

Defining Characteristics: Pulmonary symptoms are dose related, such as dyspnea and tachypnea. Pulmonary edema may occur with hypoxia because of fluid shifts.

Nursing Implications: Assess baseline cardiopulmonary status every 4 hours during therapy, noting rate, rhythm, depth of respirations, presence of dyspnea, and breath sounds (presence of wheezes, crackles, rhonchi). Identify patients at risk: those with preexisting cardiac or pulmonary disease, prior treatment with cardio-or pulmonary-toxic drugs or radiation, and smoking history. Instruct the patient to report cough, dyspnea, or change in respiratory status. Strictly monitor I/O, total fluid balance, and daily weight. Discuss abnormalities with physician, as well as the need for oxygen, diuretics, or transfer to ICU.

V.   POTENTIAL ALTERATION IN NUTRITION, LESS THAN BODY
     REQUIREMENTS, related to NAUSEA/VOMITING, DIARRHEA,
     MUCOSITIS, ANOREXIA

Defining Characteristics: Nausea and vomiting are mild and are effectively controlled by antiemetics. Diarrhea is common and can be severe. Stomatitis is common but mild.

Nursing Implications: Assess the patient's baseline nutritional status. Administer antiemetics as ordered. Teach the patient potential side effects and self-care measures, including oral hygiene, and encourage patient to eat favorite high-calorie, high-protein foods. Teach self-administration of prescribed antiemetics and antidiarrheals as needed. Refer to the dietitian as appropriate.

VI. POTENTIAL ALTERATION IN ELIMINATION related to RENAL
     DYSFUNCTION, HEPATOTOXICITY

Defining Characteristics: IL-2 causes decreased renal blood flow with cumulative doses. Oliguria, proteinuria, increased serum creatinine and BUN, and increased LFTs (bili, AST, ALT, LDH, alk phos) may occur. Anuria occurs in 5% of patients; renal dysfunction is reversible after drug discontinuance. Hepatomegaly and hypoalbuminemia may occur.

Nursing Implications: Assess baseline renal and hepatic functions and monitor during treatment. Assess fluid and electrolyte balance, urine output hourly, and total body balance. Dipstick urine for protein. Discuss abnormalities with physician and revise plan.

VII. POTENTIAL FOR FATIGUE AND BLEEDING related to ANEMIA,
     THROMBOCYTOPENIA

Defining Characteristics: Anemia occurs in 29% of patients and may require RBC transfusion. Thrombocytopenia occurs commonly but rarely requires transfusion.

Nursing Implications: Assess baseline CBC and platelet count and signs/symptoms of fatigue, severe anemia, bleeding. Instruct the patient to report signs/symptoms immediately and to manage self-care (alternate rest/activity, minimize bleeding by avoidance of OTC aspirin-containing medicines). Transfuse red cells and platelets as ordered.

VIII. POTENTIAL ALTERATION IN SKIN INTEGRITY related to DIFFUSE RASH

Defining Characteristics: Patients may develop diffuse erythematous rash, which may desquamate (soles of feet, palms of hands, between fingers). Pruritus may occur with or without rash.

Nursing Implications: Assess baseline skin integrity. Teach patient to report signs and symptoms. Discuss/teach symptomatic management, including the use of mild soaps and rinsing skin thoroughly after bathing. Encourage the use of alcohol-free, oil-based moisturizers on skin and the protection of desquamated areas.

Drug: darbepoetin alfa (Aranesp)

Class: Cytokine, CSF.

Mechanism of Action: Recombinant DNA protein that is an erythropoiesis-stimulating protein, closely resembling erythropoietin. Drug is produced in the Chinese hamster ovary. Drug stimulates erythropoiesis in the same way that endogenous erythropoietin does in response to hypoxia. Darbepoetin alfa interacts with progenitor stem cells to stimulate red blood cell production.

Metabolism: Following subcutaneous administration of Aranesp to patients with CKD (receiving or not receiving dialysis), absorption was slow and C_{max} occurred at 48 hours (range: 12 to 72 hours). In patients with CKD receiving dialysis, the average t1/2 was 46 hours (range: 12 to 89 hours), and in patients with CKD not receiving dialysis, the average t1/2 was 70 hours (range: 35 to 139 hours). Aranesp apparent clearance was approximately 1.4 times faster on average in patients receiving dialysis compared to patients not receiving dialysis. The bioavailability of Aranesp in patients with CKD receiving dialysis after subcutaneous administration was 37% (range: 30% to 50%).

Indication: For the treatment of anemia due to (1) effects of concomitant myelosuppressive chemotherapy, and upon initiation, there is a minimum of 2 additional months of planned chemotherapy; (2) chronic kidney disease in patients on dialysis and patients not on dialysis. Drug has not been shown to improve quality of life, fatigue, or patient well-being.

   Not Indicated: For use (1) in patients with cancer receiving hormonal agents, biologic products, or RT, unless also receiving concomitant myelosuppressive chemotherapy; (2) in patients with cancer receiving myelosuppressive chemotherapy when the anticipated outcome is cure; (3) as a substitute for RBC transfusions in patients who require immediate correction of anemia.

Contraindications: Patients with (1) uncontrolled hypertension; (2) pure red cell aplasia that begins after treatment with darbapoietin or other erythropoietin protein drugs; (3) serious allergic reactions to darbapoietin.

Dosage/Range:

- Only prescribers and hospitals enrolled in the ESA APPRISE Oncology Program may prescribe or dispense Aranesp. Prior to each new course of Aranesp, prescribers and patients must provide written acknowledgment of a discussion of Aranesp risks.
- Use the *lowest dose* of darbepoetin alfa necessary to avoid RBC transfusion. Should not be used if goal is cure.
- Cancer patients receiving chemotherapy: initiate only if Hgb < 10 g/dL and there is a minimum of 2 additional months of planned chemotherapy:
  - 2.25 micrograms/kg subcutaneously q week until completion of a chemotherapy course, OR
  - 500 micrograms every 3 weeks subcutaneously until completion of a chemotherapy course.

- Modifications:
  - If Hgb increases by > 1.0 g/dL in 2-week period or when Hgb reaches level to avoid RBC transfusion, reduce dose by 40% of the prior dose when using weekly or every 3-week schedule.
  - If Hgb > level to avoid RBC transfusion, hold dose until Hgb falls to point where transfusion may be needed and restart at 40% below previous dose, when using weekly or every 3-week schedule.
  - If Hgb increases by < 1 g/dL and remains < 10 g/dL after 6 weeks of therapy, increase dose to 4.5 micrograms/kg/week when given weekly, but not when given every 3 weeks.
  - If there is no response as measured by Hgb levels or if RBC transfusions are still required after 8 weeks of therapy, or following completion of a chemotherapy course, discontinue Aranesp whether weekly or every 3-week schedule is being used.
- Dose increases should not occur more frequently than once a month.
- Goal is to prevent or treat deficit of oxygen-carrying capacity (NCCN, 2014): (1) if asymptomatic, in hemodynamically stable chronic anemia without acute coronary syndrome (ACS), goal is Hgb 7–9 g/dL; (2) symptomatic anemia: (a) acute hemorrhage with evidence of hemodynamic instability or inadequate oxygen delivery: transfuse to correct; (b) Hgb < 10 g/dL with tachycardia, postural hypotension, goal is maintain Hgb 8-10 g/dL; (c) anemia with ACS or acute MI: transfusion goal to maintain Hgb ≥ 10 g/dL.
- Chronic renal failure patients: 0.45 micrograms/kg IV or SC q weekly, OR 0.75 mcg/kg IV, or SQ every 2 weeks. IV is recommended for patients on dialysis. Recommended starting dose for patients not on dialysis is 0.45 mcg/kg IV, or SQ at 4-week intervals.
  - If increase in Hgb is < 1.0 g/dL over 4 weeks and iron stores are adequate, increase dose by 25% of the previous dose; dose may be increased at 4-week intervals until Hgb is 10–12 g/dL; dose increase no more frequently than once a month.
  - If Hgb rises rapidly (>1 g/dL in any 2-week period), reduce the dose by 25%; if the Hgb continues to increase, hold the dose until Hgb starts to decline, and reinstitute drug at 25% less than prior dose.
  - If Hgb increases by > 1 g/dL in 2-week period, decrease dose by 25% to maintain the lowest hemoglobin to avoid red blood cell transfusion, not to exceed 12 g/dL.
  - Convert from epoetin alfa to darbepoetin alfa (see Special Considerations).
- NCCN alternative regimens (NCCN, 2014).
  - Darbepoetin 100 mcg/week fixed dosing—titrate up to 150–200 micrograms fixed dose weekly subcutaneously.
  - Darbepoetin 200 mcg every 2 weeks fixed dosing—titrate up to 300 mcg fixed dose every 2 weeks subcutaneously.
  - Darbepoetin 300 mcg every 3 weeks fixed dosing—titrate up to 500 mcg fixed dose every 3 weeks subcutaneously.
- Contraindicated in uncontrolled HTN, pure red cell aplasia, or if patient has serious allergic reactions to Aranesp.

Drug Preparation:
- Drug available in single-dose vials containing: 25, 40, 60, 100, 200, 300, and 500 mcg/mL and 150 mcg/0.75 mL.

- Single-dose prefilled syringes containing: 25 mcg/0.42 mL, 40 mcg/0.4 mL, 60 mcg/ 0.3 mL, 100 mcg/0.5 mL, 150 mcg/0.3 mL, 200 mcg/0.4 mL, 300 mcg/0.6 mL, or 500 mcg/1mL.
- Do not shake drug, as it may denature it; keep out of bright light; do not dilute; visually inspect drug for discoloration or particulate matter prior to parenteral administration, and discard if found.
- Store at 2–8°C (36–46°F). Do not freeze or shake, and protect from light.

Drug Administration:
- Administer weekly to start, subcutaneously or intravenously, and may be able to give every 2 weeks, depending upon response to drug.

Drug Interactions:
- No studies have been performed.

Lab Effects/Interference:
- Increased hemoglobin and hematocrit.
- Rare pure red-cell aplasia, severe anemia related to neutralizing antibodies.

Special Considerations:
- Black-box warning: Darbepoetin and other erythropoiesis-stimulating agents (ESAs) increased the risk for death and for serious cardiovascular events when given to a target hemoglobin of > 11 g/dL in cancer patients.
  - Shortened the time to tumor progression in patients with advanced head and neck cancer receiving radiation therapy when given to a target hemoglobin > 12 g/dL.
  - Shortened overall survival and increased deaths attributed to disease progression at 4 months in patients with metastatic breast cancer receiving chemotherapy when given to a target hemoglobin > 12 g/dL.
  - Increased risk of death when given to a target hemoglobin > 12 g/dL in patients with active malignant disease receiving neither chemotherapy nor radiation therapy (not indicated for this population).
  - Patients receiving ESAs preoperatively to reduce the need for allogeneic blood cell transfusions had a higher incidence of deep venous thrombosis if not also receiving prophylactic anticoagulation; darbepoetin is not indicated for this condition.
- Drug may increase the risk of cardiovascular events in patients with chronic renal failure (CRF) due to high hemoglobin, and risk increased in patients who had a rise of 1 g/dL or more in a 2-week period.
- Once starting drug, weekly hemoglobin should be monitored until stabilized and main-tenance dose has been established; once dose has been adjusted, the hemoglobin should be monitored weekly for at least 4 weeks until stabilization occurs; once maintenance established, hemoglobin should be monitored at regular intervals.
- Rarely, patients may develop antibodies that neutralize the effect, which can lead to red cell aplasia. If a patient loses response to darbepoetin alfa, evaluation should be done to find cause, including presence of binding and neutralizing antibodies to darbepoetin alfa, native erythropoietin, and any other recombinant erythropoietin administered to the patient.

- The possibility that darbepoetin alfa can stimulate tumor growth, especially as a growth factor of myeloid malignancies, has not been studied.
- Iron status should be assessed before and during treatment to ensure effective erythropoiesis; supplemental iron is recommended for patients with serum ferritin < 100 mcg/L or whose serum transferring saturation is < 20%. If patient does not respond to darbepoetin alfa, folic acid and vitamin B_{12} levels should also be assessed and deficiencies corrected.
- No studies have been performed on use of the drug in pregnant women. Drug should be used only if potential benefit outweighs risk to the fetus; it is unknown whether the drug is excreted in human milk, so caution should be used if given to a nursing mother.
- Rarely, allergic reactions can be severe, including skin rash and urticaria. Drug should be discontinued if serious allergic or anaphylactic reactions occur.
- Patients who have controlled hypertension should have regular assessment of blood pressure. Patients should be encouraged to be compliant with their antihypertensive medication regimen.
- See package insert for conversion from epoietin alfa to darbapoietin.

Potential Toxicities/Side Effects and the Nursing Process

I.   ACTIVITY INTOLERANCE related to FATIGUE

Nursing Implications: Assess baseline activity and energy levels. Assess baseline fluid.

II.   ALTERATION IN SKIN INTEGRITY, POTENTIAL, related to PERIPHERAL EDEMA, RASH

Nursing Implications: Perform baseline skin assessment, assess baseline weight and presence of edema. Teach patient to report development of peripheral edema. Teach patient self-assessment of skin, weight, and peripheral edema, and to report rash right away. Assess degree of peripheral edema if it develops, and discuss significant edema with physician to determine etiology and management. Teach patient local skin care, including avoidance of tight clothing and shoes, keeping skin moisturized to prevent cracking, and local comfort measures. If rash develops, assess extent, presence of urticaria, and implications regarding allergic reaction and drug discontinuance.

III.   ALTERATION IN COMFORT related to HEADACHE, DIZZINESS, FEVER, MYALGIA, ARTHRALGIA

Nursing Implications: Teach patient that bone pain may occur and discuss use of nonsteroidal anti-inflammatory drugs with patient and physician for symptom management. Teach patient to remain seated or lying down if feeling dizzy, and when dizziness has resolved, to change position gradually. Monitor hemoglobin weekly during dose determination period, and weekly for at least 4 weeks after each dose adjustment. Teach patient that headache, fever, dizziness, myalgia, and arthralgia may occur and to report them if they do not respond to usual management strategies.

IV. ALTERATION IN ELIMINATION related to DIARRHEA

Nursing Implications: Assess baseline patient bowel elimination pattern. Teach patient to report these side effects so that they can be evaluated. Teach patient self-care measures, including dietary modification, local comfort measures, and OTC antidiarrheal medication. Teach patient to report symptoms that persist, and discuss with physician possible other etiologies and management plan.

V. KNOWLEDGE DEFICIT related to SELF-ADMINISTRATION TECHNIQUE

Defining Characteristics: Drug is administered once weekly, or if response is adequate, may be given once every 2 weeks.

Nursing Implications: Assess baseline psychomotor ability, knowledge, and willingness to learn technique of self-injection. Teach how to refrigerate drug, self-administer using prefilled syringes, activate needle guard, and safely collect used syringes for proper disposal. Drug insert has "Information for Patients and Caregivers." Use written and video supplements to teach process and have patient correctly demonstrate technique prior to performing at home. Make referral to visiting-nurse agency to reinforce teaching if needed. Teach patient telephone number and whom to call if questions or problems arise, and ensure that patient can correctly repeat information.

Drug: eltrombopag (Promacta)

Class: Thrombopoietin (TPO) receptor agonist.

Mechanism of Action: Small-molecule TPO-receptor antagonist that binds to the human TPO receptor to initiate signaling cascades; it tells the bone marrow progenitor cells to initiate megakaryocyte (platelet precursors) proliferation and differentiation.

Metabolism: At least 52% of drug is absorbed from GI tract with peak concentration in 2–6 hours. Drug absorption is significantly decreased when taken with a high-fat meal or with antacids. 50–79% of drug is found in blood cells and is highly bound to human plasma proteins (> 99%). Drug is extensively metabolized via cleavage, oxidation (involving CYP1A2, -2C8), and glucuronidation (involving UGT1A1 and UGT1A3). Plasma elimination half-life is 26–35 hours in ITP patients. Drug is principally excreted in the feces (59%), with 31% in the urine. Drug exposure is about 70% higher in some East Asian patients (e.g., Japanese, Chinese, Taiwanese, and Korean ancestry) compared to non-Asian patients with ITP.

Indication: For the treatment of (1) thrombocytopenia in patients with chronic immune (idiopatic) thrombopoietin (ITP) who have had an insufficient response to corticosteroids, immunoglobulins, or splenectomy; and (2) thrombocytopenia in patients with chronic hepatitis C to allow the initiation and maintenance of interferon-based therapy.

Limitations of Use: Eltrombopag should be used only in patients (1) with ITP whose degree of thrombocytopenia and clinical condition increase the risk for bleeding, and NOT to try to normalize platelet counts; (2) with chronic hepatitis C whose degree of thrombocytopenia prevents the initiation interferon-based therapy or limits the ability to maintain interferon-based therapy. Safety and efficacy have not been established in combination with direct-acting antiviral agents used without interferon for treatment of chronic hepatitis C infection.

Dosage/Range:
- Chronic ITP: Starting dose is 50 mg PO daily for most patients; starting dose is 25 mg PO daily for patients of East Asian ancestry or patients with hepatic impairment. Take on an empty stomach.
- Adjust daily dose to achieve and maintain a platelet count equal to or greater than 50,000/mm³ in order to reduce the risk of bleeding.
  - After 2 weeks on eltrombopag, if the platelet count is less than 50,000/mm³, increase daily dose to a maximum of 75 mg daily.
  - If the platelet count is between 200,000–400,000/mm³ at any time, decrease the daily dose by 25 mg daily; wait 2 weeks to assess the effects of this change and any subsequent dose adjustments.
  - If platelet count is > 400,000/mm³, STOP eltrombopag, and assess the platelet count twice weekly; once the platelet count is < 150,000/mm³, reinitiate therapy at a daily dose reduced by 25 mg.
  - If platelet count is > 400,000/mm³ after 2 weeks of therapy at the lowest dose of eltrombopag, permanently discontinue eltrombopag.
- DO NOT EXCEED dose of 75 mg PO daily, and do not dose more than once daily.
- Discontinue eltrombopag if the platelet count does not increase after 4 weeks at the maximum dose; also discontinue drug for important liver test abnormalities or for excessive platelet count response.
- Chronic heptitis-C associated thrombocytopenia: Begin at 25 mg once daily for all patients; adjust dose to achieve platelet count required to initiate antiviral therapy; do not exceed dose of 100 mg. Take on an empty stomach.
- Serum ALT, AST, and bilirubin should be monitored baseline prior to starting therapy, every 2 weeks during dose adjustment phase, then monthly following establishment of a stable dose. If bilirubin is elevated, the test should be repeated with fractionation.
  - Evaluate abnormal serum liver tests with repeat testing within 3–5 days; if the abnormality is confirmed, monitor serum LFTs weekly until abnormality resolves, stabilizes, or returns to baseline level.
  - Discontinue eltrombopag if ALT increases to or is greater than 3 times ULN and is progressive or persistent for 4 weeks or more, is accompanied by increased direct bilirubin, or is accompanied by clinical symptoms of liver injury or evidence of hepatic decompensation.
- Monitor CBC, including platelet count and peripheral blood smears baseline prior to initiation of therapy, then weekly during dose adjustments, and monthly after the patient has been placed on a stable eltrombopag dose. Monitor CBC, including platelet count and peripheral blood smear when eltrombopag is discontinued, and monitor weekly

CBC/platelet count for 4 weeks after drug cessation as discontinuation may worsen thrombocytopenia. Thrombocytopenia may be more severe than that prior to starting therapy with eltrombopag.
* Patients should have a baseline ocular exam for cataracts, and during therapy to identify new or worsened cataracts.

Drug Preparation:
* None, oral tablet available as 12.5-mg, 25-mg, 50-mg, and 100-mg tablets.

Drug Administration:
* Administer on an empty stomach (e.g., 1 hour before or 2 hours after a meal).
* Allow a 4-hour interval between eltrombopag dose and other medications, foods, or supplements containing iron, calcium, aluminum, magnesium, selenium, or zinc.
* Monitor CBC, including platelet count, peripheral blood smears baseline prior to initiation of therapy, then weekly during dose adjustments, and monthly after the patient has been placed on a stable eltrombopag dose. Monitor CBC, including platelet count and peripheral blood smear when eltrombopag is discontinued, and monitor weekly CBC/platelet count for 4 weeks after drug cessation, as discontinuation may worsen thrombocytopenia.
* Monitor ALT, AST, bilirubin baseline every 2 weeks during dose adjustment phase, then monthly following establishment of stable dose.

Drug Interactions:
* Polyvalent cations (e.g., iron, calcium, aluminum, magnesium, selenium, and zinc) significantly reduce oral absorption of drug; do not take drug within 4 hours of other medications or products containing polyvalent cations such as antacids, dairy products, and mineral supplements.
* Eltrombopag is an inhibitor of OATP1B1 transporter. Monitor patients closely for signs and symptoms of excessive exposure to the drugs that are substrates of OATP1B1 (e.g., rosuvastatin, benzylpenicillin, atorvastatin, fluvastatin, pravastatin, methotrexate, nateglinide, repaglinide, rifampin), and consider reduction of the dose of these drugs.
* Coadministration with moderate or strong inhibitors of CYP1A2 (e.g., ciprofloxacin, fluvoxamine) and CYP2C8 (gemfibrozil, trimethoprim); inducers of CYP1A2 (tobacco, omeprazole) and CYP2C8 (rifampin); or other substrates of these CYP enzymes may cause increased serum levels of eltrombopag with increased toxicity. Monitor patient closely for side effects of eltrombopag.
* Coadministration with acetaminophen, opioids, NSAIDs: assess for toxicity of acetaminophen, opioids, NSAIDs as coadministration with eltrombopag decreases their metabolism with subsequent increased serum levels. Eltrombopag is an inhibitor of UGT1A1, -1A3, -1A4, -1A6, -1A9, UGT2B7, and UGT2B15 (UDP-glucuronosyltransferases, UGTs).

Lab Effects/Interference:
* Increased serum aminotransferase levels and bilirubin.
* Development of reticulin fiber deposition in the bone marrow with abnormal red cells in the peripheral smear (e.g., teardrop or nucleated RBC, or immature WBCs).

• Increased platelet count.
• Decreased platelet count on discontinuation of drug.

Special Considerations:
• In clinical studies, platelet counts generally increased within 1–2 weeks after starting eltrombopag; platelet counts decreased within 1–2 weeks after stopping eltrombopag.
Warnings and Precautions: Eltrombopag may cause hepatotoxicity with increased serum transaminases and bilirubin; monitor LFTs baseline and every 2 weeks during dose adjustment phase, then monthly after establishing a stable dose:
   • Administer at a reduced dose for patients with moderate or severe hepatic dysfunction. Monitor patients with any hepatic impairment closely.
   • Eltrombopag inhibits UGT1A1 and OAT1B1, which may lead to indirect hyperbilirubinemia; if bilirubin is elevated, perform fractionation.
   • Evaluate abnormal serum LFTs within 3–5 days. If abnormalities confirmed, monitor LFTs weekly until resolved or stabilized.
   • Discontinue drug if ALT levels increase to $\geq 3 \times$ ULN in patients with normal liver function; or $\geq$ baseline in patients with pretreatment elevations in transaminases and are progressively increasing or persistent for ≥ 4 weeks; or accompanied by increased direct bilirubin; or accompanied by clinical symptoms of liver injury or evidence of hepatic decompensation.
   • If potential benefit of reinitiating drug is greater than the risk for hepatotoxicity during the dose adjustment phase, cautiously reintroduce drug and assess LFTs weekly during this phase. Hepatotoxicity may recur; if LFTs worsen or abnormalities recur, permanently discontinue eltombopag.
• Hepatic decompensation in patients with chronic hepatitis C: decrease eltombopag if antiviral therapy is discontinued.
• Thrombotic/thromboembolic complications: portal vein thrombosis has been reported in patients with chronic liver disease, but arterial events may also occur in patients receiving eltrombopag.
   • Monitor platelet counts regularly, as complications may result from increases in platelet count.
   • Patients with known risk factors for thromboembolism are those with Factor V Leiden, ATIII deficiency, antiphospholipid syndrome, chronic liver disease.
   • Goal for therapy is equal or greater than $50,000/mm^3$ to reduce the risk of bleeding.
• Cataracts may develop or worsen. Patient should have a baseline ocular examination prior to drug initiation, during therapy, and assess for signs and symptoms of cataracts.
• The most common side effects of eltrombopag in (1) ITP patients ($\geq 3\%$) are nausea, vomiting, diarrhea, URI, increased ALT, myalgia, UTI, oropharyngeal pain, increased AST, pharyngitis, back pain, influenza, parasthesias, and rash; (2) patients with chronic hepatitis C ($\geq 10\%$ and greater than placebo) most common side effects were anemia, pyrexia, fatigue, headache, nausea, diarrhea, decreased appetite, influenza-like illness, asthenia, insomnia, cough, pruritus, chills, myalgia, alopecia, and peripheral edema.
• Eltrombopag may cause fetal harm. Pregnant patients should be enrolled in the PROMACTA pregnancy registry (1-888-825-5249). Nursing mothers should discontinue the drug or nursing, depending on how important the drug is to the mother's health.

Potential Toxicities/Side Effects (Dose- and Schedule-Dependent) and the Nursing Process

I. POTENTIAL FOR BLEEDING

Defining Characteristics: Menorrhagia occurred in 4% of patients, ecchymosis in 2%, and conjunctival hemorrhage in 2%.

Nursing Implications: Assess baseline platelet count, weekly during dose adjustment, and monthly when dosing is stable. Also assess weekly for 4 weeks following dose cessation as severe thrombocytopenia may occur. Teach patient to report any bleeding right away, and then assess platelet count.

II. POTENTIAL ALTERATION IN NUTRITION related to HEPATOTOXICITY, NAUSEA, VOMITING

Defining Characteristics: Two percent of patients had increased ALT and AST; 6% of patients developed nausea, and 4% vomiting.

Nursing Implications: Assess LFTs baseline, weekly during dose adjustments, and monthly when on a stable dose. Teach patients that nausea and vomiting can rarely occur and to report them. Teach patients dietary strategies to minimize nausea and vomiting. Discuss antiemetics if necessary with physician.

III. POTENTIAL ALTERATION IN SENSORY PERCEPTION related to CATARACTS, PARESTHESIA

Defining Characteristics: Eight percent of patients in clinical trials developed cataracts or cataracts worsened on therapy; in an extension study of patients who had baseline ocular exams, the incidence of new or worsened cataracts was 4%. Paresthesias may occur in 3% of patients.

Nursing Implications: Patients should have a baseline ocular exam, which should be repeated during therapy for the development of new or worsened cataracts. Teach patient to report symptoms of cataracts right away: clouded, blurred, or dim vision; increased difficulty in seeing at night (night vision); sensitivity to light and glare; halos around light; new need for more or brighter light when reading; frequent changes in prescriptions for vision; fading or yellowing of colors; double vision in one eye. If these occur, the patient should have an ocular exam to assess the development or worsening of existing cataracts. Teach patient that rarely paresthesias may occur, and to report them.

Drug: epoetin alfa (Epogen, erythropoietin, Procrit)

Class: Cytokine, colony-stimulating factor (CSF).

Mechanism of Action: Stimulates the division and differentiation of erythrocyte stem cells in the bone marrow and is a hormone produced by recombinant DNA techniques. Has a naturally occurring counterpart, erythropoietin. Results in the release of reticulocytes into the bloodstream in 7–10 days, where they mature into erythrocytes, taking 2–6 weeks to increase hemoglobin.

Metabolism: Following SC injection, 21–31% of drug is bioavailable, with rapid distribution to tissues. Drug is taken up in the liver, kidneys, and bone marrow. Onset of action in a few days to 2 weeks; peak effect in 2–3 weeks. Half-life is 4–13 h. Eliminated via the liver and urine (10% unchanged drug).

Indication: (A) Treatment of anemia due to (1) chronic kidney disease in patients on or not on dialysis; (2) zidovudine in HIV-infected patients; (3) the effects of concomitant myelosuppressive chemotherapy and upon initiation, there is a minimum of 2 additional months of planned chemotherapy; and (B) reduction of allogeneic RBC transfusions in patients undergoing elective, noncardiac, nonvascular surgery.

Limitations of Use: Procrit has not been shown to improve quality of life, fatigue, or patient well-being.

Contraindications: Patients with (1) uncontrolled hypertension; (2) pure red cell aplasia that begins after treatment with erythropoietin-stimulating drugs; (3) serious allergic reaction to the drug; (4) use of multidose vials in neonates, infants, pregnant women, and nursing mothers.

Dosage/Range:
- Only prescribers and hospitals enrolled in the ESA APPRISE Oncology Program may prescribe or dispense Procrit. Prior to each new course of Procrit, prescribers and patients must provide written acknowledgment of a discussion of Procrit risks.
- Use the *lowest dose* of epoietin alfa that will gradually increase the hemoglobin concentration to the lowest level sufficient to avoid the need for red blood cell transfusion.
- Cancer patients receiving chemotherapy (nonmyeloid, noncurative) with Hgb < 10 g/dL, and at least 2 months of additional chemotherapy are planned:
  - Initial adult dose is 150 U/kg subcutaneous three times weekly or 40,000 U subcutaneously weekly.
  - Initial pediatric dose 600 units/kg IV weekly until completion of a chemotherapy course.
  - Reduce dose by 25% when Hgb approaches a level sufficient to avoid RBC transfusion or Hgb increases > 1 g/dL in any 2-week period.
  - Hold dose if Hgb > level needed to avoid RBC transfusion and resume at 25% below previous dose.
  - Increase dose if after 4 weeks of erythropoietin therapy Hgb increases by < 1 g/dL AND remains < 10g/dL:
    - Three times weekly: increase dose to 300 U/kg three times weekly in adults.
    - Weekly: increase to 60,000 U weekly in adults.
    - Weekly (children): 900 units/kg (maximum 60,000 units).
    - After 8 weeks of therapy, if there is no response by Hgb or RBC transfusions are required, discontinue drug.
  - Discontinue Procrit after the completion of a chemotherapy course.

- Goal is to prevent or treat deficit of oxygen-carrying capacity (NCCN, 2014): (1) if asymptomatic, in hemodynamically stable chronic anemia without acute coronary syndrome (ACS), goal is Hgb 7–9 g/dL; (2) symptomatic anemia: (a) acute hemorrhage with evidence of hemodynamic instability or inadequate oxygen delivery: transfuse to correct; (b) Hgb < 10 g/dL with tachycardia, postural hypotension, goal is maintain Hgb 8–10 g/dL; (c) anemia with ACS or acute MI: transfusion goal to maintain Hgb ≥ 10 g/dL.
- Surgery patients (preoperative use for reduction of allogeneic red blood cell transfusion):
  - Assess Hgb: must be > 10–13 g/dL.
  - Dose is 300 U/kg/day subcutaneously × 15 days (10 days before surgery, on the day of surgery, and for 4 days after surgery) or 600 units/kg subcutaneously in 4 doses administered 21, 14, and 7 days before surgery, and on the day of surgery.
  - All patients should receive adequate iron supplementation to start at least by the beginning of epoetin alfa therapy.
  - Patients should also receive prophylactic anticoagulation to prevent DVT.
- Chronic renal failure:
  - Ensure adequate patient iron stores (transferrin saturation at least 20%, ferritin at least 100 ng/mL).
  - 50–100 U/kg tiw (adult) or 50 U/kg tiw (pediatric) to maintain Hgb between 10–12 g/dL.
  - Reduce dose by 25% if Hgb approaches 12 g/dL; if Hgb continues to increase, hold dose until Hgb begins to decline, and then reinstitute drug at dose 25% less than previous dose.
  - Reduce dose by 25% if Hgb increases by > 1 g/dL in a 2-week period.
  - Increase dose by 25% if Hgb does not increase by 2 g/dL after 8 weeks of therapy, or Hgb rise is > 1 g/dL over 4 weeks, and iron stores are adequate (transferrin saturation > 20%); do not increase dose more frequently than once a month; monitor Hgb twice weekly for 2–6 weeks after dose increase.
  - Maintain lowest dose to avoid red blood cell transfusion but not to exceed 12 g/dL.
- Zidovudine-treated HIV-infected adult patients:
  - Adult starting dose is 100 units/kg IV or SQ three times per week.
  - Increase dose if Hgb does not increase after 8 weeks of therapy, by 50–100 U/kg three times weekly subcutaneously, or IV and evaluate response every 4–8 weeks thereafter, and adjust dose in 50–100 U/kg increments three times a week SQ, or IV to a dose that reaches a level to avoid RBC transfusions or 300 U/kg.
  - Hold drug if Hgb > 12 g/dL until Hgb < 11 g/dL, and then resume drug with a 25% dose reduction of previous dose.
- Discontinue erythropoietin if an increase in Hgb does not occur at a dose of 300 U/kg for 8 weeks.
- Alternative regimens (NCCN, 2014):
  - Epoetin alfa 80,000 units every 2 weeks subcutaneously.
  - Epoetin alfa 120,000 units every 3 weeks subcutaneously.

Drug Preparation:
- DO NOT SHAKE vial, as it may denature the glycoprotein.
- Available as preservative-free, single-dose vials for injection in 2,000 U/mL, 3,000 U/mL, 4,000 U/mL, 10,000 U/mL, and 40,000 U/mL vials. These must be refrigerated, and unused portions should be discarded.
- Multidose injection vials, preserved with benzyl alcohol: available as 10,000 U/mL (2 mL) and 20,000 U/mL (1 mL); discard 21 days after initial entry.
- Store at 2–8°C (36–46°F).
- Do not dilute or administer with other drugs.
- Subcutaneous administration: At the time of injection, may admix in the syringe, bacteriostatic 0.9% sodium chloride injection USP with benzyl alcohol 0.9% (bacteriostatic saline) to the preservative-free epoetin from single-use vial to reduce injection-site discomfort.

Drug Administration:
- Subcutaneous or IV (chronic renal failure on dialysis at end of dialysis) injection.

Drug Interactions:
- None reported.

Lab Effects/Interference:
- Expect increase in Hgb/HCT in 2–6 weeks.

Special Considerations:
Warnings and Precautions:
- Erythropoiesis-stimulating agents (ESAs) increased the risk for death, myocardial infarction, stroke, venous thromboembolism, thrombosis of vascular access when using ESAs to target a Hgb > 11 g/dL.
- Increased mortality and/or increased risk of tumor progression or recurrence in cancer patients.
- Shortened overall survival and/or increased the risk of tumor progression or recurrence in clinical studies of patients with breast, NSCLC, head and neck cancer, lymphoid, and cervical cancers.
- Hypertension (HTN): control HTN prior to initiating and during drug therapy.
- Seizures: drug increases the risk for seizures in patients with chronic kidney disease.
- Pure red cell aplasia: if severe anemia and low reticulocyte count develop, hold drug and evaluate patient for neutralizing antibodies to erythropoietin. Permanently discontinue drug if pure red cell aplasia is diagnosed.
- Prescribers and hospitals must enroll in and comply with the ESA APPRISE Oncology Program to prescribe and/or dispense PROCRIT to patients with cancer.
- Use the lowest dose to avoid RBC transfusions.
- Use ESAs only for anemia from noncurative, myelosuppressive chemotherapy.
- Discontinue following the completion of a chemotherapy course.

- Patients receiving ESAs preoperatively to reduce the need for allogeneic blood cell transfusions had a higher incidence of deep venous thrombosis if not also receiving prophylactic anticoagulation. DVT prophylaxis is recommended.
- Iron stores need to be assessed and replaced to maximize response to therapy.

Potential Toxicities/Side Effects (Dose- and Schedule-Dependent) and the Nursing Process

I.   ALTERATION IN COMFORT related to PYREXIA, FATIGUE, HEADACHE

Defining Characteristics: May be due to HIV disease, rather than drug, and occurs in 20–25% of patients. Allergic reactions including urticaria may occur. Anaphylaxis has not been reported.

Nursing Implications: Assess baseline T and energy level. Instruct patient to report signs/symptoms, and discuss measures to increase comfort.

II.   POTENTIAL ALTERATION IN OXYGENATION related to POLYCYTHEMIA

Defining Characteristics: Polycythemia may result if target range is exceeded with consequent complications (Hgb > 12 g/dL).

Nursing Implications: Monitor weekly Hgb until stable dose is achieved. Dose should be interrupted if Hgb approaches 12 g/dL and then resumed at 75% dose once HCT is < 11 g/dL. When Hgb has stabilized, discuss monitoring Hgb with physician (e.g., testing).

III.   KNOWLEDGE DEFICIT related to SELF-ADMINISTRATION TECHNIQUE

Defining Characteristics: Most often drug is administered subcutaneously three times per week or weekly.

Nursing Implications: Assess baseline psychomotor ability, knowledge, and willingness to learn technique of self-injection. Teach how to prepare drug, self-administer, and safely collect used syringes for proper disposal. Use written and video materials as supplements to teaching process and have patient correctly demonstrate technique prior to performing at home. Make referral to visiting-nurse agency to reinforce teaching.

Drug: filgrastim (Neupogen, G-CSF)

Class: Cytokine, CSF.

Mechanism of Action: Recombinant DNA protein (G-CSF) that regulates the production of neutrophils in the bone marrow (proliferation, differentiation, activation of mature neutrophils). Drug is produced by the insertion of the human G-CSF gene into *Escherichia coli* bacteria.

Metabolism: Elimination half-life is 3.5 hours.

Indication: (1) To decrease the incidence of infection (febrile neutropenia) in patients with nonmyeloid malignancies receiving myelosuppressive anti-cancer drugs associated with a significant incidence of severe neutropenia with fever; (2) reducing time to neutrophil recovery and duration of fever, following induction or consolidation chemotherapy in adults with AML; (3) to reduce the duration of neutropenia and neutropenia-related clinical sequelae (e.g., febrile neutropenia) in patients with nonmyeloid malignancies undergoing myeloablative chemotherapy followed by marrow transplantation; (4) mobilization of hematopoietic progenitor cells into the peripheral blood for collection by leukapheresis, as this increases the numbers of progenitor cells capable of engraftment; (5) chronic administration to reduce the incidence and duration of sequelae of neutropenia (e.g., fever, infections, oropharyngeal ulcers).

Contraindications: Patients with known hypersensitivity to *E. coli*-derived proteins, filgrastim, or any component of the product.

Dosage/Range:

- Starting dose 5 µg/kg/day subcutaneous or IV; dose increase by 5 µg/kg for each chemotherapy cycle, based on duration and severity of neutropenia at nadir.
- BMT: After BMT, 10 µg/kg/day as IV infusion of 4 or 24 hours, or as a continuous subcutaneous, 24-hour infusion, and then titrated based on ANC.
- Mobilization of peripheral blood progenitor cells (PBPC) is 10 µg/kg/day subcutaneous at least 4 days until the first leukapheresis procedure, and continued until the last leukapheresis. Modify dose if WBC > 100,000/mm³.
- Patients with acute myeloid leukemia receiving induction or consolidation: 5 µg/kg/day subcutaneous beginning 24 hours after last dose of chemotherapy until ANC > 1,000/mm³ for 3 consecutive days.

Drug Preparation:

- Drug available in refrigerated single-dose.
- Vials of 300 mcg/mL or 480 mcg/mL in dispensing packs of 10. Teach patient to discard unused portions.
- Single-dose, preservative-free, prefilled syringe (SingleJect) with 27-gauge, 1/2-inch needle with an UltraSafe Needle Guard in 300 mcg/0.5 mL (600 mcg/mL) or 480 mcg/ 0.8 mL (600 mcg/mL), in dispensing packs of 1 or 10.
- Needle cover of prefilled syringes contains dry natural rubber, a derivative of latex.
- Filgrastim should be stored in the refrigerator at 2–8°C (36–46°F).
- Avoid shaking.
- Remove from refrigerator 30 minutes prior to injection. Discard if left out > 6 hours.

Drug Administration:

- Subcutaneous or intravenously daily, beginning at least 24 hours post-administration of chemotherapy, continuing up to 2 weeks or until ANC > 10,000/mm³.
- Teach patient/caregiver to prepare and self-administer filgrastim. See patient education material in package insert.
- Assess CBC/differential/platelet count baseline, then 2×/week during filgrastim therapy; discontinue filgrastim when ANC ≥ 10,000/mm³ after the expected chemotherapy-induced nadir.

- BMT: assess CBC/platelet counts at a minimum 3×/week following marrow infusion to monitor the recovery of marrow reconstitution.

Drug Interactions:
- None significant.

Lab Effects/Interference:
- Increased WBC and neutrophil counts.
- Increased LDH, uric acid, alkaline phosphatase.

Special Considerations:
- Warnings:
  - Allergic reactions may occur on initial or subsequent treatment characterized by symptoms in two body systems, such as skin (rash, urticaria, facial edema), respiratory (wheezing, dyspnea), and cardiovascular (hypotension, tachycardia). Most often occur within 30 minutes of administration, especially if given IV. Administration of corticosteroids, antihistamines, bronchodilators and/or epinephrine brings rapid resolution of symptoms. More than half of patients rechallenged had recurrent symptoms.
  - Splenic rupture: immediately evaluate patients who report LUQ and/or shoulder tip pain for an enlarged spleen or splenic rupture.
  - ARDS has been reported, probably as a result of an influx of neutrophils to the site of lung inflammation. If patient develops fever, lung infiltrates, or respiratory distress, immediately evaluate for ARDS; if diagnosed, hold drug until resolution or discontinue and give appropriate medical management of ARDS.
  - Alveolar hemorrhage and hemoptysis have been reported in patients undergoing PBPC mobilization, which is not an approved indication of the drug.
  - Sickle cell disorders: severe sickle cell crisis has occurred, sometimes fatal. Drug should be administered to these patients only after careful consideration of risks and benefits by a sickle cell expert physician.
  - Patients with severe chronic neutropenia: may develop MDS or AML during Neupogen therapy. If a patient with severe chronic neutropenia develops abnormal cytogenetics or myelodyspasia, risks and benefits of continuing Neupogen should be carefully considered.
- Studies showed no statistical difference between Neupogen or placebo group in complete remission rate, disease-free survival, time to disease progression, or overall survival when used in patients with acute myeloid leukemia after induction or consolidation therapy.
- Rarely, drug may exacerbate preexisting psoriasis, Sweet's syndrome (neutrophilic dermatitis), and cutaneous vasculitis.
- Do not administer drug within 24 hours of chemotherapy administration (within 24 hours before and 24 hours after). Simultaneous use of Neupogen with chemotherapy and radiation therapy should be avoided.
- Filgrastim is a growth factor for neutrophils, but it is unknown if also can act as a growth factor for tumor cells.
- Thrombocytopenia has been reported in patients receiving filgrastim. Monitor platelet counts during therapy.

Potential Toxicities/Side Effects (Dose- and Schedule-Dependent) and the Nursing Process

I.   ALTERATION IN COMFORT related to SKELETAL PAIN

Defining Characteristics: Patients (22%) may report transient skeletal pain, believed due to the expansion of cells in the bone marrow in response to G-CSF.

Nursing Implications: Teach patient that this may occur, and discuss use of NSAIDs with patient and physician for symptom management. Monitor WBC and ANC twice weekly during therapy; dose should be discontinued when ANC > 10,000/mm³.

II.   KNOWLEDGE DEFICIT related to SELF-ADMINISTRATION TECHNIQUE

Defining Characteristics: Drug is administered daily for up to 2 weeks by subcutaneous injection (outpatients).

Nursing Implications: Assess baseline psychomotor ability, knowledge, and willingness to learn technique of self-injection. Teach how to prepare drug, self-administer, and safely collect used syringes for proper disposal. Use written and video supplements to teaching process, and have patient correctly demonstrate technique prior to performing at home. Make referral to visiting-nurse agency to reinforce teaching. Patient instructions in English are on package insert. Video and more detailed patient education are available from Amgen (Thousand Oaks, CA) representative.

Drug: filgrastim-sndz (Zarxio)

Class: Granulocyte colony-stimulating growth factor (G-CSF) (Biosimilar to filgrastim [Neupogen]).

Mechanism of Action: Glycoprotein that binds to the cell surface receptors of hematopoietic cells to stimulate proliferation, differentiation, and activation of some end cell functions.

Metabolism: Exhibits nonlinear pharmacokinetics, and clearance depends on the filgrastim concentration and neutrophil count. Clearance is decreased by the presence of neutropenia, and the drug is cleared by the kidneys.

Indications: Filgrastim-sndz is indicated to (1) decrease the incidence of infection (febrile neutropenia) in patients with nonmyeloid malignancies receiving myelosuppressive anticancer drugs associated with a significant incidence of severe neutropenia with fever; (2) reduce the time to neutrophil recovery and the duration of fever, following induction or consolidation chemotherapy treatment of patients with acute myeloid leukemia (AML); (3) reduce the duration of neutropenia and neutropenia-related clinical sequelae (e.g., febrile neutropenia), in patients with nonmyeloid malignancies undergoing myeloablative chemotherapy followed by bone marrow transplantation; (4) mobilize autologous hematopoietic progenitor cells into the peripheral blood for collection by leukapheresis; and (5) reduce the incidence and duration of sequelae of severe neutropenia (e.g., fever, infections, oropharyngeal ulcers) in symptomatic patients with congenital neutropenia, cyclic neutropenia, or idiopathic neutropenia.

Contraindication: Patients with a history of serious allergic reactions to human G-CSFs such as filgrastim or pegfilgrastim products.

Dosage/Range:
* **Patients with cancer receiving myelosuppressive chemotherapy or induction and/or consolidation chemotherapy for AML:** 5 mcg/kg/day SQ, short IV infusion (15–30 min), or continuous IV infusion. Assess CBC/platelet count before administering, and monitor twice weekly. Administer at least 24 hours after chemotherapy dose(s), daily, until ANC > 10,000/mm³ after the expected nadir, or up to 2 weeks.
* **Patients with cancer undergoing bone marrow transplantation (BMT):** 10 mcg/kg/day given as an IV infusion no longer than 24 hours. Give first dose at least 24 hours after cytotoxic chemotherapy and at least 24 hours after the bone marrow infusion. Monitor CBC/platelet count frequently following BMT. During neutrophil recovery, titrate the daily dosage against the neutrophil response (see package insert).
* **Patients undergoing autologous peripheral blood progenitor cell collection and therapy:** 10 mcg/kg/day SQ. Administer drug for at least 4 days before the first leukapheresis procedure and continue until the last leukapheresis. Administration of filgrastim for 6–7 days with leukapheresis on days 5, 6, and 7 has been found safe and effective. Monitor ANC after 4 days of filgrastim-sndz, and discontinue drug if WBC count > 100,000/mm³.
* **Patients with severe chronic neutropenia:** 6 mcg/kg SQ twice daily. If patient has cyclic neutropenia, dose is 5 mcg/kg SQ once daily. See package insert for dosage adjustments.

Drug Preparation:
* Injection: 300 mcg/0.5 mL in a single-use prefilled syringe with BD UltraSafe Passive Needle Guard.
* Injection: 480 mcg/0.8 mL in a single-use prefilled syringe with BD UltraSafe Passive Needle Guard.
* Direct administration of less than 0.3 mL is not recommended owing to the high potential for dosing errors.

Drug Administration:
SQ injection: Administer in outer areas of upper arms, abdomen, or thighs, or in upper outer areas of buttock. If appropriate, teach the patient or caregiver hand hygiene, keeping the needle sterile, injection technique, and disposal of sharps, and have the patient or caregiver provide a return demonstration. If unable to successfully return the demonstration, the patient or caregiver may not be the appropriate choice to administer the drug. See patient information in the package insert. The needle cap contains latex, so it should not be used to administer the drug in patients with a latex allergy.

IV infusion: Dilute in 5% dextrose injection USP to a concentration between 5 mcg/mL and 15 mcg/mL; protect from adsorption to plastic materials by adding albumin (human) to a final concentration of 2 mg/mL. When diluted in 5% dextrose injection USP or 5% dextrose plus albumin (human), the drug is compatible with glass, polyvinylchloride, polyolefin, and polypropylene. *Do not* dilute with saline at any time, as the product may *precipitate*. Diluted filgrastim-sndz solution can be stored at room temperature for up to 24 hours, including time during room temperature storage of the infusion solution and the duration of the infusion.

Drug Interactions: None significant.

Lab Effects/Interference:
- Leukocytosis (rarely 100,000/mm³ or greater)
- Thrombocytopenia
- Increased LDH, alkaline phosphatase
- Positive bone-imaging changes (transient) related to increased hematopoietic activity in bone marrow

Special Considerations:
Warnings and Precautions:
- Fatal splenic rupture: Assess for left upper abdominal or shoulder pain for enlarged spleen or splenic rupture, and manage urgently.
- Acute respiratory distress syndrome (ARDS): Evaluate patients with fever and lung infiltrates, or respiratory distress for ARDS. If confirmed, discontinue the drug.
- Serious allergic reactions, including anaphylaxis: Provide emergent medical support and discontinue the drug.
- Fatal sickle cell crisis: May occur with the use of filgrastim in patients with sickle cell anemia; use cautiously and monitor the patient closely.
- Alveolar hemorrhage and hemoptysis: Have occurred in healthy donors undergoing peripheral blood progenitor cell collection (PBPC) mobilization; hemoptysis resolved with discontinuation of filgrastim. This drug is *not* approved for PBPC mobilization in healthy donors.
- Capillary leak syndrome (CLS): Characterized by hypotension, hypoalbuminemia, edema, and hemoconcentration; may be life threatening if not treated immediately. Closely monitor patients with CLS, including ICU monitoring as needed.
- Patients with severe, chronic neutropenia have rarely developed MDS and AML. IF the patient develops abnormal cytogenetics of myelodysplasia, risks and benefits of continuing filgrastim should be carefully considered.
- Thrombocytopenia: May occur; monitor platelet counts.
- Leukocytosis: May occur. Discontinue filgrastim if ANC > 10,000/mm³ after the chemotherapy nadir has occurred (50% decrease in ANC in 1–2 days, with return to pretreatment levels in 1–7 days in patients who have had myelosuppressive chemotherapy). Monitor WBC/differential twice weekly during therapy. In patients with cancer undergoing PBPC mobilization, discontinue filgrastim if leukocyte count > 100,000/mm³.
- Cutaneous vasculitis: Occurs in patients treated with filgrastim, especially those receiving long-term filgrastim therapy. Hold the drug if cutaneous vasculitis occurs; the drug may be resumed at a reduced dose when symptoms have resolved and ANC has decreased.
- Potential effect on malignant cells: G-CSF receptors have been found on tumor cell lines.

- Simultaneous use with chemotherapy and radiation therapy: Not recommended. Do not administer filgrastim in the period 24 hours before through 24 hours after the administration of cytotoxic chemotherapy.
- Pregnancy category C: Use filgrastim-sndz during pregnancy only if the potential benefit justifies the potential risk to the fetus. Caution should be exercised if filgrastim-sndz is administered to women who are breastfeeding.

Potential Toxicities/Side Effects (Dose- and Schedule-Dependent) and the Nursing Process

I.   ALTERATION IN COMFORT related to PAIN, FATIGUE, AND FEVER

Defining Characteristics: In studies of patients receiving myelosuppressive chemotherapy, pyrexia occurred in 48% of participants, chest pain in 13%, pain in 12%, fatigue in 20%, back pain in 15%, arthralgia in 9%, and bone pain in 7%.

Nursing Considerations: Assess baseline comfort level, and monitor during therapy. Teach patient that these effects may occur, and to report them. Teach patient self-care strategies to improve comfort, and to report them if they persist or become worse. Monitor CBC/platelet count twice weekly; the drug should be discontinued when ANC > 10,000/mm³.

II.   KNOWLEDGE DEFICIT related to SELF-ADMINISTRATION TECHNIQUE

Defining Characteristics: Drug is administered daily for up to 2 weeks by SQ injection (outpatients).

Nursing Considerations: Assess baseline psychomotor ability, knowledge, and willingness to learn technique of self-injection. Teach how to sanitize hands, prepare drug, self-administer, and safely collect used syringes for proper disposal. Use written and video supplements for the teaching process, and have the patient correctly demonstrate the technique prior to performing it at home. See the package insert and website for teaching resources. Call the patient at home the next day to assess progress.

Drug: imiquimod 5% topical cream (Aldara)

Class: Immune response modifier.

Mechanism of Action: Stimulates the immune system to release cytokines, including interferon, which stimulate Langerhans cells to kill skin cancer cells. Has been shown to reduce the expression of Bcl-2 (a protein that causes the cell to avoid apoptosis, or programmed cell death, by preventing the activation of the proapoptotic proteins called capases) and increase apoptosis of basal skin cancer cells.

Metabolism: Unknown.

Indications: For the topical treatment of patients with (1) actinic keratosis, (2) superficial basal cell carcinoma, (3) external genital warts.

Dosage/Range: Imiquimod 5% topical cream is applied to the superficial basal cell carcinoma (sBCC) lesion (must be 2 cm or less in diameter), including a 1-cm margin around the lesion, as shown in the table below.

Target Tumor Diameter	Size of Cream Droplet to Be Used (diameter)	Amount of Imiquimod Cream Used
0.5 cm–<1.0 cm	4 mm	10 mg
≥ 1.0 cm–<1.5 cm	5 mm	25 mg
≥ 1.5 cm–2.0 cm	7 mm	40 mg

Available in single-use packets, supplied 12 per box.

Drug Preparation: Wash hands before and after application of cream, and wear gloves. Wash skin area(s) with mild soap and water, then dry thoroughly before application, and again, after 8 hours application. Apply cream to lesion with an additional 1 cm surrounding the lesion(s), at bedtime leaving the cream on at least 8 hours, 5 nights a week, for 6 weeks.

Drug Interactions: Unknown.

Lab Effects/Interference: None known.

Special Considerations:
- Indicated for the treatment of superficial basal cell carcinoma (sBCC) on the body, neck, arms, or legs (not the face, hands, or feet) when surgical removal is not an option.
- Drug is also used for the treatment of external genital and nongenital warts, molluscum contagiosum, solar keratoses.

Potential Toxicities/Side Effects (More Severe with Higher Dosing) and the Nursing Process

I.   POTENTIAL ALTERATION IN SKIN INTEGRITY AND COMFORT related to SKIN IRRITATION

Defining Characteristics: Redness, swelling, development of a sore or blister, peeling, itching, and burning are common application-site reactions. Response to therapy cannot be determined until the skin reaction resolves, sometimes up to 12 weeks.

Nursing Implications: Explain to the patient that these side effects may occur. Teach patient to wash skin prior to application, and again after 8 hours. Teach patient to assess skin reactions, and to report any symptoms that interfere with activities of daily living, as a rest period of a few days may be necessary if symptoms are severe. In addition, instruct patient to stop cream and report infection in the application area right away.

II.   KNOWLEDGE DEFICIT related to SELF-ADMINISTRATION OF CREAM

Defining Characteristics: Treatment is for 6 weeks and must be applied properly for adequate tumor exposure.

Nursing Implications: Teach patient self-administration of the cream, and to keep a diary to keep track of the application schedule. Teach patient to wash hands before and after application. Teach patient verbally and through demonstration to wash treatment area with mild soap and water, then to dry prior to application. Cream should be applied to extend 1 cm beyond the lesion borders, and rubbed into the treatment area until no longer visible. Keep cream away from eyes. Cream should be on for at least 8 hours, and then removed using mild soap and water.

Drug: interferon alfa (2α) (alpha interferon, IFN, interferon alpha-2a, rIFN-A, Roferon A)

Class: Cytokine (interferon).

Mechanism of Action: Antiviral, antiproliferative, and immunomodulatory effects. Activates prenatural killer cells, increases cytotoxicity of NK cells, and enhances immune response.

Metabolism: Well absorbed following subcutaneous or IM injection with 90% bioavailability after subcutaneous injection. Drug peaks at 6–8 hours, and has an elimination half-life of 2 hours (IM/IV) and 3 hours (subcutaneous). Renal filtration and tubular reabsorption as catabolites; minor hepatic metabolism and biliary excretion.

Indications: For the treatment of patients with (1) chronic hepatitis C, (2) hairy-cell leukemia in adults age 18 and over; (3) chronic phase, Philadelphia chromosome (Ph) positive chronic myelogenous leukemia (CML) who are minimally pretreated (within 1 year of diagnosis).

Contraindications: Patients with (1) hypersensitivity to Roferon-A or any of its components; (2) autoimmune hepatitis; (3) hepatic decompensation (Child-Pugh class B and C) before or during treatment; also contraindicated in neonates and infants, as it contains benzyl alcohol.

Dosage/Range:
- Hepatitis C: 3 million international units 3X (tiw) a week SQ for 12 months (48–52 weeks) OR induction dose of 6 million international units tiw for the first 3 months (12 weeks) followed by 3 million international units tiw for 9 months (36 weeks).
  - Normalization of serum ALT usually occurs within a few weeks of initial dose; about 90% of patients who respond to Roferon A do so within the first 3 months of treatment.
  - If the patient has no response in the first 3 months, drug discontinuation should be considered.
- CML: 9 million international units daily subcutaneous for up to 18 months.
  - Short-term tolerance is improved by gradually increasing the dose over the first week from 3 million international units daily for 3 days, to 6 million international units

daily for 3 days, then to the target dose of 9 million international units for the rest of the treatment period.

- Median time to a complete hematologic response was 5 months in one study, but may take up to 18 months. Treatment should be continued until disease progression.
- If severe side effects occur, interrupt treatment or reduce dose or frequency of injections to achieve the individual maximally tolerated dose.

- Hairy-cell leukemia: Induction 3 million international units daily for 16–24 weeks SQ; maintenance 3 million international units 3 times per week for 6–24 months.

  - If dose reductions needed for severe adverse reactions, reduce dose by one-half or hold individual doses. Do not exceed doses higher than 3 million international units.
  - Patient should be evaluated for response to therapy by assessment of peripheral blood and bone marrow for hairy cells monthly. If patient does not respond within 6 months, treatment should be discontinued.

Drug Preparation:
- Available for subcutaneous administration as prefilled syringes:
  - 3 million international units/0.5 mL per syringe, in boxes of 1 or 6.
  - 6 million international units/0.5 mL per syringe in boxes of 1 or 6.
  - 9 million international units/0.5 mL per syringe in boxes of 1 or 6.
  - Store in refrigerator at 2°– 8°C (36°–46°F). Do not shake or freeze. Store in refrigerator and protect from light during storage.

Drug Administration: Intramuscular, subcutaneous, or intravenous.
- Assess CBC/platelet counts and clinical chemistry tests baseline then periodically during therapy. Carefully monitor any patients with ANC < 1,500/mm^3, platelet count < 75,000/mm^3, Hgb < 10g/dL, and creatinine > 1.5 mg/dL. Also, monitor patients with leukemia closely during the initial phase of treatment for severe BMD.
- Assess ECG baseline and during therapy in patients with preexisting cardiac abnormalities and/or in advanced stages of cancer.
- Assess LFTs in patients with chronic hepatitis C: serum ALT baseline, then at week 2 and monthly thereafter.
- Assess TSH baseline and every 3 months in patients with preexisting thyroid abnormalities, as they can be treated with the drug as long as TSH is normal.
- Assess triglycerides baseline and during therapy, and manage medically as needed. If patient has consistently elevated triglycerides (e.g., >1,000 mg/dL) associated with symptoms of pancreatitis (abdominal pain, nausea, or vomiting), drug should be discontinued.

Drug Interactions:
- May decrease elimination of aminophylline by 33–81% via inhibition of cytochrome P450 enzyme system.
- Increased effects of CNS depressants.
- Increased bone marrow suppressant effects with zidovudine (AZT).
- Drug may affect P450 oxidative metabolic process.
- Drug may increase neurotoxic, hematotoxic, or cardiotoxic effects of prior or concomitant drugs.

- IL-2 given concomitantly with Roferon-A, potentiation of risk for developing renal failure.
- Hyperglycemia.

Lab Effects/Interference:
- Dose-dependent; leukopenia, thrombocytopenia, anemia; elevated liver serum transaminases.
- Elevated triglycerides.

Special Considerations: Warnings:
- Neuropsychiatric disorders: Depression and suicidal behavior have been reported, including suicide attempts.
  - Use drug with extreme caution in patients with a history of depression, and follow patient closely if used. Teach patient to report depression or suicidal thoughts immediately.
  - Psychiatric intervention and/or drug cessation should be considered for depressed patients, but suicides have occurred after the drug was stopped.
  - CNS adverse reactions have been reported: Decreased mental status, dizziness, impaired memory, agitation, manic behavior, psychotic reactions, and rarely coma. Most were reversible with dose reduction or drug cessation within a few days–3 weeks. Use drug cautiously in patients with a seizure disorder or compromised CNS function.
- Cardiovascular disorders: Use drug cautiously in patients with cardiac disease, as drug may exacerbate preexisting cardiac disease; rarely, MI and cardiomyopathy have occurred.
- Cerebrovascular disorders: Ischemic and hemorrhagic cerebrovascular events have occurred.
- Hypersensitivity: May rarely occur (e.g., urticaria, angioedema, bronchoconstriction, anaphylaxis) as well as skin rashes. If a serious reaction occurs, drug must be discontinued and appropriate emergency medical care instituted. Transient rash does not necessitate drug interruption.
- Hepatic disorders: Transient liver abnormalities have been reported in patients with hepatitis C; if the patient has poorly compensated liver disease, results in ascites, hepatic failure, or death.
- GI disorders: Ulcerative and hemorrhagic/ischemic colitis have been reported within 12 weeks of starting therapy (characterized by abdominal pain, bloody diarrhea, fever); drug should be immediately discontinued if this occurs, and colitis usually resolves within 1–3 weeks of drug discontinuance.
- Infections: Must distinguish between fever as part of flulike symptomatology versus fever and infection, especially if patient has neutropenia. Serious bacterial, viral, fungal infections have occurred; if this happens, appropriate antimicrobial therapy should be instituted and interferon therapy discontinued.
- Bone marrow toxicity: Drug suppresses bone marrow function, resulting in cytopenias and anemia, which may be severe. Assess CBC baseline and routinely during therapy. Discontinue drug if ANC < 500 cells/mm^3 or platelets < 25,000 cells/mm^3.

• Endocrine disorders: Drug causes or exacerbates hypothyroidism and hyperthyroidism. Hyperglycemia has occurred. Diabetic patients may require adjustment of their antidiabetic medications. Assess baseline glucose and monitor during therapy, especially in diabetic patients.
• Pulmonary disorders may be induced or exacerbated; monitor for dyspnea, pulmonary infiltrates, pneumonia, bronchiolitis obliterans, interstitial pneumonitis, and sarcoidosis; evalute promptly. If patient develops persistent or unexplained pulmonary infiltrates or impaired pulmonary function, interferon should be discontinued.
• Ophthalmologic disorders: Patients should have baseline eye exam; if patient has preexisting ophthalmologic disorders (e.g., diabetic or hypertensive retinopathy), they should receive ongoing periodic exams during interferon therapy. If patient develops symptoms, this should prompt a complete eye exam, and drug should be discontinued if new or worsening ophthalmologic disorders occur.
• Pancreatitis: Marked triglyeride elevation is a risk factor. Drug should be interrupted if symptoms arise, and drug discontinued if the diagnosis of pancreatitis is confirmed.
• Most common adverse effects were: (1) in patients with chronic hepatitis C (3 million international unit dose): flulike symptoms (fatigue, myalgia/arthralgia, fever, chills, asthenia, sweating, leg cramps, malaise), headache, nausea, vomiting, diarrhea, injection-site reaction; (6 million international unit dose): higher incidence of severe psychiatric events. Fewer adverse events occur in the second 6 months of treatment than in the first 6 months; (2) patients with CML: fever, asthenia, or fatigue, myalgia, chills, arthalgia/bone pain, headache, anorexia, nausea/vomiting, diarrhea, headache, depression; (3) patients with hairy-cell leukemia: fever, fatigue, headache, chills, weight loss, skin rash, myalgia, anorexia, nausea/vomiting, diarrhea, dizziness.
• Roferon-A should be used in pregnant women only if the potential benefit justifies the potential risk to the fetus. Teach females of reproductive potential and men to use effective contraception during interferon therapy.
• Nursing mothers should make a decision whether to discontinue nursing or discontinue the drug, taking into account the importance of the drug to the mother's health.

Potential Toxicities/Side Effects (More Severe with Higher Dosing) and the Nursing Process

I.   ALTERATION IN COMFORT related to FLULIKE SYNDROME

Defining Characteristics: Chills 3–6 hours after dose in 40–60% of patients; fever (74–98% of patients) with onset 30–90 minutes after chill, lasting up to 24 hours. Temperature 39–40°C (102–104°F), tachyphylaxis (decrease in severity/occurrence after successive treatments) common. Fatigue (89–95% of patients) and malaise are cumulative and dose-limiting. Headache, myalgias occur in 60–70% of patients, as well as arthralgias (5–24% of patients).

Nursing Implications: Assess baseline T, VS, neurologic status, and comfort level; monitor every 4–6 hours if patient is in hospital. Discuss with physician premedication and regular dosing of antipyretic (e.g., acetaminophen ± diphenhydramine, NSAID). Teach patient self-care measures, including monitoring T, comfort level, self-administration of prescribed medications prior to dose and regularly postdose, as well as the use of heat or cold for myalgias, arthralgias. Encourage patient to increase oral fluids and alternate rest and activity periods. If patient is in hospital and experiences rigor, discuss with physician IV meperidine (25 mg IV q 15 min to maximum 100 mg in 1 hour) and monitor BP for hypotension. Teach patient to alternate rest and activity periods.

II. POTENTIAL FOR INFECTION AND BLEEDING related to NEUTROPENIA AND THROMBOCYTOPENIA

Defining Characteristics: Although uncommon, increased risk with increased dose; dose-limiting thrombocytopenia; reversible. Onset usually in 7–10 days, nadir at day 14, but may be delayed in hairy-cell leukemia (20–40 days); recovery in 21 days.

Nursing Implications: Assess baseline CBC, WBC, differential, and platelet count, and signs/symptoms of infection or bleeding. Discuss any abnormalities with physician before drug administration. Teach patient signs/symptoms of infection and bleeding, and to report them immediately. Teach patient self-care measures to minimize infection and bleeding, including avoidance of OTC aspirin-containing medications, and oral hygiene regimen.

III. ALTERATION IN NUTRITION, LESS THAN BODY REQUIREMENTS, related to NAUSEA, DIARRHEA, ANOREXIA

Defining Characteristics: Anorexia occurs (46–65% of patients) and is cumulative and dose-limiting. Nausea (32–51% of patients) is mild with tachyphylaxis after one week. Diarrhea (29–42% of patients) is mild, and vomiting is rare (10–17% of patients). Taste alterations and xerostomia may occur.

Nursing Implications: Assess baseline nutritional status. Teach patient potential side effects and self-care measures, including oral hygiene. Encourage patient to prepare favorite high-calorie, high-protein foods ahead of time so able to snack when hungry. Teach self-administration of prescribed antiemetics and antidiarrheals as needed. Refer to dietitian as appropriate.

IV. SENSORY/PERCEPTUAL ALTERATION related to CNS EFFECTS

Defining Characteristics: Dizziness (21–41% of patients), confusion (8–10% of patients), decreased mental status (17% of patients), and depression (16% of patients). Somnolence, irritability, poor concentration, seizures, paranoia, hallucinations, psychoses may occur in 70% of patients but are reversible. Use drug cautiously in patients with history of seizures or CNS dysfunction.

Nursing Implications: Assess baseline mental status and neurologic status prior to drug administration. Assess patient for changes (impaired memory/attention, disorientation, slow/vague responses to questions, increased lethargy) during treatment. Instruct patient to report signs/symptoms; provide information and emotional support, as well as interventions to ensure safety if signs/symptoms occur.

V. POTENTIAL ALTERATION IN CARDIAC OUTPUT related to TACHYCARDIA, CHEST PAIN, DYSRHYTHMIAS

Defining Characteristics: Uncommon but dose-related with increased risk in elderly and patients with preexisting cardiac dysfunction: tachycardia, pallor, cyanosis, chest pain, orthostatic hypotension or hypertension arrhythmias, CHF, syncope.

Nursing Implications: Assess baseline cardiopulmonary status and risk (elderly, preexisting cardiac dysfunction). EKG testing is done baseline and during treatment for high-risk individuals. Monitor VS and I/O, every 4 hours while receiving drug in hospital. Teach patient to report signs/symptoms of dyspnea, chest pain, edema, or other abnormalities immediately.

VI. POTENTIAL ALTERATION IN ELIMINATION related to RENAL AND HEPATIC DYSFUNCTION

Defining Characteristics: Dose-related increased BUN, creatinine, LFTs (increased AST 42–46%) may occur, as well as proteinuria. Patient may develop interstitial nephritis.

Nursing Implications: Assess baseline renal and hepatic function studies and urinalysis prior to drug initiation, and periodically during therapy. Discuss abnormalities with physician.

VII. POTENTIAL FOR SEXUAL DYSFUNCTION related to IMPOTENCE, MENSTRUAL IRREGULARITIES

Defining Characteristics: Impotence and decreased libido, menstrual irregularities, and increased spontaneous abortions have occurred. Drug is excreted in breastmilk.

Nursing Implications: Assess patient's baseline sexual patterns and discuss potential alterations. Provide information, emotional support, and referral as appropriate and needed. Encourage patient to use contraceptive measures; mothers receiving the drug should not breastfeed.

VIII. POTENTIAL ALTERATION IN SKIN INTEGRITY related to RASH, PARTIAL ALOPECIA, DRYNESS

Defining Characteristics: Partial alopecia (8–22% of patients), rash (11–18% of patients), throat dryness (15% of patients), as well as skin dryness, flushing, pruritus, and irritation at injection site may occur.

Nursing Implications: Assess baseline skin integrity. Instruct patient to report signs/symptoms. Discuss/teach symptomatic management, including the use of mild soaps and rinsing skin thoroughly after bathing. Encourage patient to use alcohol-free, oil-based moisturizers on skin.

IX. KNOWLEDGE DEFICIT related to SELF-ADMINISTRATION TECHNIQUE

Defining Characteristics: Often patients must receive daily dosing or thrice weekly dosing in the home setting by subcutaneous injection, and they are unfamiliar with technique.

Nursing Implications: Assess baseline psychomotor ability, knowledge, and willingness to learn technique of self-injection. Teach how to prepare drug, self-administer, and safely collect used syringes for proper disposal. Use written and video materials as supplements to teaching process and have patient correctly demonstrate technique prior to performing at home. Make referral to visiting-nurse agency to reinforce teaching.

Drug: interferon alfa-2b (Intron A, IFN-alpha-2b recombinant, β-2-interferon, rIFN-β-2)

Class: Cytokine (interferon).

Mechanism of Action: Antiviral, antiproliferative, and immunomodulatory effects. Activates prenatural killer cells, increases cytotoxicity of NK cells, and enhances immune response.

Metabolism: Well absorbed following subcutaneous or IM injection with 90% bioavailability after subcutaneous injection. Drug peaks at 6–8 hours, and has an elimination half-life of 2 hours (IM/IV) and 3 hours (subcutaneous). Renal filtration and tubular reabsorption as catabolites; minor hepatic metabolism and biliary excretion.

Indications: For the treatment of (1) adults 18 years or older with hairy-cell leukemia; (2) adults age 18 years or older with malignant melanoma, who are free of disease but at high risk for systemic recurrence, within 56 days of surgery; (3) adults age 18 years or older with clinically aggressive follicular NHL in conjunction with anthracycline-containing combination chemotherapy (efficacy in patients with low-grade, low-tumor burden follicular NHL has not been demonstrated); (4) selected adults age 18 years or older with condylomata acuminata involving external surfaces of the genital and perianal areas; (5) selected adults age 18 years or older with AIDS-related Kaposi's sarcoma (response is more likely in patients without systemic symptoms, limited lymphadenopathy, and relatively intact immune system, as indicated by total CD4 count); (6) adults age 18 years or older with chronic hepatitis C with compensated liver disease who have a history of blood or blood-product exposure and/or are HCV antibody positive (studies show clinically meaningful effects [e.g., normalization of ALT and reduction in liver necrosis and degeneration]; compensated liver disease is defined as (i) absence of history of decompensation [e.g., hepatic encephalopathy, variceal bleeding, ascites], (ii) bilirubin stable and WNL,

(iii) PT < 3 seconds prolonged, (iv) WBC ≥ 3,000/mm³, and platelets ≥ 70,000/mm³); (7) patients 1 year of age or older with chronic hepatitis B with compensated liver disease [serum HBsAg positive for at least 6 months and have evidence of HBV replication (serum HBeAg positive) with elevated serum ALT].

Contraindications: Patients with (1) hypersensitivity to interferon alpha or any product component, (2) autoimmune hepatitis, (3) decompensated liver disease. Intron A and Rebetol combination therapy is contraindicated in (1) patients with hypersensitivity to ribavirin or any other product component, (2) pregnant women, (3) men whose female partners are pregnant, (4) patients with hemoglobinopathies (e.g., thalassemia major, sickle cell anemia), (5) patients with creatinine clearance < 50 mL/min.

Dosage/Range:

- Hairy-cell leukemia: IFN-α2b: 2 million international units (MIU)/m² IM or subcutaneous three times per week for 2–6 months.
  - If platelet count is < 50,000/mm³, drug should be administered SQ not IM.
  - Dosage forms: powder: 10 million international units/mL; solution 18 million international units multidose; solution 25 million international units multidose.
  - If severe reactions, dose-reduce 50% or temporarily interrupt therapy until resolve, then resume at 50% dose (e.g., 1 million international unit/m² tiw).
  - If severe reactions recur, discontinue drug.
  - Discontinue drug if progressive disease or failure to respond after 6 months of treatment.
- Malignant melanoma: Induction: 20 million international units/m² IV infusion over 20 minutes, on days 1–5 weekly for 4 weeks.
  - Use powder ONLY: 10 million international units (10 million international units/mL), 18 million international units/mL, 50 million international units/mL. Reconstituted drug is preservative-free and single-use only.
  - Dose modifications: Hold drug for severe adverse reactions, including ANC > 250/mm³ but < 500/mm³ or ALT/AST > 5–10 × ULN, until adverse effects abate, then resume at 50% of the previous dose.
  - Permanently discontinue drug for persistent toxicity, severe adverse effects that recur on a reduced dose, or if ANC is < 250/mm³ or ALT/AST > 10 × ULN.
  - Maintenance: 10 million international units/m² subcutaneous three times per week for 48 weeks.
    - Use powder ONLY: 10 million international units (10 million international units/mL), 18 million international units/mL single dose, 18 million international units multidose (6 million international units/mL), or 25 million international units/mL (10 million international units/mL). Reconstituted drug is preservative-free and single-use only.
    - Dose modifications: Hold drug for severe adverse reactions, including ANC > 250/mm³ but < 500/mm³ or ALT/AST > 5–10 × ULN, until adverse effects abate, then resume at 50% of the previous dose.
    - Permanently discontinue drug for persistent toxicity, severe adverse effects that recur on a reduced dose, or if ANC is < 250/mm³ or ALT/AST > 10 × ULN.

- Follicular NHL: 5 million international units SQ three times a week (tiw) for up to 18 months in conjunction with an anthracycline-containing regimen and following completion of chemotherapy.
  - Powder: 10 million international units single dose; Solution: 18 million international unit multidose (6 million international unit/mL), 25 million international units (10 million international unit/mL).
  - Dose adjustment: CHOP chemotherapy doses were reduced 25% and cycle length increased by 33% from full dose when alpha-interferon was added to the regime. Delay chemotherapy cycle if ANC < 1,500/mm^3 or platelet count < 75,000/mm^3.
  - Permanently discontinue Intron A if AST > 5 × ULN or serum creatinine is > 2.0 mg/dL.
  - Hold Intron A for ANC < 1,000/mm^3 or platelet count < 50,000/mm^3.
  - Reduce Intron A dose by 50% (2.5 million international units tiw) for ANC > 1,000/mm^3 but < 1,500/mm^3; dose may be re-escalated to starting dose of 5 million international units tiw after resolution and ANC > 1,500/mm^3.
- Condylomata Acuminata: 1 million international unit per lesion in a maximum of 5 lesions in a single course. The lesions should be injected three times weekly on alternate days for 3 weeks. An additional course may be administered at 12–16 weeks.
  - DO NOT use the 18 million international units or 50 million international unit powder or the 18 million international unit multidose solution for this indication.
  - Use powder 10 million international units (single-dose), or solution 25 million international units multidose (10 million international units/mL).
  - See package insert for injection technique.
- AIDS-related Kaposi's sarcoma: IFN-α2b: 30 million international units/m^2 per dose subcutaneous or IM three times per week, until disease progression or maximal response achieved after 16 weeks of treatment. Dose reduction is frequently needed.
  - Use powder 50 million international units (50 million international units/mL). DO NOT use solution for injection. Reconstituted powder does not contain preservatives and is a single-use vial.
  - Dose adjustment: Reduce dose 50% for severe adverse reactions; resume at this lower dose after reactions abate with dosing interruption. Drug should be permanently discontinued if severe reactions persist or recur at the reduced dose.
- Chronic Hepatitis C: 3 million international units three times a week (tiw) SQ or IM. Patients tolerating therapy with normalization of ALT at 16 weeks of treatment can have treatment extended to 18–24 months, same dose, to improve the response rate.
  - If patient does not normalize ALT or have persistently high HCV RNA levels after 16 weeks, it is unlikely that he or she will get a sustained response with continued treatment; consider drug discontinuance.
  - Intron A combined with Rebetol: see package insert.
  - Dose adjustment: Dose-reduce 50% for severe adverse reactions, or therapy should be temporarily discontinued.
- Chronic Hepatitis B: Adults: 30–35 million international units per week SQ or IM, either as 5 million international units daily (QD) or as 10 million international units three times a week (tiw) for 16 weeks. Pediatrics: see package insert.

• Use dosage forms: Powder 10 million international units (single-dose) or solution 25 million international units multidose (10 million international units/mL). Reconstituted powder is preservative-free, so is a single-use vial.
• Dose adjustment: Severe adverse effects or laboratory abnormalities: 50% dose reduction, or discontinue drug as appropriate. If WBC < 1,500/mm³, ANC < 750/mm³, OR platelet count < 50,000/mm³: reduce dose 50%. If WBC < 1,000/mm³, ANC < 500/mm³, or platelet count < 25,000/mm³, permanently discontinue drug. Intron A therapy was resumed at up to 100% of the initial dose when WBC, ANC, and platelet counts returned to normal or baseline values. See package insert.

Drug Preparation:
• IFN-α2b (Intron A): Available in (1) powder for injection/reconstitution and (2) solution for injection vials. Not all dosage forms and strengths are appropriate for some indications.
• Powder for injection is preservative-free, so vial must be discarded after reconstitution and withdrawal of a single dose.
• See package insert.
• Allow solution to come to room temperature before using.

Drug Administration:
• Administer in the evening to enhance tolerability. Acetaminophen may also be administered at the same time.
• Intramuscular, subcutaneous, or IVB, intermittent or continuous infusion.
• Ensure patient has adequate hydration, especially during treatment for malignant melanoma; this may require IV hydration.
• Assess baseline CBC/differential/platelet count, blood chemistries including LFTs and TSH, electrolytes, and results of periodic assessment during therapy.
• Assess ECG of patients with preexisting cardiac abnormalities or advanced cancer baseline and periodically during therapy.
• Malignant melanoma induction: Assess differential WBC count, LFTs weekly, and then monthly during maintenance.

Drug Interactions:
• May decrease elimination of aminophylline by 33–81% via inhibition of cytochrome P450 enzyme system.
• Increased effects of CNS depressants.
• Increased bone marrow suppressant effects with zidovudine (AZT).
• Increased risk of peripheral neuropathy when combined with vinblastine.

Lab Effects/Interference:
• Dose-dependent; leukopenia; elevated liver serum transaminases.

Special Considerations:
Warnings:
• Alpha interferons, including Intron A, can cause or aggravate fatal or life-threatening neuropsychiatric, autoimmune, ischemic, and infectious disorders. Monitor patients

closely using clinical exam and laboratory evaluations. If patient has persistently severe or worsening signs or symptoms of these conditions, Intron A therapy should be withdrawn.

- Flulike symptoms can be severe and should be used cautiously in patients with debilitating medical conditons, (e.g., COPD, or DM prone to acidosis) or patients with coagulation disorders (thrombophlebitis, PE) or severe myelosuppression.
- Cardiovascular disorders: Use cautiously in patients with a history of MI or arrhythmia disorders who should be monitored closely, as drug can cause HTN, hypotension, arrhythmia, tachycardia ≥ 150 beats/min, and rarely, cardiomyopathy.
- Cerebrovascular disorders: Ischemic and hemorrhagic cerebrovascular events have occurred.
- Neuropsychiatric disorders: Depression and suicidal behavior, including suicidal ideation, have occurred.
  - If the patient develops psychiatric problems, including clinical depression, patient should be carefully monitored during treatment and in the 6-month follow-up period.
  - Drug should be used cautiously in patients with a history of psychiatric disorders and should be discontinued in any patient developing a severe psychiatric disorder during treatment. These effects usually reverse promptly after drug discontinuance, but full resolution may take up to 3 weeks.
  - If psychiatric symptoms persist or worsen, or suicidal ideation or aggressive behavior toward others occurs, drug should be discontinued and patient followed with psychiatric intervention until resolved.
  - Preexisting symptoms of psychiatric disorders may be exacerbated; if patient has a history of substance abuse, consider need for drug screening and periodic health evaluation, including psychiatric symptom-monitoring.
- Bone marrow toxicity: Drug suppresses bone marrow function and may cause cytopenias, including aplastic anemia. Monitor CBC baseline and routinely during treatment. Discontinue drug if ANC < 500 cells/mm^3 or platelet count < 25,000/mm^3.
- Ophthalmologic disorders: May be induced or aggravated; patients should have a comprehensive eye exam baseline, and if preexisting disorders (e.g., diabetic or hypertensive retinopathy), should receive periodic ophthalmologic exams. If a patient presents with ocular symptoms, a prompt and complete eye exam should be done. If the patient develops a new or worsening ophthalmologic disorder, interferon alfa-2b treatment should be discontinued.
- Endocrine disorders: Infrequently, patients may develop hypo- or hyperthyroidism. Assess baseline TSH, and repeat if patients develop symptoms of thyroid dysfunction. If the patient has a preexisting thyroid abnormality and normal thyroid function cannot be managed, Intron A should not be administered. Diabetes may occur; if it is unable to be controlled, drug should be stopped.
- GI disorders: Hepatotoxicity may occur. Monitor patients with liver function abnormalities closely, and discontinue drug if needed.
- Pulmonary disorders: May be induced or worsened (e.g., dyspnea, pulmonary infiltrates, pneumonia, bronchiolitis obliterans, interstitial pneumonitis, pulmonary hypertension, sarcoidosis). If a patient presents with fever, cough, dyspnea, or other respiratory

symptoms, a CXR should be assessed. If there are pulmonary infiltrates, or evidence of pulmonary function impairment, monitor the patient closely and discontinue drug as appropriate.

- Autoimmune disorders: May occur (e.g., thrombocytopenia, vasculitis, RA, lupus erythematosius, rhabdomyolysis). If a patient develops an autoimmune disorder during therapy, monitor the patient closely and discontinue drug if appropriate.
- Human albumin is used in the drug manufacture and carries a theoretical, remote risk of Creutzfeldt-Jakob disease (CJD).
- AIDS-related Kaposi's sarcoma: Drug should not be used if patient has rapidly progressive visceral disease. Patients receiving zidovudine and Intron A may have synergistic effect, with a higher incidence of neutropenia. Monitor the WBC closely.
- Chronic hepatitis C and chronic hepatitis B: Drug should not be used in patients with decompensated liver disease, autoimmune hepatitis, a history of autoimmune disease, or patients who are immunosuppressed transplant recipients.
- Peripheral neuropathy: Has been reported when drug is administered with telbivudine.
- Use with ribavirin (Rebetol) may cause birth defects and/or death of unborn child. Confirm a negative pregnancy test immediately before planned initiation of therapy. Teach female patients to use at least 2 forms of contraception and have monthly pregnancy tests. Combination with ribavirin may also cause hemolytic anemia, with anemia occurring within 1–2 weeks of starting ribavirin.
- Acute serious hypersensitivity reactions (e.g., urticaria, angioedema, bronchoconstriction, anaphylaxis) may rarely occur. Provide appropriate medical care as ordered, and drug should be discontinued for acute reactions.
- Elevated triglycerides may occur and may result in pancreatitis. If patient has persistently elevated triglycerides > 1,000 mg/dL, drug should be discontinued.

Potential Toxicities/Side Effects (More Severe with Higher Dosing) and the Nursing Process

I. ALTERATION IN COMFORT related to FLULIKE SYNDROME

Defining Characteristics: Chills 3–6 hours after dose in 40–60% of patients; fever (74–98% of patients) with onset 30–90 minutes after chill, lasting up to 24 hours. Temperature 39–40°C (102–104°F); tachyphylaxis (decrease in severity/occurrence after successive treatments) common. Fatigue (89–95% of patients) and malaise are cumulative and dose-limiting. Headache, myalgias occur in 60–70% of patients, as well as arthralgias (5–24% of patients).

Nursing Implications: Assess baseline T, VS, neurologic status, and comfort level; monitor every 4–6 hours if patient is in hospital. Discuss with physician premedication and regular dosing of antipyretic (e.g., acetaminophen ± diphenhydramine, NSAID). Teach patient self-care measures, including monitoring T, comfort level, self-administration of prescribed medications prior to dose and regularly postdose, as well as the use of heat or cold for myalgias, arthralgias. Encourage patient to increase oral fluids and alternate rest and activity periods. If patient is in hospital and experiences rigor, discuss with physician

IV meperidine (25 mg IV q 15 min to maximum 100 mg in 1 hour) and monitor blood pressure for hypotension. Teach patient to alternate rest and activity.

II. POTENTIAL FOR INFECTION AND BLEEDING related to NEUTROPENIA AND THROMBOCYTOPENIA

Defining Characteristics: Although uncommon, increased risk with increased dose; dose-limiting thrombocytopenia, reversible. Onset in 7–10 days, nadir in 14 days (may be delayed 20–40 days in patients with hairy-cell leukemia), and recovery at day 21.

Nursing Implications: Assess baseline CBC, white blood count, differential, and platelet count, and signs/symptoms of infection or bleeding. Discuss any abnormalities with physician before drug administration. Teach patient signs/symptoms of infection and bleeding, and to report them immediately. Teach patient self-care measures to minimize infection and bleeding, including avoidance of OTC aspirin-containing medications, and oral hygiene regimen.

III. ALTERATION IN NUTRITION, LESS THAN BODY REQUIREMENTS, related to NAUSEA, DIARRHEA, ANOREXIA

Defining Characteristics: Anorexia occurs (46–65% of patients) and is cumulative and dose-limiting. Nausea (32–51% of patients) is mild with tachyphylaxis after 1 week. Diarrhea (29–42% of patients) is mild, and vomiting is rare (10–17% of patients). Taste alterations and xerostomia may occur.

Nursing Implications: Assess baseline nutritional status. Teach patient potential side effects and self-care measures including oral hygiene. Encourage patient to prepare favorite high-calorie, high-protein foods ahead of time so able to snack when hungry. Teach self-administration of prescribed antiemetics and antidiarrheals as needed. Refer to dietitian as appropriate.

IV. SENSORY/PERCEPTUAL ALTERATION related to CNS EFFECTS

Defining Characteristics: Dizziness (21–41% of patients), confusion (8–10% of patients), decreased mental status (17% of patients), and depression (16% of patients). Somnolence, irritability, poor concentration, seizures, paranoia, hallucinations, psychoses may occur in 70% of patients but are reversible. Use drug cautiously in patients with history of seizures or CNS dysfunction.

Nursing Implications: Assess baseline mental status and neurologic status prior to drug administration. Assess patient for changes (impaired memory/attention, disorientation, slow/vague responses to questions, increased lethargy) during treatment. Instruct patient to report signs/symptoms; provide information and emotional support, as well as interventions to ensure safety if signs/symptoms occur.

V.   POTENTIAL ALTERATION IN CARDIAC OUTPUT related to TACHYCARDIA, CHEST PAIN, DYSRHYTHMIAS

Defining Characteristics: Uncommon but dose-related with increased risk in elderly and patients with preexisting cardiac dysfunction: tachycardia, pallor, cyanosis, chest pain, orthostatic hypotension or hypertension arrhythmias, CHF, syncope.

Nursing Implications: Assess baseline cardiopulmonary status and risk (elderly, preexisting cardiac dysfunction). ECG testing is done baseline and during treatment for high-risk individuals. Monitor VS and I/O every 4 hours while receiving drug in hospital. Teach patient to report signs/symptoms of dyspnea, chest pain, edema, or other abnormalities immediately.

VI.   POTENTIAL ALTERATION IN ELIMINATION related to RENAL AND HEPATIC DYSFUNCTION

Defining Characteristics: Dose-related increased BUN, creatinine, LFTs (increased AST in 42–46%) may occur, as well as proteinuria. Patient may develop interstitial nephritis.

Nursing Implications: Assess baseline renal and hepatic function studies and urinalysis prior to drug initiation, and periodically during therapy. Discuss abnormalities with physician.

VII.   POTENTIAL FOR SEXUAL DYSFUNCTION related to IMPOTENCE, MENSTRUAL IRREGULARITIES

Defining Characteristics: Impotence and decreased libido, menstrual irregularities, and increased spontaneous abortions have occurred. Drug is excreted in breastmilk.

Nursing Implications: Assess patient's baseline sexual patterns and discuss potential alterations. Provide information, emotional support, and referral as appropriate and needed. Encourage patient to use contraceptive measures; mothers receiving the drug should not breastfeed.

VIII.   POTENTIAL ALTERATION IN SKIN INTEGRITY related to RASH, PARTIAL ALOPECIA, DRYNESS

Defining Characteristics: Partial alopecia (8–22% of patients), rash (11–18% of patients), throat dryness (15% of patients), as well as skin dryness, flushing, pruritus, and irritation at injection site may occur.

Nursing Implications: Assess baseline skin integrity. Instruct patient to report signs/symptoms. Discuss/teach symptomatic management, including the use of mild soaps and rinsing skin thoroughly after bathing. Encourage patient to use alcohol-free, oil-based moisturizers on skin.

IX. KNOWLEDGE DEFICIT related to SELF-ADMINISTRATION TECHNIQUE

Defining Characteristics: Often patients must receive daily dosing or thrice weekly dosing in the home setting by subcutaneous injection, and they are unfamiliar with technique.

Nursing Implications: Assess baseline psychomotor ability, knowledge, and willingness to learn technique of self-injection. Teach how to prepare drug, self-administer, and safely collect used syringes for proper disposal. Use written and video materials as supplements to teaching process and have patient correctly demonstrate technique prior to performing at home. Make referral to visiting-nurse agency to reinforce teaching.

Drug: interferon gamma (Actimmune, IFN-gamma [γ], rIFN-gamma)

Class: Cytokine (Interferon).

Mechanism of Action: Actimmune is interferon gamma-1b. It has antiviral, antiproliferative, and immunomodulatory effects. Activates phagocytes and appears to generate toxic oxidative metabolites in phagocytes; interacts with interleukins to orchestrate immune effect, and enhances antibody-dependent cellular cytotoxicity, NK activity, and mounting of antigen on monocytes (Fc expression).

Metabolism: Slowly absorbed following subcutaneous or IM injection, with 89% bioavailability. Peaks in 4–13 hours following IM injection, and 6–7 hours after subcutaneous injection. Elimination half-lives for IV injection are 30–60 minutes, and 2–8 hours for IM or subcutaneous injection. Renal filtration and tubular reabsorption as catabolites; minor hepatic metabolism and biliary excretion.

Indication: (1) For reducing the frequency and severity of serious infections associated with chronic granulomatous disease (CGD), and (2) delaying time to progression in patients with severe, malignant osteopetrosis.

Contraindications: Patients with known or developed hypersensitivity to interferon-gamma, *E. coli* derived products, or any product components.

Dosage/Range:
- CGD and severe malignant osteopetrosis:
  - BSA > 0.5 m²: 50 mcg/m² (1 million international units)/m² SQ three times a week (e.g., M, W, F).
  - BSA < 0.5 m²: 1.5 mcg/kg/dose.
  - Dose modification: dose-reduce 50% for severe adverse reactions, or interrupt dose until reaction abates.

Drug Preparation:
- May use either sterilized glass or plastic disposable syringes.
- Drug is clear, colorless in a single-use vial for subcutaneous injection. Each 0.5 mL of Actimmune contains 100 mcg (2 million international units). It is available as a single vial or in cartons of 12.

- Vials should be stored in a refrigerator at 2–8°C (36–46°F) immediately upon receipt. DO NOT FREEZE. Avoid vigorous shaking. An unentered vial of Actimmune should not be left at room temperature for a total time > 12 hours prior to use; if it is left out for > 12 hours, it should be discarded.

Drug Administration:
- SQ in the right or left deltoid, or anterior thigh.
- Teach patient or caregiver SQ technique, aseptic technique, safe handling, and disposal of hazardous waste.
- In addition to indicated tests for each diagnosis, the following tests are recommended for patients receiving interferon-gamma baseline and every 3 months while on therapy:
  - CBC/differential/platelet count.
  - Blood chemistries (including renal, LFTs); in patients < 1 year of age, LFTs should be assessed monthly.
  - Urinalysis.

Drug Interactions:
- May decrease elimination of aminophylline by 33–81% via inhibition of cytochrome P450 enzyme system.
- Increased effects of CNS depressants.
- Increased bone marrow suppressant effects with zidovudine (AZT), other bone marrow suppressive agents.

Lab Effects/Interference:
- Dose-dependent, leukopenia; elevated liver serum transaminases.
- Increased serum creatinine, BUN, proteinuria.

Special Considerations:
Warnings:
- Cardiovascular disorders: Acute and transient flulike syndrome (fever, chills) may exacerbate preexisting cardiac problems. Use drug cautiously in patients with ischemia, CHF, or arrhythmia.
- Neurologic disorders: Abnormal neurological symptoms may occur but are reversible soon after drug discontinuation. Most are mild and include decreased mental status, gait disturbance, dizziness. Use drug cautiously in patients with a history of seizures.
- Bone marrow toxicity: Reversible neutropenia and thrombocytopenia may occur and be severe.
- Hepatic toxicity: May occur with elevations of AST and/or ALT (up to 25-fold). This occurs more often in children younger than 1 year, compared to older children; these children should have monthly LFT assessment. Elevated values are reversible with dose reduction or drug interruption.

Precautions:
- Acute serious hypersensitivity reactions may occur; if so, discontinue the drug and provide appropriate medical intervention as ordered.

- Drug should be used during pregnancy only if the potential benefit justifies the potential risk to the fetus.
- Nursing mothers should make a decision to discontinue nursing or to discontinue the drug, taking into consideration the importance of the drug to the mother's health.

Potential Toxicities/Side Effects (More Severe with Higher Dosing) and the Nursing Process

I. ALTERATION IN COMFORT related to FLULIKE SYNDROME

Defining Characteristics: Chills 3–6 hours after dose in 14% of patients; fever (52% of patients), with onset 30–90 minutes after chill. Tachyphylaxis (decrease in severity/occurrence after successive treatments) common. Fatigue (14% of patients) and myalgia (6%) can occur. Headache occurs in 33% of patients.

Nursing Implications: Assess baseline T, VS, neurologic status, and comfort level; monitor every 4–6 hours if patient is in hospital. Discuss with physician premedication and regular dosing of antipyretic (e.g., acetaminophen ± diphenhydramine, NSAID). Teach patient self-care measures, including monitoring temperature, comfort level, self-administration of prescribed medications prior to dose and regularly postdose, as well as the use of heat or cold for myalgias, arthralgias. Encourage patient to increase oral fluids and alternate rest and activity periods. If patient is in hospital and experiences rigor, discuss with physician IV meperidine (25 mg IV q 15 min to maximum 100 mg in 1 hour) and monitor blood pressure for hypotension. Teach patient to alternate rest and activity.

II. POTENTIAL FOR INFECTION AND BLEEDING related to NEUTROPENIA AND THROMBOCYTOPENIA

Defining Characteristics: Although uncommon, increased risk with increased dose; dose-limiting thrombocytopenia; reversible.

Nursing Implications: Assess baseline CBC, white blood count, differential, and platelet count, and signs/symptoms of infection or bleeding. Discuss any abnormalities with physician before drug administration. Teach patient signs/symptoms of infection and bleeding, and to report them immediately. Teach patient self-care measures to minimize infection and bleeding, including avoidance of OTC aspirin-containing medications, and oral hygiene regimen.

III. ALTERATION IN NUTRITION, LESS THAN BODY REQUIREMENTS, related to NAUSEA, DIARRHEA

Defining Characteristics: Nausea (10% of patients) is mild with tachyphylaxis after 1 week. Diarrhea (14% of patients) is mild, and vomiting is rare (13% of patients).

Nursing Implications: Assess baseline nutritional status. Teach patient potential side effects and self-care measures, including oral hygiene. Encourage patient to prepare favorite high-calorie, high-protein foods ahead of time so able to snack when hungry. Teach self-administration of prescribed antiemetics and antidiarrheals as needed. Refer to dietitian as appropriate.

IV.   KNOWLEDGE DEFICIT related to SELF-ADMINISTRATION TECHNIQUE

Defining Characteristics: Often patients must receive daily dosing or thrice weekly dosing in the home setting by subcutaneous injection, and they are unfamiliar with technique.

Nursing Implications: Assess baseline psychomotor ability, knowledge, and willingness to learn technique of self-injection. Teach how to prepare drug, self-administer, and safely collect used syringes for proper disposal. Use written and video materials as supplements to teaching process, and have patient correctly demonstrate technique prior to performing at home. Make referral to visiting-nurse agency to reinforce teaching.

Drug: oprelvekin (Neumega)

Class: Biologic (interleukin).

Mechanism of Action: IL-11 is a thrombopoietin growth factor that directly stimulates the bone marrow stem cells and megakaryocyte progenitor cells so that the production of platelets is increased. Produced by recombinant DNA technology. Results in higher platelet nadir and accelerates time to platelet recovery postchemotherapy.

Metabolism: Peak serum concentrations reached in approximately 3 ± 2 hours, with a terminal half-life of approximately 7 ± 1 hours. Bioavailability is $< 80\%$. Clearance decreases with age, and drug is rapidly cleared from the serum, distributed to organs with high perfusion, metabolized, and excreted by the kidneys. Little intact drug is found in the urine.

Indications: For the prevention of severe thrombocytopenia and the reduction in the need for platelet transfusions after myelosuppressive chemotherapy in adult patients with non-myeloid malignancies who are at high risk of severe thrombocytopenia.

Contraindication: Patients with a history of hypersensitivity to Neumega or any component of the product. Drug is NOT indicated following myeloablative chemotherapy, as there is increased toxicity.

Dosage/Range:
• Adults: 50 µg/kg subcutaneous daily.

Drug Preparation:
• Available as single-use vial containing 5 mg of oprelvekin as a lyophilized, preservative-free powder. This is reconstituted with 1 mL sterile water for injection, USP, gently swirled to mix, and results in a concentration of 5 mg/1 mL in a single-use vial. NOTE: 5 mL of diluent is supplied, but only 1 mL should be withdrawn to reconstitute drug.

Drug should be used within 3 hours of reconstitution. If not used immediately, store reconstituted solution in refrigerator or at room temperature, but DO NOT FREEZE OR SHAKE.

Drug Administration:
- The drug should be administered subcutaneously every day (abdomen, thigh or hip, or upper arm). Begin daily administration 6–24 hours after the completion of chemotherapy, and continue until the postnadir platelet count is equal to or greater than 50,000 cells/mL.
  - Do not give for more than 21 days, and stop at least 2 days before starting the next planned cycle of chemotherapy.
  - Drug has *not* been evaluated in patients receiving chemotherapy regimens longer than 5 days, nor has it been shown to cause delayed myelosuppression (e.g., mitomycin C, nitrosoureas).
- Assess for allergic reactions (e.g., edema of face, tongue, larynx); SOB, wheezing, chest pain, hypotension including shock; dysarthria, loss of consciousness; mental status changes; rash; urticaria; flushing and fever. Drug should be discontinued if patient develops an allergic or hypersensitivity reaction.

Drug Interactions:
- Unknown.

Lab Effects/Interference:
- Increase in platelet count.
- Anemia associated with increased circulating plasma volume.

Special Considerations:
- Allergic reactions including anaphylaxis have occurred.
- Increased toxicity following myeloablative therapy for which the drug is not indicated.
- Causes fluid retention, so must be used with caution in patients with CHF or in patients receiving chronic diuretic therapy.
- Monitor platelet count frequently during oprelvekin therapy, and at the time of the expected nadir to identify when recovery will begin.
- Drug should not be used during pregnancy or by nursing mothers.

Potential Toxicities/Side Effects and the Nursing Process

I.   ALTERATIONS IN FLUID AND ELECTROLYTE BALANCE related to FLUID RETENTION

Defining Characteristics: Most patients develop mild to moderate fluid retention (peripheral edema, dyspnea on exertion) but without weight gain. Fluid retention is reversible in a few days after drug is stopped. Patients with preexisting pleural effusions, pericardial effusions, or ascites may develop increased fluid, and may require drainage. Patients receiving chronic administration of potassium-excreting diuretics should be monitored extremely closely, as there are reports of sudden death due to severe hypokalemia in patients receiving ifosfamide and chronic diuretic therapy. Capillary leak syndrome has *not* been reported. Dilutional anemia has occurred.

Nursing Implications: Assess baseline fluid and electrolyte balance, and weight prior to beginning drug. Assess presence of history of cardiac problems, or CHF, and risk of developing fluid volume overload. If diuretic therapy is ordered, monitor fluid and electrolyte balance very carefully, and replete electrolytes as indicated and ordered. Teach patients that mild-to-moderate peripheral edema and shortness of breath on exertion are likely to occur during the first week of treatment and will disappear after treatment ends. If the patient has CHF or pleural effusions, instruct to report worsening dyspnea to their nurse or physician.

II.   ALTERATION IN CIRCULATION related to ATRIAL FIBRILLATION

Defining Characteristics: Some patients (10%) experience transient arrhythmias, including atrial fibrillation or flutter, after treatment with oprelvekin; it is believed to be caused by increased plasma volume rather than the drug itself. Arrhythmias may be symptomatic, are usually brief in duration, and are not clinically significant. Some patients have spontaneous conversion to a normal sinus rhythm, while others require rate-controlling drug therapy. Most patients can receive drug without recurrence of the atrial arrhythmia. Risk factors for developing atrial arrhythmias are (1) advancing age, (2) use of cardiac medications, (3) history of doxorubicin exposure, and (4) history of atrial arrhythmia. Other cardiovascular events include tachycardia, vasodilatation, palpitations, and syncope.

Nursing Implications: Assess baseline risk. If patient has history or presence of atrial arrhythmias, discuss with the physician potential benefit versus risk, and monitor very closely. Monitor baseline heart rate and other vital signs at each visit. Instruct patient to report immediately palpitations, lightheadedness, dizziness, or any other change in condition, especially if patient has any risk factors.

III.   ALTERATION IN SENSORY PERCEPTION related to VISUAL BLURRING

Defining Characteristics: Transient, mild visual blurring has been reported, as has papilledema in 1.5% of patients. Dizziness (38%), insomnia (33%), and infection of conjunctiva (19%) may also occur.

Nursing Implications: Assess risk for papilledema (existing papilledema, CNS tumors); assess for changes in pupillary response in these patients. Teach patients that dizziness and insomnia may occur; tell them to change positions slowly and to hold onto supportive structures. If insomnia is severe, discuss sleep medications with physician.

IV.   ALTERATION IN NUTRITION, LESS THAN FULL BODY REQUIREMENTS, related to GI SYMPTOMS

Defining Characteristics: Nausea, vomiting, mucositis, and diarrhea may occur, although percentage was not significantly greater than placebo control. Oral candidiasis occurred in 14% of patients, and this was significantly greater than control.

Nursing Implications: Instruct patient to report changes, and assess impact on nutrition. Inspect oral mucosa and teach patient how to inspect it. Because patient is receiving myelosuppressive chemotherapy, teaching should include oral hygiene regimen and frequent self-assessment by patient.

V. ALTERATIONS IN BREATHING PATTERN, INEFFECTIVE, POTENTIAL, related to DYSPNEA, COUGH

Defining Characteristics: Dyspnea (48% of patients), rhinitis (42%), increased cough (29%), pharyngitis (25%), and pleural effusions (10%) may occur.

Nursing Implications: Assess baseline pulmonary status and presence of pleural effusions. Instruct patient to report dyspnea and any other changes. Discuss significant changes with physician.

Drug: palifermin (Kepivance)

Class: Mucocutaneous epithelial (Keratinocyte) growth factor.

Mechanism of Action: Palifermin is a keratinocyte growth factor (KGF) produced by recombinant DNA technology, similar to the naturally occurring, endogenous KGF. Once EGF binds to its receptor found on epithelial cells—including those of the tongue, buccal mucosa, mammary gland, skin (hair follicles and sebaceous gland), lung, liver, and the lens of the eye—it stimulates proliferation, differentiation, and migration of epithelial cells. KGF decreases the incidence and duration of severe stomatitis in patients with hematologic malignancies who undergo high-dose chemotherapy and radiation therapy with stem cell rescue.

Metabolism: Palifermin has an elimination half-life of 4.5 hours (average).

Indication: To decrease the incidence and duration of severe oral mucositis in patients with hematologic malignancies receiving myelotoxic therapy requiring hematopoietic stem cell support; indicated as supportive care for preparative regimens predicted to result in ≥ WHO grade 3 mucositis in the majority of patients.

Safety and efficacy of drug have not been established in patients with nonhematologic malignancies. Drug is not recommended for use with melphalan 200 mg/m^2 as a conditioning regimen.

Dosage/Range:
- 60 mcg/kg/day IV bolus for 3 consecutive days before and 3 consecutive days after myelotoxic therapy, for a total of 6 doses.
  - The first 3 doses prior to chemotherapy, with the third dose 24–48 hours before myelotoxic therapy.

- Administer the last 3 doses after myelotoxic therapy with the first of the doses on the day of hematopoietic stem cell infusion after the infusion is completed, and more than 4 days after the most recent administration of palifermin.

Drug Preparation:
- Available as 6.25-mg lyophilized powder in a single-use vial.
- Reconstitute Kepivance lyophilized powder with sterile water for injection USP, aseptically, by slowly injecting 1.2 mL sterile water for injection USP to yield final volume of 5 mg/mL. Do not shake or agitate the vial.
- Protect from light.
- Drug should be used immediately. If not, reconstituted solution may be refrigerated in its carton for up to 24 hours at 2–8°C (36–46°F); prior to injection, may leave at room temperature for up to 1 hour protected from light. Inspect for discoloration or particulates; if found, do not use. The drug contains no preservatives, so any unused portion should be discarded.
- Do not filter drug during reconstitution or administration.
- Prior to administration, allow palifermin to reach room temperature for a maximum of 1 hour protected from light. Discard drug if left at room temperature > 1 hour.

Drug Administration:
- Administer IV bolus; if heparin used to maintain an IV line, rinse the line with saline prior to and after palifermin administration.
- Premyelotoxic therapy: The third dose should be 24–48 hours before myelotoxic chemotherapy is administered.
- Postmyelotoxic therapy: The first of the three doses should be given after, but on the same day of the hematopoietic stem cell infusion, and at least 4 days after the most recent administration of palifermin.

Drug Interactions:
- Heparin: Palifermin binds to heparin, so drugs should not be used concomitantly; flush central line well with saline prior to administration of palifermin.
- Myelotoxic chemotherapy: If given with chemotherapy, KGF increases the severity and duration of oral mucositis. Palifermin should NOT be administered within 24 hours before, during infusion of, or after the administration of myelotoxic chemotherapy.

Lab Effects/Interference:
- Increase in serum amylase and lipase.

Special Considerations:
- Potential for stimulation of tumor growth may exist in nonhematologic malignancies.
- Drug is embryotoxic to lab animals when given in higher doses; drug should be used in pregnant women only when the potential benefit to the mother exceeds the risk to the fetus.
- Nursing mothers should make a decision to discontinue nursing or to discontinue the drug, taking into account the importance of the drug to the patient's health.

• Most common adverse reactions are skin toxicities (rash, erythema, edema, pruritis), oral toxicities (dysesthesia, tongue discoloration, tongue thickening, alteration of taste), pain, arthralgias, and dysesthesia (usually localized to the perioral area).

Potential Toxicities/Side Effects and the Nursing Process

I. POTENTIAL ALTERATION IN SKIN INTEGRITY related to SKIN RASH

Defining Characteristics: Skin rash was the most common serious adverse reaction and occurred in 62% of patients in clinical studies. Skin toxicity was manifested by rash, erythema (32%), edema (28%), pruritus (35%). Median time to onset was 6 days after the first of three doses, and lasted a median of 5 days.

Nursing Implications: Teach patient that skin changes may occur and to report them. Teach patient self-care strategies to promote comfort and reduce the risk of infection.

II. ALTERATION IN NUTRITION AND COMFORT related to ORAL TOXICITIES

Defining Characteristics: Dysesthesia, tongue discoloration, tongue thickening, alterations in taste occur related to the increased keratin layer on the lining of the oral cavity.

Nursing Implications: Inform patient that these side effects may occur. Teach patient systematic oral cleansing after meals and at bedtime. Inform patient to report discomfort or inability to chew or swallow, and develop plan with measures to promote comfort and nutrition. Many patients are already receiving TPN. If taste alterations are bothersome, suggest dietitian referral for measures to stimulate taste.

III. ALTERATION IN COMFORT related to PAIN, ARTHRALGIAS, AND DYSESTHESIAS

Defining Characteristics: Dysesthesia, pain, and arthralgias may occur and affect about 12% of patients.

Nursing Implications: Assess baseline comfort, as well as existing arthralgias and dysesthesias. Perform a basic neurologic assessment. Inform patient these side effects may occur and to report them if they occur. Develop a plan of care that includes self-care activities to promote comfort, such as the use of heat or cold for arthralgias. If pain related to stomatitis is severe, then patient-controlled analgesia may be necessary. Teach patient to report any dysesthesias, hyperesthesias, hypoesthesias, or paresthesias that occur. Develop a plan to minimize discomfort, such as keeping sheets off feet if patient has hyperesthesias.

Drug: pegfilgrastim (Neulasta)

Class: Cytokine, CSF.

Mechanism of Action: Recombinant DNA protein (G-CSF) that regulates the production of neutrophils in the bone marrow (proliferation, differentiation, activation of mature neutrophils). Drug is produced by the insertion of the human G-CSF gene into *Escherichia coli* bacteria. Drug has longer half-life and different excretion pattern as compared to the parent drug, filgrastim.

Metabolism: Clearance of drug decreases with increased dose and body weight, and is directly related to the number of neutrophils so that as neutrophil recovery begins after myelosuppressive chemotherapy, serum concentration of pegfilgrastim declines rapidly. In patients with increased body weight, systemic exposure to the drug was higher, despite dose normalized for body weight. Pharmacokinetics are variable, with a half-life of 15–80 hours after subcutaneous injection. Pharmacokinetics did not vary with age (elderly) or gender.

Indication: To decrease the incidence of infection, as manifested by febrile neutropenia, in patients with nonmyeloid malignancies receiving myelosuppressive anti-cancer drugs associated with a clinically significant incidence of febrile neutropenia.

Contraindication: Patients with a history of serious allergic reactions to pegfilgrastim or filgrastim.

Dosage/Range:

- 6 mg subcutaneous once per chemotherapy cycle in adults. Do not administer between 14 days before and 24 hours after administration of cytotoxic chemotherapy.

Drug Preparation:

- Drug available in refrigerated 6-mg (0.6-mL) prefilled syringes with UltraSafe Needle Guards.
- Unopened vials should be stored in the refrigerator at 2–8°C (36–46°F) in the original carton to protect from light.
- Avoid shaking. Screen for visible particulate matter or discoloration and do not use if found.
- Remove from refrigerator 30 minutes prior to injection, but drug may be left at room temperature for up to 48 hours.
- If drug accidentally freezes, allow to thaw in the refrigerator prior to administration; if frozen a second time, discard.
- Needle cover on the single-use prefilled syringe contains dry natural rubber (latex), so individuals with latex allergies should not administer the product.

Drug Administration:

- Subcutaneous × 1 *at least 14 days prior to or more than 24 hours after* chemotherapy administration.

- Pegfilgrastim is administered as a subcutaneous injection as a single prefilled syringe either (1) via manual injection or (2) via the On-Body Injector for Neulasta, which is co-packaged with a single prefilled syringe.
- Following injection, activate UltraSafe Needle Guard by holding hands behind the needle and sliding the guard forward until the needle is completely covered and guard clicks into place. If no click is heard, drop entire syringe/needle into sharps disposal container.
- Needle cover on the single-use prefilled syringe contains dry natural rubber (latex), so individuals with latex allergies should not administer the product.

Drug Interactions:
- Lithium: may potentiate the release of neutrophils from the bone marrow; monitor neutrophil count more frequently.

Lab Effects/Interference:
- Increased white blood cell count and neutrophil count.

Special Considerations:
- Indicated to decrease the incidence of infection (febrile neutropenia) in patients with nonmyeloid malignancies receiving myelosuppressive anticancer therapy associated with a significant incidence of febrile neutropenia.
- Contraindicated in patients with known hypersensitivity to *E. coli*-derived proteins, pegfilgrastim, filgrastim, or any product component; contraindicated in peripheral blood progenitor cell (PBPC) mobilization, as the drug has not been studied in this population.
- Splenic rupture has been reported in patients receiving the parent drug, filgrastim, for PBPC. If a patient receiving pegfilgrastim complains of left upper abdominal or shoulder tip pain, patient should be evaluated immediately for an enlarged spleen or splenic rupture.
- On-Body Injector: A healthcare provider must fill the injector with Neulasta using the prefilled syringe, then apply the injector to the patient's skin (abdomen or back of arm). The back of the arm can be used only if a caregiver will monitor the status of the injector. Approximately 27 hours after the On-Body Injector is applied to intact, non-irritated skin, Neulasta will be administered over 45 minutes.
  - A healthcare provider may apply the injector to the patient's skin on the same day as chemotherapy is administered as long as the injector delivers Neulasta no less than 24 hours after the chemotherapy is administered.
  - The co-packaged prefilled syringe contains additional solution to compensate for loss during delivery, so the syringe can be used *only with the injector*. If the syringe is used for manual administration, the patient will receive an overdose of Neulasta. If a manual prefilled syringe is used for the injector, the patient will be underdosed.
  - If a dose is missed due to failure or leakage of the injector, a new dose should be administered as soon as possible once detected.
  - See the healthcare provider instructions for use of the On-Body Injector for Neulasta for complete information.

- Teach patient the following: (1) avoid traveling, driving, or operating heavy machinery during hours 26–29 following application of the injector (including the 45-minute delivery period plus an hour post delivery); (2) have a caregiver nearby for first use of the injector; (3) review the patient instructions for use of the Neulasta On-Body Injector with the patient and caregiver and ensure understanding of when the dose delivery of Neulasta will begin, how to monitor the On-Body Injector for completed delivery, and how to identify signs of malfunction of the injector.
- Adult respiratory distress syndrome (ARDS) has been reported in neutropenic patients with sepsis receiving the parent drug filgrastim, probably related to the influx of neutrophils to inflamed pulmonary sites. Neutropenic patients receiving pegfilgrastim who develop fever, lung infiltrates, or respiratory distress should be immediately evaluated for ARDS. If ARDS is suspected, pegfilgrastim should be stopped until ARDS resolves with appropriate medical care.
- Severe sickle cell crisis, rarely fatal, has been reported in patients with sickle cell disease (homozygous sickle cell anemia, sickle/hemoglobin C disease, sickle/ -thalassemia) who received filgrastim, the parent drug. Pegfilgrastim should be used in this population only when the potential benefit outweighs the risk, and patients should be well hydrated and closely monitored for sickle cell crisis, with immediate intervention.
- Pegfilgrastim should not be administered within *14 days prior to* and *for 24 hours after chemotherapy administration* because of the potential for an increase in sensitivity of rapidly dividing myeloid cells to the chemotherapy.
- Allergic reactions to pegfilgrastim, including anaphylaxis, skin rash, and urticaria, have been reported, most often on initial exposure to the drug but in some instances after the drug was stopped. If a serious allergic reaction occurs, the drug should be discontinued and the patient closely monitored for several days.
- Drug may exacerbate preexisting psoriasis, Sweet's syndrome (neutrophilic dermatitis), and cutaneous vasculitis.
- G-CSF receptor to which drug binds is also found in tumor cell lines (some myeloid, T-lymphoid, lung, head and neck, and bladder cancer), and the potential for the drug to be a tumor growth factor exists.
- Drug should not be used for peripheral blood progenitor cell mobilization.
- Drug should be used in pregnant women only when the potential benefit outweighs risk of fetal harm, as there are no adequate controlled studies in pregnant women, and laboratory animals had increased number of abortions and wavy ribs in fetuses.

Potential Toxicities/Side Effects (Dose- and Schedule-Dependent) and the Nursing Process

I.   ALTERATION IN COMFORT related to SKELETAL PAIN, HEADACHE, MYALGIA, ABDOMINAL PAIN, ARTHRALGIA

Defining Characteristics: Patients (26%) may report transient mild-to-moderate skeletal pain believed due to the expansion of cells in the bone marrow in response to G-CSF. About 12% used nonopioid analgesics, and less than 6% required opioid analgesics. Leukocytosis of more than $100–10^9$/L occurred in < 1% of patients. Other pain related to headache, myalgia and arthralgia, and abdominal pain may occur less commonly, but is easily managed.

Nursing Implications: Teach patient that bone pain may occur, and discuss use of non-steroidal anti-inflammatory drugs with patient and physician for symptom management. Monitor WBC, hematocrit, and platelet count as appropriate prior to each cycle of chemotherapy. Teach patient that headache, myalgia, arthralgia, abdominal pain may occur and to report them if they do not respond to usual management strategies.

II.   ALTERATION IN NUTRITION, POTENTIAL, related to NAUSEA, VOMITING, CONSTIPATION, DIARRHEA, ANOREXIA, STOMATITIS, MUCOSITIS

Defining Characteristics: Nutritional symptoms are rarely reported and may be related to the underlying malignancy.

Nursing Implications: Perform baseline patient nutritional assessment, history of nausea and vomiting, bowel elimination pattern, oral assessment, and usual appetite. Teach patient to report these side effects so that they can be evaluated. Teach patient self-care measures, including dietary modification and local comfort measures, as well as pharmacologic management as determined by the nurse/physician team. Teach patient to report symptoms that persist and do not respond to the planned therapy.

III.   ALTERATION IN SKIN INTEGRITY, POTENTIAL, related to PERIPHERAL EDEMA, ALOPECIA

Defining Characteristics: Peripheral edema and alopecia are rarely reported, and may be related to other factors, such as the chemotherapy agents administered.

Nursing Implications: Perform baseline skin and scalp assessment. Teach patient to report development of peripheral edema, hair loss. If hair loss occurs, discuss acceptable management strategies with patient, depending upon impact of hair loss. Assess degree of peripheral edema if it develops, and discuss significant edema with physician to determine etiology and management. Teach patient local skin care, including avoidance of tight clothing and shoes, keeping skin moisturized to prevent cracking, and local comfort measures.

IV.   KNOWLEDGE DEFICIT related to SELF-ADMINISTRATION TECHNIQUE

Defining Characteristics: Drug is administered once per chemotherapy cycle, more than 14 days prior to chemotherapy administration or more than 24 hours after chemotherapy is given.

Nursing Implications: Assess baseline psychomotor ability, knowledge, and willingness to learn technique of self-injection. Teach how to refrigerate drug, self-administer using prefilled syringes, activate needle guard, and safely collect used syringes for proper disposal. Drug insert has "Information for Patients and Caregivers." Use written and video supplements in teaching process, and have patient correctly demonstrate technique prior to performing at home. Make referral to visiting-nurse agency to reinforce teaching if needed. Teach patient telephone number and whom to call if questions or problems arise, and ensure that patient can correctly repeat information.

Drug: peginterferon alfa-2b (Sylatron)

Mechanism of Action: Drug is a pleiotropic cytokine. The exact mechanism of anti-melanoma effect is unknown, but it relates to immune effects. Interferon alfa-2b has antiviral, antiproliferative, and immunomodulatory effects. In addition, it activates pre-natural killer (NK) cells, increases cytotoxicity of NK cells, and enhances immune response.

Metabolism: After subcutaneous injection, the mean terminal half-life was about 51 hours in clinical study. The mean terminal half-life is about 43 hours. Drug is metabolized by cytochrome P-450 enzymes (CYP2C9 and CYP2D6). In patients with renal dysfunction, the AUC increased by 1.3-, 1.7-, and 1.9-fold in mild, moderate, and severe renal impairment.

Indication: For the adjuvant treatment of melanoma with microscopic or gross nodal involvement within 84 days of definitive surgical resection, including complete lymphadenectomy.

Contraindication: Patients with (1) history of anaphlyaxis to peginterferon alfa-2b or interferon alfa-2b; (2) autoimmune hepatitis; (3) hepatic decompensation (Child-Pugh score > 6 [class B and C]).

Dosage/Range:
- 6 mcg/kg/week subcutaneously for 8 doses, followed by 3 mcg/kg/week subcutaneously for up to 5 years. Premedicate with acetaminophen 500–1,000 mg orally 30 minutes prior to first dose, and as needed for subsequent injections.

Dose Modifications:
- Permanently discontinue drug for:
  - Persistent or worsening severe neuropsychiatric disorders
  - Grade 4 nonhematologic toxicity
  - Inability to tolerate a dose of 1 mcg/kg/wk
  - New or worsening retinopathy
- Withhold drug dose for any of the following:
  - ANC < 0.5×10^9/L
  - Platelet count < 50×10^9/L
  - ECOG performance status (PS) > 2 (see below)
  - Non-hematologic toxicity > grade 3
- Resume dosing at a reduced dose when ANC > 0.5×10^9/L, platelet count > 50×10^9/L, ECOG PS 0–1, nonhematologic toxicity has completely resolved or improved to grade 1. SYLATRON

Dose Modifications:

Starting Dose	Dose Modifications for Doses 1–8
6 mcg/kg/week	1st dose modification: 3 mcg/kg/week
	2nd dose modification: 2 mcg/kg/week
	3rd dose modification: 1 mcg/kg/week
	If unable to tolerate 1 mcg/kg/week, permanently discontinue drug
3 mcg/kg/week	1st dose modification: 2 mcg/kg/week
	2nd dose modification: 1 mcg/kg/week
	If unable to tolerate 1 mcg/kg/week, permanently discontinue drug

Drug Preparation:
- Drug is available in 200 mcg, 300 mcg, and 600 mcg of deliverable lyophilized powder per single-use vial. Reconstitute vial with 0.7 mL of Sterile Water for Injection USP. Upon reconstitution, the final concentration of the drug will be.
  - 200 mcg in 0.5 mL (final concentration 40 mcg per each 0.1 mL) of peginterferon alfa-2b (Sylatron)
  - 300 mcg in 0.5 mL (final concentration 60 mcg per each 0.1 mL) of peginterferon alfa-2b (Sylatron)
  - 600 mcg in 0.5 mL (final concentration 120 mcg per each 0.1 mL) of peginterferon alfa-2b (Sylatron)
- Swirl gently to dissolve the lyophilized powder. DO NOT SHAKE. Visually inspect the solution for particulate matter, cloudiness, or discoloration, and discard if present.
- Do not withdraw > 0.5 mL of reconstituted solution from each vial. If reconstituted solution is not used immediately, store at 2–8°C (36–46°F) for no more than 24 hours. Discard remaining solution after 24 hours. DO NOT FREEZE. For single-use only. Discard any unused portion.

Drug Administration:
- Administer subcutaneously. Rotate injection sites.
- Teach patient/caregiver self-administration, drug preparation, safe handling, and waste disposal of hazardous drug.
- Assess labs including CBC/differential/platelets; monitor hepatic function with serum bilirubin, ALT, AST, alkaline phosphatase, and LDH at 2 weeks and 8 weeks, and 2 and 3 months following initiation of drug, then every 6 months while receiving the drug.
- Assess baseline TSH, chemistries.

Drug Interactions:
- Drugs metabolized by CYP2C9 (e.g., glyburide, glipizide, indocin, phenobarbital, phenytoin) or CYP2D6 (e.g., SSRIs, TCAs, beta-blockers, Type 1A antiarrythmics); therapeutic effect of these drugs may be altered.

Lab Effects/Interference:
- Increased: ALT or AST, alkaline phosphatase, GGT, serum triglycerides.
- Proteinuria, anemia.

Special Considerations:

Warnings and Precautions:

- Depression and other serious neuropsychiatric adverse reactions may occur, including suicide, suicidal ideation, homicidal ideation, depression, and an increased risk of relapse of recovering drug addicts.
  - Teach patient/caregivers to report immediately symptoms of depression or suicidal thoughts.
  - Assess for signs and symptoms of depression and other psychiatric problems every 3 weeks for the first 8 weeks of treatment, then at least every 6 months.
  - Monitor patients during treatment and for at least 6 months after therapy ends, and discuss concerns with physician, NP/PA.
  - Drug should be permanently discontinued if persistent or worsening psychiatric symptoms or behaviors occur; refer for psychiatric evaluation.
- Cardiovascular adverse reactions: MI, bundle branch block, tachycardia, and supraventricular arrhythmias occurred in 4% of patients. Drug should be permanently discontinued for new onset of ventricular arrhythmias or cardiovascular decompensation.
- Drug can cause a decrease in visual acuity or blindness due to retinopathy.
  - Retinal and ocular changes include macular edema, retinal artery or vein thrombosis, retinal hemorrhages and cotton wool spots, optic neuritis, papilledema, and serous retinal detachment; they can be induced or aggravated by treatment with peginterferon alfa-2b.
  - Although rare, patients should receive an eye examination that includes assessment of visual acuity and indirect ophthalmoscopy or fundus photography at baseline in patients with preexisting retinopathy, and at any time during treatment.
  - Teach patients to report any changes in vision IMMEDIATELY. Permanently discontinue drug in patients who develop new or worsening retinopathy.
- Hepatic failure: Drug increases the risk of hepatic decompensation and death in patients with cirrhosis.
  - Monitor hepatic function with serum bilirubin, ALT, AST, alkaline phosphatase, and LDH at 2 weeks and 8 weeks, and 2 and 3 months following initiation of drug, then every 6 months while receiving the drug.
  - Permanently discontinue the drug if evidence of severe (grade 3) hepatic injury or hepatic decompensation (Child-Pugh score > 6 [class B and C]).
- Drug can cause new onset or worsening of hypothyroidism, hyperthyroidism, and diabetes mellitus. Overall incidence of endocrinopathies was 2% compared to < 1% in the observation group. Obtain TSH level 4 weeks prior to the start of peginterferon alfa-2b, at 3 and 6 months following initiation, and every 6 months thereafter. The drug should be permanently discontinued in patients who develop hypothyroidism, hyperthyroidism, or diabetes mellitus that cannot be effectively managed.
- Drug should be used during pregnancy only when the potential benefit justifies the potential hazard to the fetus.
- Nursing mothers should decide to discontinue nursing or to discontinue the drug, taking into consideration the importance of the drug to the mother's health.
- FDA approval based on an open-label, multicentered randomized trial evaluating the safety and efficacy of peginterferon alfa-2b in 1256 patients with surgically resected stage III

melanoma within 84 days of lymph node dissection (Eggermont et al., 2008). The primary endpoint was relapse-free survival (RFS). Median RFS for the peginterferon alfa-2b group was 34.8 months compared to 25.5 months in the observation group. Secondary endpoint was OS. There was no statistically significant difference in survival between the treatment and observation arms. Some patients (16%) did not continue on the 3 mcg/kg/week regimen. Patients (52%) had dose reductions, and 70% required dose delays (average delay 2.2 weeks). Some patients (33%) discontinued treatment due to adverse reactions.

Grade	ECOG
0	Fully active, able to carry on all predisease performance without restriction.
1	Restricted in physically strenuous activity but ambulatory and able to carry out work of a light or sedentary nature, e.g., light housework, office work.
2	Ambulatory and capable of all self-care but unable to carry out any work activities. Up and about more than 50% of waking hours.
3	Capable of only limited self-care, confined to bed or chair more than 50% of waking hours.
4	Completely disabled. Cannot carry on any self-care. Totally confined to bed or chair.
5	Dead.

*As published in *Am. J. Clin. Oncol.*:
Source: Oken, M.M., Creech, R.H., Tormey, D.C., et al. Toxicity and Response Criteria of the Eastern Cooperative Oncology Group. *Am J Clin Oncol.* 5:649–655, 1982.

The ECOG Performance Status is in the public domain, therefore available for public use. To duplicate the scale, please cite the reference above and credit the Eastern Cooperative Oncology Group, Robert Comis.

Potential Toxicities/Side Effects and the Nursing Process

I. ALTERATION IN COMFORT related to FLULIKE SYNDROME

Defining Characteristics: Most commonly patients experienced fatigue (94%), pyrexia (75%), headache (70%), myalgia (68%), nausea (64%), and chills (63%). Joint pain also occurred. Fatigue was severe in 7%, pyrexia in 3%.

Nursing Implications: Assess baseline T, VS, neurologic status, and comfort level and teach patient/caregiver to report severe symptoms. Teach patient to premedicate with acetaminophen 30 minutes prior to the first dose, and as needed prior to subsequent doses. Teach patient to take dose at bedtime. Teach patient self-care measures, including hydration of one 8-oz. glass of fluid every hour while awake to minimize risk of dehydration, self-assessment and monitoring of temperature, comfort level, self-administration of prescribed medications prior to dose, as well as the use of heat or cold for myalgias, arthralgias. Encourage patient to increase oral fluids and alternate rest and activity periods, medications, and oral hygiene regimen.

II.   ALTERATION IN NUTRITION, LESS THAN BODY REQUIREMENTS, related to NAUSEA, VOMITING, DIARRHEA, ANOREXIA

Defining Characteristics: Anorexia (69%) occurs and is cumulative. Nausea (64%) is mild with tachyphylaxis after 1 week. Diarrhea (37%) is mild, and vomiting (26%) may occur. Aphthous stomatitis, pancreatitis, and colitis were reported post-marketing.

Nursing Implications: Assess baseline nutritional status. Teach patient potential side effects and self-care measures, including oral hygiene. Encourage patient to prepare favorite high-calorie, high-protein foods ahead of time to be able to snack when hungry. Teach self-administration of prescribed antiemetics and antidiarrheals as needed. Refer to dietitian as appropriate.

III.   SENSORY/PERCEPTUAL ALTERATION related to CNS EFFECTS, DEPRESSION, SUICIDAL IDEATION

Defining Characteristics: Depression occurred in 59% of patients compared to 24% in the observation group. It was severe or life-threatening in 7% of patients receiving peginterferon alfa-2b, compared to < 1% in observation group. These effects are reported up to 6 months after discontinuation of the drug. Drug can also result in aggressive behavior, psychoses, hallucinations, bipolar disorders, mania, and encephalopathy. Patients also reported headache (70%), dysgeusia (38%), dizziness (35%), olfactory nerve disorder (23%), and paresthesias (21%).

Nursing Implications: Assess baseline mental status and neurologic status prior to drug administration. Assess patient for changes (depression, impaired memory/attention, change in behavior, disorientation, slow/vague responses to questions, increased lethargy) during treatment. Instruct patient to report signs/symptoms, provide information and emotional support, as well as interventions to ensure safety if signs/symptoms occur. Teach patients and their caregivers to report immediately any symptoms of depression or suicidal ideation to their healthcare provider. Monitor and evaluate patients for signs and symptoms of depression and other psychiatric symptoms every 3 weeks during the first 8 weeks of treatment, and every 6 months thereafter. Monitor patients during treatment and for at least 6 months after the last dose of peginterferon alfa-2b. Permanently discontinue drug for persistent severe or worsening psychiatric symptoms or behaviors and refer for psychiatric evaluation.

IV.   POTENTIAL ALTERATION IN CARDIAC OUTPUT related to TACHYCARDIA, CHEST PAIN, DYSRHYTHMIAS

Defining Characteristics: In the clinical trial, cardiac adverse reactions, including MI, bundle-branch block, ventricular tachycardia, and supraventricular tachycardia occurred in 4% of patients compared with 2% in the observation group. In post-marketing, patients reported hypotension, cardiomyopathy, and angina pectoris.

Nursing Implications: Assess baseline cardiopulmonary status and risk (elderly, preexisting cardiac dysfunction). Discuss EKG testing, baseline and during treatment, for high-risk individuals. Monitor vital signs at each visit. Teach patient to report signs/symptoms of palpitations, dyspnea, chest pain, edema, or other abnormalities immediately. Drug should be permanently discontinued for new onset of ventricular arrhythmias or cardiovascular decompensation.

V. POTENTIAL ALTERATION IN ELIMINATION related to RENAL AND HEPATIC DYSFUNCTION

Defining Characteristics: Dose-related increased ALT or AST occurred in 77% of patients, GGT in 8%, and increased alkaline phosphatase in 23% of patients. Drug increases the risk of hepatic decompensation and death in patients with cirrhosis. Proteinuria may occur.

Nursing Implications: Monitor hepatic function with serum bilirubin, ALT, AST, alkaline phosphatase, and LDH baseline, at 2 weeks and 8 weeks, and 2 and 3 months following initiation of drug, then every 6 months while receiving the drug. The drug should be permanently discontinued if evidence of severe (grade 3) hepatic injury or hepatic decompensation (Child-Pugh score > 6 [class B and C]).

VI. POTENTIAL ALTERATION IN SKIN INTEGRITY related to RASH, PARTIAL ALOPECIA, DRYNESS

Defining Characteristics: Injection-site reaction occurs in 62% of patients. Exfoliative rash occurred in 36% of patients and alopecia in 34%.

Nursing Implications. Assess baseline skin integrity. Instruct patient to report signs/symptoms. If skin site is painful, try applying ice to the site 5–10 minutes prior to the injection. Discuss/teach symptomatic management, including the use of mild soaps and rinsing skin thoroughly after bathing. Encourage patient to use alcohol-free, oil-based moisturizers on skin. Teach patient to report any severe symptoms, and discuss management with physician/midlevel.

VII. KNOWLEDGE DEFICIT related to SELF-ADMINISTRATION TECHNIQUE

Defining Characteristics: Patient or caregiver must administer drug weekly in the home setting by subcutaneous injection and is unfamiliar with technique.

Nursing Implications: Assess baseline psychomotor ability, knowledge, and willingness to learn technique of self-injection. Teach how to prepare drug, self-administer, and safely collect used syringes for proper disposal. Use written and video materials as supplements to teaching process and have patient correctly demonstrate technique prior to performing at home. Make referral to visiting-nurse agency to reinforce teaching if needed.

Drug: plerixafor (Mozobil, AMD3100)

Class: Hematopoietic stem cell mobilizer.

Mechanism of Action: Plerixafor inhibits CXCR4 chemokine receptor and blocks it from binding to its ligand, stromal cell-derived factor-1α (SDF-1α). SDF-1α and CXCR4 play a role in telling human hematopoietic stem cells (HSCs, CD34+ cells) where to travel, thus attracting and moving HSCs to the bone marrow. They also help them anchor to the marrow matrix so that they stay put. By inhibiting CXCR4, increased numbers of HSCs remain in the peripheral blood where they can be harvested for bone marrow transplant. CD34+ cells mobilized by plerixafor are capable of engraftment with long-term repopulating capacity up to 1 year in dog models.

Metabolism: Peak mobilization of CD34+ cells is 6–9 hours after administration; a sustained elevated CD34+ level was seen from 4–18 hours after drug administration, with a peak CD34+ count between 10–14 hours. Drug shows linear kinetics, and follows a two-compartment model. The distribution half-life is 0.3 hours, and terminal half-life 3–5 hours. The drug exposure (AUC) increases with increasing patient weight. Plasma protein binding is 58%, and drug is mainly distributed in the extravascular fluid. Drug is principally excreted unchanged in urine within 24 hours, so that patients with decreased creatinine clearance have decreased clearance of drug and should be dose reduced.

Indication: In combination, with granulocyte-colony stimulating factor (G-CSF) to mobilize hematopoietic stem cells (HSCs) to the peripheral blood for collection and subsequent autologous transportation in patients with NHL and multiple myeloma.

Dosage/Range:
- Drug is begun after the patient has received G-CSF once daily for 4 days; administer plerixafor SQ approximately 11 hours prior to initiation of apheresis for up to 4 consecutive days.
- Plerixafor dose is 0.24 mg/kg (actual body weight, maximum dose 40 mg/day) administered by subcutaneous injection.
- Dose-reduce by 33% for reduced renal function (creatinine clearance $\leq$ 50 mL/min): dose is 0.16 mg/kg (not to exceed 27 mg/day).
- Leucocytosis occurs when plerixafor is used with G-CSF as both WBC and HSCs are mobilized; discuss with the physician whether patient should receive ordered dose of plerixafor when the neutrophil count is > 50,000/mm^3.
- White blood cell and platelet count should be monitored daily.

Drug Preparation:
- Single-use vial containing 1.2 mL of a 20 mg/mL solution.
- Aseptically withdraw ordered dose.
- Stored at 25°C (77°F), drug can be used until the manufacturer's expiration date; drug can tolerate short-term exposure to 15–30°C (59–86°F).

Drug Administration:
- Administer via subcutaneous injection.

Drug Interactions:
- None.

Lab Effects/Interference:
- Increases CD34+ cells in the peripheral blood; leukocytosis; thrombocytopenia.

Special Considerations:

- Drug is indicated, in combination with G-CSF, to mobilize hematopoietic stem cells to the peripheral blood for collection and subsequent autologous transplantation in patients with NHL and multiple myeloma.
- Stem cell mobilization in leukemia patients with plerixafor may mobilize leukemic cells and should not be used in this patient population.
- Potential for tumor cell mobilization exists so that tumor cells are released from the bone marrow during HSC mobilization.
- Patients may rarely develop splenic rupture; teach patients to tell the provider right away if they develop pain in the abdomen, shoulder, or scapula. The provider should evaluate emergently any patient who complains of left upper abdominal and/or scapular or shoulder pain.
- Drug may cause fetal harm as it is teratogenic and fetotoxic in animals; female patients who are of childbearing age and who are sexually active should use effective contraception. Nursing mothers should decide whether to discontinue nursing or the drug, depending on the importance of the drug to the mother.
- Most common side effects are diarrhea, nausea, fatigue, injection-site reactions, headache, arthralgia, dizziness, and vomiting.
- Rarely, allergic reactions may occur during or after plerixafor injection manifested by urticaria, periorbital swelling, dyspnea, or hypoxia. Teach patient to report any signs or symptoms right away and institute emergency measures right away.
- Thrombocytopenia can occur with plerixafor treatment; platelet count should be monitored during and after mobilization.

Potential Toxicities/Side Effects and the Nursing Process

I.   ALTERATION IN COMFORT related to INJECTION-SITE REACTION, FATIGUE, ARTHRALGIA, HEADACHE, DIZZINESS, INSOMNIA

Defining Characteristics: Injection-site reactions occur in 34% of patients, and can include erythema, hematoma, hemorrhage, induration, inflammation, irritation, pain, paresthesia, pruritus, rash, swelling, and urticaria. Rarely, mild-to-moderate allergic reactions occurred (< 1% of patients), about 30 minutes after the injection, consisting of urticaria, periorbital swelling, dyspnea, or hypoxia, which responded to antihistamines, corticosteroids, hydration, supplemental oxygen, or resolved spontaneously. Rarely, vasovagal reactions and orthostasis may be associated with subcutaneous injection, occurring within 1 hour of the injection. Fatigue occurs in 27% of patients, arthralgia 13%, headache 22%, dizziness 11%, and insomnia 7%.

Nursing Implications: Teach patient to report any changes during the injection or within 1 hour afterward, such as rash, shortness of breath, dizziness when changing position, or swelling of the face. Discuss immediate management with physician. Discuss self-care strategies to promote comfort, such as use of NSAIDs with patient for arthralgias, pain, headache, and myalgias. Teach patient to change position slowly if dizzy, and to report worsening dizziness. Teach patient strategies to promote sleepiness if insomnia is a problem, such as reading before bedtime, warm milk, or other strategies.

II.   ALTERATION IN NUTRITION, POTENTIAL, related to NAUSEA, VOMITING, DIARRHEA, FLATULENCE

Defining Characteristics: Diarrhea occurs in about 37% of patients, nausea 34%, vomiting 10%, and flatulence 7%.

Nursing Implications: Teach patient that these side effects may occur and to report them. Discuss self-care strategies such as OTC preparations for symptoms and dietary modification, and if unsuccessful, discuss alternative medications with physician, such as antidiarrheals for diarrhea and antiemetics for nausea, vomiting.

Drug: romiplostim (Nplate)

Class: Thrombopoietin receptor agonist, a thrombopoietin-stimulating agent (peptibody or peptide antibody).

Mechanism of Action: Drug is an engineered peptibody composed of two parts: an Fc receptor of an antibody and a peptide that is fused to the antibody constant domain (Fc). Binds to and activates the thrombopoietin (TPO) receptor, mimicking natural TPO to stimulate the growth and maturation of megakaryocytes (platelet precursors). This results in increased platelet production in the body.

Metabolism: Peak serum concentration 7–50 hours after the dose with a median time of 14 hours; half-life 1–34 days, with a median of 3.5 days. Serum concentration does not correlate with the dose. Elimination depends to some degree on the platelet TPO receptors.

Indication: Treatment of thrombocytopenia in patients with chronic immune thrombocytopenia (ITP) who have had an insufficent response to corticosteroids, immunoglobulins, or splenectomy. NOT indicated for the treatment of thrombocytopenia due to MDS or any cause other than chronic ITP. Drug should be used only in patients with ITP with thrombocytopenia and clinical risk for increased bleeding; drug should not be used to normalize platelet counts.

Dosage/Range:
- Initial dose 1 mcg/kg subcutaneously once weekly to achieve/maintain a platelet count $\geq 50 \times 10^9$/L as needed to reduce bleeding risk.
- Adjust weekly dose by increments of 1 mcg/kg.
- Do not exceed maximum weekly dose of 10 mcg/kg, and do not dose if platelet count is > 400×10^9/L.
- Discontinue drug if platelet count does not increase after 4 weeks at the maximum dose (10 mcg/kg); monitor CBC, platelet count weekly.
- Discontinue drug if the patient develops new or worsening morphologic abnormalities or cytopenia(s), and consider a bone marrow biopsy, including staining for fibrosis. Monitor CBC, platelet count weekly for at least 2 weeks after drug discontinuation.
- The prescribed dose may be a very small volume. Use a syringe containing 0.01 mL gradations only.

Drug Preparation:
- To prevent medication errors, follow preparation and administration instructions exactly (see package insert).
- Available in 250 mcg and 500 mcg single use vials.
- Calculate dose and reconstitute with the correct volume of sterile water for injection, USP:
  - Add 0.72 mL diluents to the 250 mcg romiplostim vial, resulting in 250 mcg per 0.5 mL (or 500 mcg/mL);
  - Add 1.2 mL diluents to the 500 mcg vial, resulting in 500 mcg/1 mL.
- Gently swirl the contents of the vial; do not shake during reconstitution. Protect reconstituted drug from light, and administer within 24 hours.
- Draw up dose using a syringe with graduations to 0.01 mL, as the injection volume is so small.
- Drug can be kept at room temperature (25°C/77°F) or refrigerated at 2–8°C (36–46°F) for up to 24 hours prior to administration.
- Vial is single use; discard any unused drug.
- Available in 250 µg and 500 µg of romiplostim in single-use vials.

Drug Administration:
- Weekly subcutaneous injections.
- Assess CBC/platelet count weekly during dose-adjustment phase, then monthly once a stable dose is found. Assess CBC/platelet count weekly for at least 2 weeks after drug is discontinued.

Drug Interactions:
- No formal drug interactions studies have been done.

Lab Effects/Interference:
- Increased platelet count.
- Decreased platelet count after drug cessation.

Special Considerations:
- Overall platelet increase occurred in 78.6% of patients receiving romiplostim compared with 0 in the placebo group (Kuter, 2008).
- Most common side effects (> 5%) are myalgia, dizziness, pain (extremity, abdomen, shoulder), arthralgia, insomnia, dyspepsia, headache, and paresthesia.
- Monitor CBC, including platelet count and peripheral blood smears baseline prior to initiation of therapy, then weekly during dose adjustments, and monthly after the patient has been placed on a stable romiplostim dose. Monitor CBC, including platelet count monthly, and upon discontinuation of romiplostim, monitor CBC/platelet count for 2 weeks after drug cessation.
- May increase risk of hematologic malignancies, especially in patients with MDS.
- If platelet count is allowed to rise excessively, thrombotic or thromboembolic complications may occur; do not use romiplostim to normalize platelet counts, and dose to achieve and maintain a platelet count of 50,000/mm³.

- Hyporesponsiveness or initial response, then failure to maintain the platelet response, should prompt evaluation of the formation of neutralizing antibodies to romiplostim or bone marrow fibrosis. Call Amgen (1-800-772-6436) to obtain details on submitting blood samples to test for antibodies to romiplostim or TPO. Discontinue drug if platelet count does not increase to a level sufficient to avoid significant bleeding after 4 weeks at the highest weekly dose of 10 mcg/kg.
- Drug should be used in pregnant patients only if potential benefit to the mother justifies potential risk to the fetus (e.g., thrombocytosis, postimplantation loss, and increased mortality in lab animals). A pregnancy registry has been established to collect information. Physicians can register their patients, or pregnant patients can enroll by calling 1-877-Nplate1 (1-877-675-2831).

Potential Toxicities/Side Effects and the Nursing Process

I.   ALTERATION IN COMFORT related to MYALGIA, ARTHRALGIA, PAIN, DIZZINESS, INSOMNIA, HEADACHE

Defining Characteristics: Transient skeletal pain and headache may occur. Arthralgias occurred in 26% of patients compared to 20% in placebo group; dizziness in 17% (vs 0%), insomnia in 16% (vs 7%), myalgia in 14% (vs 2%), pain in extremity in 13% (vs 5%), abdominal pain in 11% (vs 0%), shoulder pain in 8% (vs 0%), paresthesia in 6% (vs 0%), and dyspepsia in 7% (vs 0%).

Nursing Implications: Teach patient that these may occur, and discuss use of NSAIDs with patient and physician for symptom management for arthralgias, pain, headache, and myalgias. Teach patient to change position slowly if dizzy and to report worsening dizziness. Teach patient strategies to promote sleepiness if insomnia is a problem, such as reading before bedtime, warm milk, or other strategies. Monitor CBC, platelet count, peripheral smear baseline weekly during dose adjustment phase, then monthly when stable; monitor at termination of therapy, and platelet count for 2 weeks following cessation of therapy.

Drug: sargramostim (Leukine, GM-CSF)

Class: Cytokine (GM-CSF, granulocyte macrophage growth factor).

Mechanism of Action: Granulocyte-macrophage colony-stimulating factor that regulates growth of all levels of granulocytes and stimulates production of monocytes and macrophages; GM-CSF induces synthesis of other cytokines and enhances cytotoxic action. Manufactured using recombinant DNA technology.

Metabolism: Peak serum levels 2–3 hours after injection. Initial half-life 12–17 minutes, with a terminal half-life of 1.6–2.6 hours.

Indication: (1) Following induction chemotherapy in older adult patients with acute myelogenous leukemia (AML) to shorten time to neutrophil recovery and to reduce incidence of severe and life-threatening infection, and infections resulting in death; (2) mobilization of hematopoietic progenitor cells into peripheral blood for leukapheresis collection; (3) acceleration of myeloid recovery in patients with NHL, acute lymphoblastic leukemia (ALL), and Hodgkin's disease undergoing autologous bone marrow transplantation (BMT); (4) acceleration of myeloid recovery in patients undergoing allogeneic BMT from HLA-matched related donors (myeloid reconstitution after allogeneic bone marrow transplantation); (5) in bone marrow transplantation failure or engraftment delay in patients who have undergone allogeneic or autologous BMT.

Contraindication: In patients with (1) excessive leukemic myeloid blasts in the bone marrow or peripheral blood ($\geq$ 10%); (2) known hypersensitivity to GM-CSF, yeast-derived products, or any product component; for concomitant use with chemotherapy and radiotherapy.

Dosage/Range:
- *Neutrophil recovery following chemotherapy in AML:* 250 mcg/m^2/day as a 4-hour infusion, beginning approximately on day 11 or 4 days after the completion of induction chemotherapy, if the day 10 bone marrow is hypoplastic with < 5% blasts.
  - Continue therapy until ANC > 1,500 cells/mm^3 for 3 consecutive days or a maximum of 42 days.
  - Discontinue drug immediately if leukemic regrowth occurs.
  - If a severe reaction occurs, dose can be reduced by 50% or interrupted until the reaction abates.
  - To prevent excessive leukocytosis (WBC > 50,000 cells/mm^3 or ANC > 20,000 cells/mm^3) assess CBC/differential twice weekly during therapy. Drug should be interrupted or dose-reduced by half if the ANC > 20,000 cells/mm^3.
- *Mobilization of peripheral blood progenitor cells:* 250 μg/m^2/day IV over 24 hours or SQ once daily. Continue same dose through the period of PBPC collection. Saragramostim dose should be reduced by 50% if WBC > 50,000 cells/mm^3.
- *Postperipheral blood progenitor cell transplantation:* 250 μg/m^2/day IV over 24 hours or SQ once daily, beginning immediately following infusion of progenitor cells and continuing until an ANC > 1,500 cells/m^3 is attained for 3 consecutive days.
- *Myeloid reconstitution after autologous or allogeneic bone marrow transplantation:* 250 μg/m^2/day IV over 2 hours beginning 2–4 hours after bone marrow infusion, and not less than 24 hours after the last dose of chemotherapy or radiotherapy.
  - Do not give until the postmarrow infusion ANC is < 500 cells/mm^3; continue sargramostim until an ANC > 1,500 cells/mm^3 for 3 consecutive days occurs.
  - If a severe adverse reaction occurs, sargramostim dose can be 50% dose-reduced or interrupted until reaction abates. Discontinue the drug immediately if blast cells appear or disease progression occurs.
  - To prevent excessive leukocytosis (WBC > 50,000 cells/mm^3 or ANC > 20,000 cells/mm^3), assess CBC/differential twice weekly during therapy. Drug should be interrupted or dose-reduced by half if the ANC > 20,000 cells/mm^3.
- *Bone marrow transplantation or engraftment delay:* 250 μg/m^2/day IV over 2 hours for 14 days; dose can be repeated after 7 days off therapy if engraftment has not occurred.

- If engraftment still has not occurred, a 3rd course of 500 mcg/m²/day IV for 14 days may be tried after 7 days off therapy.
- If there is still no improvement, it is unlikely that an increased dose will be successful.
- If a severe adverse reaction occurs, sargramostim dose can be 50% dose-reduced or interrupted until reaction abates. Discontinue the drug immediately if blast cells appear or disease progression occurs.
- To prevent excessive leukocytosis (WBC > 50,000 cells/mm³ or ANC > 20,000 cells/mm³), assess CBC/differential twice weekly during therapy. Drug should be interrupted or dose-reduced by half if the ANC > 20,000 cells/mm³.

Drug Preparation:
- Liquid Leukine is preserved with benzyl alcohol injectable solution (500 mcg/mL) in a vial. Once entered, the vial can be stored up to 20 days at 2–8°C. Discard any remaining solution after 20 days.
- Lyophilized Leukine is preservative-free (250 mcg) that requires reconstitution with 1 mL Sterile Water for Injection, USP, or 1 mL Bacteriostatic Water for Injection, USP. When reconstituted with Bacteriostatic Water for Injection, reconstituted solution can be stored up to 20 days at 2–8°C. Discard any remaining solution after 20 days. Bacteriostatic water containing solutions should not be used for neonates. See package insert for reconstitution directions.
- SQ administration: do not further dilute.
- IV administration requires further dilution in 0.9% sodium chloride. If final concentration is < 10 µg/mL, human albumin at a final concentration of 0.1% should be added to the saline prior to adding Leukine to prevent absorption of drug in IV container and tubing. (To obtain a final concentration of 0.1% albumin [human], add 1 mg albumin per 1 mL 0.9% sodium chloride injection USP [e.g., use 1 mL 5% albumin (human) in 50 mL 0.9% sodium chloride injection USP.])
- Do *not* use an in-line membrane filter when administering drug IV.
- Store liquid and reconstituted lyophilized Leukine under refrigeration at 2–8°C (36–46°F); do not freeze.

Drug Administration:
- Administer SQ or IV per Dosage/Range section.
- CBC twice a week during therapy; monitor renal and hepatic function in patients with baseline impairment in either system biweekly during therapy. Monitor body weight and hydration status closely during therapy.
- DO NOT administer sargramostim simultaneously with cytotoxic chemotherapy or radiotherapy, or within 24 hours preceding or following chemotherapy or radiotherapy.

Drug Interactions:
- Corticosteroids, lithium: may increase myeloproliferation.

Lab Effects/Interference:
- Increased stem cell, granulocyte, macrophage production.
- Serum glucose, BUN, cholesterol, bili, creatinine, ALT, alk phos; ↓ serum albumin, Ca.
- Leukocytosis, eosinophilia.

Special Considerations:
• Produces fever more commonly than G-CSF.

Warnings:
• *Fluid retention:* Edema, capillary leak syndrome, pleural and/or pericardial effusion have been described. Usually these are reversible after drug interruption or dose reduction with or without diuretic therapy. Use drug cautiously in patients with preexisting fluid retention, pulmonary infiltrates, or CHF, and monitor patient closely. Assess patient closely during and immediately after infusions, especially in patients with preexisting lung disease.
• *Respiratory symptoms:* Sequestration of granulocytes in pulmonary circulation has occurred, resulting in dyspnea. If patient develops dyspnea during the infusion, slow infusion rate by 50%; if respiratory symptoms worsen despite slowing infusion, discontinue drug. Subsequent infusions can be given per standard dose schedule with careful monitoring. Use cautiously and monitor closely hypoxic patients.
• *Cardiovascular symptoms:* Occasional supraventricular arrhythmia has occurred, especially in patients with a history of arrhythmias. This is reversible after drug discontinuation.
• *Renal and hepatic dysfunction:* Monitor lab values baseline and during treatment.
• Stop drug when WBC > 50,000 cells/mm^3, ANC > 20,000 cells/mm^3, or platelets > 500,000 cells/mm^3.
• Administer > 24 hours after last chemotherapy (usually 4 days following completion of induction chemotherapy).
• Drug should be administered to pregnant women or nursing mothers only if clearly needed.

Potential Toxicities/Side Effects (Dose- and Schedule-Dependent) and the Nursing Process

I. ALTERATION IN COMFORT related to FLULIKE SYNDROME

Defining Characteristics: Fever, myalgias, chills, rigors, fatigue, and headache may occur.

Nursing Implications: Assess baseline T, VS, neurologic status, and comfort level, and monitor q 4–6 hours if patient in hospital. Discuss with physician premedication and regular dosing of antipyretic (e.g., acetaminophen ± diphenhydramine, NSAID). Teach patient self-care measures, including monitoring temperature, comfort level, self-administration of prescribed medications prior to dose and regularly postdose, as well as the use of heat or cold for myalgias, arthralgias. Encourage patient to increase oral fluids and alternate rest and activity periods. If patient is in hospital and experiences rigor, discuss with physician IV meperidine (25 mg IV every 15 minutes to maximum 100 mg in 1 hour) and monitor blood pressure for hypotension.

II. ALTERATION IN COMFORT related to SKELETAL PAIN

Defining Characteristics: Transient skeletal pain may occur and is believed to be due to bone marrow expansion in response to GM-CSF.

Nursing Implications: Teach patient this may occur and discuss use of NSAIDs with patient and physician for symptom management. Monitor WBC, absolute neutrophil count (ANC) twice weekly during therapy; dose reduction or discontinuation depends on purpose of drug.

III. POTENTIAL ALTERATION IN SKIN INTEGRITY related to RASH, FLUSHING, INJECTION-SITE REACTION

Defining Characteristics: Facial flushing, generalized rash, and inflammation at injection site may occur.

Nursing Implications: Teach patient that these may occur, and instruct to report rash, inflammation. Teach patient to rotate injection sites. Assess rash, and teach symptomatic management.

IV. POTENTIAL ALTERATION IN OXYGENATION related to DYSPNEA AND FLUID RETENTION

Defining Characteristics: Some patients developed dyspnea during initial 2–6 hours of continuous infusion GM-CSF, thought to be due to migration of neutrophils in the lung. Fluid retention may also occur.

Nursing Implications: Assess baseline pulmonary and fluid status. Teach patient to monitor weight daily and instruct to report any changes in weight, breathing (e.g., dyspnea).

Drug: tbo-filgrastim (Granix, Neutroval)

Class: Colony stimulating factor, Granulocyte (G-CSF).

Mechanism of Action: Tbo-filgrastim binds to G-CSF receptors and stimulates neutrophil proliferation, differentiation commitment, and other actions that increase neutrophil number and activity.

Metabolism: After subcutaneous dosing, bioavailability is 33%, median time to maximal concentration is 4–6 hrs, and median elimination half-life is 3.2–3.8 hours. Peak serum levels (C_{max}) are reached between days 3–5, returning to baseline at day 21.

Indication: For the reduction in the duration of severe neutropenia in patients with nonmyeloid malignancies receiving myelosuppressive anti-cancer drugs associated with a clinically significant incidence of febrile neutropenia.

Dosage/Range:
- 5 mcg/kg/day administered subcutaneously.
- Administer first dose at least **24 hours after** myelosuppressive chemotherapy;

- Continue with daily dosing until the expected neutrophil nadir has passed, and neutrophil count has recovered to the normal range.
- Do not administer within 24 hours prior to chemotherapy.
- Monitor CBC/differential prior to chemotherapy and twice per week until recovery.

Drug Preparation:
- Tbo-filgrastim is available in:
  - 300 microgram/0.5 mL in single-use prefilled syringe.
  - 480 microgram/0.8 mL in single-use prefilled syringe.

Drug Administration:
- Drug should be administered by a healthcare professional.
- Visually inspect parenteral drug products for particulate matter and discoloration prior to administration; do not use if found.
- Ensure correct volume for prescribed dose.
- Administer a single-use, prefilled syringe subcutaneously; recommended sites are abdomen (> 2 inches from navel), front of the middle thigh, upper outer area of buttock, and upper back portion of upper arm. Rotate sites daily.
- Avoid areas that are tender, red, bruised, hard, or have scars or stretch marks.

Drug Interactions:
- Drugs that may potentiate release of neutrophils (e.g., lithium); use with caution.

Lab Effects/Interference:
- Increased neutrophil count.

Special Considerations:
Warnings and Precautions:
- Splenic rupture can occur after administration of G-CSFs. Evaluate patients who have upper abdominal or shoulder pain after receiving tbo-filgrastim for enlarged spleen or splenic rupture, and discontinue drug.
- Acute respiratory distress syndrome (ARDS) can occur in patients receiving G-CSFs. Evaluate any patient receiving tbo-filgrastim who develops fever and lung infiltrates or respiratory distress for ARDS, and discontinue drug.
- Allergic reactions (e.g., angioneurotic edema, dermatitis allergic, drug hypersensitivity, hypersensitivity, rash, pruritic rash, urticaria) may occur.
- Sickle cell crisis can be precipitated by G-CSF, which may be fatal. Patients with sickle cell disease should weigh the risks and benefits. Do not admininister to patients in sickle cell crisis.
  - Do not administer tbo-filgrastim to patients who have a history of serious allergic reactions to filgrastim or pegfilgrastim.
  - Reactions can occur with first dose.
  - If a serious allergic reaction occurs, antihistamines, steroids, bronchodilators, or epinephrine may reduce reaction severity.
- G-CSF receptors have been found on tumor cells, raising the possibility that tbo-filgrastim can act as a growth factor for any tumor type. The drug is not approved for use in myeloid malignancies or myelodysplasia.

- Most common adverse reaction is bone pain.
- Drug should be used during pregnancy only if the potential benefit justifies the potential risk to the fetus. Caution should be used if drug is used in nursing mothers, as it is not known if drug is secreted in human milk.
- Safety and effectiveness has not been established in patients < 18 years old.

Potential Toxicities/Side Effects (Dose- and Schedule-Dependent) and the Nursing Process

I.   ALTERATION IN COMFORT related to BONE PAIN

Defining Characteristics: Patients may report bone pain, believed to be due to the expansion of cells in the bone marrow in response to G-CSF. The incidence in cycle 1 during clinical trials was 3.4%.

Nursing Implications: Teach patient that this may occur, and discuss use of NSAIDs with patient and physician for symptom management. Monitor WBC and ANC twice weekly during therapy; dose should be discontinued when ANC has recovered to the normal range.

Drug: thyrotropin alfa for injection (Thyrogen)

Class: Recombinant hormone (human thyroid-stimulating hormone) for tumor remnant ablation.

Mechanism of Action: Patients with thyroid cancer normally have surgery (subtotal or total thyroidectomy) followed by radioactive iodine to remove remaining normal tissue and any malignant cells. In order to stimulate the thyroid to take up the iodine, the TSH level has to be elevated. This drug binds to thyroid stimulating hormone (TSH) receptors on remaining normal thyroid epithelial cells and differentiated thyroid cancer cells, stimulating the uptake of iodine and organification, as well as synthesis and secretion of thyroglobulin (T_g), triiodothyronine (T_3), and thyroxine (T_4). An alternative to increasing the TSH level to destroy tumor remnant is to stop taking thyroid hormone replacement therapy, but this has significant side effects. Thyrotropin alfa for injection allows patients to continue to take their hormone replacement therapy with significantly higher quality of life (Genzyme, 2008; Pacini et al., 2002). This drug is also used as a diagnostic tool in assessment of well-differentiated thyroid cancer recurrence.

Metabolism: After a single 0.9-mg IM dose, mean peak concentrations were reached in 3 to 24 hours (median 10 hours). The mean elimination half-life is 25 ± 10 hours. The drug appears to be metabolized and excreted by the liver and kidneys.

Indication: (1) Diagnostic: adjunctive tool for serum thyroglobin testing with or without radioiodine imaging in the follow-up of patients with well-differentiated thyroid cancer who have undergone thyroidectomy; (2) use as adjunctive treatment for radioiodine ablation of thyroid tissue remnants in patients who have undergone a near-total or total thyroidectomy for well-differentiated thyroid cancer and who do not have evidence of distance metastases.

Dosage/Range:
* 2-injection regimen: 0.9 mg IM followed by a second 0.9 mg injection 24 hours later. If remnant ablation is performed, radioiodine will be administered 24 hours after the second injection of THYROGEN.
* In dialysis-dependent patients with ESRD, drug elimination is slower, resulting in prolonged TSH level elevation; expect that these patients may have an increased risk for headache and nausea.

Drug Preparation:
* Reconstitute with provided 1.2-mL sterile water for injection, resulting in a 0.9-mg thyrotropin alfa in 1.0 mL-solution immediately prior to administration.
* If necessary, reconstituted solution can be stored for 24 hours, protected from light, at 2–8°C (36–46°F).

Drug Administration:
* Administer IM ONLY, in the buttock.
* Give 0.9 mg thyrotropin alfa for injection IM daily × two doses 24 hours apart.
* Consider pretreatment with glucocorticosteroids in patients who may develop local tumor extension or swelling that could compromise vital structures (trachea, CNS brain or spinal metastases, extensive macroscopic lung metastases).
* Use cautiously and closely monitor older patients with functional thyroid tumors, as they may experience palpitations or cardiac rhythm disturbances (atrial).
* Consider hospitalization for administration and monitoring post-drug dose for patients with known heart disease, extensive metastases, or known serious underlying disease.
* For radioiodine imaging or remnant ablation, give radioiodine 24 hours after the second (final) thyrotropin alfa injection. Diagnostic scanning should be done 48 hours after the radioiodine administration; post-therapy scanning can be delayed additional days (to allow background activity to decline).
* For serum T_g testing, obtain a sample 72 hours after the second (final) injection.

Drug Interactions:
* None known.
* When used for radioiodine imaging in euthyroid patients, clearance of radioiodine is increased 50% compared with hypothyroid patients and should guide selection of the radioiodine used.

Lab Effects/Interference:
* Euthyroid patients for whom the drug is used for diagnostic imaging will have a significant, transient rise in TSH.
* No patients developed antibodies to thyrotropin alfa.

Special Considerations:
* Drug is indicated as an adjunctive.
* Use cautiously in patients who have previously received bovine TSH and those patients who have had hypersensitivity reactions to TSH administration in the past.

- It is unknown whether the drug is toxic to a fetus and thus should be given to a pregnant woman only when clearly needed; mothers should not breastfeed when receiving the drug.
- Successful ablation can be inferred when thyrogen-stimulated serum T_g level is < 2 ng/mL.
- Rarely, patient may develop hypersensitivity to the injection, characterized by urticaria, rash, pruritus, flushing, and respiratory symptoms; treat symptomatically.

Warnings and Precautions:
- Drug causes a transient but significant rise in serum thyroid hormone when given to patients who still have substantial remaining thyroid tissue; use cautiously, and monitor closely those patients with heart disease.
- Stroke has occurred within 72 hours of drug administration in patients with known CNS metastases.
- Sudden rapid tumor enlargement or distant metastases can occur after treatment with the drug with symptoms dependent upon the anatomical location of the tissue: acute hemiplegia, hemiparesis, and loss of vision 1–3 days after drug administration.
  - Laryngeal edema, pain at metastatic tumor site, and respiratory distress requiring tracheostomy have also occurred.
  - Pretreatment with glucocorticoids should be considered for patients at risk for tumor expansion that may compromise vital anatomic structures.

Potential Toxicities/Side Effects (Dose- and Schedule-Dependent) and the Nursing Process

I.   ALTERATION IN COMFORT related to FLULIKE SYMPTOMS

Defining Characteristics: Transient flulike symptoms can occur lasting < 48 hours, characterized by fever, chills, myalgia, arthralgia, fatigue, asthenia, malaise, headache, and chills.

Nursing Implications: Assess baseline T, VS, and comfort level, and teach patient that this may occur and how to manage uncomfortable side effects (e.g., acetaminophen). Teach patient self-care measures, including monitoring temperature, comfort level, the use of heat or cold for myalgias, arthralgias. Encourage patient to increase oral fluids and alternate rest and activity periods.

II.   POTENTIAL ALTERATION IN NUTRITION, LESS THAN BODY REQUIREMENTS, related to NAUSEA, VOMITING

Defining Characteristics: Nausea is mild and occurs in 11.9%, with vomiting in 2.3% of patients. Nausea and vomiting were severe when the dose was inadvertently given intravenously.

Nursing Implications: Assess baseline nutritional status. Teach patient that nausea may occur and that vomiting is rare; self-care measures, including oral hygiene and preparing favorite high-calorie, high-protein foods ahead of time so that the patient can snack when hungry. Teach the patient to report unrelieved nausea and vomiting if it occurs.

III.   ALTERATION IN COMFORT related to HEADACHE

Defining Characteristics: Headache occurs in 7.3%.

Nursing Implications: Assess baseline comfort, and teach patient that these side effects may occur. Teach local comfort measures to minimize local injection reactions.

Drug: zoster vaccine live (Zostavax)

Class: Vaccine.

Mechanism of Action: Initially, varicella zoster virus (VZV) produces chickenpox (varicella). The virus remains dormant in dorsal root or sensory ganglia until reactivation, when zoster occurs. In the body, as the VZV-specific immunity decreases, the virus can become reactivated. The person develops painful, vesicular lesions along a dermatome distribution of the body (on one side). Pain can occur during the prodrome, acute eruptive phase, and the post-herpetic phase, which is called post-herpetic neuralgia. Serious complications of herpes zoster, besides pain, include cranial and motor palsies, encephalitis, visual impairment, hearing loss, and death. The vaccine increases the immune system to prevent the reactivation of VZV.

Metabolism:
• Unknown.

Indication: For the prevention of herpes zoster (shingles) in individuals 50 years of age and older.

Contraindication: Patients (1) with a history of anaphylactic/anaphylactoid reaction to gelatin, neomycin, or any other component of the vaccine; (2) with immunosuppression or immunodeficiency; (3) who are pregnant.

Dosage/Range:
• Entire contents (0.65 mL) of reconstituted vaccine lyophilized vial containing at least 19,400 PFU (plaque-forming units) of OKA/Merck strain VZV.

Drug Preparation:
• Remove the lyophilized vaccine powder from the freezer, and immediately and aseptically reconstitute using the provided diluent (stored at room temperature), using a sterile syringe and needle. Inject the entire volume of diluent, and gently agitate the vial to mix thoroughly. When reconstituted, is a semi-hazy to translucent, off-white powder to pale yellow liquid. Use within 30 minutes of reconstitution. Draw up entire contents of vial, and inject subcutaneously into subcutaneous tissue of upper arm (preferable). Vaccine lyophilized powder should be stored in the freezer at −15°C (+5°F) or colder, and protect from light. Diluent can be stored at room temperature or in the refrigerator.

Drug Interactions:
• None known.

Lab Effects/Interference:
* None known.

Special Considerations:
* Drug is not indicated for the treatment of herpes zoster or post-herpetic neuralgia, or for the prevention of primary varicella infection (chickenpox).
* Drug is a live, attenuated virus, which may cause more extensive vaccine-associated rash in patients who are immunosuppressed; the drug's efficacy in patients receiving immunosuppressive drugs, inhaled, oral low-dose, or topical corticosteroids, has not been studied.

Warnings and Precautions:
* Hypersensitivity reactions, including anaphylaxis, have occurred.
* Transmission of vaccine virus may occur between vaccines and susceptible contacts.
* If acute illness (e.g., fever) or in patients with active untreated TB, deferral should be considered.
* Avoid pregnancy for 3 months following vaccination.
* Most common adverse effects (occurring in < 1% of patients) were injection-site reactions and headache.
* Overall vaccine efficacy is 51% (64% in those aged 60–69; 41% in those aged 70–79; and 18% for those patients aged ≥ 80).
* Drug is NOT a substitute for the vaccine VARIVAX (Varicella Virus Live Vaccine).
* Patients should be taught there is a theoretical risk of transmitting the live vaccine to varicella-susceptible individuals.

Potential Toxicities/Side Effects (Dose- and Schedule-Dependent) and the Nursing Process

I.   ALTERATION IN COMFORT related to INJECTION-SITE REACTIONS, RASH, AND HEADACHE

Defining Characteristics: Injection-site reactions included erythema (34%), pain/tenderness (34%), swelling (24%), and pruritus (7%). Headache occurred in 1.4% of patients. Rarely, patients can develop varicella rash.

Nursing Implications: Assess baseline comfort, and teach patient that these side effects may occur. Teach local comfort measures to minimize local injection reactions. Teach patient to report rash right away, and to avoid contact with varicella-sensitive individuals, especially pregnant women.

Chapter 3
Cytoprotective Agents

Advances in the development of effective, new chemotherapeutic agents have been slow, although a number of excellent agents have recently been approved for use. All traditional chemotherapeutic agents work by interfering with DNA and RNA replication, and protein synthesis, causing cell death or stasis. Unfortunately, unless attached to a targeted vehicle, such as a monoclonal antibody, the chemotherapy is non-selective and also damages normal cells. Often, the dose-limiting toxicity is myelosuppression, but organ toxicity specific to the chemotherapy agent may limit the drug's usefulness. Specific organ toxicity that can occur includes neurotoxicity (e.g., cisplatin, oxaliplatin, the taxanes), cardiotoxicity (e.g., anthracyclines, alone or together with trastuzumab), bladder toxicity (e.g., high-dose cyclophosphamide, ifosfamide), and nephrotoxicity (e.g., cisplatin). Thus, both doses and duration of treatment are often limited by these organ toxicities. This can compromise optimal treatment, as well as quality of life. Similarly, radiation therapy causes cell damage (e.g., ionization causes the formation of free radicals, which, in the presence of oxygen, cause damage to DNA, leading to cell death when the cell tries to replicate). Again, normal tissue in the radiation port also is damaged, such as the bone marrow in the skull, sternum, and heads of long bones, and can lead to side effects such as bone marrow depression, which results in the need for treatment breaks and less-than-optimal radiotherapy.

In an effort to protect normal cells from treatment toxicity and to limit organ toxicities, a number of agents have been developed that offer cyto (cell) or organ protection, and even more are being studied (investigational agents). Agents that are currently approved for use are leucovorin calcium, mesna, and dexrazoxane (Zinecard, a chelating agent). Amifostine has shown "broad spectrum" activity in protecting multiple organ systems, such as the kidneys, bone marrow, and nerves. In addition, it protects the parotid glands from radiation damage. Amifostine is indicated for the reduction of cumulative nephrotoxicity from cisplatin in patients with advanced ovarian and NSCLC, as well as for reducing the incidence of moderate-to-severe xerostomia in patients with head and neck cancer whose radiation port covers the parotid glands. Mesna is included in this chapter because it protects the bladder from the toxic effects of high-dose cyclophosphamide and ifosfamide. Leucovorin is also a classic cytoprotectant in that it "rescues" normal cells from methotrexate toxicity (bone marrow and mucosal cells). This chapter also discusses dexrazoxane (Totect), which has been FDA-approved to neutralize potential damage from anthracycline extravasation (Totect).

Shortages of cytoprotective drugs or drugs that increase response, have led to many questions about substitutions or rethinking what is needed. For example, leucovorin is in very short supply, but is a necessary part of the treatment regimens FOLFOX (folinic acid, 5-FU, oxaliplatin) and FOLFIRI (leucovorin, 5-FU, irinotecan) for colorectal cancer.

In reviewing the many clinical trials, the NCCN recommends reconsideration of smaller doses of leucovorin (studies have shown equivalence in doses ranging from 20 mg/m^2 to 500 mg/m^2) (NCCN, v.3, 2014) or using levoleucovorin (200 mg/m^2 is equivalent to standard leucovorin 400 mg/m^2) (NCCN, v.3, 2014). Totect is not currently available, but studies have now shown that dexrazoxane (generic or Zinecard) can be used equally well (Arroyo et al., 2010; Conde-Estevez et al., 2010).

One organ toxicity that has received increased attention is neurotoxicity. Many highly effective agents are limited in both dose and duration of treatment by the development of peripheral neuropathy, such as the taxanes and platinums. This side effect can be one of the most clinically challenging problems for oncology nurses. See Table 3.1 for a list of antitumor agents that cause neurotoxicity. Peripheral neuropathy is defined as the injury, inflammation, or degeneration of any nerve outside the central nervous system. Chemotherapy may cause damage to the sensory and motor axons. Symptoms of sensory damage include tingling, pricking or numbness of the extremities, a sensation of wearing an invisible glove

Table 3.1   Chemotherapy Agents Likely to Cause Neurotoxicity

High Incidence (very common, > 80% incidence)	
Cisplatin	Interleukin-2 (if patient develops capillary leak syndrome)
	Interferon (especially at HD)
Moderate Incidence (common, 20–80% incidence)	
Albumin-bound paclitaxel	L-asparaginase
Arsenic trioxide	Methotrexate (IT, HD)
Bortezomib	Oxaliplatin, ormaplatin
Cabazitaxel	Paclitaxel
Carmustine (intra-arterial)	Procarbazine
Cytosine arabinoside (HD)	Suramin
Docetaxel	Thalidomide
	Tretinoin
Hexamethylmelamine	Vincristine, vinblastine
Ifosfamide	Vinorelbine
Uncommon (< 20% incidence)	
Busulfan	Fludarabine
Capecitabine	5-fluorouracil
Cladribine	Pentostatin
Etoposide	Teniposide

IT = intrathecal; HD = high dose
Data from: Armstrong T, Rust D, Kohtz JR (1997); Cheson BD, Vena DA, Foss FM, Sorensen JM (1994); Furlong TG (1993); Weiss RB (2001); Hershman et al. (2014).

or sock and thus the term *stocking-and-glove* distribution; burning or freezing pain; sharp, stabbing, or electric shock–like pain; and extreme sensitivity to touch. Patients, in some cases, will be reluctant to admit to these symptoms because they believe that if they do, their chemotherapy drug will be stopped. If the motor neurons are affected, then symptoms include muscle weakness and loss of balance or coordination. In many instances, peripheral neuropathy may be reversible, although it may take many months for this to occur. Unfortunately, damage to peripheral nerves can have long-term effects on quality of life and cause much discomfort, injury, and distress. In addition, while the exact percentage of patients with cancer who experience peripheral neuropathy is unknown, the economic cost of treatment is considerable.

Nurses have been pivotal in performing assessments of sensory and motor function, and assessing the impact of peripheral neuropathy on the patient's safety and quality of life, making them strong advocates for patients. Nurses monitor and document patients' neurologic status prior to each treatment and between treatment cycles. The exam should include a history, such as the questionnaire developed by Hausheer and shown in Figure 3.1.

For each of the following 2 items, please indicate by placing a check in the box that best describes how you have felt over the past 4 weeks.

1. ☐ I have no numbness, pain, or tingling in my hands or feet.
   ☐ I have mild tingling, pain, or numbness in my hands or feet. This does not interfere with my activities.
   ☐ I have moderate tingling, pain, or numbness in my hands or feet. This interferes with some of my activities.
   ☐ I have moderate to severe tingling, pain, or numbness in my hands or feet. This interferes with my activities of daily living.
   ☐ I have severe tingling or numbness in my hands or feet. It completely prevents me from doing most activities.
2. ☐ I have no weakness in my arms or legs.
   ☐ I have a mild weakness in my arms or legs. This does not interfere with my activities.
   ☐ I have moderate weakness in my arms or legs. This interferes with some of my activities.
   ☐ I have moderate to severe weakness in my arms or legs. This interferes with my activities of daily living.
   ☐ I have severe weakness in my arms or legs. It completely prevents me from doing most activities.

To help you complete this form, listed below are some examples of activities of daily living:

Dressing:	Button blouse/shirt, put on earrings, tie shoes, put in contact lenses
Eating:	Use knife, fork, and spoon or chopsticks
Mobility:	Walk, climb stairs
Communication:	Write, type on a keyboard
Other:	Sleep, drive, operate remote controls

Figure 3.1 Patient Neurotoxicity Questionnaire

Source: Hausheer F, Berghorn E. Bionumerik Patient Neurotoxicity Questionnaire. San Antonio, TX, Bionumerik Pharmaceuticals, Inc., 2000. Reprinted by permission.

Patients are asked if they have difficulties in performing their normal activities of daily living, such as buttoning a shirt or holding a fork to eat (fine motor movement), mobility in terms of difficulty going up or down stairs, and communicating. A physical exam of gait, motor, and sensory systems, as well as testing of reflexes, should also be done. *Appendix 2* gives directions to access the National Cancer Institute (NCI) Common Toxicity Criteria, which is commonly used to grade peripheral neuropathy; however, it does not capture the subjective patient experience. At this time, there is no standardized chemotherapy-induced peripheral neuropathy (CIPN) assessment tool that has been used consistently to study agents that might ameliorate CIPN (Wilkes, 2014).

The American Society of Clinical Oncology (ASCO, 2014) recently completed a systematic review of the literature and found that there were no agents that prevent CIPN. They found that many of the randomized controlled trials were small and heterogenous and underpowered so that they were unable to detect clinically important differences, and most studies were not directly comparable as they used different measurements, instruments, and outcomes. Conflicting studies often exist, some showing potential benefit of agents and others that are negative, such as the study of amifostine and glutamine, found in this chapter. However, in terms of treating neuropathic pain, duloxetine has been shown to significantly reduce CIPN-induced pain (Smith et al., 2013). See *Chapter 9*.

References

Armstrong T, Rust D, Kohtz JR. Neurologic, Pulmonary, and Cutaneous Toxicities of High-Dose Chemotherapy. *Oncol Nurs Forum* 1997; 24 (Suppl 1) 23–33.

Arroyo PA, Perez RU, Feijoo MAF, Hernandez MAC (2010). Good clinical and cost outcomes using dexrazoxane to treat accidental epirubicin extravasation. *J Ca Research and Therapeutics* 6:573–574.

Baxter Healthcare Corporation. Mesnex (mesna) [package insert]. Deerfield, IL, March 2014.

Berghorn E, Hausheer F. Bionumerik Patient Neurotoxicity Questionnaire. San Antonio, TX: Bionumerick Pharmaceuticals, Inc.; 2000.

Boyle FM, Wheeler HR, Shenfield GM. Glutamine Ameliorates Experimental Vincristine Neuropathy. *J Pharmacol Exp Ther* 1996; 279(1) 410–415.

Boyle FM, Wheeler HR, Shenfield GM. Amelioration of Experimental Cisplatin and Paclitaxel Neuropathy with Glutamate. *J Neuro-Oncol* 1999; 41107–41116.

Calhoun EA, Fishman DA, Roland PY, Lurain JR, Bennett CL. Total Cost of Chemotherapy-Induced Hematologic and Neurologic Toxicity. *Proc Am Soc Clin Oncol* 1999; 18A 1606.

Cassidy J, Bjarnason GA, Hickish T. Randomized Double Blind (DB) Placebo (Plcb) Controlled Phase III Study Assessing the Efficacy of Xaliproden (X) in Reducing the Cumulative Peripheral Sensory Neuropathy (PSN) Induced by the Oxaplatin (Ox) and 5-FU/LV Combination (FOLFOX4) in First-Line Treatment of Patients (pts) with Metastatic Colorectal Cancer (MCRC). *Proceedings from the 42nd Annual Meeting of the American Society of Clinical Oncology* Atlanta, GA. June 2006; Abstract #3507.

Cheson BD, Vena DA, Foss FM, Sorensen JM. Neurotoxicity of Purine Analogues: A Review. *J Clin Oncol* 1994; 12(10) 2216–2228.

Conde-Estevez D, Saumell S, Salar A, Mateu-de Antonio J. (2010). Successful dexrazoxane treatment of a potentially severe extravasation of concentrated doxorubicin. *Anti-Cancer Drugs,* 21: 790–794.

Furlong TG. Neurologic Complications of Immunosuppressive Cancer Therapy. *Oncol Nurs Forum* 1993; 20(9) 1337–1352.

Hensley ML, Schuchter LM, Lindley C. American Society of Clinical Oncology Clinical Practice Guidelines for the Use of Chemotherapy and Radiotherapy Protectants. *J Clin Oncol* 1999; 17(10) 3333–3355.

Hershman DL, Lacchetti C, Dworkin RH et al. (2014). Prevention and management of chemotherapy-induced peripheral neuropathy in survivors of adult cancers: American Society of Clinical Oncology clinical practice guideline. *J Clin Oncol* 32: 1941–1967.

Liu T, Liu Y, He S, et al. Use of Radiation With or Without WR-2721 in Advanced Rectal Cancer. *Cancer* 1992; 69(11) 2820–2825.

Mouridsen HT, Langer SW, Buter J, et al. Treatment of Anthracycline Extravasation with Savene (dexrazoxane): Results from Two Prospective Clinical Multicentre Studies. *Ann Oncol* 2007; 18 546–555.

National Comprehensive Cancer network (NCCN). NCCN Guidleines Version 3.2014 Colon Cancer. Available at http://www.nccn.org/professionals/physician_gls/pdf/colon.pdf. Accessed August 13, 2014.

Pfizer. Zinecard (dexrazoxane) [package insert]. New York, NY, April 2014.

Savarese D, Boucher J, Corey B. Glutamine Treatment of Paclitaxel-induced Myalgias and Arthralgias [letter]. *J Clin Oncol* 1998; 16(12) 3918–3939.

Schuchter LM, Luginbuhl WE, Meropol NJ. The Current Status of Toxicity Protectants in Cancer Therapy. *Semin Oncol* 1992; 19(6) 742–751.

Schulmeister L. Totect: A New Agent for Treating Anthracycline Extravasation. *Clin J Oncol Nurs* 2007; 11(3) 387–395.

Smith EM, Pang H, Cirrincione C et al. (2013). Effect of dulocetineon pain, function, and quality of life among patients with chemotherapy-induced painful peripheral neuropathy. *JAMA* 309;(13): 1359–1367.

Suoman E. Xaliproden Lessens Oxaliplatin-Mediated Neurotoxicity. *Lancet Oncol* 2006; 7(4) 288.

Viele CS, Holmes BC. Amifostine: Drug Profile and Nursing Implications of the First Pancytoprotectant. *Oncol Nurs Forum* 1998; 25(3) 515–523.

Weiss RB. Miscellaneous Toxicities. In DeVita VT Jr Hellman S Rosenberg, SA (eds). *Principles and Practice of Oncology*, 5th ed. New York, NY: Lippincott-Raven Publishers; 1997; 2802.

Weiss RB. Miscellaneous Toxicities, Adverse Effects of Treatment. In DeVita VT Jr Hellman S Rosenberg SA (eds). *Principles and Practice of Oncology*, 6th ed. New York, NY: Lippincott-Raven Publishers; 2001: Chapter 55.

Wilkes GM. Peripheral Neuropathy. In Yarbro CH, Wujuk D, Gobel BH (eds). *Cancer Symptom Management*, 4th ed. Burlington, MA: Jones & Bartlett Learning, 2014; 457–493.

Drug: allopurinol sodium (Aloprim, Zyloprim, Zurinol)

Class: Xanthine oxidase inhibitor.

Mechanism of Action: Drug inhibits xanthine oxidase, the enzyme necessary for conversion of hypoxanthine (natural purine base) to xanthine, and then xanthine to uric acid, without affecting biosynthesis of purines. This lowers serum and urinary uric acid levels.

Metabolism: Well absorbed orally and IV with comparable oxypurinol (major pharmacologic component) serum levels with the relative bioavailability of oxypurinol 100%. Time to peak serum concentration is 30–120 minutes, with half-life of allopurinol 1–3 hours, and of oxypurinol 18–30 hours. Drug metabolized in liver to active metabolite oxypurinol, and excreted by kidneys and enterohepatic circulation.

Indication: For the management of patients with (1) signs and symptoms of primary or secondary gout (acute attacks, tophi, joint destruction, uric acid lithiasis, and/or nephropathy); (2) leukemia, lymphoma, and malignancies who are receiving cancer chemotherapy, which causes elevations of serum and urinary uric acid levels; drug should be stopped when potential for uric acid overproduction is no longer present; and (3) recurrent calcium oxalate calculi whose daily uric acid excretion > 800 mg/day in male patients, and > 750 mg/day in female patients; therapy should be assessed initially and reassessed periodically to determine that treatment continues to be beneficial and that benefits outweigh the risks.

Dosage/Range:
- Gout: 200–300 mg/day (mild) or 400–600 mg/day (moderately severe) in a single or divided doses, maximum dose 800 mg).
- Prevention of uric acid nephropathy in cancer treatment.
  - Oral: 600–800 mg/day for 2–3 days with hydration (dose-reduce if creatinine clearance is < 60 mg/mL).
  - IV: in management of patients with leukemia, lymphoma, and solid tumors receiving cancer therapy expected to cause elevated serum and urinary uric acid levels and who cannot tolerate oral therapy.
  - Adults: 200–400 mg/m^2/day, maximum 600 mg/day as a single dose or in divided doses every 6, 8, or 12 hours; optimally begin allopurinol 24–48 hours prior to chemotherapy.
  - Dose-reduce for renal dysfunction based on creatinine clearance (10–20 mL/min = 200 mg/day; 3–10 mL/min = 100 mg/day).

Drug Preparation:
- Oral: available in 100-mg and 300-mg tablets.
- IV: available as 30-mL vial containing 500 mg allopurinol lyophilized powder, which is stable at room temperature (25°C, 77°F).
- Reconstitute by adding 25 mL sterile water for injection.
- The ordered dose should be withdrawn, and further diluted in 0.9% NS injection or 5% dextrose for injection to achieve a final concentration of no greater than 6 mg/mL.
- Store at 20–25°C (68–77°F) for up to 10 hours after reconstitution.
- Do not refrigerate reconstituted or diluted product.

Drug Administration:
- Oral: give with food or immediately after meals to decrease gastric irritation.
- IV: administer over appropriate period of time given volume of diluted drug.

Drug Interactions:
- Dicoumarol: PT may be prolonged due to prolonged half-life; monitor PT closely and adjust dose as needed.
- Mercaptopurine/azathioprine: allopurinol decreased drug metabolism, so dose of mercaptopurine or azathioprine must be reduced to 1/3 or 1/4 the usual dose, and then subsequent dose adjusted based on clinical response.

- Uricosuric agents: decrease the inhibition of xanthine oxidase by oxypurinol and increase the urinary excretion of uric acid. Avoid concomitant use.
- Ampicillin/amoxicillin: increased frequency of skin rash; use together cautiously.
- Chlorpropamide: allopurinol may prolong half-life of drug, as both drugs compete for excretion in renal tubule; monitor closely for hypoglycemia if drugs used concomitantly in a patient with renal dysfunction.
- Cyclosporin: cyclosporine levels may be increased, so drug levels should be monitored closely, and dose of cyclosporine adjusted accordingly.
- Theophylline: prolonged half-life when used together; monitor theophylline levels closely and adjust dose accordingly.

Physical incompatibilities with IV allopurinol:
- Amikacin sulfate, amphotericin B, carmustine, cefotaxime sodium, chlorpromazine HCl, cimetidine HCl, clindamycin phosphate, cytarabine, dacarbazine, daunorubicin HCl, diphenhydramine HCl, doxorubicin HCl, doxycycline hyclate, droperidol, floxuridine, gentamicin sulfate, haloperidol lactate, hydroxyzine HCl, idarubicin HCl, imipenem-cilastatin sodium, mechlorethamine HCl, meperidine HCl, metoclopramide HCl, methylprednisolone sodium succinate, minocycline HCl, nalbuphine HCl, netilmicin sulfate, ondansetron HCl, prochlorperazine edisylate, promethazine HCl, sodium bicarbonate, streptozocin, tobramycin sulfate, vinorelbine tartrate.

Lab Effects/Interference:
- Increased alk phos, AST, ALT, bili.

Special Considerations:
- Dose reduction necessary in renal dysfunction.
- Contraindicated in patients hypersensitive to drug (even mild allergic reaction).
- Use cautiously with patients on diuretics, as may decrease renal function and increase serum levels of allopurinol.
- Allopurinol hypersensitivity syndrome may occur rarely and is characterized by fever, chills, leukopenia or leukocytosis, eosinophilia, arthralgias, rash, pruritus, nausea, vomiting, renal and hepatic compromise.
- Drug MUST be discontinued immediately if rash develops; stop drug at first sign of rash.
- To prevent tumor lysis syndrome, patient should receive aggressive IV hydration with or without urine alkalinization, together with allopurinol.

Potential Toxicities/Side Effects and the Nursing Process

I.   POTENTIAL SENSORY/PERCEPTUAL ALTERATIONS related to CNS EFFECTS

Defining Characteristics: Drowsiness, chills, and fever have been reported in > 10% of patients. Headaches and somnolence occur in 1–10% of patients. Rarely, seizure, myoclonus, twitching, agitation, mental status changes, cerebral infarction, coma, paralysis, and tremor can occur. If fever and chills are associated with rash, eosinophilia, nausea, vomiting, they are most likely related to rare allopurinol hypersensitivity reaction.

Nursing Implications: Assess baseline neurologic status, including mental status, and periodically during treatment. If any abnormalities, discuss with physician right away. Teach patient to report chills, fever, drowsiness, or any changes, if they occur. If they do occur, teach patient self-management strategies and to report whether they are ineffective. If so, discuss management strategies with physician. If fever and chills are associated with rash, eosinophilia, nausea, vomiting, they are most likely related to rare allopurinol hypersensitivity reaction and should be discussed with the physician immediately drug should be discontinued.

II.   ALTERATION IN SKIN INTEGRITY, POTENTIAL, related to RASH, STEVENS-JOHNSON SYNDROME

Defining Characteristics: More than 10% of patients develop maculopapular rash, often associated with urticaria and pruritus; may be exfoliative. Less common but more severe, 1–10% of patients develop Stevens-Johnson syndrome or toxic epidermal necrolysis, which may be fatal. For IV administration, local injection-site reactions may occur. Alopecia has been reported in 1–10% of patients.

Nursing Implications: Assess baseline skin integrity and intactness of scalp hair. Teach patient that rash may occur, and to report it right away, as drug must be discontinued. Teach patient self-care strategies, including skin cream to moisturize the skin and to prevent itching. Discuss drug discontinuance and management with physician. Teach patient to report any hair loss. If it occurs, discuss impact on patient, self-care strategies, and if severe, discuss drug discontinuance with physician.

Drug: amifostine for injection (Ethyol, WR-2721)

Class: Cytoprotectant; free-radical scavenger, metabolized to a free thiol.

Mechanism of Action: Drug is phosphorylated by alkaline phosphatase bound in tissue membranes, producing free thiol. Inside the cell, free thiol binds to and detoxifies reactive metabolites of cisplatin and other chemotherapeutic agents, thus neutralizing the chemotherapy drug in normal tissues so that cellular DNA and RNA are not damaged. Normal cells are protected because of differences in cell physiology (higher alkaline phosphatase concentrations and tissue pH, as well as more effective vascularity in normal cells as compared to malignant cells) and transport mechanisms that promote the preferential uptake of free thiol into normal tissues. Free thiol may also scavenge reactive free-radical reactive oxygen molecules resulting from chemotherapy or radiotherapy. Free thiol may also upregulate p53 expression, so that cells accumulate in the G_1–S cell cycle phase, enabling DNA repair.

Metabolism: Drug is rapidly metabolized to an active free-thiol metabolite and cleared from the plasma, so the drug should be administered 30 minutes prior to drug dose.

Indication: To reduce the (1) cumulative renal toxicity associated with repeated administration of cisplatin in patients with advanced ovarian cancer, (2) incidence of moderate-to-severe xerostomia in patients undergoing post-operative RT for head and neck cancer, where the radiation port includes a substantial portion of the parotid glands.

Dosage/Range:
- Chemoprotectant: 910 mg/m^2 in 50 mL 0.9% NS administered IV over 15 minutes, 30 minutes prior to beginning chemotherapy.
- Radioprotectant: 200 mg/m^2/day IVP over 3 minutes, 15 minutes prior to standard fraction radiation therapy (1.8–2.0 Gy).

Drug Preparation:
- Available in 10-mL vials containing 500 mg of drug; store at room temperature.
- Use only 0.9% sodium chloride.
- Reconstitute vial with 9.7 mL of sterile 0.9% sodium chloride.
- Further dilute with sterile 0.9% sodium chloride to total 50 mL.
- Stable at 5 mg/mL to 40 mg/mL for 5 hours at room temperature, and for 24 hours if refrigerated.

Drug Administration:
- Hypertension medicines should be stopped 24 hours prior to drug administration.
- Ensure that patient has been adequately hydrated prior to drug administration, and keep patient in supine position. Monitor BP every 5 minutes during infusion and then as clinically indicated.
  - Administer combination antiemetics:
    - Administer IV antiemetic medication 1 hour prior, and oral antiemetic 2 hours prior to amifostine administration.
  - Generally, patients should be hydrated with 1 L 0.9% NS prior to amifostine when used as a chemoprotectant.
  - Infuse amifostine IV over 15 minutes, beginning 30 minutes prior to chemotherapy or IVP 15–30 minutes prior to radiotherapy.
  - Monitor BP baseline, immediately after amifostine infusion and as needed until BP returns to baseline.
  - Resume diuretic(s) and/or antihypertensive medications 30 minutes after amifostine infusion is complete as long as patient is normotensive.

Drug Interactions:
- Antihypertensive and diuretic medications may potentiate hypotension.

Lab Effects/Interference:
- May cause hypocalcemia.

Special Considerations:
- Patients unable to tolerate cessation of antihypertensive medications are not candidates for the drug.
- Studies have shown no decrease in cisplatin drug efficacy when given with first-line therapy in ovarian cancer, and no other studies have been conducted as to tumor protection by drug.

- Effectiveness of RT has not been studied when using the drug, and it should not be used in patients receiving definitive radiotherapy, except in the context of a clinical trial.
- Offers significant protection of kidneys.
- Offers protection of bone marrow and nerves.
- Drug has been shown to protect skin, mucous membranes, and bladder and pelvic structures against late moderate-to-severe radiation reactions.

Potential Toxicities/Side Effects and the Nursing Process

I.   ALTERATION IN NUTRITION, LESS THAN BODY REQUIREMENTS, related to NAUSEA AND VOMITING, HYPOCALCEMIA

Defining Characteristics: Incidence is frequent, and nausea and vomiting may be severe. These are preventable by using serotonin antagonist and dexamethasone. Hypocalcemia noted in trials using higher doses.

Nursing Implications: Administer serotonin antagonist (e.g., granisetron, ondansetron, or dolasetron) and dexamethasone 20 mg IV prior to amifostine. Encourage small, frequent meals of cool, bland foods and liquids. Teach patient self-management tips and to avoid greasy or heavy foods. Instruct patient to report nausea and/or vomiting that is not resolved by antiemetics. Teach patient to maintain oral hydration as tolerated. Identify patients at risk for hypocalcemia, i.e., nephrotic syndrome and depletion from many courses of cisplatin. Check baseline calcium and albumin, and monitor during therapy. Assess for signs/symptoms of hypocalcemia. Patients may receive calcium supplements as needed.

II.   ALTERATION IN OXYGENATION related to HYPOTENSION, POTENTIAL

Defining Characteristics: Drug causes transient, reversible hypotension in 62% of patients at a dose of 910 mg/m^2. Hypotension is usually manifested by a 5- to 15-minute transient decrease in systolic BP of $\geq$ 20 mm Hg. Incidence is less when dose is 740 mg/m^2, and infused over 5 minutes.

Nursing Implications: Assess patient's medication profile. Antihypertensives should be stopped 24 hours prior to drug administration. Assess baseline BP, heart rate, and hydration status. Ensure that patient is well hydrated, and per physician, administer 1 L of 0.9% NS IV prior to amifostine if needed to assure euhydration; if dehydrated, patient may require 2 L. Place patient in supine position during administration of drug, and monitor BP q 5 min during administration, immediately after administration, and as needed postinfusion. If the BP falls below threshold (see following table), interrupt infusion and give an IVB of 0.9% NS per physician order. If BP comes back above threshold (returns to threshold within minutes and patient is asymptomatic), then resume infusion and give full dose. If BP does not return to threshold within 5 minutes, infusion should be terminated and IV hydration fluids administered per physician, and patient placed in Trendelenburg position, if symptomatic. If BP does not return to normal in 5 minutes, dose should be reduced in next cycle. Manufacturer recommends the following thresholds for supine BP:

Systolic BP (SBP)	Threshold SBP in mm Hg
< 100	< 80
100–119	75–94
120–139	90–109
140–179	100–139
≥ 180	≥ 130

III.   ALTERATION IN COMFORT related to FLUSHING CHILLS, DIZZINESS, SOMNOLENCE, HICCUPS, AND SNEEZING

Defining Characteristics: These effects may occur during or after drug infusion and are mild. Allergic reactions are rare, ranging from skin rash to rigors, but anaphylaxis has not been reported.

Nursing Implications: Assess comfort level, and ask patient to report these symptoms. Discuss comfort measures with patient.

Drug: dexrazoxane for injection (Totect)

Class: Anthracycline extravasation neutralizer.

Mechanism of Action: Drug is a derivative of edetic acid (EDTA) and is a metal ion chelator that protects against free radical tissue damage from extravasated anthracycline chemotherapy. It appears that by binding iron it is unavailable for oxygen; most likely it is due to the drug's activity as a free radical scavenger. Theoretically, it may antagonize the chemotherapeutic effect of previously administered drug.

Metabolism: Biphasic elimination with mean initial elimination half-life of 30 minutes and a mean terminal half-life of 2.8 hours; 42% of the dose is excreted in the urine. No plasma protein binding of drug. Dose-reduce in patients with renal dysfunction.

Indication: Drug is indicated for the treatment of adults who have an anthracycline extravasation (e.g., doxorubicin, daunorubicin, epirubicin, idarubicin).

Dosage/Range:
- Given IV infusion for 3 consecutive days, beginning as soon as possible after anthracycline extravasation but within 6 hours of the extravasation.
- Days 1 and 2: 1,000 mg/m^2 IV infusion (max 2,000 mg).
- Day 3: 500 mg/m^2 IV infusion (max 1,000 mg).
- Dose-reduce by 50% in patients with creatinine clearances < 40 mL/min.

Drug Preparation:
- Available as a Totect kit with ten 500-mg vials of dexrazoxane HCl.
- Reconstitute drug with provided diluent (50-mL vials), forming a solution of drug 10 mg/mL. Use immediately.
- Stable 4 hours after reconstitution refrigerated.
- Store unopened vials of drug powder and diluent at room temperature and protected from light and heat.
- USE SAFE CHEMOTHERAPEUTIC AGENT HANDLING PRECAUTIONS!
- Totect (dexrazoxane) is the only FDA-approved antidote for anthracycline administration, but studies have shown that dexrazoxane is effective (Mouridsen et al., 2007). Generic dexrazoxane (Bedford Labs) and Totect are reconstituted with sodium lactate, but Zinecard (dexrazoxane) must be reconstituted with sterile water.

Drug Administration:
- Give as soon as possible following anthracycline extravasation but within 6 hours of the extravasation. Give at approximately the same time each day (e.g., 24 hours apart).
- Administer IV infusion over 1 to 2 hours in an area or extremity other than that with the extravasation.
- DO NOT use with other extravasation management strategies (e.g., topical dimethyl sulfoxide application), as this may worsen tissue injury.
- Remove topical cooling applications at least 15 minutes before and during drug administration.
- USE CHEMOTHERAPY personal protective equipment when preparing and administering drug.

Drug Interactions:
- None known.

Lab Effects/Interference:
- Neutropenia and thrombocytopenia.
- Increased LFTs.

Special Considerations:
- In two prospective European studies, dexrazoxane proved to be effective and well tolerated and prevented the need for surgical resection in 53 of 54 patients.
- When Zinecard (dexrazoxane) is used as a cardioprotectant, drug may reduce the response from 5-FU, doxorubicin, and cyclophosphamide (FAC) chemotherapy when given concurrently on the first cycle of therapy (48% response rate vs. 63% without the drug, and shorter time to disease progression). There is no evidence that Totect decreases tumor response.
- DRUG REQUIRES SAFE CHEMOTHERAPEUTIC AGENT HANDLING PRECAUTIONS! Also, patient side effects include bone marrow suppression, nausea, and vomiting.
- Most common side effects are neutropenia, thrombocytopenia, fever, infusion-site reactions, nausea, and vomiting.

Potential Toxicities/Side Effects and the Nursing Process

I. POTENTIAL FOR INJURY related to BONE MARROW DEPRESSION

Defining Characteristics: Drug may cause neutropenia and thrombocytopenia.

Nursing Implications: Monitor WBC, HCT/Hgb, and platelets baseline and monitor after injections. Instruct patient in self-assessment for signs/symptoms of infection and bleeding and how to report them. Teach patient self-care measures to minimize risk.

II. POTENTIAL ALTERATION IN METABOLISM related to HEPATIC AND RENAL ALTERATIONS

Defining Characteristics: Possible elevations in liver function studies are reversible.

Nursing Implications: Assess hepatic and renal function tests (bili, BUN, creatinine, and alk phos), baseline and before each treatment. Notify physician of any abnormalities. Dose should be reduced 50% if 24-hour creatinine clearance is < 40 mL/min.

III. ALTERATION IN COMFORT related to PAIN AT INJECTION SITE, FEVER

Defining Characteristics: Pain at the injection site may occur, as may fever.

Nursing Implications: Assess site during and after infusion. Instruct patient to notify nurse if discomfort arises. Apply local measures to reduce discomfort. Teach patient that fever may occur, to check temperature, and if necessary to take acetaminophen and report if the fever does not resolve.

IV. ALTERATION IN NUTRITION, LESS THAN BODY REQUIREMENTS, related to NAUSEA/VOMITING

Defining Characteristics: Nausea and vomiting may occur. Drug is an antineoplastic agent.

Nursing Implications: Assess baseline nutritional status. Premedicate before initial treatment and then give as needed for days 2 and 3. Encourage small, frequent meals and liquids. Teach patient to avoid greasy, fried, or fatty foods. Encourage patient to report onset of nausea/vomiting.

Drug: dexrazoxane for injection (Zinecard)

Class: Cardioprotector.

Mechanism of Action: Enters easily through cell membranes, but the exact mechanism of cardiac cell protection is unclear. A possible mechanism is that the drug becomes a chelating agent within the cell and interferes with iron-mediated free-radical formation that otherwise would cause cardiotoxicity from anthracyclines. Drug is a derivative of edetic acid (EDTA).

Metabolism: 42% of the dose is excreted in the urine. No plasma protein binding of drug.

Indication: Cytoprotective agent indicated for reducing the incidence and severity of cardio-myopathy associated with doxorubicin administration in women with metastatic breast cancer who have received a cumulative doxorubicin dose of 300 mg/m^2 and who will continue to receive doxorubicin therapy to maintain tumor control. Do not use Zinecard with doxorubicin initiation. Do not use Zinecard with nonanthracycline- containing chemotherapy regimens.

Dosage/Range:
- 10:1 ratio of dexrazoxane to doxorubicin (i.e., 500 mg/m^2 of dexrazoxane to 50 mg/m^2 of doxorubicin).
- Renal Impairment: Dose-reduce by 50% for patients with CrCl < 40mL/min.
- Hepatic Impairment: Since a doxorubicin dose reduction is recommended in presence of hyperbilirubinemia, reduce Zinecard dose proportionately (maintain the 10:1 ratio).

Drug Preparation:
- Available in 250- or 500-mg lyophilized vials.
- Reconstitute 250-mg drug with 25 mL Sterile Water for Injection, USP; and 500-mg vial with 50 ml Sterile Water for Injection, USP (resulting solution will contain 10 mg/mL). Following reconstitution with Sterile Water for Injection USP, drug in vial is stable for 30 minutes at room temperature and up to 3 hours when refrigerated (2°–8°C (36°– 46°F). pH of diluted drug is 1.0–3.0. Discard any unused solution.
- Further dilute in Lactated Ringer's Injection USP to a concentration of 1.3–3.0 mg/mL in IV infusion bags.
- The diluted infusion solution is stable for 60 minutes at room temperature or up to 4 hours when refrigerated (2°–8°C (36°–46°F). pH of diluted infusion solution is 3.5–5.5.
- USE SAFE CHEMOTHERAPEUTIC AGENT HANDLING PRECAUTIONS!

Drug Administration:
- Inspect solution for particulate matter and discoloration, and if precipitate for cloudiness seen, do not use.
- Give IV infusion over 15 minutes (NOT IVP); administer doxorubicin within 30 minutes after the completion of Zinecard infusion.

Drug Interactions:
- None known.

Lab Effects/Interference:
- May increase myelosuppression of concomitant doxorubicin, with leukopenia, neutrope-nia, and thrombocytopenia.

Special Considerations:
- DO NOT USE Zinecard with initiation of chemotherapy, as drug may interfere with tumor response. Drug may reduce the response from 5-FU, doxorubicin, and cyclophosphamide

(FAC) chemotherapy when given concurrently on the first cycle of therapy (48% response rate vs 63% without the drug, and shorter time to disease progression) [Pfizer, 2014].
- Zinecard does not completely eliminate the risk of anthracycline-induced cardiac toxicity. Monitor cardiac function baseline and periodically during anthracycline therapy to assess LVEF. If LVEF decreases, continued therapy should be carefully considered against risk of producing irreversible cardiac damage.
- Drug may increase the myelosuppression effects of chemotherapy.
- Secondary malignancies (e.g., AML and MDS) have been reported in studies of pediatric patients who have received Zinecard in combination with chemotherapy. Zinecard is not indicated for use in pediatric patients. Some adults have also developed AML or MDS when receiving Zinecard in combination with anti-cancer agents known to be carcinogenic.
- Drug can cause embryo-fetal toxicity as well as maternal toxicity if used during pregnancy. Teach female patients of reproductive potential to use highly effective contraception to avoid pregnancy.
- DRUG REQUIRES SAFE CHEMOTHERAPEUTIC AGENT HANDLING PRECAUTIONS!

Potential Toxicities/Side Effects and the Nursing Process

I. POTENTIAL FOR INJURY related to ENHANCED BONE MARROW DEPRESSION

Defining Characteristics: Drug may increase doxorubicin-induced bone marrow depression.

Nursing Implications: Monitor WBC, HCT/Hgb, and platelets baseline and prior to each dose. Instruct patient in self-assessment for signs/symptoms of infection and bleeding, and how to report them. Teach patient self-care measures to minimize risk.

II. POTENTIAL ALTERATION IN METABOLISM related to HEPATIC AND RENAL ALTERATIONS

Defining Characteristics: Possible elevations in liver and renal function studies may occur. Incidence did not differ from patients who received same chemotherapy (FAC) without the protector.

Nursing Implications: Assess hepatic and renal function tests (bili, BUN, creatinine, and alk phos), baseline and prior to each treatment. Notify physician of any abnormalities.

III. ALTERATION IN COMFORT related to PAIN AT INJECTION SITE

Defining Characteristics: Pain at the injection site may occur.

Nursing Implications: Assess site during and after infusion. Instruct patient to notify nurse if discomfort arises. Apply local measures to reduce discomfort.

Drug: leucovorin calcium (folinic acid, Citrovorum Factor)

Class: Water soluble vitamin in the folate group (folinic acid).

Mechanism of Action: Potentiates antitumor activity of 5-FU when given prior to or concurrently with 5-FU, ± XRT. Acts as an antidote for methotrexate and other folic acid antagonists. Circumvents the biochemical block of the enzyme inhibitors (e.g., dihydrofolate reductase [DHFR]) to permit DNA and RNA synthesis.

Metabolism: Leucovorin is metabolized to polyglutamates that are more effective in potentiating 5-FU tumor cell kill. Metabolized primarily in the liver, 50% of the single dose is excreted in 6 hours in the urine (80–90%) and stool (8% of the dose).

Indication: (1) After high-dose methotrexate (MTX) therapy in osteosarcoma to rescue normal cells; (2) to diminish the toxicity and counteract the effects of impaired MTX elimination and of inadvertent over-dosages of folic acid antagonists; (3) treatment of megaloblastic anemias due to folic acid deficiency when oral therapy is not feasible; (4) in combination with 5-fluourouracil (5-FU) to prolong survival in the palliative treatment of patients with advanced colorectal cancer (CRC). Drug should not be mixed in the same infusion as 5-FU, as a precipitate will form.

Contraindication: Patients with pernicious anemia and other megaloblastic anemias secondary to the lack of vitamine B^{12}.

Dosage/Range:

Advanced CRC: Either of the following regimens:
- Leucovorin 200 mg/m^2 by slow IV injection over a minimum of 3 minutes followed by 5-FU at 370 mg/m^2 IV repeated daily × 5 days, and cycle repeated every 28 days; dose-reduce 5-FU for hematologic or GI toxicity.
- Leucovorin 20 mg/m^2 IV followed by 5-FU 425 mg/m^2 repeated daily × 5 days, and cycle repeated every 28 days; dose-reduce 5-FU for hematologic or GI toxicity.
- Commonly used in FOLFOX or FOLFIRI regimens:
  - FOLFOX4 every 2 weeks:
    - Day 1: Oxaliplatin 85 mg/m^2 IV infusion in 250–500 mL D$_5$W and leucovorin 200 mg/m^2 IV infusion in D$_5$W, each over 2 hours simultaneously in separate bags using a Y-line, followed by 5-FU 400 mg/m^2 IVB over 2–4 minutes, followed by 5-FU 600 mg/m^2 in 500 mL D$_5$W as a 22-hour continuous infusion.
    - Day 2: Leucovorin 200 mg/m^2 IV infusion over 2 hours, followed by 5-FU 400 mg/m^2 IVB over 2–4 minutes, followed by 5-FU 600 mg/m^2 in 500 mL D$_5$W as a 22-hour continuous infusion.
  - FOLFIRI: FOLFIRI day 1: Irinotecan 180 mg/m^2 IV over 90 minutes, at the same time as leucovorin 200 mg/m^2 IV over 2 hours through separate arms of a Y-tubing, followed by 5-FU 400 mg/m^2 IVB and then 23-hour 5-FU 1200 mg/m^2 IV continuous infusion (CI), days 1 and 2. Total 5-FU CI dose is 2400 mg/m^2 over 46–48 hours. Repeat q 2 weeks.

- FOLFIRI: Repeat q 2 weeks.
  - Day 1: Irinotecan 180 mg/m² IV over 90 minutes, at the same time as leucovorin 200 mg/m² IV over 2 hours through separate arms of a Y-tubing, followed by 5-FU 400 mg/m² IVB and then 5-FU 2400 mg/m² IV continuous infusion (CI) over 46–48 hours.

Leucovorin rescue after high-dose methotrexate therapy (12–15 g/m²):
- DO NOT ADMINISTER LEUCOVORIN INTRATHECALLY.
- Serum creatinine and MTX levels should be determined at least once daily. Continue leucovorin administration, hydration, and urinary alkalization (to keep urine pH of 7.0 or greater) until the MTX level is < 5 × 10⁻⁸ M (0.05 micromolar).
- Guidelines for leucovorin dosage and administration: Dose of drug and duration of rescue dependent on serum methotrexate levels.
  - *Normal MTX elimination:* Lab: serum MTX level approximately 10 micromolar at 24 hr after administration, 1 micromolar at 48 hr, and < 0.2 micromolar at 72 hr; leucovorin10 mg/m² IV, PO, or IM every 6 hours × 10 doses, starting EXACTLY 24 hours after beginning of MTX infusion.
  - *Delayed late MTX elimination:* Lab: serum MTX level > 0.2 micromolar at 72 hr, and > 0.05 micromolar at 96 hr after administration; continue leucovorin10 mg/m² IV, PO, or IM every 6 hours × 10 doses, until MTX level < 0.05 micromolar.
  - *Delayed early MTX elimination and/or evidence of acute renal injury:* Lab: serum MTX level of 50 micromolar or more at 24 hr, or 5 micromolar more at 48 hr after administration, OR a 100% or greater increase in serum creatinine level at 24 hr after MTX administration (e.g., an increase from 0.5 mg/mL to a level of 1 mg/dL or more); leucovorin 150 mg IV every 3 hr, until MTX level is < 1 micromolar; then 15 mg IV every 3 hr until MTX level < 0.05 micromolar. These patients likely will develop reversible renal failure and need to have continuing hydration, urinary alkinization, close monitoring of fluid and electrolyte status, until serum MTX level is acceptable and renal failure has resolved.

Drug Preparation:
- Drug is supplied in ampules or vials.
- Reconstitute vials with sterile water for injection.
- Dilute reconstituted vials or ampules further with 5% dextrose or 0.9% sodium chloride.

Drug Administration:
- With 5-FU, in a variety of combinations: e.g., leucovorin 500 mg/m²/week for 6 weeks as a 2-hour infusion; 5-FU: 500–600 mg/m²/week for 6 weeks IVB midway through leucovorin infusion, then 2- week rest, then repeat 6-week cycle.
- High dose MTX: Administered starting EXACTLY 24 hours after the first methotrexate dose is given. Dose every 6 hours for up to 10 doses; then continue per table above if MTX level unacceptable.
- First dose is given IV; others can be given IM or PO when given as methotrexate rescue and able to keep oral liquids down, unless otherwise indicated in table above.
- IV doses are given as boluses over 15 min unless otherwise specified.
- When given as a rescue dose, leucovorin must be given exactly on time in order to rescue normal cells from severe methotrexate toxicity.

Drug Interactions:
- 5-FU potentiation.
- Folic acid: provides folinic acid so cells can make DNA (antagonizes drug effect).
- Phenobarbital, phenytoin, primidone: decreased anticonvulsant action when leucovorin given in high doses; monitor patient closely and increase anticonvulsant dose as needed.

Lab Effects/Interference:
- None.

Special Considerations:
- It is imperative that the patient receive leucovorin on schedule to avoid fatal methotrexate toxicity (when given as rescue). Notify the physician if the patient is unable to take the dose orally, as it then must be administered IV.
- Usually free of side effects, but allergic and local pain may occur.

Potential Toxicities/Side Effects and the Nursing Process

I. POTENTIAL FOR INJURY related to HYPERSENSITIVITY, DRUG INTERACTIONS

Defining Characteristics: Allergic sensitization has been reported: facial flushing, itching. Leucovorin in large amounts may counteract the antiepileptic effects of phenobarbital, phenytoin, and primidone.

Nursing Implications: Monitor patient for signs/symptoms of allergic reaction. Diphenhydramine is effective for relieving symptoms of allergic reaction. Monitor patient for symptoms of increased seizure activity if taking anticonvulsants; monitor antiepileptic drug levels.

II. ALTERED NUTRITION, POTENTIAL, LESS THAN BODY REQUIREMENTS, related to NAUSEA, VOMITING

Defining Characteristics: Oral leucovorin rarely causes nausea or vomiting.

Nursing Implications: Administer oral leucovorin with antacids, milk, or juice if needed.

Drug: levoleucovorin (Fusilev, d, 1-leucovorin)

Class: Folate analog.

Mechanism of Action: Drug is the pharmacologically active isomer of 5-formyl tetrahydrofolic acid that does not require further reduction by the enzyme dihydrofolate reductase in order to use folate. Acts as an antidote for methotrexate and other folic acid antagonists. Circumvents the biochemical block of the enzyme inhibitors (e.g., dihydrofolate reductase

(DHFR) to permit DNA and RNA synthesis. Potentiates antitumor activity of 5-FU when given before or concurrently.

Metabolism: After an IV dose of 15 mg, peak serum levels were reached in 0.9 hr. Mean terminal half-life was 5–6.8 hr.

Indications: (1) Rescue after high-dose methotrexate (MTX) therapy in osteosarcoma; (2) diminishing the toxicity and counteracting the effects of impaired MTX elimination and of inadvertent overdosage of folic acid antagonists; (3) use in combination chemotherapy with 5-fluouracil (5-FU) in the palliative treatment of patients with advanced metastatic colorectal cancer (CRC). Drug is not approved for pernicious anemia and megaloblastic anemias.

Dosage/Range:
- Levoleucovorin is dosed at one-half the usual dose of racemic d,l-leucovorin.
- Do NOT administer intrathecally.

Rescue after high-dose MTX therapy:
- Based on a MTX dose of 12 g/m^2 administered IV over 4 hours: 7.5 mg (5 mg/m^2) every 6 hr × 10 doses starting exactly 24 hours after the beginning of methotrexate infusion.
- Determine serum creatinine and MTX levels at least once daily.
- Continue levoleucovorin administration, hydration, and urinary alkalinization (pH > 7.0) until MTX level < 5 × (10)$^{-8}$ [0.05 micromolar].
- The levoleucovorin dose may need to be adjusted.

Clinical Situation	Laboratory Findings	Levoleucovorin Dosage/Duration
Normal MTX elimination	Serum MTX level 10 micromolar at 24 hr after administration, 1 micromolar at 48 hr, and < 0.2 micromolar at 72 hr	7.5 mg IV q 6 hr for 60 hr (10 doses starting at 24 hr after start of MTX infusion)
Delayed late elimination	Serum MTX level > 0.2 micromolar at 72 hr, and > 0.05 micromolar at 96 hr after administration	Continue 7.5 mg IV q 6 hr until MTX level is < 0.05 micromolar
Delayed early MTX elimination and/or evidence of acute renal injury	Serum MTX level at ≥ 50 micromolar at 24 hr, or ≥ 5 micromolar at 48 hr after MTX administration, OR ≥ 100% increase in serum creatinine level at 24 hr after MTX administration (e.g., an increase from 0.5 mg/dL to a level of 1 mg/dL or more)	75 mg IV q 3 hr until MTX level is < 1 micromolar; then 7.5 mg IV q 3 hr until MTX level is < 0.05 micromolar

Levoleucovorin in combination with 5-FU:
- Levoleucovorin 100 mg/m^2 by slow IV injection over a minimum of 3 minutes, followed by 5-FU at 370 mg/m^2 IV, daily × 5 days, repeat cycle every 28 days; dose-reduce 5-FU or delay for hematologic and other toxicity. See 5-FU.

- Levoleucovorin 10 mg/m^2 by slow IV injection over a minimum of 3 minutes, followed by 5-FU at 425 mg/m^2 IV, daily × 5 days, repeat cycle every 28 days; dose-reduce 5-FU or delay for hematologic and other toxicity. See 5-FU.
- Commonly used in FOLFOX (together with 5-FU and oxaliplatin) and FOLFIRI (irinotecan and 5-FU); see drug information for oxaliplatin and irinotecan for regimens.

Drug Preparation:
- Drug available in 50-mg single-use vial as a lyophilized powder with 50-mg mannitol.
- Reconstitute with 5.3 mL of sterile 0.9% sodium chloride for injection USP, resulting in a 10 gm/mL solution.
- May further dilute to concentration of 0.5 mg/mL to 5 mg/mL in 0.9% sodium chloride USP (stable for 12 hours at room temperature) or 5% dextrose injection USP (stable for 4 hours at room temperature).

Drug Administration:
- Administer IVP, not faster than 16 mL (160 mg)/min because calcium content limits speed of injection, or as a short IV infusion.

Lab Effects/Interference:
- None known.

Drug Interactions:
- 5-FU: increased toxicity.
- Trimethoprim-sulfamethoxazole (Bactrim, used to treat PCP in HIV-infected patients). Coadministration resulted in increased rates of treatment failure in one study.

Special Considerations:
- Do not administer intrathecally.
- Dosed at one-half the usual dose of leucovorin calcium (folinic acid citrovorum factor).
- Contraindicated in persons who have had a prior allergic reaction to folic acid or folinic acid.
- When given with 5-FU weekly in older patients, has caused severe enterocolitis, diarrhea, and dehydration, resulting in death.

Potential Toxicities/Side Effects and the Nursing Process

I.   POTENTIAL FOR INJURY related to HYPERSENSITIVITY, DRUG INTERACTIONS

Defining Characteristics: Allergic sensitization has been reported: facial flushing, itching.

Nursing Implications: Monitor patient for signs/symptoms of allergic reaction. Diphenhydramine is effective for relieving symptoms of allergic reaction.

II. ALTERED NUTRITION, POTENTIAL, LESS THAN BODY REQUIREMENTS, related to NAUSEA, VOMITING

Defining Characteristics: Levoleucovorin causes vomiting in 38% of patients, stomatitis in 38%, and nausea in 19% after high-dose MTX therapy. Oral leucovorin rarely causes nausea or vomiting.

Nursing Implications: Discuss need to continue antiemetics after high-dose MTX therapy with physician. Assess oral mucosa, teach patient self-assessment and to report any abnormalities. Teach patient to rinse oral mucosa after meals and at bedtime with oral rinse, such as salt water or sodium bicarbonate solution, per institutional policy and procedure.

Drug: mesna for injection (Mesnex)

Class: Sulfhydryl.

Mechanism of Action: Used to prevent ifosfamide-induced hemorrhagic cystitis. Drug is rapidly metabolized to the metabolite dimesna. In the kidney, dimesna is reduced to mesna, which binds to the urotoxic ifosfamide and cyclophosphamide metabolites acrolein and 4-hydroxyfosfamide, resulting in their detoxification.

Metabolism: Rapidly metabolized, remains in the intravascular compartment, and is rapidly eliminated by the kidneys. The drug is eliminated in 24 hours as mesna (32%) and dimesna (33%). Majority of the dose is eliminated within 4 hours. Oral mesna has 50% bioavailability of IV dose.

Indication: As a prophylactic agent in reducing the incidence of ifosfamide-induced hemorrhagic cystitis. Not indicated to reduce the risk of hematuria due to other pathological conditions, such as thrombocytopenia.

Dosage/Range:
- Initial dose should be given IV.
- Recommended IV-IV-IV: Clinical dose 20% of the mesna dose IV bolus 15 minutes before (or at the same time as the ifosfamide), 4 hours and 8 hours after ifosfamide or cyclophosphamide dose. Mesna dose is 20% of ifosfamide or cyclophosphamide dose, with total daily dose 60% of the ifosfamide or cyclophosphamide dose.
- IV-oral-oral: Mesna is given as an IV bolus injection in a dosage equal to 20% of the ifosfamide dosage at the time of ifosfamide administration. Mesna tablets are given orally in a dosage equal to 40% of the ifosfamide dose at 2 and 6 hours after each dose of ifosfamide. The total daily dose of mesna is 100% of the ifosfamide dose.
- Schedules:
  - IV dosing: Ifosfamide dose is 1.2 g/m^2 IV at 0 hours, with mesna 240 mg/m^2 IV at 0 hours; mesna 240 mg/m^2 IV at 4 hours and at 8 hours post-ifosfamide.

- IV and oral dosing: Ifosfamide dose is 1.2 g/m^2 IV at 0 hours, with mesna 240 mg/m^2 IV at 0 hours; mesna PO 480 mg/m^2 IV at 4 hours and at 8 hours post-ifosfamide.
- Maintain sufficient urinary output as required for ifosfamide treatment; assess urine for blood.
- The efficacy and safety of this ratio of IV-oral-oral mesna has not been established as being effective for daily doses of ifosfamide higher than 2.0 gm/m^2 for 3–5 days.
- For continuous ifosfamide infusions, mesna is mixed with ifosfamide in equal amounts (1:1 mix). Prior to initiating continuous infusion, mesna is given IVB (10% of total ifosfamide dose). Following completion of the infusion, mesna alone should be infused for 12–24 hours to protect against delayed drug excretion activity against the bladder.
- Oral mesna: Dose is 40% of ifosfamide or cyclophosphamide dose (not recommended for initial dose if the patient experiences nausea and vomiting).

Drug Preparation:
- Drug available as Mesnex injection 1 g multidose vial (100 mg/mL), and as tablets (400 mg mesna tablets).
- Dilute mesna with 5% dextrose, 5% dextrose/0.2% Sodium Chloride Injection USP, 5% dextrose/0.33% Sodium Chloride Injection USP, 5% dextrose/0.45% Sodium Chloride Injection USP, 0.9% Sodium Chloride Injection USP, or Lactated Ringer's Injection USP to create a designated fluid concentration.
- For continuous ifosfamide infusion, mesna should be mixed together in the same infusion bag with the ifosfamide.
- Stability: Mesnex injection multidose vials may be stored and used for up to 8 days after initial puncture. Store diluted solutions at 25°C (77°F); use diluted solutions within 24 hr.
- Do not mix Mesnex with epirubicin, cyclophosphamide, cisplatin, carboplatin, or nitrogen mustard.
- The benzyl alcohol contained in mesnex injection vials can reduce the stability of ifosfamide. Ifosfamide and mesna can be mixed in the same bag, provided the final concentration of ifosfamide is not > 50 mg/mL. Higher concentrations of ifosfamide may not be compatible with mesna and may reduce the stability of ifosfamide.

Drug Administration:
- IV: Inspect solution bag for particulate matter and discoloration; do not use if either found. Administer as IV bolus injection.
- Oral: Tablet: Patients who vomit within 2 hours of taking oral mesna should repeat the dose or receive IV mesna.

Drug Interactions:
- Ifosfamide: Mesna binds to drug metabolites; it is given concurrently for bladder protection.

Lab Effects/Interference:
- Can cause false-positive result on urinalysis for ketones.

Special Considerations:
* At clinical doses, mild nausea, vomiting, and diarrhea are the only side effects expected.

Potential Toxicities/Side Effects and the Nursing Process

I. POTENTIAL FOR INJURY related to MAINTENANCE OF BLADDER MUCOSAL INTEGRITY

Defining Characteristics: Mesna uniquely concentrates in the bladder and has a very low degree of toxicity, making it the uroprotector of choice against ifosfamide-related urotoxicity.

Nursing Implications: Assess daily urinalysis. Assess for hematuria per hospital policy and procedure. Hydrate vigorously.

II. ALTERATION IN NUTRITION, LESS THAN BODY REQUIREMENTS, related to NAUSEA/VOMITING, DIARRHEA

Defining Characteristics: Nausea and vomiting are minor in incidence and severity. Diarrhea is mild if it occurs.

Nursing Implications: Assess baseline nutritional status. Usual antiemetics for ifosfamide or cyclophosphamide-induced nausea/vomiting protect against mesna contribution. Encourage small, frequent meals and liquids. Teach patient to avoid greasy, fried, or fatty foods. Encourage patient to report onset of nausea/vomiting or diarrhea.

Chapter 4
Molecularly Targeted Therapies

The new millennium has brought exciting promise to patients with cancer and to their nurses. As a better understanding of the process of carcinogenesis and metastasis has emerged, with it has come identified molecular and immune flaws that can be therapeutically targeted. Vogelstein et al. (2013) describe the genomic successes in identifying a few common mutations in many cancer types, as well as a larger number of mutations in individual tumor types that are less commonly mutated. Of the approximately 140 mutated genes that drive tumorigenesis, two to eight "driver" mutations are found in each tumor. The driver genes can be categorized into 12 signaling pathways, regulating cell fate, cell survival, and genome maintenance (Vogelstein et al., 2013). Signaling pathways commonly mutated control **cell survival** [TGF-β, MAPK, STAT, PI3K, RAS, cell cycle/apoptosis]; **cell fate** [NOTCH, Hedgehog, APC, chromatin modification, transcriptional regulation]; **genome maintenance** [DNA damage control] (Vogelstein et al., 2013). Driver genes that are epigenetic are not mutated, but they can also be expressed in tumors, often inactivating tumor suppressor genes, and they can be targeted to turn the tumor suppressor genes back on.

Today, research scientists from different institutions and professions are working in teams to identify tumor-specific mutations and flawed signaling pathways to target, as well as targeted agents (Saporito, 2013). One example is the Stand Up To Cancer (SU2C) Dream Team, which is targeting the PI3K pathway that is commonly mutated in women's cancers.

For the past decades, systemic and local therapies have provided cure, disease stabilization, and palliation for many patients with cancer. However, the physical cost of these benefits was often significant and included bone marrow depression with increased risk of infection, bleeding, and nausea and/or vomiting. The "magic bullet" was always sought so that benefit could be achieved with minimal toxicity. Today, many molecularly targeted agents and a few immune targeted agents have been FDA-approved and thousands more are undergoing clinical testing.

This chapter lays the groundwork for a sound understanding of the molecular basis of cancer, the identified and potential molecular and immune flaws and targets, and the agents that target them. As our knowledge of carcinogenesis expands, the question arises why the immune system is unable to mount a sustained attack against the tumor-expressed antigens. In some way, malignant transformation is able to also suppress the immune response. A new subsection of this chapter addresses what has been learned about tumor evasion of the immune system and ways to harness this knowledge in the development of immune checkpoint inhibitors to stop tumor cells from "being invisible" to the immune system. Our understanding of the complexities of both the immune system and how cancer subverts it is just beginning, and new developments occur continually. Decades ago, immunotherapy appeared to offer the secret to cancer cure and control, but disappointments followed. Today, our knowledge of the immune system—when it is healthy, as well as when cancer attacks it—is much more precise. We now have a new class of immunotherapeutic drugs called "immune checkpoint inhibitors."

Dr. Andrew von Eschenbach, MD, former NCI Director, described the future of cancer care in 2003, and it still remains true:

"Today we understand cancer as both a genetic disease and a cell signaling failure. Genes that control orderly replication become damaged, allowing the cells to reproduce without restraint. A single cell's progress from normal, to malignant, to metastatic, appears to involve a series of interactive processes, each controlled by a different gene or set of genes. These altered genes produce defective protein signals, which are, in turn, mishandled by the cell. This understanding of the biology of cancer is enabling us to design interventions to preempt the cancer's progression to uncontrolled growth."

Today, oncology nurses and their patients are moving from "one size fits all" therapies (e.g., for breast cancer) into "individualized cancer treatment," where patient tissue is analyzed for mutations and more precise cell type, which can help categorize the tumor and direct appropriate therapy. Called "precision medicine," therapies depend on precision genomics to identify the cellular flaws that first led to tumor formation and then continue to sustain it (Jones et al., 2015). Targeted molecular and biologic/immunological are the key therapies. The nurse helps patients and their families to (1) understand their potential treatment choices in concert with the oncologist/hematologist, the drug's side effects, and patient's self-care requirements; (2) identify and intervene early when adverse effects occur, by assessing patients frequently and establishing a trust relationship so the patient calls/reports issues early, in consultation with physician or NP/PA. In this regard, the nurse also facilitates communication among the members of the oncology team, as the nurse has a regular presence in the patient's care (Rubin, 2012). The nurse must be articulate in the language of targeted therapies and be effective as a patient/family educator so that the patient takes the medicine correctly, adheres to the plan, and reports toxicity early. The nurse must understand the potential drug toxicities and their differences; for example, EGFRI-induced diarrhea from erlotinib (Tarceva) is very different in management and threat to the patient from that of ipilimumab (Yervoy), which is immune-related and may be life-threatening. The nurse must assess the patient's ability to comply with medication self-administration instructions. For example, certain drugs must be taken on an empty stomach 1–2 hours before or 2 hours after a meal; if these directions are not followed, the bioavailability of the drug is increased many times with severe adverse events (e.g., nilotinib (Tasigna) and erlotinib (Tarceva)).

In order to better understand targeted molecular and biological therapy, the nurse must understand the molecular basis of cancer. For this, it is important to recall early courses in biology and genetics. The following will be reviewed: basic cell biology; genetic mutations; communication within the cell (signal transduction); malignant transformation; mutations in proto-oncogene, suppressor, and DNA repair genes; cell cycle regulation; loss of apoptosis; acquisition of telomerase activity; invasion; angiogenesis; and metastasis. In addition, epigenetics is discussed.

BASIC CELL BIOLOGY

Cancer is a disease of the cell. The nucleus of the cell is where the genetic material, or deoxyribonucleic acid (DNA), is located. DNA is the building block of life, an incredibly simple yet complex double helix in which each strand is made up of millions of chemical bases, and each chemical base attaches to its complementary partner to pair in a specific way (cytosine with guanine, thymine with adenosine). See Figure 4.1.

Genes are a subunit of DNA, and each gene contains a code or recipe for a specific product, such as a protein or enzyme. Scientists have now identified all the 21,000 or so genes in the human genome. These genes can each make multiple proteins. In addition, thousands of noncoding RNA molecules have been discovered that regulate the protein coding genes (NHGRI, 2012). Genes carry the blueprint of who we are. All cells have the genetic blueprint, but only the genes we need are "turned on" or expressed, such as the color for blue eyes. The genes we don't need at the moment are "turned off." In early fetal growth, many genes are turned on, and then when the embryo develops into a baby, these genes are no longer necessary and the genes are turned off. Unfortunately, it appears that cancer is able to turn back on a number of genes that should remain off, such as those that permit unlimited cell division, and for cells to change from epithelial cells to mesenchymal cells to migrate and invade neighboring tissues. Genes code for specific proteins and are contained in a chromosome. Humans have 46 chromosomes: 22 autosomal pairs and 1 pair of sex chromosomes. As research gives us greater understanding of the small RNAs, which play such a large role in regulating gene expression and function, the knowledge about their role in cancer, as well as how to manipulate them to halt tumor cell proliferation and metastases, will enable clinicians to individualize therapy for each patient based on the tumor's genetic fingerprint (Leberman, 2013).

CELL SIGNALING AND SIGNAL TRANSDUCTION
Protein Kinases
When the body needs to make a specific protein or enzyme, or to make more cells, this requirement message is sent to the cell as a growth factor or ligand. The ligand attaches to a receptor, such as receptor tyrosine kinase (RTK), on the outside of the cell membrane. Once attached, the receptor asks a neighbor receptor to pair up with it (dimerize), or the receptor can activate itself (autostimulation) to activate the receptor. The RTK is made up of 3 components: the extracellular receptor on the outside of the cell, the transmembrane portion that connects the outside with the inside portions of the receptor, and the cytoplasmic portion that is just inside the cell membrane. Dimerization activates the phosphorylation function, which sends the message like a bucket brigade, through the cell membrane and into the cytoplasm to the cell nucleus. Another way to think of this is like being in a dark room. You flip on the light switch, and the light comes on. What has happened is that the light switch is attached to a wire; when it is turned on, it sends energy in the form of electricity to the overhead light, and it is turned on. Similarly, when the ligand attaches to the receptor, after dimerization, the message goes from the receptor outside the cell, through the membrane, to inside the membrane. There, the message is attached to a tyrosine kinase, which communicates to other tyrosine kinases to carry the message

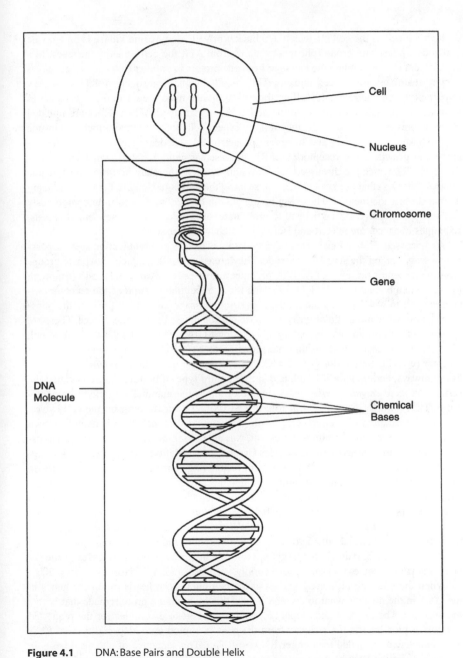

Figure 4.1   DNA: Base Pairs and Double Helix

Source: Artwork originally created for the National Cancer Institute. Adapted with permission of the artist, Jeanne Kelly. © 2013.

through the cell to the cell nucleus like a bucket brigade. A tyrosine kinase is an enzyme that adds a phosphate group (phosphorylation) from ATP, the cell's energy currency, to a protein next in line, sending the message from one protein to another so the message moves "downstream" toward the cell nucleus. This is called signal transduction. RTKs are very important in sending messages telling the cell to divide, make new blood vessels such as in wound healing, and to die when the cell is old or damaged. When RTKs are mutated or overexpressed on tumor cells, they tell the cancer cells to proliferate, move and invade nearby tissue, metastasize, and to ignore programmed cell death signals. Examples are epidermal growth factor receptor (EGFR) and vascular endothelial growth factor receptor (VEGFR), which are discussed below. Within the cell, there are non-receptor tyrosine kinases (NRTKs) that are key elements in sending the message along to the nucleus, using the bucket brigade method. These can be mutated in cancer, so they turn on continuously and send the message telling the cell to proliferate, or invade, or make new blood vessels. Examples in cancer are mTOR and Bcr-Abl, which are discussed below.

As discussed, protein kinases are key regulators of a cell's communication system, passing messages along the signaling cascade. They are enzymes that attach phosphate groups to serine/threonine proteins, or tyrosine proteins, and effectively carry the message through the cell like a bucket brigade. RTKs include the extracellular portion of the receptor outside the cell to which the ligand binds to start the message and which leads to the phosphorylation of the intracellular tyrosine kinase portion inside the cell membrane. There are 19 families of receptor tyrosine kinases, including EGFR, VEGF, platelet-derived growth factor (PDGF), insulin and insulin-like growth factor (IGF1) receptors, and stem factor receptor (c-KIT). Ten families of NRTKs in the cytoplasm regulate communication along key pathways, and include Jak, abl, and src. The third type of protein kinase is called the *serine/threonine protein kinase.* One example of this is the mammalian target of rapamycin (mTOR), which plays a central role in cell proliferation (turning on the cell cycle), cell metabolism, and regulating cell growth and angiogenesis. mTOR was named as such because Rapamycin, an immunosuppressant, was able to inhibit this kinase in organ transplant patients. mTOR acts like New York's Grand Central Station, integrating multiple signals from essential pathways, such as growth factors (e.g., insulin and insulin-like growth factor), nutrients (e.g., glucose, amino acids), hormones, and stress (e.g., starvation, hypoxia, DNA damage) (Watanabe et al., 2011). It regulates protein turnover, cell growth and differentiation, cell survival, energy balance, and the cell's response to stress. It is often dysregulated in cancer, and it is a key target (Watanabe et al., 2011). Targeted therapies that block the receptor on the outside of the cell are generally monoclonal antibodies and are large molecules, while drugs that target the tyrosine or serine/threonine kinases inside the cell are small molecules that can be given orally, such as tyroskine kinase inhibitors (TKIs).

When the message ultimately arrives at the cell nucleus, it needs to tell the genes in the DNA in the nucleus what to do, and it does this by having a protein made that brings the message. The DNA strands separate, exposing the gene that codes for the requested enzyme or protein, and information from the gene is copied onto a special type of RNA or ribonucleic acid, called messenger RNA (mRNA). The sequence of chemical bases in the gene is copied base by base onto a new strand of mRNA so that the complementary recipe is shown on the mRNA. This piece of mRNA then travels out of the nucleus into the cytoplasm of the cell to the ribosomes, which are the cell's "protein factories." Here, the complementary copy of the protein recipe is recopied onto a ribosome by transfer RNA (tRNA) so that it is exactly like the DNA copy. Now the ribosome is told to make the specific protein. Amino acids are then assembled into a completed protein molecule. See Figure 4.2.

Mutations
The body is very careful that cell birth always equals cell death so that no cell can divide unless the body needs it. When a cell needs to divide to make another cell (proliferation) to replace a damaged or dead cell, such as a cell lining the gastrointestinal tract, the cell's nucleus receives a message from a growth factor to divide. We know that the GI tract sloughs over 80,000,000 cells a minute during digestion, so it is easy to see why the body needs to replace used-up, dead, or damaged cells. Recall the process of cell division in terms of the cell cycle, as discussed in *Chapter 1*. When each cell prepares to divide, the DNA is copied during the synthesis (S) phase to make a duplicate set of DNA so that each of the daughter cells will have identical DNA. Millions of coded genes are copied during cell division. Occasionally a mistake is made, such as when one chemical base is not correctly copied. Often this is quickly fixed, but sometimes a mutation can result in the production of an abnormal protein, enzyme, or product. Figure 4.3 shows how a mutation can lead to the production of an abnormal protein. Different types of mutations are shown in Figure 4.4. If the mutation occurs near or on a proto-oncogene or a tumor suppressor gene, then it can potentially (1) turn on cell division when the body does not need more cells (i.e.,

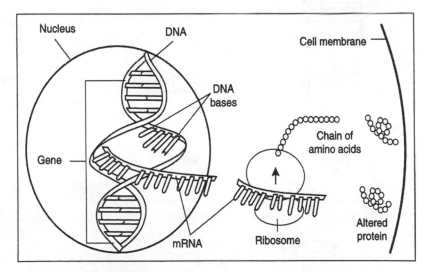

Figure 4.2　　Protein Synthesis
Source: Artwork originally created for the National Cancer Institute. Adapted with permission of the artist, Jeanne Kelly. © 2013.

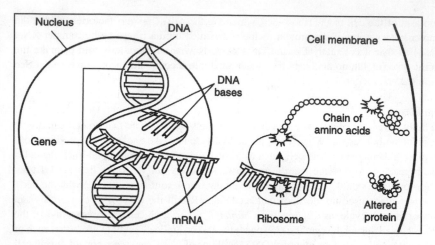

Figure 4.3   Mutation Leading to Abnormal Protein Production
Source: Artwork originally created for the National Cancer Institute. Adapted with permission of the artist, Jeanne Kelly. © 2013.

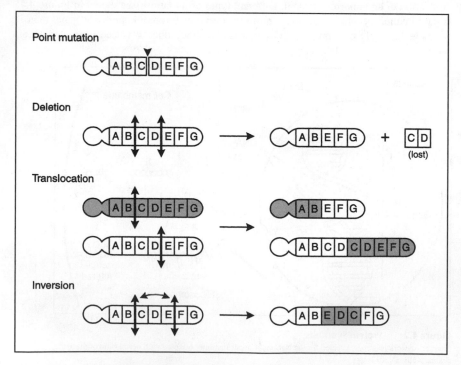

Figure 4.4   Types of Chromosomal Mutations

proto-oncogene becomes a cancer-causing oncogene), or (2) silence a tumor suppressor gene so that it does not stop uncontrolled cell division. In other words, in cancer, the onco-gene is like the accelerator of a car that is stuck, driving cell division when cells are not needed, whereas the tumor suppressor gene, when silenced, is like the brakes of a car that are failing and unable to stop the car.

One example of a serious mutation is the reciprocal translocation between chromo-some 9 and 22, forming an extra-long chromosome 9. The other chromosome is short, called the Philadelphia chromosome (Ph¹), which contains the fused ABL-BCR gene, and is shown in Figure 4.5. This genetic abnormality occurs in 90% of patients with chronic myelogenous leukemia (CML) and results in the formation of an abnormal tyrosine kinase, which can turn on continually and tell the cell nucleus to make more (leukemic) cells. Imatinib mesylate (Gleevec), a tyrosine kinase inhibitor that selectively targets this flaw, has been FDA-approved due to its extraordinary ability to block the action of this mutation.

It appears that almost all malignancies are caused by mutations in DNA; however, knowledge of epigenetic changes is evolving and helps explain why this may not always be true. Mutations continue to be very important, and it usually takes at least four mutations to cause malignant transformation. This is shown in Figure 4.6.

Approximately 10% of these mutations are inherited or carried in the DNA of reproduc-tive cells in individuals whose parents carry the gene, while 90% of mutations are acquired and considered sporadic. Usually, an inherited mutation does not result in cancer; rather, it increases the risk that the person will develop cancer in the course of his or her lifetime. Sporadic mutations develop during the course of one's life, due to exposure to carcinogens,

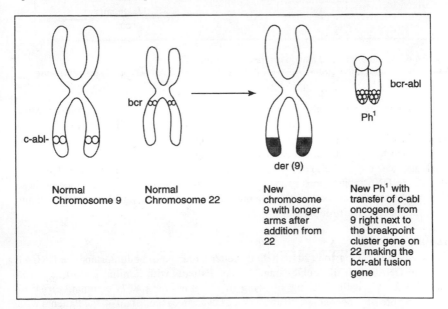

c-abl-	bcr	der (9)	bcr-abl Ph¹
Normal Chromosome 9	Normal Chromosome 22	New chromosome 9 with longer arms after addition from 22	New Ph¹ with transfer of c-abl oncogene from 9 right next to the breakpoint cluster gene on 22 making the bcr-abl fusion gene

Figure 4.5   Philadelphia Chromosome

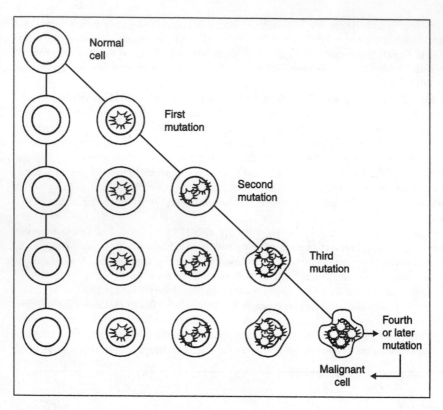

Figure 4.6   Mutations and Malignant Transformation
Source: Artwork originally created for the National Cancer Institute. Adapted with permission of the artist, Jeanne Kelly. © 2013.

and are related to relationships among and between genes and the environment. Most cancers are not inherited, although two examples of inherited vulnerability to cancer are (1) women who have mutations in the BRCA1 and/or BRCA2 gene (who represent 5% or so of women who develop breast cancer), and (2) individuals with hereditary polyposis in which one gene copy (allele) of the APC tumor suppressor gene is silenced. BRCA1 and BRCA2 are DNA repair genes and are considered tumor suppressor genes. One of these genes can be mutated not only in a few women with breast cancer, but also in some patients with ovarian, pancreatic, or prostate cancer.

DNA Repair
O'Donovan and Livingston (2010) help us better understand the importance of BRCA1 and -2 in DNA repair of double-strand breaks. Patients with familial germ-line mutations in BRCA1, with resulting silencing of the gene, have 80% cumulative risk of developing breast cancer at age 70 and a risk of ovarian cancer of 30–40%. Patients with

a germ-line mutation in BRCA2 have a cumulative risk of 50% of developing breast cancer at age 70 and between 10–15% risk of developing ovarian cancer. BRCA1 and -2 help to maintain the integrity of the genome not only by repairing DNA but also by helping to control the cell cycle at the checkpoints and regulating key mitotic or cell division steps.

The human genome is under constant stress caused from internal (e.g., reactive oxygen species, cytosine deamination resulting from metabolism) and external (e.g., UV, ionizing radiation, including cancer RT; and chemicals, including chemotherapy) stressors that damage the cell's DNA. This damage can be either single- or double-strand DNA breaks. The double-strand breaks are more toxic to the cell because there is no "normal" or correct DNA strand to serve as a repair template. If the cell cannot repair the DNA strand breaks, then the cell undergoes apoptosis. If the cell is not repaired correctly, it can lead to serious mutations or rearrangement of the chromosomes (e.g., translocations and deletions) each time the cell divides.

With continued cell divisions with the misrepaired DNA, cancer may evolve. In addition, many genes on the damaged DNA are tumor suppressor genes, so these may now be ineffective or silent. Given that within the human body, cells undergo millions of mitotic cell divisions each day to replace dead or damaged cells, it is easy to see that multiple cell divisions with damaged DNA can lead to genomic instability and cancer.

Thus, the cells have evolved a very sophisticated way to repair the DNA errors, especially the double-strand breaks, so that the human genome remains intact. The two major pathways to repair DNA double-strand breaks are called (1) nonhomologous end-joining (NHEJ, the primary mechanism where the ends of a double-strand break are directly religated) and (2) homologous recombination (HR, an error-free mechanism). BRCA1 and -2 repair DNA double-strand breaks by using the HR mechanism. Other repair pathways are those for single-strand DNA repair: base excision repair, nucleotide excision repair, or mismatch repair (Ford et al., 2010). If single-strand breaks or nicks are not repaired and are allowed to go through cell division, the breaks become double-strand DNA breaks. The most commonly used mechanism for DNA repair is base excision repair (BER), which refers to cutting out the damaged base or bases and replacing them (cut and patch) by using the complementary DNA as a template to synthesize the correct base or base sequence in the damaged strand (Ford et al., 2010). Remember that DNA is made up of two strands of nucleotides with a backbone of sugar and phosphate groups. The two strands are tied together by paired bases (adenine, guanine, cytosine, thymine) that attach to a sugar. A base forms a bond with another base to make a base pair: adenine always with thymine and cytosine always with guanine. The sequence of the paired bases attached to the sugar spell out the recipe or code for the protein to be made (instructions to the cell for a specific function, such as for the cell to divide). This recipe is read by messenger RNA and taken out to the cytoplasm to make the protein on the ribosome.

When DNA is damaged, a nuclear enzyme called poly (ADP-ribose) polymerase or PARP is activated in the nucleus of the cell. PARP1 is the most abundant member of this large family; this enzyme helps the chromatin relax, and it calls in the BER proteins to the DNA break so that it can fix it. If the double-strand break genes are damaged or nonfunctional, then the BER proteins will be their backup to repair the DNA.

Thus, if a patient has a BRCA1 or -2 mutation, PARP enzymes are critical to the survival of a cell with damaged DNA. Normally, if the damaged DNA cannot be repaired, the cell is told to die or to undergo apoptosis (programmed cell death). An important example is a cancer cell trying to recover from radiation or chemotherapy. Investigators believe that by giving chemotherapy and also blocking PARP1, they can kill the cancer cell by forcing it to undergo apoptosis. This is called *synthetic lethality,* when the cell can get along with a mutation in either of the repair pathways, but not in both pathways, which causes the cell to die (Fong et al., 2009) (Figure 4.7). Thus, PARP1 inhibition represents a new direction in cancer drug development (Iglehart & Silver, 2009). Interestingly, PARP enzymes are "upregulated" or increased due to overexpression of the PARP1 gene in many cancers, and it is believed that this confers acquired resistance to some chemotherapy agents when the patient originally responded to the drug(s) and then, after a few treatments, no longer responds (O'Connor and Breen, 2008).

PARP inhibitors confer chemosensitization and radiosensitization. Additionally, cancer cells that do not have a functional PTEN tumor suppressor gene or gene product (protein) appear sensitive to PARP inhibition because there is downregulation of a critical component of HR function (Rad51). When PTEN does not work (loss-of-function mutations), the cancer cell message to divide is amplified via P13K signaling, which promotes tumorigenesis (Hanahan and Weinberg, 2011). A number of aggressive cancers, including some prostate cancers, have PTEN defects, so this will be an important niche for treatment (Ana et al., 2009). Normal cells do not divide as frequently as cancer cells, and as they still have functional HR, they are relatively spared and therefore survive while the cancer cells are forced into programmed cell death. Hence, this is a selective way to kill cancer cells. In addition, women with triple negative breast cancer often carry BRCA1 mutations, making it a difficult-to-treat cancer that is aggressive in behavior. Olaparib (Lynparza) has been FDA approved for use in women with *BRCA*-mutated advanced ovarian cancer, and many other PARP inhibitors are undergoing clinical trials.

Another example is inherited familial adenomatous polyposis (FAP). The adenomatous polyposis coloni (APC) gene is located in the intraepithelial cells of the intestines and functions as a tumor suppressor gene. A person with FAP inherits one copy of the gene (called an allele) that is mutated and one allele that is normal. When the second allele becomes mutated, the gene no longer functions as a tumor suppressor gene and is "silent," so that it does not stop uncontrolled cell division. Thousands of polyps are formed, and many can progress to malignancy. Fortunately, cyclo-oxygenase 2 (COX-2) inhibitors appear to prevent many of the polyps from forming. This also suggests that COX-2 is an important mediator not only of inflammation, but also of malignant transformation. Scientists are studying the process of inflammation to see why it is such an essential part of malignant transformation. COX-2 is overexpressed in many premalignant and malignant tumors: colorectal adenomas and cancer, pancreatic cancer, oral leucoplakia and head and neck cancer, prostate intraepithelial neoplasia and prostate cancer, ductal carcinoma in situ, and breast cancer. Specifically, it appears that COX-2 plays a role in angiogenesis, apoptosis, inflammation, immunosuppression, and invasiveness (Dannenberg et al., 2001). However, because the COX-2 inhibitors carry a cardiovascular risk, COX-2 inhibitors are now being studied in lower doses and combined with dietary changes to prevent FAP progression.

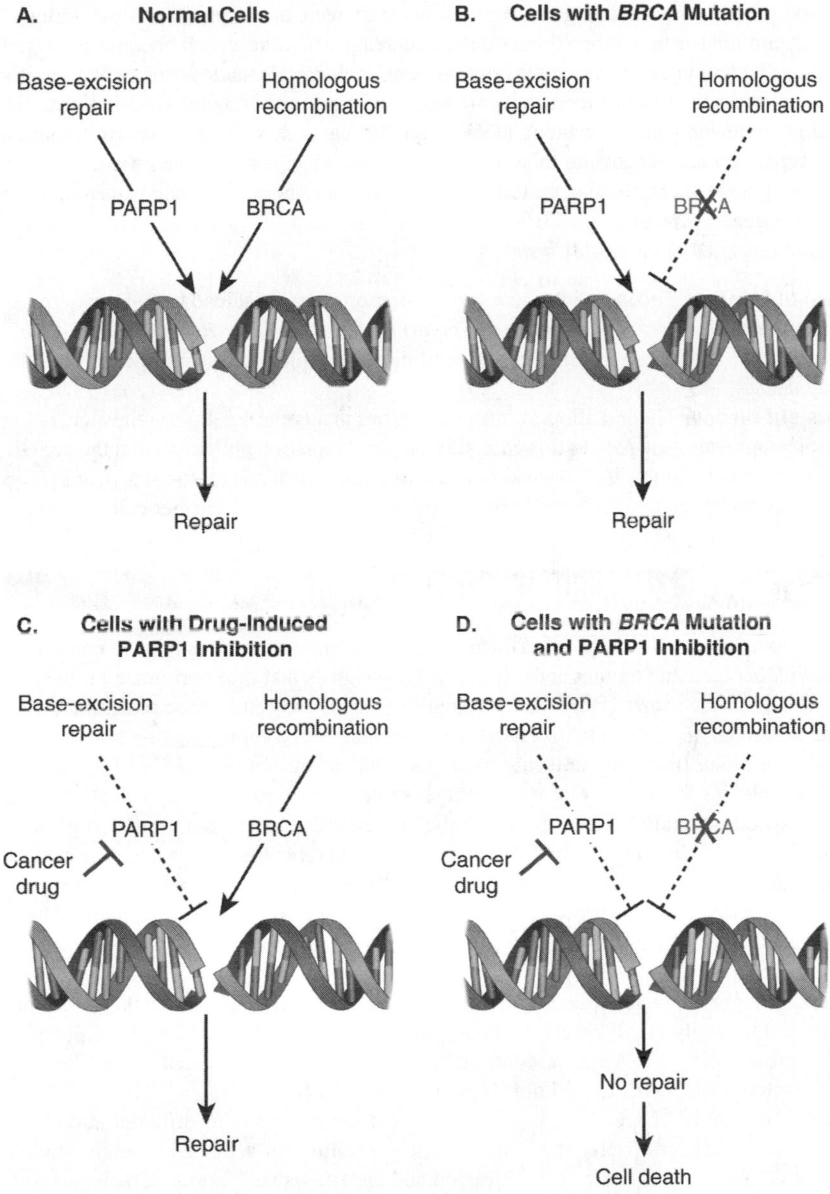

A.   Normal Cells

Base-excision   Homologous
repair   recombination

PARP1   BRCA

Repair

B.   Cells with *BRCA* Mutation

Base-excision   Homologous
repair   recombination

PARP1   BRCA

Repair

**C.   Cells with Drug-Induced
      PARP1 Inhibition**

Base-excision   Homologous
repair   recombination

PARP1   BRCA

Cancer
drug

Repair

**D.   Cells with *BRCA* Mutation
      and PARP1 Inhibition**

Base-excision   Homologous
repair   recombination

PARP1   BRCA

Cancer
drug

No repair

Cell death

Figure 4.7   PARP Inhibitors and Synthetic Lethality
Reproduced from "Targeting the Microenvironment: Bone Metastasis, Apoptosis, DNA Repair, and Mitosis,"
in Wilkes GM, *Targeted Cancer Therapy: A Handbook for Nurses*. Sudbury, MA: Jones & Bartlett Publishers,
2011, p. 279.

Thus, people who have a genetic mutation start with one mutation. Most cancers, however, are related to acquired mutations, occurring when the genes become damaged during one's lifetime by factors in the environment or chemicals made in the cells. Genetic errors may be added during cell division when enzymes are copying DNA so that the mutation is copied into permanent DNA. Usually the body's DNA repair mechanism (DNA repair genes) catches the mistake, and if unable to repair it, causes the cell to die (apoptosis). Sometimes, the system fails; the error becomes permanent and is passed on to successive generations of cells.

Mutations in DNA can result from:

- **Gain of function:** The mutation activates one or more genes that lead to malignant transformation, such as with the *Ras, Myc, Epidermal Growth Factor Receptor* family. This results in the speeding up of cell growth and division, which makes more cells than the body needs.
- **Loss of function:** The mutation(s) inactivate genes that control cell growth, such as the tumor suppressor gene p53. In this case, there are no "mutation police" so that the genetic mutation is not caught, the DNA is not repaired, the cell is not destroyed if unable to repair the mutation, and the genetic flaw is perpetuated with each further cell division.

TARGETS IN CELL COMMUNICATION (SIGNAL TRANSDUCTION)

We have seen how a cell is told to perform a function. Signal transduction is the communication link between and among cells. It depends on signals that often originate on the cell surface, such as the growth factors or hormones that attach to cell surface receptors called *ligands*. Once the receptor dimerizes and activates phosphorylation, tyrosine kinases pass the message along from one molecule to another, like a "bucket brigade" or "signal cascade" (Weinberg, 1996). This way, the message is relayed "downstream" to the cell nucleus or down specific signaling pathways to get the desired effect, such as normal cell growth, cell division, differentiation (specialization), or cell death (apoptosis). It is a precise system and has many redundant parallel pathways. As the understanding of the complexity of cell signal transduction has grown, the many potential targets for anticancer therapy have skyrocketed. Figure 4.8 and Figure 4.9 show schemas of cell signals resulting in important cell functions.

Important growth factors that initiate the message for a cell to divide are the epidermal growth factor family (EGF or erB-1, erB-2 or HER-2-neu, erB-3, and erB-4), platelet-derived growth factor (PDGF), vascular endothelial growth factor (VEGF), transforming growth factor alpha (TGF-α), and fibroblast growth factor (FGF).

The EGF family of receptors is very important for cell growth, differentiation, and survival. Many cancers overexpress this receptor, resulting in a more aggressive tumor behavior with increased tendency for invasion and metastases and shorter patient survival. The HER-2-neu receptor (EGFR2) has become well known because it is amplified or over-expressed in about 20% of patients with breast cancer, again conferring a poor prognosis. A number of monoclonal antibodies have been developed to block the external domain of the EGFR-1 receptor (cetuximab or Erbitux, panitumumab or Vectibix), the HER-2

Receptors can be

1. Receptor kinases that extend through the plasma membrane with intrinsic enzyme activity. Enzymes can activate the message by passing it to the next protein using a phosphate group, or autophosphorylate (attach directly to the phosphate group). Examples are receptor tyrosine kinases (RTK), which attach to a tyrosine residue, or serine-threonine kinase, which attach to a serine or threonine residue. (ATP → ADP gives energy transfer.)

2. Receptors that couple inside the cell to GTP binding or hydrolyzing proteins (G-proteins). G-protein lies in the cell near the receptor. When the receptor is activated by the ligand, the G-protein adds a phosphate, going from GDP (resting) to GTP (active), turns "on," and sends the message downstream as the G-protein hydrolyzes itself from GTP to GDP. Having lost a phosphate, it shuts itself off.

3. Receptors inside the cell that are activated when the ligand binds to the cell. Receptor ligand complex goes to the nucleus to alter gene transcription.

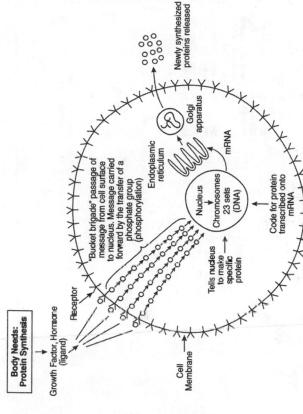

Body Needs: Protein Synthesis

Growth Factor, Hormone (ligand)

Receptor

Cell Membrane

"Bucket brigade" passage of message from cell surface to nucleus. Message carried forward by the transfer of a phosphate group (phosphorylation)

Endoplasmic reticulum

Golgi apparatus

mRNA

Nucleus Chromosomes 23 sets (DNA)

Tells nucleus to make specific protein

Code for protein transcribed onto mRNA

Newly synthesized proteins released

Figure 4.8   Signal Transduction

(Figure modified and redrawn from "Cell Communication: The Inside Story," Scott JD and Pawson T. *Scientific American*, June 2000.)

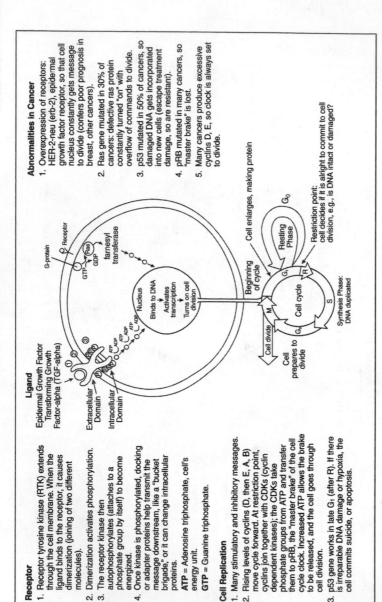

Receptor
1. Receptor tyrosine kinase (RTK) extends through the cell membrane. When the ligand binds to the receptor, it causes dimerization (joining of two different molecules).
2. Dimerization activates phosphorylation.
3. The receptor kinase then autophosphorylates (attaches to a phosphate group by itself) to become energized.
4. Once kinase is phosphorylated, docking or adapter proteins help transmit the message downstream, like a "bucket brigade," or it can change intracellular proteins.

ATP = Adenosine triphosphate, cell's energy unit.
GTP = Guanine triphosphate.

Cell Replication
1. Many stimulatory and inhibitory messages.
2. Rising levels of cyclins (D, then E, A, B) move cycle forward. At restriction point, cyclins join together with CDKs (cyclin dependent kinases); the CDKs take phosphate groups from ATP and transfer them to pRB, the "master brake" of the cell cycle. Increased ATP allows the brake to be released, and the cell goes through cell division.
3. p53 gene works in late G_1 (after R). If there is irreparable DNA damage or hypoxia, the cell commits suicide, or apoptosis.

Abnormalities in Cancer
1. Overexpression of receptors: HER-2-neu (erb-2), epidermal growth factor receptor, so that cell nucleus constantly gets message to divide (confers poor prognosis in breast, other cancers).
2. Ras gene mutated in 30% of cancers; defective ras protein constantly turned "on" with overflow of commands to divide.
3. p53 mutated in 50% of cancers, so damaged DNA gets incorporated into new cells (escape treatment damage, so are resistant).
4. pRB mutated in many cancers, so "master brake" is lost.
5. Many cancers produce excessive cyclins D, E, so clock is always set to divide.

Figure 4.9 Epidermal Growth Factor Receptor and Its Role in Signal Transduction and Tumor Progression

(Modified from Huang SM, Harari PM. Epidermal growth factor receptor inhibition in cancer therapy: Biology, rationale, and preliminary clinical results. *Invest New Drugs.* 2000 17: 259–269.)

receptor (trastuzumab or Herceptin), and the internal domain of EGFR-1 by tyrosine kinase inhibitors such as erlotinib (Tarceva). Today, many tyrosine kinase inhibitors are multitargeted, inhibiting more than one receptor or pathway, such as lapatinib (Tykerb), which blocks both EGFR-1 and -2 receptor kinases. It may be beneficial to combine a monoclonal antibody from outside of the cell, such as trastuzumab, with a small molecule that blocks the tyrosine kinase portion inside the cell, such as lapatinib (Tykerb), which can cross the blood–brain barrier, and trials in HER-2-neu–positive women with breast cancer have been conducted, such as the adjuvant ALLTO trial (Adjuvant lapatinib and/or trastuzumab Treatment Optimisation), which compared the adjuvant use of trastuzumab alone, trastuzumab followed by lapatinib, or both drugs given simultaneously after breast cancer surgery. The lapatinib-alone arm was discontinued. Results presented at the American Society of Clinical Oncology June 2014 meeting showed that in the **adjuvant** setting, there was no difference between the trastuzumab-only group compared to the lapatinib-plus-trastuzumab group (Piccart-Gebhart et al., 2014). This is in contrast to the earlier "sister" NeoALLTO trial, which compared patients in the **neoadjuvant** setting, who received both drugs, plus paclitaxel chemotherapy, to the control arm patients who received one of the drugs plus paclitaxel chemotherapy in the neoadjuvant setting. Data presented at the 2013 San Antonio Breast Cancer Symposium showed that patients receiving the dual blockade combination had a statistically higher rate of achieving a pathological complete response (CR) (51%) compared to those receiving lapatinib plus paclitaxel (25%) or trastuzumab plus paclitaxel (30%). At 4 years, a pathologic CR correlated significantly with survival (Piccart-Gebhart et al., 2013).

As more targets in signaling pathways are discovered, drugs are being developed to target them. Because in most instances multiple pathways are involved, we may eventually see "cocktails" of multiple drugs as clinical trials define their usefulness. This chapter presents drugs currently FDA-approved.

MALIGNANT TRANSFORMATION

How exactly does malignant transformation occur? Hanahan and Weinberg (2011) identified 10 hallmarks of cancer and targeted therapeutic approaches. These include the 6 original hallmarks (2001): (1) self-sufficiency in growth signals, (2) insensitivity to anti-growth signals, (3) evasion of apoptosis, (4) sustained angiogenesis, (5) tissue invasion and metastasis, and (6) limitless replication potential. Two additional hallmarks added in 2011 are (7) avoiding immune destruction, and (8) deregulating cellular energetics [reprogramming of energy metabolism (e.g., inefficient energy production using glycolysis)]. The final two are labeled as "Enabling Characteristics" and are (9) tumor-promoting inflammation, and (10) genome instability and mutations (e.g., mutated repair mechanisms).

In addition, the tumor microenvironment or stroma has gained increasing importance. Cancer cells recruit normal-appearing cells in the tumor microenvironment that contribute to malignant transformation. Signals from cells in the microenvironment may start the malignant process, and they are key figures in supporting invasion and metastases (Hanahan and Weinberg, 2011). Necrotic cell death releases pro-inflammatory signals into the microenvironment. Stromal cells in the microenvironment are involved in angiogenesis.

It is also possible that the leading edge of the tumor that is invading neighboring tissue receives signals from the microenvironment for those cells to undergo epidermal mesenchymal transition (EMT) transformation (Weinberg, 2013). Epidermal cells cannot invade and metastasize, while mesenchymal cells can migrate to different sites. Finally, the microenvironment plays an important role in helping newly landed metastatic cells make a niche and succeed to start further metastases (Hanahan and Weinberg, 2011).

SELF-SUFFICIENCY IN GROWTH SIGNALS, INSENSITIVITY TO ANTIGROWTH SIGNALS, LIMITLESS REPLICATION POTENTIAL, AND GENOME INSTABILITY AND MUTATIONS

Normally, cell division occurs only when the tissue needs to replace lost or dead cells and the body has many mechanisms to make sure that cell birth equals cell death. Proto-oncogenes are normal cells that encourage cell growth. They are kept in check by tumor suppressor genes that not only tell the cell nucleus not to divide if cells are not needed, but they also prevent injured or mutated cells from going through cell division and then passing on genetic errors to their progeny. Mutations occur in both proto-oncogenes and suppressor genes to get malignant transformation, as well as DNA repair genes that normally repair the mutations in DNA, or direct the damaged cell to undergo apoptosis or programmed cell death. For example, a mutation in a proto-oncogene can start the process. This is because proto-oncogenes often produce the protein molecules in the bucket brigade. As a result, when the proto-oncogene is mutated to form an oncogene, the oncogene keeps sending the message to the nucleus for the cell to divide over and over again, leading to uncontrolled cell division. Other oncogenes can also lead to the overproduction of growth factors. PDGF or TGF-α can repeatedly tell the cell to divide, while HER-2-neu overexpression (more than the normal number of copies of a single gene) causes proliferation of cell surface receptors that flood the cell with signals to divide, again leading to uncontrolled cell division.

Proto-oncogenes code for other molecules in the signal cascade, such as the *ras* family of proto-oncogenes that include the H-ras gene, the K-ras-gene, and the N-ras gene (Weinberg, 1996). Normally, the *ras* gene, a proto-oncogene, codes for proteins that bring the message from the cell surface growth factor receptors to other protein messengers further down the signal cascade as part of the bucket brigade, activating downstream effectors such as the Raf-1/mitogen-activating protein kinase (MAPK) pathway. Normally, once the message is sent to the nucleus, the ras protein is turned "off" and remains off until recruited again to the cell membrane to bring another message from the extracellular growth factor outside to inside the cell, and down to the cell nucleus. If the ras proto-oncogene is mutated and then activated, it becomes locked in an "on" position, and keeps sending the message to divide, even when there is no growth factor binding to the surface receptor and no message was actually generated. In order to become activated and to attach to the inner surface of the cell membrane, ras has a molecule added called farnesyl isoprenoid; it depends upon an enzyme called farnesyltransferase (FTase) to catalyze this addition. If the enzyme is inhibited, then the ras protein is blocked, and in many tumor studies, causes cells to undergo programmed cell death (apoptosis). If farnesylation is not blocked and the ras protein goes to the cell membrane, then Raf-1 kinase is activated and phosphorylates two MAPK kinases (MEK$_1$ and MEK$_2$ that are also known as extracellular signal-regulated kinases 1 and 2).

Once phosphorylated (activated), the MAPKs move to the nucleus, where they start a chain reaction leading to cell proliferation (Rowinsky et al., 1999). Trametinib (Mekinist) is a reversible inhibitor of MEK_1 and MEK_2 activation and kinase activity; it is indicated for the treatment of metastastic melanoma with BRAF V600E or V600K mutations. The MEK proteins are upstream of the extracellular signal-related kinase (ERK pathway), which stimulates cell proliferation. In BRAF V600E mutation-positive melanoma, the mutation causes the BRAF pathway, which includes $MEK_{1 \text{ and } 2}$, to continually tell the cell nucleus to make melanoma cells. Turning $MEK_{1 \text{ and } 2}$ off with trametinib halts melanoma growth that is dependent upon this mutation. In addition, trametinib is indicated in combination with dabrafenib (Tafinlar), which further decreases cell proliferation. Dabrafenib targets the BRAF V600E and other kinases, so each of the drugs targets different tyrosine kinases (GlaxoSmithKline, Mekinist package insert, 2014). Another drug, sorafenib (Nexavar), is a multitargeted protein kinase inhibitor that inhibits Raf-kinase, as well as two kinases involved in angiogenesis (VEGFR-2, PDGF-β). Sorafenib is FDA-approved for the treatment of the following cancers: metastatic renal cell, unresectable hepatocellular, and differentiated thyroid. It is estimated that 33% of all cancers have a mutated *ras* proto-oncogene (forming the *ras* oncogene), especially cancers of the colon, pancreas, and lungs (Weinberg, 1996). These oncogenes, or their products, are therapeutic targets being studied in clinical trials to block their function so that, for example, the abnormal *ras* proteins are not produced.

Another key pathway that appears to play an important role in cancer is the STAT (signal transducers and activators of transcription) pathway. Any message that reaches the cell nucleus telling the cell to divide must be transcribed (e.g., the part of the DNA where the gene is located opens up, and the gene is copied onto mRNA). STAT proteins are necessary for activating transcription, and thus are important targets. This pathway is made up of proteins in the cytoplasm of the cell that join together (dimerize) when activated by tyrosine phosphorylation (Haura et al., 2005). This causes the activated STAT proteins to move into the cell nucleus, then into the DNA where they bind to gene promoters and regulate the expression of certain genes involved in malignancy. Some STAT proteins are activated by themselves (constitutively) without normal growth regulation. The STAT proteins are active during malignant transformation, and regulate pathways such as cell cycle progression, programmed cell death (apoptosis), angiogenesis, invasion, metastases, and evasion of the immune system by tumor (Haura et al., 2005). Many tumors have dysregulation of Stat 3, Stat 4, and loss of Stat 1 function. Agents are being studied to target the flaws in the STAT signaling pathway. STAT 3 is an example. It is a cytokine transcription factor normally present in all tissues, but not always turned on. However, in many cancer cells it is persistently turned on, driving cell growth and survival. If it is inhibited, the cancer cell will undergo programmed cell death or apoptosis (Lavecchia et al., 2011). It is now recognized that the STAT pathway is part of the interleukin 6 (IL-6) and Janus kinase (JAK) pathway. The IL-6/JAK/STAT pathway straddles the boundaries between the immune system and malignancy (Munoz et al., 2014). Somatic STAT mutations are found in lymphocytic leukemia, aplastic anemia, and myelodysplastic syndrome (MDS), and they may have a role in some lymphomas (Munoz et al., 2014). STAT 3 inhibitors are being studied for these tumor types.

Via an analogous bucket brigade of inhibitory signals from the cell surface to the nucleus, the normal cell nucleus also receives messages from tumor suppressor genes, telling the cell not to divide unless the body tissues need more cells. This normally prevents the oncogene from causing uncontrolled cell growth, and can be thought of as "putting brakes on" the cell division process. However, tumor suppressor genes also become mutated, effectively silencing them, and this must occur in order for the malignant transformation to happen. The most famous of these tumor suppressor genes is p53, which appears to be mutated in over 50% of human cancers (Soussi and Wiman, 2007).

Once there are mutations in both the proto-oncogene and tumor suppressor genes, then there is no longer balance between cell birth and cell death. Instead, there is uncontrolled cell growth. How does this happen? Again, recall the **cell cycle** as shown in Figure 4.9 and Figure 4.10. Normally, the nucleus activates the cell cycle by putting the cell into cell division mode only when the stimulatory signals are greater than the inhibitory signals. When this happens, levels of cyclins rise (cyclin D, followed by E, A, and B) as the cell moves through the phases of the cell cycle.

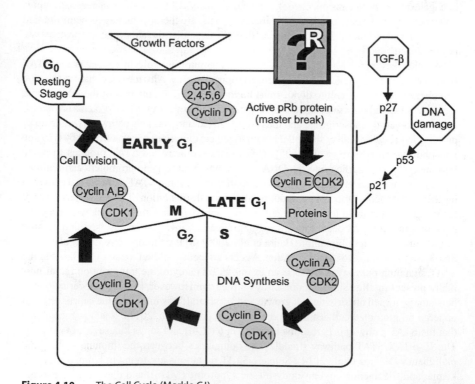

Figure 4.10   The Cell Cycle (Merkle CJ)

Reproduced from Merkle CJ, Loescher LJ. The Biology of Cancer. In Yarbro CH, Frogge MH, and Goodman M, (eds). *Cancer Nursing: Principles and Practice*, 6th ed. Sudbury, MA: Jones and Bartlett; 2005;15

During the G_1 phase, the cell produces new proteins that will make DNA in preparation for cell division. The cell enlarges, and the time spent in this phase is highly variable. If division is not needed or if the cellular conditions are not right (the cell is too small or there are insufficient nutrients), then the cell goes into a resting phase called G_0. Near the end of G_1, the cell decides whether to commit to cell division, and this is called a *restriction point*. Weinberg (2013) describes this as a time when the molecular switch needs to be moved from the "off" mode to "on" mode, as follows: Cyclins D then E combine/activate cyclin-dependent kinases, enzymes that then transfer phosphate groups from adenosine triphosphate (ATP), the energy molecule, to the retinoblastoma protein (pRB), which is the "master brake" of the cell cycle. If no phosphate groups are added to pRB, the brake keeps the cell cycle in the "off" position; however, the brake is lifted when sufficient phosphate groups are added.

When the brake is lifted, transcription factors are released that interact with genes (turns them on or off) so that proteins are actively synthesized for moving the cell cycle through its stages. Studies have helped us better understand the role of cyclin D1 in breast cancer. Normally, the BRCA1 gene is a tumor suppressor gene that acts to protect against cancer by making a protein that binds to the BRCA1 docking site on the estrogen receptor. Cyclin D1 binds to the same estrogen receptor alpha as the BRCA1 protein, and it antagonizes or competes with the BCRA1 protein. Unfortunately, in 30–40% of breast cancer patients, cyclin D1 is overexpressed. This overexpression takes over the ER-alpha binding, thus negating BRCA1's repression of estrogen-responsive genes (Pestell et al., 2005). Overexpression of cyclin D1 correlates with resistance to tamoxifen in postmenopausal women with breast cancer (Stendahl et al., 2004), and to a poor prognosis in ER-alpha positive breast cancer. This makes cyclin D1 an excellent therapeutic target.

Well, what other factors can turn a gene on or off, besides transcription factors, which are regulated by genes that can mutate? Most mutations as discussed involve changes in DNA that silence (tumor suppressor) or activate (oncogene) genes. Epigenetics can help explain how the environment can influence gene expression. Epigenetics refers to the fact that there is an extra layer of instructions in the chromosome that influences which genes get turned off or are silenced without altering the DNA sequence. This silencing of genes without mutational changes in DNA (that occur during cell division or mitosis) is becoming more important and has been linked to the silencing of tumor suppressor genes in a number of malignancies. This can occur through DNA methylation and histone deacetylation (Claus and Lubbert, 2003). These two exciting areas offer new targets, and we have already seen the success of azacytidine (Vidaza) and decitabine (Sprycel) in the treatment of myelodysplastic syndrome (MDS). Let's take a moment to look at these mechanisms.

DNA Methylation
Whether or not the DNA is methylated influences gene transcription. DNA methylation means that a methyl group is added to part of the chemical structure (cytosine ring), and this methyl group sticks out into a major groove of the DNA helix so it inhibits or stops transcription of the gene located on that part of the DNA (Herman and Baylen, 2003). This occurs mostly in CpG-rich islands, as they are called, located near promoter regions of genes. At least 50% of the human genes, including housekeeping genes, have these CpG island-containing promoter regions, but they are generally unmethylated

(Jones, 2005). Hypermethylation occurs in myelodysplastic syndrome and acute leukemia, and the activity of two hypomethylating agents has led to their FDA approval for treating MDS: 5-azacitidine and decitabine, found in *Chapter 1*. These agents get into the DNA and trap methyltransferases (enzymes that help put the methyl into the DNA) on the DNA strand so that there can be no further methylation when the cell goes to divide again. However, they do not remove methyl groups from existing genes. As expected, unlike chemotherapy, which kills or stops the growth of cancer cells right away, hypomethylating agents probably require prolonged therapy to get the optimal efficacy.

Histone Deacetylation

Another exciting group of agents in the arsenal is the histone deacetylase (HDAC) inhibitor class. The chromosomal DNA is wrapped around histones, a specific type of protein. The histones determine how tightly the chromatin or DNA is wrapped: If it is tightly wrapped, the gene is turned off or silenced; if it is loosely wrapped, the gene is turned on. Imagine a coiled Slinky® toy. When the Slinky coils are on a flat surface, the coils lie tight against one another; this is analogous to the histones tightly packing the DNA so that the DNA cannot open and express the gene. The gene is thus turned off. In contrast, when the Slinky is placed on a step and slides down to the next step, the space between the Slinky rings is open; this is analogous to the histone being loosely coiled, so that the DNA is open, and the gene can be expressed or turned on.

Normally, HDACs combine with cell regulatory proteins to regulate gene transcription (copying the recipe for that gene's protein onto mRNA to be taken outside of the nucleus to the ribosome, or protein synthesis factory) and are key components of cell proliferation, angiogenesis, apoptosis, and cell differentiation. Histone deacetylators remove the acetyl groups from proteins, such as histones and transcription factors, causing the chromatin to be tightly wrapped, thus shutting off the genes. Some cancer cells have overexpression of HDACs, or they recruit extra HDACs to oncogene transcription factors, causing hypoacetylation. This results in tightening of the chromatin structure and gene silencing. HDAC inhibitors cause hyperacetylation, which decreases expression of oncogenes such as BCR-ABL and HER-2, stops the cell cycle, induces apoptosis, and stops angiogenesis and cell motility (George et al., 2005). HDAC inhibitors are intended to help malignant cells become normal again, since they target and accumulate in malignant cells. Examples of HDAC inhibitors are vorinostat (Zolinza) and romidepsin (Isodax), FDA-approved for the treatment of progressive or recurrent symptoms of cutaneous T-cell lymphoma (CTCL), and belinostat (Beleodaq), FDA-approved for the treatment of patients with relapsed or refractory peripheral T-cell lymphoma (PTCL).

AVOIDANCE OF APOPTOSIS (PROGRAMMED CELL DEATH)

Mutations can also occur in the genes that make important inhibitory proteins that would otherwise stop the cell cycle from progressing forward, specifically p53, pRB, p16, and p15. This is important because the cell's DNA is examined by DNA repair genes to see whether there are any mutations or mistakes and, if so, whether they can be repaired. If the DNA cannot be repaired, p53 causes the cell to go into "programmed cell death," or apoptosis. This normally eliminates any abnormal cells from the body so that the cells undergoing cell division all have intact DNA. However, in cancer, mutations often occur in the DNA repair genes. Unfortunately, in over 50% of cancers, p53 is inactive. In some cancers, such as cervical cancer, both p53 and pRB are inactivated (Weinberg, 1996), and in small-cell lung cancer and retinoblastoma, pRB is lost. Other proteins such as the cyclins or cyclin-dependent kinases (CDK), which can be synthesized in greater number, or loss of CDK inhibitors, can move the cell through the cell cycle relentlessly. Most cancers have some abnormalities in the cell cycle machinery, and each of these becomes a molecular flaw that can be targeted.

Many of the genes mutated during malignant transformation are those responsible for control of the mTOR pathway; for example, a loss of PTEN, a tumor suppressor gene, activates mTOR signaling. mTOR is a member of the phosphatidylinositide kinase (PIK) subgroup of serine/threonine protein kinases. The other members of this family act as checkpoints in controlling DNA damage repair while mTOR controls nutrient and energy signaling and exists as two distinct complexes. The first, mTOR Complex 1, is sensitive to rapamycin and has three proteins: regulatory associate protein of mTOR (raptor), G-protein b-subunit-like protein (GbL), and praline-rich PKB/Akt substrate 40 kDa (PRAS40). The second, mTOR Complex 2, is not rapamycin-sensitive and has four proteins: GbL, rapamycin-insensitive companion of mTOR (rictor), mammalian stress-activated protein kinase (SAPK)–interacting protein-1 (mSin1), and protein observed with rictor (protor) (Dann et al., 2007). While the two pathways are controlled by growth factors (VEGFs, PDGF, EGF, IGF-1) and hormones (such as insulin, estrogen, progesterone), mTOR Complex 1 is also under the control of input about nutrients (glucose, amino acids, oxygen) and available energy (Shaw and Canthley, 2006). Many tumors make ATP using inefficient anaerobic glycolysis rather than aerobic or oxidative phosphorylation in the mitochondria (Warburg effect); therefore, the tumors need to import more glucose to provide energy (Dennis et al., 2001).

Activation of mTOR Complex 1 is often involved in malignant transformation (e.g., breast, colon, kidney, lung, neuroendocrine, lymphoma, sarcoma, and glioblastoma). It is activated by oncogene-stimulated pathways PI3K, PKB/Akt, and Ras. A number of tumor suppressor genes are located upstream of mTOR Complex 1 to turn down signaling to mTOR such as PTEN, and some are also located downstream of mTOR Complex 1. mTOR signaling is necessary for estrogen-induced breast cancer cellular proliferation (Boulay et al., 2005). As discussed, one of the characteristics of cancer is uncontrolled cell proliferation. The cell cycle is responsible for cell proliferation, and cyclin-dependent kinases (CDKs) regulate cells moving through the cell cycle. Cyclins regulate the activity of CDKs. mTOR controls cell proliferation by controlling cyclin D_1, which in turn controls key CDKs (4 & 6) that are responsible for moving the cell through the G_1-S restriction point. Cyclin D_1 is involved in transcribing genes, cell metabolism, and cell migration (Fu et al., 2004). Thus, malignant transformation and mutations in upstream signaling proteins can "turn on" mTOR, resulting in overexpression of Cyclin D_1 and cell proliferation in a number of cancers (breast, colon, prostate, and melanoma). Cancer cells damaged by chemotherapy are either able to repair the damaged DNA or are able to tell the cell to ignore the fact that the DNA is damaged. Normally, cells without intact DNA that cannot be repaired undergo programmed cell death (apoptosis). Activated mTOR controls p21, a gene product that stops the cell cycle so that the damaged DNA can be repaired.

Additionally, mTOR plays a central role in angiogenesis, as it controls production of hypoxia-inducible factor (HIF) proteins HIF1-α and HIF1-β. HIF is a critical transcription factor that allows the expression of genes whose products (proteins) are involved in angiogenesis, as well as cell proliferation, motility, adhesion, and survival—all qualities necessary for tumor progression and metastases (Semenza, 2003). HIF induces gene expression to produce VEGF (which stimulates endothelial cells to proliferate and migrate toward the tumor in a new tube) and angiopoietin-2 (destabilizes existing blood vessels so they can develop the tube extension in concert with VEGF and then will grow toward the tumor). Angiogenesis is tightly controlled. Hypoxia tips the balance toward angiogenesis to increase the oxygen delivered to tissues and is mediated by hypoxia inducible factor (HIF), which is controlled by the von Hippel-Linday (VHL) protein, a tumor suppressor. During hypoxia, HIF is released so new blood vessels can be stimulated, and when tissue is oxygenated, HIF is rapidly broken down. In the presence of very high levels of HIF, apoptosis occurs (Semenza, 2003). When tumors subvert the upstream signaling pathways, mTOR is activated, and high levels of HIF are produced; if HVL protein is mutated or lost, HIF is not broken down, and high levels persist. This way the tumor can get the proteins and essential nutrients it needs to continue to proliferate and have adequate energy even in hypoxic conditions (Shaw, 2006). Activated mTOR also upregulates VEGF-C, which is associated with lymphangiogenesis (Kobayashi et al., 2007).

Clearly, if mTOR Complex 1 can be blocked, this theoretically will turn off cell proliferation and survival. Analogues (or "rapalogues") of rapamycin (sirolimus) are temsirolimus and everolimus. Temsirolimus (Torisel) is the first FDA-approved mTOR inhibitor and is indicated for the treatment of patients with advanced renal cell cancer, as its study endpoint of increased survival was met. Many of these patients had poor prognostic features. Everolimus (Afinitor) is FDA-approved for treatment of patients with postmenopausal advanced hormone receptor positive, HER2 negative breast cancer together with exemestane, advanced renal cell cancer, advanced pancreatic neuroendocrine tumor (PNET), and also patients with subependymal giant cell astrocytoma (SEGA). This is especially interesting because inhibition of mTOR Complex 1 primarily results in a cytostatic response rather than a cytotoxic one. It is expected that these agents may be combined with cytotoxic chemotherapy or other agents. PI3K (phosphatidylinositide 3-kinases) is a family of intracellular signaling proteins that are important in many cell functions, such as cell migration, proliferation, differentiation, and survival. PI3K is part of the PI3K-AKT (also known as protein kinase B)-mTOR pathway. PI3K-delta is expressed on white blood cells, but it is critical for signaling, development, migration, and survival of B-lymphocytes. Idelalisib (Zydelig) inhibits proliferation of malignant B-lymphocytes, as well as cell signaling (B-cell receptor, CXCR4, CXCR5), which is involved in telling B-lymphocytes how to migrate to the lymph nodes and bone marrow (e.g., trafficking and homing in to the lymph nodes and bone marrow). It is FDA-approved for treatment of patients with (1) relapsed CLL together with rituximab, (2) relapsed follicular B-cell NHL after at least 2 prior systemic therapies, and (3) relapsed small lymphocytic lymphoma after at least 2 prior systemic therapies (Gilead, 2014).

The genes that produce p53 and pRB are also active in regulating normal cell aging or senescence, leading to programmed cell death. All somatic cells have a finite life of 50–60 doublings, after which the cell dies. At the end of the chromosomes, caps called *telomeres* count each of the cell divisions and snip off a piece of the chromosome with each division. After 50–60 divisions, the chromosome is too short to divide again. In a developing embryo, where there is rapid cell division, the chromosome is protected from being snipped off with each division by the enzyme telomerase, which replaces each snipped piece. This enzyme is not found in normal cells after the embryo develops into a fetus but is found in all tumor cells. If there is a mutation that inactivates either of these genes, the cells can use telomerase to replace each of the snipped off pieces of chromosome to become immortal. Again, telomerase becomes a molecular target.

As dividing cells progress through the cell cycle, at specific restriction points, the DNA is assessed for fidelity in copying as the DNA is replicated. If there are errors, specific repair genes attempt to correct the mistakes (mutations). If the mutation cannot be corrected, the cell is directed by p53 to undergo programmed cell death (apoptosis). Poly ADP-ribose polymerase (PARP) enzymes play a central role in DNA repair in cancer cells, and as such are considered excellent targets for therapy. These enzymes are also very important in repairing the damage from chemotherapy, which causes damage to DNA. BRCA1 and BRCA2 are also involved in repair of DNA damage from chemotherapy. Patients with mutations in BRCA1/BRCA2 depend upon PARP1 to repair DNA damage. Thus, as discussed, PARP inhibitors are being studied in patients with triple negative breast cancer, which appears to share some similar molecular features as those with BRCA1/BRCA2 mutations, and thus is also dependent upon PARP1 for repair of DNA damage. While much fanfare accompanied reports of success with PARP inhibitors, unfortunately, in a phase III trial in women with metastatic triple negative breast cancer, the PARP1 inhibitor BSI-201 did not add value when added to gemcitabine/carboplatin (G/C), compared to those women receiving G/C alone (OS 11.1 vs 11.8, $p = 0.284$) (O'Shaughnessy et al., 2011).

In the last decade, we have seen many new targeted agents. Bortezomib (Velcade) is the first of the proteasome inhibitor class that is FDA-approved for cancer therapy, specifically multiple myeloma, as it interferes with the interaction of the myeloma cells with the bone marrow microenvironment; now a second-generation proteasome inhibitor is approved (carfilzomib, Kyprolis). Proteasomes are enzyme complexes that are housekeeping enzymes, which degrade or break down proteins in the cell nucleus that are no longer needed, and turn off key processes such as the cell cycle. The proteins are recycled and used again. They are found in every cell of the body. The proteasomes know which proteins to degrade because they are tagged with ubiquitin, a small protein. The ubiquitin-proteasome pathway regulates protein homeostasis within the cell (Kemple, 2003). Proteasome inhibitors block this process from occurring, so the cell gets conflicting signals about cell regulation. The high volume of the conflicting messages that the cell nucleus receives causes malignant cells to go into apoptosis or programmed cell death, while normal cells are less sensitive to this overload and can recover.

Specifically, three pathways are affected by proteasome inhibition: the cell cycle (proteins active in the cell cycle such as cyclins, cyclin-dependent kinase inhibitors, and the tumor suppressor p53 protein), apoptosis (proteins that inhibit apoptosis like XIAP, cIAP, and Bcl-2 proteins), and Nuclear Factor-kappa B dependent signaling (inhibitor of this pathway is I kappa

B-alpha) (Glickman and Ciechanover, 2002). Nuclear Factor (NF)-kappa B is a transcription factor that has been found to regulate a number of genes that control malignant transformation and metastases. Inactive proteins p50, p65, I kappa B-alpha, and NF-kappa B are found in the cytoplasm of the cell (outside the nucleus). When NF-kappa B is activated by carcinogens, tumor promoter factors, inflammatory cytokines, and some chemotherapy agents, I kappa B-alpha is broken down and the other two proteins move into the nucleus. They attach to DNA in the nucleus at a promoter region and activate the gene. Once NF-kappa B is activated, it can stop apoptosis, which leads to tumor formation and resistance to chemotherapy. There is much excitement about using chemoprevention strategies to block activation of NF-kappa B by inhibiting its signaling pathway, much as the proteasome does. In addition, it theoretically increases tumor sensitivity to chemotherapy (Bharti and Aggarwal, 2002). One such preventive approach is with non-steroidal anti-inflammatory drugs (NSAIDs), such as aspirin. Aspirin appears to induce signal-specific I kappa-B-alpha degradation, followed by NF-kappa B nuclear translocation, leading to apoptosis, in colorectal cancer cells (Din et al., 2004).

A number of agents are being investigated that target Bcl-2 or other proteins that may suppress apoptosis. Since Bcl-2 protein inhibits apoptosis and makes the cells resistant to treatment with standard chemotherapy, drugs such as antisense oligonucleotides can disable Bcl-2 and restore responsiveness to chemotherapy. As more is known about the pathophysiology of apoptosis, new drugs will emerge. Apo2L/TRAIL agents are being studied. (TRAIL stands for tumor necrosis factor (TNF)–related apoptosis-inducing ligand; it activates two cell-death pathways, resulting in apoptosis of cancer cells while normal cells are relatively resistant, and it is synergistic with chemotherapy). Tumor cells also have been found to have a protein called Programmed Death-1 (PD-1) that allows them to escape apoptosis; drugs are being tested to block this, such as lambrolizumab and nivolumab. This is discussed further under the section on "Avoiding Immune Destruction."

Turning Back on Embryologic Features

Interestingly, many of the events that occur in embryogenesis are reactivated during carcinogenesis. Normally, the "software" that guides embryogenesis is turned on when needed; then when the fetus is formed, it is turned off. Apparently, however, the "software" is still present in all cells, so when the cell transforms into a malignant cell, the software can become activated again (Weinberg, 2013). To appreciate how powerful this pathway is, one must understand that the migration of embryologic tissue to the right anatomic area depends upon Hedgehog signaling. For example, the neural tissue that becomes the spinal cord has to migrate to the center of the body. The arms and legs have to form, and the fingers and toes have to be oriented perfectly so the thumb is where it should be and the baby finger in the right place. This is all dependent upon the Hedgehog signaling pathway. The Hedgehog genes code for a soluble secreted protein that ensures that the developing embryologic tissues reach the correct size, location, and cellular content. After the fetus is formed and the baby is born, the Hedgehog signaling software is largely turned off; however, the software is still in our cells. In the case of basal cell cancer formation, the Hedgehog pathway becomes reactivated and leads to malignant transformation in the skin. In fact, more than 90% of patients with basal cell cancer have mutations in one of two genes, turning the Hedgehog pathway back on. Normally, the pathway is turned off. In the resting state, the Patched

(PTCH) receptor prevents the activation of the pathway by inhibiting the second protein, Smoothened (SMO). When the Hedgehog ligand is secreted, it binds to and inactivates PTCH. Without PTCH control, SMO is activated and signaling events begin, resulting in the transcription of Hedgehog target genes: those involved in cell proliferation, development, and tissue maintenance, including stem cells. The tumor microenvironment can also secrete Hedgehog ligands that support tumor growth. Vismodegib (Erivedge) is the first Hedgehog pathway inhibitor to be FDA-approved. This drug binds to and inhibits SMO, so signal transduction is shut down.

TUMOR-PROMOTING INFLAMMATION

The relationship between cancer and chronic inflammation has been widely publicized. For example, *Helicobacter pylori* and chronic gastritis are causal agents of adenocarcinoma of the stomach, human papillomavirus has been found to cause cervical cancer, and hepatitis B virus can cause hepatocellular carcinoma. As more is learned about these relationships, it appears that recurrent or persistent inflammation may induce or promote cancer through DNA damage, leading to cell proliferation in an effort to heal the area, as well as creating a stromal "soil" rich in cytokines and growth factors ideal for a malignant cell to flourish (Schottenfeld and Beebe-Dimmer, 2006). To combat cervical cancer, the FDA approved vaccines for the prevention of cervical cancer, which kills millions of women worldwide each year. Hepatitis B vaccines are used to prevent the infection, with resulting liver cirrhosis, liver failure, and hepatocellular cancer of the liver.

AVOIDING IMMUNE DESTRUCTION

There is great attention to the immune system now and to immunotherapeutic approaches to cancer control. Recently, with more research enhancing our understanding of how the immune system is circumvented by cancer, new drugs are being developed to target these events when the immune system's T-lymphocytes become overwhelmed or tricked by cancer cells. The following is a simplified overview of the immune system and its elements, and the reader is directed to articles or texts in the reference list for more information. It is important for oncology nurses to be conversant about elements of the immune system so they can teach patients and their families about them. There is an urgent need, and most nurses do not have a working knowledge of the immune system.

The immune system is responsible for identifying invading microorganisms and abnormal cells that might harm the body. It uses immune surveillance to accomplish this, distinguishing self from nonself by markers on the cell surface that match the person's major histocompatibility complex (MHC) proteins, also called human leukocyte antigens (HLA). Normally, the immune system is quiet or tolerant as it encounters cells with the correct MHC proteins. However, when a microorganism invades, or a cell without the MHC protein is found, the immune system is turned on to destroy it.

Our bodies are protected by both an **innate** immune response and an **adaptive** immune response, which are both interconnected. The innate immune response is immediate, as when you get the flu. You may develop fever, malaise, and other symptoms. The innate immune response is the first line of defense, and while immediate, it is not antigen-specific, nor is there immunological memory. Of note, there are natural killer (NK) cells activated by the innate response that kill any potential target it recognizes as "nonself" that does not have an MHC protein. It is not antigen-specific. An antigen is any substance that can evoke an immune response and that itself subsequently reacts with the products of the response (Male, 2013).

In contrast, the adaptive immune response takes longer to evolve initially, is antigen-specific, and your body's immune system remembers the antigen, so the next time the antigen is seen, the adaptive response is much more swift and potent. In the adaptive immune system, the immune cells are able to distinguish self from nonself, to remember the "foreign" antigens to which they have been exposed (memory T and B cells), and to mount an immune attack to eliminate the foreign antigen. When the antigen is encountered again, the immune system will mount a rapid and increasingly more potent defense against the antigen. It does this by activating specific immune cells. Once an antigen is recognized as not belonging to self, dendritic cells (a type of B-lymphocyte) digest the foreign cell and mount a peptide fragment of the antigen on its cell surface to teach the T-lymophocyte cells to recognize the foreign antigen and to attack it. This type of cell is called an antigen-presenting cell, or APC. Key immune warriors can be activated by the dendritic cells: cytotoxic T-lymphocytes, B-lymphocytes, and NK cells. First, the dendritic cell activates helper T-lymphocytes cells, which produce cytokines that activate the appropriate B-lymphocyte and/or T-lymphocyte to seek and destroy the antigen(s) marked for destruction. These helper T-lymphocytes may be activated to differentiate into cytotoxic T-lymphocytes, which proliferate rapidly against the specific antigen(s) and kill the cell containing the antigen. Second, B-lymphocytes can recognize APCs, and then seek and destroy the cells with this cell surface antigen. Third, NK cells can attack and destroy cells based on identifying the cell as nonself.

The three key cell types in the immune fight against cancer are B-(cell) lymphocytes, T-(cell) lymphocytes, and antigen presenting cells, or APCs. Cytokines allow the cells to talk to each other and orchestrate the immune reaction.

- APCs: When a foreign organism invades the body, macrophages and dendritic cells will find the organism, engulf and digest it, and then remove a peptide fragment containing the antigen and mount it on their cell surface to show the target to T-lymphocytes and other immune cells. These cells are therefore called antigen-presenting cells or APCs. Dendritic cells have great potential in recognizing and orchestrating an immune attack against tumor cell antigens; however, they must mature before they can activate T-lymphocytes. After the dendritic cell recognizes the foreign antigen on the surface of the tumor cell, it infiltrates into the tumor, processes intracellular proteins and/or antigens, and matures so that it can express fragments of the antigen on its surface to present to the T-lymphocytes. The mature dendritic cell uses the major histocompatibility complex (MHC) to present the foreign antigen; when bound to the T-lymphocyte, a signal is sent to make more T-lymphocytes: the B7 costimulatory molecule on the dendritic cells binds to the CD28 receptor on the T-lymphocyte, which then signals T-lymphocyte replication. The resulting activated T-lymphocytes should be able to seek and destroy tumor cells expressing that particular antigen. First, the dendritic cell activates helper T-lymphocytes cells, which produce cytokines that activate the appropriate B-lymphocyte and/or T-lymphocyte to seek and destroy the antigen(s) marked for destruction. These helper T-lymphocytes may be activated to differentiate into cytotoxic T-lymphocytes, which proliferate rapidly against the specific antigen(s). Second, B-lymphocytes can recognize APCs and then seek and destroy the cells with this cell surface antigen. Third, NK cells can attack and destroy cells that do not have an MHC protein.

- B-lymphocytes: These cells are involved in innate as well as humoral or antibody-mediated immunity. Once taught by the APC, B-lymphocytes make antibodies against the invading antigen. Antigen containing cells are killed in one of two ways: (1) antibody-dependent cell-mediated cytotoxicity (ADCC), or (2) complement-dependent cytotoxicity (CDC). In ADCC, B-lymphocytes become activated and begin manufacturing antibodies against the specific antigen presented by the APCs. The upper Y section of the antibody is the variable region; it matches the antigen shape exactly, and it binds to the antigen to mark the cell for attack, while the stem of the Y is the constant region (Fc), which calls in the effector cells of the immune system to kill the antigen-containing cell (e.g., natural killer cells, macrophages). The natural killer (NK) cells release cytotoxic granules, along with cytokines, which kill the cell by digesting the cell membrane and entering the cell, causing apoptosis. In CDC, B lymphocytes bind to the antigen and activate complement, which triggers the completement cascade. The antigen-containing cell is coated with complement, which "punches" holes in the cell membrane, killing the cell (Weinberg, 2011). Complement is a very powerful cell-killing mechanism, and normal cells protect themselves from it by expressing anti-complement proteins on their cell membranes. Unfortunately, some cancer cells have been found to overexpress membrane-bound complement regulatory proteins, which protect them from CDC (Weinberg, 2013).

  Monoclonal antibodies are similar in that they are manufactured to target a single antigen and bind tightly to that antigen like a key in a lock.

- T-lymphocytes: These cells are involved in the cell-mediated (cytotoxic) immune response and are divided into helper [CD4+ (T4), which help activated B-lymphocytes make antibody] and cytotoxic T- cells [CD8+ (T8), which kill invading organisms or cancer cells], among others. In order for the cytotoxic T-lymphocytes to function, they must be activated, which stimulates them to proliferate and then mature so that they are directed only against the invading antigen (containing cell) which they will kill (Melman, 2013). CD8 T-lymphocytes can be either cytotoxic, which can kill identified antigen-specific cells or regulatory, which help to turn down the immune response after the invading organism has been neutralized. Because the immune reaction can be so powerful, there has to be a way to turn down the immune system so that the person's organs are not attacked, such as with autoimmune diseases. These are called immune checkpoints. This is one place malignant cells co-opt the immune system and turn down the cytotoxic T-lymphocyte response.

- Cytokines: These are messengers secreted by immune cells that provide communication between and among the cells. Cytokines regulate the intensity and duration of the immune response to an invading microorganism and are critical to the orchestration of the immune response. Cytokines include interleukins, interferons, and colony-stimulating factors; they are discussed in *Chapter 2*.

Cancer evades the immune system in a number of ways that are known today, and many other processes that are awaiting discovery. Zielinski et al. (2013) describes four ways the immune system is circumvented. First, tumors may reduce expression of the class-I MHC molecules so that they are not detected as nonself and an immune response is not activated; the tumor antigen cannot be seen by cytotoxic T-lymphocytes. Second, they can turn down (down-regulate) the innate immune system's cancer-fighting natural killer (NK) cells. Third, they can avoid apoptosis by down-regulating Fas receptor cell surface expression so they are invisible to NK and cytotoxic T-lymphocytes. Fourth, they can promote an anti-inflammatory state favoring tumor growth through secretion of growth factors that are immunosuppressive to T-lymphocytes and macrophages.

Dunn (2006) describes a theory of immunoediting that spans from immune surveillance to tumor escape. Initially, cancer cells are identified and totally eliminated. Equilibrium may occur, where cancer growth is controlled, but not all cancer cells are eliminated. Last, tumor escape occurs, when the immune system is exhausted, overwhelmed, and metastases occurs.

Finally, cancer cells evade the immune system by suppressing immune cells locally; in the microenvironment, they can also make the immune system tolerant to the cancer antigens by co-opting the inhibitory immune checkpoints and by using immune editing described above (Schreiber et al. (2011), Zou (2006), and Pardoll (2012)).

CTLA-4 is expressed on T-lymphocytes, and its ligand is CD80 (Quezada and Peggs, 2013). The CTLA-4 cell surface protein is a negative regulator of T-lymphocyte function and activation, and it turns down the powerful T-lymphocyte immune response after the pathogen is eliminated to protect normal tissues from the ravages of the immune response (Wolchok and Saenger, 2008). Most malignant cells express CTLA-4 (CD152) and use it to escape cytotoxic T-lymphocyte attack. Blockade of CTLA-4 results in anti-tumor immunity (Wolchok and Saenger, 2008).

Other reasons include the tumor's ability to interfere with dendritic cell maturation, and/or it may block signaling between the costimulatory molecules B7 and CD28, which is required for maturation of activated T-lymphocytes. Without this signaling, cytokines are not produced, such as IL-2, which is necessary for full activation of T-lymphocytes, and the proliferating T-lymphocytes are not fully activated (Scandella and Ludewig, 2005).

For decades, different clinical trials explored ways to stimulate and/or augment immune function. The immune response can be very powerful and threaten normal tissues, so there are immune checkpoints that sense when it is time to turn down or off the immune response, principally the activity of activated cytotoxic T-lymphocytes. Cancer cells have learned that if they co-opt or make the patient's immune system develop immune tolerance to the antigen, the cancer antigen is not recognized as foreign and does not ramp up the immune response against it.

Ipilimumab (Yervoy) is an immune checkpoint inhibitor that is FDA-approved for the treatment of unresectable or metastatic melanoma. Ipilimumab is a monoclonal antibody directed against cytotoxic T-lymphocyte-associated antigen 4 (CTLA-4), designed to augment cytotoxic T-cell function. CTLA-4 acts as the "off" switch to depress T-lymphocyte activation and function as the immune response is winding down. Cancer cells co-opt this process by releasing CTLA-4 and turning off/down activated T-lymphocyte function. Ipilimumab blocks CTLA-4 so no inhibitory protein is sent; T-cell proliferation, activation, and IL-2 production continue so that the cytotoxic T-lymphocytes attack the tumor antigen identified by the APCs (Ribas, 2012). Side effects are immune-related and may be very serious; they include rash, diarrhea, adrenal insufficiency, and hepatitis.

Another important immune checkpoint is the Programmed Death-1 (PD-1) receptor and its ligand PD-L1, which tumor cells co-opt and use to become invisible to the immune system (Pardoll, 2012). Many cells express ligands for PD-1; when bound to the PD-1 receptor on T-lymphocytes, PD-1 turns down/off activated T-lymphocyte immune response. PD-1 is also expressed by T-lymphocytes when they are exposed to antigens for a long time, which may explain gradual immune tolerance to tumor antigen(s). PD-1's role is to protect the peripheral tissues from autoimmunity. Drugs such as nivolumab and pembrolizumab, which are monoclonal antibodies, block the PD-1 receptor so that it cannot be stimulated by its ligand, and the activated T-lymphocytes continue their war against the cells with cancer antigens. Both have been FDA approved. See the drug information in the text.

Immunotherapy uses techniques to develop a large population of immune cells that can seek out and destroy cancer cells carrying that antigen. Immunotherapy techniques not only increase the number but also often increase the effectiveness of the immune cells in killing cancer cells. T-lymphocyte-adoptive therapies (called chimeric antigen receptor (CAR) therapy), use the patient's own genetically modified T-lymphocytes that are treated so that they seek and attack the patient's specific tumor antigen when reinjected back to the patient. Clinical trials of CAR therapy are showing promising results, so it will be exciting to see their future unfold (Lipowska-Bhalla et al., 2012).

Currently, there is one vaccine, sipuleucel-T (Provenge), an autologous cellular immunotherapy agent that is indicated for the treatment of asymptomatic or minimally symptomatic metastatic, castrate-resistant, prostate cancer. See drug information.

Cytotoxic T lymphocytes (CTLs) are highly specific and powerful effector cells, being able to destroy tumor cells. However, they cannot attack free antigens. The CTL has a protein complex on its cell membrane called a T-cell receptor (TCR), which interacts with APCs. An important protein in the TCR is CD3, which regulates signal transduction to activate T cells, allowing them to recognize and kill this specific (tumor) antigen. Bispecific T-cell Engager (BiTE) technology uses monoclonal antibodies to bind together CTLs and the malignant antigen. One MAb binds to CTLs via the CD3 receptor, and the other MAb binds to a tumor-specific antigen. Once linked, the CTL produces dissolving substances like perforin and granzymes; when released into the tumor cell, they cause the tumor cell to undergo apoptosis. Blinatumomab (Blincyto) is the first bispecific CD19-directed CD3 T-cell engager to receive FDA approval; it is indicated for the treatment of Philadelphia-chromosome–negative relapsed or refractory B-cell precursor ALL (Amgen, 2014).

INVASION AND METASTASIS

Once mutation of an epithelial cell occurs, further development and transformation into malignancy occurs in stages. For example, the first mutation causes hyperplasia or increased proliferation of normal-appearing cells, and the second leads to dysplasia. The cells now appear abnormal. A third mutation may cause a change to carcinoma in situ, in which the cells are transformed and malignant, but they remain within normal tissue boundaries. If allowed to continue, the cells may again mutate and develop invasiveness, allowing them to invade underlying tissue and enter blood and lymphatic vessels. As cells are shed, they travel via the blood or lymph system to distant sites. This is called *metastasis*. It initially seemed that metastasis begins after the development of a detectable tumor, but it is now clear that, with some tumors, metastasis can begin even before the primary tumor is detectable. In general, a tumor cannot grow beyond a size of 2 mm (the head of a pin) unless it forms new blood vessels (angiogenesis), as the diffusion distance of oxygen, a critical cell nutrient, is only 1–2 mm (Folkman, 1986).

However, not all cancers invade or metastasize. The explosion of scientific discovery about cell function and the molecular processes of metastasis have led to clinical trials of numerous molecularly targeted therapies, including agents that interrupt different steps in the metastasis process. Fortunately, it appears that the metastatic process is highly inefficient, especially in late disease; in addition, each of the steps is "rate limiting," so that if one step is not achieved, the process cannot move forward (Stetler-Stevenson and Kleiner, 2001).

Stetler-Stevenson and Kleiner (2001) identify eight steps in the "metastatic cascade," each controlled by a number of gene products in the malignant cell. Some aggressively permit invasion, and others subvert the normal body's defenses against metastases. These steps include the detachment of cells from the primary tumor, invasion of the underlying basement membrane and extracellular tissue, movement of cells into blood vessels, and survival in the venous or lymphatic circulation until reaching a capillary bed. There the malignant cell must attach to the basement membrane of the blood vessel, enter the tissue of the organ fed by the capillary bed, respond to local growth factors, begin cell division to form a small tumor, and begin the formation of local blood vessels to support growth beyond 2 mm. More recently, Chaffler and Weinberg (2011) describe a two-phase process: (1) physical translocation of a cancer cell to a distant organ, and (2) development of a metastatic site in a distant site.

As seen, a cell undergoes multiple mutations during malignant transformation. A single cell (clone) that goes through multiple mutations usually results in cells that are not all alike (heterogenous). Some of the cells have aggressive qualities and are more likely to invade and metastasize than others, such as cancer stem cells (CSCs). CSCs have the ability to self-renew (make more cancer stem cells) and also to initiate tumors (proliferate tumor cells); in addition, these cells also have qualities critical to invasion and metastasis: motility, invasiveness, and resistance to apoptosis (Chaffler and Weinberg, 2011).

Activation of the *ras* oncogene turns a malignant cell into one that invades and metastasizes, and there appears to be a survival advantage for more aggressive cells that respond to local growth factors. The new, tiny tumor gets nourishment by simple diffusion. However, once the tumor reaches 2 mm, it can grow no larger until it gets its own blood supply to increase the delivery of nutrients and remove waste products. The microenvironment helps give the necessary growth factors and nourishment.

As the tumor grows, the cells on the outside get nourishment (e.g., oxygen), but the cells in the inside (core) become hypoxic. This causes the activation of an "angiogenic switch," involving secretion of angiogenic growth factors (e.g., vascular endothelial growth factor, VEGF) and suppressing normal inhibitors of angiogenesis (e.g., angiostatin). The blood vessels that form are leaky but have an invasiveness not seen in normal new blood vessels. If the tumor grows near an existing vessel, it may invade and use existing vessels before making its own. Unfortunately, studies have shown that turning on the angiogenic switch is associated with increased frequency of metastases, disease recurrence, and shorter patient survival (Weidner, 1998).

Cells continue to mutate in the primary tumor, and a clone of cells emerges that is superior in growth and is highly invasive. This clone of cells turns down (down-regulates) the activity of substances that keep normal cells sticking to their neighboring cells (cell–cell adhesion molecules called *cadherins*, and in epithelial cells, *E-cadherin*) and to the extracellular matrix (integrins). Thus, the tumor cells become mobile and can separate from the rest of the primary tumor. Stromolysin-1 is a matrix metalloproteinase (MMP) that can degrade E-cadherin, and it is associated with tumor progression.

More and more, the microenvironment has taken center stage in our understanding of invasion and metastases. The microenvironment is composed of the extracellular matrix, growth factors, fibroblasts, and immune and endothelial cells, and it begins a critical interaction with premalignant cells. This interaction is necessary for malignant transformation, as well as for invasion and metastases.

The tumor cell then uses enzymes (e.g., MMPs) to destroy the integrity of the basement membrane that the tumor lies on, as well as the extracellular matrix. Imagine it as a tank destroying the area ahead so that the invading army can move forward. Now the malignant cells can invade neighboring normal tissue and the newly made leaky blood vessels or nearby thin-walled lymph vessels.

Normal epithelial cells must remain attached to the extracellular matrix or they die. It is unclear how malignant cells can overcome this. It is believed that the microenvironment or stroma surrounding the tumor sends signals telling the tumor cells on the outer edges of the epithelial mass to undergo a change from epithelial cells to mesenchymal cells, called the epithelial mesenchymal transition (EMT). Mesenchymal cells are less tightly woven together so that they can separate easily; in the embryo, they also have the ability to migrate. TGF-β helps transmit these stromal signals, as do TNF-α, EGF, HGF or scatter factor, and IGF-1. In addition, if the ras oncogene is mutated, this also helps activate EMT. Once activated, these cells make their own TGF-β, which helps to keep the mesenchymal phenotype. Cancer cells recruit "normal" cells into the surrounding stroma, such as fibroblasts, granulocytes, macrophages, and mesenchymal stem cells, which create a "reactive stroma," or inflammatory environment, resulting in signals that lead to EMT (Chaffler and Weinberg, 2011). It now appears that the EMT process also can induce non-CSCs to acquire the traits of CSCs, which enables these cells to disseminate from the primary tumor, enter the blood circulation, and form distant metastatic sites (Chaffler and Weinberg, 2011).

Integrins are critical molecules in the extracellular matrix and also have a role in cell signal transduction and cell growth. Changes in integrin-mediated signaling allow the malignant cell to become invasive and to migrate. Integrin attached to the extracellular matrix gives the malignant cell adhesive traction. As the actin filaments in the cell's cytoskeleton contract, the cell body is propelled forward. Proportionate to the age and size of the primary tumor, huge numbers and clumps of malignant cells can be shed into the bloodstream. The clinical effect depends on whether the embolized cells reach a favorable environment and can achieve the steps in metastasis. The role of the microenvironment of this metastatic site is critical in the establishment of a metastatic site. One integrin inhibitor, cilengitide, is being studied in patients with poor prognosis glioblastoma (unmethylated MGMT-promoter), together with radiation therapy and temozolomide or cetuximab (Verschaeve et al., 2011).

Individual cells or clumps of cells are carried in the blood or lymph circulation, and many do not survive. The cells need to survive the turbulence of blood flow as well as the circulating cell-mediated and humoral immune cell elements (e.g., cytotoxic and killer lymphocytes). Most die. Fidler (2003) described the attributes of cells that survive and find their ultimate niche in his "seed and soil" hypothesis; in addition, he showed that metastatic landing sites that flourish are not random.

Cells that survive the ride to distant organs or lymph nodes either get stuck in the microcirculation or attach to specific endothelial cells in capillaries or lymph vessels. In addition, they may attach to an exposed basement membrane of the organ or lymph node.

The cells "extravasate" from the blood or lymph vessel into the extracellular tissue and either grow in response to growth factors or stay dormant in this secondary site. Malignant cells migrate to find a "favorable" site. Many die. In order to respond to the growth signals from this microenvironment or stroma, the tumor cells must revert back to epithelial cells, and thus, they undergo a mesenchyme-to-epithelial transition, or MET (Weinberg, 2013).

If successful in finding a hospitable local environment, after some growth to 2 mm, the tumor cells release angiogenic growth factors to build blood vessels in this secondary site. This increases the ability of the metastatic cells to metastasize again.

How the metastatic cells evade the body's host immune responses is not well known, but it is likely through immune tolerance after chronic exposure to cancer antigens.

ANGIOGENESIS

Many similarities exist between angiogenesis and tumor invasion and, as a result, they may have similar molecular targets. The body normally needs the ability to make new blood vessels for processes such as wound healing, female menstruation, rebuilding the endometrial lining, or making the placenta during pregnancy. The body maintains a fine balance between turning angiogenesis on and turning it off. When there are more factors favoring angiogenesis than opposing it (inhibitors), angiogenesis occurs. Angiogenic growth factors are shown in Table 4.1. When cells are hypoxic or lacking oxygen, they release vascular endothelial growth factor (VEGF), also known as vascular permeability factor. VEGF initiates new blood vessel growth and causes the release of nitric oxide (NO) from the endothelial cells lining the blood vessel, which causes them to dilate. Malignant blood vessels are flawed: they are leaky, they are disorganized and may have blind channels that do not connect with other vessels, and they have many different diameters so that parts of the tumor fed by narrow vessels with low blood flow remain hypoxic and resistant to chemotherapy, as chemotherapy does not reach that area.

VEGF and its receptor on the endothelial cell are essential for angiogenesis. VEGF is a family of glycoproteins: VEGF-A is essential for blood vessel formation, and it is commonly referred to as VEGF (Takahashi and Shibuy, 2005). VEGF-B may be a redundant ligand; VEGF-C and VEGF-D appear to be involved with lymphangiogenesis. The VEGF ligands bind to VEGFR (receptors) 1, 2, and 3 (Flt-4), which then stimulate a signaling cascade, resulting in endothelial cell (vascular or lymphangenic) proliferation, migration, and survival. VEGFR2 is most commonly associated with VEGF-A, but VEGFR-1 also may be linked to VEGF-A. In developing agents to target the ligand VEGF or the receptor

VEGFR, some agents are selective for VEGF, like the monoclonal antibody bevacizumab (Avastin), whereas others are oral, small molecule tyrosine kinase inhibitors that target VEGF receptors (VEGFR), such as axitinib (VEGFR-1, 2, 3). Other agents are multitargeted for VEGF, as well as other related or unrelated targets, such as the more well-known sorafenib (Nexavar), which inhibits VEGFR-2, PDGFR-β, and Raf-kinase; and sunitinib (Sutent), which inhibits (VEGFR-1, 2, 3), stem cell factor receptor (KIT), fms-like tyrosine kinase-3 (FLT-3), colony-stimulating factor receptor type 1 (CSF-1R), and the glial cell-line-derived neurotrophic factor receptor (RET). It is becoming clear that angiogenesis occurs earlier in the malignant process, as it is necessary in the microenvironment to help selected transformed cells invade and metastasize.

The most important VEGFR appears to be VEGFR-2. When the ligand VEGF attaches to VEGFR (receptor) on the endothelial cell, the receptor dimerizes (comes together as partners with another cell surface receptor, which activates the message sending), and the message for proliferation and migration of endothelial cells is sent via a tyrosine kinase system. Neuropilin, a nontyrosine kinase receptor, is hypothesized to be a survival factor for tumors (Parikh et al., 2004).

Antiangiogenesis agents can be divided into at least three categories based on their mechanism of action. (1) Agents that prevent VEGF from reaching their receptors on the endothelial cell (e.g., bevacizumab (Avastin), and the VEGF trap aflibercept (Zaltrap)); (2) agents that block signaling within the endothelial cell so the nucleus of the endothelial cell never gets the message to proliferate and migrate to form the new blood vessel (e.g., small molecule tyrosine kinase inhibitors sunitinib (Sutent) and sorafinib (Nexavar)); and (3) agents that interfere with signals from the stroma asking for more blood vessels (e.g., thalidomide (Thalomid), lenalidomide (Revlimid), and pomalidomide (Pomalyst), all immunomodulatory agents). Other antangiogenic agents include interferon alfa (Intron A, Roferon), imiquimod (Aldara 5% cream, Zyclara 3.75% cream), and alitretinoin (Panretin 0.1% gel) (Angiogenesis Foundation, 2014).

Bevacizumab prevents VEGF (the ligand) from binding to VEGFR-2 (the receptor). Two multitargeted tyrosine kinase inhibitors that block the message in the endothelial cell (initiated by the VEGF-receptor 2) are sunitinib (Sutent) and sorafinib (Nexavar). Integrins, specifically α5β1 integrin, are proteins on the proliferating endothelial cell. The sprouting endothelial tube has to migrate or move toward the tumor, and it does this by having the integrin on the endothelial cell attach to fibronectin in the extracellular matrix. The integrins then act like grappling hooks to move the new blood vessel tube to the tumor. New agents are being developed to block integrin binding so that the new blood vessel sprout cannot move toward the tumor; the proliferating endothelial cell cannot bind to fibronectin, and thus, it undergoes apoptosis (programmed cell death).

Of interest, clinical trials with bevacizumab (Avastin) showed not only the cessation of tumor angiogenesis and growth, but also tumor regression, suggesting that when combined with chemotherapy, antiangiogenesis agents alter the tumor blood flow so that the chemotherapy is more effective in killing tumor cells. Thus, the mechanism of bevacizumab is thought to be twofold: blocking (1) development of new blood vessels and (2) VEGF, which is necessary for the maintenance of existing malignant blood vessels, so existing blood vessels actually normalize; this then increases blood flow within the tumor so that concomitantly administered chemotherapy can now enter the tumor more uniformly.

In addition, it is now believed that there are VEGF-receptors on tumor cells that are involved in tumor cell migration and invasion; thus, antiangiogenesis agents appear to directly affect tumor cells (Fan et al., 2005).

Mancuso et al. (2006) have shown in the laboratory that antiangiogenesis agents reduce the tumor blood vessels by 50–60%, but the empty sleeves of the blood vessels in the basement membrane remain, along with nonmalignant-appearing pericytes (provide strength to the new blood vessel, but can also differentiate into a fibroblast, smooth muscle cell, or macrophage if needed). One day after the antiangiogenesis drug was stopped, new blood vessels sprouted in the empty sleeves in the basement membrane, connected to nearby capillaries, and by 7 days after the drug was stopped, tumors were fully revascularized and protected with tumor-related pericytes. However, when the tumor was again retreated with an antiangiogenesis drug, the regrown vasculature regressed as much as it did the first time. This suggests that the empty sleeves of the basement membrane, as well as the pericytes, should be targeted by anticancer therapies; it also suggests that perhaps antiangiogenic drugs should be continued after tumor progression with just a change in the chemotherapy. New agents with ability to target multiple receptors are being developed.

Platelet-derived growth factor is necessary for the pericytes, which give the newly formed blood vessel stability, much like the shingles of a house give it protection.

Table 4.1   Natural Factors That Stimulate or Inhibit Angiogenesis

Factors Stimulating Angiogenesis	Factors Inhibiting Angiogenesis
Angiopoietin-1	Angiostatin, Antiangiogenic antithromin III (aaATIII)
Fibroblast growth factors	
Granulocyte-colony stimulating factor (G-CSF)	Cartilage-derived inhibitor (CDI)
Hepatocyte growth factor (HGF)/scatter factor	CD59 complement fragment
Interleukin-8 (IL-8)	Endostatin (collagen XVIII fragment)
Tumor necrosis factor (TNF) alpha	Fibronectin fragment
Transforming growth factor (TGF) alpha and beta	Heparanases
	Human chorionic gonadotropin (hCG)
Platelet-derived growth factor (PDGF) BB	Kringle 5 (plasminogen factor)
Pleiotrophin (PTN)	Interferon (alpha, gamma)
Transforming growth factors- alpha and beta	Interleukin-12
Tumor Necrosis Factor (TNF)-alpha	2-Methoxyestradiol
VEGF, also known as vascular permeability factor (VPF)	Plasminogen activator inhibitor
	Platelet factor-4
	Retinoids
	Tissue inhibitors of metalloproteinases called TIMPs
	Thrombospondin-1
	Troponin 1
	Vasculostatin

Data from The Angiogenesis Foundation, http://www.angio.org/understanding/growth.php, accessed October 25, 2013

Sorafenib (Nexavar), a multiple-targeted protein tyrosine kinase inhibitor, appears to block the Raf kinase step in the ras pathway, VEGFR-2 and PDGF-β.

Drugs such as bevacizumab (Avastin) neutralize vascular endothelial growth factor (VEGF), which is released by tumors to start the process of angiogenesis. This drug, in combination with chemotherapy, has produced statistically significant increased response rates, increased time to progression, and overall survival in patients with metastatic colon, rectal, and lung cancers. It was thought that giving patients adjuvant chemotherapy and bevacizumab for stage II/III colon cancer would prevent metastasis and increase the cure rate. However, the NSABP C-08 results reported that at 3 years, there was no statistical difference in DFS or OS. However, the patients received adjuvant chemotherapy with bevacizumab for 6 months, then bevacizumab alone for 6 months. During this time, there was a 40% reduction in disease progression that was statistically significant ($p < .0004$), which disappeared after the first year. The implication is that while this was a negative study, it may also indicate that the bevacizumab needed to be continued for 3 years to make a significant difference in DFS and as a surrogate, OS. Studies looking at this are planned (Wolmark, 2009).

The Angiogenesis Foundation illustrates the process of angiogenesis in Figure 4.11 (Angiogenesis Foundation, 2014). A simplified process is as follows:

Normal blood vessels supply oxygen and nutrients to a cell and remove waste products. Blood vessels have an inner lining that is made up of endothelial cells that are tightly joined with their neighbors, surrounded by a basement membrane containing pericytes, which act like shingles on a house to protect the endothelial cells. Blood vessels have sensors that identify when more oxygen is needed by the tissue (e.g., oxygen and hypoxia-induced sensors or receptors). The blood vessel can then dilate to allow more blood to come to the tissue.

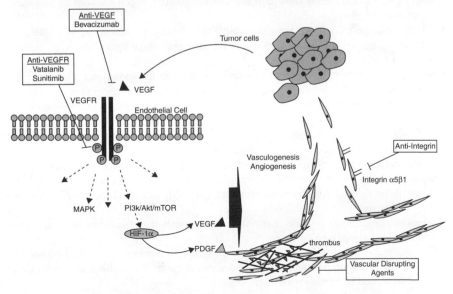

Figure 4.11   The Angiogenesis Cascade

Hypoxia, as well as some other signals, can activate cells to release angiogenic growth factors, such as VEGF, Ang-2, FGF, and chemokines, which stimulate new blood vessel capillaries to grow from nearby existing blood vessels, a process called angiogenesis. For example, solid tumors cannot grow beyond 2 mm without building new blood vessels, as this is the diffusion distance of oxygen, so they release VEGF, among other substances, to build more blood vessels.

The process of angiogenesis is usually tightly controlled:

- Hypoxia causes angiogenic growth factors to be released to promote new blood vessel capillary growth.
- Pericytes detach from the vessel (resulting from Ang-2 signaling).
- The growth factors bind to receptors on the endothelial cells of a nearby blood vessel, activating the endothelial cells. Once activated, the endothelial cells move away from their neighboring endothelial cells as the blood vessel dilates (VE-cadherin is responsible for the tight endothelial junctions, so VE-cadherin signaling allows the endothelial cells to loosen their junctions).
- Once activated, the endothelial cells send a signal from the cell membrane into the cell nucleus telling the nucleus (genes) to make new molecules, including enzymes, such as matrix metalloproteinases (MMPs), which dissolve tiny holes in the basement membrane of the blood vessels.
- The endothelial cells are stimulated to divide, making more endothelial cells that migrate through the holes in the basement membrane and move toward the injured tissue or malignant cells that released the growth factor, like tiny sprouting new blood vessels.
- The tip cell, at the end of the sprout, is selected (by VEGF/VEGFR, NOTCH/DLL4, neuropilin, and JAGGED1 signaling) and releases MMPs, which remodel the extracellular matrix.
- The tip cells are guided by filopodia (cytoplasmic projections that act as small feet) as the sprout migrates toward the area where the antigenic signal came from (e.g., tumor-releasing VEGF).
- Stalk cells follow the tip cell and proliferate, extending the sprout and releasing substances like EGFL7 (epidermal growth factor-like domain containing protein 7, vascular endothelial statin), which help it to bind to the extracellular matrix, and also regulate the formation of the lumen of the blood vessel. Tip cells do not proliferate.
- Adhesion molecules (integrins αvβ3, αvβ5) act like little grappling hooks and pull the sprouting new blood vessels forward toward the tumor.
- Additional enzymes (matrix metalloproteinases, MMPs) are made that dissolve the tissue in front of the sprouting blood vessel so that it can continue to move toward the tumor. After the blood vessel moves forward, the MMPs remodel the tissue to anchor the blood vessel.
- When two tip cells of neighboring sprouts come together, the vessels fuse to form a continuous blood vessel tube or lumen.
- Extracellular matrix is used to make a basement membrane to stabilize the new vessel; endothelial cells stop proliferating, and pericytes are attached to also stabilize the new vessel (recruited by PDGFR/PDGF-B, Ang-1).

- Blood begins to flow from the parent blood vessel to the new blood vessel loops; oxygen in the blood vessel turns off the oxygen sensors in the endothelial cell and turns down angiogenic stimuli (VEGF expression), so building stops and the blood vessel becomes quiescent.

Table 4.2 lists agents currently FDA-approved as antiangiogenic agents. In addition, altering the dose and administration schedule of some standard chemotherapy agents appears to change the mechanism of action. As illustrated in the complex steps of metastasis, there are many opportunities for interruption, causing the arrest of the metastatic cascade.

Drugs that inhibit angiogenesis, either by neutralizing the binding of the ligand VEGF to its receptor (e.g., bevacizumab) or by blocking signaling within the endothelial cell (e.g., sunitinib or sorafinib), or the response to hypoxia (e.g., mTOR inhibitors), may all cause (drug) class-related effects. These include hypertension, believed related to the blockade of nitric oxide, which is necessary for the walls of arterioles and other resistance vessels to relax; rare gastrointestinal perforation with unknown relationship; and bleeding events (epistaxis) with rare hemorrhage. Hypertension is usually amenable to treatment; now, angiotensin-converting enzyme (ACE) inhibitors or angiotensin II receptor blockers are preferred treatment, as they have low interaction potential with angiogenesis inhibitors, help reduce proteinuria, and prevent the expression of plasminogen-activator inhibitor-1 (which may be stimulated by angiogenesis inhibitors and increases the risk of thrombosis) [Izzedine et al., 2009; Wang & Lockhart, 2012]. Maitland et al. (2010) on behalf of a consensus group made recommendations for the initial assessment, surveillance, and management of patients receiving VEGF signaling pathway inhibitors. Recommendations included controlling preexisting hypertension before initiation of a VEGF pathway inhibitor, actively monitoring BP during treatment, especially at the beginning of treatment in the first cycle, targeting a BP goal of < 140/90 (lower in patients with cardiovascular risk

Table 4.2   Targeted Agents That Inhibit Angiogenesis

I. Monoclonal antibodies that bind to proangiogenic growth factors or their receptors: bevacizumab (Avastin), ziv-aflibercept (Zaltrap).

II. Tyrosine kinasse inhibitors that block single or multiple proangiogenic growth factor receptor signals: cabozantinib (Cometriq), pazopanib (Votrient), regorafenib (Stivarga), sorafenib (Nexavar), sunitinib (Sutent), vandetanib (Caprelsa).

III. mTOR (mammalian target of rapamycin) inhibitors that block the response to hypoxia: everolimus (Afinitor), temsirolimus (Torisel).

IV. Agents that may indirectly inhibit angiogenesis through mechanisms not completely understood: the immunomodulatory agents thalidomide (Thalomid), lenalidomide (Revlimid), pomalidomide (Pomalyst).

Data from The Angiogenesis Foundation, http://www.angio.org/understanding/growth.php, accessed May 22, 2014; Chau CH, Figg WD. Antiangiogenesis Agents. *Chapter 47* in DeVita VT, Lawrence TS, Rosenberg SA (eds.) *Cancer: Principles & Practice of Oncology,* 9th ed. Philadelphia, PA: Wolters Kluwer/Lippincott Williams & Wilkins, 2011.

factors), maximizing the dose of each antihypertensive agent and adding agents based on the individual risk and comorbidities, and adding dietary and exercise interventions appropriate to the patient's clinical status. Another important issue that arises with the tyrosine protein kinases sunitinib and sorafinib is a possible reduction in left ventricular ejection fraction (LVEF).

Blockade of an angiogenesis growth factor/signaling pathway may make tumor growth worse over time, as alternate pathways for angiogenesis emerge. Theoretically, by normalizing tumor blood vessels, the tumor cells remain oxygenated, may be less likely to metastasize, and be more responsive to antitumor chemotherapy. Histidine-rich glycoproteins (HGP) are found in the tumor stroma, and they appear to be able to normalize tumor blood vessels and decrease tumor progression (Rolny et al., 2011). The actual mechanism of HGPs may be polarizing tumor-associated macrophages, leading to decreased tumor growth and metastases (Huang et al., 2011).

FINDING AND ESTABLISHING A METASTATIC SITE

First, in order to be embolized, malignant epithelial cells must overcome two types of adhesion, which keeps normal cells adhering to one another and attached to the protein meshwork around it (extracellular matrix), especially in epithelial tissue. This is important because most cancers are epithelial, arising from the epithelial cells covering the outer layer of skin or outer layer and lining of many organs, such as the gut and lungs.

Cell-to-cell adhesion molecules keep normal cells orderly. One molecule is especially important, E-cadherin, which ensures intercellular adhesion. Early studies show that when this molecule is manipulated in cancer cells, it changes a cell from a noninvasive cell to an invasive cell capable of forming tumors. When functional E-cadherin is restored, this tendency can be reversed. Malignant cells are able to inactivate E-cadherin and are released from this requirement of cell-to-cell adhesion.

In addition, for cell survival and reproduction, normal cells must adhere to the extracellular matrix. In laboratory tests, cells in culture cannot grow unless they attach to a surface or achieve *anchorage dependence* (Ruoslahti and Reed, 1994). The molecules on the cell surface that actually do the attachment are *integrins*. Integrins must be intact for cell growth and cell division. It appears that integrins influence a protein in the cell nucleus called cyclin E-CDK2 complex (cyclin-dependent kinase [CDK]), which is necessary for the cell cycle clock to move toward cell growth and division. When cells do not adhere to the extracellular matrix, the lack of integrin adherence causes inhibition of cyclin E-CDK2 in the cell nucleus; the cell cycle clock stops; and the cell commits suicide (apoptosis). Unfortunately, cancer cells are able to circumvent this process, to become *anchorage independent* so cyclin E-CDK2 stays active whether or not the cell is attached, and cells keep growing and dividing, thus avoiding programmed death. In addition, with only a few exceptions (e.g., neutrophils), normal cells cannot penetrate the underlying basement membrane on which they rest, or go through basement membranes of blood vessels (endothelial lining). Like neutrophils, malignant cells release the enzymes called *matrix metalloproteinases (MMPs)* that dissolve parts of the basement membrane, as well as the extracellular matrix, so that like a military tank, the cells can migrate away from the primary tumor and into the neighboring tissue and blood vessels for the process of metastasis.

Once in the blood vessel, it is estimated that only one cell in 10,000 is successful in setting up a new metastatic site distant from the primary tumor. As stated, it must attach to the inner lining of capillaries and dissolve holes in the blood vessel basement membrane to escape into the extravascular tissue. It appears that most cells get trapped in the nearest capillary bed they encounter after leaving the primary tumor. Metastatic cells tend to be large and easily trapped, and many secrete clotting factors that cause platelets to aggregate around them. The primary destination for venous blood from most organs is the lungs; thus, this is the most common metastatic site. Venous blood leaves the gut and goes to the liver first; the liver is the most common metastatic site for intestinal tumors. While this is true, it appears that, in addition, the cell surface adhesion molecules are directed to specific organ locations, via a code much like telephone area codes, so that malignant cells migrate to specific areas, such as prostate cancer to bone. This was further defined by Muller et al. (2001). It also appears that there is "metastatic inefficiency"; some cells go to places without "area codes," or cells from a primary tumor that lack metastatic qualities undergo apoptosis (Wong et al., 2001). The microenvironment of the metastatic site is critical, and it releases growth factors to help the newly arrived metastatic cell survive.

By studying neutrophils, normal cells that migrate where needed to fight infection, Muller et al. (2001) were able to demonstrate that chemokines, soluble substances that carry messages between cells, are responsible for directing breast cancer cells to the primary organs where breast cancer metastasizes: lymph nodes, bone marrow, lung, and liver. Chemokines are small molecules that resemble cytokines and connect with specific receptors on the cell surface, causing rearrangement of the cell's cytoskeleton. This allows cells to adhere firmly to endothelial cells (lining blood vessels) and migrate in a specific direction. Chemokines work with integrins and other proteins on the surface of the cell to direct the breast cancer cells to specific organs. The authors found that breast cancer cells have functionally active chemokine receptors. When these receptors are activated by binding with a ligand (a substance that binds to a receptor on the cell surface and that turns on signal transduction within a cell), the cell activates actin (which gives structure to a cell) polymerization with the formation of pseudopods (fake feet) that allow the cell to migrate and invade tissue. The tissues in which these ligands are overexpressed are the primary metastatic sites in breast cancer. Further, in studies, by neutralizing interactions between the chemokines and their receptors, metastases to lymph nodes and lung could be inhibited. As more is learned about the process of metastases, new agents can be developed to inhibit each of the critical steps, thus preventing the process.

Reprogramming of Energy Metabolism
Most body cells use glucose for an energy source, providing a high number of ATP, the energy currency of the cell, by mitochondrial oxidative phosphorylation. If there is insufficient oxygen, for example, in hypoxic conditions, anaerobic glycolysis is normally used. Cancer cells, however, use glycolysis as their primary energy process, whether there is enough oxygen or not. Glycolysis is very inefficient, and the number of ATP generated is 18 times less than if the cancer cell used glucose as an energy source

(Hanahan and Weinberg, 2011). The end product of this process is lactate. This is called the Warburg effect, after Otto Warburg who first identified this metabolic abnormality. Of course, using such an inefficient system, cancer cells need more glucose, especially as they continue to proliferate, so they increase the number of glucose receptors (GLUT1) to import more glucose into the cells (Hanahan and Weinberg, 2011). Some cancers have this metabolic energy system but also have another, for cells that are better oxygenated, which import and use the lactate as the primary energy source (Hanahan and Weinberg, 2011). As discussed in the angiogenesis section, tumor blood vessels are poorly made, with areas of hypoxia and others of oxygenation. Having two systems would be useful if the tumor cells had sections that were hypoxic and others that were better oxygenated.

TARGETED MOLECULAR AND BIOLOGICAL/IMMUNOLOGICAL AGENTS

As the 21st century unfolds, there is tremendous momentum in transforming cancer care. The human genome project and other molecular research have given great insight into the process of carcinogenesis, metastasis, and molecular flaws that can be targeted to provide cytostatic and cytocidal effects. In addition, genomics has enabled the identification of molecular signatures of different cancers, and this will lead to individualized therapy tailored to the individual tumors of patients. Also, pharmacogenomics has helped to identify which tumor types are responsive to which drugs or therapies, as well as which patients have difficulty metabolizing certain drugs. This chapter presents FDA-approved agents in which an agent targets one or more molecular flaws, thus interrupting the malignant process. If investigational agents are remarkable, they will be included as well.

Targeted molecular therapy is directed at the molecular flaws in the cell, from the receptor tyrosine kinase on the cell membrane, such as EGFR and VEGFR, to the protein kinases passing the message along like a bucket brigade, within the cell, to the cell nucleus.
Targets
Principal signaling pathways and other targets within the cell that are targeted include (Ma and Aijai, 2009; Wilkes, 2011):

- Membrane-bound receptor kinase pathways: EGFR, HER2, hepatocyte growth factor (HGF/c-Met), insulin-like growth factor receptor.
- Intracellular signaling kinase pathways: P13K/Akt/mTOR, mitogen-activated protein kinase (MAP-K), RAF-MEK-RAS, sonic Hedgehog pathway.
- Tumor vasculature and microenvironment: VEGF, VEGFR, integrins, hypoxia inducible factor (HIF).
- Apoptosis pathways.
- Epigenetic abnormalities: DNA methyltransferase, histone deacetylase.
- Protein dynamics: ubiquitin-proteasome system, heat shock protein HSP-90.

Agents that target these molecular and biological flaws can be thought of as large or small molecules. Large molecules are the monoclonal antibodies (MAbs) that must be administered IV, while the small molecules are protein kinase inhibitors that are given

Table 4.3　Quick Tips on Understanding Monoclonal Antibody Names

1st syllable	Name unique to the product	Tras
2nd syllable	Target, e.g., tumor = tu	tu
3rd syllable	Identifies the source, where	zu
	o = mouse	
	zu = humanized	
	xi = chimeric (mouse and human)	
4th syllable	mab = monoclonal antibody	mab
X and z	Consonants to link syllables	Trastuzumab

orally. Table 4.3 gives some quick tips on understanding how MAb names are formed. Small molecules also have a rule: If the drug has an *ib* at the end of the name, the drug has protein inhibitory properties (e.g., imatinib, bortezomib). If the agent has *tin* in it, it is a tyrosine kinase inhibitor (e.g., erlotinib, ponatinib).

Groups of agents that are described in this chapter by generic drug name are: (1) protein kinase inhibitors, both tyrosine and serine-threonine kinase inhibitors; (2) angiogenesis inhbitors; (3) proteasome inhibitors; (4) mTOR inhibitors; (5) Hedgehog pathway inhibitor; and (6) immune checkpoint inhibitors.

The following examples of drugs are based on their mechanism of action that (1) inhibit (target); (2) bring a weapon to destroy the cell (antibody-drug conjugate or ADC, or antibody radio isotope conjugate); or (3) modulate the immune system (iMIDs):

- The abnormal protein kinase BCR-ABL, used to treat CML: bosutinib, dasatinib, imatinib mesylate, nilotinib, ponatinib.
- Epidermal growth factor receptor (EGFR): afatnib, cetuximab, erlotinib, lapatinib, panitumumab.
- HER2: ado-trastuzumab emtansine (ADC), lapatinib, pertuzumab, trastuzumab.
- Angiogenesis: (zif-) aflibercept, axitinib, bevacizumab, ramucirumab.
- mTOR (mammalian target of rapamycin): everolimus, temsirolimus.
- BRAF: dabrafinib, vemurafenib.
- MEK: trametinib.
- PI3K: idelalisib.
- Bruton tyrosine kinase: ibrutinib.
- Multiple targets: Cabozantinib (MET, VEGFR-1, -2, -3, others), ceritinib (ALK, IGF-1R, InsR), crizotinib (ALK, cMET, HGFR), pazopanib (VEGFR-1, -2, -3; PDGFR), regorafenib (VEGFR-1, -2, -3; PDGFR, Raf), sorafenib (VEGFR-2, PDGFR, Raf), sunitinib (VEGFR-1, -2, -3; PDGFR; others), vandetanib (VEGFR-1, -2, others).
- Proteasome Pathway: bortezomib, carfilzomib.
- Hedgehog Pathway: vismodegib.
- Histone deacetylase (HDAC): belinostat, romidepsin for injection, vorinostat.
- Janus-associated kinases (JAKs): ruxolitinib.
- Immune checkpoint: ipilimumab (CTLA-4), pembrolizumab (PD-1).

- CD$_{20}$: rituximab, obinutuzumab, ofatumumab; ibritumomab (antibody-radioisotope conjugate).
- CD$_{30}$ (ADC): brentuximab vedotin.
- CD$_{52}$: alemtuzumab.
- Interleukins: aldesleukin (IL-2), denileukin diftitox (IL-2/diptheria toxin), siltuximab (IL6).
- IMIDs: thalidomide, lenalidomide, pomalidomide.

As targets are identified, they can often be directly attacked by specifically engineered drugs, such as with the fusion protein denileukin diftitox (Ontak), which carries the diphtheria toxin directly to high-affinity IL-2 receptors containing a CD$_{25}$ component, such as activated T- and B-cell lymphocytes. The drug is indicated in the treatment of persistent or recurrent CD$_{25}$, expressing cutaneous T-cell lymphoma (CTCL or mycoses fungoides).

The uses of MAbs include:

- Blocking a receptor so that the ligand cannot bind to it, such as Erb-B1 or EGFR1 (Cetuximab [Erbitux] or panitumumab [Vectibix], or EGFR2 or HER-2-neu [trastuzumab (Herceptin)]), which prevent overexpressed growth factor receptors from sending the signal for cell division.
- Attaching to a cell receptor to bring the body's immune system to kill the cell, such as rituximab (Rituxan), which targets B-lymphocytes that express the CD20 antigen.
- Conjugated MAbs, which carry chemotherapy or radioisotopes like a Trojan horse, which, when internalized into the cell, cause cell death, such as ado-trastuzumab emtansine (Kadcyla) and 90Y ibritumomab (Zevalin).

Figure 4.12 shows mechanisms of MAb therapy. As can be seen, chimeric MAbs contain more mouse than humanized or human MAbs, so premedication is usually required to prevent infusion reactions.

In developing the monoclonal antibody (MAb), the isotype (reflecting the immunoglobulin skeleton of the MAb) of a monoclonal antibody is a deliberate design element. IgG$_1$ MAbs stimulate host immune response and complement activation, and they stimulate antibody-dependent cell-mediated cytotoxicity (ADCC) when the MAb attaches to an antigen. ADCC mobilizes immune elements that can destroy cancer cells, such as NK cells and macrophages. Examples of MAbs that are isotype IgG$_1$ are bevacizumab, trastuzumab, cetuximab, and ipilimumab. IgG$_2$ MAbs activate host defenses mildly, if at all; they do activate complement, but they do not activate ADCC. An example of an IgG$_2$ MAb is panitumumab. Research continues to improve the structural form of MAbs to try to increase effectiveness.

Matrix metalloproteases (MMPs) have been shown to be overexpressed in breast, lung, and prostate cancers, and it appears that certain MMPs are necessary for the formation of new capillaries (angiogenesis), movement of the cancer cells into neighboring tissue (invasion), and metastasis. Normally, the extracellular matrix provides structure between cells, with basement membranes that separate subdivisions within tissues. This matrix prevents aberrant cells from invading other tissues or moving into the bloodstream to go elsewhere in the body.

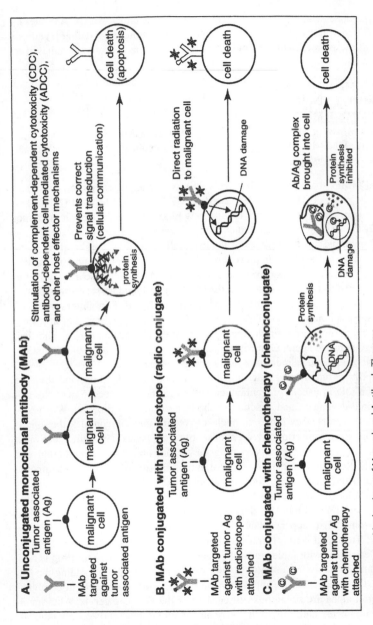

Figure 4.12 Mechanisms of Monoclonal Antibody Therapy

Source: Modified from Wyeth-Ayerst Laboratories, Antibody-Targeted Chemotherapy, 1999, p. 3. Reprinted by permission of Pfizer, Inc.

MMPs are zinc-dependent enzymes that maintain the extracellular matrix of tissues by breaking down different parts of the matrix as needed for ongoing remodeling (synthesis and breakdown of these proteins) over time. There are five main subcategories, based on their site of action:

- Collagenases (MMP-1, MMP-8, MMP-13).
- Gelatinases (MMP-2, MMP-9).
- Stromelysins (MMP-3, MMP-7, MMP-10).
- Membrane-type MMPs or MT-MMPs (MMP-14, MMP-15, MMP-16, MMP-17).
- Others (MMP-11, MMP-12, MMP-18) (Agouron Pharmaceuticals, 1999; Chambers and Matrisian, 1997).

The principal MMPs that appear to be involved in tumor angiogenesis, invasion, and metastasis are gelatinase A (MMP-2), gelatinase B (MMP-9), and MT-MMP-1 (MMP-14). It is known that tumors larger than 2 mm require new blood vessels to nourish the tumor cells and support tumor growth. As the tumor grows, it releases MMPs to enable cells to break from the tumor and attach to pieces of the extracellular matrix, then to break down the extracellular matrix so the cells can move through the tissue compartments, and, finally, to move through the created openings to invade blood and lymphatic vessels and travel to distant sites. It is hoped that through inhibiting the MMPs, new blood vessel growth (angiogenesis), invasion, and metastases can be prevented. Currently, MMP inhibitors (MMPIs) can be specific, such as inhibiting MMP-2 and MMP-9, or broad spectrum; they are being clinically tested either alone as a single agent, or together with chemotherapy, and then continued as a maintenance agent. Clinical studies with MMPIs have been disappointing, and this book will be updated as more promising agents appear.

Retinoids appear to function by interfering with tumor differentiation, and they are believed to have a role in cancer prevention as well as in therapy. Receptors in the cell nucleus are retinoid-dependent and function in the transcription of proteins. When retinoids bind to the receptors, they dimerize nuclear proteins, and the complex then binds to DNA, which results in transcription of a number of target genes. Thus, these activated retinoid receptors regulate the expression of genes responsible for differentiation and replication of cells. Retinoids have been effective in treating superficial Kaposi's sarcoma lesions (alitretinoin) and acute promyelocytic leukemia (tretinoin).

In acute promyelocytic leukemia (APL), there is a translocation of a gene called retinoic-receptor alpha (RAR-alpha) on chromosome 17 that is switched with a gene called PML on chromosome 15. It appears that this translocation of RAR-alpha is part of the etiology of APL. Treatment with all-trans-retinoic acid induces the primitive leukemic blast cells to differentiate, with replacement by normal myelocyte cells. This drug is now indicated for induction remission in patients with APL with subtype 3, including the M3 variant of AML. Other cancers that appear sensitive to 13-*cis* retinoic acid in combination with interferon alpha are squamous cell cancers of the skin and cervix. Alitretinoin (9-*cis*-retinoic acid) occurs naturally in the body and is able to bind and activate intracellular retinoid receptors. It has been shown to inhibit the growth of Kaposi's sarcoma when used topically and is now indicated for topical treatment of cutaneous lesions in patients with AIDS-related Kaposi's sarcoma who do not require systemic therapy.

As more is learned about the pathways involved in malignant transformation, targets are selected and agents developed to target these molecularly flawed pathways. Many patients do well. It is very humbling to realize the plethora of pathways involved, the interrelatedness, and the redundant pathways. As more patients are studied, it is becoming clear that cancer is a dynamic process, and initial responses may over time give way to loss of control as tumor cells mutate and find different pathways to communicate the demands of cancer: proliferation, blood vessels, invasiveness, and immortality.

This raises the question about anticipating the emergence of resistance and adding that drug to the regimen. For example, Batchelor et al. (2007) in a phase II study of the investigational drug cediranib (AZD2171) also combined biomarker and imaging; the investigators were able to visualize impressive normalization of blood vessels in patients with recurrent glioblastoma, leading to reduced cerebral edema, a steroid-sparing effect, as well as almost a doubling of PFS compared with historic controls. However, as most of these patients eventually progressed, biomarkers revealed that the tumor was now using fibroblast growth factor (bFGF) and a new growth factor, chemokines-stroma-cell-derived factor Ia (SDF1a), to build new blood vessels. The authors stated that this underscores the need for multitargeted agents to treat the multiple pathways.

Similarly, patients who respond to erlotinib (Tarceva) in the treatment of lung cancer have specific mutations in the EGFR gene, but ultimately, the tumor becomes resistant to the drug. Pao et al. (2005) described the finding of a new, second mutation that prevented the drug from binding to the EGFR in the same way. Engleman (2007) identified that a subset of patients who did not develop the second mutation developed resistance because the tumor cells found a different pathway to go around the drug-inhibited tyrosine protein kinase—they sent the message via the *MET* oncogene, which now became amplified, and it reactivated the same, mutated signaling pathway that had been shut off by the drug by going through ERBB3. *MET* tyrosine kinases are normally activated by hepatocyte growth factor, but in cancer, they are associated with metastasis.

Another exciting advance accompanying the understanding of different signaling pathways and tumor (signature) mutational pathways is the use of proteonomics and genomics to guide individualized treatment planning. For example, it is now clear that the EGFRI Mabs cetuximab and panitumumab are only effective in patients with colorectal (CRC) tumors that have the wild-type or normal K-RAS/RAS genes and are ineffective in patients with a mutant gene, as K-RAS and other RAS proteins are downstream from the EGFR receptor and their action is unaffected by EGFRI blockade (Benvenuti et al., 2007; Finocchiaro et al., 2007). In addition, they must also have a wild-type BRAF gene.

We are learning more and more about the importance of specific mutational sequences in breast cancer, which correspond to different types of breast cancer that can be used to guide individualized treatment plans (Chaitlanya et al., 2008). Similarly, with K-RAS/RAS in CRC, we can use gene testing of K-RAS/RAS to guide the use of cetuximab and panitumumab, as patients with mutations will not benefit from the therapy.

Yet, it is still a very exciting time in cancer care as the paradigms of care change. Genetic microarrays are being perfected, thus improving diagnosis and treatment and promising to pave the way for individualized multidimensional therapy. It may be possible in the near future to prevent tumors from enlarging beyond 2 mm, prevent metastases, and if patients are not cured of their cancer, contain cancer as a chronic disease much like diabetes, since most patients die from metastasis, not from the primary tumor. Given world politics and individual lifestyle choices, it is probably not possible to eliminate environmental carcinogens. However, the future looks promising that cancer, if not cured, will become a chronic, not terminal, disease over time.

TARGETED THERAPY: NEW ISSUES AND TOXICITIES

Cost

While it is encouraging to see the possibilities of targeted therapy, the cost is of major concern. Today we are in a healthcare economic crisis. For example, a course (3 treatments) of sipuleucel-T (Provenge) costs $93,000 with a resulting median increase in survival of 4.1 months (patients with minimal disease prostate cancer) (Anassi and Ndefo, 2011), while four treatments with ipilimumab (Yervoy) costs $120,000 resulting in a median 3.7-month increase in survival in patients with metastatic melanoma (Fellner, 2012). In contrast, treatment with oral, small molecule Bcr-Abl TKIs results in improved 10-year survival from 20% (no treatment) to 80%, but the cost of imatinib (Gleevec) is $92,000 for a year of therapy (Kantarjian et al., 2013).

Kantarjian and 120 leukemia experts published an article stating that the high price of cancer drugs, in particular, TKIs approved for the management of CML, were harming patients (Kantarjian et al., 2013). The group's concern is patient-centered and documents that up to 10% of patients do not take their prescribed CML medication due to cost, reducing their chances for survival. In addition, the cost of targeted CML drugs is 50–100% higher in the United States as compared to all other countries; for example, in the United States, Gleevec costs $92,000/year, while in Australia and Canada it costs $46,500. This article may stimulate Congressional hearings on the high price of cancer drugs.

Nurses must participate with physicians to help patients and their families understand the cost of treatment options and their copayments for each of the treatment options, as well as help them find resources, such as pharmaceutical drug benefit plans.

Adherence to and Persistence with Oral Anticancer Therapy

The tremendous growth in oral agents has helped nurses refocus on concordance or patient adherence to a prescribed regimen and identify strategies to help patients manage self-administration, calling the provider when specific signs and symptoms of toxicity occur; they must also be knowledgeable about insurance coverage and other resources for paying for oral agents or their copays. As much of patient teaching comes from the nurse in the infusion room, few patients receiving oral agents alone receive this education. This leaves a large gap in nursing care, and many opportunities to improve patient adherence (e.g., following the prescribed instructions exactly) and persistence (e.g., ability to continue taking the medication for a long period after the drug is started) are lost. Fortunately, today nurse practitioners or PAs are providing much of patient teaching and adherence monitoring. Predictors of nonadherence include (Ruddy et al., 2009) pill counts showing too many pills, complex treatment regimens, cognitive impairment, depression or psychological issues, treatment of asymptomatic disease, inadequate follow-up or discharge planning, poor patient-provider relationships, missed appointments, and expensive drugs that have limited drug coverage.

Thus, reasons that patients may not adhere to the drug prescription include cost (some drugs may cost $10,000 a month) and complex instructions or regimen (e.g., taking one drug on an empty stomach and another within 30 min of a meal, such as lapatinib and capecitabine). Nurses should monitor patient adherence by (Moore and Brandt, 2010): (1) asking about missed doses and any problems; (2) managing side effects early to avoid more toxicity and problems; (3) telephoning the patient, especially initially after starting therapy and for the first few weeks; (4) encouraging the patient to do the problem-solving; and (5) giving the patient a treatment calendar and a phone number to call, as well as encouraging patient to report side effects.

Drug Class Effects

Now, as new categories of targeted therapies emerge, many class effects are common denominators for agents in that class, in addition to some drug-specific potential toxicities that relate to other signaling pathways affected. Specific classes of drugs and their class effects include:

- EGFR inhibitors (EGFRIs): sterile inflammatory rash and related skin changes, interstitial lung disease (ILD), diarrhea, and with the MAbs, hypomagnesemia.
- VEGF inhibitors: HTN, bleeding, gastrointestinal perforation, wound-healing complications.
- mTOR inhibitors: metabolic abnormalities, infection, HSRs, gastrointestinal perforation, wound healing complications, and renal failure.

This chapter reviews three groups of adverse side effects that can be challenging to nurses: EGFRI rash, risk of cardiotoxicity from TKIs, and immune-mediated side effects from CTLA-4 inhibitors. There are few evidence-based interventions in the care of patients with new toxicities from targeted therapy; however, nurses across the country share anecdotal successes that may lead to prospective clinical trials. In addition, evidence-based interventions used to manage chemotherapy-related toxicities have been found successful in the management of similar toxicities resulting from similar targeted therapy drugs, such as diarrhea. However, it is important to remember that diarrhea resulting from a CTLA-4 inhibitor (e.g., ipilimumab) is very different in management and threat to life compared to EGFRI-induced diarrhea. As a class, tyrosine kinase inhibitors affect signaling pathways and, as the heart cannot be spared, have some degree of cardiotoxicity, which is discussed here later.

Rash and Related Skin Problems

With the promise of epidermal growth factor receptor inhibitors (EGFRIs), the dose-limiting toxicities of skin rash and diarrhea are clearly within the domain of nursing practice. The degree of rash predicts response, with increased likelihood of response with increased intensity of rash (Saltz et al., 2001). It is also known that patients with mutated *K-RAS/RAS* genes do not respond to EGFRI therapy, so that therapy can be tailored to prevent side effects from a drug to which the patient will not respond (Lièvre et al., 2008). As responding patients need to consider this treatment as chronic therapy, the challenge to nurses is to help patients minimize and manage symptoms and to maximize quality of life.

A number of authors have described effective approaches, including Lynch et al. (2007), who reported the results of a consensus group, as did MASCC (2011) and Alberta Health Services in their evidence-based Clinical Practice Guideline (2012). The following describes the pathophysiology of EGFR toxicity.

EGFRs are located in the epidermis (skin keratinocytes, hair follicles, and sweat and sebaceous glands) and lining of the gastrointestinal tract where EGF is important in stimulating replacement cells and repair of gut mucosal injury. Blockade of EGF pathways in skin results in an inflammatory, sterile rash that then crusts and looks like acne but is pathologically quite distinct. Skin rash is more intense with MAbs such as cetuximab and panitumumab, whereas the rash with small molecular oral TKIs (e.g., erlotinib) may last longer, and dark-skinned patients such as African Americans may have fewer rashes than lighter-skinned patients. In addition, rash does not appear in previously irradiated skin, thought to be due to depletion of the EGFRs, but EGFRIs are radiosensitizers (Lynch et al., 2007). Blockade of EGFR in the gut results in diarrhea. EGFRs are also located in the ascending limb of the loop of Henle in the glomerulus (kidney) (Schrag et al., 2005), where 70% of magnesium is resorbed; EGFR blockade most likely causes the hypomagnesemia associated with monoclonal antibody EGFRIs.

Normally, when skin epidermis is damaged or aged, it is replaced by underlying keratinocytes that have differentiated and migrated to the skin surface. The skin is the primary protective barrier for the body and helps to keep in moisture. Lacouture (2006) describes the pathophysiology; thinking of the pathophysiology in phases can help understand the skin toxicity related to EGFRIs.

Phase I: weeks 0–1, erythema and edema like a sunburn. EGFR inhibition in the skin stops the keratinocytes from differentiating and migrating, and they are arrested. The body senses that they should not be there and thus causes them to undergo apoptosis. The dead keratinocytes cause the release of chemokines, which recruit neutrophils to the area as part of the sterile, inflammatory response. The patient feels a sunburn-like reaction (erythema, tenderness, slight swelling) on the face and areas that have previously been exposed to the sun. The goal is to preserve skin integrity, minimize discomfort, and prevent infection. Key patient teaching includes (1) use skin cream with emollients to keep the skin from drying out; (2) avoid sun exposure, using a sunblock of SPF 30 or higher, with a zinc base; (3) use a mild soap with active ingredients that reduce skin drying, such as pyrithione zinc (Head & Shoulders); (4) consider applying aloe gel to red, tender areas; (5) report distressing tenderness, as pramoxine (lidocaine topical anesthetic) may help; (6) keep fingernails clean and trimmed; and (7) apply zinc ointment to rectal mucosa after washing (Walker and Lacouture, 2006).

Lacouture et al. (2010) studied whether beginning preventive treatment before the rash occurs could decrease severity of panitumumab-related rash. They found that grade 2 or higher rash and other skin changes were significantly reduced in patients who received daily moisturizer, sunscreen, topical hydrocortisone, and oral doxycycline compared to a control group; there was no difference in tumor response.

Phase II: weeks 1–3, paulopustules appear: This sterile inflammatory process results in death of the keratinocytes (undergo apoptosis) and the formation of debris, which causes a papular rash on the skin. At the same time, the skin is no longer fortified by healthy keratinocytes, and thus, it thins and is unable to preserve water in the body, leading to skin dryness (xerosis) and itching. The rash begins within 7–10 days of starting therapy and peaks in intensity in 2–3 weeks and then gradually gets better. The goal is to prevent infection, promote healing, and maximize comfort and coping. See drug information in this chapter, as well as drug package inserts for specific information on holding or discontinuing drug for severe dermatologic adverse effects.

Management should be as follows:

- **Grade 1/mild rash,** which is localized, does not interfere with ADLs, and is not infected (Lynch et al., 2007): Maintain current drug dose, observe or give topical hydrocortisone 1% or 2.5% or clindamycin 1% gel (anti-inflammatory benefit); reassess in 2 weeks.
- **Grade 2/moderate,** which is generalized, has mild symptoms, minimal effect on ADLs, and no infection: Continue EGFRI dose; use topicals (hydrocortisone 2.5% or clindamycin 1% gel). If pustules are present, also add doxycycline 100 mg PO twice daily or minocycline 100 mg PO twice daily (give antimicrobial and anti-inflammatory effect); and reassess after 2 weeks.
- **For grade 3 or severe rash,** which is generalized, severe, has a significant impact on ADLs, and increased risk of infection: Interrupt dose for up to 21 days or until rash is improved to grade 2. Treat rash with topicals (hydrocortisone 2.5% or clindamycin 1% gel), and patient should receive doxycycline 100 mg PO twice daily or minocycline 100 mg PO twice daily, along with methylprednisolone (Medrol dose pack); reassess after 2 weeks. Restart treatment based on manufacturer's recommendation. Interrupt or discontinue drug if rash worsens (Lynch et al., 2007). If the rash appears infected (exudate, vesicular formation, different appearance), obtain C+S, treat empirically until sensitivity received, and/or obtain dermatology consult.
- **Grade 4,** generally drug is discontinued.

The rash develops into pustules with crusting related to the drying of the cellular debris (keratinocytes, neutrophils, fibrin, serum) in about 4–6 weeks after the initial EGFRI drug dose; the skin tenderness goes away. Use the same algorithm for management as in phase II. Patient deaths have been reported related to infected skin lesions, so prevention of infection is a primary goal.

Phase III: weeks 3–5, lesions crust. The skin becomes drier (xerosis) with pruritus and the formation of telangiectasias (dilated capillaries in the skin). The skin flakes and itches. For flaking skin, keratolytics such as lactic acid, salicylic acid, or urea-containing topicals such as 12% Lac-Hydrin or other exfoliating lotions can be helpful. Topical agents for itch include Sarna Ultra Anti-Itch Cream, Aveeno Anti-Itch Concentrated Cream, and Regenecare gel for the body and for the scalp, Clobetasol propionate (Olux foam) or fluocinolone acetonide and topical shampoo, 0.01% (Capex shampoo) (O'Keefe et al., 2006; Walker and Lacouture, 2006). Itching may require pharmacologic management: diphenhydramine 25–50 mg PO and cetirizine 10–20 mg PO daily, and for resistant itch, pregabalin (Porzio et al., 2006) and doxepin (Greene et al., 1985) have shown impressive results.

Phase IV: weeks 5–8, persistent dry skin, erythema, other skin/hair changes. EGFR blockade of the hair follicles and nail beds results in hair changes (hair thinning or alopecia on scalp but increased hair growth on the eyelids (trichomegaly) or face (hypertrichosis)). The hair texture can change (changes in texture and strength). Paronychia (periungual inflammation) can develop with crusted lesions on nail folds and tenderness. Painful skin fissures on the fingers can develop. For paronychia, treat with emollients, and consider flurandrenolone (Cordran) for wrapping around the finger. Consider flurandrenolone as well for fissures (O'Keefe et al., 2006). It is important to assess eyelashes, and if they are long, they can fold back and irritate the conjunctiva; refer to an ophthalmologist for redirection as needed (Borkar et al., 2013). The STEPP trial demonstrated that the intensity of EGFRI rash could be reduced, with a significant decrease in grade 3 rash when prophylactic treatment was begun prior to starting therapy with the EGFRI drug. This RCT compared patients who received doxycycline 100 mg PO twice daily steroid cream to external skin areas and SPF when going outside prior to starting treatment with panitumumab, to patients who received intervention only when they developed a rash. There was a significant difference between groups, and many practitioners are beginning to administer prophylactic agents (Lacouture, 2009).

Skin-related problems from the multitargeted TKIs sunitinib and sorafinib are a bit different, as their targets are different from EGFR. Sorafinib can cause facial erythema, splinter subungual hemorrhage, with or without alopecia, whereas sunitinib can cause hair depigmentation (white when on therapy, and dark during treatment break), splinter subungual hemorrhage, with or without periorbital edema (Widakowich et al., 2007). Both agents can cause hand-foot syndrome (acral erythema) involving the palms of the hands and soles of the feet and are characterized by symmetrical red, swollen skin that may have dysesthesia or paresthesia and may progress to pain and desquamation. Specific nursing interventions are discussed under the specific drug.

Cardiotoxicity
Tyrosine kinases (TKs) transduce signals from the outside of, or within, the cell and send the message to the cell nucleus to stimulate or inhibit cell functions. Tyrosine kinase inhibitors (TKIs) can block receptor TKs or their ligands (MAbs) outside the cell or inside the cell by small molecule TKIs, which prevent phosphylation; thus, this message, for cell proliferation or other survival functions, never reaches the cell nucleus. TKs in the heart are blocked as well, however, which leads to damage to myocytes and, in some individuals, altered heart function. Because cardiac function is not a clinical endpoint of the drug trials and many of the drugs are nonselective in some of their targets, it is difficult to know the exact risk and incidence of cardiotoxicity except for the well-studied trastuzumab and lapatinib. Force et al. (2007) describe our understanding of the TKI-specific cardiotoxicity. The authors point out that cardiac myocytes have a very high demand for energy (ATP) and are thus especially susceptible to agents that alter mitochondrial function.

The first and most widely studied drug is trastuzumab (Herceptin), a MAb-directed against EGFR2 (HER-2), which had an incidence of cardiotoxicity of 4–7% as a single agent, increasing to 27% when combined with an anthracycline, and manifested first as a decrease in LVEF (left ventricle pumping ability) and later as symptomatic CHF. Thus, an anthracycline chemotherapy agent should not be given at the same time as trastuzumab. Lapatinib blocks both EGFR1 and EGFR2 but in contrast only has a small risk of lowering LVEF below normal values of 50–70%. EGFR2 (HER-2) is an important pathway in cardiomyocyte development and function. In addition, HER-2 dimerizes with EGFR3 and EGFR4 receptor tyrosine kinases and is a coreceptor for their ligands the neuregulins, which are all expressed in cardiac tissue. HER-2 (EGFR2)–EGFR4 signaling is essential to myocardial contractility in the adult. The authors hypothesize that by blocking the HER-2 receptor, dimerization does not occur, with loss of signaling leading to changes in mitochondrial membrane polarization, ATP depletion, and loss of contractility. Mitochondria are the energy factory and storehouse of ATP, the energy currency of the cell. Other factors enhancing cardiotoxicity might be mediated by ADCC, as trastuzumab is an IgG_1 MAb.

Force et al. (2007) also discuss cardiotoxicity related to TKIs. Imatinib (Gleevec) has rarely caused CHF, and in those patients, electron microscopy of the heart has shown nonspecific mitochondrial abnormalities. When cardiomyocytes are studied in culture with imatinib, there is significant damage to the mitochondria resulting in cell death and declines in ATP stores. The active myocardium uses tremendous amounts of energy in the form of ATP to contract, and if these are inadequate, the heart fails. Other hypotheses include the fact that this drug and others like the related dasatinib inhibit ABL, which may be protecting the heart from oxidative stress. Dasatinib has an incidence of 4% LVEF dysfunction or CHF when taken for 6 months or longer. The multitargeted TKIs sorafinib and sunitinib may cause myocardial injury as collateral effects. Patients receiving sunitinib reportedly have an 11% incidence of declines in LVEF < 50% when taken for 6 months, which may have been compounded by possible drug-induced hypothyroidism. The drug inhibits PDGFa/b, which are also expressed on cardiomyocytes and believed important in cardiomyocyte survival; however, the exact cause is unknown. Patients taking sorafinib have a 2.9% incidence of acute coronary syndrome (compared to 0.4% in the placebo arm). Sorafinib inhibits PDGFRs as well as RAF1 and BRAF, which are important in oxidative stress-induced injury. In addition, when RAF1 is deleted in a mouse heart, it develops a dilated, hypocontractile heart with fibrosed and dead cardiomyocytes; however, the actual mechanism of cardiotoxicity with these drugs is still unclear. Although there is some provocative evidence that statins may provide not only some degree of cardioprotection, but also specific antitumor effects, focused research on this and other agents needs to be done to define any potential benefit or interaction (Popat and Smith, 2008). Future targeted therapy studies need to consider possible influences on the heart cells, either directly or indirectly.

QT Prolongation

A number of targeted anticancer agents cause prolongation of the QT interval and may be associated with sudden death. It is important to understand how prolongation of the QT interval on the EKG can be life-threatening. See Figure 4.13 for the cardiac cycle. An EKG is the capture of electrical activity in the heart over time. The QT interval measures the time or duration of ventricular activation (depolarization) and recovery (repolarization). On the EKG, the QT interval is the time from the start of the Q wave (beginning of ventricular depolarization) to the end of the T wave (ventricular repolarization). If the

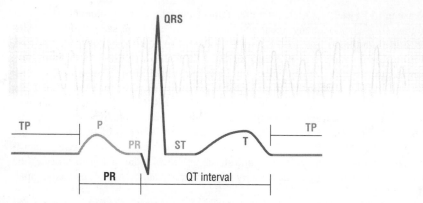

Figure 4.13   Basic Components of the ECG Complex
(*From 12-Lead ECG: The Art of Interpretation,* courtesy of Tomas B. Garcia, MD)

heart is beating rapidly, the QT interval will be short, as compared to a slower heartbeat, where the QT interval will be longer. Because this period of time is affected by how fast the heart beats, it is corrected by a mathematical formula called Bazett's formula, and the interval is called the QTc, or corrected QT interval. The QTc = QT interval divided by the square root of R-R (interval from the onset of one QRS complex to the next), measured in seconds. Fortunately, the QTc is available from many Internet sources, such as Up-To-Date. The normal QTc is 0.2–0.4 seconds (or 200 to 400 ms). Normal corrected QTc intervals are < 0.44 seconds (440 ms). Since 2005, the FDA has required all drugs to be tested for their effect on the QT interval (FDA, 2005). This is because when the QTc is prolonged, it sets up a risk for tachyarrythmia, and, more worrisome, a special type of ventricular tachycardia called torsades de pointes, which on EKG looks like the ventricular beats are twisting around the isoelectric line (see Figure 4.14). This can quickly progress to ventricular fibrillation and sudden cardiac death. The risk is further increased by hypomagnesemia, hypokalemia, and hypocalcemia (Strevel et al., 2007). In addition, patients can have familial QT prolongation syndrome, or take drugs that prolong the QTc.

Table 4.4 shows drugs that can prolong the QTc interval, and a more complete list can be found at http://www.azcert.org/medical-pros/drug-lists/drug-lists.cfm, the website of Arizona Center for Education and Research on Therapeutics. Table 4.5 shows the NCI CTCAE grading of QTc prolongation. In addition, oncology patients have comorbidities, which increase the risk, such as older age and preexisting cardiac disease. Often they take concomitant medications that increase the risk, such as antidepressants, antiemetics, antibiotics, antihistamines, antifungals, and perhaps antipsychotics or methadone (Brell, 2010).

Oncology nurses should understand the danger of QTc prolongation and work collaboratively with physicians and midlevel practitioners to reduce the risk of adverse events. For example, although MAbs themselves do not cause QT prongation, the MAbs cetuximab and

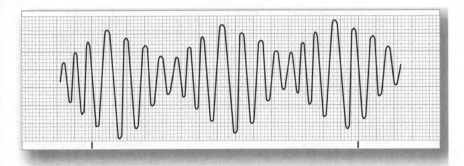

Figure 4.14 Torsades de Pointes
(*From Arrhythmia Recognition: The Art of Interpretation,* courtesy of Tomas B. Garcia, MD)

Table 4.4 Selected Drugs Causing QTc Prolongation

Antiarrythmics: amiodarone*, bepridil*, disopyramide*, dofetilide*, dronedarone, flecainide, ibutilide*, isradipine, mibefradil, nicardipine, procainamide*, quinidine*, ranolazine, sematilide, sotalol*

Psychotropics: amitriptyline, chlorpromazine*, desipramine, doxepin, haloperidol*, lithium, mesoridazine*, olanzapine, paliperidone, pimozide*, quetiapine, risperidone, thioridazine*, sertindole, venlafaxine, ziprasidone

Antimicrobials: azithromycin, chloroquine*, clarithromycin*, erythromycin*, gatifloxacin, gemifloxacin, halofantrine mefloquine*, levofloxacin, moxifloxacin, ofloxacin, pentamidine*, sparfloxacin*, spiramycin, telithromycin, voriconazole

Antihistamines: astemizole*, terfenadine*

Anticancer drugs: arsenic trioxide*, dasatinib, lapatinib, nilotinib, romidepsin, sorafinib, sunitinib, tamoxifen, vandetanib, vorinostat

Other drugs: alfuzosin, amantadine, atazanavir, chloral hydrate, cisapride*, dolasetron, droperidol*, felbamate, ganisetron, foscarnet, fosphenytoin, hydrochlorothiazide, indapamide, levomethadyl*, methadone*, octreotide, ondansetron, oxytocin, perflutren lipid microspheres, quinine, tacrolimus, vardenadil, vasopressin

*Risk of torsades de pointes

Source: Data from Force T, et al. Cardiotoxicity of Tyrosine-Kinase Targeting Drugs. *Nat Rev Cancer* 2007; 7 332–344; Strevel EL, et al. Molecularly Targeted Oncology Therapeutics and Prolongation of the QT Interval. *J Clin Oncol* 2007; 35 3362–3372; Arizona CERT, http://www.azcert.org, accessed June 20, 2010.

panitumumab cause hypomagnesemia. If this becomes severe, the patient is at significant risk for torsades de pointes. Anticancer agents that are associated with increased incidence of QT prolongation include the histone deacetylase inhibitors vorinostat (Zolinza, 3.5–6%) and romidepsin (Istodax, 2–63%); and the tyrosine kinase inhibitors dasatinib (Sprycel, < 1–3%), lapatinib (Tykerb, 16%), nilotinib (Tasigna, 1–10%), sunitinib (Sutent, dose dependent), and vandetanib (Vandetanib, 14%) (Yeh and Bickford, 2009; Bello et al., 2007).

Table 4.5   National Cancer Institute CTCAE Version 4.0 Grading Criteria for QTc Prolongation

Grade	Definition
I	QTc > 450–480 ms
II	QTc > 481–500 ms or > 60 ms above baseline
III	QTc > 501 ms
IV	QTc > 501 ms; life-threatening signs of symptoms (e.g., arrhythmia, CHF, hypotension, shock, syncope, torsades de pointes)
V	Death

Source: Data from Common Terminology Criteria for Adverse Events (CTCAE) Version 4.0. Published: May 28, 2009 (v4.03: June 14, 2010). U.S. DEPARTMENT OF HEALTH AND HUMAN SERVICES National Institutes of Health National Cancer Institute. Available at: http://evs.nci.nih.gov/ftp1/CTCAE/CTCAE_4.03_2010-06-14_QuickReference_8.5x11.pdf

As more targeted therapies are investigated and FDA-approved, oncology nurses will have more agents that require monitoring of the QTc interval baseline and regularly during therapy, especially in patients with a history of cardiovascular disease or who are also taking other agents that potentially could prolong the QTc interval. Strevekl et al. (2007) describe a number of investigational agents in the following classes that have potential to cause prolongation of the QTc interval: HDAC inhibitors (depsipeptide, LBH589, LAQ824), multitargeted TKIs (ZL647), vascular disrupting agents CA4P, farnesyl protein transferase inhibitors (L-778123, lonafarnib), and the protein kinase C inhibitors enzastaurin. In most cases, the effect of the QTc prolongation is insignificant and without sequelae. Key nursing measures, however, include (1) identifying patient's risk for prolongation of QTc over and above that conferred by the agent (e.g., hypokalemia, hypomagnesemia, congenital long QT syndrome, taking antiarrhythmic medications, cumulative high-dose anthracycline therapy, and history of cardiovascular heart disease); and (2) identifying and correcting hypokalemia, hypomagnesemia, and hypocalcemia, if they exist, prior to administration of the targeted agent. In addition, as ordered by the physician or midlevel practitioner, monitor EKGs with QTc calculation baseline and regularly during therapy. A number of drug serum levels are affected by food or other interacting drugs. The nurse should review with the patient how the drug is self-administered and also what other drugs the patient is taking, either prescribed, over-the-counter, or "health food supplements." The nurse should also know the specific management of patients if they develop changes in their QTc interval. For example, with nilotinib, if a patient develops a QTc of > 480 ms, the drug is withheld, the patient's serum potassium and magnesium are checked, and if below the LLN, these electrolytes are repleted, bringing them to normal limits. The patient's concomitant medications are also reviewed. If the QTc returns to < 450 ms and to within 20 ms of baseline within 2 weeks, the drug is resumed at the prior dose. If the QTc is between 450 and 480 ms after 2 weeks, the nilotinib dose is reduced to 400 mg once daily. If, following dose reduction to 400 mg once daily, the QTc returns to > 480 ms, nilotinib is discontinued. An EKG with calculation of the QTc is repeated about 7 days after all dose adjustments (Tasigna package insert, 2010).

Although rare, if torsades de pointes does develop, the first treatment is IV magnesium sulfate 2 g, regardless of the patient's serum magnesium level (Yeh and Bickford, 2009).

Defibrillation is indicated if fibrillation or sustained ventricular tachycardia occur, and overdrive transvenous pacing can be used to shorten the QTc (Yeh and Bickford, 2009). The patient's serum potassium should be maintained in the high-normal range, and any QT-prolonging medications should be discontinued, along with other drugs interfering with the patient's metabolism (Yeh and Bickford, 2009).

Immune-Mediated Adverse Effects of Immune Checkpoint Inhibitors
The immune checkpoint inhibitors [ipilimumab (Yervoy), nivolumab (Opdivo), pembro-lizumab (Keytruda)] have potential toxicities related to their effect on specific organs. The T-lymphocyte hyperactivated immune response damages normal organ tissue, such as the gut (colitis), liver (hepatitis), or endocrine organs (e.g., thyroid). Patients require close monitoring during therapy and for 6 months following completion of therapy (Weber et al., 2015). Almost all immune toxicities can be reversed by administration of corticosteroids, which should be used only for grade 3–4 toxicity, or prolonged grade 2 immune adverse effects (Weber et al., 2015). Patients receiving PD-1 inhibitors may take a longer time to fully respond than patients receiving ipilimumab, so they require long-term monitoring (Weber et al., 2015). In general, patients receiving immune checkpoint inhibitors may experience fevers, chills, and lethargy; maculopapular skin toxicity; diarrhea and colitis; elevated LFTs; and hypophysitis, thyroiditis, and adrenal insufficiency.

Ipilimumab (Yervoy), the first immune checkpoint inhibitor, was FDA approved using a Risk Evaluation and Mitigation Strategy (REMS) to ensure that providers, patients, and pharmacists are well versed in the potential immune-related adverse effects. The drug enhances and prolongs the activation and proliferation of cytotoxic T-lymphocytes so that the immune system can identify and kill the cancer cells. Normally, CTLA-4 slows/stops this immune response after the invading pathogen has been neutralized to protect normal body tissue from the effects of the powerful immune system. Most patients (70–88%) experience adverse effects, which can occur during therapy or be delayed in onset. It is important for the nurse and patient/family to know that adverse reactions, as well as the patient tumor response to ipilimumab, can take months to occur (Rubin, 2011). Skin reactions typically occur after 3–4 weeks (after first or second drug dose), GI tract adverse effects occur 6.5–7 weeks after starting therapy, liver toxicity occurs after 9–10 weeks, and endocrine effects occur after 3–9 weeks (Rubin, 2011; Weber et al., 2012).

As part of the REMS program, nursing assessment, guide for management, and checklist are available, as well as a patient wallet card from the drug-specific website. Early side effects that can occur during the infusion or up to 24–72 hours or more after the infusion are fatigue, nausea, vomiting, diarrhea, fever, headache, dizziness, rash, and pruritus (Fecher et al., 2013). The most immune-related adverse effects are enterocolitis, hepatitis, dermatitis, neuropathy, and endocrinopathy (Yervoy package insert, 2013). Most reactions begin during treatment, but some may occur weeks to months after the drug has been stopped. Early identification of toxicity is critical, so that early intervention can follow and minimize the effect. Most low-grade immune-related adverse effects are managed with supportive care, while moderate or severe toxicity is managed by drug interruption and high-dose steroids followed by a taper

Table 4.6   Assessment and Management of Immune-Related Adverse Effects

Adverse Effect	Nursing Assessment/ Management	Medical Management
Skin: Erythematous and/or maculopapular rash (**10–30% BSA**) may occur; dry skin; pruritus (localized or diffuse, intermittent); vitiligo.	• Inspect for rash (trunk, hands, feet), assess extent, skin dryness, other changes. • Assess use/teach use of prophylactic emollients or moisturizers. • Cold washcloth or oatmeal baths, tepid baths for pruritus.	**Mild** (grade 1): moisturizers, topical interventions as needed, monitor, continue drug. **Moderate** (grade 2) topical steroids, antihistamines, or other antipruritic agents, consider course of oral steroids if symptoms persist after 1-2 weeks, consider dermatology consult if persists; continue drug if improved/resolved.
Skin: Erythematous rash (> 30% BSA); pruritus diffuse and constant; blisters, ulceration, bullae, necrotic or hemorrhagic lesions; toxic epidermal necrolysis.	Inspect for rash, assess extent, skin dryness, and other changes. • Teach patient to call if symptoms develop. • Assess use/teach use of prophylactic emollients or moisturizers. • Cold washcloth or oatmeal baths, tepid baths for pruritus.	**Severe** (grade 3–4): systemic steroids (IV or PO); taper over ≥ 4 weeks once symptoms controlled; consider hospitalization; dermatology consult +/− biopsy. Discontinue ipilimumab (if grade 3 rash improves to grade 1 or less, consider resuming drug).
GI: Diarrhea, blood or mucus in stool, abdominal cramping or pain, nausea or vomiting, constipation, fever. Rule out other causes (e.g., infection, progression).	• Assess baseline bowel elimination pattern prior to starting drug, then monitor. • Teach patient to report right away any changes in bowel pattern, indigestion, bloating, gas, or cramping. • Teach patient to purchase OTC anti-diarrheal agents (e.g., loperamide). • If diarrhea occurs, teach patient to increase hydration, dietary modifications, and to call MD/RN. • Teach patient/family how to obtain immediate medical attention if needed.	**Mild** (grade 1, < 4 stools/day over baseline): symptomatic treatment, no steroids, monitor closely; continue drug. **Moderate** (grade 2, 4–6 stools/day over baseline, abdominal pain, blood, or mucus): symptomatic treatment, no steroids, monitor closely. • If improves to ≤ grade 1, continue ipilimumab. • If persistent symptoms > 5–7 days, start oral steroids, once symptoms controlled taper steroids over ≥ 4weeks; hold drug until ≥ grade 1. **Severe** (grade 3–4, ≥ 7 stools/day over baseline, severe or persistent abdominal pain; fever; ileus; peritoneal signs; life threatening): hig-dose IV steroids, consider hospitalization, GI consult,

Table 4.6 *(Continued)*

Adverse Effect	Nursing Assessment/ Management	Medical Management
		endoscopy, evaluate for perforation as indicated, use analgesics cautiously; discontinue drug.
		• Persistent symptoms or relapse with taper, consider infliximab or other immunosuppressive agent.
		• Avoid infliximab if perforation or sepsis.
		• Reevaluate for other causes.
		• Discontinue ipilimumab.
Hepatic dysfunction: Elevated AST/ALT, bilirubin; jaundice; abdominal, RUQ pain; nausea or vomiting; fever; encephalopathy.	• Assess LFTs baseline and before each treatment. • Assess for nausea, vomiting, pain, jaundice. • Liver toxicity may be insidious as it is often asymptomatic. • Teach patient to report symptoms right away.	**Mild** AST/ALT < 3 × ULN and/or total bilirubin <1.5 × ULN (or < 2 baseline): monitor, consider assessing more frequently; continue ipilimumab.
Rule out other causes (e.g., medications, infection, disease progression).		**Moderate** AST/ALT 3–8 × ULN (or ≥ 2 baseline): increase monitoring daily × 3 days or every 3 days; consider autoimmunity workup, consider imaging-disease progression.
		• Improves to ≤ grade 1, continue ipilimumab.
		• No improvement: initiate steroids (PO/IV), consider hospital admission, monitor LFTs daily, consider GI/hepatology consult, taper steroids over ≥ 4 weeks if LFTs normalized; hold ipilimumab until resolved.
		Severe (AST/ALT > 8 × ULN +/or total bilirubin > 5 × ULN): high dose IV steroids, hospital admission, daily LFTs; hepatology/GI consult, consider liver biopsy; discontinue ipilimumab
		• If relapse with steroid taper: Increase steroid until improvement; then slow taper.
		• If persistently refractory to steroid taper OR no response to high-dose steroids in 3–5 days, consider additional immunosuppressive agent.

(continued)

Table 4.6 *(Continued)*

Adverse Effect	Nursing Assessment/ Management	Medical Management
Endocrine dysfunction: abnormal electrolyes, fatigue, malaise, headache, vision changes or field cuts, nausea or vomiting, abdominal pain, impotence, loss of libido, cardiac arrhythmia, hypotension, mental status changes. Suspect adrenal crisis. Workup: serum studies (TSH, free T4, total and free T3, AM cortisol, ACTH) • Consider LH, FSH, prolactin, testosterone (in men). • MRI brain with and without contrast with pituitary cuts. • Evaluate for other causes (e.g., medications, infection, brain metastases, disease progression).	• Assess for signs/symptoms of hypopituitarism: headache, worsening fatigue, lethargy. • Assess for less common symptoms: weakness, memory loss, personality changes, visual field changes (uveitis), nausea and vomiting, fever, hypotension, impotence, decreased TSH or cortisol. • Assess for uncommon symptoms resulting from hypophysitis, panhypopituitarism, hypothyroidism, pancreatitis, adrenal insufficiency. • If patients have a change in symptoms, they must be screened for endocrinopathies (e.g., worsening fatigue, new nausea/vomiting). • Assessment is often difficult, as patient disease-related symptoms may be present.	**Normal results:** no further intervention, continue to monitor and repeat labs; continue ipilimumab. **Moderate:** abnormal findings; symptomatic, no evidence of adrenal crisis: • Initiate steroids (PO/IV) • Endocrine consult • Hold ipilimumab **Severe:** hypotension, hemodynamic instability, altered mental status, shock: • High-dose IV steroids • Evaluate for sepsis, treat if indicated • Hospitalization • Supportive care • Endocrine consult • Discontinue ipilimumab • Once stabilized • Consider steroid taper; may need permanent steroid replacement therapy. • Coinsider need for additional hormone replacement therapy. • Additional workup as indicated.

(Fecher et al., 2013; Yervoy package insert, 2013). Algorithms are available for toxicity management (Fecher et al., 2013). The drug is discontinued if steroids cannot be tapered to 7.5 mg prednisone/equivalent/day, or failure to complete the full treatment course within 16 weeks from first dose.

Early identification and intervention are key components to patient safety, and the nurse must be knowledgeable about the potential adverse effects and key points to teach patients and their families. It is important to reassure patients that most side effects are mild to moderate and can be effectively managed (Rubin, 2012). However, it is critical that the patient/family report any symptoms as they occur, and the nurse should assess the patient in a systematic fashion at each visit. With each potential toxicity, medical management (Fecher et al., 2013) and nursing management (Rubin, 2012) is indicated in Table 4.6.

SUMMARY OF SELECTED ISSUES AND NURSING CARE

EGFRI-Related Rash

Nursing care focuses on minimizing symptoms and helping patients maximize their quality of life. Nursing priorities have been highlighted in each of the phases, and treatment options may overlap as symptoms occur earlier or later. Patient educational materials are available, including CancerCare Connect: Tips for managing treatment-related rash and dry skin at http://www.cancercare.org/publications/tagged/rash; (attached) MASCC: Caring for your skin, hair, and nails when on targeted therapy, at http://www.mascc.org/assets/documents/skin_toxicity_egfri_patientbrochure. pdf. All patients should be taught to keep their skin well moisturized using a water-based emollient, avoiding sun exposure and using a sunblock (at least SPF 30, and zinc-based), and staying well hydrated (Lynch et al., 2007). There is much opportunity for nurses to become involved in nursing research to test different approaches to minimizing rash and optimizing quality of life. For example, Hetherington et al. (2007) reported a case report of a patient receiving cetuximab 500 mg/m^2 every other week. The patient developed a grade 2 rash on her face and thorax, but when she received local cooling before and during her treatment, she developed only a grade 1 rash. Studies are beginning to look at quality of life. Zachariae et al. (2003) found that dermatologic disease-related impairment of quality of life predicted psychological symptoms. Molinari et al. (2005) found that 5 of 13 patients in a study of cetuximab-induced rash felt the rash had significant impact on their quality of life. Wagner et al. (2007) reported that the most commonly distressing aspects of skin toxicity on patients receiving EGFRIs are pain, irritation, pruritus, dryness, hair changes, interference with activities (work or hobbies), and the emotional impact (feeling depressed, frustrated, isolated). Fortunately, in a study by Humblet (2007), patients with the most severe rash also tended to have the highest response rate; patients who were most bothered by skin toxicity also had the highest quality-of-life scores and fewest symptoms from cancer. Nurses need to assess the impact of skin changes on patients in terms of function, emotion, social, and physical, such as pain or tenderness.

Cytokine Release/Hypersensitivity

MAbs continue to have a role in targeted therapy. The nurse should be cognizant of the drug risk for causing infusion reactions (cytokine release syndrome or grades 1–2 hypersensitivity), should premedicate the patient before infusion as ordered, and should monitor the patient closely during treatment. Other MAbs may cause severe hypersensitivity reactions (HSRs), either anaphylactoid (nonimmune mediations, no prior sensitization) or hypersensitivity (IgG E-mediated, prior sensitization) reactions, and the reader is referred to *Chapter 1* for a review of assessment and management of HSRs.

Class-related toxicities have been identified and are highlighted with each drug. For example, the EGFRIs all cause skin toxicity to some degree, diarrhea, and risk of interstitial lung disease as the function of EGFRs is blocked. EGFRI MAbs block the EGFRs in the distal loop of Henle responsible for reabsorption of magnesium, and thus, these drugs are associated with significant hypomagnesemia. Angiogenic inhibitors block the action of VEGF to stimulate VEGFRs. VEGF appears to be necessary for nitric oxide, a vasodilator, and thus, all angiogenic inhibitors are associated with hypertension. As more experience is gained in the treatment of patients, more class-related side effects will be identified, helping the nurse to anticipate side effects.

Drug Interactions of TKIs

Many of the TKIs are metabolized by the P450 microenzyme system in the liver and have significant side effects with other drugs or substrates. The cytochrome P450 microenzyme system is a very important protection pathway for humans and has evolved over the millennia. It is a superfamily of isoenzymes that are found in the endoplasmic reticulum and mitochondrial membranes within cells and serve to detoxify poisons that are ingested or inhaled. They are found in the cells lining the nose, kidneys, lungs, small intestines, and liver and in the saliva. The P450 system is responsible for the metabolism of 75% of all drugs that are metabolized. Within this family, isoenzymes also synthesize estrogen and testosterone. CYP refers to cytochrome and is followed by a number, which refers to the family, then a letter, which refers to a subfamily, and then a final number, which refers to a subfamily gene. These genes regulate the proteins used to metabolize drugs. Individuals can have polymorphisms, or different copies of the gene, causing differences in how effectively liver enzymes detoxify the drugs. Sometimes this is an ethnic variation, and sometimes it is just due to an inherited gene copy. There are four classifications for how well people metabolize drugs: (1) **Ultra-rapid** metabolizers break down the drug quickly so the serum drug levels are low, and the person may need higher drug doses to get the intended drug effect; (2) **extensive** metabolizers metabolize the drug normally; (3) **intermediate** metabolizers are slightly less effective than extensive metabolizers, and the drug dose is usually effective; and (4) **poor** metabolizers break down the drug very slowly, resulting in higher serum drug levels as the drug is not completely metabolized, with more toxicity.

The CYP3A4 is the most important pathway in drug metabolism. If a drug is metabolized, it is called a **substrate**. If a drug inhibits the enzyme's activity so that the substrate is incompletely metabolized, it is called an **inhibitor**. If a drug increases the drug's metabolism, it is called an **inducer** (e.g., St. John's wort induces the CYP3A4 system, as does smoking). Induction will decrease the drug's effectiveness, making drug serum levels too low. Table 4.7 describes key drug interactions of targeted therapies.

Table 4.7   Important Drug Interactions Between P450 Isoenzyme Pathways and Targeted Therapies

Drug	P450 Isoenzyme	Inducer, Inhibitor, Substrate
Afatinib (Gilotrif)	P-glycoprotein (P-gp)	**Not** metabolized by P450; but transported by P-glycoprotein (P-gp). **Pgp inhibitors:** Increase afatinib systemic exposure: amiodarone, cyclosporine A, erythromycin, Itraconazole, ketoconazole, nelfinavir, quinidine, ritonavir, saquinavir, tacrolimus, verapamil. Avoid coadministration; if must coadminister, reduce afatinib dose by 10 mg/day if not tolerated. **Pgp inducers:** Decrease afatinib systemic exposure: carbamazepine, phenytoin, phenobarbital, rifampicin, St. John's wort. If must coadminister, consider increasing afatinib dose by .10mg/day as tolerated. Teach patient to avoid St. John's wort.
Axitinib (Inlyta)	CYP3A4/5	**Inhibitors of CYP3A4:** The following are examples of strong inhibitors that may increase serum levels of axitinib: atazanavir, clarithromycin, ketoconazole, indinavir, itraconazole, nefazodone, nelfinavir, ritonavir, saquinavir, telithromycin, voriconazole; do not coadminister, but if necessary, decrease axitinib dose by 50%. Dose may be increased or decreased based on safety and tolerability. If coadministration of the strong inhibitor is discontinued, axitinib dose should be returned (after 3–5 half-lives of the inhibitor) to that used before initiating the CYP3A4/5 inhibitor. Teach patient to avoid grapefruit and grapefruit juice. **Inducers of CYP3A4:** Strong inducers may decrease serum axitinib concentrations and coadministration should not be done: carbamazepine, dexametasone, phenytoin, phenobarbital, rifampin, St. John's wort. Avoid coadministration if possible. If coadministered with a moderate inducer (e.g., bosentan, efavirenz, etravirine, modafinil, nafcillin), axitinib serum levels may be reduced, so avoid coadministration if possible.
Bexarotene (Targretin)	CYP3A4	**Inhibitors of CYP3A4:** The following may increase serum levels of bexarotene: ketoconazole, itraconazole, erythromycin, gemfibrozil, grapefruit, grapefruit juice; also (strong) atazanavir, indinavir, nefazodone, nelfinavir, ritonavir, saquinavir, telithromycin, voriconazole; (moderate) amprenavir, aprepitant, diltiazem, fluconazole, verapamil; and (weak) cimetidine. DO NOT give together with gemfibrozil, as dangerous bexarotene levels result; avoid coadministration with other drug(s) if possible or monitor closely for drug side effects.

(continued)

Table 4.7 *(Continued)*

Drug	P450 Isoenzyme	Inducer, Inhibitor, Substrate
		Inducers of CYP3A4: May decrease serum bexarotene concentrations: rifampin, phenytoin, phenobarbital; also carbamazepine, dexamethasone, efavirenz, griseofulvin, modafinil, nafcillin, nevirapine, primidone, rifabutin, St. John's wort. Avoid coadministration if possible. If coadministered, assess need for increased bexarotene dose. Studies have not been done. Do NOT give together with St. John's wort.
		Other: Bexarotene decreases tamoxifen plasma concentration by 35%; decreases atorvastin AUC by 50%; may also decrease serum levels of systemic hormonal contraceptives. Avoid coadministration if possible, and use two types of contraception, including one type of barrier contraceptive. When given with carboplatin/paclitaxel, bexarotene AUC is increased by 2-fold; administer together cautiously, if at all.
Bortezomib (Velcade)	CYP3A4; 2C19; 1A2 CYP3A4 CYP3A4 CYP3A4	**CYP3A4 Inhibitors:** May increase serum levels of bortezomib: ketoconazole, and (strong inhibitors) atazanavir, clarithromycin, indinavir, itraconazole, grapefruit, grapefruit juice, nefazodone, nelfinavir, ritonavir, saquinavir, telithromycin, voriconazole; (moderate) amprenavir, aprepitant, diltiazem, fluconazole, verapamil; and (weak) cimetidine. If strong inhibitor coadministered, assess for increased bortezomib toxicity. Melphalan-prednisone coadministration increased bortezomib serum levels, but this is not thought to be clinically relevant.
		CYP3A4 Inducers: Can theoretically lower bortezomib levels: rifampin, carbamazepine, phenytoin, St. John's wort. Do not coadminister, but if must, assess for efficacy of bortezomib and need for increased drug dose. Do NOT give together with St. John's wort.
		CYP2C9 Inhibitor: Omeprazole coadministration did not affect bortezomib serum levels.
Bosutinib (Bosulif)	CYP3A4	**CYP3A4 Inhibitors:** Decreased metabolism of bosutinib by strong inducers can increase bosutinib AUC (boceprevir, clarithromycin, conivaptan, indinavir, itraconazole, ketoconazole, nefazodone, nelfinavir, posaconazole, ritonavir, saquinavir, telaprevir, telithromycin, voriconazole) and moderate CYP3A4 inhibitors (aprepitant, amprenavir, atazanavir, ciprofloxacin, crizotinib, darunavir, diltiazem, erythromycin, fluconazole, fosamprevir, grapefruit and grapefruit juice, imatinib, verapamil), also increase bosutinib plasma concentrations; do not give concurrently. For example, coadministration with ketoconazole increased bosutinib plasma concentrations and AUC 8.6-fold, compared to bosutinib alone.

Table 4.7 *(Continued)*

Drug	P450 Isoenzyme	Inducer, Inhibitor, Substrate
		CYP3A4 Inducers: Increased metabolism of bosutinib can significantly decrease bosutinib serum level by strong inducers (carbamazepine, dexamethasone, phenytoin, phenobarbital, rifabutin, rifampin, St. John's wort) and moderate CYP3A4 inducers (bosentan, efavirenz, etravirine, modafinil, nafcillin); do not give concurrently. For example, coadministration with rifampin decreased bosutinib AUC by 94%.
		Proton Pump Inhibitors (PPIs): May decrease bosutinib serum levels; avoid concurrent use, and consider using short-acting antacids instead.
		Substrates of p-glycoprotein (P-gp): Bosutinib may increase the plasma concentration of P-gp substrates, such as digoxin. Monitor patient closely for toxicity, or serum drug levels if available.
Cabozantinib (Cometriq)	CYP3A4	**CYP3A4 Inhibitors:** Strong inhibitors decrease metabolism of cabozantinib and can increase cabozantinib AUC (atazanavir, clarithromycin, indinavir, itraconazole, ketoconazole, nefazodone, nelfinavir, ritonavir, saquinavir, telithromycin, voriconazole). Avoid concomitant administration. Teach patient to avoid grapefruit juice and fruit.
		CYP3A4 Inducers: Strong inducers can increase metabolism of cabozantinib and decrease cabozantinib serum level (carbamazepine, dexamethasone, phenytoin, phenobarbital, rifabutin, rifampin, rifapentine, St. John's wort). Avoid coadministration.
Ceritinib (Zykadia)	CYP3A4	**CYP3A Inhibitors:** Strong inhibitors may increase ceritinib plasma levels. Avoid concurrent use with strong inhibitors (atazanavir, clarithromycin, indinavir, itraconazole, ketoconazole, nefazodone, nelfinavir, ritonavir, saquinavir, telithromycin, troleandomycin, voriconaze); grapefruit and grapefruit juice. If must coadminister with ceritinib, reduce ceritinib dose by 33%, rounded to the nearest capsule strength.
		CYP3A Inducers: May decrease ceritinib plasma concentration; avoid concurrent use with strong inducers (e.g., carbamazepine, phenobarbital, phenytoin, rifabutin, rifampin, St. John's wort).
		CYP3A4, CYP2C9 Substrates: Avoid concurrent use of drugs that are substrates of CYP3A4 and CYP2C9 and have a narrow therapeutic window (e.g., CYP3A4: alfentanil, cyclosporine, dihydroergotamine, ergotamine, fentanyl, pimozide, quinidine, sirolimus, tacrolimus); CYP2C (phenytoin, warfarin).

(continued)

Table 4.7 *(Continued)*

Drug	P450 Isoenzyme	Inducer, Inhibitor, Substrate
Crizotinib (Xalkori)	CYP3A4	**CYP3A Inhibitors:** May increase crizotinib plasma concentration. Avoid concurrent use with strong inhibitors (atazanavir, clarithromycin, indinavir, itraconazole, ketoconazole, nefazodone, nelfinavir, ritonavir, saquinavir, telithromycin, troleandomycin, voriconaze); grapefruit and grapefruit juice; use caution if concomitant use of moderate CYP3A inhibitors. **CYP3A Inducers:** May decrease crizotinib plasma concentration; avoid concurrent use with strong inducers (e.g., carbamazepine, phenobarbital, phenytoin, rifabutin, rifampin, St. John's wort). **CYP3A4 Substrates:** Coadministered drugs that are metabolized by CYP3A4 may need to be dose-reduced, if narrow therapeutic window (e.g., alfentanil, cyclosporine, dihydroergotamine, ergotamine, fentanyl, pimozide, quinidine, sirolimus, tacrolimus).
Dabrafenib (Tafinlar)	CYP3A4; CYP2C8	**CYP3A Inhibitors:** Strong inhibitors may increase dabrafenib plasma concentration. Avoid concurrent use with strong inhibitors (atazanavir, clarithromycin, indinavir, itraconazole, ketoconazole, nefazodone, nelfinavir, ritonavir, saquinavir, telithromycin, troleandomycin, voriconaze); grapefruit and grapefruit juice. **CYP3A Inducers:** May decrease dabrafenib plasma concentration; avoid concurrent use with strong inducers (e.g., carbamazepine, phenobarbital, phenytoin, rifabutin, rifampin, St. John's wort). **CYP2C8 Inhibitors:** Strong inhibitors such as gemfibrozil may increase dabrafenib serum levels; do not coadminister. **Substrates of CYP3A4, CYP2C8, CYP2C9, CYP2C19, CYP2B6 That Are Sensitive:** Coadministration may result in loss of efficacy (e.g., midazolam is a CYP3A4 substrate, dabrafenib decreases midazolam C_{max} and AUC by 61% and 74% respectively). **Drugs That Increase Gastric pH:** May alter drug solubility and reduce bioavailability; drug serum levels, and effectiveness. Studies have not been done (e.g., PPIs, H2-receptor antagonists, antacids). **Other Drug Effects:** WARFARIN, dexamethasone, hormonal contraceptives: serum levels may be decreased with loss of efficacy; avoid use and substitute with alternative drug/method of contraception.

Table 4.7 *(Continued)*

Drug	P450 Isoenzyme	Inducer, Inhibitor, Substrate
Dasatinib (Sprycel)	CYP3A4	**CYP3A4 Inhibitors:** The following may decrease metabolism of dasatinib, resulting in increased serum concentrations of dasatinib: (strong) atazanavir, clarithromycin, erythromycin; grapefruit juice, grapefruit, indinavir, itraconazole, ketoconazole, nefazodone, nelfinavir, ritonavir, saquinavir, telithromycin, voriconazole; (moderate) amprenavir, aprepitant, diltiazem, fluconazole, verapamil; and (weak) cimetidine. Avoid coadministration; if must give together, monitor closely for drug toxicity and consider reducing dasatinib dose to 20 mg daily (if taking 100 mg/day, or 40 mg if taking 140 mg/day). **CYP3A4 Inducers:** May decrease dasatinib serum levels (e.g., rifampin decreased dasatinib levels by 82%); others: carbamazepine, dexamethasone, phenobarbital, phenytoin, St. John's wort. If must coadminister, assess efficacy of dasatinib and need for increased drug dose. Do NOT give together with St. John's wort. **Antacids:** May decrease dasatinib levels; avoid coadministration or administer at least 2 hours before or after the dasatinib dose. **H₂-Antagonists/Proton Pump Inhibitors:** May decrease dasatinib serum levels; use antacids instead. **CYP3A4 Substrates:** Drug is a time-dependent inhibitor of CYP3A4 and may decrease metabolism of drugs primarily metabolized by CYP3A4, such as alfentanil, astemizole, terfenadine, cisapride, cyclosporine, ergotamine, fentanyl, pimozide, quinidine, sirolimus, tacrolimus, or ergot alkaloids. Avoid coadministration or monitor drug closely for side effects; single dose of dasatinib with simvastatin increases simvastatin (AUC) serum level by 37%.
Erlotinib (Tarceva)	CYP3A4; CYP1A2	**CYP3A4 Inhibitors** (may decrease metabolism of erlotinib and increase its plasma concentration when coadministered with strong inhibitors): e.g., atazanavir, clarithromycin, indinavir, itraconazole, ketoconazole, nefazodone, nelfinavir, ritonavir, saquinavir, telithromycin, trcleandomycin (TAO), voriconazole, or grapefruit (fruit or juice). Consider dose reduction of erlotinib if severe reactions occur. **CYP3A4 Inducers** (may increase metabolism of erlotinib and decrease its plasma concentration): rifapentine, rifabutin, rifampicin, carbazepine, phenytoin, phenobarbital, St. John's wort; avoid if possible, otherwise may need to increase dose of erlotinib.

(continued)

529

Table 4.7 *(Continued)*

Drug	P450 Isoenzyme	Inducer, Inhibitor, Substrate
		Rifampicin decreased erlotinib AUC by 66% to 80%: use alternative drug that does not induce CYP3A4 or consider erlotinib dose escalation every 2 weeks while monitoring the patient, to a maximum dose of 450 mg. If the erlotinib dose is increased, and rifampicin (or other inducer) is discontinued, reduce erlotinib dose immediately to the indicated starting dose.
		CYP3A4 and CYP1A2 Inhibitor (e.g., ciprofloxacin): Increased erlotinib AUC 39%; avoid coadministration.
		CYP3A4 Substrate: Midazolam dose was reduced by 24% when given prior to and together with erlotinib.
		CYP1A2 Inducers: May decrease erlotinib plasma concentrations.
		pH-Altering Drugs: Erlotinib solubility is pH dependent. Drugs that alter the pH of the upper GI tract may alter erlotinib solubility and its absorption. There is risk of low erlotinib serum levels if the drug is given in combination with drugs that change GI pH, such as omeprazole (a proton pump inhibitor) or ranitidine (an H^2 receptor antagonist); avoid if possible. If antacids are used, antacids should be separated by several hours from the dose of erlotinib. If an H2 receptor antagonist like ranitidine is required, erlotinib must be taken 10 hours AFTER the dose, and at least 2 hours before the next dose of H2 receptor antagonist.
		Warfarin: Increased International Normalized Ratio (INR) and bleeding is possible; monitor INR and patient bleeding, and decrease warfarin dose as needed.
		Cigarette smoking: Reduced erlotinib serum levels; teach patient to quit smoking, and if not possible, consider titrating erlotinib dose upwards; if the patient is able to quit after the dose increase, return dose to the indicated starting dose. It is unknown if nicotine in nicotine patches interacts with erlotinib.
		Food: Increases bioavailability of erlotinib by 100%; give drug on empty stomach, at least 1 hour before or 2 hours after a meal.
Everolimus	CYP3A4	**CYP3A4 Inhibitors:** Strong inhibitors may increase everolimus serum levels: e.g., atazanavir, clarithromycin, indinavir, itraconazole, ketoconazole, nefazodone, nelfinavir, ritonavir, saquinavir, telithromycin, voriconazole; AVOID coadministration; teach patient to avoid grapefruit, grapefruit juice.

Table 4.7   (Continued)

Drug	P450 Isoenzyme	Inducer, Inhibitor, Substrate
		Moderate CYP3A4 Inhibitors and/or Pgp Inhibitors: Use cautiously if at all, together with (moderate) amprenavir, aprepitant, diltiazem, fluconazole, verapamil, CYP3A4 inhibitors. If must be coadministered, reduce dose of everolimus. If the interacting drug is discontinued, give a washout period of 2–3 days before increasing the everolimus dose back to the dose prior to initiation of the moderate CYP3A4 or Pgp inhibitor. Assess closely for increased everolimus toxicity.
		CYP3A4 Inducers: Can lower everolimus serum levels if coadministered with carbamazepine, fosphenytoin, dexamethasone, phenytoin, phenobarbital, primidone, rifabutin, rifampin, St. John's wort. Avoid coadministration. If coadministration is necessary, increase the everolimus dose; if/when the interacting drug is discontinued, give a washout period of 3–5 days before decreasing the everolimus dose back to the dose prior to initiation of the strong CYP3A4 inducer. Teach patient NOT to take St. John's wort.
		CYP3A4 Substrates: Everolimus is a substrate of CYP3A4 and a substrate and moderate inhibitor of P-glycoprotein efflux pump; it is also a competitive inhibitor of CYP3A4 and a mixed inhibitor of CYP2D6.
Ibrutinib (Imbruvica)	CYP3A4	**CYP3A4 Inhibitors:** Strong inhibitors may increase ibrutinib serum levels: e.g., atazanavir, clarithromycin, indinavir, itraconazole, ketoconazole, nefazodone, nelfinavir, ritonavir, saquinavir, telithromycin, voriconazole; AVOID coadministration; teach patient to avoid grapefruit, grapefruit juice.
		Moderate CYP3A4 Inhibitors: Use cautiously if at all together with moderate CYP3A4 inhibitors: e.g., amprenavir, aprepitant, diltiazem, fluconazole, verapamil. If must be coadministered, reduce dose of ibrutinib to 140 mg. See dose modifications. Assess closely for increased toxicity.
		CYP3A4 Inducers: Can lower ibrutinib serum levels if coadministered with carbamazepine, fosphenytoin, dexamethasone, phenytoin, phenobarbital, primidone, rifabutin, rifampin, or St John's wort. Avoid coadministration. Teach patient NOT to take St. John's wort.
		Antiplatelet or Anticoagulation Therapy: Increased risk of bleeding; monitor patients and lab work closely.

(continued)

Table 4.7 *(Continued)*

Drug	P450 Isoenzyme	Inducer, Inhibitor, Substrate
Imatinib mesylate (Gleevec)	CYP3A4; CYP2C9 (warfarin)	**CYP3A4 Inhibitors:** May increase serum levels of imatinib mesylate: (strong) atazanavir, clarithromycin, indinavir, itraconazole, grapefruit, grapefruit juice, ketoconazole, nefazodone, nelfinavir, ritonavir, saquinavir, telithromycin, voriconazole; AVOID coadministration; use cautiously if at all together with (moderate) amprenavir, aprepitant, diltiazem, fluconazole, verapamil, and (weak) cimetidine CYP3A4 inhibitors. If must be coadministered, assess closely for increased imatinib toxicity. **CYP3A4 Inducers:** Can lower imatinib serum levels if coadministered with carbamazepine, fosphenytoin, dexamethasone, phenytoin, phenobarbital, primidone, rifabutin, rifampin, St. John's wort. Avoid coadministration. Do NOT give together with St. John's wort. **CYP3A4 Substrates:** Imatinib interferes with CYP3A4 metabolism of the following drugs: • Simvastatin levels: increases simvastatin levels; monitor LDL and reduce simvastatin dose if needed. • Cyclosporine, pimozide: increased plasma concentrations; avoid concurrent administration. • Triazolobenzodiazepines, dihydropyridine calcium channel blockers, and HMG-CoA reductase inhibitors: may have increased serum levels; use cautiously and monitor patient closely. • Eletriptan (Relpax): do not administer within 72 hr of imatinib; monitor VS closely. **Interference with Drugs Metabolized by CYP2D6:** If drugs metabolized by CYP2D6 are coadministered with imatinib, serum levels of these drugs will be elevated; coadminister cautiously and monitor closely. **Warfarin:** Do not coadminister; use low molecular weight heparin (LMWH). **Acetaminophen:** May increase serum acetaminophen levels.
Lapatinib (Tykerb)	CYP3A4; CYP2C8	**CYP3A4 Inhibitors:** The following may decrease metabolism of lapatinib, resulting in increased serum concentrations of lapatinib: (strong) atazanavir, clarithromycin, grapefruit juice, grapefruit, indinavir, itraconazole, ketoconazole, nefazodone, nelfinavir, ritonavir, saquinavir, telithromycin, voriconazole. Avoid coadministration; if must give together with strong inhibitor, monitor closely for drug toxicity and consider reducing lapatinib dose. Use cautiously if at all, and monitor patient closely if coadministered with (moderate) amprenavir, aprepitant, diltiazem, fluconazole, verapamil; and (weak) cimetidine CYP3A4 inhibitors.

Table 4.7 *(Continued)*

Drug	P450 Isoenzyme	Inducer, Inhibitor, Substrate
		CYP3A4 Inducers: May decrease lapatinib serum levels: carbamazepine, dexamethasone, phenytoin, phenobarbital, rifabutin, rifampicin, St. John's wort. If must coadminister, assess efficacy of lapatinib and need for increased drug dose. Do NOT give together with St. John's wort.
		CYP3A4 and CYP2C8 Substrates: Lapatinib inhibits both pathways, so assess for toxicity in coadministered drugs that are metabolized by either pathway: **p-glycoprotein (Pgp) metabolism** (transport system)—lapatinib coadministered with Pgp substrates (e.g., loperamide, dexamethasone): Assess for toxicity from increased substrate concentration. Conversely, lapatinib is also a substrate of Pgp so that if given with an inhibitor of Pgp (e.g., quinidine), lapatinib drug levels are likely to be elevated; assess for lapatinib toxicity.
		CYP3A4, P-pg Substrates: Midazolam AUC increases by 22–45% when coadministered. Paclitaxel (CYP2C8 and p-gp substrate): increased paclitaxel AUC by 23%; digoxin (P-pg substrate): increased digoxin AUC by twofold; monitor digoxin serum levels, and reduce dose by half f concentration is greater than 1.2 mg/mL.
Nilotinib (Tasigna)	CYP3A4	**CYP3A4 Inhibitors:** The following may increase serum levels of nilotinib: (strong) atazanavir, clarithromycin, grapefruit, grapefruit juice, indinavir, itraconazole, ketoconazole (increases nilotinib levels threefold), nefazodone, nelfinavir, ritonavir, saquinavir, telithromycin, voriconazole. AVOID coadministration with strong inhibitors; if must coadminister, consider dose reduction of nilotinib and monitor patient closely for toxicity, including QT intervals on EKG.
		Coadminister cautiously, if at all, drugs that are moderate (amprenavir, aprepitant, diltiazem, erythromycin, fluconazole, verapamil) or weak (cimetidine) inhibitors of CYP3A4; monitor closely for drug side effects.
		Inducers of CYP3A4: May decrease serum nilotinib concentrations: carbamazepine, dexamethasone, phenytoin, phenobarbital, rifabutin, rifampicin (decreased nilotinib levels by 80%), rifapentin, St. John's wort. Avoid coadministration if possible. If coadministered, assess need for increased nilotinib dose by 50%. Do NOT give together with St. John's wort.

(continued)

Table 4.7 *(Continued)*

Drug	P450 Isoenzyme	Inducer, Inhibitor, Substrate
		Drugs That Affect Gastric pH: Proton Pump Inhibitors (PPIs): Nilotinib has pH-dependent solubility, and is less soluble if gastric pH is high (e.g., with PPIs, e.g., omeprazole decreased nilotinib AUC by 34%); avoid coadministration if possible, and if not, separate doses of nilotinib and PPI or antacid by at least several hours.
		Drugs That Prolong QTc: Avoid coadministration.
		Food: Increases serum levels of nilotinib; patient should take nilotinib on an empty stomach, 1 hour before or 2 hours after the drug dose.
		Substrates:
		• Nilotinib is an inhibitor of CYP3A4, CYP2C8, CYP2C9, CYP2D6.
		• Nilotinib may induce CYP2B6, CYP2C8, CYP2C9.
		• Warfarin: Nilotinib is a competitive substrate, so INR needs to be monitored closely and dose adjusted frequently. (Warfarin is metabolized by CYP2C9 and CYP3A4, so warfarin should be avoided if possible.)
		• Nilotinib is a substrate of the efflux transporter p-glycoprotein (Pgp). If administered with Pgp inhibitors (e.g., quinidine), serum concentration of nilotinib will be increased; avoid coadministration.
Olaparib (Lynparza)	CYP3A4	**CYP3A inhibitors** may increase olaparib serum levels: *Avoid coadministration with* **strong inhibitors** (e.g., itraconazole, telithromycin, clarithromycin, ketoconazole, voriconazole, nefazodone, posaconazole, ritonavir, lopinavir/ritonavir, indinavir, saquinavir, nelfinavir, boceprevir, telaprevir) and **moderate inhibitors** (e.g., amprenavir, aprepitant, atazanavir, ciprofloxacin, crizotinib, darunavir/ritonavir, diltiazem, erythromycin, fluconazole, fosamprenavir, imatinib, verapamil). See dose modification if drug must be coadministered with olaparib. Teach patient to avoid grapefruit and Seville oranges while taking olaparib as this may also increase olaparib serum levels and toxicity.
		CYP3A4 inducers may decrease olaparib serum levels: *Avoid* concomitant administration of **strong inducers** (e.g., rifampicin, phenytoin, carbamazepine, St. John's Wort) as this may decrease serum level of olaparib by up to 87%. Avoid coadministration with **moderate inducers** (e.g., bosentan, efavirenz, etravirine, modafinil, nafcillin) but if unavoidable, assess for decreased olaparib efficacy.

Table 4.7 *(Continued)*

Drug	P450 Isoenzyme	Inducer, Inhibitor, Substrate
Palbociclib (Ibrance)	CYP3A4	**CYP3A inhibitors:** may increase serum palbociclib levels and increasing toxicity (e.g., itraconazole increases Cmax 70% and AUC 87%). Avoid co-administration of strong inhibitors, and drug is essential, consider dose reduction of palbociclib. **CYP3A4 inducers** may decrease palbociclib serum levels (e.g., rifampin decreased Cmax 70% and AUC 85%): *Avoid* concomitant administration of **strong inducers** (**e.g.**, rifampicin, phenytoin, carbamazepine, St. John's Wort) and moderate inducers. **CYP3A substrates** (e.g., midazolam) When coadministered with palbociclib, midazolam Cmax increased 37%, and AUC 61%. If substrate is sensitive and has a narrow therapeutic window, consider dose reduction of substrate. **Gastric pH elevating medicines:** In fasting patient, PPI given concomitantly, reduces Cmax by 80% and AUC 62%. If given to a patient who is eating, there is no significant interaction.
Panobinostat (Farydak)	CYP3A4	Drug is a CYP3A substrate, and it inhibits CYP2D6. **CYP3A inhibitors:** May increase serum panobinostat levels; avoid concomitant use or decrease panobinostat dose. Teach patients to avoid star fruit, pomegranate juice, and grapefruit/grapefruit juice. If coadministered with a strong CYP3A inhibitor (e.g., boceprevir, clarithromycin, conivaptan, indinavir, itraconazole, ketoconazole, lopinavir/ritonavir, nefazodone, nelfinavir, posaconazole, ritonavir, saquinavir, telaprevir, telithromycin, voriconazole), reduce panobinostat dose to 10 mg. **CYP3A4 inducers:** Decrease serum panobinostat level by up to 70%; avoid concomitant use. **CYP2D6 substrates:** Panobinostat may increase the Cmax and AUC of sensitive substrate by 80% and 60% respectively (e.g., atomoxetine, desipramine, dextromethorphan, metoprolol, nebivolol, perphenazine, tolterodine, venlafaxine) or CYP2D6 substrates with a narrow therapeutic window (e.g., thioridazine, pimozide); avoid coadministration. If must coadminister, monitor patients closely for toxicity. **Drugs that prolong the QT interval** (e.g., anti-arrhythmic medicines amiodarone, disopyramide, procainamide, quinidine, sotalol; other drugs such as chloroquine, halofantrine, clarithromycin, methadone, moxifloxacin, bepridil, pimozide). If anti-emetic agents that prolong the QT interval are used (e.g., dolasetron, ondansetron, tropisetron), monitor ECG and QTc frequently.

(continued)

Table 4.7 *(Continued)*

Drug	P450 Isoenzyme	Inducer, Inhibitor, Substrate
Pazopanib (Votrient)		**CYP3A Inhibitors:** Increase pazopanib concentrations, and risk for toxicity; avoid coadministration (e.g., atazanavir, clarithromycin, indinavir, itraconazole, ketoconazole, nefazodone, nelfinavir, ritonavir, saquinavir, telithromycin, voriconazole). If must co administer, reduce pazopanib dose. Teach patients not to eat/drink grapefruit/grapefruit juice.
		CYP3A Inducers: Decrease pazopanib concentrations and effectiveness (e.g., carbamazepine, dexamethasone, phenytoin, phenobarbital, rifabutin, rifampin, St. John's wort). If coadministration of a strong inducer cannot be avoided, do not give pazopanib. Teach patient not to take St. John's wort.
		CYP3A4 Substrates: If narrow therapeutic window, do not coadminister as they create potential for serious adverse events.
		Other Drugs: Simvastatin: concomitant use increases incidence of ALT elevations (e.g., 27% vs 14%); if used together and elevated ALT occurs, follow dosing guidelines or consider an alternative to pazopanib.
Pomalidomide (Pomalyst)	CYP1A2 and CYP3A4/5	**CYP1A2 Strong Inhibitors:** (e.g., ciprofloxacin, fluvoxamine) in the presence of a strong CYP3A4/5 inhibitor (ketoconazole): may increase pomalidomide serum level: DO NOT coadminister; if medically necessary, reduce pomalidomide dose.
		Drug is a substrate for P-gP.
		Smoking: May reduce pomalidomide serum level due to CYP1A2 induction; teach patient to stop smoking, as smoking may reduce the drug's effectiveness.
Ponatinib (Iclusig)	CYP3A4/5; CYP2C8; CYP2D6	**CYP3A4 Inhibitors:** Strong inhibitors may increase ponatinib serum levels: e.g., atazanavir, clarithromycin, indinavir, itraconazole, ketoconazole, nefazodone, nelfinavir, ritonavir, saquinavir, telithromycin, voriconazole. AVOID coadministration with strong inhibitors; if must coadminister, consider ponatinib dose reduction and monitor patient closely for toxicity. Teach patient to avoid grapefruit and grapefruit juice.
		Inducers of CYP3A4: Strong inducers may decrease serum panatinib concentrations: e.g., carbamazepine, dexamethasone, phenytoin, phenobarbital, rifabutin, rifampicin, rifapentin, St. John's wort. Avoid coadministration if possible. If coadministered, assess efficacy of ponatinib. Teach patient NOT to take St. John's wort.

Table 4.7 (Continued)

Drug	P450 Isoenzyme	Inducer, Inhibitor, Substrate
		Drugs That Affect Gastric pH: Ponatinib has pH-dependent solubility, and is less soluble if gastric pH is high, e.g., with proton pump inhibitors (PPIs), which reduce bioavailability. Avoid coadministration if possible; if not, separate doses of ponatinib and PPI or antacid by at least several hours, and assess ponatinib efficacy.
		Drugs That Are Substrates of P-gp (e.g., aliskiren, ambrisentan, colchicine, dabigatran, etexilate, digoxin, everolimus, fexofenadine, imatinib, lapatinib, maraviroc, nilotinib, posaconazole, ranolazine, saxagliptin, sirolimus, sitagliptin, tolvaptan, topotecan) or **ABCG2 transport system:** have not been studied; do not coadminister.
Regorafenib (Stivarga)	CYP3A4	**CYP3A4 Inhibitors:** Strong inhibitors may increase regorafenib serum levels: e.g., atazanavir, clarithromycin, indinavir, itraconazole, ketoconazole, nefazodore, nelfinavir, ritonavir, saquinavir, telithromycin, voriconazole. AVOID coadministration with strong inhibitors. Teach patient to avoid grapefruit and grapefruit juice.
		Inducers of CYP3A4: Strong inducers may decrease serum regorafenib concentrations: e.g., carbamazepine, dexamethasone, phenytoin, phenobarbital, rifabutin, rifampicin, rifapentin, St. John's wort. Avoid coadministration. Teach patient NOT to take St. John's wort.
		CYP3A4 Inhibitors: No interaction.
Sorafenib (Nexavar)	CYP3A4; UGT1A9; CYP2C9 (warfarin)	**CYP3A4 Inducers:** May increase the metabolism of sorafenib and decrease its serum level; carbamazepine, dexamethasone, phenytoin, phenobarbital, rifabutin, rifampin (decreases sorafenib AUC by 37%), rifapentin, St. John's wort. Avoid coadministration if possible. If coadministered, assess need for increased sorafenib dose. Do NOT give together with St. John's wort.
		Substrates:
		• No increased systemic exposure to concomitant administered drugs: Midazolam (CYP3A4), dextromethorphan (CYP2D6 substrate), omeprazole (CYP2C9 substrate).
		• CYP2C9 substrate: Warfarin: potential increased INR; monitor and correct warfarin dose frequently.
		Other Interactions:
		• Neomycin 1 gm tid for 5 days: decreased sorafenib AUC by 54%.
		• Drugs that increase gastric pH: sorafenib solubility if pH dependent by concomitant administration of omeprazole did not make a clinically significant change.

(continued)

Table 4.7 *(Continued)*

Drug	P450 Isoenzyme	Inducer, Inhibitor, Substrate
Sunitinib (Sutent)	CYP3A4	**CYP3A4 Inhibitors: Strong inhibitors** may increase serum levels of sunitinib: atazanavir, clarithromycin, grapefruit, grapefruit juice, indinavir, itraconazole, ketoconazole, nefazodone, nelfinavir, ritonavir, saquinavir, telithromycin, voriconazole; AVOID coadministration with strong inhibitors; if must coadminister, consider dose reduction of sunitinib to 37.5 mg PO daily and monitor patient closely for toxicity and effect. Coadminister cautiously, if at all, with drugs that are moderate (amprenavir, aprepitant, diltiazem, erythromycin, fluconazole, verapamil) or weak (cimetidine) inhibitors of CYP3A4; monitor closely for drug side effects. Teach patient to avoid grapefruit and grapefruit juice.

Inducers of CYP3A4: May decrease serum sunitinib concentrations: carbamazepine, dexamethasone, phenobarbital, phenytoin, rifabutin, rifampin, rifapentin, St. John's wort. Avoid coadministration if possible. If coadministered, assess need for increased sunitinib dose to a maximum of 87.5 mg PO daily. Teach patient NOT to take St. John's wort. |
| Temsirolimus (Torisel) | CYP3A4 | **Strong CYP3A4 Inhibitors:** Strong inhibitors may increase serum temsirolimus levels: atazanavir, clarithromycin, grapefruit, grapefruit juice, indinavir, itraconazole, ketoconazole, nefazodone, nelfinavir, ritonavir, saquinavir, telithromycin, and voriconazole. Avoid co administration; if must be given together, consider temsirolimus dose decrease to 12.5 mg weekly; when interacting drug discontinued, allow 1-week washout period, then resume dose taking prior to adding interactive drug. Teach patient to avoid grapefruit juice and grapefruit.

Strong Inducers: May decrease serum temsirolimus level: carbamazepine, dexamethasone, phenobarbital, phenytoin, rifabutin, rifampin, rifampicin. If must give together, consider temsirolimus dose increase to 50 mg weekly; when interacting drug is discontinued, resume dose given prior to adding interacting drug. Teach patient NOT to take St. John's wort. |

538

Drug	P450 Isoenzyme	Inducer, Inhibitor, Substrate
Tretinoin (ATRA, Vesanoid, All-Trans Retinoic Acid)	CYP3A4; 2C8; 2E	**Other Drugs:** Sorafenib: Combination resulted in dose-limiting toxicity; live vaccines (e.g., intranasal influenza, measles, mumps, rubella, oral polio, BCG, yellow fever, varicella, and TY21a typhoid vaccines): do not use, and teach patient to avoid contact with people immunized with live vaccines. **Strong CYP3A4 Inhibitors:** Strong inhibitors may increase serum tretinoin level: e.g., atazanavir, clarithromycin, grapefruit, grapefruit juice, indinavir, itraconazole, ketoconazole, nefazodone, nelfinavir, ritonavir, saquinavir, telithromycin, and voriconazole; also erythromycin, cimetidine, verapamil, diltiazem, and cyclosporine: No data exist to show increased or decreased effect. However, ketoconazole was shown to increase tretinoin plasma AUC by 72%. Use together cautiously, if at all. Teach patient to avoid grapefruit and grapefruit juice.
Vandetanib (Caprelsa)		**Strong CYP3A4 Inhibitors:** No clinically significant interaction. **Strong CYP3A4 Inducers:** May decrease serum vandetanib level: carbamazepine, dexamethasone, phenobarbital, phenytoin, rifabutin, rifampin; avoid concomitant administration. St. John's wort may decrease vandetanib unpredictably so should be avoided. **Drugs That Prolong the QTc Interval:** Avoid coadministration (e.g., anti-arrhythmic drugs amiodarone, disopyramide, procainamide, sotalol, dofetilide; and other drugs such as chloroquine, clarithromycin, dolasetron, granisetron, haloperidol, methadone, moxifloxacin, and pimozide).

Source: Modified from Wilkes GM. Drug Essentials: The Cytochrome P450 Microenzyme System and Targeted Therapies. *ONCOLOGY Nurse Edition* 2009;22(11):52–57; updated 6.1.13.

In 2012, a study by Medco Research Institute found that 23%–74% of patients taking TKIs were also taking a drug with a potential drug-drug interaction. They found that the more pathways involved in the TKIs metabolism, the higher the risk for drug interaction (Bowlin, 2012). In general, **CYP3A4 inhibitors** are amiodarone, amprenavir, aprepitant, atazanavir, clarithromycin, conivaptan, cyclosporine, darunavir, delaviridine, diltriazem, erythromycin, gemfibrozil, indinavir, itraconazole, ketoconazole, nelfinavir, posaconazole, quinupristin-dalfopristin, rionavir, saquinavir, telithromycin, verapamil, voriconazole, grapefruit, or grapefruit juice. **CYP3A4 inducers** are bosentan, carbamazepine, dexamethasone, efavirenz, fosphenytoin, nafcillin, nevirapine, oxcarbazepine, phenobarbital, phenytoin, primidone, rifabutin, rifampin, rifapentine, St. John's wort.

References

Abbas AK, Lichtman AH. *Basic Immunology*. Philadelphia, PA: Saunders Elsevier, 2011; pp. 80–113.

Anassi E, Ndefo UA. (2011). Sipuleucei-T(Provenge) injection. P&Te 36(4):197–202.

Acharya CR, Hsu DS, Anders CK, et al. Gene expression signatures, clinicopathological features and individualized therapy in breast cancer. *J Am Med Assoc* 2008; 299(13) 1574–1587.

Adjei AA, Hidalgo M. Intracellular signal transduction pathway proteins as targets for cancer therapy. *J Clin Oncol* 2005; 23 5386–5403.

Alberta Health Services (2012). Prevention and treatment of rash in patients treated with EGFR inhibitor therapies. Clinical Practice Guidelines Supp-003. Alberta CA: Alberta Health Services.

Amgen, Inc. Blincyto (blinatumomab) [package insert]. Thousand Oaks, CA, December 2014.

Amgen Inc. Vectibix (panitumumab) [package insert]. Thousand Oaks, CA, May 2014.

Ariad Pharmaceuticals, Inc. Iclusig (ponatinib) [package insert]. Cambridge, MA, July 2014.

Ana MMP, Sarah AM, Rachel B, et al. Synthetic lethality targeting of PTEN mutant cells with PARP inhibitors. *EMBO Mol Med* 2009; 1 315–322.

Angiogenesis Foundation. The Angiogenesis Process. Available at http://www.angio.org/learn/angiogenesis/. Accessed August 20, 2014.

AstraZeneca. Caprelsa (vandetanib) [package insert]. Wilmington, DE, April 2014.

AstraZeneca, Inc. Lynparza (olaparib) capsules [package insert]. Wilmington, DE, December 2014.

AstraZeneca Pharmaceuticals, Inc. Iressa (gefitinib) [package insert]. Wilmington, DE, July 2015.

Badros AZ, Vij R, Martin T, et al. Phase II study of carfilzomib in patients with relapsed/refractory multiple myeloma and renal insufficiency. *J Clin Oncol* 18; 15s, 2010 (suppl; abstr 8128).

Bang Y, Kwak EL, Shaw AT, et al. Clinical activity of the oral ALK inhibitor PF-02341066 in ALK-positive patients with non-small cell lung cancer (NSCLC). *J Clin Oncol* 2010; 28(7S) (suppl; abstr 3).

Bartlett JB, Dredge K, Dalgleish AG. The evolution of thalidomide and its IMiD derivatives as anti-cancer agents. *Nat Rev Cancer* 2004; 4(4) 314–322.

Baselga J, Cortes J, Kim SB et al. *N Engl J Med* 2012 366 109–119. Pertuzumab plus trastuzumab plus docetaxel for metastatic breast cancer.

Batchelor TT, Sorensen AG, diTomaso E. AZD2171, a Pan-VEGF Receptor Tyrosine Kinase Inhibitor, Normalizes Tumor Vasculature and Alleviates Edema in Glioblastoma Patients. *Cancer Cell* 2007; 11(1) 83–95.

Becher OJ, Trippett TM, Kolesar J, et al. Phase I Study of Single-agent Perifosine for Recurrent Pediatric Solid Tumors. *J Clin Oncol* 2010; 28(15S) (suppl, abstr 9540).

Becker M. Honing in on Chemoresistance Pathways: P13k/Akt/Mtor's Role in Disease Progression and Drug Resistance Needs to Be Ascertained. *Genetic Engineering & Biotechnology News* 2008; 28(11) 1–3.

Beck KE, Blansfield JA, Tran KQ, et al. Enterococolitis in Patients with Cancer After Antibody Blockade of Cytotoxic T-Lymphocyte–Associated Antigen 4. *J Clin Oncol* 2006; 24 2283–2289.

Bello Cl, Mulay M, Huang X, et al. Electrocardiographic Characterization of the Qtc Interval in Patients with Advanced Solid Tumors: Pharmacokinetic-Pharmacdynamic Evaluation of Sunitinib. *Clin Cancer Res* 2009; 15(22) 70 45–52.

Benvenuti S, Sartore-Bianchi A, DiNicolantonio F, et al. Oncogenic Activation of RAS/RAF Signaling Pathway Impairs the Response of Metastatic Colorectal Cancers to Anti-Epidermal Growth Factor Receptor Antibody Therapies. *Cancer Res* 2007; 67 2643–2648.

Bernier J, Bonner J, Vermorken JB, et al. Consensus Guidelines for the Management of Radiation Dermatitis and Coexisting Acne-Like Rash in Patients Receiving Radiotherapy Plus EGFR Inhibitors for the Treatment of Squamous Cell Carcinoma of the Head and Neck. *Ann Oncol* 2008; 19(1) 142–149.

Bharti AC, Aggarwal BB. Nuclear Factor-kappa B and Cancer: Its Role in Prevention and Therapy. *Biochem Pharmacol* Sept 2002; 64(5–6) 883–888.

Blansfield JA, Beck KE, Tran K, et al. Cytotoxic T-lymphocyte–Associated Antigen-4 Blockage Can Induce Autoimmune Hypophysitis in Patients with Metastatic Melanoma and Renal Cancer. *J Immunotherapy* 2005; 28 593–598.

Boehringer Ingelheim Pharmaceuticals, Inc. Gilotrif (afatinib) [package insert]. Ridgefield, CT, April 2014.

Borkar DS, Lacouture ME, Basti S. (2013) Spectrum of ocular toxicities from epidermal growth factor receptor inhibitors and their intermediate-term follow-up: A five-year review. *Support Care Cancer* 1(4):1167–74.

Bowlin S. Drug interactions significantly reduce targeted therapy efficacy. Presented at the 2012 American Society for Clinical Pharmacology and Therapeutics (ASCPT) Annual Meeting National Harbor, MD, on March 16, 2012.

Brell JM. Prolonged QTc interval in cancer therapeutic drug development: Defining arrhythmic risk in malignancy. *Prog Cardiovasc Dis* 53(2): 164–172, 2010.

Bristol-Myers Squibb Co. Opdivo (nivolumab) injection [package insert]. Princeton, NJ, March 2015.

Bristol Myers Squibb Company. Sprycel (dasatinib) [package insert]. Princeton, NJ, May 2014.

Burchert A, Wang Y, Cai D, et al. Compensatory P13-Kinase/Akt/mTOR Activation Regulates Imatinib Resistance Development. *Leukemia* 2005; 19 1774–1782.

Cardinale D, Colombo A, Torrisi R, et al. Trastuzumab-induced Cardiotoxicity: Clinical and Prognostic Implications of Troponin I Evaluation. *J Clin Oncol* 2010; 28(25): 390–391.

Celgene Corporation. Pomalyst (pomalidomide) [package insert]. Summit, NJ, May 2014.

Cella D, Escudier B, Rini BI, et al. Patient-reported Outcomes (PROs) in a Phase III AXIS Trial of Axinitinib versus Sorafenib as Second-line Therapy for Metastatic Renal Cell Carcinoma (mRCC). *J Clin Oncol* 2011; 29 (suppl; abstr 4504).

Chabner BA. Approval after Phase I: Ceritinib runs the three-minute mile. *The Oncologist* 2014; 19:1–2.

Chanan-Khan A, Sonneveld P, Schuster MW, et al. Analysis of Herpes Zoster Events Among Bortezomib-Treated Patients in the Phase III APEX Study. *J Clin Oncol* 2008; 26(29) 4784–4791.

Chang F, Lee JT, Navolanic PM, et al. Involvement of P13K/Akt Pathway in Cell Cycle Progression, Apoptosis, and Neoplastic Transformation: A Target for Cancer Chemotherapy. *Leukemia* 2003; 17(3) 590–603.

Chapman PB, Hauschild A, Robert C, et al. Improved Survival with Vemurafenib in Melanoma with BRAF V600E Mutation. *New Engl J Med* 2011; 10.1056/NEJMoa1103782 (published June 5, 2011) at NEJM.org.

Chung CC, Mirakhur B, Chan E et al. (2008). Celuximab-induced anaphylaxis and IgE specific for galactose-a- 1,3-galactose. *N Engl J Med* 358(11): 1109–1117.

Dann SG, Selvaraj A, Thomas G. mTOR Complex-1-S6K1 Signaling: At the Crossroads of Obesity, Diabetes, and Cancer. *Trends Mol Med* 2007; 13 252–259.

Dannenberg AJ, Altorki NK, Boyle JO. Cyclo-oxygenase 2: A Pharmacological Target for the Prevention of Cancer. *Lancet Oncol* 2001; 2(9) 544–551.

Deininger M, Buchdunger E, Druker BJ. The Development of Imatinib as a Therapeutic Agent for Chronic Myeloid Leukemia. *Blood* 2005; 105 2640–2653.

Demetri GD, Reichardt P, Kang Y-K, Blay J-Y, Joensuu H, Maki RG, et al. 2012; *J Clin Oncol* 2012 (suppl; abstr LBA 10008). Randomized phase III trial of regorafenib in patients (pts) with metastatic and/or unresectable gastrointestinal stromal tumor (GIST) progressing despite prior treatment with at least imatinib (IM) and sunitinib (SU): GRID trial.

Dent RA, Lindeman GJ, Clemons H, et al. Safety and Efficacy of the Oral PARP Inhibitor Olaparib (AZD2281) in Combination with Paclitaxel for the First- or Second-Line Treatment of Patients with Metastatic Triple Negative Breast Cancer: Results from the Safety Cohort of a Phase I/II Multicenter Trial. *J Clin Oncol* 2010; 28(7s) (Suppl; Abstr 1018).

Department of Health and Human Services. Understanding Gene Testing. Washington, DC, National Cancer Institute, NIH Publication. 1995; 96–390.

Digel W, Lubbert M. DNA Methylation Disturbances as Novel Therapeutic Target in Lung Cancer and Clinical Results. *Crit Rev Oncol Hematol* 2005; 55 1–11.

Din FNV, Dunlop MG, Stark LA. Evidence for Colorectal Cancer Cell Specificity of Aspirin Effects on NF Kappa B Signaling and Apoptosis. *Br J Cancer* 2004; 91 381–388.

Divino CM, Chen SH, Yang W. Anti-tumor Immunity Induced by Interleukin-12 Gene Therapy in a Metastatic Model of Breast Cancer Is Mediated by Natural Killer Cells. *Breast Cancer Res Treat* 2000; 60(2) 129–134.

Dunn GP, Koebel CM, Schreiber RD. Interferons, immunity, and immunoediting. *Nat Rev Immunol* 2006; 6(11):836–848.

Eli Lilly and Company. Cyramza (ramucirumab) [package insert]. Indianapolis, IN, April 2015.

Easai Inc. Lenvima (lenvatinib) capsules [package insert]. Woodcliff Lake, NJ, February 2015.

Fakih M. Management of Anti-EGFR-Targeting Monoclonal Antibody-Induced Hypomagnesemia. *Oncology* 2008; 22(1). Accessed at http://cancernetwork.com/showArticle.jhtml?articleId= 205900749, 14 July 2008.

Fan F, Wey JS, McCarty MF. Expression and Function of Vascular Endothelial Growth Factor Receptor 1 on Human Colorectal Cancer Cells. *Oncogene* 2005; 24 2647–2653.

Fecher LA, Agarwala SS, Hodi FS, Weber JS. Ipilimumab and its toxicities: A multidisciplinary approach. *The Oncologist* 2013; 18(6):733–743.

Feliner C. (2012). Ipilimumbab (Yervoy) prolongs survival in advanced melanoma. *P&Te* 37(9): 503–530.

Fidler IJ. The pathogenesis of cancer metastasis: The 'seed and soil' hypothesis revisited. *Nat Rev Cancer* 2003; 3(6):453–458.

Fiocari S, Brown WS, McIntyre BW et al. The PI3-kinase delta inhibitor idelalisib (GS-1101_ targets I integrin-mediated adhesion of chronic lymphocytic leukemia (CLL) cell to endothelial and marrow stromal cells. *PLoS One* 2013; 8(12):e83830, published online 12.23.13, doi: 10.1371/journal.pone.0083830.

Fink K, Mikkelsen T, Nabors LB, et al. Long-term Effects of Cilengitide, a Novel Integrin Inhibitor, in Recurrent Glioblastoma: A Randomized Phase IIa Study. *J Clin Oncol* 2010; 28: 15s (suppl; abstr 2010).

Folkman J. Pharmacology of Cancer Biotherapeutics: Antiangiogenesis Agents DeVita VT, Hellman S, Rosenberg SA. *Principles and Practice of Oncology*, 6th ed. Philadelphia, PA: Lippincott, Williams & Wilkins 2001; 509–521.

Folkman J. How is blood vessel growth regulated in normal and neoplastic tissue? A GHA Memorial Award Lecture. *Cancer Res* 1986; 46:467–473.

Fong PC, Boss DS, Yap TA, et al. Inhibition of Poly (ADP-ribose) Polymerase in Tumors from BRCA Mutation Carriers. *N Engl J Med* 2009; 36 123–134.

Food and Drug Administration (FDA). FDA Drug Safety Communication: Ongoing Safety Review of Revlimid (Lenalidomide) and Possible Increased Risk of Developing New Malignancies, April 8, 2011. Available online at http://www.fda.gov/Drugs/DrugSafety/ucm250575.htm.

Food and Drug Administration. Pfizer Volunarily Withdraws Cancer Treatment Mylotarg from US Market. Available at http://www.fda.gov/newsevents/newsroom/pressannouncements/ucm216448.htm.

Food and Drug Administration/US Department of Health and Human Services. Guidance for Industry: E14 Clinical Evaluation of QT/Qtc Interval Prolongation and Proarrhythmic Potential for Non-antiarrhythmic Drugs, October 2005. Available at http://www.fda.gov/downloads/regulatoryinformation/guidelines/UCM129357.Pdf.

Force T, Krause DS, VanEtten RA. Molecular Mechanisms of Cardiotoxicity of Tyrosine Kinase Inhibition. *Nature Rev Cancer* 2007; 7 332–344.

Ford JM, Helleday T, Curtin NJ. DNA Damage Signaling and Repair in Cancer: Therapeutic Potential. *ASCO 2010 Educational Book.* Alexandria, VA: American Society of Clinical Oncology; 2010, 467–474.

Fox LP. Pathology and Management of Dermatologic Toxicities Associated with Anti-EGFR Therapy. *Oncology* 2006; 20 26–34.

Fu M, Wang C, Li Z, Sakamaki T, Pestell RG. Minireview: Cyclin D1: Normal and Abnormal Functions. *Endocrinology* 2004; 145 5439–5447.

Fuchs CS, Tomasek J, Yong CJ et al. Ramucirumab monotherapy for previously treated advanced gastric or gastro-oesophageal junction adenocarcinoam (REGARD): An international, randomized, multicentre, placebo-controlled, phase 3 trial. *Lancet* 2014; 383(9911): 31–39.

Gainor JF, Shaw AT. Novel targets in non-small cell lung cancer: ROS1 and RET fusions. *The Oncologist.* 2013; 18: 865–875.

Genentech Inc. Avastin (bevacizumab) [package insert]. South San Francisco, CA: Genentech Inc., August 2014.

Genentech Inc. Gazyva (obinutuzumab) [package insert]. South San Francisco, CA: Genentech Inc., June 2014.

Genentech Inc. Perjeta (pertuzumab) [package insert]. South San Francisco, CA: Genentech Inc., September 2013.

Genentech, Inc. Zelboraf (vemurafenib) [package insert]. South San Francisco, CA: Genentech Inc., March 2014.

Genentech Inc. Kadcyla (ado-trastuzumab emtansine) [package insert]. South San Francisco, CA: Genentech Inc., July 2014.

Genentech Inc. Avastin (bevacizumab) [package insert]. South San Francisco, CA: Genentech Inc., December 2013.

Genentech Inc. Tarceva (erlotinib) [package insert]. South San Francisco, CA: Genentech Inc., April 2014.

Genentech Inc. Herceptin (trastuzumab) [package insert]. South San Francisco, CA: Genentech Inc., June 2014.

Genentech Inc. Rituxan (rituximab) [package insert]. South San Francisco, CA: Genentech Inc., August 2014.

Gilead Sciences, Inc. Zydelig (idelalisib) [package insert]. Foster City, CA: Gilead Sciences, Inc., July 2014.

GlaxoSmithKline. Tafinlar (dabrafenib) [package insert]. Research Triangle Park, NC: GlaxoSmithKline, January 2014.

GlaxoSmithKline. Mekinist (trametinib) [package insert]. Research Triangle Park, NC: GlaxoSmithKline, January 2014.

GlaxoSmithKline. Arzerra (ofatumumab) [package insert]. Research Triangle Park, NC: GlaxoSmithKline, April 2014.

Greene SL, Reed CE, Schroeter AL. Double Blind Crossover Study Comparing Doxepin with Diphenhydramine for the Treatment of Chronic Urticaria. *J Am Acad Derm* 1985; 12 669–675.

Grothey A, Sobrero AF Siena S, et al. 2012; Results of a phase III randomized, double-blind, placebo controlled, multicenter trial (CORRECT) of regorafenib plus best supportive care (BSC) in patients (pts) with metastatic colorectal cancer (mCRC) who have progressed after standard therapies. *J Clin Oncol* 30 2012 (suppl 4; abstr LBA385).

Grothey A, Sugrue M, Hedric kE, et al. Association Between Exposure to Bevacizumab (BV) Beyond First Progression and Overall Survival (OS) in Patients (pts) with Metastatic Colorectal Cancer (mCRC): Results from a Large Observational Study (BriTE). *J Clin Oncol* 2007 ASCO Annual Meeting Proceedings Part I. Vol 25, No. 18S, (June 20 Supplement), 4036.

Gupta S, Takebe N, LoRusso P, et al. *2010; Ther Adv in Med Oncol* 2 (4) 237–250 Review: Targeting the Hedgehog pathway in cancer.

Hamid O, Robert C, Daud A et al., Safety and tumor responses with lambrolizumab (Anti-PD-1) in melanoma. *The New Engl J Med* 2013; 369:134–144; DOI: 10.1056/NEJMoa1305133.

Hanahan D, Folkman J. Patterns and Emerging Mechanisms of the Angiogenic Switch During Tumorigenesis. *Cell* 1996; 86 353–358.

Hanahan D, Weinberg RA. Hallmarks of Cancer: The Next Generation. *Cell* 2011; 144(5) 646–674.

Hanahan D, Weinberg RA. The Hallmarks of Cancer. *Cell* 2000; 100 57–100.

Haouala A, Widmer N, Duchosal MA et al. (2011). Drug interactions with the tyrosine kinase inhibitors imatinib, dasatinib, and nilotinib. *Blood* 117(8): e75–e87.

Hapani S, Chu D, Wu S. Risk of Gastrointestinal Perforation in Patients with Cancer Treated with Bevacizumab: A Meta-analysis. *Lancet Oncol* 2009 doi 10.1016/S1470-2045(09)70112-3 early online publication 25 May 2009.

Harari PM, Huang SM. Modulation of Molecular Targets to Enhance Radiation. *Clin Cancer Res* 2000; 6 323–325.

Haura EB, Turkson J, Jove R. Mechanisms of Disease: Insights into the Emerging Role of Signal Transducers and Activators of Transcription in Cancer. *Nat Clin Pract Oncol* 2005; 2(6) 315–324.

Henriks RW, Yuvaraj S, Kil LP. Targeting Bruton's tyrosine kinase in B cell malignancies. *Nat Rev Cancer* 2014; 14, 219–232.

Herman JG, Baylin SB. Gene Silencing in Cancer in Association with Promoter Hypermethylation. *New England J Med* 2003; 349 2042–2054.

Hershman DL, Lacchetti C, Dworkin RH et al. Prevention and management of chemotherapy-induced peripheral neuropathy in survivors of adult cancers: American Society of Clinical Oncology Practice Guidelines. *J Clin Oncol* April 14, 2014, published online before print. DOI: 10.1200/JCO.2013.54.0914.

Hetherington J, Andrews C, Vaynshteyn Y, Fishel R. Managing Follicular Rash Related to Chemotherapy and Monoclonal Antibodies. *Commun Oncol* 2007; 4(3) 157–162.

Hidalgo M, Siu LL, Neumanitis J. Phase I and Pharmacologic Study of OSI-774, an Epidermal Growth Factor Receptor Tyrosine Kinase Inhibitor, in Patients with Advanced Solid Malignancies. *J Clin Oncol* 2001; 19(13) 3267–3279.

Huang Y, Snuder lM, Jain RK. Polarization of Tumor-associated Macrophages: A Novel Strategy for Vascular Normalization and Antitumor Activity. *Cancer Cell* 2011; 19(1) 1–2.

Humblet Y, Peeters M, Siena S. Association of Skin Toxicity (ST) Severity with Clinical Outcomes and Health-Related Quality of Life (HRQoL) with Panitumumab. *J Clin Oncol* 2007 ASCO Annual Meeting Proceedings Part I. Vol 25, No. 18S (June 20 Supplement), 2007; 4038.

Iglehart JD, Silver DP. Synthetic Lethality—A New Direction in Cancer-Drug Development. *New Engl J Med* 2009; 361(2) 189–191.

Infante JR, Falchook GS, Lawrence DP, et al. Phase I/II Study to Assess Safety, Pharmacokinetics, and Efficacy of the Oral MEK 1/2 Inhibitor GSK1120212 (GSK212) Dosed in Combination with the Oral BRAF Inhibitor GSK2118436 (GSK436). *J Clin Oncol* 2011; 29: 2011 (suppl; abstr CRA8503).

Isakoff SJ, Overmoyer B, Tung M, et al. A Phase II Trial of the PARP Inhibitor Veliparib (ABT888) and Temozolomide for Metastatic Breast Cancer. *J Clin Oncol* 2010; 2(7S) (suppl; abstr 1019).

Ismael G, Hegg R, Muehlbauer S, et al. Subcutaneous versus intravenous administration of (neo) adjuvant trastuzumab in patients with HER2 positive, clinical stage I-III breast cancer (HannaH study): A phase 3, open-label, multicentre, randomized trial. *Lancet Oncology* 9 August 2012, doi:10.1016/S1470-2045(12)70329-7.

Izzedine H, Ederhy S, Goldwasser F, et al. Mangement of hypertension in angiogenesis inhibitor treated patients. *Ann Oncol* 2009; (20) 807–815.

Janssen Biotech Inc. Sylvan (siltuximab) [package insert]. Horsham, PA, April 2014.

Jones P. *DNA Methylation and Cancer.* Presented at: Breakthroughs in Therapeutic Epigenetics: An Emerging Clinical Approach, symposium held in conjunction with the 41st Annual Meeting of the American Society of Clinical Oncology, Orlando, FL, May 2005.

Jones S, Anagnostou V, Lytle K, et al. Personalized genomic analyses for cancer mutation discovery and interpretation. *Sci Transl Med* 2015; 7(283) 283. DOI:10.1126/scitranslmed.aaa7161

Kamba T, McDonald DM. Mechanisms of Adverse Effects of Anti-VEGF Therapy for Cancer. *Br J Cancer* 2007; 96 1788–1795.

Kantarjian H and Experts in CML. The price of drugs for chronic myeloid leukemia (CML); A reflection of the unsustainable prices of cancer drugs: From the perspective of a large group of CML experts. *Blood* prepublished online April 25, 2013; doi: 10.1182/blood-2013-03-490003.

Keefe DL. Trastuzumab-Associated Cardiotoxicity. *Cancer* 2002; 95(7) 1592–1600.

Kobayashi S, Kishimoto T, Kamata S, Otsuka M, Miyazaki M, Ishikura H. Rapamycin, a Specific Inhibitor of the Mammalian Target of Rapamycin, Suppresses Lymphangiogenesis and Lymphatic Metastasis. *Cancer Sci* 2007; 98 726–733.

Kollmannsberger C, Bjarnason G, Burnett P, et al. Sunitinib in Metatastic Renal Cell Carcinoma: Recommendations for Management of Non-cardiovascular Toxicities. *The Oncologist* 2011; 16 543–553.

Krop IE, Beeram M, Modi B, et al. Phase I Study of Trastuzumab-DM1, an HER2 Antibody-Drug Conjugate, Given Every 3 Weeks to Patients with HER2-Positive Metastatic Breast Cancer. *J Clin Oncol* 2010; 28(16) 2698–2704.

Kwak EL, Camidge DR, Clark J, et al. Clinical Activity Observed in a Phase I Dose Escalation Trial of an Oral C-Met and ALK Inhibitor, PF-02341066. *J Clin Oncol* 2009; 27(15S) (suppl; abstr 3509).

Lacouture ME. Prevention and treatment of multikinase inhibitor-induced hand-foot syndrome. *ASCO POST* 3(18): 1(2012).

Lacouture ME, Anadkat MJ, Bensadoun R-J et al., (2010). Clinical practice guidelines for the prevention and treatment of EGFR inhibitor-associated dermatologic toxicities. *Support Care Cancer* 19: 1079–1095, 2011.

Lacouture ME, Basti S, Patel J, Benson A. The SERIES Clinic: An Interdisciplinary Approach to the Management of Toxicities of EGFR Inhibitors. *J Support Oncol* 2006; 4 236–238.

Lacouture ME, Lai SE. The PRIDE (Papulopustules and/or Paronychia, Regulatory Abnormalities of Hair Growth, Itching, and Dryness Due to Epidermal Growth Factor Receptor Inhibitors) Syndrome. *Br J Dermatol* 2006; 155 852–854.

Lacouture ME, Mitchel EP, Piperdi B et al. Skin toxicity evaluation protocol with panitumumab (STEPP), a phase II, open-lavel, randomized trial evaluating the impact of a preemptive skin treatment regimen on skin toxicities and quality of life in patients with metastatic colorectal cancer. *J Clin Oncol* 2010; 28(8): 1351–7.

Lacouture ME, Anadkat MJ, Bensadoun RJ, Bryce J et al. Clinical practice guidelines for the prevention and treatment of EGFR inhibitor-associated dermatologic toxicities. Support Cancer Care 19(8):1079–1095 (2011).

Lacouture ME. Mechanisms of Cutaneous Toxicities to EGFR Inhibitors. *Nat Rev Cancer* 2006; 6 803–812.

Lavecchia A, DiGiovanni C, Novellino E. Stat-3 inhibitors: State of the Art and New Horizons for Cancer Treatment. *Curr Med Chem* 2011; 18(16) 2359–2375.

Levy C, *Detect and Manage Adverse Events Associated with Ipilimumab.* Targeted and Biological Therapies SIG Newsletter May 2007. Accessed 14 July 2008, at http://onsopcontent.ons.org/ Publications/SIGNewsletters/tbt/tbt18.1.html.

Li C, Alvey C, Bello A, et al. Pharmacokinetics (PK) of Crizotinib (PF-02341066) in Patients with Advanced Non-small Cell Lung Cancer (NSCLC) and Other Solid Tumors. *J Clin Oncol* 2011; 29: 2011 (suppl. abstr e13065).

Li F. Angiogenesis. *The Angiogenesis Foundation* 2000 (http://www.angio.org).

Lieberman J. Noncoding RNAs and cancer: Knockout punch for cancer. *Cell* 2013; 153:9–10.

Linderholm B, Grankvist K, Wilking N. Correlation of Vascular Endothelial Growth Factor Content with Recurrences, Survival, and First Relapse Site in Primary Node-positive Breast Carcinoma after Adjuvant Treatment. *J Clin Oncol* 2000; 18 1423–1431.

Lipowska-Bhalla G, Gilham DE, Hawkins RE, Rothwell DG. Targeted immunotherapy of cancer with CAR T cells: Achievements and challenges. *Cancer Immunol Immunother* 2012; 61(7): 953–962.

List A, Kurtin S, Roe DJ. Efficacy of Lenalidomide in Myelodysplastic Syndromes. *N Eng J Med* 2005; 352 549–557.

Liu ET. Tumor Suppressor Genes: Changing Concepts. ASCO Educational Book. 35th Annual Meeting, Atlanta, GA: 1999.

Lièvre A, Bachet J-B, Boige V, et al. KRAS Mutations as an Independent Prognostic Factor in Patients with Advanced Colorectal Cancer Treated with Cetuximab. *J Clin Oncol* 2008; 26 374–379.

Lundin J, Kimby E, Bjorkholm M. Phase II Trial of Subcutaneous Anti-CD52 Monoclonal Antibody Alemtuzumab (Campath-1H) as First-Line Treatment for Patients with B-Cell Chronic Lymphocytic Leukemia (B-CLL). *Blood* 2002; 100(3) 768–773.

Lynch TJ, Kim ES, Eaby B, Garey J, West DP, Lacouture ME. Epidermal Growth Factor Receptor Inhibitor-Associated Cutaneous Toxicities: An Evolving Paradigm in Clinical Management. *Oncologist* 2007; 12(5) 610–621.

Ma WW, Adjei AA. Novel agents on the horizon for cancer therapy. *CA Cancer J Clin* 2009; 59(2):111–137.

Maitland ML, Bakris GL, Black HR, et al. 2010; *J Natl Cancer Inst* 102 9596–9604 Initial assessment, surveillance, and management of blood pressure in patients receiving vascular endothelial growth factor signaling pathway inhibitors.

Male D, Brostoff J, Roth DB, Toit IM. *Immunology*, 8th ed. Philadelphia, PA: Elsevier Saunders, 2013, pp. 50–60.

Mancuso MR, Davis R, Norberg SM. Rapid Vascular Regrowth in Tumors After Reversal of VEGF Inhibition. *J Clin Invest* 2006; 116 2610–2621.

Mavragani CP, Vlachoyiannopoulos PG, Kosmas N, et al. A Case of Reversible Posterior Leucoencephalopathy Syndrome After Rituximab Infusion: Letter to the Editor. *Rheumatology* 2004; 43(11) 1450–1451.

Melman I. Dendritic cells: Master regulators of the immune response. *Ca Immunol Res* 2013; doi: 10.1158/2326-6066. CIR-13-0102.

Merck & Co., Inc. Keytruda (pembrolizumab) [package insert]. Whitehouse Station, NJ, January 2015.

Merkle CJ, Loescher LJ. The Biology of Cancer. In: Yarbro CH, Frogge MH, Goodman M. *Cancer Nursing: Principles and Practice,* 6th ed. Sudbury, MA: Jones and Bartlett Publishers; 2005: 15.

Millennium Pharmaceuticals, Inc. Velcade (bortezomib). [package insert]. Cambridge, MA, August 2014.

Moore S, Brandt ML. Adherence to oral therapies. Pittsburgh, PA: ONS, 2010. Available at http:// www.ons.org/ClinicalResources/OralTherapies/media/ons/docs/clinical/AdherenceToolkit/ oraladherencetoolkit-print.pdf, accessed 5.29.13.

Morabito A, Piccirillo MC, Falasconi F, et al. Vandetanib (ZD6474), a Dual Inhibitor of Vascular Endothelial Growth Factor (VEGFR) and Epidermal Growth Factor Receptor (EGFR) Yyrosine Kinases: Current Status and Future Directions. *Oncologist* 2009; 14 378–390.

Moreau P, Pylpenko H, Grosicki S, et al. Subcutaneous versus Intravenous Administration of Bortezomib in Patients with Relapsed Multiple Myeloma: A Randomised, Phase 3, Noninferiority Study. *Lancet Oncol* 2011; 12 431–440.

Morrow PK, Wulf GM, Booser DJ, et al. Phase I/II Trial of Everolimus (RAD001) and Trastuzumab in Patients with Resistant HER2 Overexpressing Breast Cancer. *J Clin Oncol* 2010; 28(15S) (suppl; abstr 1014).

Muller A, Homey B, Soto H. Involvement of Chemokine Receptors in Breast Cancer Metastases. *Nature* 2001; 410 50–56.

Munoz J, Dhillon N, Janku F et al. STAT3 inhibitors: Finding a home in lymphoma and leukemia. *The Oncologist* 2014; 19:536–544.

Murray JL, Witzig TE, Wiseman GA, *Zevalin Therapy Can Convert Peripheral Blood bcl-2 Status from Positive to Negative in Patients with Low-grade, Follicular, or Transformed Non-Hodgkin's Lymphoma (NHL)*. Proc ASCO 2000 19 22a (77) New Orleans, LA: May 20–23, 2000.

National Cancer Comprehensive Network (NCCN). Clinical Practice Guidelines in Colon Cancer, Version 3.2014; http://www.nccn.org. Accessed June 1, 2014.

National Human Genome Research Institute (NHGRI). Is the exact number of genes in the human genome known? Available online at https://www.genome.gov/DNADay/q.cfm?aid=2&year=2012. Accessed May 31, 2014.

Niu G, Carter WB. Human Epidermal Growth Factor Receptor 2 Regulates Angiopoietin-2 Expression in Breast Cancer Via AKT and Mitogen-Activated Protein Kinase Pathways. *Cancer Res* 2007; 67 1487–1493.

Novartis Pharmaceuticals Corporation. Afinitor (everolimus) Tablets [package insert]. East Hanover, NJ: Novartis Pharmaceuticals Corporation, March 2009.

Novartis Pharmaceuticals Corporation. Tasigna (Nilotinib) Tablets [package insert]. East Hanover, NJ, Novartis Pharmaceuticals Corporation, January 2011.

Novartis Pharmaceuticals Corporation. Zykadia (ceritinib) Tablets [package insert]. East Hanover, NJ, Novartis Pharmaceuticals Corporation, April 2014.

Novartis Pharmaceuticals Corporation. Afinitor (everolimus) Tablets [package insert]. East Hanover, NJ: Novartis Pharmaceuticals Corporation, February 2014.

Novartis Pharmaceuticals Corporation. Tasigna (nilotinib) Tablets [package insert]. East Hanover, NJ, Novartis Pharmaceuticals Corporation, January 2014.

Novartis Pharmaceuticals Corp. Farydak (panobinostat) capsules [package insert]. East Hanover, NJ, February 2015.

Novartis Pharmaceuticals Corporation. Odomzo (sonidegib) [package insert]. East Hanover, NJ, July 2015.

O'Brien NA, Wang YH, Chow L, et al. Increased P13K/AKT Activity, Which Confers Resistance to Trastuzumab, Can Be Overcome by Lapatinib. *American Association for Cancer Research 101st Annual Meeting, 2010* Poster Session 23, Abstract 613, presented in Washington, DC, April 17–21, 2010.

O'Connor R, Breen L. Resistance to Chemotherapy Drugs. In Missailidis S (ed). *Anticancer Therapeutics*. New York, NY, John Wiley & Sons, 2008.

O'Day, Weber JS, Wolchok JD, et al. Effectiveness of Treatment Guidance on Diarrhea and Colitis Across Opilimumab Studies. *J Clin Oncol* 2011; 29 2011 (suppl; abstr 8554).

O'Donovan PJ, Livingston DM. BRCA-1 and BRCA-2: Breast/Ovarian Cancer Susceptibility Gene Products and Participants in DNA Double-Strand Break Repair. *Carcinogenesis* 2010; 31(6) 961–967.

O'Keefe P, Parrilli M, Lacouture ME. Toxicity of Targeted Therapy: Focus on Rash and Other Dermatologic Side Effects. *ONCOLOGY Nurse Ed* 2006 (Suppl 13) 1–6.

O'Shaughnessy J, Blackwell KL, Burstein H, et al. A Randomized Study of Lapatinib ± Trastuzumab in Patients with Heavily Pretreated HER2+ Metastatic Breast Cancer Progressing on Trastuzumab Therapy. *J Clin Oncol* 2008; 26 (May 20 suppl; abstr 1015).

O'Shaughnessy J, Osborne C, Pippen J, et al. Final Results of a Randomized Phase II Study Demonstrating Efficacy and Safety of BSI-201, a Poly (ADP-Ribose) Polymerase (PARP)

Inhibitor, in Combination with Gemcitabine/Carboplatin (G/C) in Metastatic Triple Negative Breast Cancer (TNBC) Cancer Research 69 (Meeting Abstract Supplement), 3122, December 15, 201. Doi: 1158/0008-5472: SABCS-09-3122. Presented at the 32nd Annual CTRC-AACR San Antonio Breast Cancer Symposium Dec 10–13, 2009, San Antonio, TX. *J Clin Oncol* 27; 18s, 2009 (suppl; abstr 3).

O'Shaughnessy J, Schwartzberg LS, Danso MA, et al. A Randomized Phase III Study of Iniparib (BSI-201) in Combination with Gemcitabine/Carboplatin (G/C) in Metastatic Triple-negative Breast Cancer (TNBC). *J Clin Oncol* 29: 2011 (suppl; abstr 1007).

Pao W, Miller VA, Politi KA. Acquired Resistance of Lung Adenocarcinomas to Gefitinib or Erlotinib Is Associated with a Second Mutation in the EGFR Kinase Domain. *PLoS Medicine* 2005; 2(3) 225–235 http://www.plosmedicine.org. Accessed 11 June 2007.

Pardoll DM. The blockade of immune checkpoints in cancer immunotherapy. *Nat Rev Cancer* 2012; 12:252–264.

Perez EA, Suman VJ, Davidson NE, et al. Results of Chemotherapy Alone, with Sequential or Concurrent Addition of 52 Weeks of Trastuzumab in the NCCTG N9831 HER2 Positive Adjuvant Breast Cancer Trial. *Cancer Res* 2009; 69(24 suppl) (abstract 80).

Pestell. Cyclin D1 Nullifies BRCA1' Tumor Suppressive Function. *Cancer Res* 2005; 65 6557–6566.

Pharmacyclics, Inc. Imbruvica (ibrutinib) (prescribing information). Sunnyvale, CA, July 2014.

Piccart-Gebhart MJ. First Results of the HERA Trial. *Proc Am Soc Clin Oncol* 2005; Scientific Session presented at the 41st American Society of Clinical Oncology Annual Meeting. May 16, 2005. Orlando, FL.

Pfizer Labs. Ibrance (palbociclib) capsules [package insert]. New York, NY, February 2015.

Pfizer Labs. Sutent (sunitinib) [package insert]. New York, New York, June 2014.

Piccart-Gebhart M, Holmes AP, de Azambuja E, et al. The association between event-free survival and pathological complete response to neoadjuvant lapatinib, trastuzumab, or their combination in HER2-positive breast cancer study. Survival follow-up analysis of the Neo ALLTO study, presented at the 36th Annual San Antonio Breast Cancer Symposium, December 10–14, 2013; San Antonio, TX. Abstract S1-01.

Piccart-Gebhart M, Holmes AP, Baselga J, et al. First results from the phase III ALTTO trial (BIG 2-06; NCCTG [Alliance] N063D) comparing one year of anti-HER2 therapy with lapatinib alone (L), trastuzumab alone (T), their sequence (T→L), or their combination (T+L) in the adjuvant treatment of HER2-positive early breast cancer (EBC). *J Clin Oncol* 32:5s, 2014 (suppl; abstr LBA4).

Popat S, Smith I E. Therapy Insight: Anthracyclines and Trastuzumab: The Optimal Management of Cardiotoxic Side Effects. *Nat Clin Pract Oncol* 2008; 5(6) 324–335.

Porzio G, Aielli F, Verna L. Efficacy of Pregabalin in the Management of Cetuximab-Related Itch. *J Pain Symptom Manage* 2006; 32(5) 397–398.

Quezada SA, Peggs KS. Exploiting CTLA-4, PD-1, and PD-L1 to reactivate the host immune response against cancer. *Br J Ca* 2013; 108:1560–1565.

Ranpura V, Hapani S, Wu S, et al. Treatment-related Mortality with Bevacizumab in Cancer Patients: A Meta-Analysis. *JAMA* 2011; 305 487–494.

Rehman S, Qian ZR, Wang EL, et al. Mir-21 Upregulation in Breast Cancer Cells Leads to PTEN Loss and Herceptin Resistance. *American Association for Cancer Research 101st Annual Meeting, 2010* abstract 4033, presented in Washington, DC, April 17–21, 2010.

Reidy DL, Chung KY, Imoney JP, et al. Bevacizumab 5 mg/kg Can Be Infused Safely Over 10 Minutes. *J Clin Oncol* 2007; 28(19) 2691–2695.

Ribas, A. Tumor immunotherapy directed at PD-1. *N Engl J Med* 2012; 366(26):2517–2519.

Rini BI, Cohen DP, Lu DR. Hypertension as a Biomarker of Efficacy in Patients with Metastatic Renal Cell Carcinoma Treated with Sunitinib. *J Natl Cancer Inst* 2011; 103 763–773.

Rini BI, Escudier B, Tomczak P, et al. Axitinib versus Sorafenib as Second-Line Therapy Metastatic Renal Cell Carcinoma (mRCC): Results of Phase III AXIS Trial. *J Clin Oncol* 29: 2011 (suppl; abstr 4503).

Robert C, Ribas A, Wolchok JD et al., Anti-programmed-death-receptor-1 treatment with pembrolizumab in ipilimumab-refractory advanced melanoma: a randomised dose-comparison cohort of a phase 1 trial. *The Lancet.* Early online publication, 15 July 2014. Doi: 10.1016/SO140-6736(14)60958-2.

Rolny C, Mazzone M, Tugues S, et al. HRG Inhibits Tumor Growth and Metastases by Inducing Macrophage Polarization and Vessel Normalization Through Downregulation of PlGF. *Cancer Cell* 2011; 19(1) 31–44.

Rowinsky EK, Windle JJ, VonHoff DD. Ras Protein Farnesyltransferase: A Strategic Target for Anticancer Therapeutic Development. *J Clin Oncol* 1999; 17(11) 3631–3652.

Rubin K. Managing immune-related adverse events to ipilimumab: A nurse's guide. *Clin J Oncol Nurs* 16(2):E69–E75.

Ruddy K, Mayer E, Partridge A. Patient adherence and persistence with oral anticancer treatment. *CA A Cancer J Clin* 2009; 59: 56–66.

Ruoslahti E, Reed JC. Anchorage Dependence, Integrins, and Apoptosis. *Cell* 1994; 77(4) 477–478.

Ruoslahti E. How Cancer Spreads. *Scientific American (Sept 1996)* 1996; 275(3) 72–77.

Sabnis G, Brodie A. Trasntuzumab Sensitizes ER Negative, HER2 Positive Breast Cancer Cells (Skbr-3) to Endocrine Therapy. *ENDO* 2009 (abstract OR38-02).

Saltz L, Rubin MS, Hochster H, et al. Acne-like Rash Predicts Response in Patients Treated with Cetuximab (IMC-C225) Plus Irinotecan (CPT 11) in CP1-11 Refractory Colorectal Cancer (CRC) That Expresses Epidermal Growth Factor Receptor (EGFR). *Clin Cancer Res* 2001; 7 3766s. Abstract 559.

Sandler AB, Blumenschein GR, Henderson T. Phase I/II Trial Evaluating the Anti-VEGF MAb Bevacizumab in Combination with Erlotinib, a HER1/EGFR-TK Inhibitor, for Patients with Recurrent Non-small Cell Lung Cancer. 2004 ASCO Annual Meeting Proceedings, Post Meeting Edition. *J Clin Oncol* 2004; 22(14S) 2000.

Saporito B. How to cure cancer. *Time* 4.1.13, available at http://healthland.time.com/2013/04/01/the-conspiracy-to-end-cancer/. Accessed May 12, 2013.

Sausville EA, *Cyclin Dependent Kinases: Novel Targets for Cancer Development.* ASCO 1999 Educational Book 35th Annual Meeting, Atlanta: 1999.

Scandella E, Ludewig B. Dendridic Cells and Autoimmunity. *Transfusion Med Hemotherapy* 2005; 32(6) 363–368.

Schlom J, Gulley JL, Arlen PM. Paradigm Shifts in Vaccine Therapy. *Exp Biol Med* 2008; 233(5) 522–534.

Schottenfeld D, Beebe-Dimmer J. Chronic Inflammation: A Common and Important Factor in the Pathogenesis of Neoplasia. *CA Cancer J Clin* 2006; 5669–5683.

Schrag D, Chung KY, Flombaum C, Saltz L. Cetuximab Therapy and Symptomatic Hypomagnesemia. *J Natl Cancer Inst* 1997; (16) 1221–1224.

Schreiber RD, Old LJ, Smyth MJ. Cancer immunoediting: Integrating immunity's roles in cancer suppression and promotion. *Science* 2011; 331: 1565–1570.

Segaert S, VanCutsem E. Clinical Management of EGFRI Dermatological Toxicities: The European Perspective. *Oncology (Williston Park)* 2007; 21(11 Suppl 5) 22–26.

Segaert S, VanCutsem E. Clinical Signs, Pathophysiology and Management of Skin Toxicity During Therapy with Epidermal Growth Factor Receptor Inhibitors. *Ann Oncol* 2005; 16 1425–1433.

Semenza GL. Targeting HIF-1 for Cancer Therapy. *Nat Rev Cancer* 2003; 3721–3731.

Shah NT, Kris MG, Pao W, et al. Practical management of patients with non–small-cell lung cancer treated with gefitinib. *J Clin Oncol* 2005; 23 165–174.

Shaw AT, Yeap BY, Solomon BJ, et al. Impact of Crizotinib on Survival in Patients with Advanced ALK-positive NSCLC Compared with Historical Controls. *J Clin Oncol* 2011; 29 2011 (suppl. abstr 7507).

Shaw AT, Kim DW, Mehra R et al., Ceritinib in ALK-rearranged non-small cell lung cancer. *N Engl J Med* 2014; 370:1189–1197.

Shaw RJ, Cantley LC. Ras, PI(3)K and mTOR Signaling Controls Tumour Cell Growth. *Nature* 2006; 441 424–430.

Shaw RJ. Glucose Metabolism in Cancer. *Curr Opin Cell Biol* 2006; 18 598–608.

Siegel JA. Revised Nuclear Regulatory Commission Regulation for Release of Patients Administered Radioactive Materials: Outpatient Iodine-131 Anti-B1 Therapy. *J Nucl Med* 1998; 39(8) 285–335.

Slamon D, Eiermann W, Robert N, et al. BCIRG 006: 2nd Interim Analysis Phase III Randomized Trial Comparing Doxorubicin and Cyclophosphamide Followed by Docetaxel (AC → T) with Doxorubicin and Cyclophosphamide Followed by Docetaxel and Trastuzumab (AC → TH) with Docetaxel, Carboplatin, and Trastuzumab (TCH) in Her2neu Positive Early Breast Cancer Patients. Paper presented at: 29th Annual San Antonio Breast Cancer Symposium; December 14-17, 2006; San Antonio, TX. Abstract 52. Available at http://www.abstracts2view.com/ sabcs06/view.php?nu=SABCS06L_78. Accessed June 21, 2008.

Smith EML. Pang H, Cirrincione C et al. (2012). A phase III double blind trial of duloxetine to treat painful chemotherapy-induced peripheral neuropathy (CIPN). *J Clin Oncol* 20(suppl), abstract CRA 9013.

Soda M, Choi YL, Enomoto M, et al. Identification of the Transforming EML4-ALK Fusion Gene in Non-small Cell Lung Cancer. *Nature* 2007; 448(7153) 561–566.

Soussi T, Wiman KG. Shaping genetic alterations in human cancer: The p53 mutation paradigm. *Cancer Cell* 2007; 12(4): 303–12.

Spectrum Pharmaceuticals, Inc. Beleodaq (belinostat) for injection. [package insert]. Irvine, CA: Spectrum Pharmaceuticals, Inc, July 2014.

Stendahl M, Kronblad A, Ryden L. Cyclin D1 Overexpression Is a Negative Predictive Factor for Tamoxifen Response in Postmenopausal Breast Cancer Patients. *Br J Cancer* 2004; 90 1942–1948.

Stetler-Stevenson WG, Kleiner DE. Molecular Biology of Cancer: Invasion and Metastases. In DeVita VT, Hellman S, Rosenberg SA. Principles and Practice of Oncology, 6th ed. Philadelphia, PA: Lippincott, Williams & Wilkins; 2001 123–137.

Strevel E L, Ing DJ, Siu LL. Molecularly Targeted Oncology Therapeutics and Prolongation of the QT Interval. *J Clinc Oncol* 2007; 25(22) 3362–3371.

Swan JT, Zaghloul H, Wagner J, et al. Safety of a Rapid, 90-minute Rituximab Infusion Protocol. *J Clin Oncol* 29: 2011 (suppl; abstr e18551).

Takahashi H, Shibuy M. The Vascular Endothelial Growth Factor (VEGF)/VEGF Receptor System and Its Role Under Physiologic and Pathologic Conditions. *Clin Sci* 2005; 109 227–241.

Tan W, Winer KD, Bang Y, et al. Pharmacokinetics (PK) of PF-02341066, a Dual ALK/MET Inhibitor after Multiple Oral Doses to Advanced Cancer Patients. *J Clin Oncol* 2010; 28(7S), 2010 (suppl; abstr 2596).

Tejpar S, Peeters M, Humblet Y, et al. Relationship of Efficacy with KRAS Status (Wild-Type Versus Mutant) in Patients with Irinotecan-Refractory Metastatic Colorectal Cancer (mCRC), Treated with Irinotecan (q 2 wk) and Escalating Doses of Cetuximab (q 1 wk): The EVEREST Experience (Preliminary Data). *J Clin Oncol* 2008; 26 (May 20 suppl: abstract 4001).

Tutt A, Robson M, Garber JE, et al. Phase II Trial of the Oral PARP Inhibitor Olaparib in BRCA-Deficient Advanced Breast Cancer. *J Clin Oncol* 2009; 27 (suppl 18) CRA501.

VanCutsem E, Lang I, D'haens G, et al. KRAS Status and Efficacy in the First-Line Treatment of Patients with Metastatic Colorectal Cancer (mCRC) Treated with FOLFIRI with or without Cetuximab: The CRYSTAL Experience. *J Clin Oncol* 2008; 26 (May 20 suppl: abstr 2).

VanUmmersen L, Binger K, Volkman J, et al. A Phase I Trial of Perifosine (NSC 639966) on a Loading Dose/Maintenance Dose Schedule in Patients with Advanced Cancer. *Clin Cancer Res* 2004; 10 7450–7456.

Verschaeve V D'Hondt LA, Verbeke LM, et al. CeCil: A Randomized, Noncomparative Phase II Clinical Trial of the Effect of Radiation Therapy (RT) plus Temozolomide (TMZ) Combined with Cilengitide or Cetuximab on the 1-year Overall Survival of Patients with Newly Diagnosed MGMT-promoter Unmethylated Glioblastoma. *J Clin Oncol* 29; 2011 (suppl; abstr TPS134).

Vogelstein B, Papdopoulous N, Velculescu V, et al. (2013). Cancer genome landscapes. *Science* 229: 1546–1558.

VonEschenbach. *Keynote Presentation: Summit Series on Cancer Clinical Trials* Executive Summary VIII: Retooling the System: Implementing Solutions. September 29–October 1, 2003.

Wagner LI. *Psychological Impact and Quality of Life Issues Associated with Therapy-Induced Rash.* Presentation ONS Ancillary Event, April 25, 2007, Las Vegas, NV.

Walker S, Lacouture ME. Wall Chart Featuring Skin-Related Toxicities of Targeted Therapies. *Oncology* 2006; 20 (suppl 7).

Wang T-F, Lockhart AC, 2012; *Clin Med Insights: Oncology* 6, 19–30 Aflibercept in the treatment of metastatic colorectal cancer.

Weber J. Review: Anti-CTLA-4 Antibody Ipilimumab: Case Studies of Clinical Response and Immune-Related Adverse Events. *Oncologist* 2007; 12 864–872.

Weber JS, Kahler KC, Hauschild A. Management of immune-related adverse events and kinetics of response with ipilimumab. *J Clin Oncol* 2012; 30(21):2691–7.

Weidner N. Tumoral Vascularity as a Prognostic Factor in Cancer Patients: The Evidence Continues to Grow. *J Pathol* 1998; 184 119–120.

Weinberg RA. Fundamental Understandings: How Cancer Arises. *Sci Am* Sept 1996; 275(3) 62–72.

Weinberg RA. *The Biology of Cancer,* 2nd ed. London, UK: Garland Science. Taylor and Francis Group LLC; 2013.

Watanabe R, Wei L, Huang J, 2011. mTOR signaling, function, novel inhibitors, and therapeutic targets. *J Nucl Med* 52(4):497–500.

Weber JS, Yang JC, Atkins MB, Disis ML. Toxicities of immunotherapy for the practitioner. *J Clin Oncol* 2015 [Epub ahead of print April 27, 2015]. DOI:10.1200/JCO.2014.60.0379

Wilkes GM, Barton-Burke M. *Oncology Nursing Drug Handbook.* Burlington, MA: Jones & Bartlett Learning, 2015.

Wilkes GM. *Targeted Cancer Therapy: A Handbook for Nurses.* Sudbury, MA: Jones & Bartlett Publishing, 2011.

Wolmark N, Yothers G, O'Connell MJ, et al. A Phase III Trial Comparing mFOLFOX6 to mFOLFOX6 Plus Bevacizumab in Stage II and III Carcinoma of the Colon: Results of NSABP Protocol C-08. *J Clin Oncol* 27; 18s 2009 (suppl; abstr LBA4).

Wong RS, Casper C, Munshi N, et. al. A multicenter, randomized, double-blind, placebo-controlled study of the efficacy and safety of siltuximab, an anti-Interleukin-6 monoclonal antibody, in patients with multicentric Castleman's disease. *Blood* 2013; 122(21):505. Oral presentation presented at 55th American Society of Hematology (ASH) Annual Meeting; December 7–11, 2013; New Orleans, LA.

Wood LS, Gornell S, Rini BI, 2012; Maximizing clinical outcomes with axitnib therapy in advanced renal cell carcinoma through proactive side effect management *Comm Oncol* 9 (2) 46–55.

Wood LS. Managing the side effects of sorafenib and sunitinib. *Commun Oncol* 2006; 3(9) 558–562.

Wyeth-Ayerst Laboratories. *Antibody-Targeted Chemotherapy: Coming of Age.* Philadelphia, PA: Wyeth-Ayerest Laboratories; 1999.

Wyeth Pharmaceuticals Inc. Torisel (temsirolimus) [package insert]. Philadelphia, PA, May 2014.

Yeh ETH, Bickford CL. Cardiovascular Complications of Cancer Therapy: Incidence, Pathogenesis, Diagnosis, and Management. *J Am Coll Cardiol* 2009; 53 2231–2247.

Zachariae R, Zachariae C, Ibsen HHW. Psychological Symptoms and Quality of Life of Dermatology Outpatients and Hospitalized Dermatology Patients. *Acta Dermatol-Venereol* 2003; 84(3) 205–212.

Zielinski C, Knapp S, Mascaux C, Hirsch F. Rationale for targeting the immune system through checkpoint molecule blockade in the treatment of non-small cell lung cancer. *Annals of Oncol* 2013; 24:1170–1179.

Zou W. Regulatory T-cells, tumor immunity, and immunotherapy. *Nat Rev Cancer* 2006; 6:295–307.

Drug: ado-trastuzumab emtansine (Kadcyla)

Class: Antibody-drug conjugate, HER2-targeted.

Mechanism of Action: HER2-targeted monoclonal antibody (trastuzumab) with microtubule-inhibitor conjugate. The cellular poison DM1 (emtansine), a micro-tubular inhibitor, is linked to trastuzumab. Like a Trojan horse, when the drug attaches to an HER2 receptor, the poison is internalized in the HER2 positive cell, and the poison released intracellularly. Then, MD1 (emtansine) binds to tubulin, preventing cell division, which results in cell cycle arrest and programmed cell death (apoptosis). The drug appears also to inhibit HER2 receptor signaling, mediate antibody-dependent cell-mediated cytotoxicity (ADCC), and prevent shedding of the HER2 extracellular domain in human, HER2 positive, breast cancer cells.

Metabolism: Maximal serum levels occur near the end of the infusion. DM1 is about 93% plasma protein bound, and DM1 is a substrate of P-glycoprotein (P-gp). DM1 is metabolized by CYP3A4 primarily and by CYP3A5 to a lesser degree, but does not inhibit or induce major CYP450 enzymes. The elimination half-life of the drug is about 4 days. Renal impairment (mild or moderate) does not affect clearance.

Indications: Drug is indicated as a single agent for the treatment of patients with HER2 positive, metastatic breast cancer who previously received trastuzumab and a taxane, separately or in combination. Patients should have received prior therapy for metastatic disease or developed disease recurrence during or within 6 months of completing adjuvant therapy.

Dosage/Range:

- Recommended dose is 3.6 mg/kg given as an IV infusion every 3 weeks (21-day cycle), until disease progression or unacceptable toxicity. Initial dose is 3.6 mg/kg (actual body weight) IV infusion over 90 minutes; subsequent doses are 3.6 mg/kg IV over 30 min. Do not exceed dose of 3.6 mg/kg.
- Drug is not recommended for patients who have previously had trastuzumab permanently discontinued due to infusion-related reactions or hypersensitivity reactions.
- Dose interruption, reduction, or treatment discontinuation for management of increased LFTs, decreased LVEF, thrombocytopenia, ILD, peripheral neuropathy: See full prescribing information.
  - Starting dose: 3.6 mg/kg. First dose reduction = dose level 3 mg/kg; second dose reduction = dose level 2.4 mg/kg; if further dose reductions needed, discontinue drug.
  - Increased Liver Function Tests
  - Increased serum transaminases (AST/ALT): grade 2 (> 2.5 to ≤ 5 × ULN = treat at same dose level); grade 3 (> 5 to ≤ 20 X ULN): hold ado-trastuzumab emtansine until AST/ALT recovers to grade ≤ 2, and then reduce one dose level; grade 4 (> 20 × ULN): permanently discontinue drug.
  - Hyperbilirubinemia: grade 2 (> 1.5 to ≤ 3 X ULN): hold drug until total bilirubin recovers to ≤ grade 1, then treat at same dose level; grade 3 (> 3 to ≤ 10 × ULN): hold drug until total bilirubin recovers to ≤ grade 1, then reduce one dose level; grade 4 (> 10 × ULN): permanently discontinue drug.

- Permanently discontinue drug in patients with transaminases > 3 × ULN and concomitant total bilirubin > 2 × ULN.
- Permanently discontinue drug in patients diagnosed with nodular regenerative hyperplasia (NRH).
- Left Ventricular Dysfunction:
- Symptomatic CHF: discontinue ado-trastuzumab emtansine.
- LVEF < 40%: do not administer ado-trastuzumab emtansine; repeat LVEF assessment within 3 weeks. If LVEF < 40% is confirmed, discontinue drug.
- LVEF 40% to ≤ 45% and decrease is ≥ 10% points from baseline: hold ado-trastuzumab emtansine. Repeat LVEF assessment within 3 weeks. If LVEF has not recovered to within 10% points from baseline, discontinue drug.
- LVEF 40% to ≤ 45% and decrease is < 10% points from baseline, continue treatment with drug; repeat LVEF assessment within 3 weeks.
- LVEF > 45%: continue treatment with ado-trastuzumab emtansine.
- Thrombocytopenia
- Grade 3 (platelets 25,0000/ mm^3 to < 50,000/mm^3): hold drug until platelet count recovers to ≤ grade 1 (≥ 75,000/mm^3) and then treat at same dose level.
- Grade 4 (platelets < 25,000/mm^3): hold drug until platelet count recovers to ≤ grade 1 (≥ 75,000/ mm^3), then reduce one dose level.
- Pulmonary Toxicity: Permanently discontinue drug in patients diagnosed with ILD or pneumonitis.
- Peripheral Neuropathy: Temporarily discontinue drug in patients experiencing grade 3 or 4 peripheral neuropathy until it resolves to ≤ grade 2.
- DO NOT re-escalate dose after a dose reduction is made.
- If a planned dose is delayed or missed, it should be administered as soon as possible; do not wait until the next planned cycle. The treatment schedule should be adjusted to maintain a 3-week interval between doses, at the dose and rate the patient tolerated in most recent infusion.
- Kadcyla Access Solutions available to assist patients in specific access and reimbursement issues, including copay assistance for underinsured patients and free medication for uninsured patients (1-888-249-4918).

Drug Preparation:

- Drug is available in single-use 100-mg and 160-mg sterile lyophilized powder containing vials. Double-check label to ensure that drug is Kadcyla (ado-trastuzumab emtansine). Do not substitute Herceptin (trastuzumab) for this drug.
- Using a sterile syringe, aseptically add 8 mL Sterile Water for Injection into the 160-mg vial, or 5 mL to the 100-mg vial. Vials reconstitute to 20mg/mL.
- Gently swirl the vial until solution is completely dissolved. Solution should be colorless to pale brown. Do not shake or freeze. Do not use if visible particulate matter or if the solution is cloudy or discolored.
- Aseptically draw up calculated dose volume, and add reconstituted solution to an infusion bag containing 250 mL 0.9% Sodium Chloride Injection. Mix by gentle inversion of infusion bag. DO NOT USE Dextrose (5%) solution.

- Do not mix or dilute the drug with any other drugs.
- Reconstituted vials should be used immediately, or may be stored in a refrigerator at 2° C–8° C (36° F–46° F) for up to 24 hours prior to use. Do not freeze. Diluted drug infusion bags may be stored in a refrigerator at 2° C–8° C (36° F–46° F) for up to 24 hours prior to use. This storage time is additional to the time allowed for the reconstituted vials. Do not freeze or shake.
- Drug contains no preservatives and is for single use only. Discard any unused solution after 4 hours.

Drug Administration:
- Prior to administration: Assess LFTs prior to each cycle, LVEF baseline and at least every 3 months during treatment.
- Administer via 0.22 micron in-line, non-protein adsorptive polyethersulfone (PES) filter. Do not use Dextrose (5%) solution; do not administer by IVP or IV bolus.
- Administer initial dose over 90 minutes; subsequent doses over 30 min (if prior infusions were well tolerated), at 3-week intervals. Observe patient **during** and following infusion (at least 90 minutes **following** initial dose, and for at least 30 min **following** subsequent doses) for flushing, fever, chills, dyspnea, hypotension, wheezing, bronchospasm, and tachycardia, or other infusion-related reactions.
  - The infusion rate should be slowed or interrupted if an infusion reaction occurs.
  - Incidence in Study 1 was 1.4%, and most reactions resolved over the course of several hours to a day after the infusion was terminated. One patient had severe infusion reaction/anaphylaxis. Emergency equipment and medications should be immediately available.
  - Permanently discontinued drug if life-threatening infusion-related reactions occur.
- Monitor infusion site for possible subcutaneous infiltration during drug administration. Avoid extravasation. Reactions, generally within 24 hours of drug administration, have been reported characterized by erythema, tenderness, skin irritation, pain, and swelling at the infusion site. These were usually mild.

Drug Interactions:
- Incompatible with Dextrose (5%) solutions.
- Strong CYP3A4 inhibitors (e.g., atazanavir, clarithromycin, indinavir, itraconazole, nefazodone, nelfinavir, ritonavir, saquinavir, telithromycin, voriconazole) may increase drug serum level and increase toxicity. Avoid concomitant administration. If concomitant use is unavoidable, consider delaying ado-trastuzumab emtansine until the strong CYP3A4 inhibitor has cleared from the circulation (about 3 elimination half-lives of the CYP3A4 inhibitor). Assess for signs/symptoms of toxicity.

Lab Effects/Interference:
- Increased LFTs: bilirubin (17%), increased AST (98%), increased ALT (82%).
- Decreased platelet (83%), and neutrophil (39%) counts; decreased hemoglobin (60%).
- Decreased potassium (33%).

Special Considerations:
- Ensure patient is HER2 positive (overexpression or gene amplification) using an FDA-approved test by laboratories with demonstrated proficiency.

- Hepatotoxity: serious hepatotoxicity has been reported, including liver failure and death, in patients treated with ado-trastuzumab emtansine.
  - Monitor serum transaminases and bilirubin prior to initiation of ado-trastuzumab emtansine treatment and prior to each ado-trastuzumab emtansine dose. Reduce dose or discontinue drug as appropriate in cases of increased serum transaminases or total bilirubin.
  - Nodular regenerative hyperplasia (NRH) has affected 3 patients out of 884 treated patients, but it can be confirmed only by histopathology. Consider NRH in patients with clinical symptoms of portal hypertension but with normal transaminases and no manifestations of cirrhosis.
- Cardiac toxicity: ado-trastuzumab emtansine increases risk of LVEF dysfunction. In Study 1, incidence of LVEF dysfunction occurred in 1.8% of patients. Evaluate LVEF in all patients prior to and during treatment (e.g., every 3 months) with ado-trastuzumab emtansine. If at routine monitoring, LVEF is < 40%, or is 40% to 45% with a 10% or greater absolute decrease below the pretreatment value, hold drug and repeat LVEF assessment within approximately 3 weeks. Permanently discontinue ado-trastuzumab emtansine if the LVEF has not improved or has declined further.
- Embryo-fetal toxicity: Embryo-fetal death or birth defects can occur following exposure to ado-trastuzumab emtansine. Verify pregnancy status prior to the initiation of ado-trastuzumab emtansine. Advise patients of these risks and the need for effective contraception during and after treatment. If the drug is administered during pregnancy or if a patient becomes pregnant while receiving the drug, report exposure immediately to the Genentech Adverse Event Line (1-888-835-2555). Encourage women who may be exposed during pregnancy to enroll in the MotHER Pregnancy Registry by contacting 1-800-690-6720.
- Interstitial lung disease (ILD) may occur, including pneumonitis (incidence 0.8%–1.2%), possibly leading to acute respiratory distress syndrome. Evaluate symptoms if they arise (e.g., dyspnea, cough, fatigue, and pulmonary infiltrates) and permanently discontinue drug if ILD or pneumonitis is diagnosed. Patients with dyspnea at rest due to complications of advanced cancer and comorbidities may be at increased risk for pulmonary toxicity.
- Infusion-related reactions, hypersensitivity reactions: Drug was not studied in patients with prior hypersensitivity or serious infusion reactions to/from trastuzumab, so drug is not recommended in this group of patients. In clinical studies, incidence of infusion-related reactions was 1.4%, and in most patients, reactions resolved in hours to a day after the infusion. Drug should be permanently discontinued if a life-threatening infusion-related reaction occurs. Patients should be closely monitored during and after treatment (e.g., monitor patient 90 minutes and 30 minutes after initial and subsequent infusions, respectively). Emergency resuscitation and medication should be immediately available in the infusion area.
- Thrombocytopenia occurred in 31.2% of patients overall. Nadir occurred by day 8, and generally improved to grade 0-1 by the next scheduled dose. Grade 3 or higher thrombocytopenia occurred in 14.5% of patients (45.1% in Asian patients), so platelet count should be monitored closely (baseline and prior to each dose); modify dose accordingly. Patients with thrombocytopenia (< 100,000/mm^3) and patients on anticoagulant treatment should be closely monitored.

• Fatal hemorrhage has occurred, in patients with and without risk factors.
  • Overrall frequency of hemorrhage was 32% in clinical trials in the Kadcyla group (1.8% grade 3–4) vs 16.4% (0.8% grades 3–4) in the lapatinib+capecitabine treated group.
  • Use cautiously in patients with thrombocytopenia or receiving anticoagulation or antiplatelet therapy if drug is medically necessary, and monitor patient very closely.
• Peripheral neuropathy occurred in 21.2% of patients overall in Study 1; it was mainly grade 1 and sensory. Greater than grade 3 peripheral neuropathy occurred in 2.2% of patients. Assess for signs/symptoms baseline and before each dose. Drug should be interrrupted until peripheral neuropathy has resolved to ≤ grade 2.
• Most common side effects (frequency > 25%) are nausea, fatigue, musculoskeletal pain, thrombocytopenia, increased liver transaminases, headache, constipation. Most common grade 3–4 adverse effects in clinical trials were thrombocytopenia, increased transaminases, anemia, hypokalemia, peripheral neuropathy, and fatigue.

Potential Toxicities/Side Effects and the Nursing Process

I.   POTENTIAL FOR BLEEDING, INFECTION AND FATIGUE related to BONE MARROW SUPPRESSION

Defining Characteristics: Thrombocytopenia occurs in 31.2% (14.5% grade 3–4, while in Asian patients it was 45.1%), anemia in 14.3%, and neutropenia in 6.7%. Fatigue occurs in 36.3%. Epistaxis occurs in 22.5%. Platelet nadir occurs by day 8 and usually returns to grade 0 or 1 by the next scheduled dose. In clinical trials, the incidence of thrombocytopenia was higher in Asian patients.

Nursing Implications: Assess CBC/differential and platelet count baseline and prior to each treatment. Hold drug if platelet count < 75,000 cells/mm³ and dose-modify per physician/prescribing information. Teach patient to report bleeding, signs/symptoms of bleeding, right away. Teach patient to self-assess for signs/symptoms of infection, bleeding, or severe fatigue. Teach patient to avoid aspirin-containing OTC medications and NSAIDs. Teach patient strategies to manage fatigue and conserve energy, such as alteration of rest and activity amd organizing chores.

II.   POTENTIAL FOR SENSORY/PERCEPTUAL ALTERATIONS related to NEUROLOGICAL TOXICITY

Defining Characteristics: Peripheral neuropathy occurs in 21.2% (2.2% grades 3-4), dizziness 10.2%, headache in 28.2% of patients.

Nursing Implications: Teach patient that these side effects may occur and to report them. Assess sensory/perceptual changes (e.g., numbness, tingling, weakness) baseline and prior to each drug administration. Assess one side versus the other side, and note extent of paresthesias if present (stocking glove distribution), starting at fingertips or tips of toes, and progressing proximally to wrist/ankle like a glove and stocking, and document. Assess patient's ability to do ADLs, and impact of neuropathy on functioning. Discuss grade with NP/PA or physician and need to dose-modify or interrupt (hold drug for grade 3–4). Assess for presence of dizziness and risk for falls, and discuss strategies to minimize risk of falling. Assess for headache and discuss self-care strategies to prevent/manage them.

III. ALTERATION IN NUTRITION related to DYSPEPSIA, STOMATITIS, DRY MOUTH, ABDOMINAL PAIN, VOMITING, DIARRHEA, CONSTIPATION, NAUSEA, DYSGEUSIA, INCREASED LFTs

Defining Characteristics: Dyspepsia occurs in 9.2% of patients, stomatitis in 14.1%, dry mouth 16.7%, abdominal pain (18.6%), diarrhea (24.1%), constipation (26.5%), nausea (39.8%), increased transaminases (28.8%), and hypokalemia (10.2%).

Nursing Implications: Assess baseline nutritional status, lab findings, especially LFTs (transaminases, bilirubin), and serum potassium. Discuss abnormalities with physician or NP/PA and understand dose interruption or modification per prescribing information. Teach patient that nutritional impact symptoms may occur and to report them. Discuss with the patient medication and self-care strategies to manage nausea, vomiting, diarrhea, constipation, dyspepsia, and stomatitis if they occur. Discuss dietary modifications as needed. If the patient has persistent diarrhea, discuss lab testing of serum potassium and need for repletion and hydration with physician or NP/PA. If symptoms persist, discuss pharmacologic plan revision with NP/PA or physician.

IV. ALTERATIONS IN COMFORT related to MYALGIAS, ARTHRALGIAS, MUSCULOSKELETAL PAIN

Defining Chracteristics: Myalgias occur in 14.1% of patients, arthralgias in 19.2%, and musculoskeletal pain in 36% of patients.

Nursing Implications: Teach patient that these symptoms may occur and to report them. Assess baseline comfort, and teach self-care strategies, such as application of heat or local cooling to manage symptoms. If they persist, discuss pharmacologic management with NP/PA or physician.

Drug: afatinib (Gilotrif)

Class: Tyrosine kinase inhibitor of the epidermal growth factor receptor.

Mechanism of Action: Drug is a 4- anilinoquinazoline. It binds to the kinase domains of EGFR1, HER2, and HER4, thus irreversibly preventing the tyrosine kinase from auto-phosphorylation and downstream signaling to the cell nucleus. It prevents cell proliferation by inhibiting wild-type EGFR, as well in as cells expressing EGFR exon 19 deletion mutations, exon 21 L858R mutations, and some with a secondary T790 M mutation. It also inhibits proliferation in cell lines overexpressing HER2.

Metabolism: After oral dosing, time to peak afatinib plasma concentration (Tmax) is 2–5 hrs. Drug is 95% protein bound. A high-fat meal decreases AUC by 39%, and maximal concentration (Cmax) by 50%. Drug is excreted via the biliary system and the feces (85%), with 4% recovered from the urine. Elimination half-life is 37 hours with repeat dosing, and steady state is reached within 8 days. Median trough plasma concentrations are 27% higher in patients with mild renal dysfunction (Cr Cl 60–89 mL/min) and 85% higher in patients with moderate renal dysfunction (CrCl 30–59 mL/min) compared to patients with normal renal function (Cr Cl > 90 mL/min). While there is no effect on mild to moderate hepatic dysfunction on drug excretion, the drug has not been studied in patients with severe hepatic dysfunction.

Indication: Treatment of patients with metastatic NSCLC whose tumor has an EGFR exon 19 deletion or exon 21 (L858R) substitution. Mutations must be detected by an FDA-approved test. Drug safety and efficacy are not established for other EGFR mutations in NSCLC.

Dosage/Range:
* 40-mg orally once daily until disease progession or intolerance.

Dose Modifications:
* Hold drug for (1) any grade 3 or higher toxicity; (2) grade 2 or higher diarrhea persisting for 2 or more consecutive days while taking anti-diarrheal medication; (3) grade 2 cutaneous reactions that last for > 7 days or are intolerable; and (4) grade 2 or higher renal dysfunction.
* Resume drug when toxicity fully resolved, returns to baseline, or improves to grade 1. Reduce dose by 10 mg less per day than the dose being taken when toxicity occurred.
* Permanently discontinue drug for (1) life-threatening bullous, blistering, or exfoliative skin lesions; (2) confirmed interstitial lung disease (ILD); (3) severe, drug-induced hepatic impairment; (4) persistent ulcerative keratitis; (5) symptomatic left ventricular dysfunction; (6) severe or intolerable adverse reactions at any dose.

Drug Preparation:
* None, oral. Available in 40-mg, 30-mg, and 20-mg tablets.

Drug Administration:
* Teach patient to take tablet on empty stomach, at least 1 hour before or 2 hours after a meal, and not to make up a dose, if missed, if it is within 12 hours of the next dose.

Drug Interactions:
* P-glycoprotein **inhibitors** (e.g., ritonavir): administered 1 hour before afatinib increased systemic exposure by 48%; do not coadminister. Other inhibitors are cyclosporine A, ketoconazole, itraconazole, erythromycin, verapamil, quinidine, tacrolimus, nelfinavir, saquinavr, amiodarone. If must give concomitantly, reduce afatinif dose by 10 mg/day if not tolerated.

TREATMENT

- P-glycoprotein **inducers** (e.g., rifampicin): may decrease afatinib exposure (up to 34%). Do not coadminister. Other inducers are carbamazepine, phenytoin, phenobarbital, St John's wort. If must coadminister, increase afatinib dose by 10 mg/day as tolerated. Teach patient to avoid St. John's wort.

Lab Effects/Interference:
- Decreased serum potassium.
- Increased serum AST, ALT.

Special Considerations:
- Diarrhea is common (incidence 96%); occurs during the first 6 weeks of treatment but may be severe in 15% (grade 3–4). It may rarely result in dehydration, with or without renal impairment, and be fatal. Renal impairment as a result of diarrhea occurred in 6.1% of patients in clinical trials. Hold drug for grade 2 prolonged (> 48 hours) or grade 3 diarrhea (see dose modification). Teach patient to take anti-diarrheal medicine (e.g., loperamide) at onset of diarrhea and to continue until no bowel movements occur for 12 hours.
- Drug has not been studied in patients with renal dysfunction. Closely monitor patients with moderate (CrCl 30–59 mL/min) to severe (CrCl < 30 mL/min), and adjust afatinib dose as needed if not tolerated.
- Grade 3 bullous and exfoliative skin dsorders may occur rarely; drug should be discontinued if life-threatening. See dose modifications.
- ILD characterized by lung infiltrates, pneumonitis, ARDS, or allergic alveolitis occurred in 1.5% of patients in clinical trials. Risk may be higher in Asian patients (2.1%). Hold drug if ILD suspected, and discontinue if ILD confirmed.
- Hepatic toxicity: Monitor LFTs baseline and periodically during treatment, closely monitoring patients with severe liver dysfunction. Ten percent of patients across clinical trials had abnormalities; 0.18% were fatal. Hold drug in patients with worsening LFTs, and discontinue in patients who develop severe hepatic impairment. As drug has not been studied in patients with severe liver impairment (Child Hugh C), closely monitor patients with severe liver impairment, and adjust afatinib dose if not tolerated.
- Keratitis characterized by worsening or acute eye inflammation, lacrimation, light insensitivity, blurred vision, eye pain; red eye may occur. Incidence across clinical trials was 0.8%. Hold drug if keratitis is suspected, and interrpt/discontinue drug if ulcerative keratitis is confirmed. Use drug cautiously, if at all, in patients with a history of keratitis, ulcerative keratitis, or severe dry eye. Closely monitor patients who wear contact lenses, as this is a risk factor for keratitis and ulceration.
- Drug is embryotoxic. Teach women of childbearing age to use highly effective contraception to prevent pregnancy during and for at least 2 weeks after the last dose of afatinib. Nursing mothers should discontinue drug or nursing.
- Afatinib should not be used in combination with vinorelbine in the treatment of HER2 positive metastatic breast cancer, as this may increase mortality as well as toxicity in those patients receiving the combination (Boehringer Ingelheim, 2014).
- Most common side effects are diarrhea, rash/dermatitis, stomatitis, paronychia, dry skin, decreased appetite, and pruritus.

Potential Toxicities/Side Effects and the Nursing Process

I.   ALTERATION IN ELIMINATION PATTERN related to DIARRHEA

Defining Characteristics: Diarrhea affects approximately 96% of patients with 15% of patients experiencing grade 3 diarrhea. Diarrhea usually occurs in the first 6 weeks. Six percent of patients developed renal impairment as a complication of diarrhea. Grade 2 persisting > 48 hours, or grade 3 requires drug interruption.

Nursing Implications: Assess bowel elimination pattern baseline and regularly during therapy. Teach patient to report diarrhea; teach patient self-care strategies to manage diarrhea, such as dietary modification and self-administration of loperamide and to continue loperamide until the patient has no loose bowel movement in 12 hours; teach patient to minimize potential complications, such as dehydration and electrolyte depletion. Identify patients at risk for dehydration and follow closely, such as patients with renal insufficiency, diabetes, congestive heart failure, or the older population. If diarrhea does not resolve or is severe, discuss with physician dose interruption, as well as fluid and electrolyte replacement. If diarrhea is refractory or difficult to manage, patient may become dehydrated and will be at risk for acute renal failure, which may be fatal. If the patient is dehydrated and at risk for renal impairment (e.g., preexisting renal disease, disease or medications that may lead to renal disease, advancing age), the drug should be temporarily discontinued while the patient is rehydrated. Renal function should be assessed at baseline and periodically during therapy, more closely if the patient has diarrhea and is at risk for dehydration. Hold drug for prolonged grade 2 diarrhea (> 48 hours) or grade 3, or diarrhea unresponsive to therapy, until diarrhea resolves to < grade 1, and reduce dose.

II.   ALTERATION IN SKIN INTEGRITY related to RASH

Defining Characteristics: As expected, because EGFR is important in skin function, this is the area of major toxicity. Rash, erythema, and caneiform rash affect 90% of patients, with an incidence of grade 3 of 16%. Incidence of grades 1–3 palmar-plantar erythrodysesthesia was 7%. Rarely, bullous, blistering, and exfoliative lesions have occurred (0.15%). Pruritus affects 21%, dry skin 31%, and paronychia 58%, with 11% grade 3 or higher.

Nursing Implications: Assess skin integrity of face, neck, arms, and upper trunk, baseline and regularly during treatment. Teach patient that rash may occur, explain the rash's usual course, and teach self-care measures for comfort. Emphasize the need to keep skin with rash clean to prevent infection. Teach patient that skin may become dry and to use skin emollients or moisturizers. Assess body image intactness; if rash develops, assess its threat to body image. Encourage patient to verbalize feelings; provide emotional support and individualize care plan to patient response. For rash management, refer to the introduction in this chapter. Teach all patients to (1) use a water-based emollient frequently during the day to prevent dryness, (2) stay hydrated, (3) avoid sun exposure, and (4) wear SPF 30 (zinc-based). Do not use anti-acne medications. Tetracycline analogues provide anti-inflammatory benefit. **Grade 1/mild rash** (localized, does not interfere with ADLs, and is not infected): Goal is to preserve skin integrity, minimize discomfort, and prevent infection. Key patient teaching includes (1) use a mild soap with active ingredients that reduce skin drying, such as pyrithione zinc (Head & Shoulders), (2) consider applying aloe gel to red, tender areas, (3) report distressing tenderness, as pramoxine (lidocaine topical anesthetic) may help, (4) keep fingernails clean and trimmed, and (5) apply zinc ointment to rectal mucosa after washing. Management: maintain current drug dose, observe or give topical hydrocortisone 1% or 2.5% or clindamycin 1% gel (anti-inflammatory benefit), reassess in 2 weeks. **For grade 2/moderate,** which is generalized, mild symptoms, has minimal effect on ADLs, and no infection: Goal is to prevent infection and promote comfort. Continue EGFRI dose; use topicals (hydrocortisone 2.5% or clindamycin 1% gel) and consider adding doxycycline 100 mg PO twice daily or minocycline 100 mg PO twice daily (give antimicrobial and anti-inflammatory effect); reassess after 2 weeks. **Interrupt drug** if patient develops prolonged grade 2 cutaneous reactions (lasting > 7 days), or if intolerable. **For grade 3–4 or severe rash** (generalized, severe, has a significant impact on ADLs, and increased risk of infection): The goal is to prevent infection or identify it early to minimize complications and to promote effective coping. **Interrupt drug.** Treat rash with topicals (hydrocortisone 2.5%, or clindamycin 1% gel,), doxycycline 100 mg PO twice daily or minocycline 100 mg PO twice daily, and methylprednisolone (Medrol dose pack); reassess after 2 weeks. Resume drug when rash improved to grade 2, at full or reduced dose (Lynch et al., 2007; Lacouture et al., 2011). If rash appears infected (exudate, vesicular formation, different appearance), obtain culture and sensitivity, treat empirically until sensitivity value determined, and/or obtain dermatology consult. Hold drug for severe rash that does not respond to medical intervention. If the drug is interrupted, afatinib can be resumed at a lower dose once skin reaction has resolved to a grade 1 or less. Teach patient to stop drug and to report the development of bullous lesions, blisters, or desquamation right away.

III. SENSORY/PERCEPTUAL ALTERATION, POTENTIAL, related to CONJUNCTIVITIS, EYE DRYNESS, KERATITIS

Defining Characteristics: Conjunctivitis and eye dryness may occur and are generally mild to moderate (grades 1 to 2). Rarely, keratitis and corneal ulceration may occur. Incidence of conjunctivitis is 11%, and keratitis is 0.8% across all studies.

Nursing Implications: Teach patient to report symptoms of keratitis (e.g., any new or worsening eye irritation, lacrimation, light sensitivity, blurred vision, eye pain, red eye) or change in visual acuity. Teach patient to use artificial tears to keep eyes lubricated. Refer patient to ophthalmologist immediately for any acute signs or symptoms, such as red eye or eye pain. Teach patient to stop drug if these occur and to report them immediately. Drug is interrupted if keratitis is suspected and if ulcerative keratitis is confirmed, drug interruption should continue or drug should be discontinued. Drug should be used cautiously in patients with a history of keratitis, ulcerative keratitis, severe dry eye, or in patients who wear contact lens.

IV. POTENTIONAL ALTERATION IN NUTRITION, LESS THAN BODY REQUIREMENTS, related to MUCOSITIS, HEPATOTOXICITY, ANOREXIA, NAUSEA, VOMITING

Defining Characteristics: Stomatitis is common, occurring in 71% of patients receiving afatinib, with grade 3–4 occurring in 9% of patients. Cheilitis occurs in 12% of patients. Decreased appetite occurs in 19%, with 4% grade 3–4. Hepatotoxicity may occur. ALT and AST elevated in 11% and 8% of patients respectively.

Nursing Implications: Assess oral hygiene practices and status of oral mucosa, gums, and teeth baseline and regularly throughout therapy. Assess nutritional status and weight baseline and regularly during treatment. Teach patient to report stomatitis, and to use a systematic cleansing regimen as determined by institutional policy. Assess baseline LFTs, and monitor LFTs and patient tolerance very closely during therapy if abnormal at baseline. If a patient develops worsening LFTs, discuss with physician dose interruption or discontinuance (see dose modifications). Teach patient to report irritation of lips (cheilitis) and loss of appetite.

Drug: alemtuzumab (campath-1H anti-CD52 monoclonal antibody, humanized IgG1 MAb)

Class: Monoclonal antibody.

Mechanism of Action: Humanized monoclonal antibody, which targets the CD52 antigen present on the surface of most normal human lymphocyte cells, as well as malignant T-cell and B-cell malignant lymphocytes (lymphomas). Most monocytes, macrophages, NK cells, some granulocytes, and CD4$^+$ cells, also have the CD52 antigen. Once the monoclonal antibody binds with the CD52 antigen, it initiates antibody-dependent cellular cytotoxicity (ADCC) and complement binding, which then lead to apoptosis, or programmed cell death, and activation of normal T-cell cytotoxicity against the malignant cells.

Metabolism: When given subcutaneously or intravenously, pharmacokinetics appear similar, but the absorption is much slower with subcutaneous administration. It takes a higher cumulative dose (an additional 6 weeks) to achieve a therapeutic level. The mean half-life is 11 hours after the first 30-mg dose, 6 hours after the last 30-mg dose, but steady-state plasma levels are not reached until week 6. Levels appear to correlate with the number of circulating CD52-positive cells. Drug clearance decreases with repeated dosing as more leukemic cells are killed. Given subcutaneously, CLL cells were cleared from the blood in 95% of patients in a median time of 21 days (Lundin et al., 2002). Host antibodies may develop 14–21 days after the first dose and theoretically can decrease lymphocyte killing.

Indication: Indicated as a single agent for the treatment of B-cell chronic lymphocytic leukemia (B-CLL).

Dosage/Range:
- Initial dose is 3 mg IV infusion over 2 hours, daily, with dose escalated to 10 mg daily when well tolerated (side effects are grade 2 or less).
- When dose of 10 mg is well tolerated, the dose is increased to 30 mg and becomes the maintenance dose, 30 mg/day, given three times a week (e.g., Monday, Wednesday, and Friday) for up to 12 weeks. Total duration of therapy, including dose escalation, is 12 weeks. Dose escalation to 30 mg usually takes 3–7 days.
- Subcutaneous administration is better tolerated and results in similar efficacy (Lundin et al., 2002).

Dose Modification for Neutropenia or Thrombocytopenia:
- ANC < 250/μL and/or platelet count ≤ 25,000/μL.
  - First occurrence: hold alemtuzumab; resume alemtuzumab at 30 mg when ANC ≥ 500/μL and platelet count ≥ 50,000/μL.
  - Second occurrence: hold alemtuzumab; resume alemtuzumab at 10 mg when ANC ≥ 500/μL and platelet count ≥ 50,000/μL.
  - Third occurrence: discontinue alemtuzumab.
- ≥ 50% decrease from baseline in patients initiating therapy with a baseline ANC ≤ 250/μL and/or a baseline platelet count ≤ 25,000/μL.
  - First occurrence: hold alemtuzumab; resume alemtuzumab at 30 mg upon return to baseline value(s).
  - Second occurrence: hold alemtuzumab; resume alemtuzumab at 10 mg upon return to baseline value(s).
  - Third occurrence: discontinue alemtuzumab.
- If the delay between dosing is ≥ 7 days, initiate therapy at alemtuzumab 3 mg and escalate to 10 mg and then to 30 mg as tolerated.

Drug Preparation:
- Available in single-use vials containing 30 mg alemtuzumab in 1 mL of diluent.
- Use a syringe calibrated in increments of 0.01 for 3-mg and 10-mg doses. Use a syringe calibrated in 0.1 mL increments for the 30-mg dose. Draw up ordered dose, and dilute in 100 mL sterile 0.9% Sodium Chloride USP or 5% Dextrose in water. Gently invert IV bag to mix. Use within 8 hours after dilution. Store at room temperature or refrigerated; protect from light.
- Drug is compatible with polyvinylchloride (PVC) infusion bags and PVC or polyethylene-lined PVC administration sets. Do not add or simultaneously infuse other drug substances through the same IV line.
- Drug is available only through the Campath Distribution Program, free of charge (1-877-422-6728); it requires healthcare provider documentation and compliance with certain requirements.

Drug Administration:
- IV infusion over 2 hours. Initial dose is 3mg; repeat daily until infusion reactions are less than or equal to grade 2; then administer 10 mg daily until infusion reactions are less than or equal to grade 2; then administer the 30-mg dose as below (subsequent dosing).

- Premedicate with acetaminophen 650 mg and diphenhydramine 50 mg 30 min prior to beginning each infusion.
- Assess CBC/differential weekly during alemtuzumab therapy, more frequently if cytopenias.
- Stop drug immediately if a reaction develops during the infusion.
- Severe reactions may require hydrocortisone 200 mg. If drug requires slower infusion, repeat premedications at 4 hours.
- Institute appropriate medical management for infusion reactions as needed (e.g., steroids, epinephrine, meperidine).
- Subsequent dosing: 30 mg IV over 2 h three times per week, for a minimum of 4 weeks, but may continue up to 12 weeks (total duration of therapy is 12 weeks, including dose escalation). Give on Monday, Wednesday, and Friday.
- If dose held more than 7 days, reinstitute gradually with dose escalation as with initial dose.
- Give IV hydration (at least 500 mL D_5W or 0.9% NS) before and after drug dose (Williamson, 2001).
- *Anti-infective prophylaxis recommended*, starting on day 8 and continuing for 2 months after treatment completed/stopped, or CD4+ count ≥ 200 cells/μL, whichever occurs later:
  - PCP prophylaxis with trimethoprim and sulfamethoxazole (Bactrim) DS/twice daily, three times a week (or equivalent);
  - Herpes prophylaxis: an antiviral such as famciclovir 250 mg twice daily (or equivalent). Stop the drug immediately if a serious infection occurs.
  - Dose-reduce if ANC < 250/μL and/or platelet count ≤ 25,000/μL. See package insert.
  - Single doses > 30 mg or cumulative doses > 90 mg weekly increase the risk of pancytopenia.

Drug Interactions:
- No formal drug studies have been done.

Lab Effects/Interference:
- An immune response to the drug may interfere with subsequent serum laboratory tests using antibodies.
- Decreased WBC, lymphocyte, red blood cell, and platelet counts.

Special Considerations:
- Cytopenias: severe, including fatal auroimmune anemia and thrombocytopenia; prolonged myelosuppression have been reported. In addition, hemolytic anemia, pure red cell aplasia, bone marrow aplasia, and hypoplasia have been reported after treatment with alemtuzumab at the recommended dose. Hold drug for cytopenias (except lymphpenia); discontinue for autoimmune cytopenias or recurrent/persistent severe cytopenias.
- The drug may cause serious infusion reactions during or shortly after drug infusion, characterized by pyrexia, chills/rigors, nausea, hyptension, urticaria, dyspnea, rash, emesis, and bronchospasm. In clinical trials, the highest frequency of infusion reactions was during the first week of treatment. Monitor for signs/symptoms and hold infusion for

grade 3–4 reactions. Post-marketing reports have described reactions including syncope, pulmonary infiltrates, adult respiratory distress syndrome (ARDS), cardiopulmonary arrest, myocardial infarction, acute cardiac insufficiency, angioedema, and anaphylaxis. The drug dose must be gradually increased at the initiation of therapy or if therapy is interrupted for 7 or more days; in addition, the patient should receive premedication prior to dosing. Institute medical management (e.g., glucocorticoids, epinephrine, meperidine) as needed and ordered.

- Patients who have received multiple courses of chemotherapy prior to campath-1H are at increased risk for bacterial, viral, and other opportunistic infections.
- Drug-related immunosuppression results in severe and prolonged lymphopenia, with increased risk of opportunistic infections. Administer PCP and herpes viral prophylaxis during alemtuzumab therapy and for a minimum of 2 months after completion of alemtuzumab therapy or until CD4+ count is ≥ 200 cells/ μL, whichever occurs later. Prophylaxis does not eliminate these infections. Drug may reactivate herpes simplex infections.
  - Routinely monitor patients for cytolomegalovirus (CMV) infection during therapy and for 2 months after therapy is completed.
  - Hold drug for serious infections and during antiviral treatment for CMV infection or confirmed CMV viremia (PCR positive CMV in ≥ 2 consecutive samples obtained 1 week apart. Administer therapeutic ganciclovir or equivalent for CMV infection or confirmed CMV viremia.
  - Administer ONLY irradiated blood products to avoid transfusion associated Graft versus Host Disease (TAGVHD), unless emergency.
  - After receiving alemtuzumab for initial CLL therapy, recovery of CD4+ counts to ≥ 200cells/μL occurred by 6 months post-treatment (median at 2 months was 183 cells/μL). In previously treated patients, median time to recovery of CD4+ counts to ≥ 200cells/μL was 2 months; full recovery to baseline CD4+ and CD8+ may take > 12 months.
  - Assess CBC/differential weekly or more frequently if cytopenias; assess CD4+ counts after treatment until recovery to ≥ 200cells/μL.
- DO NOT administer live viral vaccines to patients who have recently received alemtuzumab. Nursing mothers should make a decision whether to discontinue nursing or alemtuzumab, taking into account the elimination half-life of alemtuzumab and the importance of the drug to the mother's health.
- Subcutaneous and intravenous have similar efficacy and effect.
- Following three-times-a-week therapy, destruction of CLL cells takes about 14 days before being removed from the peripheral blood, with no cells detectable at 5 weeks (Solimandro et al., 2000). Bone marrow clearance takes 6–12 weeks, and bulky lymphadenopathy takes considerably longer.
- It is not known if alemtuzumab causes fetal harm. Women of reproductive potential should avoid pregnancy. Drug should be given to a pregnant woman only if clearly needed.
- Most common side effects are infusion reactions (pyrexia, chills, hypotension, urticaria, nausea, rash, tachycardia, dyspnea), cytopenias (neutropenia, lymphopenia, thrombocytopenia, anemia), infections (CMV viremia, CMV infection, other infections),

gastrointestinal symptoms (nausea, emesis, abdominal pain), and neurological symptoms (insomnia, anxiety). The most common, serious reactions are cytopenias, infusion reactions, and immunosuppression infections.

Potential Toxicities/Side Effects (Dose- and Schedule-Dependent) and the Nursing Process

I.   POTENTIAL FOR INJURY related to INFUSION REACTIONS, HYPERSENSITIVITY REACTION DURING INFUSION

Defining Characteristics: Infusion reactions are common and require premedication to prevent them. Symptoms occur during or shortly after drug infusion (pyrexia, chills/rigors, nausea, hypotension, urticaria, dyspnea, rash, emesis, and bronchospasm) with highest incidence the first week of therapy. Hypotension occurs in 15%, rash in 30%, nausea in 47%, vomiting in 33%, drug-related fever 83%, and rigors in 89% of patients. Infusion reactions usually resolve after 1 week of therapy. Subcutaneous dosing significantly reduces the risk of allergic reactions. Rarely, syncope, pulmonary infiltrates, ARDS, respiratory arrest, cardiac arryhthmias, MI, acute cardiac insufficiency, cardiac arrest, angioedema, and anaphylactoid shock have been described in post-marketing reports.

Nursing Implications: Assess vital signs baseline and frequently during infusion, especially during dose escalation. Teach patient that reactions may occur and to tell nurse or physician immediately. Administer premedication as ordered, usually 500–1,000 mg acetaminophen and 50 mg diphenhydramine 30 minutes prior to infusion. Provide adequate hydration, as this seems to decrease the incidence of infusion reactions (e.g., at least 500 mL before and after dose). Dose is begun low at 3 mg, then gradually increased based on patient tolerance to 10-mg dose, then to a 30-mg dose. If the patient has a treatment break of 7 days or more, then it is necessary to reintroduce drug at the lower dose and gradually escalate dose. Assess skin for integrity and presence of rash. Teach patient to report this, and discuss management with physician. Teach patient that nausea may develop and to report it right away. Discuss antiemetic agent with physician, and administer as ordered. If reaction happens, stop infusion but keep main IV line open, notify physician, and, if rigors, give meperidine and any other medications ordered by physician. Expect reaction to resolve in 20 minutes or so, and gradually resume infusion per physician order. Withhold drug for grade 3–4 infusion reactions; give glucocorticoids and/or epiphephrine per physician order when needed. Emergency equipment should be available; rarely, reaction can be severe.

II.   POTENTIAL FOR INFECTION AND BLEEDING related to BONE MARROW DEPRESSION

Defining Characteristics: Drug kills lymphocytes, plus other infection fighting cells of the immune system (e.g., monocytes, macrophages, NK cells). Severe lymphopenia and a rapid and sustained decrease in lymphocyte subsets occur after drug is given. In previously untreated patients, $CD4^+$ count was 0 cells at 1 month after treatment (normal is 500–1,500 cells/µL), recovering to 238/µL at 6 months. All patients develop leukopenia, with approximately 99% lymphopenic, and 85% of patients developing neutropenia. The incidence of thrombocytopenia is 71% with platelet recovery weeks 7 to 12; incidence of anemia is 76%. There is a dramatic fall in WBC during the first week. As both T- and B-cell lymphocytes are killed, patients are at an increased risk for bacterial, viral, and other opportunistic infections. Most patients require prophylactic antimicrobials with/without antiviral therapy, especially heavily pretreated patients. Most common pulmonary infections are opportunistic: *Pneumocystis jiroveci (carinii)* pneumonia (PCP), cytomegalus virus (CMV) pneumonia, and pulmonary aspergillosis. Commonly, there is reactivation of herpes simplex infections and development of oral candidiasis. Rarely, pancytopenia, marrow aplasia, autoimmune anemia, severe autoimmune thrombocytopenia, and prolonged myelosuppression have occurred and may be fatal.

Nursing Implications: Assess baseline leukocyte, platelet, and Hgb/HCT; monitor before each treatment, during therapy at least weekly, and more often as needed. Ensure that a single drug dose does not exceed 30 mg, and that the cumulative weekly drug total does not exceed 90 mg. Hold drug for ANC < 250/µL or platelets ≤ 25,000/µL. See package insert for dose modifications. Teach that patient is at risk for opportunistic infections, to take medications as prescribed, and to report any problems or changes right away. Teach patient about recommended antimicrobials as ordered: trimethoprim/sulfamethoxazole DS twice daily three times a week (PCP prophlyaxis), and famociclovir 250 mg twice daily as herpetic prophylaxis. Assess risk for infection and integrity of skin and mucous membranes, pulmonary status, and ability to clear secretions, as well as history of past infections, baseline and prior to each treatment. Teach patient to self-administer prophylactic antibiotics, antiviral, and antifungal agents as ordered by physician. Ensure that patient has coverage or can purchase antimicrobial medications. Teach patient to self-administer oral antifungal agent if oral candidiasis develops. Teach patient to self-assess for signs/symptoms of infection, and to call provider immediately or come to the emergency room if temperature > 100.5°F, shaking chills, or rash, productive cough, burning on urination, or any signs/symptoms of infection or bleeding. Teach self-care strategies to minimize risk of infection and bleeding, including avoidance of OTC aspirin-containing medications. Following completion of therapy, assess and follow CD4 counts until recovery greater than or equal to 200cells/µL. If serious infection develops, drug should be interrupted until infection resolves. Patient should NOT receive live vaccines, during or recently after Campath treatment. The drug should be permanently discontinued for autoimmune or severe hematologic adverse reactions.

III. ALTERATION IN OXYGENATION, POTENTIAL, related to HYPOTENSION, HYPERTENSION, TACHYCARDIA

Defining Characteristics: Hypotension is common, affecting 32% of patients in clinical studies, while 11% had hypertension. 11% of patients also had sinus or supraventricular tachycardia.

Nursing Implications: Assess baseline cardiac status, including blood pressure and heart rate, noting rhythm and rate. Assess past medical history for arrhythmia, hypertension. If heart rate irregular, document rhythm on EKG, monitor blood pressure for evidence of decompensation, and discuss management with physician. If hypertension noted, discuss management with physician. If hypotension noted, assess patient tolerance and need for intervention; discuss management with physician.

Drug: alitretinoin gel 0.1% (Panretin)

Class: Retinoid.

Mechanism of Action: A 9-*cis*-retinoic acid, alitretinoin is a naturally occurring, endogenous retinoid necessary for regulation of gene expression responsible for cell differentiation and replication. 9-*cis*-retinoic acid binds to and activates intracellular retinoid receptors that enable transcription of these genes. Alitretinoin has been found to inhibit the growth of Kaposi's sarcoma (KS) cells directly.

Metabolism: Drug is used topically, without any detectable plasma concentrations or metabolites.

Indication: Indicated for TOPICAL treatment of cutaneous KS lesions in patients with AIDS. It should not be used when systemic therapy for KS is necessary (> 10 KS lesions in prior month, or symptomatic lymphedema, pulmonary KS, or visceral involvement).

Dosage/Range:
• Sufficient gel applied to cover the lesion with generous coating.
• Available in 60-gram tube.

Drug Preparation:
• None.
• Gel tube should be stored at room temperature.

Drug Administration:
• Use glove to apply generous coating of gel to lesions bid, avoiding surrounding skin.
• DO NOT APPLY on or near mucosal surfaces.
• Allow to dry for 3–5 minutes before covering with clothing.
• Gradually increase applications to 3–4 per day.
• If severe skin irritation develops, stop application for a few days until irritation resolves.
• DO NOT USE an occlusive dressing over gel.

Drug Interactions:
• DEET (*N, N*-diethyl-*m*-toluamide) insect repellent or products containing DEET, as gel increases DEET toxicity.
• No testing has been done to assess possible interactions between systemic antiretroviral agents, or other agents used in the systemic management of HIV infection.

Lab Effects/Interference:
• None known.

Special Considerations:
• Responses may be seen in 2 weeks, but most often take longer, rarely 14 weeks. Gel should be used as long as there is clinical benefit. Contraindicated in patients having hypersensitivity to retinoids.
• Women of childbearing age should use contraception to prevent pregnancy, as it is unknown whether topical gel can modulate endogenous 9-*cis*-retinoic levels. 9-*Cis*-retinoic acid is teratogenic.
• Drug SHOULD NOT BE USED by nursing mothers; mothers must discontinue nursing prior to using the drug.
• Drug may increase photosensitivity, so patients should be taught to AVOID sunlamps and to minimize sunlight exposure.
• Safety testing has not been done in pediatric or geriatric (> 65 yr) populations.
• Toxicity almost exclusively related to skin reactions at the application site.

Potential Toxicities/Side Effects and the Nursing Process

I. ALTERATION IN COMFORT AND SKIN INTEGRITY, POTENTIAL, related to APPLICATION SITE REACTIONS

Defining Characteristics: Toxicity begins as erythema. This may increase, and edema may develop with continued application. Most of reactions are mild to moderate, but in some patients (10%), severe reactions may occur with intense erythema, edema, and formation of vesicles. Other skin reactions occurring in > 5% of patients are rash, pain, pruritus, exfoliative dermatitis, cracking, crusting, drainage, oozing, stinging, or tingling.

Nursing Implications: Assess baseline skin integrity and condition of KS cutaneous lesions. Teach patient to apply gel only to lesions and AVOID surrounding skin, as irritation will occur. Teach patient to assess and report any changes in the lesions, such as erythema, and edema. Teach patient to reduce frequency of application if skin reaction occurs, to stop use of the gel if severe reactions occur, and to report this as soon as possible.

Drug: axitinib (Inlyta, AG-013736)

Class: Receptor tyrosine kinase inhibitor of VEGFR; angiogenesis inhibitor.

Mechanism of Action: Potent, and selective inhibitor of vascular endothelial growth factor (VEGF) receptors 1, 2, 3 on the endothelial cells lining blood vessels. VEGFR inhibition prevents VEGF (ligand) from binding to the receptor on the endothelial cells, thus preventing the blood vessel endothelial cells from proliferating and migrating to form capillary tubes (angiogenesis) to send to the tumor. The tumor cannot grow beyond 2 mm without angiogenesis. Blockade of these receptors helps to inhibit tumor growth and progression.

Metabolism: After oral dosing, bioavailability is 58%. Peak serum levels are reached in 2.5–4.1 hours, and steady-state is achieved within 2–3 days of dosing. Drug solubility is pH dependent, with a higher pH resulting in lower solubility. Drug is highly protein bound (> 99%). Plasma half-life of drug is 2.5–6.1 hours. Drug is primarily metabolized by the liver (CYP3A4/5, and to a lesser degree CYP1A2, CYP2C19, UGT1A1). Drug is excreted in the feces (41%, with 12% as unchanged drug) and urine (23%).

Indication: Drug is FDA-approved for treatment of patients with advanced renal cell cancer after failure of one prior systemic therapy.

Dosage/Range:
- Initial dose: 5 mg orally, twice daily 12 hours apart, with or without food; swallow tablet whole with a glass of water.
- Dose adjustments made based on tolerability and individual safety.
  - If the patient tolerates axitinib for at least 2 consecutive weeks without adverse effects > grade 2, is normotensive, and not receiving antihypertensive medication, the dose may be increased (e.g., if increased from 5 mg twice daily, it may be increased to 7 mg twice daily, and further to 10 mg twice daily using the same criterion).
  - Some adverse drug reactions require temporary interruption or dose reduction. If dose reduction from 5 mg twice daily is required, the recommended dose is 3 mg twice daily. If additional dose reduction is required, the recommended dose is 2 mg twice daily.
- If the patient is taking a strong CYP3A4/5 inhibitor, decrease axitinib dose by approximately 50%. Subsequent doses can be increased or decreased based on safety and tolerability. If coadministration of the strong inhibitor is discontinued, the axitinib dose should be returned (after 3–5 half-lives of the inhibitor) to that used prior to the initiation of the strong CYP3A4/5 inhibitor.
- Patients with moderate hepatic impairment should start at approximately 50% of the dose, or 2.5 mg orally, twice daily. Drug has not been studied in patients with severe liver impairment.

Drug Preparation:
- None, oral. Available as 1-mg and 5-mg tablets.

Drug Administration:
- Oral. Teach patient to take tablet every 12 hours, morning and evening. Swallow tablet whole with a glass of water. Tablet may be taken with or without food.
- If the patient vomits or misses a dose, an additional dose should not be taken. The next dose should be taken at the usual time.
- Stop drug 24 hours prior to scheduled surgery.
- Prior to starting axitinib therapy:
  - Assess thyroid function tests baseline, then periodically during axitinib therapy.
  - Assess urine for protein baseline, then periodically during axitinib therapy.
  - Assess LFTs (ALT, AST, bilirubin) baseline, then periodically during axitinib therapy.
  - Assess BP; BP should be well controlled before starting axitinib.

- If bleeding occurs and requires medical intervention, temporarily interrupt axitinib therapy.
- Drug has not been studied in patients with evidence of untreated brain metastases or recent active GI bleeding, and should not be used in these patients (hemorrhagic events including fatal events have occurred).

Drug Interactions:
- Strong CYP3A4/5 inhibitors (e.g., ketoconazole, itraconazole, clarithromycin, atazanavir, indinavir, nefazodone, nelfinavir, ritonavir, saquinavir, telithromycin, and voriconazole; grapefruit or grapefruit juice): increased serum level of axitinib; avoid concurrent administration; if must give together, reduce axitinib dose by 50%.
- Strong CYP3A4/5 inducers (e.g., rifampin, dexamethasone, phenytoin, carbamazepine, rifabutin, rifapentin, phenobarbital, St. John's wort): reduced axtinib serum level: do not give concurrently. Moderate inducers (e.g., bosentan, efavirenz, etravirine, modafinil, nafcillin): may decrease serum level: avoid concurrent administration if possible.

Lab Effects/Interference:
- Decreased soluble VEGFR-2 and VEGFR-3 and increased VEGF in blood.
- Decreased hemoglobin, lymphocytes, white blood cells, platelets.
- Increased serum creatinine, glucose, lipase, amylase, ALT, ALP, sodium, potassium, TSH.
- Decreased serum bicarbonate, calcium, albumin, glucose, sodium, phosphated, T4.
- Proteinuria.

Special Considerations:
- Most common toxicities (≥ 20%) are diarrhea, HTN, fatigue, decreased appetite, nausea, dysphonia, palmar-plantar erythrodysesthesia (hand-foot syndrome, HFS), decreased weight, vomiting, asthenia, and constipation.
- Hypothyroidism was reported in 19% of patients, while hyperthyroidism was reported 1%. Hypothyroidism requiring thyroid hormone replacement was also reported. Assess thyroid function before starting axitinib, and periodically during therapy. Of patients who had a TSH < 5 microU/mL before treatment, 32% had elevations of TSH to ≥ 10 microU/mL on axitinib. Monitor TSH baseline before starting axitinib, then periodically during treatment.
- Hypertension, including hypertensive crisis, has occurred. BP should be well controlled prior to starting axitinib. Monitor for hypertension and treat as needed. If hypertension is persistent despite antihypertensives, reduce axitinib dose.
- Arterial (TIAs, CVA, MI, retinal artery occlusion) [ATE] and venous thrombotic (PE, DVT) [VTE] events have been observed and can be fatal. Use with caution in patients at increased risk of thrombotic events. Incidence of grade 3–4 ATEs was 1%. Incidence of VTEs was 3%, with grade 3–4 (3%). Drug should be used cautiously in patients who are at risk for or who have a history of thrombotic events. Drug has not been studied in patients who had a venous thrombotic event in the prior 6 months, or arterial thrombotic event within the past 12 months.

- Hemorrhagic events, including fatal events, have been reported in 16% of patients, with only 1% grade 3–4. Drug has not been studied in patients with untreated brain metastases, or recent GI bleed, and should not be used in these patients. Stop drug 24 hours before scheduled surgery. If any bleeding requires medical intervention, temporarily interrupt the axitinib dose.
- GI perforation and fistula have occurred in < 1% of patients; some fatalities have occurred. Use cautiously in patients with risk for GI perforation or fistula. Monitor for symptoms of GI perforation or fistula periodically throughout axitinib treatment.
- Reversible posterior leukoencephalopathy syndrome (RPLS) has been observed in < 1% of patients receiving axitinib. Signs/symptoms are headache, seizure, lethargy, confusion, blindness, and other visual and neurological disturbances. Mild to severe hypertension may also be present. MRI is necessary to confirm a diagnosis of RPLS. Discontinue axitinib in patients who are developing RPLS and the safety of reinitiating axitinib threrapy is unknown.
- Proteinuria may occur. In studies, incidence is about 11%, with 3% having grade 3–4. Assess baseline urine for protein before starting axitinib, then monitor periodically during treatment. If moderate to severe proteinuria occurs, reduce dose or temporarily hold drug.
- Elevation of LFTs has occurred (22%). Monitor ALT, AST, and bilirubin baseline prior to starting drug, then periodically during treatment.
- Patients with moderate hepatic dysfunction (Child-Pugh Class B) should start treatment at a 50% reduced dose. The drug has not been studied in patients with severe hepatic impairment (Child-Pugh Class C).
- Wound-healing complications: stop treatment with axitinib at least 24 hours prior to scheduled surgery. The decision to resume axitinib therapy after surgery should be based on clinical judgment of adquate wound healing.
- Drug can cause fetal harm. Women of childbearing age/potential should be advised to use effective birth control measures to avoid pregnancy. Nursing mothers should make the decision whether to discontinue nursing or discontinue the drug, taking into account the importance of the drug to the mother.
- Drug can cause hoarseness/dysphonia: assess impact on patient, communication ability, and need for assistance.
- Drug compared to sorafinib in the treatment of patients with clear cell advanced RCC and found to extend median PFS (6.7 months vs 4.7 months, with a delayed deterioration in quality of life (Rini et al., 2011; Cella et al., 2011).

Potential Toxicities/Side Effects and the Nursing Process

I.   POTENTIAL ALTERATION IN CIRCULATION related to HYPERTENSION

Defining Characteristics: Axitinib increases the incidence and severity of hypertension, a class effect of all angiogenesis inhibitors believed caused by the influence of VEGF on nitric oxide and blood vessel dilation. Overall incidence of hypertension was 40%, with 16% grade 3–4. Hypertensive crisis was reported in < 1% of patients. Median time to onset of hypertension (SBP > 150 mm Hg, DBP > 100 mm Hg) was within the first month of therapy, but starting as early as day 4. Hypertension was effectively managed with standard antihypertensive therapy, and < 1% of patients discontinued therapy due to hypertension.

Nursing Implications: Assess baseline BP prior to starting axitinib, and during treatment at each clinic visit. BP should be well controlled prior to starting axitinib. If the patient has a history of hypertension, monitor BP more closely, although hypertension develops over time. If needed, teach patient and family how to measure BP at home, and to record measurements and bring diary to clinic at each visit. Blood pressure should continue to be monitored after patient has stopped the drug. Teach patient drug administration, potential side effects, and self-care measures if prescribed antihypertensive medication, such as angiotensin-converting enzyme inhibitors, or angiotensin receptor blockers (antagonists). If patient has persistent hypertension despite standard antihypertensive therapy, the dose of axitinib should be reduced. Drug should be permanently discontinued if (1) hypertension is persistent despite antihypertensives and dose reduction, or (2) the patient develops hypertensive crisis (diastolic blood pressure > 120 mm Hg). Drug can be temporarily suspended in patients with severe hypertension until BP can be controlled with medical management. If axitinib therapy is interrupted, patients receiving antihypertensive drug(s) should be monitored closely for hypotension.

II.   ALTERATION IN COMFORT AND ACTIVITY INTOLERANCE, POTENTIAL, related to FATIGUE

Defining Characteristics: Fatigue occurs in 39% of patients, and 11% had grade 3–4 fatigue. Asthenia occurred in 21%, 5% grade 3–4. Hypothyroidism may also occur so should be evaluated.

Nursing Implications: Assess comfort and presence of discomfort, fatigue, inability to do ADLs baseline and before each treatment. Assess thyroid function tests and discuss any abnormalities with physician or nurse practitioner. Teach patient that these side effects may occur and to report them. Teach patient local comfort measures as well as energy conservation, calling in other members of the family to assist with performing energy-draining functions, and discuss management plan with physician if ineffective.

III.   ALTERATION IN NUTRITION, LESS THAN BODY REQUIREMENTS, related to DIARRHEA, DECREASED APPETITE, NAUSEA, WEIGHT DECREASE, CONSTIPATION, DYSGEUSIA, DYSPEPSIA

Defining Characteristics: Diarrhea was the most common side effect, occurring in 55% of patients, 11% grade 3–4. The following other symptoms also occurred in the descending incidence: decreased appetite (34%, 5% grade 3–4), nausea (34%, 3% grade 3–4), decreased weight (25%, 2% grade 3–4), vomiting (24%, 3% grade 3–4), constipation (20%, 1% grade 3–4), stomatitis (15%, 1% grade 3–4), dysgeusia (11%, 3% grade 3–4), dyspepsia (10%).

Nursing Implications: Assess baseline weight, nutritional status, elimination status, and monitor at each visit. Assess oral mucosa. Teach patient that these side effects may occur and to report them. Develop symptom management plan, including dietary modification, increased fluids, self-administration of symptom management medications. For patients with diarrhea, teach self-administration of antidiarrheal medicines, and to call if diarrhea persists > 24 hours. Teach patients with anorexia and weight loss to use small plates with small amounts of food frequently during the day, and to include a bedtime snack of high-calorie high-protein foods. If taste changes impact eating, identify them and develop a plan to circumvent it; for example, as if the patient has a metallic taste, suggest eating with plastic utensils. For all symptoms that are unrelieved, teach patient to call nurse/ provider and revise symptom management plan. If diarrhea is grade 3–4, teach patient to stop drug and contact health provider. Discuss the drug interruption or dose reduction with physician.

IV.   ALTERATION IN SKIN INTEGRITY AND COMFORT, POTENTIAL, related to HAND-FOOT SYNDROME

Defining Characteristics: Hand-foot syndrome (palmar-plantar erythrodysesthesia syndrome) occurred in 27% of patients, and was grade 3–4 in 5%.

Nursing Implications: Assess baseline skin integrity, including soles of feet and palms of hands, and teach patient that HFS may occur, and to report erythema, swelling, tingling, rash, peeling of palms of hands or soles of feet, or pain. Teach patient self-care measures including: (1) assess all skin areas, especially areas under pressure, and to report symptoms; (2) use topical creams/moisturizers to apply to hands and feet daily starting with day 1 of axitinib therapy, (3) wear cotton gloves/socks after applying moisturizer to hands and feet; (4) wear loose-fitting clothing and shoes, and elevate hands and feet when sitting or lying down; (5) apply ice packs or cool compresses indirectly to hands or feet for up to 20 min; (6) gently pat skin dry after bathing or washing; (7) avoid exposure to hot water (e.g., sauna or hot tub) or direct sunlight, activities causing pressure and friction on hands and feet (e.g., jogging), and contact with harsh laundry detergents or cleaning products.

Drug: belinostat for injection (Beleodaq)

Class: Histone deacetylase inhibitor (HDAC).

Mechanism of Action: HDACs catalyze the removal of acetyl groups from histones, thereby stopping the enzyme activity of histone deacetylase. This leads to the accumulation of acetylated histones, and other proteins, which stops cell division (cell cycle arrest) and forces some transformed cells to die via apoptosis (programmed cell death). Belinostat causes more cell death in tumor cells than in normal cells.

Metabolism: Drug elimination half-life is 1.1 hours, and there is limited body tissue distribution. Drug is highly protein bound, and primarily metabolized by the hepatic enzyme UGT1A1. Drug undergoes hepatic metabolism by hepatic microenzymes including CYP2A6, CYP2C9, CYP3A4 enzymes, forming belinostat amide, belinostat acid, and other metabolites. Drug is eliminated primarily through metabolism, with < 2% of drug excreted unchanged in the urine. Major metabolites are excreted in the urine within the first 24 hours after drug administration.

Indication: For the treatment of patients with relapsed or refractory peripheral T-cell lymphoma (PTCL). Accelerated drug approval made by FDA based on tumor response rate, and duration of response. Continued approval may be contingent upon demonstrated clinical benefit in the confirmatory trial, such as improvement in survival or disease-related symptoms (Spectrum Pharmaceuticals, 2014).

Dosage/Range:
- 1,000mg/m^2 IV infusion over 30 min once daily on days 1–5 of a 21-day cycle. Cycles can be repeated until disease progression or unacceptable toxicity.
- If patient has reduced UGT1A1 activity (e.g., homozygous for UGT1A1*28 allele), initial dose should be 750 mg/m^2.
- Adverse reactions: may require treatment discontinuation or interruption with or without a 25% dose reduction.

Drug Preparation:
- Available as a 500-mg, lyophilized powder, single-use vial for reconstitution.
- Aseptically reconstitute each vial by adding 9 mL Sterile Water for Injection, USP so final concentration is 50 mg belinostat per mL. Swirl contents until fully dissolved. Reconstituted drug may be stored for up to 12 hours at ambient temperature (15–25°C; 59–77°F).
- Aseptically withdraw ordered amount, and transfer to a 250 mL 0.9% sodium chloride for injection infusion bag. Once diluted, the drug containing bag may be stored at ambient room temperature (15–25°C; 59–77°F), for up to 36 hours, including infusion time.
- Visually inspect for particulate matter, cloudiness; if found, do not use.
- Connect infusion bag to an infusion set with a 0.22 μm in-line filter and prime under the hood.

Drug Administration:
- Assess CBC/differential baseline and weekly; assess chemistries including renal and hepatic function tests prior to start of the first dose of each cycle.
- Ensure ANC ≥ 1.0 × 10^9/L, and platelets ≥ 50 × 10^9/L prior to the start of each cycle and prior to resuming treatment after treatment interruption for toxicity; ensure toxicity has recovered to grade 2 or less, and the patient has no signs/symptoms of infection.
- Consider antiemetic prior to belinostat administration.
- IV infusion over 30 minutes, daily × 5, repeated every 21 days. If patient complains of infusion site pain, extend infusion time to 45 minutes.

- Discuss need for dose modification with physician.
  - ANC ≥ 0.5 × 10^9/L, and platelet count ≥ 25 × 10^9/L: No change in dose.
  - ANC < 0.5 × 10^9/L with any platelet count, or platelet count < 25 × 10^9/L (any nadir count): decrease dose by 25% (e.g., if prior dose full dose, to 750 mg/m^2).
  - Recurrent ANC nadirs < 0.5 × 10^9/L and/or platelet count nadirs < 25 × 10^9/L after 2 dose reductions: discontinue drug.
  - For nausea, vomiting, diarrhea: use modified dose only if duration is > 7days with supportive management.
  - Any grade 3 or 4 (CTCAE) adverse reaction: decrease dose by 25% (e.g., if prior dose full dose, to 750 mg/m^2).
  - Recurrence of CTCAE grade 3 or 4 adverse reaction: discontinue drug.

Drug Interactions:
- UGT1A1 inhibitors: drug is primarily metabolized by UGT1A1, so concomitant administration with a UGT1A1 inhibitor will increase belinostat serum levels, and risk of toxicity. Do not administer with strong UGT1A1 inhibitors (e.g., atazanavir, gemfibrozil, indinavir, ketoconazole; herbals *silybum marianum, Valeriana officinalis*).
- Drug and its metabolites inhibit metabolic activities of CYP2C8, and CYP2C9. Drug coadministration with warfarin did not significantly change warfarin AUC or C$_{max}$.

Lab Effects/Interference:
- Thrombocytopenia, neutropenia, lymphopenia, anemia.
- Elevated LFTs, LDH.
- Hypokalemia.
- Decreased serum creatinine.
- Prolonged QT interval.

Special Considerations:
- Dose-reduce in patients with UGT1A1*28 polymorphism as this decreases belinostat metabolism and increases risk of belinostat toxicity. UGT1A1*28 polymorphism (homozygous for the UGT1A1*28 allele) is found in 20% of blacks, 10% of whites, and 2% of Asians.
- Serious infections may occur, and may be fatal (e.g., pneumonia, sepsis). Do not give belinostat to patients with active infection. In addition, patients with a history of extensive or intensive chemotherapy treatment may be at greater risk of life-threatening infections.
- Hepatotoxicity may occur. Monitor LFTs, and discuss dose modification or hold for abnormalities. Dose-modify, interrupt, or discontinue belinostat for hepatotoxicity.
- Tumor lysis syndrome (TLS) may occur in patients with advanced disease and/or a high tumor burden. Discuss TLS prophylaxis with physician or NP/PA prior to initial dose.
- Consider premedication with antiemetic to prevent nausea and vomiting, and teach patient the use of antidiarrheals in case diarrhea develops.
- Drug may cause embryo-fetal toxicity. Counsel women of reproductive potential to use effective contraception to avoid pregnancy while receiving the drug.
- Nursing mothers should not breastfeed while receiving the drug. Nursing mothers should make a decision whether to discontinue nursing or to discontinue the drug, taking into account the importance of the drug to the mother's health.

- Drug may impair male fertility.
- Most common adverse reactions were nausea, fatigue, anemia, and vomiting.

Potential Toxicities/Side Effects and the Nursing Process

I.   POTENTIAL FOR INFECTION AND BLEEDING related to BONE MARROW SUPPRESSION

Defining Characteristics: Infections included pneumonia and sepsis. Pyrexia occurred in 37% of patients, and was grade 3–4 in 5%; cough occurred in 19%, and chills in 16%. Thrombocytopenia occurred in 16% (7% grade 3–4), and anemia occurred in 32% with 11% of patients having grade 3–4.

Nursing Implications: Assess CBC/differential and platelet counts baseline and weekly as ordered during therapy. Assess skin integrity, potential for infection, and teach patient measures to prevent infection (e.g., keeping skin intact, avoiding sources of infection, good hand-washing). Teach patient to report any signs/symptoms of infection (e.g., redness, heat, exudate on skin, temperature ≥ 100.4°F, cough, sputum production, dysuria). Assess for signs/symptoms of infection during therapy and at each visit. If a patient develops an infection, discuss with physician or midlevel practitioner interrupting or discontinuing drug, and beginning appropriate antimicrobial treatment Teach the patient that thrombocytopenia may occur, to avoid situations that could increase bleeding, and to report any signs or symptoms of bleeding right away. Review medication profile, and discuss discontinuance of aspirin or NSAIDs with patient and physician or NP/PA. Follow HGB/HCT and assess patient's tolerance, and need for supportive measures.

II.   POTENTIAL ALTERATION IN NUTRITION, LESS THAN BODY REQUIREMENTS, related to NAUSEA, VOMITING, DIARRHEA, HEPATOTOXICITY

Defining Characteristics: In clinical studies, nausea occurred in 43% of patients (grade 3–4 in 1%), vomiting in 29% (1% grade 3–4), diarrhea in 23% (2% grade 3–4), constipation in 23%, decreased appetite in 15%, and hypokalemia in 12%.

Nursing Implications: Assess baseline nutritional and elimination status, and appetite. Assess serum chemistries including renal and hepatic function, baseline and prior to each belinostat cycle. Assess patient tolerance of chemotherapy and need for premedication with antiemetics. Teach the patient to report nausea and/or vomiting that is not relieved by prescribed antiemetics. Teach patient that diarrhea or constipation may occur, dietary modifications for each problem, and to call nurse or physician for diarrhea, nausea, or vomiting that does not resolve within 24 hours with recommended over-the-counter or prescription medicines. Notify physician of any abnormalities, and discuss implications and management.

Drug: bevacizumab (Avastin)

Class: Recombinant humanized monoclonal antibody targeted against vascular endothelial growth factor (VEGF); angiogenesis inhibitor.

Mechanism of Action: VEGF binds to receptors on endothelial cells, turning on the cell surface receptors KDR and Flt-1, which then function as tyrosine kinases sending the message to the cells to proliferate and migrate. This leads to the establishment of new blood vessels (neovascularization) in tumors. Studies show that tumors that express VEGF tend to be more aggressive, more invasive, and more likely to metastasize. Bevacizumab binds to all human forms of VEGF-A, thus preventing it from binding to its receptors on the endothelial cells. This theoretically prevents one step in the process of angiogenesis from occurring. In addition, it appears that VEGF is necessary to maintain existing tumor blood vessels, and when blocked by bevacizumab, these blood vessels normalize, reducing tumor interstitial pressure, and allowing normal blood flow throughout the tumor. When given with chemotherapy, this theoretically results in increased chemotherapy penetrating the tumor, and cell kill. Bevacizumab may augment the body's antitumor immune response by helping dendritic cells function more effectively. Finally, bevacizumab is an IgG$_1$ monoclonal antibody that theoretically recruits immune effector cells such as natural killer cells and macrophages, which attack tumor cells (antibody-dependent cellular cytotoxicity), as well as stimulating complement-mediated killing of tumor cells.

Metabolism: Humanized via recombinant technologies resulting in a 93% human monoclonal antibody. It is widely distributed throughout the body and has a terminal half-life of approximately 20 days (range 11–50 days). It appears to reach steady state in 100 days. Drug clearance varies by body weight, gender, and tumor burden: men and patients with a large tumor burden have higher clearances than females, but this does not appear to decrease drug efficiency. Drug clearance has not been studied in patients with either renal or hepatic impairment, but it appears that there is minimal drug clearance by these organs. Concurrent administration of 5-fluorouracil, carboplatin, doxorubicin, cisplatin, or paclitaxel does not affect pharmacokinetics of the drug.

Indication: FDA-approved for (1) first- or second-line treatment of patients with metastatic cancer of colon or rectum in combination with IV fluorouracil-based regimen; (2) second-line, in combination with fluoropyrimidine-irinotecan- or fluoropyrimidine-oxaliplatin-based chemotherapy, in patients with metastatic CRC, who have progressed on a first-line bevacizumab-containing regimen; (3) first-line treatment of patients with unresectable, locally advanced, recurrent or metastatic, nonsquamous NSCLC in combination with carboplatin and paclitaxel; (4) treatment of glioblastoma with progressive disease in adult patients following prior therapy, as a single agent; (5) treatment of metastatic renal cell carcinoma in combination with interferon alfa; (6) cervical cancer, in combination with paclitaxel and cisplatin or paclitaxel and topotecan in persistent, recurrent, or metastatic disease; (7) platinum-resistant recurrent epithelial ovarian, fallopian tube, or primary peritoneal cancer, in combination with paclitaxel, pegylated liposomal doxorubicin, or topotecan.

Dosage/Range:
- Metastatic CRC: 5 mg/kg IV every 2 weeks with bolus-IFL.
- Metastatic CRC: 10 mg/kg IV every 2 weeks with FOLFOX4.
- Metastatic CRC: 5 mg/kg every 2 weeks or 7.5 mg/kg every 3 weeks when used in combination with a fluoropyrimidine-irinotecan or fluoropyrimidine-oxaliplatin based chemotherapy regimen in patients who have progressed on a first-line Avastin containing regimen.
- Non-squamous NSCLC: 15 mg/kg every 3 weeks when combined with carboplatin and paclitaxel.
- Glioblastoma: 10 mg/kg IV every 2 weeks.
- Metastatic renal cell cancer (mRCC): 10 mg/kg IV every 2 weeks with interferon-alfa.
- Persistent, recurrent, or metastatic cervical cancer: 15 mg/kg every 3 weeks with paclitaxel/cisplatin or paclitaxel/topotecan.
- Platinum-resistant recurrent epithelial ovarian, fallopian tube, or primary peritoneal cancer: (a) 10 mg/kg IV every 2 weeks with paclitaxel, pegylated liposomal doxorubicin, or weekly topotecan; (b) 15 mg/kg IV every 3 weeks with topotecan given every 3 weeks.
- Drug is NOT indicated for the adjuvant treatment of colon cancer.
- Discontinue bevacizumab for:
  - GI perforation, fistula formation involving an internal organ or GI tract, non- GI fistula.
  - Wound dehiscence and wound-healing complications requiring medical intervention.
  - Serious hemorrhage requiring medical intervention.
  - Severe arterial thromboembolic events.
  - Hypertensive crisis or hypertensive encephalopathy.
  - Reversible posterior leukoencephalopathy syndrome (RPLS).
  - Nephrotic syndrome.
- Temporarily suspend bevacizumab for:
  - At least 4 weeks (28 days) prior to elective surgery; do not reinitiate for at least 28 days after surgery and until the surgical wound is fully healed.
  - Severe hypertension not controlled with medical management.
  - Moderate to severe proteinuria pending further evaluation (e.g., ≥ 2 grams of proteinuria/24 hours).
  - Severe infusion reactions.

Drug Preparation:
- Single-use vials contain 4 mL to deliver 100 mg, and 16 mL to deliver 400 mg per vial. Use within 8 hours of opening. Store at 2–8°C (36–46°F). Protect from light. Do not freeze or shake.
- Further dilute in 100 mL 0.9% normal saline for injection. Discard unused portions of the vial.

Drug Administration:
- Do not administer as an IV push or bolus.
- Do not initiate bevacizumab for 28 days following major surgery and until surgical wound is fully healed.

- Patients with active hemoptysis (≥ ½ tsp of red blood) should not receive the drug.
- Administer IV over 90 minutes for the first infusion.
  - Subsequent infusions. If first infusion tolerated well (e.g., without fever and/or chills), administer second dose over 60 minutes; if this is well-tolerated, administer all subsequent doses as a 30-minute infusion.
  - Bevacizumab 5 mg/kg has been shown to be safely infused over 10 minutes (Reidy et al., 2007).

Drug Interactions:
- Paclitaxel/carboplatin combination: may decrease paclitaxel exposure after 4 cycles of treatment (day 63).
- Incompatible with dextrose solutions.

Lab Effects/Interference:
- Thrombocytopenia.
- Proteinuria.
- Leukopenia and neutropenia.
- Hypokalemia.
- Bilirubinemia.

Special Considerations:
- Bevacizumab is **not** indicated for adjuvant treatment of colon cancer.
- Black box warnings discuss risk of (1) gastrointestinal perforations (incidence in patients with CRC was 2.4%, NSCLC 0.9%), sometimes associated with intra-abdominal abscesses, and fistula formation; (2) complications of wound healing; and (3) hemorrhage (fatal hemoptysis occurred in 5 patients with NSCLC—incidence was 31% in patients with squamous cell and 2.3% in patients with adenocarcinoma histology).
- *Warnings include:*
  - Gastrointestinal perforation (GI perforation, intra-abdominal abscesses and/or fistula formation) occurs in up to 3.2% of patients, and highest incidence was in patients with cervical cancer and who had received prior pelvic radiation.
    - Presentation may include abdominal pain, nausea, emesis, constipation, and fever; generally occurs within the first 50 days of bevacizumab therapy.
    - Perforation can be complicated by intra-abdominal abscess, fistula formation, and the need for diverting ostomies.
    - GI fistula can occur; in patients with cervical cancer, the incidence of GI-vaginal fistulae was 8.2% in the bevacizumab treated group, compared to 0.9% in the control patients, all patients had had prior pelvic radiation.
    - Permanently discontinue drug if GI perforation occurs.
  - Non-GI fistula formation (tracheoesophageal, bronchopleural, biliary, vaginal, renal, bladder sites). Most events occurred within the first 6 months of therapy. Permanently discontinue drug if patient develops a tracheoesophageal (TE) fistula; or any grade 4 fistula; or if a fistula forms involving an internal organ.
  - Surgical and wound-healing complications: Incidence of patients with mCRC who underwent surgery during bevacizumab therapy was 15% vs 4% in those who did not. Suspend drug at least 28 days before elective surgery, and do not initiate drug for at least 28 days after surgery and until the surgical wound is fully healed. Discontinue

drug for wound healing complications requiring medical intervention. Necrotizing fasciitis, most commonly related to wound healing complications, GI perforation or fistula formation have occurred and some cases have been fatal. Discontinue drug in patients who develop necrotizing fasciitis.

- Hemorrhage: There are two patterns of bleeding: (a) minor hemorrhage, most commonly grade 1 epistaxis, and (b) serious hemorrhagic events (e.g., hemorrhage, hemoptysis, GI bleeding, hematamesis, CNS hemorrhage, epistaxis, vaginal hemorrhage), which in some cases were fatal. The incidence of grade $\geq$ 3 in bevacizumab patients was 1.2–6.9%.
  - Drug is not indicated in NSCLC patients with squamous histology, as the incidence of serious or fatal pulmonary hemorrhage was 31% in these patients. In NSCLC patients with CNS metastases who had completed RT and surgery > 4 weeks prior to the start of bevacizumab, the incidence of grade 2 CNS hemorrhage was documented in 1.2% of patients. Intracranial hemorrhage in patients with previously treated glioblastoma was 8/163 patients.
  - Do NOT give bevacizumab to patients with recent hemoptysis of $\geq$ 1/2 teaspoon of red blood; discontinue bevacizumab in patients with hemorrhage.
- Arterial thromboembolic events (ATE) with increased risk of cerebral infarction, myocardial infarction, transient ischemic attacks, and angina have occurred compared to control patients (grade $\geq$ 3 2.6%, vs 0.8% in control).
  - The risk of developing ATE increased in patients with a history of arterial thromboembolism, diabetes, age > 65 years.
  - Permanently discontinue drug if a severe ATE occurs. Safety of resuming bevacizumab after resolution of an ATE has not been studied.
- Hypertension (HTN): Monitor BP and treat HTN. The incidence of grade 3–4 HTN was 5–18% in bevacizumab patients. Continue to monitor BP regularly in patients with bevacizumab-induced or exacerbated HTN after bevacizumab is discontinued. Temporarily suspend bevacizumab if HTN not medically controlled. Permanently discontinue drug if hypertensive crisis or encephalopathy occurs.
- Posterior Reversible Encephalopathy Syndrome (PRES) has an incidence of < 0.5%, with signs and symptoms of headache, seizure, lethargy, confusion, blindness, and other visual changes occurring from 16 hours to 1 year after bevacizumab was begun. It may be associated with mild-moderately severe HTN. Confirm diagnosis of PRES with MRI. Discontinue drug in patients developing PRES. Symptoms likely resolve or improve within days, although some patients have ongoing neurological sequelae.
- Proteinuria and rare nephrotic syndrome: Monitor urine protein by urine dipstick/ urinalysis baseline and serially during bevacizumab therapy; if the urine dipstick is 2+ or greater, perform a 24-hour urine sample for protein.
  - Suspend drug for moderate proteinuria ($\geq$ 2 grams of protein per 24 hours in a 24-hour urine) and resume when 24-hour urine for protein is < 2gm/24 hr. Discontinue drug if nephrotic syndrome develops.
  - There is a poor correlation between urine protein/creatinine ratio (UPCR) and the 24-hour urine protein, so a 24-hour urine collection is necessary.
- Infusion reactions may occur rarely (< 3%, with 0.2% severe) manifested by hypertension, hypertensive crisis associated with neurologic signs and symptoms, wheezing, oxygen desaturation, grade 3 hypersensitivity, chest pain, headaches, rigors, and

diaphoresis. Stop infusion if a severe infusion reaction occurs, and treat as medically appropriate and ordered.

• Ovarian failure: Teach patients of childbearing age that this may occur (incidence in one study of premenopausal women was 34% compared to 2% in control arm). After discontinuance of bevicizumab, recovery of ovarian function occurred in 22% of these patients.

• Venous thromboembolic events (VTE): Patients with cervical cancer receiving bevacizumab with chemotherapy had an incidence of 10.6% of grade ≥ 3 VTE compared to 5.4% in patients receiving chemotherapy alone. Permanently discontinue bevacizumab in patients with life-threatening (grade 4) VTE, including pulmonary embolism.

• Drug is teratogenic. Women of childbearing age should use highly effective contraceptive measures during treatment to avoid pregnancy, and for 6 months after the drug is stopped. Bevacizumab use during pregnancy is only if the potential benefit to the pregnant woman justifies the potential risk to the fetus. Nursing mothers should decide whether to discontinue nursing, or to discontinue the drug, taking into account the half-life of bevacizumab (approximately 20 days, range 11–50 days) and the importance of the drug to the mother's health.

• The incidence of neutropenia and febrile neutropenia are increased in patients receiving bevacizumab plus chemotherapy compared to patients receiving chemotherapy alone.

• The incidence of grade ≥ 3 left ventricular dysfunction was 1% in bevacizumab patients compared to the control arm across indications.

• Most common toxicities (> 10%, twice control group incidence): epistaxis, headache, hypertension, rhinitis, proteinuria, taste alterations, dry skin, rectal hemorrhage, lacrimation disorder, back pain, exfoliative dermatitis.

• Drug toxicities that occur more commonly in the elderly (≥ 2%) were asthenia, sepsis, deep thrombophlebitis, hypertension, hypotension, myocardial infarction, congestive heart failure, diarrhea, constipation, anorexia, leukopenia, anemia, dehydration, hypokalemia, and hyponatremia. In those aged 75 or older, in addition, dyspepsia, gastrointestinal hemorrhage, edema, epistaxis, increased cough, and voice alteration occurred more commonly than those under age 65.

• Ranpura et al. (2011) performed a meta-analysis of RCTs and found that bevacizumab, in combination with chemotherapy or biological therapy compared to chemotherapy alone, was associated with increased mortality.

Potential Toxicities/Side Effects and the Nursing Process

I.   ALTERATION IN INTESTINAL AND SKIN INTEGRITY related to GASTROINTESTINAL PERFORATION, FISTULAE, AND WOUND DEHISCENCE

Defining Characteristics: Rarely, patients may develop gastrointestinal perforation, sometimes fatal. It may be associated with intra-abdominal abscesses, or fistula, and occur at variable times during the treatment. Incidence across all studies was 3.2%, and for patients with cervical cancer the highest incidence was in patients who had received prior pelvic radiation. Presenting symptoms were abdominal pain associated with nausea and constipation. Colonoscopy has a similar risk of GI perforation, so drug should be stopped 28 days before a planned colonoscopy.

It is unknown how long the interval between surgery and treatment with bevacizumab should be, but it may be greater than 2 months and the surgical incision should be completely healed; similarly, it is not known how long the interval should be between treatment with bevacizumab and elective surgery, but it certainly should be longer than the elimination time of the drug (half-life 20 days).

The incidence of GI-vaginal fistulae in the cervical cancer trial was 8.2% in the bevacizumab arm, compared to 0.9% in the control group. All patients who developed vaginal-GI fistulae had had prior pelvic RT.

The incidence of non-GI fistulae is increased but is uncommon, and generally occurs within the first 6 months of treatment.

Exfoliative dermatitis occurred in 19% of patients receiving 5-FU/LV plus bevacizumab. GI perforation has occurred in patients with NSCLC and advanced breast cancer receiving bevacizumab.

Nursing Implications: Assess baseline bowel, skin integrity, and healing of any wounds or incisions; assess for dehiscence, and integrity of skin or wound at each visit. Teach patient that very rarely GI perforation or wound dehiscence may occur and to report or come to the emergency room for severe abdominal pain associated with nausea, vomiting, constipation, or other symptoms; or problems with wound healing right away for immediate evaluation. Bevacizumab should be discontinued if perforation or wound dehiscence occurs. Bevacizumab should be held prior to elective surgery based on the drug half-life of 20 days (range, 10 50 days) and not started until at least 28 days after major surgery; the surgical incision must be fully healed. For patients who are undergoing metastectomy, the drug may be stopped 2 months before and not resumed for at least 60 days after hepatectomy. Teach patient to self-assess changes in skin or wound integrity and to report it right away. Bevacizumab should be discontinued if the patient develops GI perforation, tracheoesophageal fistula, grade 4 fistula, or fistula formation involving an internal organ.

II.   ALTERATION IN HEMOSTASIS related to BLEEDING AND THROMBOSIS

Defining Characteristics: Two patterns of bleeding may rarely occur: minor hemorrhage such as mild (grade 1) epistaxis, and serious hemorrhage. The incidence of epistaxis is 35% compared to 10% in the chemotherapy-only mCRC group. Epistaxis is easily controlled with pressure application. Of note, hemorrhage (pulmonary) occurred when drug was being studied in patients with lung cancer, with a higher incidence (31% in a small study) in patients with squamous cell histology; thus the drug is contraindicated in patients with squamous cell histology or those with hemoptysis. Many of these patients bled from a cavitation or area of necrosis in the pulmonary tumor. Rare severe hemorrhage includes hemoptysis, gastrointestinal (GI) bleeding, hematemesis, CNS hemorrhage, epistaxis, and vaginal bleeding occurred five times more frequently in the group receiving bevacizumab than the group receiving only chemotherapy. The incidence of severe (grades 3 and higher) hemorrhage was 1.2–4.6%. The incidence of grade 2 CNS hemorrhage in NSCLC patients with CNS metastasis was 1.2% in the bevacizumab arm, while intracranial hemorrhage occurred in 4.9% of patients with previously treated glioblastoma, with 1.2% grade 3–4. Thrombocytopenia may occur in 5% of patients. Deep vein thrombosis may occur in 6–9% of patients. Patients on low-dose Coumadin for implanted port patency had no increased risk of bleeding. There was an increased incidence of venous thromboembolism in patients with cervical cancer receiving bevacizumab with chemotherapy (10.6% vs 5.4% in patients receiving chemotherapy alone).

Nursing Implications: Assess baseline hematologic parameters and monitor during therapy. Teach patient that bleeding may occur and is most commonly epistaxis; but may also rarely occur as bleeding in the gastrointestinal tract, vagina in women, or elsewhere, and to report signs/symptoms of bleeding, changes in mental status, mobility, vision, weakness, or any new sign or symptom right away. Teach patient to assess for and report right away signs/symptoms of thrombosis: new swelling, pain, skin warmth, and/or change in color (e.g., erythema, mottling) on the legs or thighs; new onset pain in the abdomen; dyspnea or shortness of breath, rapid heartbeat, chest pain, or pressure that may signal a pulmonary embolism; and any changes in vision, new onset of severe headache, lightheadedness, or dizziness. Assess baseline mental status and neurologic signs, and monitor during therapy, especially in patients with brain metastasis. Teach patients to apply pressure if epistaxis occurs. Discuss any abnormalities with physician. Bevacizumab should be discontinued if the patient develops serious hemorrhage, and it should not be given to patients with recent hemoptysis (≥ ½ tsp bright red blood). Drug should be discontinued in patients who develop a severe arterial thrombotic event, or a life-threatening (grade 4) venous thrombotic event including pulmonary embolism.

III. POTENTIAL ALTERATION IN CIRCULATION related to HYPERTENSION AND CONGESTIVE HEART FAILURE

Defining Characteristics: Bevacizumab increases the incidence and severity of hypertension, a class effect of all angiogenesis inhibitors believed caused by inhibition of VEGF, which decreases nitric oxide and prevents blood vessel dilation. Across clinical studies, incidence of grade 3–4 HTN ranged from 5–18%.

Nursing Implications: Assess baseline BP prior to and during treatment, at least for the first treatment, then prior to each drug administration. BP should be monitored every 2–3 weeks during treatment. If the patient has a history of hypertension, monitor BP more closely, although hypertension develops over time rather than during the drug infusion. Blood pressure should continue to be monitored after patient has stopped the drug. Teach patient drug administration, potential side effects, and self-care measures if prescribed antihypertensive medication, such as angiotensin-converting enzyme inhibitors, beta-blockers, diuretics, and calcium channel blockers. Drug should be temporarily suspended in patients with severe hypertension until BP can be controlled with medical management. Drug should be permanently discontinued if the patient develops hypertensive crisis (diastolic blood pressure >120 mm Hg) or hypertensive encephalopathy.

IV.   ALTERATION IN RENAL FUNCTION related to NEPHROTIC SYNDROME

Defining Characteristcs: Nephrotic syndrome and proteinuria may occur. 36% of mCRC patients receiving bevacizumab developed grades 1–4 proteinuria; and 20% of patients with renal cell cancer receiving bevacizumab and IFN-α; grade 3–4 proteinuria ranged from 0.7–7.4% across studies. Median time to onset of proteinuria was 5.6 months after starting drug, and median time to resolution was 6.1 months. Proteinuria did not resolve in 40% of patients.

Nursing Implications: Assess baseline renal function and presence of protein in urine (1+ or greater by dipstick), and monitor prior to each treatment. Discuss any abnormalities with the physician. Patients with 2+ or higher proteinuria by urine dipstick should be asked to collect a 24-hour urine sample for protein. Drug should be held for proteinuria ≥ 2 g/24 h, and resume when proteinuria < 2 g/24 h. Monitor patients closely if moderate to severe proteinuria until improved or resolved. Drug should be discontinued if the patient develops nephrotic syndrome.

Drug: bexarotene (Targretin oral capsules and topical gel)

Class: Retinoid.

Mechanism of Action: Retinoid that selectively binds to and activates retinoid X receptors (RXRs), which have biologic activity distinct from retinoic acid receptors (RARs). The activated receptors can partner with receptor partners (e.g., retinoic acid receptors, vitamin D receptor, thyroid receptor), become activated, and then function as transcription factors that regulate the expression of genes, which control cellular differentiation and proliferation. The exact mechanism of action in cutaneous T-cell lymphoma is unknown.

Metabolism: Drug is well absorbed after oral administration, especially after a fat-containing meal, with a terminal half-life of 7 hours. Drug is highly protein-bound (> 99%). Drug appears to be metabolized by the cytochrome P450 CYP3A4 isoenzyme system in the liver, forming glucuronidated oxidative metabolites. Four metabolites are formed and are active, but it is unclear which metabolites or whether the parent drug is responsible for the efficacy of the drug. Probably excreted via the hepatobiliary system.

Indication: Bexarotene (Targretin) is indicated for the treatment of cutaneous manifestations of cutaneous T-cell lymphoma in patients who are refractory to at least one prior systemic therapy.

Dosage/Range:
Oral capsules:
- Indicated for the treatment of cutaneous manifestations of cutaneous T-cell lymphoma in patients who are refractory to at least one prior systemic therapy.
- Initial dose of 300 mg/m² PO per day for up to 97 weeks (maximum in clinical trials).

- Dose-reduce for toxicity to 200 mg/m² PO daily, then down to 100 mg/m² PO daily, or stop temporarily until toxicity resolves. After resolution, gradually titrate dose upward.
- Evaluate treatment efficacy at 8 weeks, and if no tumor response but the drug is well tolerated, increase dose to 400 mg/m² PO daily and monitor closely.
- Consider suspending or discontinuing drug if LFTs become elevated > 3 X ULN for AST, ALT, or bilirubin. Use drug cautiously in patients with hepatic insufficiency.

Topical gel:
- 1% gel indicated for the topical treatment of skin lesions in patients with early stage cutaneous T-cell lymphoma who have failed other therapies.

Drug Preparation:
- Available as 75-mg gelatin capsules in bottles of 100 capsules. The contents of the bottle should be protected from light, high temperatures, and humidity once opened.
- Store at 2–25°C (36–77°F).
- 1% gel available in tube. Store at 2–25°C (36–77°F).

Drug Administration:
- Assess:
  - Pregnancy test results, done within 1 week prior to beginning therapy, and repeated monthly during therapy with oral capsule.
  - Baseline serum lipid levels must be assessed prior to initiation of therapy, and any abnormalities treated so that fasting triglycerides are normal before starting therapy.
  - LFTs baseline; then at weeks 1, 2, 4 weeks of treatment; then, if stable, every 8 weeks.
  - WBC/differential and thyroid function tests baseline, then periodically during treatment.
- Oral: single daily oral dose with a meal.
- Topical gel: apply to affected areas only (NOT entire body) as needed.

Drug Interactions:
Oral capsules:
- Presumed to be related to P450 CYP3A4 isoenzyme system metabolism.
- Inhibitors of cytochrome P450 CYP3A4 enzyme system (e.g., ketoconazole, itraconazole, erythromycin, gemfibrozil, grapefruit juice) theoretically can increase serum levels of bexarotene; DO NOT GIVE GEMFIBROZIL concomitantly with bexarotene as bexarotene levels significantly raised.
- Inducers of cytochrome P450 CYP3A4 enzyme system (e.g., rifampin, phenytoin, phenobarbital, St. John's wort) may cause a decrease in serum bexarotene concentrations. These have not been studied. If used concomitantly, assess response, and increase bexarotene accordingly. Do not give together with St. John's wort.
- Theoretically, as drug is highly protein-bound, it is possible that bexarotene can displace drugs or be displaced by drugs that bind to plasma proteins (e.g., methotrexate); use together cautiously.

- Paclitaxel plus carboplatin: increased bexarotene AUC twofold.
- Bexarotene may be an inducer of CYP3A4 enzymes, and reduce serum levels of the coadministered drug, e.g., atorvastin, tamoxifen, paclitaxel, oral contraceptives.
- Tamoxifen: concomitant administration of bexarotene resulted in a 35% decrease in plasma concentrations of tamoxifen.
- Atorvastin: concomitant administration of bexarotene resulted in a 50% decrease in plasma concentrations of tamoxifen.

Lab Effects/Interference:
Oral capsules:
- CA 125 assay values in patients with ovarian cancer may be increased.
- Significantly increased serum triglycerides, total cholesterol, and decreased HDL.
- Increased LFTs.
- Decreased TSH and total T_4.
- Leukopenia and neutropenia.
- Increased LDH.

Special Considerations:
Oral capsules:
- Bexarotene is contraindicated in patients: (1) with a known hypersensitivity to bexarotene or other components of the product; (2) who are pregnant or mothers who are nursing as drug is teratogenic.
  - Women of childbearing age should use effective contraception   optimally, two forms unless abstinence is chosen.
  - Effective contraception should begin 1 month, continuously, before starting the drug, continued during therapy, and for 1 month after the completion of therapy.
  - A pregnancy test should be done within 1 week prior to beginning therapy, and repeated monthly during therapy. If pregnancy occurs, the drug must be stopped immediately and the woman counseled.
  - Bexarotene may reduce the plasma concentrations of oral or other systemic hormonal contraceptives (see drug interactions).
- Bexarotene capsules should be started on the second or third day of a normal menstrual period; no more than a one-month supply should be given so that the results of a pregnancy test are assessed, and counseling regarding avoidance of pregnancy and birth defects provided/reinforced prior to giving the prescription for the next month's bexarotene.
- Male patients with sexual partners who are pregnant, possibly pregnant, or who could become pregnant should use condoms during therapy, and for 1 month after therapy is ended.
- Patients with risk factors for pancreatitis (e.g., prior pancreatitis, uncontrolled hyperlipidemia, excessive alcohol consumption, uncontrolled diabetes mellitus, biliary tract disease, and medications known to increase triglyceride levels or to be associated with pancreatic toxicity) should generally NOT be treated with bexarotene capsules.
- Most patients have major lipid abnormalities, and one patient died of pancreatitis.
  - 70% of CTCL patients who received an initial dose of $\geq$ 300 mg/m^2/day had fasting triglyceride levels > 2.5 X ULN; about 55% had values > 800 mg/dL (median

1200 mg/dL). Elevated serum cholesterol > 300 mg/dL occurred in 60% of patients receiving an initial dose of ≥ 300 mg/m^2/day, and 75% of patients receiving a higher initial dose. High-density lipoproteins (HDL) levels were reduced to < 25 mg/dL in 55% receiving an initial dose of ≥ 300 mg/m^2/day, and 90% of patients who received a higher initial dose. The effect on lipoproteins was reversible with drug cessation and could generally be managed with dose reduction or concomitant antilipemic therapy.

- Assess fasting blood lipid levels baseline prior to therapy, then weekly for at least the next 2–4 weeks until the lipid response is established; then assess every 8 weeks. Correct fasting lipid levels prior to starting bexarotene (triglycerides: < 400 mg/dL).
- If fasting triglycerides become elevated during therapy, start antilipemic therapy, and if necessary, dose-reduce bexarotene or drug suspended. Of patients started at 300 mg/m^2/day, 60% required antilipemic therapy; atorvastin was used in 48%; DO NOT use gemfibrozil.
- Acute pancreatitis has occurred.
- Baseline laboratory assessment prior to starting drug should include WBC with differential, fasting blood glucose, thyroid function tests, fasting blood lipid profile, and liver function tests.
- Patients should limit vitamin A intake to ≤ 15,000 international units/day to avoid possible additive toxicity.
- Drug may cause increased LFTs, and decreased T4, TSH. Treatment with thyroid hormone supplements should be considered in patients with laboratory evidence of hypothyroidism. Assess baseline thyroid function tests baseline and monitor during therapy.
- Leukopenia may occur, generally occurring 4–8 weeks after starting therapy. The incidence was 18% at the recommended initial dose, and 43% in those starting at higher doses. Incidence of grade 3–4 neutropenia was 12% and 4%, respectively. Assess WBC/differential baseline and periodically during treatment.
- Drug may cause cataracts; patients who experience visual difficulties should have an ophthalmologic exam.
- Patients with diabetes mellitus: use caution in patients using insulin, agents enhancing insulin secretion (e.g., sulfonylureas), or insulin-sensitizers (e.g., thiazolidinedione class). Baroxetine may enhance the action of these agents and result in hypoglycemia.
- Patients should avoid direct sunlight and artificial ultraviolet light while taking bexarotene pills or gel, as severe sunburn and skin sensitivity reactions may occur due to photosensitization; patients should also wear SPF 30 or higher.
- No studies have been done with patients having hepatic dysfunction, but theoretically, hepatic dysfunction would greatly reduce metabolism/excretion and increase serum drug levels. Use cautiously, if at all, in this setting.
- Response rate in patients with cutaneous T-cell lymphoma who were refractory to one prior systemic therapy was 32%.
- *1% gel:*
  - Main side effects are rash, itching, and pain at application site.

Potential Toxicities/Side Effects and the Nursing Process

I.   ALTERATION IN NUTRITION, POTENTIAL, related to ABNORMAL LIPID LEVELS, PANCREATITIS, ELEVATED LFTs, AND NAUSEA (oral capsules)

Defining Characteristics: Almost all patients experience major lipid abnormalities, including elevated fasting triglycerides (70% receiving doses of ≥ 300 mg/m²/day had elevations of more than 2.5 times upper limits of normal [ULN], and 55% had values over 800 mg/dL with a median of 1200 mg/dL), elevated cholesterol (60% of patients receiving 300 mg/m²/day, and 75% of patients receiving doses of ≥ 300 mg/m²/day), and decreased levels of the protective high-density lipoproteins (HDL) to < 25 mg/dL (55% of patients receiving a dose of 300 mg/m²/day, and 90% of patients receiving a dose of > 300 mg/m²/ day). These values normalize after bexarotene is stopped. In most patients, either antilipemic medication or dose reduction of bexarotene allowed control over elevated levels. Rarely, patients with markedly elevated triglycerides (lowest level 770 mg/dL) can develop pancreatitis, which can be fatal. Patients with risk factors for pancreatitis should not receive the drug (e.g., history of pancreatitis, uncontrolled hyperlipidemia, uncontrolled diabetes mellitus, biliary tract disease, or medications known to increase triglyceride levels or to be associated with pancreatic toxicity). Uncommonly, patients may have elevated LFTs (5% of patients receiving an initial dose of 300 mg/m²/day and 7% when doses of > 300 mg/m²/day were used), but one patient developed cholestasis and died of liver failure in clinical trials. Nausea/vomiting occurs in 15%/3%, respectively, of patients receiving a dose of 300 mg/m²/day and 7%/13% of patients receiving doses of > 300 mg/m²/day. Anorexia affects 2% of patients receiving a dose of 300 mg/m²/day, and 22% of patients receiving higher doses.

Nursing Implications: Assess baseline triglyceride, cholesterol, and HDL levels. If abnormal, discuss pharmacologic management plan (e.g., atorvastatin), as fasting triglyceride level should be normal before patient begins therapy. Gemfibrozil should NOT be used. Fasting triglyceride level should then be monitored weekly until the lipid response to bexarotene is known (2–4 weeks), then at 8-week intervals. Goal is to keep fasting triglyceride level < 400 mg/dL to prevent pancreatitis. If fasting triglyceride level becomes elevated during treatment, discuss with physician antilipemic medication (e.g., atorvastatin), and if no response, discuss with physician bexarotene dose reduction or drug holiday. Teach patient about importance of testing fasting triglycerides, and monitoring level throughout treatment. LFTs should be assessed baseline, and after 1, 2, and 4 weeks of starting treatment; if stable, then assess every 8 weeks during treatment. Monitor serum LFTs, HDL, and discuss any abnormalities with physician (manufacturer recommends suspension or discontinuance of bexarotene if LFTs [SGOT/AST, SGPT/ALT, and bilirubin] > 3 times ULN). Assess baseline nutritional status; teach patient that nausea, vomiting, and anorexia may occur and to report them. If these occur, teach strategies to minimize occurrence, and if ineffective or symptoms are severe, discuss pharmacologic management with physician.

II.   ALTERATION IN ACTIVITY, POTENTIAL, related to HYPOTHYROIDISM (oral capsules)

Defining Characteristics: Bexarotene binds and activates retinoid × receptors, and can partner with thyroid receptor; once activated, the receptor functions as a transcription factor that regulates gene expression controlling cellular differentiation and proliferation. Drug induces reversible clinical hypothyroidism in about 50% of patients (decrease in TSH in 60% of patients, and total T_4 in 45% of patients at a dose of 300 mg/m^2/day), and hypothyroidism was reported in 29% of patients. Asthenia occurs in 29.8% of patients at a dose of 300 mg/m^2/day and in 45% of patients at higher doses.

Nursing Implications: Assess baseline thyroid function tests (TFTs), and discuss pharmacologic replacement of thyroid hormone with physician if values indicate hypothyroidism. Monitor TFTs during treatment. Teach patient that this may occur, importance of laboratory testing, fact that hypothyroidism induced by drug is reversible following discontinuance of drug, and to report signs/symptoms of hypothyroidism (e.g., weight gain, lethargy, slowed thinking, skin dryness, constipation, joint pain/stiffness). Teach patient to alternate rest and activity periods, and other measures to conserve energy.

III.   POTENTIAL FOR INFECTION related to LEUKOPENIA (oral capsules)

Defining Characteristics: Reversible leukopenia (WBC/mm^3 1,000–3,000) occurred in 18% of patients receiving dose of 300 mg/m^2/day, and in 43% of patients receiving higher doses. Patients receiving 300 mg/m^2/day had grade 3 (12%) and grade 4 (4%) neutropenia. Incidence of bacterial infection was 1.2% in patients receiving a dose of 300 mg/m^2/ day (overall body infection was 13%), and bacterial infection was 13% (overall infections 22%) in patients receiving higher doses. Onset of leukopenia was 4–8 weeks. Resolution of leukopenia/neutropenia occurred in 30 days with a drug dose reduction or discontinuance in most patients (82–93%). There were rare serious adverse events associated with leukopenia/neutropenia.

Nursing Implications: Assess WBC and ANC baseline and periodically during therapy. Teach patient that leukopenia may occur, and teach self-care measures, including self-assessment for infection, minimizing risk of infection, and when to notify provider. Teach patient/family signs/symptoms of infection, and how to take temperature if this is not known.

IV.   ALTERATION IN BOWEL ELIMINATION related to DIARRHEA (oral capsules)

Defining Characteristics: Diarrhea is uncommon in patients receiving × dose of 300 mg/ m^2/day, but is more common (41%) when dose is increased.

Nursing Implications: Assess baseline elimination status, and monitor throughout treatment. Teach patient that diarrhea may occur, especially if dose is > 300 mg/m²/day, and to report it. Teach patient self-care measures, including dietary modification (decreased insoluble fiber, increased soluble fiber, and increased fluid) and self-administration of OTC medicines to manage diarrhea. Teach patient to report diarrhea that does not resolve in 24 hours, or is severe, and discuss management with physician.

V. ALTERATION IN COMFORT related to HEADACHE, ABDOMINAL PAIN, CHILLS, FEVER, FLU SYNDROME, BACK PAIN, INSOMNIA (oral capsules)

Defining Characteristics: Symptoms occur with the following incidence (300 mg/m²/day dose vs higher dose): headache (30% vs 42%), abdominal pain (11% vs 4%), chills (9% vs 13%), fever (5% vs 17%), insomnia (5% vs 11%), flulike symptoms (3% vs 13%), back pain (2% vs 11%).

Nursing Implications: Assess baseline comfort status. Teach patient that these symptoms may occur and teach self-management measures. Teach patient to report fever > 100.5°F, chills, or symptoms that persist or are severe. Discuss management with physician if these occur.

VI. POTENTIAL ALTERATION IN SKIN INTEGRITY related to RASH, DRY SKIN, ALOPECIA, PERIPHERAL EDEMA (oral capsules), AND RASH, PRURITUS, PAIN AT GEL APPLICATION SITE (topical gel)

Defining Characteristics: Oral capsules: Symptoms occur with the following incidence (300 mg/m²/day vs higher dose): rash (17% vs 23%), exfoliative dermatitis (10.7% vs 9%), alopecia (3.6% vs 11%), and peripheral edema (13% vs 11%). Topical gel: Commonly, rash, pruritus, and pain at application site occur.

Nursing Implications: Oral capsules: Assess baseline skin integrity and extent of cutaneous lesions, and teach patient to report rash right away after taking capsules, especially if peeling. Discuss drug continuance with physician if this occurs. Teach patient to use skin cream to keep skin moist, to prevent cracking and peeling, and to prevent itching as directed by the physician. Teach patient to report any hair thinning, and if it occurs, assess impact on patient's body image. Discuss measures to enhance coping, such as use of scarf, measures to protect hair follicles (e.g., gentle shampoo, avoidance of hair perms, or use of curling iron), encourage patient to verbalize feelings, and provide emotional support. Teach patient to report swelling of feet or hands, to keep skin moisturized to prevent cracking or dryness, and to report skin changes that persist or are severe. Discuss management with physician. Topical gel: Assess integrity/extent of cutaneous lesions prior to patient starting therapy. Teach patient application of topical gel on areas of lesions only. Teach patient to report rash, persistent itching, or pain at application site. Teach patient self-care measures to manage itching, or pain at application site if they occur. Discuss with physician management of rash, and if severe, discontinuance of gel.

Drug: blinatumomab (Blincyto)

Class: Bispecific CD19-directed CD3 T-cell engager, first in class.

Mechanism of Action: Agent is made up of two monoclonal antibodies that bind and link together (1) CD19-expressed cells on the surface of B-lineage cells (the antigen), and (2) CD3 expressed on the surface of T lymphocytes, which in turn activates T lymphocytes. CD3 is located in the T-cell receptor. When it complexes with CD19 on benign and malignant cells, it activates the T lymphocytes, making them cytotoxic. The cytotoxic T-cells produce and release cytolytic proteins and inflammatory cytokines, and stimulate the proliferation of more T-cells, which then attack and lyse the CD19+ cells.

Metabolism: When blinatumomab was given as a 4-week continuous infusion (CI), T-cell activation occurred, with a resulting decrease in peripheral B-cells and a transient increase in cytokine levels. The metabolic pathway of the agent is unknown. Clearance is reduced in patients with moderate renal impairment.

Indication: For the treatment of Philadelphia-chromosome–negative relapsed or refractory B-cell precursor ALL. Approved under accelerated approval, and continued approval may be dependent upon verification of clinical benefit in subsequent trials.

Contraindications: Patients with known hypersensitivity to blinatumomab or to any component of the product formulation.

Dosage/Range:
- A single treatment cycle is 4 weeks of continuous infusion of blinatumomab, followed by a 2-week treatment-free interval.
- Treatment course consists of up to 2 cycles of the blinatumomab induction, followed by 3 cycles for consolidation treatment (up to a total of 5 cycles).
- Patients who weight at least 45 kg:
  - Cycle 1: 9 mcg/day for days 1–7, and 28 mcg/day on days 8–28.
  - Subsequent cycles: 28 mcg/day on days 1–28.
- *Dose modifications:*
  - Cytokine release syndrome (CRS): *Grade 3*: Withhold blinatumomab until resolved, then restart at 9 mcg/day; escalate to 28 mcg/day after 7 days if CRS does not recur. *Grade 4*: Permanently discontinue blinatumomab.
  - Neurological toxicity: (1) Seizure: Permanently discontinue blinatumomab if more than 1 seizure occurs. (2) *Grade 3*: Withhold blinatumomab until no more than grade 1 (mild) and for at least 3 days, then restart at 9 mcg/day; escalate to 28 mcg/day after 7 days if the toxicity does not recur. If the toxicity occurred at 9 mcg/day, or if the toxicity takes more than 7 days to resolve, permanently discontinue blinatumomab. *Grade 4*: Permanently discontinue blinatumomab.
  - Other clinically relevant adverse reactions: *Grade 3*: Withhold blinatumomab until no more than grade 1 (mild) and for at least 3 days, then restart at 9 mcg/day; escalate to 28 mcg/day after 7 days if the toxicity does not recur. If the toxicity takes more than 14 days to resolve, permanently discontinue blinatumomab. *Grade 4*: Consider discontinuing blinatumomab permanently.

Drug Preparation:
- Available as 35 mcg lyophilized powder in a single-use vial for reconstitution.
- Use IV solution stabilizer provided to coat the prefilled IV bag prior to the addition of reconstituted blinatumomab.
- Reconstitute with sterile water for injection, USP *only*.
- Strictly observe sterile technique, as agent does not contain antimicrobial preservatives.
- *Use specific volumes described in admixture instructions,* as dosage errors may occur.
- **Follow instructions exactly.**
  - **Gather supplies from package:** 1 package (1 vial of blinatumomab and 1 vial of IV solution stabilizer) to prepare a dose of 9 mcg/day over 24 hours at a rate of 10 mL/hr or over 48 hours at a rate of 5 mL/hr, and 28 mcg/day dose infused over 24 hours at a rate of 10 mL/hr; **or** 2 packages of drug to prepare a dose of 28 mcg/day infused over 48 hours at a rate of 5 mL/hr.
  - **Gather supplies but not included in package:** (1) sterile, single-use disposable syringes; (2) 21- to 23-gauge needles; (3) preservative-free sterile water for injection, USP; (4) 250 mL 0.9% sodium chloride IV bag (usually contains overfill with a total volume of 265–275 mL); use only polyolefin, PVC non-di-ethylhexylphthalate (non-DEHP), or ethyl vinyl acetate (EVA) infusion bags/pump cassettes; (5) polyolefin, PVC non-DEHP, or EVA IV tubing with a sterile, non-pyrogenic, low-protein-binding 0.2-micron in-line filter (ensure that tubing is compatible with infusion pump).
  - **Aseptic preparation (adhere to strict aseptic technique, as the drug contains *no* antimicrobial preservatives):**
    - The preparation must take place in a USP <797> facility; it must also be done in an ISO Class 5 laminar flow hood or better.
    - The admixture area should have appropriate environmental specifications, confirmed by periodic monitoring.
    - Personnel should be trained in aseptic manipulations and admixing oncology drugs, and wear appropriate protective clothing and gloves.
    - Gloves and surfaces should be disinfected.
  - **Special considerations**:
    - **IV** solution stabilizer is provided with the blinatumomab package; it is used to coat the prefilled IV bag prior to addition of the reconstituted blinatumomab to prevent adhesion of the IV bag and IV lines. *Add the IV solution stabilizer to the IV bag containing 0.9% sodium chloride;* **do not use the stabilizer to reconstitute blinatumomab.**
    - The entire volume of the admixed blinatumomab will be more than the volume administered to the patient (240 mL) to account for priming the IV line and to ensure the patient receives the full dose of blinatumomab.
    - When preparing the IV bag, remove air from the IV bag. This step is most important for use with an ambulatory infusion pump.
    - Use the **specific volumes described** in the admixing instructions to minimize errors in calculation.
  - **Preparation of blinatumomab solution for infusion using a prefilled 250-mL 0.9% sodium chloride IV bag:** Follow the admixture instructions for each dose and infusion time in sections 2.4.4.1–2.4.4.4 in the package insert.

- 9 mcg/day infused over 24 hours at a rate of 10 mL/hr: section 2.4.4.1
- 9 mcg/day infused over 48 hours at a rate of 5 mL/hr: section 2.4.4.2
- 28 mcg/day infused over 24 hours at a rate of 10 mL/hr: section 2.4.4.3
- 28 mcg/day infused over 48 hours at a rate of 5 mL/hr: section 2.4.4.4
- **Storage requirements (including infusion time):**
  - **Lyophilized** blinatumomab vial and IV solution stabilizer may be stored for a maximum of 8 hours at room temperature; protect both vials from light.
  - **Reconstituted** blinatumomab vial and prepared IV bag containing blinatumomab solution for infusion:
    - *Vial*: Room temperature (23–27°C [73–81°F]): 4 hours; refrigerated (2–8°C [36–46°F]): 24 hours.
    - *Prepared IV bag* containing blinatumomab solution for infusion: Room temperature (23–27°C [73–81°F]): 48 hours; refrigerated (2–8°C [36–46°F]): 8 days.
  - If the IV bag containing blinatumomab solution for infusion is not administered within the time frames and temperature indicated, discard the solution. *Do not refrigerate it again.*

Drug Administration:
- Cycles 1 and 2: Patient should be hospitalized for the first 9 days of cycle 1, and for the first 2 days of cycle 2. The infusion in the subsequent cycle starts and reinitiation, if required after a 4-hour or longer interruption, should be supervised by a healthcare professional or the patient hospitalized.
- Premedicate with dexamethasone 20 mg IV 1 hour prior to the first dose of blinatumomab in each cycle, prior to a step dose (such as cycle 1, day 8), or if the infusion is restarted after an interruption of 4 hours or more.
- Administer via an infusion pump, at a constant flow rate. The pump should be programmable, lockable, and non-elastomeric, and have an alarm.
- Administer using IV tubing that contains a sterile non-pyrogenic, low-protein-binding, 0.2-micron in-line filter.
- The IV bag should be infused over 24 or 48 hours. Infuse the total 240 mL of the blinatumomab solution according to the pharmacy label instructions, at an infusion rate of either (1) 10 mL/hr for 24 hours or (2) 5 mL/hr for 48 hours.
- Use a dedicated IV lumen.
- *Do not* **flush the blinatumomab infusion line, especially when changing infusion bags, as this may cause overdose with increased complications.**
- **Strictly follow instructions** for preparation (including admixture) and administration, as errors may occur.
- At the end of the infusion, discard any unused the blinatumomab solution in the IV bag, along with the IV lines.
- Monitor the patient closely for signs and symptoms of infection and ensure prompt treatment.
- Assess the patient's ability to drive or use machines; teach the patient to avoid driving or using hazardous machinery while blinatumomab is being administered.

Drug Interactions: CYP450 enzymes may be suppressed by transient cytokine elevation.

Lab Effects/Interference:
- Neutropenia, anemia, thrombocytopenia
- Decreased serum potassium, phosphate, and magnesium
- Increased serum ALT, AST, total bilirubin, and glucose

Special Considerations:
- Warnings: Interrupt or discontinue as needed for the following events:
  - Cytokine release syndrome, which may be fatal
  - Neurologic toxicity, which may be severe, life threatening, and fatal
- Most common adverse reactions (incidence ≥ 20%): pyrexia, headache, peripheral edema, febrile neutropenia, nausea, hypokalemia, tremor, rash, and constipation.
- Preparation and administration errors have occurred; instructions for preparation and administration should be followed exactly to minimize medication errors.
- Tumor lysis syndrome (TLS) may occur and be life threatening. Use prophylactic measures, including pretreatment nontoxic cytoreduction and on-treatment hydration to prevent TLS. Monitor for signs and symptoms of TLS and manage TLS with medication management, as well as with temporary interruption or discontinuation of blinatumomab.
- Patients are at risk for loss of consciousness (LOC) related to the potential neurologic events, including seizures, that may occur with blinatumomab administration. Advise patients *not* to drive or engage in hazardous occupations or activities such as operating heavy or potentially dangerous equipment while blinatumomab is being administered.
- Elevated liver enzymes (transient) may occur. If this effect occurs outside of CRS, the median time of onset is 15 days. Monitor LFTs closely, and interrupt blinatumomab therapy if transaminases rise to more than 5 × ULN, or if bilirubin rises to more than 3 × ULN.
- Infusion reactions may occur and may be clinically indistinguishable from CRS manifestations.
- Leukoencephalopathy has occurred in patients receiving blinatumomab, especially if they have received prior treatment with cranial irradiation and antileukemic chemotherapy, including systemic high-dose methotrexate or intrathecal cytarabine.
- Blinatumomab may cause fetal toxicity; the drug should be used during pregnancy only if the potential benefit justifies the potential risk to the fetus. Mothers should not breast-feed while receiving the drug, and should decide whether to discontinue the drug or nursing, taking into account the importance of the drug to the mother.

Potential Toxicities/Side Effects and the Nursing Process

I. ALTERATION IN COMFORT AND HOMEOSTASIS, POTENTIAL, related to CYTOKINE RELEASE SYNDROME

Defining Characteristics: Incidence is 11%. Symptom constellation may include pyrexia (62%), headache (36%), asthenia (17%), hypotension (11%), increased ALT and AST (11–12%), and increased total bilirubin. Other signs and symptoms are fever, fatigue, dizziness, nausea, vomiting, chills, face swelling, wheezing or trouble breathing, and skin rash. CRS may be rarely life threatening or fatal. Rarely, disseminated intravascular coagulation (DIC), capillary leak syndrome (CLS), and hemophagocytic lymphohistiocytosis/macrophage activation syndrome (HLH/MAS) may complicate CRS. CLS, if it occurs, is characterized by loss of vascular tone and extravasation of plasma proteins and fluid into the extravascular space. This results in hypotension and decreased organ perfusion. CLS may be associated with cardiac arrhythmias, angina, MI, respiratory insufficiency requiring intubation, GI bleeding, edema, and mental status changes. Infusion reactions may also occur and be clinically indistinguishable from CRS signs and symptoms. Hypersensitivity reactions occur in 1% of patients. Peripheral edema occurs in 25% of patients, dyspnea in 15%, and hypotension in 11%.

Nursing Implications: Assess baseline temperature, vital signs, pulmonary and neurologic status, and comfort level, and monitor every 4–6 hours when the patient is hospitalized. Assess LFTs and other laboratory tests as ordered. Teach the patient to report any difficulty breathing, or other signs and symptoms of CRS. Be prepared to institute medical orders to manage signs and symptoms, and expect that the drug may be temporarily interrupted or discontinued depending on their severity.

II.   SENSORY/PERCEPTUAL ALTERATIONS related to NEUROLOGIC TOXICITY

Defining Characteristics: Approximately 50% of patients experience neurologic toxicity, with 15% having grade 3 or higher reactions (severe, life threatening, or fatal). Mean time to development is 7 days. Toxicity may include encephalopathy, seizures, speech disorders, disturbances in consciousness, confusion, disorientation, and disorders of balance and coordination. Most events resolve with drug interruption, but some require permanent discontinuation of the drug.

Nursing Implications: Assess baseline mental status, neurologic status, and consciousness before drug administration. Assess for changes such as decreased consciousness, confusion, disorientation, loss of balance or coordination, changes in speech, or seizures; if identified, discuss with physician regarding management and interruption of drug. Teach the patient to report any changes in mental or neurologic status, or seizure occurrence.

III.   POTENTIAL FOR INJURY related to INFECTION

Defining Characteristics: Febrile neutropenia occurs in 25% of patients, with 23% having grade 3 or higher. The incidence of neutropenia is 16%, thrombocytopenia 11%, and anemia 18%. Serious infections occur in 25% of patients, including sepsis (7%), pneumonia (9%), bacteremia, opportunistic infections, and catheter-site infections. Bacterial infections account for 19% of all infections, fungal 15%, and viral 13%. Fifteen percent of patients have chills.

Nursing Implications: Assess baseline CBC, ANC, and platelet count and monitor during therapy. Assess patients for signs and symptoms of infections. Teach the patient to self-assess and to report any fever, or other signs and symptoms of infection. Teach self-care measures to minimize risk of infection and bleeding, including avoidance of OTC aspirin-containing medications. Discuss with physician/NP/PA prophylactic antibiotics and any surveillance testing as appropriate. Discuss possible signs and symptoms of infection with physician/NP/PA, and implement antimicrobial medication(s) as ordered. Discuss drug interruption with physician/NP/PA for prolonged neutropenia.

IV. POTENTIAL FOR ALTERATION IN NUTRITION, LESS THAN BODY REQUIREMENTS, related to NAUSEA, CONSTIPATION, DIARRHEA, VOMITING

Defining Characteristics: Nausea occurs in 25% of patients, constipation 20%, diarrhea 20%, and vomiting 13%. Eleven percent of patients had increased weight but 25% had peripheral edema.

Nursing Implications: Assess the patient's baseline nutritional status and weight, and monitor it during therapy. If the patient experiences weight gain, assess for peripheral edema. Teach the patient to report nausea, vomiting, or change in bowel status that does not resolve. Discuss management strategies with physician/NP/PA. Teach the patient self-care strategies to manage diet and symptoms.

Drug: bortezomib (Velcade)

Class: Proteasome inhibitor.

Mechanism of Action: A reversible inhibitor of the 26S proteasome; inhibits the breakdown of ubiquinated intracellular proteins and disrupts the ubiquitin proteasome pathway. This pathway normally regulates the intracellular concentration of specific proteins, thus controlling homeostasis. Cancer cells depend on the proteins that are available from this process to turn on the cell cycle and to make the apparatus of mitosis. When the ubiquitin–proteasome pathway is disrupted, the proteins are not available, and multiple signaling pathways within the cell are disrupted, encouraging the cell to undergo apoptosis. Cell cycle movement (cell division) stops. Cells are unable to migrate, and sensitivity to chemotherapy is increased. In addition, the drug appears to downregulate the NF-kB pathway, which is necessary for cell growth, avoidance of apoptosis, and adhesion. This may restore chemosensitivity. In multiple myeloma, it interferes with cellular adhesion molecules so that tumor cells cannot bind to the bone marrow.

Metabolism: After IV administration, the drug is rapidly cleared from the plasma, with a mean elimination half-life range of 40–193 hours after multiple dosing. Drug undergoes oxidative metabolism via cytochrome P450 enzymes 3A4, 2D6, 2C19, 2C9, and 1A2. Drug is deboronated into two metabolites that are then hydroxylated into several metabolites. Unknown elimination path.

Indication: Treatment of patients with (1) multiple myeloma, including initial treatment, and (2) mantle cell lymphoma who have received at least one prior therapy.

Dosage/Range: 1.3 mg/m^2 either as an IVB (1 mg/mL) over 3- to 5-seconds or SQ (2.5 mg/mL) injection. At least 72 hours should elapse between consecutive doses of bortezomib. Ensure drug is prepared and labeled as either an **IV or SQ medication;** each route of administration has a different reconstituted concentration. Drug **cannot be administered via IT route, as it may be fatal.**

- Previously untreated multiple myeloma: Nine 6-week treatment cycles, given with melphalan 9 mg/m^2 and prednisone 60 mg/m^2:
  - Cycles 1–4: 1.3 mg/m^2 per dose IVB or SQ **twice weekly** (days 1, 4, 8, 11) followed by a 10-day rest period, then resume on days 22, 25, 29, and 32. Cycle repeated q 6 weeks.
  - Cycles 5–9: bortezomib is given **weekly** on days 1, 8, 22, 29.
  - See package insert for melphalan and prednisone dosing and days.
  - Prior to beginning any cycle, platelet count should be ≥ 70 × 10^9/L, ANC ≥ 1.0 × 10^9/L, and nonhematologic toxicities should have resolved to grade 1 or baseline.
  - Consider the addition of an antiviral agent during treatment (incidence of herpes zoster was 13% in the bortezomib arm vs 5% high-dose dexamethasone arm, $p = .0002$, in the phase III APEX trial [Chanan-Khan et al., 2008]).
- Relapsed multiple myeloma or mantle cell lymphoma:
  - 1.3 mg/m^2 IV twice weekly x 2 weeks (days 1, 4, 8, 11) followed by a 10-day rest period (days 12–21).
  - For extended therapy of > 8 cycles, bortezomib is given on standard schedule or maintenance (once weekly x 4 weeks on days 1, 8, 15, and 22, followed by a 13-day rest period on days 23–35) every 35 days.
  - Doses should be separated by at least 72 hours to give normal cells a chance to recover.
- Retreatment for multiple myeloma in patients who had previously responded to bortezomib, and who relapsed at least 6 months after completing prior bortezomib therapy (alone or in combination): may retreat starting at the last tolerated dose.
  - Bortezomib 1.3 mg/m^{2}IVB or SQ twice weekly (days 1, 4, 8, 11) every 3 weeks for a maximum of 8 cycles.
  - Bortezomib can be given alone or in combination with dexamethasone.
- *Dosage in patients with **moderate or severe** hepatic impairment:*
  - Mild (BR ≤ 1.0 X ULN, SGOT > ULN): No dose modification; if BR > 1.0–1.5 X ULN, any AST: no dose modification.
  - **Moderate** (BR > 1.5–3 X ULN, any AST) or **Severe** (BR > 3 X ULN, any AST): Reduce starting dose to 0.7 mg/m^2 per injection during the first cycle. Consider dose escalation to 1.0 mg/m^2; or further dose reduction to 0.5 mg/m^2 may be considered based on patient tolerance.
- Dose must be individualized to prevent overdosage.
- Patients with severe preexisting PN should be treated with bortezomib only after a careful risk-benefit assessment;
  - Subcutaneous administration causes a lower incidence of peripheral neuropathy, so subcutaneous administration of bortezomib should be considered for patients with preexisting or at high risk of peripheral neuropathy.
- Drug dose is not modified for renal impairment, including patients requiring renal dialysis.

Dose Reduction to Manage Adverse Events:

Bortezomib should be held at the onset of any grade 3 nonhematologic or grade 4 hematologic toxicity excluding neuropathy. Once the symptoms of toxicity have resolved, bortezomib may be restarted at a 25% reduced dose (1.3 mg/m^2 is reduced to 1 mg/m^2).

Newly diagnosed multiple myeloma, when given with melphalan/prednisone:

- Prolonged grade 4 neutropenia or thrombocytopenia, or thrombocytopenia with bleeding: consider 25% melphalan dose reduction next cycle.
- Platelet count $\leq$ 30 x 10^9/L or ANC $\leq$ 0.75 x 10^9/L on a bortezomib dosing day (except day 1), hold bortezomib.
- If several bortezomib doses are held consecutively due to toxicity, decrease dose of bortezomib by 1 dose level, e.g., from 1.3 mg/m^2 to 1.0 mg/m^2, or from 1 mg/m^2 to 0.7 mg/m^2.
- Grade 3 or higher nonhematological toxicity: hold drug, and when resolved to grade 1 or less, resume at a dose reduced by 1 dose level. See below for dose modifications for neuropathic pain and/or peripheral neuropathy (PN).

Relapsed multiple myeloma or mantle cell lymphoma: Any grade 3 nonhematologic toxicity or grade 4 hematologic toxicity except for PN: Hold drug at onset, and when resolved to grade 1 or less, resume at 25% dose reduction (e.g., 1.3 mg/m^2/dose reduced to 1 mg/m^2/ dose; 1 mg/m^2/dose reduced to 0.7 mg/m^2/dose).

Peripheral neuropathic pain, and/or peripheral sensory or motor neuropathy:
- Consider starting patient with preexisting or at high risk of PN on bortezomib given subcutaneously; patients with preexisting severe PN should be treated with bortezomib only after careful risk benefit assessment.
- Patients experiencing new or worsening PN during bortezomib therapy may require a dose reduction and/or a less intense schedule.
  - Grade 1 without pain or loss of function (asymptomatic loss of DTRs or paresthesia): no action.
  - Grade 1 with pain or grade 2 [moderate symptoms, limiting instrumental ADLs (e.g., preparing meals, grocery or clothes shopping, using telephone, managing money)]: reduce bortezomib dose to 1 mg/m^2.
  - Grade 2 with pain or grade 3 [severe symptoms, limiting self-care ADLs (e.g., bathing, dressing and undressing, feeding self, using toilet, taking medications, not bedridden)]: withhold bortezomib therapy until toxicity resolves, then re-initiate with reduced dose of 0.7mg/m^2 once weekly.
  - Grade 4 (life-threatening, requiring urgent intervention): discontinue drug.
  - Instrumental ADLs: preparing meals, grocery shopping, using telephone, managing money; self-care ADLs: bathing, dressing, undressing, feeding self, toileting, taking medications, not bedridden.

Drug Preparation:
- Available in 10-mL vials containing 3.5 mg of bortezomib powder; store unopened vials at room temperature 25°C (77°F), and protect from light.
- Drug quantity in one 3.5 mg vial may exceed the usual dose; use caution in calculating the dose to prevent overdosage.
- Use aseptic technique, and reconstitute only with 0.9% sodium chloride. Inspect for particulate matter and discoloration; and if found, do not use.

- IV: Reconstitute each vial with 3.5 mL 0.9% sodium chloride injection USP, forming a 1 mg/mL solution that should be colorless and clear (stable for 8 hours at controlled room temperature). Label as IV.
- SQ: Reconstitute each vial with 1.4 mL 0.9% sodium chloride injection USP, forming a 2.5 mg/mL solution that should be colorless and clear (stable for 8 hours at controlled room temperature). Label as SQ.
- Make certain to use the correct reconstituted concentration for the intended route, and use caution in calcuating the volume to be administered. Make certain to have drawn-up volume and reconstituted vial double checked by another chemotherapy-competent professional.
- Carefully draw up prescribed amount, as drug in vial may exceed ordered dose (stable as reconstituted drug, or in a syringe including reconstituted time, for 8 hours).
- Apply VELCADE label to syringe containing drug indicating route of administration; drug CANNOT be given by the IT route.

Drug Administration:
- Prior to any cycle of therapy with bortezomib, melphalan, and prednisone, platelet count should be at least 70,000/mm^3 and ANC at least 1,000/mm^3; in addition, any nonhematologic toxicities must have resolved to grade 1 or baseline.
- Administer IVP over 3–5 seconds, followed by saline flush; or by SQ injection. SQ administration should be considered for patients at high risk for or preexisting PN, as incidence is reduced with SQ administration; it has been studied and is noninferior to IV administration (Moreau et al., 2011).
- Local skin irritation reported in 5% of patients, but drug is not a vesicant.
- Rotate sites for injection (thigh or abdomen), **avoiding** old sites (at least 1 inch away) and sites that are tender, bruised, erythematous, or indurated.
- If injection-site reaction occurs, use a less concentrated solution (1 mg/mL instead of the 2.5 mg/mL) or consider IV injection.
- Bortezomib, melphalan, prednisone regimen: at the beginning of each cycle, nonhematologic toxicities must have resolved to grade 1 or less.
- Drug has accidently been administered intrathecally resulting in patient death; ensure intrathecal medications are prepared and delivered separately from IV preparations, and labeled as IT administration. Bortezomib **can only be administered IV or SQ.**

Drug Interactions:
- Strong CYP3A4 inhibitors (e.g., ketoconazole, ritonavir): increased bortezomib exposure; monitor patient closely for bortezomib toxicity if drugs must be given concomitantly.
- Strong CYP3A4 inducers (e.g., rifampin, St. John's wort): decreased bortezomib exposure; avoid concomitant use.

Lab Effects/Interference:
- Decreased neutrophil, platelet, and red blood cell counts.
- Hypoglycemia and hyperglycemia in diabetic patients.
- Increased LFTs.

TREATMENT

Special Considerations:

- Contraindicated in patients with hypersensitivity to bortezomib, boron, or mannitol; IT administration is contraindicated; avoid use in pregnancy and teach patient not to breast-feed while receiving the drug.
- Use cautiously in patients with hepatic dysfunction and monitor closely; in patients with a history of CHF, peripheral neuropathy, or syncope; in patients receiving antihypertensive medications (additive hypotension); and in patients who are dehydrated.
- Bortezomib treatment causes a primarily sensory PN; however, cases of severe sensory AND motor PN have been reported. Patients with preexisting PN may experience worsening of PN.
  - Patients should be monitored closely for symptoms, such as burning sensation, hyperesthesia, hypoesthesia, paresthesia, discomfort, neuropathic pain, or weakness.
  - In the phase 3 relapsed multiple myeloma trial comparing bortezomib SQ to IV, incidence of ≥ grade 2 PN was 24% for SQ and 39% for IV administration. Grade ≥ 3 PN occurred in 6% of SQ patients and 15% of IV patients. Patients experiencing new or worsening PN during bortezomib therapy may need a dose reduction and/or a less dose-intense schedule.
  - Improvement or resolution of PN was reported in 73% of patients who discontinued due to grade 2 PN or who had ≥ grade 3 PN in the phase 2 MM studies.
- Patients with diabetes may require close monitoring of blood glucose and adjustment of antidiabetic medication.
- Drug is metabolized by liver enzymes with increased drug exposure in patients with moderate or severe hepatic dysfunction, dose-reduce initially and then titrate up or down, depending upon patient response. Monitor patient closely for toxicities.
- Moreau et al. (2011) compared IV and subcutaneous drug administration and found that patients had similar response rates of 42% ($p = 0.002$), median time to progression (10.4 months vs 9.4 months (IV)). One-year survival was similar (72.6% in subcutaneous arm vs 76.7% in IV arm). Grade 3–4 adverse events were 57% in the subcutaneous arm vs 72% in the IV arm. Incidence of drug-related peripheral neuropathy was significantly lower in the subcutaneous arm (all grades 38%, grades ≥ 2, 24%, ≥ 3, 6%) compared to the IV arm (53% all grades, $p = 0.044$; grades ≥ 2, 41% $p = 0.012$, and grades ≥ 3, 16%, $p = 0.026$) (Moreau et al., 2011).
- Rarely, CHF may worsen, and the onset of decreased LVEF has been reported. In addition, there have been rare reports of cases of QT-interval prolongation. Monitor patients with preexisting cardiac disease closely.
- Rarely, posterior reversible encephalopathy syndrome (PRES) has occurred, characterized by seizure, hypertension, headache, lethargy, confusion, blindness, and/or other visual or other neurologic disturbance. Diagnosis is confirmed with MRI. Discontinue bortezomib if PRES develops.
- GI toxicity: nausea, diarrhea, constipation, and vomiting can occur, sometimes requiring use of an antiemetic and antidiarrheal medication. Ileus can occur; administer fluid and electrolyte replacement as needed to prevent dehydration, and interrupt bortezomib for severe symptoms.
- Thrombocytopenia and neutropenia follow a cyclical pattern with nadirs occurring following the last dose of each cycle and usually recovering prior to the start of the next cycle. Mean platelet nadir in studies was 40% of baseline. CBC/platelets should be

monitored frequently, and platelets assessed prior to each dose of bortezomib. Patients who develop thrombocytopenia may require dose and schedule modification.

- Carefully consider risk–benefit ratio in patients with preexisting peripheral neuropathy, and monitor closely; dose-modify or discontinue drug as needed.
- Hypotension (postural, orthostatic, and hypotension) may occur in up to 8% of patients; monitor patients receiving antihypertensive therapy, those with a history of syncope, and dehydrated patients closely.
- There are rare reports of pulmonary hypertension in the absence of left heart failure or significant pulmonary disease. If patient develops new or worsening cardiopulmonary symptoms, consider interrupting the drug; a comprehensive diagnostic evaluation should be done.
- Tumor lysis syndrome and acute hepatic failure have been reported; consider allopurinol and hydration for newly diagnosed patients with high tumor burden.
- Women of reproductive potential should avoid pregnancy and must use effective contraception.
- Herpes virus infection may occur, so prophylaxis with acyclovir 400 mg PO bid is recommended during and for 3 months following completion of therapy with bortezomib; if patient has renal compromise, then the acyclovir dosage should be reduced.
- Teach patients to call provider (and give them telephone number) for dizziness, light-headedness, fainting spells, persistent headache, any changes in vision, swelling of the feet, ankles, legs, rash, shortness of breath or new cough, seizure, or increased blood glucose levels in diabetic patients.

Potential Toxicities/Side Effects and the Nursing Process

I.   POTENTIAL SENSORY/PERCEPTUAL ALTERATIONS related to SENSORY PERIPHERAL NEUROPATHY (PN)

Defining Characteristics: 80% of patients on clinical trials had a preexisting baseline PN. 37% of patients had new onset or aggravation of existing peripheral neuropathy (PN). 14% developed grade 3 PN overall, with 5% occurring in patients without baseline PN symptoms. There were no patients with grade 4 PN. Peripheral neuropathy improved/resolved in 51% of patients who underwent a dose adjustment for ≥ grade 2 PN and in 73% of patients who discontinued the drug. While primarily sensory, motor neuropathy can also occur. SQ injection of bortezomib resulted in grade 2 or greater PN in 24% of patients compared to 41% for those receiving IV drug.

Nursing Implications: Teach patient to report new onset or worsening of PN symptoms (numbness, pain, or burning sensation in feet or hands), any changes in sensory function (temperature sensation, knowing where body parts are in relation to the whole, etc.), functional ability (e.g., especially senses of smell and taste), and ability to carry out activities of daily living (ADLs). Assess patient for symptoms of PN (burning sensation, hypersthesia, hypoesthesia, paresthesia, discomfort, neuropathic pain, weakness) as well as severity of symptom(s) if they arise and potential for injury. If these are new symptoms or worsening of preexisting symptoms and patient is receiving drug IV, discuss with physician or midlevel changing to SQ administration. Teach patient measures to minimize symptoms and ensure safety. Review drug profile, and discuss with physician any potentially neurotoxic drugs that increase the risk of PN: amiodarone, antivirals, isoniazid, nitrofurantoin, or statins. If patient has neuropathic pain, discuss with physician use of duloxetine, as this has shown significant benefit in decreasing pain compared to placebo (59% vs 39%) (Smith et al., 2012).

Dose reductions: Grade 1 (paresthesias +/or loss of reflexes) without pain or loss of function: no action.

Grade 1 with pain or grade 2 (interfering with instrumental ADLs): decrease dose to 1.0 mg/m²/dose.

Grade 2 with pain or grade 3 (interfering with self-care ADLs): hold drug until toxicity resolves, then re-initiate with dose reduced to 0.7 mg/m² and change treatment schedule to once a week.

Grade 4 (life-threatening, urgent intervention indicated): discontinue drug.

II. POTENTIAL FOR INFECTION AND BLEEDING related to BONE MARROW DEPRESSION

Defining Characteristics: Thrombocytopenia occurred in 32% of patients (22% grade 3, 4% grade 4, with nadir day 11, and recovery by day 21) and neutropenia in 15% of patients (8% grade 3 and 2% grade 4; incidence higher in patients with multiple myeloma than mantle cell lymphoma). Febrile neutropenia occurred in < 1% of patients. Anemia incidence was 12–19%. Fever is common and higher in patients with multiple myeloma (23%) compared with mantle cell (10%).

Nursing Implications: Assess baseline leukocyte, platelet, and Hgb/HCT and monitor before each treatment, during therapy, and more often as needed. Hold drug for grade 4 hematologic toxicity (see NCI CTCAE) and dose-reduce 25%. Assess risk for infection and integrity of skin and mucous membranes, pulmonary status, and ability to clear secretions, as well as history of past infections, baseline and prior to each treatment. Teach patient to self-assess for signs/symptoms of infection, and to call provider immediately or come to the emergency room if temperature < 100.4°F, or has shaking chills, rash, productive cough, burning on urination, or any signs/symptoms of infection or bleeding. Teach self-care strategies to minimize risk of infection and bleeding, including avoidance of OTC aspirin-containing medications.

III. ALTERATION IN NUTRITION, LESS THAN BODY REQUIREMENTS, related to NAUSEA, DIARRHEA, DECREASED APPETITE, CONSTIPATION, VOMITING, AND DEHYDRATION

Defining Characteristics: Patients in clinical studies developed these symptoms with the following incidence: nausea (64%), diarrhea (51%), decreased appetite (43%), constipation (43%), vomiting (36%), dehydration (18%). Diarrhea, nausea, and vomiting occur 6–24 hours after infusion. Nausea is more common in patients with multiple myeloma. Diarrhea and constipation may occur during cycles 1 and 2, and then disappear. Patients with diabetes require close monitoring of their blood glucose and may require adjustments in their antidiabetic medication.

Nursing Implications: Assess baseline weight and nutritional status, and monitor prior to each treatment. Assess glucose, electrolytes prior to each treatment to weekly, especially serum sodium and potassium; replete as necessary and teach diet high in sodium and potassium. Teach patient that serum electrolytes may be decreased and to assess for signs/symptoms: hyponatremia (confusion, weakness, seizures), hypokalemia (muscle weakness, confusion, irregular heartbeats), hypercalcemia (constipation, thirst, confusion, muscle cramps, sleepiness), and hypomagnesemia (muscle cramps, headache, weakness). Teach patient that side effects may occur, self-care strategies, and to report them if symptoms do not resolve. Use aggressive antiemetics to prevent nausea and vomiting: serotonin antagonist IV prior to bortezomib dose and for 36 hours after each drug dose, if needed. If diarrhea develops after first treatment, teach patient to take loperamide prior to next dose of bortezomib and after every loose stool × 36 hours (not to exceed eight tablets a day), as well as to use the BRAT diet (bananas, rice, applesauce, toast). If patient develops constipation, teach preventive self-care (stool softener, flax seed oil, Milk of Magnesia, prunes, or prune juice every AM to ensure BM at least every other day). Teach patient to drink 2 quarts of fluid daily, drinking 1 glass an hour while awake to prevent dehydration. Teach patient to report dizziness, light-headedness, or fainting spells, and to avoid operating heavy machinery or driving a car if these occur. Develop symptom management plan with physician. Make referral to dietitian as appropriate. Teach diabetic patients to monitor their blood glucose closely, and discuss abnormalities and changes in their antidiabetic dose with their NP, PA, or physician.

IV.   ALTERATION IN OXYGENATION, POTENTIAL, related to HYPOTENSION

Defining Characteristics: Orthostatic hypotension/postural hypotension can affect up to 13% of patients throughout therapy.

Nursing Implications: Identify patients at risk: patients with history of syncope, dehydration, or taking medications associated with hypotension. Assess baseline cardiac status, including blood pressure and heart rate, noting rhythm and rate. Teach patient to prevent injury by gradual change in position, and to report any dizziness. Teach patients to avoid dehydration, especially in warm climates. If hypotension noted, assess patient tolerance and need for intervention; discuss management with physician. Manage orthostatic/postural hypotension with adjustment of antihypertensive doses (if patient is on them), hydration, and administration of mineralocorticoids and/or sympathomimetics.

V.   ALTERATION IN COMFORT related to ASTHENIA, PYREXIA, HEADACHE, INSOMNIA, EDEMA, DIZZINESS, RASH, MYALGIA, MUSCLE CRAMPS, BLURRED VISION

Defining Characteristics: Asthenia (characterized by fatigue, malaise, and weakness) was most common, affecting 65% of patients in clinical trials. Other symptoms included pyrexia (36%), headache (28%), insomnia (27%), arthralgias (26%), edema (26%), dyspnea (22%), dizziness (21%), myalgia (14%), pruritus (11%), and blurred vision (11%).

Nursing Implications: Assess comfort and presence of discomfort, fatigue, peripheral edema, baseline and prior to each treatment. Teach patient that these side effects may occur and to report them. Teach patient local comfort measures as well as energy conservation, and discuss management plan with physician if ineffective.

Drug: bosutinib (Bosulif)

Class: Tyrosine kinase inhibitor.

Mechanism of Action: Third-generation Bcr-Abl TKI. It inhibits many imatinib-resistant forms of Bcr-Abl. It also inhibits the Src family of kinases.

Metabolism: After oral dosing, peak concentration occurs in 4–6 hours. Taking the drug with a high-fat meal increases the C_{max} and AUC. Drug is highly protein bound (94%), and is a P-gp substrate and inhibitor in vitro. Primarily metabolized by the CYP3A4 microenzyme system to inactive metabolites, mean terminal elimination time (t1/2) is 22.5 hours. Primarily excreted in the feces (91.3%) and 3% in the urine. Hepatic impairment delays excretion with increases in C_{max} and AUC 1.9–2.3 fold, respectively.

Indication: Treatment of adult patients with chronic, accelerated, or blast phase Ph+ chronic myelogenous leukemia (CML) with resistance or intolerance to prior therapy.

Dosage/Range:
- 500 mg orally once daily with food, continued until disease progression or patient intolerance.
- Consider dose escalation to 600 mg once daily with food in patients who do not achieve a complete hematological remission by week 8 and or complete cytogenetic response by week 12 and do not have grade 3 or higher adverse reactions, and who are currently taking 500 mg daily.
- Hepatic impairment baseline (mild, moderate, severe): dose is 200 mg orally, daily with food, which approximates a similar AUC as 500-mg dose in patients without renal impairment.
- Preexisting severe renal impairment (CrCl < 30 mL/min): dose is 300 mg orally daily, with food, which approximates a similar AUC as 500-mg dose in patients without hepatic impairment.
- Dose-modify for toxicity:
  - Elevated transaminases (> 5 x institutional ULN): hold drug until recovery to ≤ = 2.5 x ULN and resume at 400 mg once daily thereafter. If recovery takes > 4 weeks, discontinue drug. If transaminase elevation ≥ 3 x ULN occurs with elevation in bilirubin greater than 2 x ULN and alkaline phosphatase is < 2 x ULN, discontinue drug. Diarrhea: grade 3–4 (≥ 7 stools/day over baseline); hold drug until recovery to grade ≤ 1; may resume at 400 mg once daily.
  - Other clinically significant, moderate, or severe nonhematologic toxicity, hold bosutinib until toxicity has resolved, then resume at 400 mg once daily. If clinically appropriate, consider re-escalating bosutinib dose to 500 mg once daily with food.

* Myelosuppression (ANC < 1,000 cells/mm^3 or platelets < 50,000 cells/mm^3): hold drug untilt ANC ≥ 1,000 cells/mm^3 AND platelets ≥ 50,000 cells/mm^3. Resume at same dose if recovery occurs within 2 weeks. If recovery occurs after 2 weeks, reduce dose by 100 mg and resume treatment. If cytopenia recurs, reduce dose again by 100 mg upon recovery and resume treatment. There is no data about doses < 300 mg/day.

Drug Preparation:
* Available in 100-mg and 500-mg tablets.

Drug Administration:
* Oral, daily as a single dose, with food.

Drug Interactions:
* Strong CYP3A4 inhibitors (boceprevir, clarithromycin, conivaptan, indinivair, itraconazole, ketoconazole, nefazodone, nelfinavir, posaconazole, ritonavir, saquinavir, telaprevir, telithromycin, voriconazole) and moderate CYP3A4 inhibitors (atazanavir, aprepitant, ciprofloxacin, crizotinib, darunavir, diltiazem, erythromycin, fluconazole, fosamprevir, grapefruit and grapefruit juice, imatinib, verapamil) increase bosutinib plasma concentrations; do not give concurrently.
* Strong CYP3A4 inducers (carbamazepine, dexamethasone, phenytoin, phenobarbital, rifabutin, rifampin) and moderate CYP3A4 inducers (bosetan, efavirenz, etravirine, modafinil, nafcillin) significantly decrease bosutinib plasma concentration; do not give concurrently.
* Proton Pump Inhibitors (PPIs) may decrease bosutinib serum levels. Avoid PPIs and consider using short-acting antacids instead.
* Substrates of p-glycoproteins (P-gp): Bosutinib may increase the plasma concentration of P-gp substrates, such as digoxin. Monitor patient closely for toxicity, and assess serum drug levels (e.g., digoxin).

Lab Effects/Interference:
* Decreased platelets, ANC, hemoglobin.
* Increased LFTs.
* Increased lipase, decreased phosphorus.

Special Considerations:
* Drug very rarely can cause hypersensitivity and anaphylaxis; then the drug is contraindicated.
* Monitor blood counts closely (e.g., CBC/differential, platelets) weekly for the first month, then monthly thereafter or as clinically indicated; LFTs baseline then monthly × 3 months, then as clinically indicated; if any of the transaminases is elevated, monitor LFTs more frequently.
    * Fluid retention may rarely occur and may be manifested as pericardial effusion, pleural effusion, pulmonary edema, and/or peripheral edema. The incidence of severe edema in clinical trials was 3%. Assess for, and interrupt, dose-reduce, or discontinue treatment and manage as necessary.

TREATMENT

- Counsel women of childbearing potential to avoid pregnancy, as drug is fetotoxic.
- Most common adverse events are diarrhea, nausea, thrombocytopenia, vomiting, abdominal pain, rash, anemia, pyrexia, and fatigue.

Potential Toxicities / Side Effects and the Nursing Process

I. POTENTIAL FOR INFECTION, BLEEDING, AND FATIGUE related to BONE MARROW DEPRESSION

Defining Characteristics: Thrombocytopenia affects 84% of patients (9% grade 3–4), anemia 33%, and neutropenia 16% of patients. Fatigue occurs in 26% of patients.

Nursing Implications: Assess CBC/differential, platelet count baseline, weekly for the first month, then monthly or more frequently as needed. Teach patient to report bleeding or signs/symptoms of bleeding right away. Teach patient to self-assess for signs/symptoms of infection, bleeding, or severe fatigue. Teach patient to avoid aspirin, NSAIDs, and aspirin-containing OTC medications. Teach patient strategies to manage fatigue and conserve energy.

II. ALTERATION IN NUTRITION, POTENTIAL, related to DIARRHEA, NAUSEA, VOMITING, ABDOMINAL PAIN, INCREASED LFTS

Defining Characteristics: Diarrhea is common, occurring in 82–84% of patients; nausea affects 46%, vomiting 37%, and abdominal pain 40%. The median time to diarrhea onset was 2 days, the median number of episodes was 3, and duration was 1 day. Decreased appetite affects 13%. Liver transaminases become elevated in 16–20% of patients.

Nursing Implications: Assess nutritional status baseline and at each visit. Teach patient that these side effects may occur, and teach self-management strategies such as antidiarrheals, antinausea medications, dietary modifications, and to report any symptoms that do not improve. Discuss prescription medication with provider to manage refractory symptoms. Teach patient tips to increase appetite (e.g., small, frequent meals, use of spices). Offer services of dietitian as appropriate. Assess and monitor LFTs baseline, then monthly × 3 months, then as clinically indicated. If transaminases become elevated, monitor LFTs more frequently.

III. ALTERATION IN COMFORT, related to PYREXIA, EDEMA, ASTHENIA, RASH, PRURITUS, HEADACHE

Defining Characteristics: Pyrexia occurred in 22%, edema in 14%, asthenia in 11%, rash in 34%, and pruritus in 11%. Rarely edema may be manifested as pericardial effusion, pleural effusion, pulmonary edema, and or peripheral edema (incidence of severe edema 3%). Headache occurs in 20% of patients.

Nursing Implications: Teach patient that these side effects may occur. Assess baseline skin integrity, weight, presence of peripheral edema, pulmonary and cardiac status. Teach patient to report fever, swelling of legs, face or other body parts, rash, itching, shortness of breath, or any changes. Assess reported symptoms and review with patient self-care management techniques. Teach patient to weigh self at least weekly, and to report increases in weight, as this may reflect edema (fluid gain). Teach patient to report right away any difficulty breathing (e.g., shortness of breath), chest pain, and discuss evaluation with physician, NP, or PA. If rash develops, assess for allergic reaction, and other accompanying symptoms. Monitor rash and teach patient strategies to prevent infection and promote healing.

Drug: brentuximab vedotin (Adcetris, SGN-35)

Class: Anti-CD30 antibody drug conjugate (ADC).

Mechanism of Action: Drug is a monoclonal antibody linked to a highly toxic antitubulin chemotherapy drug, monomethyl auristatin E (MMAE), which targets lymphoma cells expressing CD30, such as Hodgkin and anaplastic large-cell lymphomas. When the monoclonal antibody attaches to the CD30-expressing lymphocytes, it is taken inside the cell and releases the chemotherapy drug, killing the cell.

Metabolism: Maximum drug concentrations are reached at the end of the infusion, and the drug has a terminal half-life of 4–6 days. Steady state is reached in 21 days with every 3-week dosing. Only a small fraction of the released MMAE is metabolized via oxidation by CYP3A4/5 microenzyme system in the liver. Approximately 24% of the total MMAE administered is recoverable from the urine and feces (72%) over 1 week, and MMAE was largely unchanged.

Indication: Drug is FDA-indicated for the treatment of patients with
- Classical Hodgkin lympoma after failure of autologous stem cell transplant (ASCT).
- Classical Hodgkin lymphoma who are not ASCT candidates, after failure of at least 2 prior multiagent chemotherapy regimens.
- Classical Hodgkin lymphoma at risk of relapse or progression as post-auto-HSCT consolidation
- Systemic anaplastic large-cell lymphoma after failure of at least one prior multiagent chemotherapy regimen.
- Indications are based on response rate, and no data are available to show improvements in patient outcome or survival.
- Contraindications: concomitant use of brentuximab vedotin with bleomycin due to pulmonary toxicity.

Dosage/Range:
- 1.8 mg/kg as an intravenous infusion over 30 minutes every 3 weeks. Continue treatment until a maximum of 16 cycles, disease progression, or unacceptable toxicity.
- Dose for patients weighing over 100 kg should be based on a weight of 100 kg.

- Recommended starting dose for patients with mild to moderate renal impairment or mild (Child-Pugh A) hepatic impairment is 1.2 mg/kg. Avoid use in patients with severe renal impairment (CrCl < 30 mL/min), and patients with moderate or severe hepatic impairment (Child-Pugh B or C).
- Continue treatment until disease progression or unacceptable toxicity.

Dose Modifications:
- Peripheral Neuropathy (PN) using dose delay and reduction:
  - For new or worsening grade 2 or 3 PN, hold drug until PN improves to grade 1 or baseline, and then restart at 1.2 mg/kg.
  - For grade 4 PN, discontinue drug.
- Neutropenia: grade 3–4: hold drug until resolution to baseline or grade 2 or lower.
  - Consider growth factor (G-CSF) support for subsequent cycles.
  - For patients with recurrent grade 4 neutropenia despite G-CSF, discontinue drug or dose-reduce to 1.2 mg/kg.

Drug Preparation:
- Available in a 50-mg single-use vial. Calculate drug amount for patients weighing > 100 kg as 100 kg.
- Reconstitute each 50-mg vial with 10.5-mL sterile water for injection USP, to yield a single-use solution containing 5 mg/mL brentuximab vedotin.
- Gently swirl the vial to dissolve, and do not shake. Inspect solution for particulates and discoloration. Drug should be clear to slightly opalescent, colorless, and free of visible particulates.
- Following reconstitution, withdraw the ordered dose from the vial, and immediately add to an infusion bag containing a minimum of 100 mL to achieve a final concentration of 0.4 mg/mL to 1.8 mg/mL, OR store the solution at 2–8°C (36–46°F). DO NOT FREEZE. Discard any unused portion left in the vial.
- Intravenous solutions that can be used are 0.9% sodium chloride injection, 5% dextrose injection, or Lactated Ringer's injection. Gently invert the bag to mix. Do not shake.
- If the diluted infusion bag is not used immediately, store the solution at 2–8°C (36–46°F) and use within 24 hours of reconstitution. Do not freeze.

Drug Administration:
- Administer IV over 30 minutes every 3 weeks. Do not give IVP or IV bolus. Do not mix with or administer as an infusion with other medicines.
- If an infusion reaction occurs (incidence 12%), interrupt the infusion, keep IV patent with a plain solution not containing the drug, and provide appropriate medical management as ordered.
  - Most common signs/symptoms were chills, nausea, dyspnea, itching, fever, cough.
  - If a patient has had a prior infusion reaction, obtain order for premedications (acetaminophen, antihistamine, corticosteroid).
  - If anaphylaxis occurs, drug should be discontinued immediately.

Drug Interactions:
• Drug is a substrate and an inhibitor of CYP3A4/5.
• Effect of other drugs on brentuximab vedotin:
  • CYP3A4 inhibitors (e.g., ketoconazole): increased exposure to MMAE (e.g., ketoconazole, 34%): monitor patient closely for brentuximab vedotin toxicity;
  • CYP3A4 inducers (e.g., rifampin): potential reduced MMAE exposure (e.g., rifampin, 46%): do not use concurrently.
  • P-glycoprotein (P-gp) inhibitors: monitor closely for adverse reactions.
• Effect of brentuximab vedotin on other drugs: no alteration on other drugs.
• Bleomycin: severe pulmonary toxicity; DO NOT administer concurrently.

Lab Effects/Interference:
• Neutropenia, anemia, thrombocytopenia.

Special Considerations:
• MMAE exposure is increased in patients with moderate to severe hepatic impairment and severe renal impairment.
• Severe cases of hepatotoxicity have occurred, often associated with increased transaminases and/or bilirubin, after the first dose of brentuximab or upon drug rechallenge. Patients with preexisting liver disease, elevated baseline liver enzymes, or taking concomitant hepatotoxic drugs are at increased risk. Monitor liver transaminases and bilirubin, and interrupt/delay, change dose, or discontinue the drug if patient experiences new, worsening, or recurrent hepatotoxicity.
• Drug causes a predominantly sensory peripheral neuropathy (PN), although motor PN has been reported.
  • PN is cumulative, and across clinical trials, 54% of patients experienced any grade PN. Of these, 49% had complete resolution, 31% had partial improvement, and 20% had no improvement.
  • Monitor patients for PN symptoms (hypoesthesia, hyperesthesia, paresthesia, discomfort, a burning sensation, neuropathic pain, or weakness). If patients have new or worsening PN, discuss dose delay, modification, or discontinuance with physician.
• Infusion reactions may occur, including anaphylaxis.
  • Monitor the patient during the infusion. If an infusion reaction occurs, stop the infusion immediately and institute appropriate medical support.
  • The patient should receive premedication (e.g., acetaminophen, corticosteroid, and an antihistamine) for subsequent drug infusions.
  • If anaphylaxis occurs, drug should be permanently discontinued.
• Hematologic toxicities: Grade 3–4 anemia, thrombocytopenia, and prolonged (≥ 1 week) severe neutropenia can occur, as can febrile neutropenia.
  • Monitor CBC/differential prior to each dose, and more frequently for patients with grade 3–4 neutropenia.
  • Monitor patients closely for fever.
  • If grade 3–4 neutropenia develops, manage by G-CSF support, dose delays, reductions, or discontinuation.
• Serious infections and opportunistic infections: Pneumonia, bacteremia, and sepsis/septic shock have been reported, and some cases were fatal. Closely monitor patients for the

emergence of bacterial, fungal, or viral infections during treatment with brentuximab vedotin.

- Tumor Lysis Syndrome (TLS) may occur in patients with rapidly proliferating tumor or with high tumor burden. Discuss with physician measures to prevent TLS (e.g., prehydration, allopurinol) and monitor patient closely.
- Stevens-Johnson syndrome and toxic epidermal necrolysis (TEN) have been reported. If this happens, drug should be permanently discontinued, and the patient given appropriate medical therapy.
- Progressive multifocal leukoencephalopathy (PML) has been reported related to JC virus infection. Fatalities have occurred. Immunosuppressive risk factors may include prior therapies and underlying disease.
  - Consider PML in patients who present with new-onset signs/symptoms of central nervous system abnormalities.
  - Evaluation usually includes neurology consult, brain MRI, lumbar puncture, or brain biopsy.
  - Hold brentuximab vedotin If PML is suspected, and discontinue drug if the diagnosis is confirmed.
- Non-infectious pulmonary toxicity including pneumonitis, interstitial lung disease, and ARDS have occurred. Monitor patients closely for signs and symptoms, such as dyspnea and cough. Hold drug if new or worsening pulmonary symptoms occur, so that patient can be fully evaluated, and do not resume drug until symptoms improve.
- Drug is embryotoxic. Women of childbearing age should use effective contraception to avoid pregnancy. If a mother becomes pregnant during therapy, or the drug is used during pregnancy, the patient should be apprised of the potential hazard to the fetus.
- Nursing mothers: A decision should be made whether to discontinue nursing or to discontinue the drug, taking into account the importance of the drug to the mother's health.
- Most common side effects (> 20%) are neutropenia, peripheral sensory, neuropathy, fatigue, nausea, anemia, URI, diarrhea, pyrexia, rash, thrombocytopenia, cough, and vomiting.

Potential Toxicities/Side Effects and the Nursing Process

I.   POTENTIAL FOR INFECTION AND BLEEDING related to BONE MARROW DEPRESSION

Defining Characteristics: Neutropenia occurred in 54% of patients, with 15% experiencing grade 3 and 6% grade 4. 28% developed thrombocytopenia, with 7% grade 3 and 2% grade 4. Anemia affected 33% of patients.

Nursing Implications: Assess baseline CBC, including WBC, differential, and platelet count prior to dosing, as well as patient report of fever, chills, signs of infection, or bleeding. Discuss dose interruption and reduction for neutropenia or thrombocytopenia. Discuss use of growth factor support to reduce risk of neutropenia with subsequent cycles of therapy. Teach patient self-assessment of signs/symptoms of infection and bleeding (including epistaxis and development of petechiae), and instruct patient to report them right away. Teach patient self-care measures to minimize risk of infection and bleeding, including avoidance of OTC aspirin-containing medications. See section for fatigue management, which may be accentuated by anemia.

II.   POTENTIAL SENSORY/PERCEPTUAL ALTERATIONS related to SENSORY PERIPHERAL NEUROPATHY (PN)

Defining Characteristics: Drug-induced PN is predominantly sensory, but motor PN has been reported. 54% of patients on clinical trials developed any grade PN. PN is cumulative, but reversible in about half of patients (49% had complete resolution, 31% partial improvement, and 20% no improvement).

Nursing Implications: Teach patient to report new onset or worsening of PN symptoms (paresthesias, dysesthesias, hypoesthesias, discomfort, burning sensation, neuropathic pain or weakness), any changes in sensory function (temperature sensation, knowing where body parts are in relation to the whole, etc.), functional ability (e.g., especially senses of smell and taste), and ability to carry out activities of daily living (ADLs). Assess presence, extent, and severity of symptom(s), and progression over time. PN begins in fingers and toes and progresses in a stocking-glove distribution. Assess for potential for injury. If patient develops new or worsening PN, discuss with physician need for treatment delay, change in dose, or drug discontinuance. Teach patient self-care strategies to assure safety and minimize discomfort and function.

III.   ALTERATION IN NUTRITION, LESS THAN BODY REQUIREMENTS, related to NAUSEA, VOMITING, DIARRHEA

Defining Characteristics: These alterations in GI function have been reported in clinical studies: nausea 42% of patients, diarrhea 36%, vomiting 22%, and constipation 16%.

Nursing Implications: Assess baseline weight and nutritional status. Teach patient that these effects may occur and to report symptoms if uncontrolled by self-care measures or per protocol. Teach patient self-administration of antinausea medication, as well as dietary modifications for nausea, vomiting, diarrhea, and constipation as appropriate (e.g., small feedings with low-fat or nonspicy foods, BRAT diet: bananas, rice, applesauce, and toast). Assess efficacy of intervention, and revise plan as needed.

IV.   ALTERATION IN COMFORT related to FATIGUE

Defining Characteristics: Asthenia (characterized by fatigue, malaise, and weakness) was common. Fatigue was reported by 49% of patients.

Nursing Implications: Assess comfort and presence of discomfort and fatigue, baseline and at each visit. Teach patient that these side effects may occur and to report them. Teach patient local comfort measures, as well as energy conservation, and discuss management plan with physician if ineffective.

Drug: cabozantinib (Cometriq)

Class: Tyrosine kinase inhibitor of MET and VEGFR2.

Mechanism of Action: Cabozantinib is a dual tyrosine kinase inhibitor of MET (stimulated by the ligand, hepatocyte growth factor, or HGF, called scatter factor), and vascular endothelial growth factor receptor 2 (VEGFR2). It also inhibits the tyrosine kinases of RET, VEGFR1, VEGFR3, KIT, TRKB, FLT-3, AXL, and TIE-2, which are involved in normal as well as cancer processes of oncogenesis, metastasis, angiogenesis, and tumor microenvironment maintenance. MET is expressed on tumor cells, endothelial cells, and on bone cells. MET is upregulated in a number of cancers (thyroid, prostate, ovarian, and breast). Stimulation of the MET receptor by its ligand hepatocyte growth factor (HGF, scatter factor) facilitates certain cancer cells becoming more aggressive, more invasive, making more blood vessels, and escaping from the initial tumor to invade and metastasize. When some cancer therapies are used to kill the majority of cancer cells in a tumor, it is believed that stimulation of the MET-signaling pathway occurs as an escape route—certain cells become more aggressive (aggressive phenotype) and escape via their new invasive and metastatic qualities. Binding of VEGF to VEGFR2 leads to endothelial cell proliferation, migration, and the formation of blood vessels that nourish the tumor and facilitate tumor embolization. When this is blocked, reduced tumor oxygenation causes increased levels of waste products, creating hypoxia. Hypoxia further upregulates MET. In some studies, use of a VEGF or VEGFR inhibitor alone can result in tumors becoming more aggressive and invasive, as MET becomes upregulated. In the laboratory, cabozantinib is a potent antiangiogenic and antitumor drug, which also reduces tumor invasiveness and metastases. The drug was designed to block MET and VEGFR2, as well to block MET-driven tumor escape. It increases tumor apoptosis, decreases tumor and endothelial cell proliferation, decreases tumor cell invasiveness and metastases; in addition, it causes a blockade of metastatic bone lesion progression and disrupts tumor vasculature.

Metabolism: Drug half-life is approximately 55 hours after consecutive oral dosing. Median time to peak plasma concentrations (T_{max}) is 2–5 hours after dosing. A high-fat meal increases C_{max} and AUC by 41% and 57% respectively. Drug is a substrate of CYP3A4 in vitro. Drug is excreted in the feces (54%) and urine (27%).

Indication: Treatment of patients with progressive, metastatic medullary thyroid cancer.

Dosage/Range:
- 140 mg (one 80-mg and three 20-mg capsules) orally once daily on an empty stomach (no food at least 2 hours before and for at least 1 hour after taking the drug).
- Drug is not recommended for use in patients with moderate and severe hepatic impairment.

Dose Reductions:
- Hold drug for NCI CTCAE grade 4 hematologic adverse reactions, grade 3 or greater non-hematologic adverse reactions, or intolerable grade 2 adverse reactions. Upon resolution/improvement of adverse reaction (baseline or grade 1) reduce dose as follows:
  - If previously taking 140-mg daily dose, resume at 100 mg daily (one 80-mg and one 20-mg capsule).

* If previously taking 100 mg daily, resume treatment at 60 mg daily (three 20-mg capsules).
* If previously taking 60 mg daily, resume at 60 mg if tolerated; otherwise, discontinue drug.
* Permanently discontinue the drug for
  * Development of visceral perforation or fistula formation.
  * Severe hemorrhage.
  * Serious arterial thromboembolic event (e.g., MI, cerebral infarction).
  * Nephrotic syndrome.
  * Malignant hypertension, hypertensive crisis, persistent uncontrolled hypertension despite optimal medical management.
  * Osteonecrosis of the jaw.
  * Reversible posterior leukoencephalopathy syndrome.
* Patients taking strong CYP3A4 inhbitors:
  * Decrease daily dose by 40 mg (e.g., from 140 mg to 100 mg, from 100 mg to 60 mg daily).
  * After the interacting drug is discontinued, resume the dose that was used prior to initiating the CYP3A4 inhibitor 2–3 days after discontinuing the strong inhibitor.
* Patients taking strong CYP3A4 inducers:
  * Increase daily dose by 40 mg (e.g., from 140 mg to 180 mg, or from 100 mg to 140 mg daily) as tolerated.
  * Once the CYP3A4 inducer is discontinued, resume the dose that was used prior to initiating the CYP3A4 inducer 2–3 days after discontinuing that drug.

Drug Preparation/Administration:
* Available in 20-mg and 80-mg capsules.
* Teach patient to take capsules on an empty stomach (no food at least 2 hours before and for at least 1 hour after taking the drug).
* Teach patient to take drug whole, not to open capsules, and not to take a missed dose within 12 hours of the next dose. Instruct patient not to drink grapefruit juice, eat grapefruit, or take St. John's wort while taking this drug.
* Stop drug at least 28 days before scheduled surgery; resume drug after surgery based on clinical judgment of adequate wound healing.

Drug Interactions: Cabozantinib is a CYP3A4 substrate.
* CYP3A4 inhibitors (strong) (e.g., atazanavir, clarithromycin, indinavir, itraconazole, ketoconazole, nelfinavir, nefazodone, saquinavir, telithromycin, ritonavir, voriconazole, grapefruit, and grapefruit juice): increase cabozantinib serum levels; do not take concomitantly.
* CYP3A4 (strong) inducers, chronic exposure (e.g., carbamazepine, phenytoin, phenobarbital, rifabutin, rifampin, rifapentine, St. John's wort): decrease cabozantinib serum levels; do not take concomitantly.

Laboratory Effects/Interference (Incidence %):
* Increased AST (86%), ALT (86%), alkaline phosphatase (52%), bilirubin (25%).
* Lymphopenia (53%), neutropenia (35%), thrombocytopenia (35%).

TREATMENT

- Hypocalcemia (52%), hypophosphatemia (28%), hypomagnesemia (19%), hypokalemia (18%), hyponatremia (10%).
- Proteinuria (2%).

Special Considerations:
- Most common side effects are diarrhea, stomatitis, palmar–plantar erythrodysesthesia syndrome (PPES), decreased weight, decreased appetite, nausea, fatigue, oral pain, hair color changes, dysgeusia, hypertension, abdominal pain, constipation.
- Most common grade 3–4 side effects are fatigue (9%), hand-foot syndrome (13%), HTN (8%).
- Thrombotic events occurred at a higher incidence in cabozantinib-treated patients compared to control: venous thromboembolism (VTE): 6% vs 3%, and arterial thromboembolism (ATE) 2% vs 0%. Discontinue drug for MI, cerebral infarction, or other serious arterial thromboembolic events.
- Perforations and fistulas: GI perforation occurred in 3% of patients, and fistula formation in 1%. Non-GI fistulas occurred in 4% (e.g., tracheal/esophageal). Monitor patients for symptoms of perforations and fistulas. Discontinue drug if perforation or fistula occurs.
- Hemorrhage: severe, sometimes fatal, hemorrhage has occurred, including hemoptysis and GI hemorrhage. Incidence was 3%. Drug should not be given to patients with a recent history of hemorrhage or hemoptysis. Teach patient to report bleeding and how to manage nosebleeds. Monitor for signs and symptoms of bleeding, and stop drug if patient has severe hemorrhage.
- Wound complications: Stop drug at least 28 days before scheduled surgery; resume drug after surgery based on clinical judgment of adequate wound healing. Hold drug for dehiscence or complications requiring medical intervention.
- Hypertension: Stage 1 or 2 HTN (modified JNC criteria) occurred in 61% of patients. Monitor BP baseline prior to initiation of drug and regularly during treatment. Hold drug for HTN that is not adequately controlled with medical management; resume drug at a reduced dose when BP controlled. Discontinue drug for hypertensive crisis.
- Osteonecrosis of the jaw (ONJ) occurred in 1% of patients.
  - Manifested as jaw pain, osteomyelitis, osteitis, bone erosion, tooth or periodontal infection, toothache, gingival ulceration or erosion, persistent jaw pain or slow healing of the mouth or jaw after dental surgery.
  - Patient should have oral exam prior to starting drug, and periodically during treatment.
  - Teach patient good oral hygiene; if patient wants to have invasive dental procedures, drug should be stopped for at least 28 days prior to scheduled surgery.
  - If ONJ occurs, discontinue drug.
- Palmar–plantar erythrodysesthesia syndrome (PPES): Occurs in 50% of patients and was severe (≥ grade 3) in 13% of patients. Hold drug in patients who develop intolerable grade 2 PPES or grade 3–4 PPES until improvement to grade 1; resume drug at a reduced dose.
- Proteinuria was observed in 2% of patients: monitor urine protein regularly. Discontinue drug for nephrotic syndrome.
- Reversible leukoencephalopathy syndrome (RPLS): Occurred rarely (< 1%); evaluate patient for RPLS if presenting with seizures, headache, visual disturbances, confusion, or altered mental function. Discontinue drug if patient develops RPLS.

- Embryo-fetal toxicity: can cause fetal harm. Counsel women of childbearing potential to use effective contraception to prevent pregnancy. If drug is used during pregnancy, or if the patient becomes pregnant while taking the drug, patient should be apprised of the potential hazard to the fetus.
- Nursing mothers: a decision should be made whether to discontinue nursing or to discontinue the drug, taking into acocunt the importance of the drug to the mother's health.

Potential Toxicities/Side Effects and the Nursing Process

I. ALTERATION IN NUTRITION, POTENTIAL, LESS THAN BODY REQUIREMENTS, related to DIARRHEA, STOMATITIS, NAUSEA, VOMITING, DYSPHAGIA

Defining Characteristics: Nutritional impact symptoms are diarrhea (63%), stomatitis (51%), decreased appetite (46%), nausea (43%), oral pain (36%), dysgeusia (34%), constipation (27%), abdominal pain (27%), vomiting (24%), dysphagia ((13%), dyspepsia (11%), and weight loss in 48% of patients.

Nursing Implications: Assess baseline nutritional status and bowel elimination status. If patient develops nausea and/or vomiting, teach patient to self-administer antiemetics 1 hour prior to each dose, and to call if nausea/vomiting persist. Discuss with physician more effective antiemetic regimen if nausea/vomiting persist. Encourage small, frequent intake of cool, bland foods as tolerated if nausea develops. Refer to dietitian as needed for meal planning. Teach patient to report diarrhea that does not respond to OTC antidiarrheal medication, or if constipation occurs that is unresponsive to fluids, laxatives, and use of high-fiber foods. Teach self-care measures of diet modification and increased oral fluids to 2–3 L during the waking hours. If constipation occurs, teach patient self-care measures to prevent constipation. Monitor weight at each visit, and review nutritional impact symptoms with patient and caregiver that does cooking; assess need for referral to dietitian.

II. POTENTIAL ALTERATION IN CIRCULATION related to HTN

Defining Characteristics: Almost all patients developed elevated blood pressure. Overt HTN (stage I [systolic BP $\geq$ 140 mmHg or diastolic $\geq$ 90 mmHg] or II [systolic $\geq$ 160 mmHg or diastolic $\geq$ 100 mmHg]) occurred in 61% of patients in clinical trials, consistent with class effects of a VEGF inhibitor. Proteinuria occurred in 2% of patients.

Nursing Implications: Assess baseline circulation, including BP baseline and regularly during treatment. Discuss abnormalities with physician or mid-level practitioner. Hold drug if HTN not well controlled, and when well controlled, resume drug at a reduced dose. Drug should be discontinued for severe hypertension that cannot be controlled with antihypertensive therapy. Monitor urine for protein baseline and regularly during treatment. Discontinue drug if nephrotic syndrome occurs.

III. POTENTIAL ALTERATION IN SKIN INTEGRITY/COMFORT related to HAND-FOOT SYNDROME, HAIR CHANGES

Defining Characteristics: Hand–foot syndrome (Palmar-plantar erythrodysesthesia syndrome, PPES) has been described in 50% of patients studied, characterized by redness, swelling, and pain on palms of hands and soles of feet. It was severe (grades 3 or 4) in 13% of patients. Hair color changes (depigmentation, graying) occurred in 34% of patients.

Nursing Implications: Teach patient that this may occur, and to report it. Assess at each visit palms of hands, soles of feet, and any areas of constant pressure. Teach patient to keep skin areas well moisturized, and to avoid activities that cause pressure such as jogging, repeated use of palms of hands (e.g., chopping of vegetables for a long period), and activities that expose the skin of these body parts with heat (e.g., hot tub). Hold drug in patients who develop intolerable grade 2 PPES or grade 3–4 PPES until improvement to grade 1; resume drug at a reduced dose.

IV. ALTERATION IN COMFORT related to FATIGUE, ARTHRALGIAS, SENSORY SYMPTOMS

Defining Characteristics: Fatigue affected 41% of patients in clinical trials, and asthenia 21% (characterized by fatigue, malaise, and weakness). Arthralgias affected 14%, muscle spasms 12%, and musculoskeletal chest pain 9%. Sensory symptoms included headache (18%), dizziness (14%), paresthesia (7%), peripheral sensory neuropathy (7%).

Nursing Implications: Assess comfort and presence of discomfort and fatigue, baseline and at each visit. Teach patient that these side effects may occur and to report them. Teach patient local comfort measures, as well as energy conservation, and discuss management plan with physician if ineffective.

Drug: carfilzomib (Kyprolis, PR-171)

Class: Proteasome inhibitor, second generation.

Mechanism of Action: Carfilzomib is a selective proteasome inhibitor. The proteasome system is a critical system that degrades and recycles proteins, which effectively turn on and off key cell functions, such as the cell cycle and cell signaling. Carfilzomib binds irreversibly to, and inhibits the chymotrypsin-like activity of, the 20S proteasome, an enzyme responsible for degrading many cellular proteins. This results in polyubiquinated proteins accumulating, which is thought to lead to cell cycle arrest, apoptosis, and inhibition of tumor growth. In lab tests, carfilzomib appeared more potent than bortezomib, and demonstrated activity against multiple myeloma cells resistant to bortezomib. Carfilzomib demonstrates synergy when given with dexamethasone to enhance cell death (Kuhn et al., 2007).

Metabolism: Drug absorption is pH dependent. Drug is rapidly and extensively metabolized, probably via peptidase cleavage and hydrolysis. Half-life of drug is ≤ 1 hour on cycle 1 day 1. Elimination is believed to be extrahepatic, but the exact routes are unknown.

Indication: Treatment of patients with multiple myeloma: (1) in combination with lenalidomide and dexamethasone in patients who have relapsed after 1–3 prior therapies, and (2) as a single agent in patients who have receied at least 2 prior therapies including bortezomib and an immunomodulatory agent and have progressed on or within 60 days of completion of last therapy.

Dosage/Range:

* A cycle is 28 days in length, with drug given IV on two consecutive days each week for three weeks (days 1, 2, 8, 9, 15, and 16), followed by a 2-week rest period (days 17–28).
* Cycle 1 dose is 20 mg/m^2/day IV on days 1 and 2, and if well tolerated, escalate dose to a target dose of 27 mg/m^2/day on Day 8 of Cycle 1.
* Maximum BSA is 2.2 m^2. Do not adjust BSA for changes in weight ≤ 20%. Premedicate with 4 mg oral or IV dexamethasone prior to cycle 1 doses, during the first week of dose escalation, and if infusion reactions develop or reappear. Treatment may be continued until disease progression or unacceptable toxicity occurs.
* If patient is on dialysis, administer drug after the dialysis procedure.
* Modify dose based on toxicity (grade 3–4 neutropenia, grade 4 thrombocytopenia, cardiac toxicity, pulmonary hypertension, pulmonary complications, hepatotoxicity, renal toxicity, peripheral neuropathy, other toxicity). See package insert.

Preparation/Administration:

* Drug is available in a single-use vial, as 60-mg lypholyzed powder, and is refrigerated at 2°–8°C, or 36°–46°F.
  * Aseptically reconstitute each vial with 29-mL sterile water slowly injected onto the inside of the vial wall to reduce foaming. Gently swirl or invert the vial slowly for about 1 minute, until powder is completely diluted.
  * Do not shake. If foam forms, allow vial to sit for 2–5 minutes until gone. Solution should be colorless, and if not, do not use.
  * The final solution is 2 mg/mL.
  * Draw up the calculated dose. The quantity of carfilozomib contained in one single-use vial may exceed the required dose; carefully calculate and withdraw the correct ordered dose. If administering via IV bag, aseptically add to a 50-mL 5% dextrose injection USP IV bag. Discard any remaining drug in the vial.
  * Reconstituted drug is stable, refrigerated (2°–8°C, or 36°–46°F) for 24 hours in the vial, syringe, or IV bag (5% Dextrose injection, USP). Total time from reconstitution to administration should not exceed 24 hours. Vial, syringe, and IV bag are stable for 4 hours at room temperature (15°–30°C or 59°–86°F).
* Hydrate patient prior to and following each dose with 250–500 mL IV normal saline, or appropriate solution, to reduce the risk of tumor lysis syndrome and renal toxicity.
  * Monitor blood chemistries closely.
  * Monitor patients for fluid overload.

- Premedicate with 4 mg oral or IV dexamethasone prior to all cycle 1 doses, during the first week of dose escalation, and if infusion reactions develop or reappear.
- Administer IV as a 10 minute infusion on two consecutive days each week for three weeks (Days 1, 2, 8, 9, 15, 16), followed by a 12-day rest period (Days 17–28).
  - Do not administer as a bolus. Flush IV line with normal saline or 5% Dextrose USP immediately before and after drug is administered. Do not mix with, or administer as an infusion with, any other medicines.
  - Monitor patient during hydration for signs/symptoms of fluid overload.

Drug Interactions:
- Dexamethasone: synergy, used in combination in multiple myeloma.

Lab Effects/Interference:
- Decreased WBC (neutropenia 21%), RBC (47%), platelets (36%). Platelet nadir day 8 with recovery by day 28.
- Increased LFTs (AST, ALT, bilirubin), increased creatinine (24%).
- Hypokalemia (13%), hypomagnesemia (13%), hyperglycemia (12%), hypercalcemia (11%), hypophosphatemia (11%), hyponatremia (10%).

Special Considerations:
- Drug causes less peripheral neuropathy compared to bortezomib. Incidence of peripheral sensory and motor neuropathy was 14% with 1% grade 3.
- Cardiac arrest, CHF, myocardial ischemia: Heart failure and ischemia may occur and have resulted in sudden cardiac death within a day of treatment. New onset or worsened case of preexisting CHF with decreased left ventricular function or myocardial ischemia have occurred following drug administration. Cardiac failure events (e.g., CHF, pulmonary edema, decreased LVEF) were reported in 7% of clinical trial patients.
  - Monitor for cardiac complications and manage promptly.
  - Hold drug for grade 3–4 cardiac events until recovery, and consider whether to restart drug using a benefit/risk assessment.
  - Patients with New York Heart Association Class III and IV failure, MI in the preceding 6 months, or uncontrolled conduction abnormalities were not studied in clinical trials and may likely be at increased risk.
- Pulmonary arterial hypertension (PAH) has been reported in 2% of treated patients.
  - Stop drug and evaluate with cardiac imaging or other tests if signs/symptoms occur.
  - When PAH has resolved or returned to baseline, drug should be resumed only if benefit outweighs risk.
- Pulmonary complications occurred in 35% of patients on clinical trials receiving the drug; grade 3 dyspnea occurred in 5% of patients. ARDS, acute respiratory failure, and acute diffuse infiltrative pulmonary disease have occurred. Monitor and manage severe or life-threatening dyspnea immediately, and interrupt drug, until resolved or returned to baseline. See dose modifications.

- Infusion reactions, characterized by fever, chills, arthralgias, myalgia, facial flushing facial edema, vomiting, weakness, shortness of breath, hypotension, syncope, chest tightness or angina, may occur immediately following or up to 24 hours after drug administration.
  - Dexamethasone usually reduces the incidence.
  - Teach the patient to report signs/symptoms immediately during or after treatment and to seek emergency medical care if at home and symptoms are severe.
- Tumor lysis syndrome may occur in < 1% of patients, and patients with MM and a high tumor burden are at greater risk. Administer hydration prior to and after drug administration to prevent this. Encourage patients to remain well-hydrated at home, and before coming in for treatment. Monitor for signs/symptoms of TLS during treatment, and manage promptly. Interrupt drug until TLS is resolved. Discuss with physician or NP/PA other meaures to minimize risk of TLS in high-risk patients prior to initial drug administration.
- Acute renal failure: monitor serum creatinine regularly.
- Thrombocytopenia may occur. Nadir is day 8, with recovery by day 28 of each cycle. Incidence is 36%, with 10% grade 4. Monitor platelet count closely, and hold/modify dose as appropriate. See dose modifications.
- Hepatic toxicity: monitor LFTs (AST, ALT, bilirubin) baseline and frequently during therapy, as hepatic failure may occur. Hold drug for grade 3 or greater elevations of transaminases, bilirubin, or other abnormalities, until resolved or returned to baseline.
- Hypertensive crisis: Monitor BP regularly. If HT cannot be controlled, a risk-benefit decision should be made.
- Venous thrombosis: thromboprophylaxis is recommended.
- Thrombotic thrombocytopenic purpura/hemolytic uremic syndrome (TTP/HUS): Monitor for signs and symptoms of TTP/HUS. Discontinue drug if suspected.
- Posterior reversible encephalopathy syndrome (PRES): Consider MRI for onset of visual or neurological symptoms and discontinue drug if PRES is suspected.
- Drug is fetotoxic. Women of reproductive potential should use effective contraception to avoid pregnancy. If carfilzomib is used during pregnancy, or if the patient becomes pregnant while taking the drug, the patient should be apprised of the potential hazard to the fetus.
- Nursing mothers: a decision should be made whether to discontinue nursing or to discontinue the drug, taking into account the importance of the drug to the mother's health.
- Most common side effects (> 30%) are fatigue, anemia, nausea, thrombocytopenia, dyspnea, diarrhea, and pyrexia.
- Herpes zoster was reactivated in 2% of patients. Consider antiviral prophylaxis in patients with a history of herpes zoster infection.

Potential Toxicities/Side Effects and the Nursing Process

I.   ALTERATION IN OXYGENATION related to DYSPNEA

Defining Characteristics: Dyspnea occurred in 35% of patients in clinical trials. Grade 3 dyspnea occurred in 5%. ARDS, acute respiratory failure, and acute diffuse infiltrative pulmonary disease have occurred.

Nursing Implications: Assess pulmonary status including breath sounds, baseline and prior to each treatment. Teach patient to report onset of or worsening of dyspnea, and have patient evaluated promptly. Drug should be interrupted for severe or life-threatening dyspnea, and the patient evaluated.

II.   ALTERATION IN COMFORT related to FATIGUE

Defining Characteristics: Asthenia is characterized by fatigue, malaise, and weakness. Fatigue occurred in more than half of patients.

Nursing Implications: Assess comfort and presence of discomfort and fatigue, baseline and at each visit. Teach patient that these side effects may occur and to report them. Teach patient local comfort measures, as well as energy conservation, and discuss management plan with physician if ineffective.

III.   ALTERATION IN NUTRITION, LESS THAN BODY REQUIREMENTS, related to NAUSEA, DIARRHEA, CONSTIPATION, HYPOKALEMIA

Defining Characteristics: Symptoms that interfere with adequate nutrition were common. Nausea occurred in 45% of patients, vomiting 22%, diarrhea 33%, constipation 21%, and anorexia 12%. In addition, abnormal lab values occurred (see lab abnormalities). Hepatic toxicity can occur, as evidenced by changes in LFTs.

Nursing Implications: Assess baseline weight and nutritional status, as well as bowel elimination status. Teach patient that these side effects may occur and to report symptoms if uncontrolled by self-care measures. Monitor serum electrolytes, including serum potassium, before each dose and replete as needed. Monitor LFTs baseline and periodically during treatment. Teach patient self-administration of antiemetic agent, as well as antidiarrheal or cathartic as appropriate. Teach patient dietary modifications for constipation, nausea, diarrhea (e.g., small feedings with low-fat or nonspicy foods, BRAT diet: bananas, rice, applesauce, and toast). Assess efficacy of intervention, and revise plan as needed.

Drug: ceritinib (Zykadia)

Class: Kinase inhibitor.

Mechanism of Action: Kinase inhibitor that targets ALK, insulin-like growth factor (IGF-1R), insulin receptor (InsR), and ROS1 (tyrosine kinase insulin receptor). Drug is most active against ALK receptor tyrosine kinase (RTK), inhibiting autophosphorylation of ALK, ALK-mediated phosphorylation of STAT (downstream signaling protein), and ALK-dependent cancer cell proliferation. Alterations in the ALK gene have been found in 3–5% of patients with NSCLC, neuroblastoma, and rare sarcomas. The abnormality is called EMLA-ALK (echinoderm microtubule-associated protein-like 4 anaplastic lymphoma kinase) fusion gene, and it makes a protein product that turns on signaling for the cell to proliferate. In mice, ceritinib showed dose-dependent anti-tumor activity against EMLA-ALK-positive NSCLC xenografts that were resistant to crizotinib. ROS1 is an RTK related to ALK, and ROS1 gene rearrangements are found in about 1–2% of patients with NSCLC (Gainor and Shaw, 2013).

Metabolism: After a single oral dose, peak plasma levels (C_{max}) occurred 4–6 hrs after the dose, and steady state with daily dosing, in about 15 days. Systemic exposure (AUC) increased when administered with a meal: AUC increased 73% (C_{max} by 41%) with a high-fat meal, and 58% with a low-fat meal (C_{max} by 43%), compared to the fasting state. It is estimated that a 600 mg or higher dose taken with a meal will approximate a dose of 750 mg of ceritinib taken in a fasting state. Drug is 97% bound to human plasma proteins. The mean plasma terminal half-life (t1/2) was 41 hours. The drug is primarily metabolized by the hepatic microsomal enzyme CYP3A4, and 92.3% is excreted in the feces (68% unchanged drug) and 1.3% in the urine. Ceritinib exposure is similar in patients with normal and mild hepatic impairment, but it has not been studied in patients with moderate or severe hepatic impairment. Ceritinib exposure is similar in patients with normal and mild-to-moderate renal dysfunction. Patients with severe renal impairment (CrCl < 30mL/min) were not studied. Drug is a substrate of the efflux transporter P-glycprotein (P-gp).

Indications: Ceritinib (Zykadia) is indicated for the treament of patients with anaplastic lymphoma kinase (ALK)-positive metastatic NSCLC who have progressed or are intolerant to crizotinib. Indication was approved as an accelerated approval based on tumor response rate and duration of response in Phase I clinical trials. Improvement in survival or disease-related symptoms has not been established.

- Drug was designed specifically for the ALK mutation, and patients had to meet this critieria in Phase I testing. Response rates for treatment naïve patients were 58% and 56% in patients who had tumor progression on crizotinib; an additional 20% of patients of both groups had stable disease. Median PFS for patients receiving $\geq$ 400 mg/m^2 per day exceeded 7 months (Shaw et al., 2014).
- 62% of patients beginning therapy at 750 mg/m^2 per day required a dose reduction, so this may not be the optimal dose (Chabner, 2014).

Dosage/Range:
- 750 mg orally once daily on an empty stomach (2 hours or longer after a meal), until disease progression or unacceptable toxicity.
- A recommended dose has not been determined for patients with moderate to severe hepatic impairment.

Dose Modifications:
- ALT or AST elevation > 5 × ULN with **total bilirubin elevation ≤ 2 × ULN**: hold ceritinib until recovery to baseline or ≤ 3 × ULN, then resume certinib with a 150-mg dose reduction.
- ALT or AST elevation > 3 × ULN with **total bilirubin elevation > 2 × ULN**: permanently discontinue ceritinib.
- Interstitial Lung Disease (ILD, any grade): permanently discontinue ceritinib.
- QTc > 500 msec on at least 2 separate ECGs: hold until QTc is < 481 msec, or recovery to baseline if baseline QTc ≥ 481 msec, then resume ceritinib with a 150-mg dose reduction.

- QTc interval prolongation in combination with torsades de pointes, polymorphic ventricular tachycardia, or signs/symptoms of serious arrhythmia: permanently discontinue ceritinib.
- Severe or intolerable nausea, vomiting, or diarrhea despite optimal antiemetic or anti-diarrheal therapy: hold until improved; then resume ceritinib with a 150-mg dose reduction.
- Persistent hyperglycemia > 250 mg/dL despite optimal antihyperglycemic therapy: hold until hyperglycemia is adequately controlled, then resume ceritinib with a 150-mg dose reduction. If adequate hyperglycemia control cannot be achieved with optimal medical management, discontinue ceritinib.
- Symptomatic bradycardia that is not life-threatening: hold until recovery to asymptomatic bradycardia or to a heart rate of 60 bpm or above, evaluate concomitant medications known to cause bradycardia, and adjust dose of ceritinib.
- Clinically significant bradycardia requiring intervention or life-threatening bradycardia in patients taking a concomitant medication also known to cause bradycardia or a medication known to cause hypotension: hold until recovery to asymptomatic bradycardia or to a heart rate of 60 bpm or above. If the concomitant medication can be adjusted, resume ceritinib with a 150-mg dose reduction, with frequent monitoring.
- Life-threatening bradycardia in patients who are not taking a concomitant medication also known to cause bradycardia or known to cause hypotension: permanently discontinue ceritinib.
- Avoid concurrent use of strong CYP3A4 inhibitors during ceritinib therapy; if unavoidable, reduce ceritinib dose by approximately one-third, rounded to the nearest 150-mg dose strength. After discontinuation of a strong CYP3A4 inhibitor, resume the ceritinib dose that was taken prior to initiating the strong CYP3A4 inhibitor.
- Discontinue ceritinib in patients who are unable to tolerate 300 mg daily.
- An improvement in survival or disease-related symptoms has not been established. Drug approved after Phase I trials. Continued approval for this indication may be contingent upon verification and description of clinical benefit in confirmatory trials.

Drug Preparation:
- Oral. Available in 150-mg hard gelatin capsules.

Drug Administration: Teach patient to:
- Take prescribed dose once a day on an empty stomach (e.g., do not administer within 2 hours of a meal).
- Avoid grapefruit and grapefruit juice during cediranib therapy.
- Make up a missed dose of ceritinib UNLESS the next dose is within 12 hrs, then the dose should be skipped.
- Keep medication away from children or pets.

Drug Interactions:
- CYP3A4 inhibitors (strong): increase the systemic exposure of ceritinib. Avoid coadministration with strong CYP3A4 inhibitors (e.g., some antiretrovirals like ritonavir, macrolide antibiotics like telithromycin, antifungals like ketoconazole, and nefazodone). If coadministration is unavoidable, reduce ceritinib dose by 33%, rounded to the nearest 150-mg dosage strength. In addition, avoid grapefruit and grapefruit juice, as these may inhibit CYP3A4.

* CYP3A inducers (strong): decrease systemic exposure of ceritinib. Avoid concurrent use (e.g., carbamazepine, phenytoin, rifampin, St. John's wort).
* Ceritinib may inhibit CYP3A4 and CYP2C9. Avoid concurrent use of CYP3A4 and CYP2C9 substrates, which have a narrow therapeutic window, or substrates primarily metabollizd by CYP3A4 (e.g., alfentanil, cyclosporine, dihydroergotamine, ergotamine, fentanyl, pimozide, quinidine, sirolimus, tacrolimus) and CYP2C9 (e.g., phenytoin, warfarin) during treatment with ceritinib. If they must be used concurrently with ceritinib, consider dose reduction of the drug.

Lab Effects/Interference:
* Decreased Hgb, phosphate.
* Increased ALT, AST, bilirubin (total).
* Increased creatinine, glucose, lipase.

Special Considerations:
* About 60% of patients who began therapy at the recommended dose required at least one dose reduction; median time to first dose reduction was 7 weeks.
* Warnings and precautions:
  * Severe or persistent GI toxicity: Dose modification due to diarrhea, nausea, vomiting, or abdominal pain occurred in 38% of patients. Hold drug if symptoms are not responsive to antiemetics or antidiarrheals, then dose-reduce.
  * Hepatotoxicity: Ceritinib can cause hepatotoxicity. Monitor LFTs baseline and at least monthly. Hold, then dose-reduce, or permanently discontinue for hepatotoxicity. Teach patient to report these symptoms right away: fatigue, yellowing of the skin or white of the eyes, decreased appetite, itchy skin, nausea/vomiting, pain on the right side of stomach area, or if the patient bruises more easily than normal.
  * ILD: Incidence 4%. Teach patients to report these symptoms right away: trouble breathing or SOB, fever, cough with or without mucus, chest pain. Permanently discontinue ceritinib in patients diagnosed with treatment-related ILD/pneumonitis.
  * QTc interval prolongation: Ceritinib can cause QTc interval prolongation. Monitor ECG and electrolytes in patients with CHF, bradyarrhythmias, electrolyte abnormalities, or those who are taking medications known to prolong the QTc interval. Hold drug, then dose-reduce, or permanently discontinue ceritinib.
  * Hyperglycemia: Ceritinib can cause hyperglycemia. Patients at increased risk are those with diabetes, glucose intolerance, or taking corticosteroids. Monitor glucose and initiate or optimize antihyperglycemic medications as indicated. Teach patients to report increased thirst, inceased frequency of urination, increased hunger, blurred vision, headaches, tiredness, trouble thinking or concentrating, or if breath has a fruity smell. Hold, then dose-reduce, or permanently discontinue drug.
  * Bradycardia: Ceritinib can cause bradycardia. Monitor heart rate and BP regularly. Teach patients to report right away the following symptoms: new chest pain or discomfort, dizziness or light-headedness, if you feel faint, or have abnormal heartbeats. Hold, then dose-reduce, or permanently discontinue drug.
  * Ceritinib may cause fetal harm. Teach female patients of reproductive potential about the potential risk to a fetus and to use an effective method of contraception,

both during ceritinib therapy and for at least 2 weeks after stopping the drug. Nursing mothers should decide whether to discontinue nursing or discontinue use of the drug.

- Most common adverse reactions (incidence ≥ 25%) are diarrhea, nausea, elevated transaminases, vomiting, abdominal pain, fatigue, decreased appetite, and constipation.

Potential Toxicities/Side Effects and the Nursing Process

I. ALTERATION IN NUTRITION, POTENTIAL, LESS THAN BODY REQUIREMENTS, related to DIARRHEA, NAUSEA, VOMITING, DECREASED APPETITE, CONSTIPATION, HYPERGLYCEMIA

Defining Characteristics: Diarrhea, nausea, vomiting, or abdominal pain occurred in 96% patients in clinical studies, and were severe in 14%. Diarrhea occurred in 86% (6% grade 3–4), nausea 80% (4% grade 3–4), vomiting 60% (4% grade 3–4), constipation 29%, decreased appetite 34%, and abdominal pain in 54% of patients. Dose modification was necessary for 38% of patients. Hyperglycemia occurred in 49%, with 13% grade 3–4. Risk increased in patients with diabetes, glucose intolerance, or taking corticosteroids.

Nursing Implications: Assess baseline nutritional status, labs including hyperglycemia, and bowel elimination status. Teach patient that these side effects can occur and to report them if they do not resolve. Teach patient to administer antidiarrheal medication if diarrhea occurs, and to report if it does not resolve within 24 hours. Teach patient to increase oral fluid intake and to modify diet (e.g., 5–6 small meals of foods high in soluble fiber (e.g., rice, noodles, bananas, well-cooked eggs) and low in insoluble fiber (e.g., raw fruit, whole grain breads, seeds). If patient develops nausea and/or vomiting, teach patient to self-administer antiemetics 1 hour prior to each dose and to call if nausea/vomiting persists. Discuss with physician more effective antiemetic regimen if nausea/vomiting is not improved. Encourage small, frequent intake of cool, bland foods as tolerated if nausea develops. Refer to dietitian as needed for meal planning. If constipation occurs, teach patient to increase fluid intake, self-administer laxatives, and to increase the intake of high-fiber foods. Monitor baseline and blood glucose level, and discuss with physician or NP/PA the need for antihyperglycemic medication. Discuss dose interruption and dose reduction depending upon severity of symptoms. See Dose Modifications.

II. POTENTIAL FOR ACTIVITY INTOLERANCE related to FATIGUE

Defining Characteristics: Fatigue occurred in 52% of patients and was grade 3–4 in 5%. Hemoglobin was decreased in 84% of patients (5% grade 3–4).

Nursing Implications: Assess baseline activity level, and Hgb. Teach patient that fatigue may occur, and may rarely be severe. Teach patient to alternate rest and activity and teach strategies to conserve energy. If fatigue is severe, discuss if family members can take over tasks that are energy-consuming, such as grocery shopping or cleaning the house. Monitor Hgb, and discuss with physician or NP/PA strategies to minimize the effect of decreased Hgb if it occurs. Teach patient to report worsening fatigue.

III.   SENSORY ALTERATIONS, POTENTIAL, related to PERIPHERAL NEUROPATHY, VISUAL CHANGES

Defining Characteristics: Neuropathy occurred in 23% of patients and ranged from grade 1, grade 2 motor neuropathy, to grade 3 peripheral neuropathy. Dizziness (24%) and dysgeusia (13%) were common, all grades 1 and 2. Headache occurred in 13% of patients.

Nursing Implications: Teach patient that these side effects may occur and to report them. Assess for the presence of neuropathy, comparing one side of the body to the others, focusing on the hands and feet, as peripheral neuropathy starts at the toes and fingertips (longest axons), and then moves in a stocking-glove distribution. Discuss any positive findings with physician or NP/PA for a more focused neurological exam.

Drug: cetuximab (Erbitux)

Class: Chimeric (mouse/human) monoclonal antibody targeted against epidermal growth factor receptor (EGFR1).

Mechanism of Action: Epidermal growth factor receptor (EGFR, HER1) is a transmembrane glycoprotein receptor tyrosine kinase (RTK) that is turned on (constitutively expressed) in many normal epithelial tissues, such as the skin and hair follicles. Activation of this RTK is also seen in cancers in the head and neck, colon and rectum, as well as others. Cetuximab binds specifically to EGFR in normal and tumor cells, and it competitively inhibits the binding of its ligand Epidermal Growth Factor (EGF) and others, such as transforming growth factor-α. This prevents dimerization and initiation of cell signaling via receptor tyrosine kinase phosphorylation; thus, the message telling the cell to divide does not occur. In addition to cell growth inhibition, there is induction of apoptosis, and decreased matrix metalloproteinase and vascular endothelial growth factor production. As an IgG1 MAb, it may also recruit immune effector cells via antibody-dependent cellular cytotoxicity (ADCC), as well as complement activation. Drug is synergistic with chemotherapy and radiotherapy, as it appears to prevent the malignant cell from repairing DNA damage. Drug is effective only if *KRAS* gene is normal (called wild-type). If *KRAS* gene is mutated, it turns itself on and sets up an independent signaling cascade, bringing a message to the nucleus that tells the cell to divide regardless of whether or not EGFR is blocked by cetuximab. *KRAS* gene is mutated in about 30% of patients with mCRC, but rarely in patients with SCCHN.

Metabolism: Drug is an IgG_1 chimerized antibody, and it is postulated that clearance is via binding of the antibody to EGFR of hepatocytes with internalization of the cetuximab-EGFR complex. Mean elimination half-life is approximately 97 hours (range, 41–213 h). Steady state reached by third weekly infusion. Mean half-life is 112 hours. Females have a 25% lower clearance of drug than males, but there was no difference in efficacy. No differences were found related to race, age, and hepatic and renal functional impairment.

Indication: Treatment of patients with

- Head and neck cancer (1) as initial treatment of locally or regionally advanced squamous cell carcinoma in combination with radiation therapy; (2) as first-line treatment of recurrent locoregional disease or metastatic squamous cell carcinoma in combination with platinum-based therapy with 5-FU; (3) as a single agent, for the treatment of recurrent or metastatic squamous cell carcinoma in whom prior platinum-based therapy has failed.
- *K-Ras* mutation-negative (wild-type), EGFR-expressing metastatic colorectal cancer (mCRC), as determined by FDA-approved tests (1) in combination with FOLFIRI (irinotecan, 5-Fluorouracil, leucovorin) for first-line treatment; (2) in combination with irinotecan in patients refractory to irinotecan-based chemotherapy; and (3) as a single agent in patients who have failed oxaliplatin- and irinotecan-based chemotherapy, or who are intolerant to irinotecan.
- Indicated only in mCRC patients with *KRAS* wild-type tumors, as determined by an FDA-approved test. Patients with *KRAS* gene mutation in codon 12 or 13 (exon 2) have not shown a treatment benefit, so drug is not recommended in these patients. Signal transduction through the EGFR results in activation of wild-type *KRAS* protein. However, in cells with activating *KRAS* (somatic) mutations, the mutant KRAS protein is continually active and appears independent of EGFR regulation.

Dosage/Range:
Squamous cell carcinoma of the head and neck (SCCHN):

- Cetuximab in combination with radiation therapy (RT) or in combination with platinum-based therapy with 5-FU:
  - *Initial dose:* 400 mg/m^2 administered 1 week prior to the initiation of a course of RT or on the day of initiation of platinum-based therapy with 5-FU, as a 120-minute IV infusion (maximum infusion rate 10 mg/min). Complete cetuximab administration 1 hr prior to platinum-based therapy with 5-FU.
  - *Susbsequent weekly dose* (all other infusions): 250 mg/m^2 infused over 60 min (maximum infusion rate 10 mg/min) for the duration of RT (6–7 weeks), or until disease progression or unacceptable toxicity when administered in combination with platinum-based therapy with 5-FU. Complete cetuximab infusion 1 hr prior to RT or platinum-based therapy with 5-FU.
- Cetuximab monotherapy:
  - *Initial dose:* 400 mg/m^2 administered as a 120-minute IV infusion (maximum infusion rate 10 mg/min).
  - *Subsequent weekly dose* (all other infusions): 250 mg/m^2 infused over 60 min (maximum infusion rate (10 mg/min) until disease progression or unacceptable toxicity).

K-Ras/RAS Mutation-negative, EGFR-expressing Colorectal Cancer:

• Ensure *K-Ras/RAS* mutation and EGFR-expression status assessed. Only patients with *K-Ras* mutation-negative (wild-type) tumors should receive the drug.
• *Initial dose*, either as monotherapy or in combination with irinotecan, or FOLFIRI (irinotecan, 5-fluorouracil, leucovorin): 400 mg/m^2 administered as a 120-minute IV infusion (maximum infusion rate 10 mg/min); complete infusion within 1 hr prior to FOLFIRI chemotherapy.
• *Subsequent weekly dose*, either as monotherapy or with irinotecan or FOLFIRI: 250 mg/m^2 infused over 60 min (maximum infusion rate (10 mg/min) until disease progression or unacceptable toxicity).

Recommended Premedications:

• Premedicate with an H1 antagonist (e.g., 50 mg of diphenhydramine) IV 30–60 min prior to first dose; premedication should be administered for subsequent cetuximab doses based upon clinical judgment and presence/severity of prior infusion reactions.

Dose Modifications:
• Reduce the infusion rate by 50% for grade 1 or 2 infusion reactions and nonserious grade 3 infusion reactions.
• Permanently discontinue drug for serious infusion reactions requiring medical intervention and/or hospitalization.
• Severe grade 3 or 4 acneiform rash:
  • First occurrence: Delay infusion 1–2 weeks; if improvement, continue at 250 mg/m^2; if no improvement, discontinue cetuximab.
  • Second occurrence: Delay infusion 1–2 weeks; if improvement, continue at 200 mg/m^2; if no improvement, discontinue cetuximab.
  • Third occurrence: Delay infusion 1–2 weeks; if improvement, continue at 150 mg/m^2; if no improvement, discontinue cetuximab.
  • Fourth occurrence: Discontinue cetuximab.
• Drug is NOT indicated for treatment of *K-Ras* mutation-positive colorectal cancer.

Drug Preparation:
• Available in 100-mg/50-mL and 200-mg/100-mL single-use vials, with concentration of 2 mg/mL, as a sterile, injectable liquid without preservatives. Do not shake or dilute. Solution should be clear and colorless, and may contain small, white particles of cetuximab that are easily visible.
• Store vials under refrigeration at 2–8°C (36–46°F). Do not freeze. Increased particulate formation may occur at temperatures at or below 0°C. Drug contains no preservatives.
• Drug prepared in infusion containers are chemically and physically stable for 12 hours at 2–8°C (36–46°F), and for 8 hours at controlled room temperature (20–25°C or 68–77°F). Discard any remaining solution in the infusion container after 8 hours at room temperature, or 12 hours at 2–8°C (36–46°F). Discard any unused portion of the vial.

Drug Administration:
- Inspect drug for any particulate matter; solution should be clear and colorless, and it may contain small, white particles of cetuximab that are easily visible. Do not shake or dilute.
- Drug must be filtered using a low protein-binding 0.22-μm in-line filter prior to infusion.
- Administer as an IV infusion over 2 hours for a loading dose, and 1 hour for a maintenance dose, using an infusion pump or syringe pump. Do not exceed infusion rate of 10 mg/min.
- Premedicate with an antihistamine before administration, and administer at a maximum of 10 mg/min. Observe patient for 1 hour following infusion, or longer (as needed) if an infusion reaction develops.
- Flush with 0.9% saline solution at the end of the infusion.

Drug Interactions:
- Synergy with cytotoxic chemotherapy (e.g., irinotecan) or radiotherapy.
- Radiation sensitizer.

Lab Effects/Interference:
- Hypomagnesemia; also related hypocalcemia, hypokalemia.

Special Considerations:
- Incidence of severe (grade 3–4) infusion reactions low (2–5%), but may be fatal (1/1,000). Ninety percent occur during first infusion, and are characterized by rapid onset of airway obstruction (stridor, hoarseness, bronchospasm), hypotension, shock, loss of consciousness, myocardial infarction, and/or cardiac arrest. Treat with epinephrine, corticosteroids, antihistamines, bronchodilators, oxygen as needed, and keep available. Drug should be discontinued if severe reaction occurs. Mild-to-moderate reactions require infusion-rate reduction and prophylactic diphenhydramine.
- In one clinical trial of patients with squamous cell cancer of the head and neck receiving RT and cetuximab, 2% of patients experienced cardiopulmonary arrest. Carefully consider cetuximab use in combination with RT or platinum-based therapy with 5-FU in head and neck cancer patients with history of coronary artery disease, CHF, or arrhythmia. In addition, electrolytes including magnesium, calcium, and potassium should be closely monitored during and after cetuximab therapy, as low serum magnesium, calcium, and potassium increase risk of development of torsades de pointes, with subsequent ventricular tachycardia and sudden death.
- Studies show similar pharmacokinetics when drug is administered weekly or as a 500-mg/m^2 biweekly regimen.
- Very rarely (< 0.5%), interstitial lung disease (ILD) may occur, which may be complicated with noncardiogenic pulmonary edema and death. Onset is between cycle 4 and 11 of cetuximab, and is more likely in patients with preexisting fibrotic lung disease. Hold drug and evaluate patients who develop acute or worsening pulmonary symptoms. Discontinue the drug if ILD is found.
- Skin toxicity (acneform rash) is major toxicity affecting 76–88% of patients in clinical trials. Other dermatologic toxicity was skin drying and fissuring, paronychial inflammation, infectious sequelae (e.g., *S. aureus* sepsis), ocular infections (blepharitis, conjunctivitis, keratitis) and hypertrichosis (long eyelashes). Patients should be taught to wear

sunscreen and hats, as well as to limit sun exposure. Rash is not acne but a sterile, inflammatory rash (see introduction to this chapter for a complete discussion).
- Pretreatment assessment for EGFR expression is not required for patients with SCCHN, as EGFR expression is found in almost all patients. Patients with colorectal cancer in clinical trials were required to have evidence of EGFR overexpression. Response rate did not correlate with percentage of positive cells, or with the intensity of EGFR expression.
- Use of cetuximab in combination with RT and cisplatin: in a controlled study of patients with locally advanced SCCHN, the addition of cetuximab in combination with RT and cisplatin resulted in increased grade 3–4 mucositis, radiation recall syndrome, acneiform rash, cardiac events, and electrolyte disturbances in the cetuximab group compared to patients receiving RT and cisplatin alone. In addition, mortality was 4.4% in the cetuximab group vs 3% in the control arm, and the incidence of myocardial ischemia was 2% in the cetuximab arm vs 0.9% in the control arm. There was no difference in PFS, the study's main efficacy outcome.
- During clinical trials, hypomagnesemia occurred in 55% of patients and was severe (grade 3–4) in 6–17%. Onset of hypomagnesemia and accompanying electrolyte abnormalities occurred days to months after starting cetuximab. Periodically monitor patients for hypomagnesemia, hypocalcemia, and hypokalemia during treatment and for at least 8 weeks following treatment completion. Replete electrolytes as necessary.
- Women of childbearing age should use effective contraception, extending for 60 days from the last dose of cetuximab. If cetuximab is administered to a pregnant woman, it should be done only if the benefit outweighs the potential risk. Nursing mothers should discontinue nursing during cetuximab therapy for 60 days from the last dose of the drug.
- Cetuximab improved overall survival when compared with best supportive care (BSC), which led to its second indication in treatment of patients with advanced CRC: patients receiving cetuximab had a 23% improvement in OS and a 32% reduction in risk of disease progression. OS was 6 months in the cetuximab arm compared with 4.5 months in the BSC arm (Jonker et al., 2007).
- The most common (≥ 25%) adverse reactions include cutaneous adverse reactions (e.g., rash, pruritus, and nail changes), headache, diarrhea, and infection. The most serious adverse reactions are infusion reactions, cardiopulmonary arrest, dermatologic toxicity and radiation dermatitis, sepsis, renal failure, ILD, and pulmonary embolism.

Potential Toxicities/Side Effects and the Nursing Process

I.   POTENTIAL FOR INJURY related to HYPERSENSITIVITY/ANAPHYLAXIS AND INFUSION REACTION

Defining Characteristics: Across all studies, some patients (15%–21%) experienced an infusion reaction, largely (90%) with the first infusion, as evidenced by pyrexia, chills, rigors, dyspnea, bronchospasm, angioedema, urticaria, hypertension, and hypotension. Grade 3–4 reactions occurred in 2–5% of patients and were fatal in 1 patient. Severe infusion reactions can be characterized by rapid onset of airway obstruction (bronchospasm, stridor, hoarseness), hypotension, shock, loss of consciousness, myocardial infarction, and/or cardiac arrest. Treat with epinephrine, corticosteroids, anthistamines, bronchodilators, oxygen as ordered, and keep these medications close by and available. The incidence of anaphylaxis is geographically predicted, with an incidence of 20% in Tennessee to Missouri, about 11% in California, and 0.6% in Boston (Chung et al., 2008).

Nursing Implications: Ensure patient receives premedication with diphenhydramine as ordered. Assess baseline VS and mental status prior to drug administration, at 15 minutes, and periodically during infusion, as needed. Remain with patient during first 15 minutes of first infusions. Recall signs/symptoms of anaphylaxis, and if these occur, stop drug immediately, notify physician, and assess patient's vital signs. Subjective symptoms are generalized itching, nausea, chest tightness, crampy abdominal pain, difficulty speaking, anxiety, agitation, sense of impending doom, uneasiness, desire to urinate/defecate, dizziness, and chills. Objective signs are flushed appearance; angioedema of face, neck, eyelids, hands, and feet; localized or generalized urticaria; respiratory distress with or without wheezing; hypotension; and cyanosis. Review standing physician orders or nursing procedures for patient management of anaphylaxis, and be prepared to stop drug immediately and change IV to a plain NS solution to keep vein patent, notify physician, keep patent airway, monitor VS, and administer ordered medications, which may include epinephrine 1:1,000 IM in the thigh, IV hydrocortisone sodium succinate, and IV diphenhydramine. Teach patient to report any unusual symptoms. Patient should be observed for 1 hour after each treatment, and longer periods may be required if the patient experiences an infusion reaction. For mild-to-moderate infusion reactions (grade 1–2), decrease infusion rate permanently by 50%, and continue prophylactic diphenhydramine. Drug should be discontinued in patients who experience severe infusion reactions (grade 3–4).

II. POTENTIAL ALTERATION IN BODY IMAGE, SKIN INTEGRITY, COMFORT related to SKIN RASH, CHANGES IN EYES AND HAIR FOLLICLES

Defining Characteristics: Drug inhibits epidermal growth factor receptor, so major toxicity is manifested in the skin. Most patients (88–90%) develop a mild-to-moderate acne-like rash that is self-limiting. Grade 3–4 rash across all studies occurred in 9%–18% of patients. Rash is a sterile, suppurative rash with multiple follicular or pustular lesions that appear during the first 2 weeks of therapy in areas of sun exposure: face, upper chest, and back, but in some cases, it is extended to the arms. Rash maximizes within 4 weeks, and then improves. Rash also resolves when treatment is stopped. However, in 50% of patients, it takes longer than 28 days to resolve. Dry skin and itching often occur. Scratching with dirty hands or nails can lead to fissures and infection. Nail changes occur, as well as paronychia. Eye changes are related to EGFR blockade and inflammation, and include blepharitis (inflammation of eyelid), conjunctivitis, keratitis/ulcerative keratitis with decreased visual acuity, and hypertrichosis (excessive hair). Infection can be treated with topical clindamycin or oral antibiotics. It appears that patients who have significant rash also have a tumor response.

Nursing Implications: Teach patient that rash most likely will occur due to mechanism of drug action. Assess baseline skin integrity on areas of face, neck, and trunk; assess baseline comfort and satisfaction with body image, and monitor at each treatment. Teach patient to report any distress and assess extent of rash. For severe rash, first occurrence, hold drug for 1–2 weeks, and if improvement, continue drug at usual dose. For second occurrence, hold for 1–2 weeks, and then if improved, reduce dose to 200 mg/m². If third occurrence of severe rash, hold drug for 1–2 weeks, and if improvement, dose-reduce to 150 mg/m². For the fourth occurrence or if there is no improvement after holding drug for 2 weeks in prior occurrences, drug is stopped. If skin appears to be infected (exudate, vesicle formation, abnormal appearance), obtain C+S and discuss empiric treatment with physician. *For rash management, refer to introduction in this chapter.* Teach all patients to (1) use a water-based emollient frequently during the day to prevent dryness, (2) stay hydrated, (3) avoid sun exposure and wear SPF 30 (zinc-based). Do not use anti-acne medications. Tetracycline analogues provide anti-inflammatory benefit. Grade 1/mild rash (localized, does not interfere with ADLs, and is not infected): Goal is to preserve skin integrity, minimize discomfort, and prevent infection. Key patient teaching includes (1) use a mild soap with active ingredients that reduce skin drying, such as pyrithione zinc (Head & Shoulders), (2) consider applying aloe gel to red, tender areas, (3) report distressing tenderness, as pramoxine (lidocaine topical anesthetic) may help, (4) keep fingernails clean and trimmed, and (5) apply zinc ointment to rectal mucosa after washing. Management: maintain current drug dose, observe or give topical hydrocortisone 1% or 2.5% or clindamycin 1% gel (anti-inflammatory benefit), reassess in 2 weeks. For grade 2/moderate, which is generalized, mild symptoms, has minimal effect on ADLs, and no infection: Goal is to prevent infection and promote comfort. Continue EGFRI dose; use topicals (hydrocortisone 2.5% or clindamycin 1% gel) and consider adding doxycycline 100 mg PO twice daily or minocycline 100 mg PO twice daily (give antimicrobial and anti-inflammatory effect) and reassess after 2 weeks. For grade 3–4 or severe rash (generalized, severe, has a significant impact on ADLs, and increased risk of infection): The goal is to prevent infection or identify it early to minimize complications and to promote effective coping. Interrupt drug. Treat rash with topicals (hydrocortisone 2.5%, or clindamycin 1% gel,), doxycycline 100 mg PO twice daily or minocycline 100 mg PO twice daily, and methylprednisolone (Medrol dose pack); reassess after 2 weeks. Resume drug when rash improved to grade 2, at full or reduced dose. (Lynch et al., 2007; Lacouture et al., 2011). If rash appears infected (exudate, vesicular formation, different appearance), obtain C+S, treat empirically until sensitivity received, and/or obtain dermatology consult.

III.   ALTERATION IN ELECTROLYTE BALANCE related to HYPOMAGNESEMIA, POTENTIAL

Defining Characteristics: Magnesium wasting appears related to EGFR inhibition in the renal tubular epithelial cells so that excreted magnesium is not resorbed in the distal convoluted tubules. This leads to initial magnesium wasting, followed by losses of calcium and potassium. Hypomagnesemia occurs in about 55% of patients receiving the drug and is severe in 6%–17% of patients. It begins within days to months of receiving the drug, and there is much interpatient variability. There appears to be a direct relationship between the duration of cetuximab treatment and severe hypomagnesemia (Fakih, 2007). Symptoms of grade 3–4 hypomagnesemia include fatigue, cramps, and somnolence.

Nursing Implications: Assess baseline electrolyte balance before initial treatment and before each successive weekly treatment. Grade 1 is a serum level of 1.0 mg/dL LLN, grade 2 is 0.9–1.0 mg/dL, grade 3 is 0.7–0.8 mg/dL, and grade 4 is ≤ 0.6 mg/dL. Replete magnesium, calcium, and potassium as needed. Oral magnesium may be ineffective and result in diarrhea (Tejpar et al., 2007). Magnesium repletion regimens include weekly IV replacement of 4-g magnesium sulfate for grade 2. For grade 3–4, patients may be symptomatic, and magnesium replacement may involve once to twice weekly IV infusions of 6–10 grams. Provide support for patients, as magnesium replacement infusions require lengthy time in clinic, as an 8-g infusion requires 4 hours. Post-IV replacement with every other day serum magnesium monitoring is important until the patient develops a steady state (Fakih, 2007). Continue to monitor after drug has been discontinued (half-life of the drug and time drug persists, e.g., 8 weeks). Magnesium replacement in IV hydration, beginning when a patient has grade 1 hypomagnesemia, may be effective in preventing worsening hypomagnesemia. For patients who have refractory grade 4 hypomagnesemia, a stop-and-go approach has been effective where cetuximab is held for 4–8 weeks until the magnesium corrects; it is reported that grade 4 hypomagnesemia does not recur when cetuximab is then reintroduced (Fakih, 2007).

IV. ALTERATION IN NUTRITION, LESS THAN BODY REQUIREMENTS, related to NAUSEA, VOMITING, DIARRHEA, STOMATITIS/MUCOUS MEMBRANE DISORDER, CONSTIPATION, WEIGHT LOSS

Defining Characteristics: Incidence of mild-to-moderate digestive symptoms includes nausea (64% for patients across all trials, 19–64%, diarrhea (19%–66%), vomiting (0–40%), stomatitis/mucous membrane disorder (0–32%), weight loss (0–15%), anorexia (0–30%), and constipation (0–53%). Seven percent of patients develop mucous membrane disorder (MMD); 86% of patients with squamous cell cancer of the head and neck receiving concurrent RT experienced mucositis.

Nursing Implications: Assess baseline weight and nutritional status. Teach patient that these symptoms may occur, and to report them. Administer antiemetic and other symptom management medications as ordered. Teach patient self-administration of these medications at home. Monitor serum electrolytes (magnesium, calcium) prior to each dose, and replete magnesium as needed. Teach patient dietary modifications to address symptoms such as anorexia (small, frequent high-calorie, high-protein foods, stimulants as permitted by protocol); constipation (high-fiber, high-fluid, high-roughage foods, stool softeners); diarrhea (BRAT diet: bananas, rice, applesauce, and toast); nausea (avoid food preparation odors by cooking in zipped plastic bag, or having someone else cook; choose cool, soft, nonspicy, or fatty foods); mucositis (blenderized high-calorie, protein-dense foods, cold or cool soft foods, avoidance of spicy or acidic foods;

or percutaneous endoscopically placed gastrostomy (PEG) tube feedings when unable to swallow, local anesthetics to reduce oral and esophageal discomfort/pain). Assess efficacy of intervention, and revise plan as needed.

V.   POTENTIAL FOR INFECTION AND FATIGUE related to LEUKOPENIA AND ANEMIA

Defining Characteristics: Leukopenia occurs in about 25% of patients (combination vs 1% monotherapy) with 17% grade 3–4 (combination) and anemia in 16% (combination vs 10% monotherapy) with 4–5% grade 3–4.

Nursing Implications: Assess baseline WBC, hematocrit, and hemoglobin, and monitor prior to each treatment, especially if drug is given in combination with irinotecan. Teach patient to monitor temperature, and report temperature > 100.5°F. Assess level of fatigue and teach energy baseline and prior to each treatment. Teach patient that fatigue may occur due to anemia, and teach energy-conserving strategies such as alternating rest and activity periods.

Drug: crizotinib (Xalkori)

Class: Kinase inhibitor; small molecule, orally bioavailable, receptor tyrosine kinase inhibitor that blocks the tumor-specific protein ALK (anaplastic lymphoma kinase). This is a first-in-class drug.

Mechanism of Action: Drug is a selective, ATP-competitive small molecule inhibitor of the ALK and MET/HGF receptor tyrosine kinases. By blocking the ALK receptor tyrosine kinase, crizotinib blocks tumor signaling in a number of key pathways necessary for tumor cell growth and survival. Alterations in the ALK gene that makes this tumor-specific protein have been found in 3–5% of patients with NSCLC, neuroblastoma, and rare sarcomas. The abnormality is called EMLA-ALK (echinoderm microtubule-associated protein-like 4 anaplastic lymphoma kinase) fusion gene, and it makes a protein product that turns on signaling for the cell to proliferate. Crizotinib competes for ATP binding with the abnormal tyrosine kinase, so the abnormal tyrosine kinase does not bind to the receptor, the pathway is not turned on, and no message is sent to the cell nucleus telling the cell to divide. Drug also inhibits *cMET*, known as hepatocyte growth factor receptor (HGFR) tyrosine kinase. cMET/HGFR is also known as scatter factor, which plays a role in metastases. Drug serum levels may be increased in patients with severe renal impairment (cr clearance < 30 mL/min) not requiring peritoneal or hemodialysis.

Metabolism: After oral dosing, the drug bioavailability is 43%, with peak concentration in 4–6 hrs. The AUC accumulated by 4- to 5.9-fold after multiple dosing, achieving steady state in 15 days, with a terminal half-life of 42 hours. There is increased systemic exposure to the drug in Asian patients but this is not clinically significant

(Li et al., 2011). Drug is 91% bound to plasma proteins. Drug is predominantly metabolized by CYP3A4/5, with 63% (53% unchanged drug) excreted in the feces and 22% excreted in the urine.

Indication: Drug is indicated for the treatment of patients with metastatic NSCLC that is anaplastic-lymphoma-kinase- (ALK-) positive, as detected by an FDA-approved test. ALK testing should be done by an FDA-approved test performed by laboratories with demonstrated proficiency.

Dosage/Range:
- 250 mg orally twice daily with or without food, until disease progression or patient intolerance.
- For severe renal impairment (Cr Cl < 30 mL/min) not requiring dialysis: 250 mg orally once daily.

Dose Modifications:
- **Grade 3–4 toxicity may require the following dose level changes:**
  - First dose reduction: 200 mg orally twice daily.
  - Second dose reduction: 250 mg orally once daily.
  - Third/unable to tolerate crizotinib 250 mg once daily: permanently discontinue drug.
- **Hematologic (exept lymphopenia, unless associated with clinical events, e.g., opportunistic infections):**
  - **Grade 3:** hold drug until recovery to grade ≤ 2, then resume at same dose.
  - **Grade 4:** hold until recovery to grade ≤ 2, then resume at next lower dose.
- **Nonhematologic:**
  - QTc prolongation > 500 ms on at least 2 separate ECGs: hold drug until recovery to baseline or to a QTc < 481 ms, then resume drug at a reduced dose.
  - QTc > 500 ms or ≥ 60 ms change from baseline with torsades de pointes or polymorphic ventricular tachycardia or signs/symptoms of serious arrhythmia: permanently discontinue drug.
  - Bradycardia (symptomatic, may be severe and medically significant, medical intervention indicated): Hold drug until recovery to asymptomatic bradycardia or to a HR ≥ 60 bpm. Evaluate concomitant medications known to cause bradycardia, as well as antihypertensive medications. If contributing concomitant medication is identified and discontinued, or its dose adjusted, resume crizotinib at previous dose upon recovery to asymptomatic bradycardia or to a HR ≥ 60 bpm. If no contributing concomitant medication is identified, or if contributing concomitant medications are not discontinued or dose modified, resume crizotinib at a reduced dose upon recovery to asymptomatic bradycardia or to a HR ≥ 60 bpm.
  - Bradycardia that is life-threatening requiring urgent intervention: Permanently discontinue crizotinib if no contributing concomitant medication is identified. If contributing concomitant medication is identified and discontinued, or its dose is adjusted, resume crizotinib at 250 mg once daily upon recovery to asymptomatic bradycardia or to a HR ≥ 60 bpm, with frequent monitoring.
  - ALT or AST > 5 × ULN with total bilirubin ≤ 1.5 × ULN: hold crizotinib until recovery to baseline or ≤ 3 × ULN, then resume at reduced dose.

- ALT or AST > 3 × ULN with concurrent total bilirubin > 1.5 × ULN (in the absence of cholestasis or hemolysis): permanently discontinue crizotinib.
- Any grade drug-related interstitial lung disease (ILD) or pneumonitis: permanently discontinue crizotinib.

Drug Preparation/Administration:
- Oral, available as 250-mg and 200-mg hard gelatin capsules. A high-fat diet does not appear to affect pharmacokinetics (Tan et al., 2010).
- Teach patient to swallow capsules whole. If a dose is missed, make up that dose unless the next dose is due within 6 hours. If vomiting occurs after taking a dose, take the next dose at the regular time.
- Monitor CBC with differential baseline, then monthly, as clinically indicated, assessing more frequently if grade 3–4 toxicity, or if fever or infection occurs.
- Monitor LFTs baseline then every 2 weeks for first 2 months, then monthly or as indicated during crizotinib therapy.

Drug Interactions:
- Strong CYP3A inhibitors increase crizotinib plasma concentrations; do not coadminister (e.g., atazanavir, clarithromycin, indinavir, itraconazole, ketoconazole, nefazodone, nelfinavir, ritonavir, saquinavir, telithromycin, troleandomycin, voricoazole).
- Strong CYP3A4 inducers: decrease crizotinib plasma concentrations; avoid coadministration (e.g., carbamazepine, phenobarbital, phenytoin, rifabutin, rifampin, St. John's wort).
- Drugs whose plasma concentrations may be altered by crizotinib: drug appears to be a moderate CYP3A4 enzyme inhibitor (Tan et al., 2010). Avoid coadministration with CYP3A substrates having a narrow therapeutic window (e.g., alfentanil, cyclosporine, dihydroergotamine, ergotamine, fentanyl, pimozide, quinidine, sirolimus, and tacrolimus).

Lab Effects/Interference:
- Increased AST, ALT.
- Neutropenia, thrombocytopenia, lymphopenia.

Special Considerations:
- About 3–5% of patients with NSCLC have the EMLA-ALK fusion gene; they are often nonsmokers, who also do not have mutations in EGFR or KRAS gene. EMLA-ALK fusion gene is also believed to play a role in 15% of neuroblastoma in children.
- Drug-induced hepatic toxicity with fatal outcome has occurred rarely. Monitor LFTs, including ALT and total bilirubin baseline, once a month or more frequently in patients with grade 2–4 elevations, and as clinically indicated.
- Laboratory abnormalities were generally reversible on drug interruption. Transaminate elevations usually occurred within the first 2 months of therapy.
  - Monitor LFTs (including ALT and total bilirubin) baseline and every 2 weeks during first 2 months of crizotinib therapy, then once a month, and as clinically indicated.
  - If abnormalities identified, temporarily suspend, dose-reduce, or permanently discontinue drug as shown in dose modifications.

- Interstitial lung disease (ILD), any grade, occurred in 2.5% of patients across all clinical trials, and 0.9% had grade 3 or 4. Severe, life-threatening, or fatal ILD/ pneumonitis can occur.
  - Cases generally occurred within 2 months of starting treatment.
  - Monitor patients for pulmonary symptoms and exclude other possible causes. If ILD/ pneumonitis occurs, permanently discontinue drug.
- QTc prolongation has occurred in 2.7% of patients across all clinical trials, especially in patients with high risk for QTc prolongation who are taking medications that can prolong the QTc.
  - Consider periodic monitoring of ECG and serum electrolytes (e.g., potassium, magnesium, calcium) in patients with CHF, bradyarrythmias, electrolyte abnormalities, or patients who are taking medications that are known to prolong the QT interval at risk baseline; monitor periodically during treatment. Permanently discontinue drug in patients who develop grade 4 QTc prolongation. Avoid crizotinib therapy in patients with congenital long QT syndrome. See dose modifications.
- Bradycardia occurs in 11% of patients, and is usually asymptomatic. Full effect of drug on heart rate may not be apparent until several weeks after treatment has started.
  - Monitor pulse rate and BP baseline and at least monthly.
  - Avoid using drugs in combinations that cause bradycardia (e.g., beta-blockers; non-dihydropyridine calcium channel blockers such as verapamil and diltiazem; clonidine; digoxin) to prevent increased risk of symptomatic bradycardia (syncope, dizziness, hypotension).
  - If symptomatic bradycardia develops, hold drug, reevaluate the use of concomitant medications, and adjust dose.
- Most common adverse reactions (≥ 25%) are visual changes, nausea, diarrhea, vomiting, edema, and constipation. Dose-limiting toxicities are nausea, vomiting, fatigue, and diarrhea (Kwak et al., 2009).
- Drug can cause fetal harm. Teach women of reproductive potential to use effective contraception. If the drug is used during pregnancy, or if the patient becomes pregnant while taking the drug, apprise the patient of the potential hazard to the fetus.
- In 50 patients studied with NSCLC having *EML4-ALK* fusion oncogenes (ALK mutation), drug showed overall response rate of 64% and disease control rate of 90%. The median number of prior treatments for patients was three, and most patients had adenocarcinoma histology and had never smoked or were former smokers. The median duration of treatment was 25.5 weeks (Bang et al., 2010). *EML4-ALK* fusion gene results from a small inversion within chromosome 2 and involves the fusion of portions of the echinoderm microtubule-associated protein-like (EML4) gene and the anaplastic lymphoma kinase (ALK) gene in NSCLC (Soda et al., 2007).
- Shaw et al. (2011) reported 1 year OS of 77%, 2 years OS of 64%, and median OS has not been reached; this was compared to controls who at 1 year OS was a 73%, at 2 years 33%, and median OS was 20 months. Patients treated with second- and third-line crizotinib had significantly longer OS than untreated ALK+ controls: 1 year 71% vs 46%; 2 year 61% vs 9%; and med OS was not reached in crizotinib patients but 11% months for the controls.

Potential Toxicities/Side Effects and the Nursing Process

I.   ALTERATION IN NUTRITION, POTENTIAL, LESS THAN BODY REQUIREMENTS, related to NAUSEA, VOMITING, DIARRHEA, CONSTIPATION

Defining Characteristics: Nausea, vomiting, diarrhea were dose-limiting toxicities. Nausea occurred in 57% of patients, and vomiting in 45% (Bang et al., 2010). Diarrhea occurred in 49% of patients, and constipation in 38% of patients. Stomatitis occurred in 11%. Decreased appetite occurred in 27% of patients. Dysgeusia occurred in 13% of patients.

Nursing Implications: Assess baseline nutritional status and bowel elimination status. If patient develops nausea and/or vomiting, teach patient to self-administer antiemetics 1 hour prior to each dose, and to call if nausea/vomiting persist. Discuss with physician more effective antiemetic regimen if nausea/vomiting persist. Encourage small, frequent intake of cool, bland foods as tolerated if nausea develops. Refer to dietitian as needed for meal planning. Teach patient to report diarrhea that does not respond to OTC antidiarrheal medication, or if constipation occurs that is unresponsive to fluids, laxatives, and use of high-fiber foods. Teach self-care measures of diet modification and increased oral fluids to 2–3 L during the waking hours. If constipation occurs, teach patient self-care measures to prevent constipation. Assess oral mucosa, and teach patient to self-assess, perform oral rinses after meals and at bedtime with normal saline or bicarbonate in water rinses, and to report irritation or lesions.

II.   ALTERATION IN SENSORY PERCEPTION related to VISUAL CHANGES

Defining Characteristics: Patients described visual disorders 64% of the time, including diplopia, photopsia, photophobia, blurred vision, visual impairment, vitreous floaters, visual brightness, and reduced visual acuity. Changes usually started within 2 weeks of starting drug.

Nursing Implications: Assess baseline visual complaints, and teach patient to report any changes. Discuss with physician any abnormalities. Ophthalmological evaluation should be considered in patients with photopsia or new or increased vitreous floaters, as these may be signs of a retinal hole or pending retinal detachment. Teach patients to use caution when driving or operating machinery due to the risk of developing a vision disorder.

III.   POTENTIAL FOR INFECTION AND BLEEDING related to BONE MARROW DEPRESSION

Defining Characteristics: Grades 3–4 neutropenia occurred in 5.2%, thrombocytopenia in 0.4%, and lymphopenia in 11.4% of patients. Fever occurred in 12% of patients, and URIs occurred in 20% of patients.

Nursing Implications: Assess baseline CBC, including WBC, differential, and platelet count prior to dosing, as well as at least weekly during first month of treatment, at least every other week for the second month of treatment, and then as clinically indicated and ordered. Discuss dose interruption and reduction as above for neutropenia and thrombocytopenia. Teach patient self-assessment of signs/symptoms of infection and bleeding (including epistaxis and development of petechiae), and instruct patient to report them right away. Teach patient self-care measures to minimize risk of infection and bleeding, including avoidance of OTC aspirin-containing medications. Discuss dose reductions as needed.

IV.   ALTERATION IN COMFORT related to EDEMA, ARTHRALGIA, RASH

Defining Characteristics: Edema occurred in 38% of patients, arthralgia and back pain in 11% of patients, and rash in 16% of patients.

Nursing Implications: Assess baseline parameters of weight, presence of edema, pulmonary function, and monitor closely during therapy. Teach patient to monitor weight gain and edema, or the development of dyspnea. Assess skin integrity baseline and frequently during treatment. Teach patient to report rash. Develop a plan to protect skin and maintain skin integrity.

V.   SENSORY ALTERATIONS, POTENTIAL, related to PERIPHERAL NEUROPATHY, DIZZINESS, HEADACHE

Defining Characteristics: Neuropathy occurred in 23% of patients and ranged from grade 1, grade 2 motor neuropathy, to grade 3 peripheral neuropathy. Dizziness (24%) and dysgeusia (13%) were common, all grades 1 and 2. Headache occurred in 13% of patients.

Nursing Implications: Teach patient that these side effects may occur and to report them. Assess for the presence of neuropathy, comparing one side of the body to the others, focusing on the hands and feet, as peripheral neuropathy starts at the toes and fingertips (longest axons), and then moves in a stocking-glove distribution. Discuss any positive findings with physician or NP/PA for a more focused neurological exam.

Drug: dabrafenib (Tafinlar)

Class: Kinase inhibitor.

Mechanism of Action: Drug inhibits some of mutated BRAF kinases (e.g., BRAF V600E) as well as the wild-type BRAF and CRAF kinases. Mutations such as BRAF V600E can result in constituitively activated BRAF kinases that can stimulate tumor cell growth, such as melanoma.

Metabolism: After oral dosing, median time to peak plasma concentration (T_{max}) is 2 hours. Mean absolute bioavailability is 95%. If drug is administered with a high-fat mean, the C_{max} is decreased by 51%, AUC decreased by 31% and T_{max} delayed by 3.6 hour, compared to fasting state. Drug is 99.7% plasma protein bound. Drug is primarily metabolized by liver microenzymes CYP2C8 and CYP3A4 to form hydroxy-dabrafenib, an active metabolite, which is further oxidized to form another metabolite. Most of the drug and metabolites are excreted in the bile and urine. One metabolite, desmethyl-dabrafenib, may be reabsorbed from the gut and contributes to the chemical activity. Terminal half-life of dabrafenib is 8 hours. Seventy-one percent of the drug is excreted via feces, and 23% via urine (metabolites only). Mild or moderate renal impairment, and mild hepatic impairment do not effect systemic exposure of drug or its metabolites.

Indication: Drug is FDA-indicated for the treatment of patients
- With unresectable or metastatic melanoma with BRAF V600E mutation, as detected by an FDA-approved test,
- In combination with trametinib, in unresectable melanoma with BRAF V600E or V600K mutation, as detected by an FDA-approved test.

Dosage/Range:
- Confirm the presence of BRAF V600E mutation in tumor specimens, prior to starting dabrafenib as a single agent, and BRAF V600E or V600K mutations in tumor specimens prior to starting combined dabrafenib and trametinib. Mutations must be detected by an FDA-approved test.
- 150 mg orally twice daily as a single agent, or in combination with trametinib 2 mg once daily, on an empty stomach (at least one hour prior to or two hours after a meal).
- Indication for combination therapy is based on demonstration of durable response rate, but no improvement in disease-related symptoms or overall survival has been demonstrated.

Dose Modifications:
- Dose reductions:
  - First dose reduction: 100 mg orally twice daily.
  - Second dose reduction: 75 mg orally twice daily.
  - Third dose reduction: 50 mg orally twice daily.
  - If unable to tolerate 50 mg twice daily, discontinue dabrafenib.
- When trametinib is administered with dabrafenib:
  - First dose reduction of trametinib: 1.5 mg once daily.
  - Second dose reduction: 1 mg once daily.
  - Subsequent modification: permanently discontinue trametinib if unable to tolerate 1 mg once daily.
- Febrile drug reaction:
  - Temperature 101.3–104°F (38.5–40°C): hold dabrafenib, or both drugs, until reaction resolves, then resume at same dose or a reduced drug dose (see previous bullet);
  - Temperature > 104°F or fever complicated by rigors, hypotension, dehydration, or renal failure: either hold dabrafenib until reaction resolves, then resume at a reduced dose level, or permanently discontinue dabrafenib; hold trametinib until fever resolves, then resume at same or lower dose level.
- Cutaneous grade 2 toxicity, or grade 3 or 4 skin toxicity: hold dabrafenib, and trametinib if used in combination, for up to 3 weeks; if improved, resume dose at a lower dose level; if not improved, permanently discontinue.

- Cardiac:
  - Asymptomatic, absolute decrease in LVEF of ≥ 10% from baseline, and is below LLN from pretreatment values: no dose change of dabrafenib, but hold trametinib if used, for up to 4 weeks; if LVEF returns to normal, resume drug at lower dose level; if not, permanently discontinue trametinib.
  - Symptomatic CHF or an absolute decrease of ≥ 20% in LVEF from baseline that is below LLN: hold dabrafenib until LVEF improved, then resume at same dose; if LVEF does not return to normal, permanently discontinue trametinib dose.
- Venous Thromboembolism:
  - Uncomplicated DVT or PE: do not change dabrafenib but hold trametinib for up to 3 weeks; if improved to grade 0–1, resume trametinib at a lower dose level; if not improved, permanently discontinue trametinib.
  - Life-threatening PE: permanently discontinue dabrafenib and trametinib.
- Ocular Toxicities:
  - Grade 2–3 retinal pigment epithelial detachment (RPED): do not change dabrafenib dose, but hold trametinib dose for up to 3 weeks; if improved to grade 0–1, resume trametinib at a lower dose level; if not improved, permanently discontinue trametinib.
  - Retinal vein occlusion: do not change dabrafenib dose, but permanently discontinue trametinib.
  - Uveitis and iritis: hold dabrafenib for up to 6 weeks; if improved to grade 0–1, resume dabrafenib same dose; if not, permanently discontinue dabrafenib; do not modify trametinib dose.
- Interstitial Lung Disease (ILD) or pneumonitis: do not modify dabrafenib dose, but permanently discontinue trametinib.
- Other:
  - Intolerable grade 2, or any grade 3 reactions: hold dabrafenib until adverse reaction resolves to grade 1 or less, then resume at reduced dose level; if no improvement, permanently discontinue dabrafenib; hold trametinib for up to 3 weeks; if improved to grade 0–1, resume trametinib at a reduced dose level; if no improvement, permanently discontinue.
  - First occurrence of any grade 4 adverse reaction: either permanently discontinue dabrafenib or hold until reaction resolves to grade 0–1, then resume at a reduce dose; hold trametinib until toxicity improves to grade 0–1, then resume at lower dose level; if no improvement, permanently discontinue.
  - Recurrent grade 4 adverse reaction: permanently discontinue dabrafenib and trametinib if used in combination.

Drug Preparation:
- Available as 50-mg and 75-mg capsules.

Administration:
- Take drug on an empty stomach, at least one hour prior to or two hours after a meal.
- Take two times a day, about 12 hours apart.
- If receiving the combination, the patient should take the trametinib once-daily dose with either the morning or evening dose of dabrafenib at the same time each day.
- Teach patient (1) to take capsule whole without crushing, opening, or breaking the capsule; (2) to take a missed dose when remembered, but not if it is within 6 hours

of the next scheduled dose; then just take the scheduled dose. Do not make up the missed dose.

Drug Interactions:
- Drug is substrate of CYP3A4 and CYP2C8; metabolites are substrates of CYP3A4. Drug is substrate of human P-glycoprotein (Pgp).
- Drug is a moderate inducer of CYP3A4 and may induce other microenzymes.
- Strong inhibitors of CYP3A4 (e.g., ketoconazole, nefazodone, clarithromycin) or CYP2C8 (e.g., gemfibrozil): may increase serum level of dabrafenib; coadministration not recommended.
- Strong inducers of CYP3A4 (e.g., rifampin, phenytoin, carbamazepine, phenobarbital, St. John's wort) or CYP2C8 (e.g., rifampicin): may decrease serum level of dabrafenib; coadministration not recommended.
- Drugs that increase gastric pH may decrease dabrafenib concentrations (e.g., PPIs, H2-receptor antagonists, antacids).
- Concomitant use with agents that are sensitive substrates of CYP3A4, CYP2C8, CYP2C9, CYP2C19, or CYP2B6 may result in loss of efficacy of these agents; e.g., midazolam is a CYP3A4 substrate, dabrafenib decreases midazolam C_{max} and AUC by 61% and 74% respectively.

Lab Effects/Interference:
- Hyperglycemia.
- Hypophosphatemia, hyponatremia, increased alkaline phosphatase.

Special Considerations:
- Drug is not approved for treatment of patients with wild-type BRAF melanoma. BRAF inhibitors can cause increased cell proliferation and tumor promotion in BRAF wild-type melanoma.
- Drug may cause the development of new primary cutaneous malignancies (e.g., cutaneous squamous cell carcinomas and keratocanthomas; incidence 7%, with median time to first squamous cell carcinoma of 9 weeks, and to second 6 weeks in one study). Incidence of basal cell carcinoma is increased in combination therapy with trametinib (incidence 9% vs 2% with dabrafenib alone), while cutaneous squamous cell carcinoma was reduced with the combination (7% vs 19% receiving dabrafenib alone). Perform dermatologic evaluations prior to starting therapy, every two months while on therapy, and for up to six months following drug discontinuance.
- Noncutaneous malignancies in patients receiving combination: Dabrafenib can stimulate malignancies through RAS mutational activation (e.g., *KRAS* mutation-positive CRC). Discontine dabrafenib if noncutaneous RAS mutation-positive cancer occurs.
- Hemorrhage, including major hemorrhage, may occur in patients receiving the combination (incidence 16% all bleeding, and 5% serious hemorrhage, e.g., intracranial bleed).
  - Permanently discontinue dabrafenib and tramatinib for all grade 4 hemorrhage or grade 3 hemorrhage that does not improve.
  - Hold dabrafenib (and trametinib if combination used) for grade 3 hemorrhage, and if improved, resume dabrafenib (and trametinib if the combination used) at a lower dose level.

- Combined dabrafenib and trametinib therapy increases risk of venous thromboembolism. Teach patients to seek immediate medical care for symptoms of DVT or PE (e.g., shortness of breath, chest pain, swelling of arm or leg). See Dose Modifications.
- Combined dabrafenib and trametinib therapy increases risk of cardiomyopathy. Assess LVEF (ECHO or MUGA) baseline, one month after combination started, then at 2–3 monthly intervals while on combination therapy. See Dose Modifications.
- Dabrafenib can cause serious febrile drug reactions (incidence 28%); hold drug if fever ≥ 101.3°F, or complicated fever occurs (e.g., hypotension, rigors or chills, dehydration, or renal failure in absence of other identifiable cause). See Dose Modifications.
- Drug may cause uveitis and iritis; monitor patient baseline and regularly for visual symptoms (change in vision, photophobia, eye pain). Symptomatic treatment usually involves steroid and mydriatic ophhthalmic drops. See Dose Modifications.
- Retinal Pigment Epithelial Detachment (RPED) may occur rarely when dabrafenib is combined with trametinib; trametinib as a single agent can cause bilateral, multifocal RPED. See Dose Modifications.
- Combined dabrafenib and trametinib therapy may result in serious skin toxicity. Trametinib alone and in combination causes a 68% incidence of skin toxicity. Dabrafenib causes palmar-plantar erythrodysesthesia in about 20% of patients. See Dose Modifications.
- Dabrafenib may cause hyperglycemia in 50% of patients (grade 3 in 6%); assess baseline serum glucose and monitor regularly during therapy as appropriate.
  - Monitor patients with diabetes very closely, as patients may need an increase in dose of or initiation of insulin or oral hypoglycemic agent.
  - Teach patients to report symptoms of hyperglycemia (e.g., polyphagia, polyuria, polydipsia).
- Patients with Glucose-6-phosphate dehydrogenase deficiency: monitor patient closely for hemolytic anemia.
- Drug is fetotoxic. Counsel women and men of reproductive potential to use effective contraception; drug may cause hormonal contraception to be ineffective, so women should use an alternative form of contraception. Nursing mothers should discontinue nursing or not take the drug.
- Most common side effects of dabrafenib as a single agent are hyperkeratosis, headache, pyrexia, arthralgia, papilloma, alopecia, palmar–plantar erythrodysesthesia syndrome (PPES). Most common side effects of dabrafenib in combination with trametinib are pyrexia, chills, fatigue, rash, nausea, vomiting, diarrhea, abdominal pain, peripheral edema, cough, headache, arthralgia, night sweats, decreased appetite, constipation, and myalgia.

Potential Toxicities/Side Effects and the Nursing Process

I. ALTERATION IN COMFORT AND HOMEOSTASIS related to FEBRILE DRUG REACTION

Defining Characteristics: Serious drug reactions (fever or fever complicated by hypotension, rigors or chills, dehydration, or renal failure without other identifiable cause) occurred in 28% of patients. Median time to initial onset was 11 days (range 1–202 days), and median duration of fever was 3 days (range 1–129 days).

Nursing Implications: Teach patient that fever may occur and to report it or the occurrence of chills, rigors, or dizziness right away. Drug should be stopped until patient discusses symptoms with physician or NP/PA. Ensure patient has a thermometer and can read it. Teach patient that dehydration can worsen this, and to make sure the patient drinks adequate fluids daily (e.g., one 8-oz glass of fluid, excluding alcohol, every hour while awake). Drug should be held for fever of 101.3°F or greater, or for chills, rigors, hypotension, or renal failure. Prophylaxis with acetaminophen may be needed when resuming drug per physician or NP/PA.

II.   ALTERATION IN SENSORY PERCEPTION related to VISUAL CHANGES

Defining Characteristics: Uveitis, including iritis, occurred in 1% of patients.

Nursing Implications: Assess baseline visual complaints, and teach patient to report any changes (such as change in vision, photophobia, eye pain) right away. Discuss ophthalmic evaluation if symptoms arise. In clinical trials, symptoms were controlled with steroid and mydriatic ophthalmic drops.

III.   ALTERATION IN SKIN INTEGRITY, POTENTIAL, related to SKIN CHANGES, NEW CUTANEOUS MALIGNANCY, PPES

Defining Characteristics: Hyperkeratosis occurred in 37% of patients, alopecia in 22% of patients, PPES in 20% of patients, and rash in 17% of patients. Papilloma occurred in 27% of patients, and cutaneous squamous cell carcinoma in 7% of patients.

Nursing Implications: Teach patient that these side effects may occur and to report them. Examine skin of hands and feet, and areas of high pressure. Patient should have a dermatologic evaluation baseline starting therapy, every 2 months while on therapy, and for up to 6 months following drug discontinance for squamous cell cancers. Teach patient to examine skin of hand, feet, areas of pressure and to report pain, edema, numbness, stinging, dysesthesias, flat blisters with a reddish halo, peeling (desquamation), painful hyperkeratotic lesions, scaly skin calluses. Teach patient to avoid hot water and to use tepid water in shower or bath; to use a mild soap and to pat the area dry gently and not rub vigorously; to avoid constrictive clothing; to avoid prolonged pressure on feet, like jogging or long walks; to avoid repetitive hand motion (e.g., raking); to use skin moisturizer on hands and feet bid and protect from the sun exposure.

Drug: dasatinib (Sprycel)

Class: Multitargeted tyrosine kinase inhibitor.

Mechanism of Action: Inhibits the following kinases: BCR-Abl, SRC-family (SRC, LCK, YES, FYN), c-KIT, EPHA2, and PDGFR-b. Drug forms a tighter bond with Bcr-Abl kinase (300–1,000 times more potently) than imatinib mesylate (Gleevec) and binds to both active and inactive forms.

Metabolism: Drug is rapidly absorbed after oral ingestion with peak serum levels in 0.5–6 hours and an overall mean half-life of 3–5 hours. If ingested with a high-fat meal, there was a 14% increase in the mean area under the curve exposure, but this is not felt to be clinically relevant. Drug and its active metabolite bind to plasma proteins 96% and 93%, respectively. Drug is extensively metabolized by the P450 microenzyme CYP3A4. Drug is excreted in the feces (85%), and to a lesser degree the urine (4%).

Indication: Drug is indicated for the treatment of (1) newly diagnosed adults with Philadelphia chromosome-positive (Ph+) chronic myeloid leukemia (CML) in chronic phase; (2) adults with chronic, accelerated, or myeloid or lymphoid blast phase Ph+ CML with resistance or intolerance to prior therapy, including imatinib; And (3) adults with Ph+ acute lymphoblastic leukemia (Ph+ ALL) with resistance or intolerance to prior therapy.

Dosage/Range:
- Chronic phase CML: 100 mg PO once daily.
- Accelerated phase CML, myeloid, or lymphoid blast phase CML, or Ph+ ALL: 140 mg PO once daily.
- Administer orally, with or without a meal. Do not crush or cut
- Continue dasatinib until disease progression or no longer tolerated.
- Use dasatinib with caution in patients with hepatic impairment.
- Dose may be increased or decreased in 20-mg increments based on individual patient response, or coadministration with drugs that either increase or decrease dasatinib serum levels (see Drug Interactions).

Dose Modifications:
- Myelosuppression is managed by dose interruption, reduction, or discontinuance. Hematopoietic growth factor has been used in patients with resistant myelosupression. See package insert for full description.
- Dose modifications for hematologic toxicity. Monitor CBC weekly for the initial 2 months and then periodically. See table on next page.
  Dose Adjustments for Neutropenia and Thrombocytopenia: Sprycel Package Insert. Princeton, NJ: Bristol Myers Squibb Oncology, May 2014.

- **Concomitant strong CYP3A4 inducers:** CYP3A4 inducers (e.g., dexamethasone, phenytoin, carbamazepine, rifampin, rifabutin, phenobarbital) may decrease dasatinib plasma concentrations and should be avoided; St. John's wort may decrease dasatinib concentrations unpredictably and should be avoided. If a strong inducer must be coadministered with dasatinib, consider increasing dasatinib dose and monitor the patient closely for toxicity.
- **Concomitant strong CYP3A4 inhibitors:** CYP3A4 inhibitors (e.g., ketoconazole, itraconazole, atazanavir, indinavir, nefazodone, nelfinavir, ritonavir, saquinavir,

telithromycin, voriconazole; also grapefruit and grapefruit juice) may increase dasatinib plasma concentrations and should be avoided. If coadministration with a strong inhibitor must occur, consider decreasing dasatinib dose to 20 mg daily (if taking 100 mg a day) or 40 mg daily (if taking 140 mg daily), which approximates the AUC. However, there are no clinical data with these dose adjustments. If dasatinib is not tolerated after dose reduction, either the strong CYP3A4 inhibitor must be discontinued or dasatinib stopped until treatment with the inhibitor has ceased. When the strong inhibitor is discontinued, a washout period of approximately 1 week should occur before dasatinib dose is increased.

* **Severe nonhematological adverse reactions:** hold Sprycel until event resolves or improves. When resuming Sprycel, reduce dose depending upon the initial severity of the event.

Chronic Phase CML (starting dose 100 mg once daily)	ANC < 0.5 × 10⁹/L or platelets < 50 × 10⁹/L	1. Stop Sprycel until ANC > 1.0 × 10⁹/L, and platelets > or equal to 50 × 10⁹/L; 2. Resume Sprycel at the original starting dose if recovery occurs in 7 days or less; 3. If platelets < 25 × 10⁹/L or recurrence of ANC < 0.5 × 10⁹/L for > 7 days, repeat Step 1 and resume Sprycel at a reduced dose of 80 mg once daily for 2nd episode. For 3rd episode, further reduce dose to 50 mg once daily (for newly diagnosed patients) or discontinue Sprycel (for patients resistant or intolerant to prior therapy including imatinib).
Accelerated Phase CML, Blast Phase CML, and Ph+ ALL (starting dose 140 mg once daily)	ANC < 0.5 × 10⁹/L or Platelets < 10 × 10⁹/L	• Assess whether cytopenia is related to leukemia (marrow aspirate or biopsy); • If cytopenia is unrelated to leukemia, stop Sprycel until ANC ≥ equal to 1.0 × 10⁹/L, and platelets ≥ to 20 × 10⁹/L, and resume at original starting dose; • If recurrence of cytopenia, repeat Step 1 and resume Sprycel at a reduced dose of 100 mg once daily (2nd episode) or 80 mg once daily (3rd episode); • If cytopenia is related to leukemia, consider dose escalation to 180 mg once daily.

Dose Adjustments for Neutropenia and Thrombocytopenia: Sprycel Package Insert. Princeton NJ: Bristol Myers Squibb Oncology, May 2014.

Drug Preparation/Administration:
* None, oral. Available in 20-mg, 50-mg, 70-mg, 80-mg, 100-mg, and 140-mg tablets.

Drug Administration:
* Oral, once daily. Administer once in the morning OR in the evening, with or without food; do not crush or cut.
* Assess CBC/differential weekly for the first 2 months, and then monthly, or as clinically indicated.
* Assess and discuss with physician or NP/PA correction of hypokalemia or hypomagnesemia before dasatinib administration.

Drug Interactions:
- **CYP3A4 inhibitors:** These inhibitors (e.g., ketoconazole, itraconazole, erythromycin, clarithromycin, atazanavir, indinavir, nefazodone, nelfinavir, ritonavir, saquinavir, telithromycin) may decrease metabolism of dasatinib, thus increasing serum concentrations of dasatinib; avoid coadministration, and if they must be given together, decrease dose of dasatinib. See package insert: For example, if the patient is taking dasatinib 100 mg plus a strong CYP3A4 inhibitor that cannot be changed, the dasatinib dose should be decreased to 20 mg daily; if taking dasatinib 140 mg daily, the dose should be reduced to 40 mg daily. Avoid grapefruit and grapefruit juice.
- **CYP3A4 inducers:** Rifampin decreased dasatinib serum concentrations by 81%; with others (e.g., dexamethasone, phenytoin, carbamazepine, phenobarbital, St. John's wort), avoid coadministration; if they must be given together, increase dose of dasatinib and monitor for toxicity. Patients receiving dasatinib should NOT take St. John's wort.
- **Antacids (aluminum hydroxide/magnesium hydroxide):** Decrease dasatinib AUC by 55%, as drug requires acid pH; avoid concurrent administration or administer 2 hours prior to or 2 hours after dasatinib dose.
- **H₂ blockers/proton pump inhibitors:** Famotidine decreases dasatinib AUC 61%; avoid concurrent administration. Consider replacing with antacids that should be taken at least 2 hours before or after dasatinib so there is no interference with absorption.
- **Simvastatin, CYP3A4 substrates:** Dasatinib is a time-dependent inhibitor of CYP3A4 and may decrease the metabolism of drugs primarily metabolized by CYP3A4, such as alfentanil, astemizole, terfenadine, cisapride, cyclosporine, fentanyl, pimozide, quinidine, sirolimus, tacrolimus, or ergot alkaloids; decreases simvastatin AUC 37%; avoid concurrent administration or administer cautiously.

Lab Effects/Interference:
- Grades 3–4 neutropenia, thrombocytopenia, and anemia.
- Hypophosphatemia, hypocalcemia.
- Elevated ALT, AST, bilirubin.
- Elevated creatinine.
- QT/QTc prolongation on EKG.

Special Considerations:
- Severe myelosuppression (e.g., grade 3–4 thrombocytopenia, neutropenia, and anemia) may occur.
  - Occurrence is more frequent in patients with advanced phase CML or Ph+ALL than in chronic phase CML.
  - In a trial of patients with resistance or intolerance to prior imatinib therapy and chronic phase CML, grade 3–4 myelosuppression was reported less frequently in patients receiving dasatinib 100 gm once daily.
  - Myelosuppression is generally reversible and manageable with dose interruption or reduction.
  - Assess CBC/differential weekly for the first 2 months and then monthly, or as clinically indicated.

- Bleeding related events: dasatinib can cause platelet dysfunction. Severe central nervous system (CNS) bleeding occurred in 1% of patients; severe GI hemorrhage occurred in 4% and generally required drug interruption and transfusions.
  - Most patients had thrombocytopenia as well.
  - Use caution if used together with other medicines that inhibit platelet function or anticoagulants.
  - In later clinical trials, patients could also take anticoagulants, aspirin, and NSAIDs if their platelet count was > 50,000–75,000/mL.
- Drug is associated with fluid retention (including ascites, edema, pleural, and pericardial effusions), which can be severe in up to 10% of patients.
  - If a patient develops dyspnea, dry cough, suggestive of pleural effusions, evaluate by CXR. Pleural effusions may require thoracentesis, and patient may require oxygen therapy.
  - Fluid retention is manageable with supportive measures, including diuretics and a short course of steroids. In dose-optimization studies, fluid retention events occurred less frequently in patients who received once-daily dosing.
- Drug can cause QT interval (ventricular repolarization) prolongation. Administer cautiously to patients who may develop prolongation of the QTc interval (hypokalemia, hypomagnesemia, congenital long QT syndrome), patients taking anti-arrhythmic medications, or who have cumulative high-dose anthracycline therapy. Monitor and correct deficits in magnesium and potassium prior to administering dasatinib.
- CHF, left ventricular dysfunction, and myocardial infarction. Cardiac adverse reactions were reported in 7% of dasatinib patients: 1.6% cardiomyopathy, CHF, diastolic dysfunction, fatal MI, and left ventricular dysfunction. Monitor patients for signs/symptoms of cardiac dysfunction, and discuss medical management with physician.
- Pulmonary arterial hypertension (PAH): dasatinib may increase risk for developing PAH, which may be reversible upon discontinuation of dasatinib. PAH may occur any time after starting dasatinib, including > 1 year of treatment. Assess for dyspnea, fatigue, hypoxia, and fluid retention. Evaluate patients for signs/symptoms of underlying cardiopulmonary disease prior to beginning dasatinib and throughout treatment. If PAH is confirmed, permanently discontinue dasatinib.
- Drug is teratogenic and embryo-fetal toxic. Women of reproductive potential should be advised to use effective contraception to avoid pregnancy. If dasatinib is used during pregnancy, or if the patient becomes pregnant while receiving the drug, patient should be apprised of potential hazard to the fetus.
- Nursing mothers should decide to discontinue nursing or discontinue the drug, taking into account the importance of the drug to the mother's health.
- Use cautiously, if at all, in patients with hepatic dysfunction. Most common side effects (≥ 15%) in newly diagnosed CML-chronic phase patients included: myelosuppression, fluid retention, and diarrhea. Most common side effects (≥ 20%) in patients with resistance or intolerance to prior imatinib therapy included: myelosuppression, fluid retention events, diarrhea, headache, dyspnea, skin rash, fatigue, nausea, and hemorrhage.

• Assess patient drug profile; teach patient about possible interacting drugs, and instruct patient to tell nurse or physician before starting any over-the-counter or herbal medications.

Potential Toxicities/Side Effects and the Nursing Process

I. POTENTIAL FOR INFECTION AND BLEEDING related to BONE MARROW DEPRESSION

Defining Characteristics: Grades 3–4 neutropenia, thrombocytopenia, and anemia are common, especially severe in patients with advanced CML or Ph+ ALL, as compared to those in chronic phase CML. Drug can cause platelet dysfunction, resulting in rare CNS or GI hemorrhage, and are most often associated with severe thrombocytopenia. Use caution if patients are also taking medications that inhibit platelet function, or anticoagulants, and monitor very closely. Infection (bacterial, viral, fungal) occurred in 34% of patients.

Nursing Implications: Assess baseline CBC, including WBC, differential, and platelet count prior to dosing, as well as at least weekly during first month of treatment, at least every other week for the second month of treatment, and then as clinically indicated and ordered. Discuss dose interruption and reduction as above for neutropenia and thrombocytopenia. Teach patient self-assessment of signs/symptoms of infection and bleeding (including epistaxis and development of petechiae), and instruct patient to report them right away. Teach patient self-care measures to minimize risk of infection and bleeding, including avoidance of OTC aspirin-containing medications. Discuss dose reductions as needed.

II. ALTERATION IN FLUID AND ELECTROLYTE BALANCE related to FLUID RETENTION, EDEMA

Defining Characteristics: Fluid retention is common (50%). Superficial edema is most common, but pleural effusion may occur in 22% of patients. However, ascites, rapid weight gain, and pulmonary edema may develop, and in some cases, be life-threatening (pleural effusion, congestive heart failure, pulmonary hypertension, pericardial effusion, anasarca).

Nursing Implications: Assess baseline parameters of weight, presence of edema, pulmonary function, and monitor closely during therapy. Teach patient to monitor weight daily at home, and to report weight gain of 2 pounds in 1 week, development of edema, or dyspnea. Develop a plan to protect skin and maintain skin integrity, and discuss the prescription of diuretics with physician or NP.

III. ALTERATION IN NUTRITION, POTENTIAL, LESS THAN BODY REQUIREMENTS, related to NAUSEA, VOMITING, DIARRHEA

Defining Characteristics: Nausea affected 34% of patients; vomiting affected 22%. Diarrhea affected 50%, while constipation affected 14%.

Nursing Implications: Assess baseline nutritional status and bowel elimination status. If patient develops nausea and/or vomiting, teach patient to self-administer antiemetics 1 hour prior to each dose, and to call if nausea/vomiting persist.

Discuss with physician more effective antiemetic regimen if nausea/vomiting persist. Encourage small, frequent intake of cool, bland foods as tolerated if nausea develops. Refer to dietitian as needed for meal planning. Teach patient to report diarrhea that does not respond to OTC antidiarrheal medication. Teach self-care measures of diet modification and increased oral fluids to 2–3 L during the waking hours. If constipation, teach patient self-care measures to prevent constipation.

IV. ALTERATION IN COMFORT related to PAIN, HEADACHE, FATIGUE, ARTHRALGIA, AND FATIGUE

Defining Characteristics: Headache affected 40% of patients, musculoskeletal pain affected 39% of patients, fatigue 39% of patients, myalgias/arthralgias 19% of patients, and abdominal pain affected 25% of patients.

Nursing Implications: Teach patient that these events may occur and to report them. Assess baseline comfort, and monitor closely during treatment. Develop plan to assure comfort depending on symptoms reported. Discuss ineffective strategies with physician, and revise plan as needed.

Drug: denileukin diftitox (ONTAK)

Class: Fusion protein.

Mechanism of Action: Agent is recombinant DNA-derived cytotoxic protein containing diphtheria toxin fragments, and IL-2. It targets cells with high affinity for IL-2 receptors containing a CD25 component, such as activated T and B lymphocytes, and activated macrophages. The IL-2 portion of the fusion protein binds to the IL-2 receptor on malignant cells, which contain a CD25 component. The diphtheria toxin fragments are brought into the cell through the receptor (receptor-mediated endocytosis) and into the endosomal vesicles. Acidification cleaves the active fragment of diphtheria toxin, which is then actively transported into the cytoplasm. There, it catalyzes a reaction that inhibits protein synthesis and causes cell death within hours.

Metabolism: Distribution phase has half-life of 2–5 minutes, and terminal phase half-life of 70–80 minutes; the development of antibodies to denileukin diftitox significantly increases clearance 2–3 times, with a consequent decrease in mean systemic exposure of about 75%. Metabolized by proteolytic degradation and primarily excreted via the liver and kidneys; excreted material is < 25% of total dose.

Indication: ONTAK is indicated for the treatment of patients with persistent or recurrent CD25-positive cutaneous T-cell lymphoma (CTCL, or mycosis fungoides whose malignant cells express the CD25 component of the IL-2 receptor).

Dosage/Range:
- As of 10.11.14, Eisai, the manufacturer, states that there continues to be an ONTAK supply interruption. Call 1-888-274-2378 for more information.
- Confirm with physician that patient's malignant cells express CD25 before administering ONTAK.
- Premedicate with an antihistamine and acetaminophen prior to each infusion.
  - 9 or 18 µg/kg/day IV daily over 30–60 minutes daily × 5 consecutive days, repeated every 3 weeks for 8 cycles.

Drug Preparation:
- Single-use vial contains 150 µg/mL (300 µg in 2 mL).
- Thaw in refrigerator at 2–8°C (36–46°F) over less than 24 hours, or at room temperature for 1–2 hours.
- Bring ONTAK vial to room temperature (25°C or 77°F), before preparing dose. DO NOT HEAT.
- Mix by gentle swirling. DO NOT SHAKE.
- DO NOT REFREEZE DRUG after thawing.
- Inspect solution for clarity and discard if it remains hazy (will be hazy after thawing, but becomes clear when at room temperature). Use only if colorless without visible particulate matter.
- Prepare and hold diluted drug in plastic syringes or soft plastic IV bags; DO NOT use glass containers.
- Withdraw ordered dose from vial and inject into an empty IV infusion bag; add up to 9 mL of sterile saline without preservative for each 1 mL of ONTAK to the IV bag, for a final concentration of at least 15 µg/mL.
- Discard any unused portion of the drug.

Drug Administration:
- Assess serum albumin and if < 3.0 g/dL, hold ONTAK.
- Premedicate with antihistamine and acetaminophen to minimize the risk of infusion reaction.
- Give by IV infusion over 30–60 minutes. Do NOT give IV bolus.
- Slow or stop infusion if infusion reaction occurs, depending upon severity of symptoms.
- DO NOT administer with other drugs, or give through an inline filter.
- Administer prepared IV solution within 6 hours, using a syringe pump or infusion bag.
- Administer at least 500-mL 0.9% normal saline IV hydration to reduce risk of vascular leak syndrome.

Drug Interactions:
- Unknown. No studies have been performed.

Lab Effects/Interference:
- Hypoalbuminemia may occur in up to 83% of patients, with nadir 1–2 weeks after drug administration.
- Increased serum transaminases (temporary).

Special Considerations:
- Hypoalbuminemia increases risk of capillary leak syndrome. Delay administration of drug until serum albumin is ≥ 3.0 g/dL.
- There is a delay in manufacturing the drug. Contact the drug company (Eisai) for further information if the drug is difficult to obtain.
- Infusion reactions, defined as symptoms occurring within 24 hours of infusion and resolving within 48 hours of the last infusion in that course, occur in 70.5% of patients across all ONTAK studies, with 8.1% being serious. There have been post-marketing reports of infusion reactions resulting in death. Stop the infusion immediately if an infusion reaction occurs, and permanently discontinue drug if serious. Monitor patients following the infusion. The incidence in patients who complete at least 4 cycles decreases in the third and forth cycles compared to the first and second cycles. Keep resuscitation equipment available.
- Capillary leak syndrome: Defined as the occurrence of at least 2 of the following 3 symptoms: hypotension, edema, serum albumin < 3.0 g/L at any time during ONTAK therapy.
  - Incidence 32.5% of patients; onset may be delayed, occurring up to 2 weeks after infusion. Symptoms may persist or worsen after ONTAK is stopped.
  - One-third of patients required hospitalization or medical intervention to prevent hospitalization.
  - Assess patients for weight gain, development of new or worsening peripheral edema, hypotension including orthostatic hypotension, and albumin level prior to each cycle of therapy to identify early capillary leak syndrome.
  - Hold ONTAK if serum albumin is < 3.0 g/dL.
- Loss of visual acuity, usually with loss of color vision ± retinal pigment mottling, has been reported; recovery occurred in some patients, but most patients had persistent visual impairment.
- Avoid use during pregnancy unless benefit outweighs risk.
- Nursing mothers should make a decision to discontinue nursing or to discontinue ONTAK, taking into account the importance of the drug to the mother's health.
- The most common adverse reactions (≥ 20%) were pyrexia, nausea, fatigue, rigors, vomitng, diarrhea, headache, peripheral edema, cough, dyspnea, and pruritus.
- Hepatobiliary disorders: Increase in ALT or AST from baseline occurred in 84% of patients receiving ONTAK, usually during either the first or second cycle, and resolved without medical intervention.
- Monitor serum albumin prior to the start of each ONTAK treatment course. Delay administration of drug until serum albumin level is at least 3.0 g/dL.
- Teach patients to report:
  - Fever, chills, breathing problems, chest pain, tachycardia, and urticaria following infusion.
  - Rapid weight gain, edema, and orthostatic hypotension following infusion. Teach patients to weigh themselves daily.
  - Visual loss, including loss of color vision.

Potential Toxicities/Side Effects and the Nursing Process

I. POTENTIAL FOR INJURY related to INFUSION REACTIONS, HYPERSENSITIVITY OR ANAPHYLAXIS REACTIONS

Defining Characteristics: Acute hypersensitivity reactions occurred in 69% of patients during clinical trials during or within 24 hours of the ONTAK infusion, with 50% occurring during the first day of dosing of each cycle. Reactions were characterized by hypotension (50%), back pain (30%), dyspnea (28%), vasodilation (28%), rash (25%), chest pain/tightness (24%), tachycardia (12%), dysphagia or laryngismus (5%), syncope (3%), allergic reaction (1%), anaphylaxis (1%). Infusion reaction (fever, chills, asthenia, myalgias, arthralgias, headache) is easily managed. Risk of reaction decreases with premedication with acetaminophen, antihistamines, and corticosteroids (dexamethasone or prednisone 10–20 mg). Steroid premedication may also increase response rates. The incidence of infusion reactions decreases in cycles 3 and 4 for those patients who receive at least 4 cycles. Emergency equipment should be readily available.

Nursing Implications: Assess baseline VS and mental status prior to drug administration, at 15 minutes, and periodically during infusion. Remain with patient during first 15 minutes of infusion. Teach patient to report fever, chills, breathing problems, chest pain, increased heart rate, itching, or urticaria following infusion. Recall signs/symptoms of anaphylaxis and, if these occur, stop drug immediately and notify physician. Subjective symptoms are generalized itching, nausea, chest tightness, crampy abdominal pain, difficulty speaking, anxiety, agitation, sense of impending doom, uneasiness, desire to urinate/defecate, dizziness, chills. Objective signs are flushed appearance; angioedema of face, neck, eyelids, hands, feet; localized or generalized urticaria; respiratory distress with or without wheezing, hypotension, cyanosis. Review standing orders or nursing procedure for patient management of anaphylaxis and be prepared to stop drug immediately, notify physician, monitor VS, and administer ordered medications, which may include epinephrine 1:1,000, hydrocortisone sodium succinate, and diphenhydramine. Teach patient to report any unusual symptoms. Monitor patients postinfusion.

II. POTENTIAL FOR INJURY related to VASCULAR LEAK SYNDROME (VLS)

Defining Characteristics: Twenty-seven percent of patients in clinical trial testing developed VLS about 10 days after the first infusion, characterized by hypotension, edema, and hypoalbuminemia. Onset of symptoms occurs within the first two weeks of infusion and may persist or become more severe after the drug has been stopped. Patients with preexisting cardiac problems are at risk for developing myocardial infarctions. Syndrome is usually self-limiting, but may rarely require management of edema or hypotension. Low serum albumin is a predictor of development of syndrome. The incidence of VLS can be decreased by saline hydration after drug infusion (Duvic, 2006). Capillary leak syndrome is defined as two of the following three symptoms: hypotension, edema, serum albumin < 3.0 g/dL.

Nursing Implications: Monitor weight, orthostatic BP, and serum albumin levels baseline and prior to each cycle; assess for presence of edema baseline and prior to each treatment. Teach patient to report rapid weight gain, edema, and dizziness when standing following infusion. Teach patient to weigh self daily. Notify physician if new or worsening peripheral edema, hypotension, or serum albumin < 3.0 g/dL. Treatment should be delayed until serum albumin is ≥ 3.0 g/dL. Hydrate with at least 500 mL 0.9% NS after drug dose.

III.   POTENTIAL FOR INFECTION related to LYMPHOPENIA, IMMUNE SUPPRESSION OF MACROPHAGES

Defining Characteristics: Cutaneous T-cell lymphoma increases risk of cutaneous infection, together with drug-induced lymphopenia, and impaired immune function further increases risk. During clinical trials, 48% of patients developed infections (23% severe). Lymphocyte counts < 900 cells/µL occurred in 34% of patients. Counts decreased during days 1–5 (dosing period) with recovery by day 15; subsequent cycles had less lymphopenia and more rapid recovery.

Nursing Implications: Assess baseline WBC, lymphocyte count, and monitor weekly during therapy. Assess skin integrity, potential for infection, and teach patient measures to prevent infection (e.g., keeping skin intact, avoiding sources of infection, good hand-washing). Teach patient to report any signs/symptoms of infection (e.g., redness, heat, exudate on skin, T > 100.5°F, sputum production, dysuria). Assess for signs/symptoms of infection during therapy and at each visit.

IV.   ALTERATION IN COMFORT related to FLU-LIKE SYMPTOMS

Defining Characteristics: 91% of patients developed flu-like symptom complex during clinical trials, consisting of fever and chills (81%), asthenia (66%), nausea/vomiting (64%), myalgias (18%), arthralgias (8%). Dehydration occurred in 9% of patients. Symptoms developed within hours to days after having received drug infusion. Symptoms are generally mild to moderate and are responsive to symptom management.

Nursing Implications: Teach patient that flu-like symptoms may occur commonly following treatment, and teach symptom management with antipyretics (e.g., acetaminophen) and dietary modification if nausea experienced. Discuss with physician giving patient prescription for antiemetic agent in case nausea is severe or vomiting develops. Discuss use of meperidine, diphenhydramine if patient develops rigors. Teach patient to call nurse or physician if symptoms do not respond, become worse, if unable to take at least 1 qt of fluid orally per day, or new symptoms develop.

V.   ALTERATION IN NUTRITION related to DIARRHEA, ANOREXIA, NAUSEA/ VOMITING, HYPOALBUMINEMIA

Defining Characteristics: Nausea/vomiting occurs in 64% of patients as part of flu-like syndrome, anorexia occurs in 36% of patients, and diarrhea occurs in 29%.

Hypoalbuminemia occurs in 83%, weight loss in 14%, and elevated transaminases in 61%. Elevation of serum transaminases occurred during first cycle of therapy and resolved within 2 weeks. Hypocalcemia (17%) and hypokalemia (6%) have also been reported. Constipation occurred in 9%, dyspepsia in 7%, and dysphagia in 6%. Rarely, pancreatitis, hyperthyroidism, and hypothyroidism may occur.

Nursing Implications: Assess baseline nutritional status, as well as baseline LFTs and serum albumin, and monitor weekly during therapy. Teach patient to eat high-calorie, high-protein foods. Assess for occurrence of symptoms of nausea, vomiting, diarrhea, anorexia, other problems, and teach patient to report them. Teach patient self-administration of prescribed medications to manage symptoms.

VI.   ALTERATION IN COMFORT related to SKIN RASHES, PAIN AT TUMOR SITES

Defining Characteristics: During clinical trials, rash occurred in 34%, pruritus 20%, and sweating 10%. Rashes occurred during/after treatment or were delayed. They were varied, as generalized maculopapular, petechial, vesicular bullous, or urticarial, or as eczema.

Nursing Implications: Assess baseline skin integrity and presence of rashes. Assess daily during treatment and weekly thereafter; teach patient to report any skin changes. Assess need for diphenhydramine or other antihistamines for pruritus, and use of topical and/or oral corticosteroids for moderate to severe rashes and discomfort.

Drug: dinutuximab (Unituxin)

Class: Monoclonal antibody; GD2 binding.

Mechanism of Action: Dinutuximab binds to the glycolipid GD2, which is expressed on neuroblastoma cells and normal cells derived from the neuroectoderm. Through binding, the drug induces cell lysis of GD2-expressing cells through antibody-dependent cell-mediated toxicity (ADCC) and complement-dependent cytotoxicity (CDC).

Metabolism: Drug terminal half-life is 10 days.

Indication: In combination with GM-CSF, interleukin-2 (IL-2), and 13-*cis*-retinoic acid (RA) for the treatment of pediatric patients with high-risk neuroblastoma who achieve at least a partial response to prior first-line multiagent, multimodality therapy.

Contraindications: Patients who have had anaphylaxis to dinutuximab.

Dosage/Range:
- 17.5 mg/m^2 as a diluted IV infusion over 10–20 hours for 4 consecutive days for up to 5 cycles.
- Cycles 1, 3, and 5 are 24 days in duration, and are given in combination with GM-CSF.
- Cycles 2 and 4 are 32 days in duration, and are given in combination with IL-2.

Dose Modifications:
- Permanently discontinue drug for grade 3 or 4 anaphylaxis; grade 3 or 4 serum sickness; grade 3 pain, unresponsive to maximal supportive measures; grade 4 sensory neuropathy or grade 3 sensory neuropathy that interferes with daily activities for more than 2 weeks; grade 2 peripheral motor neuropathy; grade 4 hyponatremia despite appropriate fluid management; subtotal or total vision loss.
- Mild to moderate symptoms (e.g., transient rash, fever, rigors, localized urticaria that responds promptly to symptomatic treatment):
  - Onset of reaction: Reduce dinutuximab rate to 50% of previous rate, and monitor closely.
  - After resolution, gradually increase rate up to a maximum rate of 1.75 mg/m^2/hr.
- Prolonged or severe adverse reactions (e.g., mild bronchospasm without other symptoms, angioedema that does not affect the airway):
  - Onset: Immediately interrupt dinutuximab infusion.
  - After resolution, if signs and symptoms resolve rapidly, resume dinutuximab at 50% of the previous rate and monitor closely.
  - First recurrence: Discontinue dinutuximab until the following day. If symptoms resolve and continued treatment is warranted, premedicate with hydrocortisone 1 mg/kg (maximum 50 mg) IV and administer dinutuximab at a rate of 0.875 mg/m^2/hr in an ICU.
  - Second recurrence: Permanently discontinue dinutuximab.
- Capillary leak syndrome (CLS):
  - Moderate to severe but not life-threatening CLS:
    - Onset: Immediately interrupt dinutuximab.
    - After resolution: Resume dinutuximab at 50% of the previous rate.
  - *Life-threatening CLS:*
    - Onset: Discontinue dinutuximab for the current cycle.
    - After resolution: In subsequent cycles, administer dinutuximab at 50% of the previous rate.
    - First recurrence: Permanently discontinue dinutuximab.
- Hypotension (symptomatic, systolic BP [SBP] < lower limit of normal for age, or SBP decreased by more than 15% compared to baseline) requiring medical intervention:
  - Onset: Interrupt dinutuximab infusion.
  - After resolution: Resume dinutuximab infusion at 50% of previous rate. If BP remains stable for ≥ 2 hours, increase the infusion rate as tolerated up to a maximum rate of 1.75 mg/m^2/hr.
- Severe infection or sepsis: At onset of reaction, discontinue dinutuximab until resolution of infection; then proceed with subsequent cycles of therapy.
- Neurologic disorders of the eye (e.g., blurred vision, photophobia, mydriasis, fixed or unequal pupils, optic nerve disorder, eyelid ptosis, papilledema):
  - Onset of reaction: Discontinue dinutuximab until resolution.
  - After resolution: Reduce dinutuximab dose by 50%.
  - First recurrence or if accompanied by visual impairment: Permanently discontinue dinutuximab.

Drug Preparation: Available as injection solution of 17.5 mg/5 mL (3.5 mg/mL) in a single-use vial.
- Store vials in a refrigerator at 2–8°C (36–46°F). Protect from light by storing in the outer carton. *Do not freeze or shake vials.*
- Visually inspect for particulate matter and discoloration, and do not use the vial if the solution is cloudy or discolored, or contains particulate matter.
- Aseptically withdraw the required volume of dinutuximab from the single-use vial and inject into a 100-mL bag of 0.9% sodium chloride injection USP. Mix by gentle inversion. Do not shake. Discard any unused drug in the vial.
- Store the diluted dinutuximab solution under refrigeration (2–8°C [36–46°F]). Initiate infusion within 4 hours of preparation.
- Discard diluted dinutuximab solution 24 hours after preparation.

Drug Administration:
- Cycles 1, 3, and 5 are 24 days in duration; cycles 2 and 4 are 32 days in duration.
- Assess serum electrolytes daily and monitor CBC/differential closely during dinutuximab therapy.
- Assess temperature, blood pressure, respirations, neurologic vital signs (including pupil size, reactivity to light, and bilateral strengths); ask if patient has experienced any visual changes, numbness/tingling, motor weakness, or changes in ability to do ADLs. Assess for signs and symptoms of infection. Assess level of comfort and presence of pain.
- Pretreatment:
  - *IV hydration* of 10 mL/kg of 0.9% sodium chloride injection USP IV over 1 hour just prior to starting each dinutuximab infusion.
  - *Analgesics*:
    - Morphine sulfate 50 mcg/kg IV immediately prior to initiation of dinutuximab, then continue as a morphine drip at an infusion rate of 20–50 mcg/kg/hr during and for 2 hours after the completion of dinutuximab.
    - Administer additional 25 mcg/kg to 50 mg/kg IV doses of morphine sulfate as needed for pain up to once every 2 hours, followed by an increase in the morphine sulfate infusion rate in clinically stable patients.
    - Consider fentanyl or hydromorphone if morphine sulfate is poorly tolerated.
    - If pain is inadequately managed with opioids, consider gabapentin or lidocaine in conjunction with IV morphine.
  - *Antihistamines and antipyretics:*
    - Administer an antihistamine such as diphenhydramine (0.5–1 mg/kg; maximum dose of 50 mg) IV over 10–15 minutes starting 20 minutes prior to the start of dinutuximab, and as tolerated every 4–6 hours during dinutuximab infusion.
    - Administer acetaminophen (10–15 mg/kg; maximum dose of 650 mg) 20 minutes prior to each dinutuximab infusion, and every 4–6 hours as needed for fever or pain. Administer ibuprofen (5–10 mg/kg) every 6 hours as needed for control of persistent fever or pain.
- Initiate infusion at a rate of dinutuximab 0.875 mg/m^2/hr for 30 minutes. Gradually increase the rate as tolerated to a maximum rate of 1.75 mg/m^2/hr.

- Monitor patient closely for signs and symptoms of an infusion reaction during and for 4 hours after the end of the infusion. Immediately interrupt the dinutuximab infusion for severe infusion reactions, and permanently discontinue it if anaphylaxis occurs.

Drug Interactions: No drug–drug studies have been conducted.

Lab Effects/Interference:
- Hyponatremia, hypokalemia, hypocalcemia, hypoalbuminemia, hypophosphatemia, and hypomagnesemia: Immediately interrupt therapy.
- Thrombocytopenia, lymphopenia, anemia, and neutropenia.
- Hyperglycemia and hypertriglyceridemia.
- Increased ALT, AST, and serum creatinine.
- Proteinuria.

Special Considerations:
- Black box warnings:
  - Serious and potentially life-threatening infusion reactions occurred in 26% of patients; administer prehydration and premedication (including antihistamines) prior to each dinutuximab infusion. Monitor patients closely for signs and symptoms of an infusion reaction during and for 4 hours after the end of each dinutuximab infusion. Interrupt the drug for severe reactions, and permanently discontinue it if anaphylaxis occurs.
  - Severe neuropathic pain occurs in most patients during the infusion. Administer IV opioids prior to, during, and for 2 hours after the end of each infusion. Grade 3 peripheral sensory neuropathy occurred in 2–9% of patients. Severe motor neuropathy was observed in adults receiving dinutuximab, and may not resolve in all cases. The drug should be permanently discontinued for severe unresponsive pain, severe sensory neuropathy, or moderate to severe peripheral motor neuropathy.
- CLS and hypotension may occur; ensure prehydration is administered and monitor closely during infusion. To manage these effects, depending on their severity, interrupt the infusion, decrease the infusion rate, or permanently discontinue dinutuximab.
- Infection (systemic): Dinutuximab should be interrupted until infection resolves.
- Neurologic disorders of the eye: Dinutuximab should be interrupted for dilated pupils with sluggish light reflex or other visual disturbances; permanently discontinue for recurrence of eye disorder or loss of vision.
- Bone marrow suppression: Monitor peripheral blood counts during therapy.
- Electrolyte disturbances: Incidence is 25%; severe hypokalemia occurred in 37% of patients, and 23% had severe hyponatremia. Monitor serum electrolytes closely.
- Atypical hemolytic uremic syndrome (HUS): Permanently discontinue dinutuximab and provide supportive management.
- Nausea and vomiting: Incidence rates are 46% (6% grades 3–4) and 19% (2% grades 3–4) of patients, respectively. Incidence of diarrhea is 43% (13% grades 3–4).
- Dinutuximab may cause fetal harm. Teach women of reproductive potential to use effective contraception.

• Most common adverse reactions (≥25%) are pain, pyrexia, thrombocytopenia, lymphopenia, infusion reactions, hypotension, hyponatremia, increased ALT, anemia, vomiting, diarrhea, hypokalemia, CLS, neutropenia, urticarial, hypoalbuminemia, increased AST, and hypocalcemia.

• Most common serious reactions (≥5%) are infections, infusion reactions, hypokalemia, hypotension, pain, fever, and CLS.

Potential Toxicities/Side Effects and the Nursing Process

I. POTENTIAL FOR INJURY related to INFUSION-RELATED REACTIONS

Defining Characteristics: Infusion reactions usually occurred during or within 24 hours of dinutuximab infusion. Serious infusion reactions (grade 3 or 4) occurred in 26% of patients receiving dinutuximab with RA compared to 1% receiving RA alone. Urgent intervention was required for facial and upper airway edema, dyspnea, bronchospasm, stridor, urticaria, and hypotension. Signs and symptoms may overlap with hypersensitivity reactions. One patient had multiple cardiac arrests and died within 24 hours after dinutuximab infusion.

Nursing Implications: Ensure that premedications are administered prior to dinutuximab infusion. Monitor the patient closely during the infusion and for 4 hours after the infusion is completed. The clinical setting should have resources for cardiopulmonary resuscitation (medications, equipment, qualified responders) if needed. For mild to moderate infusion reactions (e.g., rash, fever, rigors, and localized urticaria) that respond promptly to antihistamines or antipyretics, reduce the infusion rate and monitor the patient closely. If severe or prolonged infusion reactions occur, immediately interrupt or permanently discontinue dinutuximab, and provide supportive management. If life-threatening effects occur, dinutuximab should be permanently discontinued. Urgent interventions for severe infusion reactions include interruption of dinutuximab, BP support, bronchodilator therapy, and corticosteroids.

II. ALTERATION IN COMFORT related to PAIN

Defining Characteristics: Up to 85% of patients experience pain despite opioid analgesic pretreatment, and it is severe (grade 3) in 51%. Pain occurs during the infusion, and is characterized as abdominal, generalized, extremity, back musculoskeletal chest pain, neuralgia, or arthralgia.

Nursing Implications: Document baseline comfort level and any analgesics used. Premedicate with analgesics (including opioids) prior to each dinutuximab dose; continue analgesics as a continuous infusion during the dinutuximab infusion, and for 2 hours after the dose is completed. If pain is severe, decrease the dinutuximab infusion rate to 0.875 mg/m^2/hr. If pain persists despite opioids, other analgesics, and infusion rate reduction, dinutuximab should be discontinued.

III.   ALTERATION IN ACTIVITY, POTENTIAL, related to NEUROPATHY

Defining Characteristics: Peripheral neuropathy occurred in 13% of patients, and 3% experienced grade 3 (severe) effects. Peripheral sensory neuropathy affected 9% of patients, with a median duration of 9 days. Peripheral motor neuropathy is more common in adult patients compared to pediatric patients.

Nursing Implications: Assess patient for signs and symptoms of peripheral sensory (e.g., paresthesias, dysesthesias) and motor neuropathy (e.g., weakness). Discuss any findings with physician/NP/PA. Dinutuximab should be permanently discontinued in patients with grade 2 peripheral motor neuropathy, grade 3 sensory neuropathy (interferes with ADLs for more than 2 weeks), or grade 4 sensory neuropathy.

IV.   ALTERATION IN SENSORY PERCEPTION, VISUAL, related to NEUROLOGIC
      DISORDERS OF THE EYE

Defining Characteristics: Incidence is 2–15%, and includes blurred vision, photophobia, mydriasis, fixed or unequal pupils, optic nerve disorder, eyelid ptosis, and papilledema. Median duration is 4 days.

Nursing Implications: Assess the patient for pupil equality in size and reaction to light; assess for ptosis. Ask if patient has experienced any changes in vision, and discuss findings with physician/NP/PA. Teach the patient to report any changes in vision immediately. Dinutuximab should be interrupted if the patient experiences dilated pupils with sluggish light reflex or other visual disturbances that do not cause visual loss. Once this reaction is resolved, dinutuximab dose should be reduced by 50% if further therapy is warranted. The drug should be permanently discontinued if the patient has recurrent signs and symptoms following dose reduction, or if the patient experiences loss of vision.

V.   INCREASED RISK OF INFECTION, BLEEDING related to BONE MARROW
      DEPRESSION

Defining Characteristics: Incidence in clinical trials was 66% for thrombocytopenia (39% grades 3–4), 62% for lymphopenia (51% grades 3–4), 51% for anemia (34% grades 3–4), and 39% for neutropenia (34% grades 3–4). Infections included sepsis (incidence 18%; 16% grades 3–4) and device-related infection (16%; 16% grades 3–4). Hemorrhage occurred in 17% of patients (6% grades 3–4).

Nursing Implications: Assess CBC/differential. Assess the patient for signs and symptoms of systemic infection and bleeding, and discuss with physician/NP/PA the possibility of drug interruption until the infection resolves. Teach the patient self-care strategies to minimize the risks of infection and bleeding, and to report any signs and symptoms of infection or bleeding right away.

VI.   ALTERATION IN HOMEOSTASIS related to CAPILLARY LEAK SYNDROME

Defining Characteristics: CLS occurred in 40% of patients and was severe (grades 3–4) in 23%. Hypotension occurred in 60% (16% grades 3–4). Hypoxia was reported by 24% of patients (12% grades 3–4). CLS is characterized by loss of vascular tone and extravasation of plasma proteins and fluid into the extravascular space. This results in hypotension and decreased organ perfusion. CLS may be associated with cardiac arrhythmias, angina, MI, respiratory insufficiency requiring intubation, GI bleeding, edema, and mental status changes.

Nursing Implications: Assess the patient at baseline and during the infusion for signs and symptoms of CLS, including hypotension. Ensure prehydration is administered. If signs and symptoms are identified, discuss interventions immediately with physician/NP/PA *as infusion should be immediately interrupted*. If the patient has mild or moderate signs and symptoms, expect that when the patient's symptoms return to baseline, the infusion will be resumed at 50% of the previous rate. If life-threatening reaction occurs, discontinue the drug for the current cycle. In addition, be prepared to implement orders for emergency, supportive management. For subsequent cycles, after life-threatening CLS has resolved, the patient should receive the dinutuximab infusion at 50% of the previous rate. If signs and symptoms of CLS recur, the drug should be permanently discontinued.

Drug: erlotinib (Tarceva)

Class: Kinase inhibitor (epidermal growth factor receptor (HER-1/EGFR1) tyrosine kinase inhibitor).

Mechanism of Action: Mechanism of antitumor activity not fully characterized. Inhibits the phosphorylation of the intracellular portion of the EGFR or tyrosine kinase domain of the EGFR. Erlotinib binding affinitiy for EGFR exon 19 deletion or exon 21 (L858R) mutation is higher than its affinity for the wild-type (normal) receptor. This inhibits the activation of cell signaling telling the nucleus of the cell to divide, to avoid programmed cell death, and to release vascular endothelial growth factor (VEGF). EGFR is expressed on the cell surface of normal as well as cancer cells.

Metabolism: Drug bioavailability is about 60% after oral administration with peak plasma concentration occurring four hours after ingestion. Erlotinib solubility is pH-dependent, with erlotinib solubility decreasing as the pH increases. Coadministration of erlotinib with omeprazole, a proton pump inhibitor, decreased erlotinib exposure (AUC) and maximum concentration (C_{max}) by 46% and 61% respectively. When erlotinib is administered 2 hrs following a dose of ranitidine 300 mg (an H2 receptor antagonist), the erlotinib AUC was reduced by 33% and C_{max} by 54%; when erlotinib was administered 10 hrs. after the previous ranitidine evening dose and 2 hrs. before the ranitidine morning dose, the erlotinib AUC and C_{max} decreased by 15% and 17%, respectively.

Drug is highly protein-bound (93%). Drug is eliminated by hepatic metabolism and biliary excretion. It is primarily metabolized by the cytochrome P450 hepatic microsomal enzyme system (CYP3A4). Excretion is primarily fecal (83%, with 1% intact parent drug), with 8% excreted in the urine. Food can increase drug bioavailability by 100%. Smoking increases erlotinib clearance by 24% and decreases erotinib serum concentration.

Indications:
- First-line treatment of patients with metastatic NSCLC whose tumors have EGFR exon 19 deletions or exon 21 (L858R) substitution mutations, as detected by an FDA-approved test.
- Maintenance treatment of patients with locally advanced or metastatic NSCLC whose disease has not progressed after 4 cycles of platinum-based first-line chemotherapy.
- Treatment of patients with locally advanced or metastatic NSCLC after failure of at least 1 prior chemotherapy regimen.
- First-line treatment of patients with locally advanced, unresectable metastatic pancreatic cancer, in combination with gemcitabine.
- Limitations of use:
  - Not recommended for use in combination with platinum-based chemotherapy.
  - Safety and efficacy have not been evaluated as first-line therapy in patients with metastatic NSCLC whose tumors have EGFR mutations other than exon 19 deletions or exon 21 (L858R) substitutions.
- FDA-approved tests for the detection of EGFR mutations in NSCLC are available at http://www.fda.gov/CompanionDiagnostics.

Dosage/Range:
- Tarceva (erlotinib) is available only through select specialty pharmacies as of 7/1/13 (www.tarceva.com).
- Non-small-cell lung cancer (NSCLC): 150 mg PO once daily on an empty stomach at least one hour before or two hours after meals. Treatment should continue until disease progression or unacceptable toxicity occurs.
- Pancreatic cancer: 100 mg PO once daily on an empty stomach at least one hour before or two hours after meals, in combination with gemcitabine. Treatment should continue until disease progression or unacceptable toxicity occurs.
- Dose-reduce in 50-mg decrements when necessary.

Dose Modifications:
- **Discontinue** erlotinib for (1) interstitial lung disease (ILD); (2) severe hepatic toxicity that does not improve significantly or resolve within three weeks; (3) GI perforation; (4) severe bullous, blistering, or exfoliating skin conditions; (5) corneal perforation or severe ulceration.
- **Hold** erlotinib (1) during diagnostic evaluation for possible ILD; (2) for severe CTCAE grade 3 or 4 renal toxicity and consider drug discontinuance; (3) in patients without preexisting hepatic impairment for total bilirubin levels > 3 × ULN or transaminases > 5 × ULN, and consider erlotnib discontinuation; (4) in patients with preexisting hepatic impairment or biliary obstruction for doubling of bilirubin or tripling of transaminases values over baseline and consider discontinuation of erlotinib; (5) for persistent severe diarrhea not responsive to medical management (e.g., loperamide); (6) for severe rash not responsive to medical management; (7) for keratitis of (NCI-CTC version 4.0) grade 3–4

or for grade 2 lasting > 2 weeks; (8) for acute/worsening ocular disorders such as eye pain, and consider erlotinib discontinuation.

- **Reduce erlotinib by 50-mg decrements:** (1) if severe reactions occur with concomitant use of strong CYP3A4 inhibitors (see drug listing in Drug Interactions) or when using an inhibitor of both CYP3A4 and CYP1A2 (e.g., ciprofloxacin), avoid concomitant use if possible; (2) when restarting therapy following withholding treatment for a dose-limiting toxicity that has resolved to baseline or grade < or equal to 1.
- **Increase erlotinib dose by 50-mg increments as tolerated for:** (1) concomitant use with CYP3A4 inducers (see drug listing in Drug Interactions, increase dose by 50-mg increments at two-week intervals to a maximum 450-mg dose. Avoid concomitant use if possible); (2) concurrent cigarette smoking, increase dose by 50-mg increments at two-week intervals to a maximum of 300 mg. Immediately reduce the dose of erlotinib to the recommended dose (150 mg or 100 mg daily) upon cessation of smoking.
- **Drugs affecting gastric pH:** (1) avoid concomitant use of proton pump inhibitors (PPI) if possible, as separation of dose may not eliminate the interaction, and as PPIs affect the pH of the upper GI tract for an extended period; (2) if treatment with an H_2 receptor antagonist like ranitidine is required, erlotinib must be taken 10 hours AFTER H_2 receptor antagonist dose, and at least 2 hours BEFORE the next dose of the H_2 receptor antagonist; (3) antacids should be taken several hours before or after erlotinib.

Drug Preparation/Administration:
- Oral, available in 150-, 100-, and 25-mg tablets.
- Dose should be taken on an empty stomach, at least one hour before meals or two hours after meals.

Drug Interactions:
- *Inducers of CYP3A4* (may increase metabolism of erlotinib and **decrease erlotinib plasma concentration**): rifampicin, rifapentine, rifabutin, phenytoin, phenobarbital, St. John's wort, carbamazepine; avoid if possible; otherwise may need to increase dose of erlotinib.
- *Rifampicin* decreased erlotinib area under the curve (AUC) by 66% to 80%: use alternative drug that does not induce CYP3A4, or consider erlotinib dose escalation every two weeks while monitoring the patient, to a maximum dose of 450 mg. If the erlotinib dose is increased and rifampicin (or other inducer) is discontinued, reduce erlotinib dose immediately to the indicated starting dose.
- *Inhibitors of CYP3A4* (may decrease metabolism of erlotinib and **increase erlotinib plasma concentration**); strong inhibitors (e.g., atazanavir, clarithromycin, indinavir, itraconazole, ketoconazole, nefazodone, nelfinavir, ritonavir, saquinavir, telithromycin, troleandomycin [TAO], voriconazole, or grapefruit [fruit or juice]): consider dose reduction of erlotinib if severe reactions occur.
- *Inhibitor of CYP3A4 and CYP1A2* (e.g., ciprofloxacin): consider dose reduction of erlotinib if severe reactions occur.
- *CYP1A2 Inducers*: may decrease erlotinib plasma concentrations.
- *CYP1A2 Inhibitors* (e.g., ciprofloxacin): may increase erlotinib plasma concentrations.

- Erlotinib solubility is pH dependent. Drugs that alter the pH of the upper GI tract may alter erlotinib solubility and its absorption. There is risk of low erlotinib serum levels if the drug is given in combination with drugs that change GI pH, such as omeprazole (a proton pump inhibitor, PPI) or ranitidine (an H_2 receptor antagonist). Avoid concomitant use of PPIs and erlotinib, as dose separation may not eliminate the drug interaction. If treatment with an H2-receptor antagonist is necessary (e.g., ranitidine), erlotinib must be taken 10 hours after the H2-receptor antagonist, and at least two hours before the next dose of ranitidine. Antacids should be separated by several hours from the dose of erlotinib.
- *Warfarin* increases International Normalized Ration (INR) and bleeding is possible; monitor INR and patient bleeding, and decrease warfarin dose as needed.
- Cigarette smoking reduces serum levels of erlotinib so drug may be ineffective in smokers; teach patients to quit; it is unclear whether nicotine patches also inactivate the drug. If the patient cannot stop smoking, the erlotinib dose may be titrated upward. However, if the patient is able to stop smoking, then the dose should be immediately reduced to the indicated starting dose.

Lab Effects/Interference:
- May increase liver function tests (serum transaminases).
- May increase INR with increased potential for bleeding.

Special Considerations:
- Drug is not recommended for use in combination with platinum-based chemotherapy. The drug's safety and efficacy have not been studied as first-line treatment of metastatic NSCLC in patients whose tumors have EGFR mutations other than exon 19 deletions or exon 21 (L858R) substitutions.
- Cases of serious ILD, including fatal cases, can occur with erlotinib. Incidence was 1.1% across all studies. This is a class effect of EGFR inhibitors.
  - Onset of symptoms between 5 days to > 9 months (median 39 days) after beginning erlotinib therapy.
  - Drug should be stopped immediately in patients who develop acute onset of new or progressive unexplained pulmonary symptoms, such as dyspnea, cough, and fever. Begin appropriate diagnostic workup to establish the cause.
  - If ILD is diagnosed, erlotinib should be discontinued.
  - Gemcitabine may also cause ILD. Contributing factors include concomitant/prior chemotherapy, prior radiotherapy, preexisting parenchymal lung disease, metastatic lung disease, and pulmonary infections.
- Acute renal failure, renal insufficiency, and hepatorenal syndrome have been reported; some cases may be fatal.
  - Renal failure may arise from exacerbation of underlying baseline hepatic impairment or severe dehydration. Incidence in NSCLC was 0.5% (vs 0.8% in control), and 1.4% in erlotinib-plus-gemcitabine arm (vs 0.4% in control).
  - Monitor renal function and electrolytes during erlotinib therapy.
  - Interrupt erlotinib in patients developing severe renal impairment until renal toxicity has resolved.
- Hepatotoxicity with or without hepatic impairment, including hepatic failure and hepatorenal syndrome, has been reported; in some cases, it may be fatal. This can occur

in patients with normal hepatic function, but risk is increased in patients with baseline hepatic impairment.

- Monitor patient LFTs (transaminases, bilirubin, alkaline phosphatase) at baseline and periodically during treatment; increase monitoring frequency in patients with preexisting hepatic impairment or biliary obstruction.
- Hold erlotinib in patients without preexisting hepatic impairment for total bilirubin > 3 × ULN or transaminases > 5 × ULN.
- Hold erlotinib in patients with preexisting hepatic impairment or biliary obstruction for doubling of bilirubin or tripling of transaminase values over baseline.
- Discontinue erlotinib if abnormal LFTs meeting above criteria do not improve significantly or resolve within 3 weeks. See package insert.
- GI perforation may occur, and some cases may be fatal.
  - Patients at risk are those receiving concomitant antiangiogenic drug(s), NSAIDs, corticosteroids, and/or taxane-based chemotherapy, or those who have a prior history of peptic ulceration or diverticular disease.
  - Incidence in erlotinib-containing arms was 0.2% in NSCLC studies (vs 0.1% in control), and 0.4% in pancreatic studies (vs 0% in control).
  - Permanently discontinue erlotinib if GI perforation occurs.
- Bullous, blistering, and exfoliative skin disorders can occur, some resembling Stevens-Johnson syndrome/Toxic epidermal necrolysis. Some cases were fatal. Incidence in erlotinib-containing arms was 1.2% in NSCLC studies (vs 0% in control), and 0.4% in pancreatic studies (vs 0% in control). Discontinue erlotinib if severe bullous, blistering, or exfoliating conditions occur
- Myocardial infarction/ischemia was reported in the pancreatic cancer trials (incidence 2.1%) in the erlotinib/gemcitabine group compared to 1.1%; incidence of cerebrovascular accident (CVA) was also increased (incidence 2.5% compared to 0% in control arm).
- Microangiopathic hemolytic anemia with thrombocytopenia has occurred in patients with pancreatic cancer receiving erlotinib/gemcitabine (incidence 1.4% vs 0% in control).
- Ocular disorders: decreased tear production, abnormal eyelash growth, keratoconjunctivitis sicca or keratitis can occur with erlotinib therapy and can lead to corneal perforation or ulceration.
  - Incidence in NSCLC studies was 17.8% in erlotinib group vs 4% in control arm, and in pancreatic cancer studies, incidence was 12.8%, vs 11.4% in control arm.
  - Interrupt erlotinib or discontinue erlotinib in patients with acute or worsening ocular disorders such as eye pain.
- Hemorrhage in patients taking warfarin: International Normalized Ratio (INR) elevations and bleeding events (including hemorrhage and fatalities) associated with warfarin administration have been reported. Closely monitor patients taking warfarin or other coumarin-derivative anticoagulants, and adjust dose of warfarin accordingly.
- Erlotinib can cause fetal harm, so women of reproductive potential should use highly effective contraception to avoid pregnancy during therapy, and for at least 2 weeks after the last dose of erlotinib.

- Advise patients to contact their healthcare provider if they become pregnant, or if pregnancy is suspected, while taking erlotinib.
- If erlotinib is used during pregnancy, or if the patient becomes pregnant while taking erlotinib, the patient should be apprised of the potential hazard to the fetus.
- Women who are nursing should decide whether to discontinue nursing or to discontinue erlotinib, taking into account the importance of the drug to the patient's health.
- Most common toxicities (≥ 20%): rash, diarrhea, anorexia, fatigue, dyspnea, cough, nausea, vomiting.
- Teach patient to report promptly (1) onset or worsening of skin rash or development of bullous lesions or desquamation; (2) severe or persistent diarrhea, nausea, anorexia, or vomiting; (3) onset or worsening of unexplained shortness of breath (SOB) or cough; and (4) eye irritation.

Potential Toxicities/Side Effects and the Nursing Process

I.   ALTERATION IN SKIN INTEGRITY related to RASH

Defining Characteristics: As expected, because EGFR is important in skin function, this is the area of major toxicity. Rash ranges from maculopapular to pustular on the face, neck, chest, back, and arms, affecting up to 75% of patients. Most rashes are mild to moderate (Sandler et al., 2004). Typically, rash begins on days 8 through 10 of therapy, maximizing in intensity by week 2, and resolving gradually on therapy (often by week 4). Skin treatments (corticosteroids, topical clindamycin, or minocycline) have been used with varying results.

Nursing Implications: Assess skin integrity of face, neck, arms, and upper trunk baseline, and regularly during treatment. Teach patient that rash may occur, its usual course, and self-care measures for comfort. Emphasize the need to keep skin with rash clean to prevent infection, and to continue taking erlotinib until told to stop by nurse or physician. Teach patient that skin may become dry, and to use skin emollients or moisturizers. Assess body image intactness, and if rash develops, its threat to body image. Encourage patient to verbalize feelings; provide emotional support, and individualize care plan to patient response. For rash management, refer to the introduction in *Chapter 5*. Teach all patients to (1) use a water-based emollient frequently during the day to prevent dryness, (2) stay hydrated, (3) avoid sun exposure and wear SPF 30 (zinc-based). Do not use anti-acne medications. Tetracycline analogues provide anti-inflammatory benefit. **Grade 1/ mild rash** (localized, does not interfere with ADLs, and is not infected): Goal is to preserve skin integrity, minimize discomfort, and prevent infection. Key patient teaching includes (1) use a mild soap with active ingredients that reduce skin drying, such as pyrithione zinc (Head & Shoulders), (2) consider applying aloe gel to red, tender areas, (3) report distressing tenderness, as pramoxine (lidocaine topical anesthetic) may help, (4) keep fingernails clean and trimmed, and (5) apply zinc ointment to rectal mucosa after washing. Management: maintain current drug dose, observe or give topical hydrocortisone 1% or 2.5% or clindamycin 1% gel (anti-inflammatory benefit), reassess in 2 weeks. **For grade 2/moderate,** which is generalized, mild symptoms, and has minimal effect on ADLs, and no infection: Goal is to prevent infection and promote comfort.

Continue EGFRI dose; use topicals (hydrocortisone 2.5% or clindamycin 1% gel) and consider adding doxycycline 100 mg PO twice daily or minocycline 100 mg PO twice daily (give antimicrobial and anti-inflammatory effect) and reassess after 2 weeks. **For grade 3–4 or severe rash** (generalized, severe, has a significant impact on ADLs, and increased risk of infection): The goal is to prevent infection or identify it early to minimize complications and to promote effective coping. Interrupt drug. Treat rash with topicals (hydrocortisone 2.5%, or clindamycin 1% gel), doxycycline 100 mg PO twice daily or minocycline 100 mg PO twice daily, and methylprednisolone (Medrol dose pack); reassess after 2 weeks. Resume drug when rash improved to grade 2, at full or reduced dose. (Lynch et al., 2007; Lacouture et al., 2011). If rash appears infected (exudate, vesicular formation, different appearance), obtain C+S, treat empirically until sensitivity received, and/or obtain dermatology consult. Hold drug for severe rash that does not respond to medical intervention.

Teach patient to report right away the development of bullous lesions or desquamation.

II. ALTERATION IN ELIMINATION PATTERN related to DIARRHEA

Defining Characteristics: Affects approximately 54% of patients and is mild to moderate, with only 6% of patients experiencing grade 3 diarrhea. Diarrhea usually begins weeks 3 through 4. Symptoms may be self-limited or require an antidiarrheal agent, such as loperamide. Severe diarrhea not responsive to antidiarrheal medication may require temporary dose interruption or adjustment if refractory.

Nursing Implications: Assess bowel elimination pattern baseline, and regularly during therapy. Teach patient to report diarrhea; teach patient self-care strategies to manage diarrhea such as dietary modification and self-administration of loperamide; teach patient to minimize potential complications such as dehydration and electrolyte depletion. Identify patients at risk for dehydration and follow closely, such as patients with renal insufficiency, diabetes, congestive heart failure, or the older population. If diarrhea does not resolve or is severe, discuss with physician dose interruption, as well as fluid and electrolyte replacement. If dose needs to be reduced, reduce in 50-mg increments. If diarrhea is refractory or difficult to manage, patient may become dehydrated and will be at risk for acute renal failure, which may be fatal. If the patient is dehydrated and at risk for renal impairment (e.g., preexisting renal disease, disease or medications that may lead to renal disease, advancing age), the drug should be temporarily discontinued while the patient is rehydrated. Renal function should be assessed at baseline and periodically during therapy, more closely if the patient has diarrhea and is at risk for dehydration. Hold drug for severe diarrhea that does not respond to medical intervention.

III. SENSORY/PERCEPTUAL ALTERATION, POTENTIAL, related to CONJUNCTIVITIS AND EYE DRYNESS

Defining Characteristics: Decreased tear production, abnormal eyelash growth, keratoconjunctivitis, or keratitis can occur. Pooled incidence of ocular disorders in three NSCLC trials was 17.8% in the erlotinib arm, and 4% in the control arm. Incidence in erlotinib/

gemcitabine arm was 12.8% and 11.4% in the control arm. Rarely, corneal ulceration or perforation may occur.

Nursing Implications: Teach patient to report any eye irritation, pain, or change in visual acuity. Teach patient to use artificial tears to keep eyes lubricated. Refer patient to ophthalmologist immediately for any acute signs or symptoms, such as red eye or eye pain. Teach patient to stop drug if these occur, and to report them immediately. Drug is discontinued for corneal perforation, ulceration, or keratitis of (NCI-CTCAE version 4.0) grade 3–4 or for grade 2 lasting > 2 weeks.

IV.   POTENTIAL ALTERATION IN NUTRITION, LESS THAN BODY REQUIREMENTS, related to MUCOSITIS, HEPATOTOXICITY, ANOREXIA, NAUSEA, VOMITING

Defining Characteristics: Stomatitis is uncommon, occurring in 17% of patients receiving erlotinib, compared with 3% receiving placebo. Grade 3–4 occurs in < 1% of patients. It is usually mild to moderate and is generally self-limited. Anorexia affects about 52% of patients, with 8% experiencing grade 3. Hepatotoxicity may occur, especially in patients with baseline hepatic impairment.

Nursing Implications: Assess oral hygiene practices, and status of oral mucosa, gums, and teeth baseline and regularly throughout therapy. Assess nutritional status and weight baseline and regularly during treatment. Teach patient to report stomatitis, and to use a systematic cleansing regimen as determined by institutional policy. Assess baseline LFTs, and monitor LFTs and patient tolerance very closely during therapy if abnormal at baseline. If a patient develops worsening LFTs, discuss with physician dose interruption or discontinuance (see Dose Modifications). Teach patient to report nausea, and/or vomiting, and discuss antiemetic therapy with physician or NP/PA; review instructions with patient along with diet modifications to minimize nasuea and/or vomiting.

Drug: everolimus (Afinitor)

Class: mTOR inhibitor.

Mechanism of Action: Everolimus inhibits mTOR, so it reduces tumor cell division, growth of blood vessel, and cell metabolism. mTOR is an intracellular serine-threonine kinase protein that regulates cell proliferation and angiogenesis. It is found in the cytoplasm and turns on and off the translation of signals that tell the cell's protein factory (ribosomes) to make proteins. Proteins control all the cell functions. Proteins that activate mTOR are growth signals from EGF, insulin-like growth factor (IGF), and VEGFs. Proteins that stop mTOR activity are tuberous sclerosis complex (TSC) 1 and 2, and if there are not enough nutrients to support more cells, mTOR activity is blocked. As an mTOR inhibitor, everolimus interferes with the central regulation of tumor cell division, metabolism, and angiogenesis. Blocking this important protein results in cell cycle arrest and cell death. mTOR is also a very important component of the P13K/AKT signaling pathway that is often dysregulated in solid tumors, as it plays a role in cell cycle regulation, and it also suppresses apoptosis (Chang et al., 2003).

Specifically, everolimus binds to an intracellular protein, FKBP-12, a protein-folding chaperone, thus inhibiting mTOR kinase activity. Everolimus also reduces the activity of downstream effectors of mTOR, which are involved in protein synthesis, inhibits the expression of hypoxia-inducible factor (HIF-1), and reduces expression of vascular endothelial growth factor (VEGF). Through these actions, everolimus reduces cell proliferation, angiogenesis, and glucose uptake (Novartis, 2009).

Drug is also used as an immunosuppressant to prevent transplanted organ rejection; it reduces incidence of chronic allograft vasculopathy in heart transplant patients (drug name Certican). Drug is a proliferation signal inhibitor and inhibits the proliferation and clonal expansion of antigen-activated T-cells, which are stimulated by cytokines IL-2 and IL-5. Cells are arrested in the G1 phase of the cell cycle.

Metabolism: Peak serum concentrations achieved in 1–2 hours after oral dosing, with steady state reached within 2 weeks with once-daily dosing. mTOR inhibition is complete after a 10-mg oral daily dose. In clinical studies, a high-fat meal reduced AUC by 16%, but the manufacturer recommends the dose be given without regard to meals. Plasma binding is about 74%. Drug is a substrate of CYP3A4 and PgP (P-glycoprotein). Everolimus is mainly metabolized by CYP3A4 in the liver and to some extent in the intestinal wall and is a substrate for the multidrug efflux pump P-glycoprotein. It is metabolized into six metabolites, which have less activity than the intact drug. The mean elimination half-life of everolimus is 30 hours, with 80% of drug excreted in the feces, and 5% in the urine. Moderate hepatic dysfunction (Child-Pugh Class B) doubles the AUC, so dose should be reduced in these patients. Oral clearance of the drug is 20% higher in African-American patients compared to Caucasian, and Japanese patients had, on average exposures, a higher drug exposure compared to non-Japanese. The implications of ethnic differences are unknown.

Indications:
Afinitor (everolimus) tablets are indicated for the treatment of:

- Postmenopausal women with advanced hormone receptor-positive, HER2-negative, breast cancer (HR+ BC) in combination with exemestane, after failure of treatment with letrozole or anastrozole.
- Adult patients with progressive neuroendocrine tumors of pancreas origin (PNET) that are unresectable, locally advanced, or metastatic disease. It is not indicated for the treatment of patients with functional carcinoid tumors.
- Adult patients with advanced renal cell carcinoma (RCC) after failure of treatment with sunitinib or sorafenib.
- Adult patients with renal angiomyolipoma and tuberous sclerosis complex (TSC).

Afinitor (everolimus) tablets and Disperz are indicated for the treatment of:

- Pediatric and adult patients with tuberous sclerosis complex (TSC) for the treatment of subependymal giant cell astrocytoma (SEGA) that requires therapeutic intervention but cannot be curatively resected.

Dosage/Range:
- Everolimus (Afinitor) is available in two dosage forms: Afinitor tablets (for all indications) and tablets for oral suspension (Afinitor Disperz, for treatment of patients with SEGA and TSC).
- See package insert for dose adjustment and management recommendations for adverse reactions.

Patients with HR+ BC, PNET, RCC, or renal angiomyolipoma with tuberous sclerosis complex (TSC):
- 10 mg once daily at the same time every day, consistently with or without food. Swallow tablet whole with a glass of water; do not crush or break tablets.
- Management of severe or intolerable adverse reactions may require temporary dose interruption (with or without a dose reduction) or discontinuation. If a dose reduction is needed, suggested dose is approximately 50% lower than the daily dose previously administered. See package insert for dose adjustment and management recommendations for adverse reactions.
- Continue treatment until disease progression or unacceptable toxicity occurs.
- Hepatic impairment increases the exposure (AUC) of everolimus: Recommended dose adjustments:
  - Mild impairment (Child-Pugh Class A): 7.5 mg PO daily for patients with; the dose may be decreased to 5 mg if not well tolerated.
  - Moderate hepatic impairment (Child-Pugh Class B): 5 mg PO daily for patients with the dose may be decreased to 2.5 mg if not well tolerated.
  - Severe hepatic impairment (Child-Pugh Class C): if the desired benefit outweighs the risk, 2.5 mg PO daily for patients. Do not exceed dose of 2.5 mg PO daily.
  - Dose adjustments should be made if a patient's hepatic (Child-Pugh) status changes during treatment.
- Avoid concomitant use of strong CYP3A4/PgP inhibitors (e.g., ketoconazole, itraconazole, clarithromycin, attazanavir, nefazodone, saquinavir, telithromycin, ritonavir, indinavir, nelfinavir, voriconazole).
  - If moderate inhibitors of CYP3A4 and/or P-glycoprotein (PgP) are required (e.g., amprenavir, fosamprenavir, aprepitant, erythromycin, fluconazole, verapamil, diltiazem), reduce the everolimus dose to 2.5 mg once daily; if tolerated, consider increasing to 5 mg once daily.
  - If the moderate inhibitor is discontinued, allow a washout period of 2–3 days before the everolimus dose is increased. The everolimus dose should be returned to the dose used prior to starting the moderate CYP3A4/PgP inhibitor.
- Avoid concomitant strong CYP3A4/PgP inducers (e.g., phenytoin, carbamazepine, rifampin, rifabutin, rifapentine, phenobarbital).
  - If coadministration with a strong CYP3A4 inducer is required, consider doubling the everolimus daily dose in 5-mg increments or less.
  - If the strong CYP3A4 drug is discontinued, allow a washout period of 3–5 days before the everolimus dose is returned to the original dose used before start of the strong CYP3A4 inducer.
- AVOID coadministration with St. John's wort, as herbal may decrease everolimus AUC unpredictably.

Subependymal Giant Cell Astrocytoma (SEGA) with TSC:
* Recommended starting dose:
  * 4.5 mg/m^2 once daily; adjust dose to attain trough concentration of 5–15 ng/mL.
  * Severe hepatic impairment or requiring moderate CYP3A4 and/or PgP inhibitors, reduce the starting dose of Afinitor tablets or Afinitor Disperz to 2.5 mg/m^2 once daily.
* Assess serum trough concentration two weeks after starting therapy, after a change in dose, a change in coadministration of CYP3A4 and/or PgP inducers or inhibitors, a change in hepatic function, or a change in dosage form between Afinitor tablets and Afinitor Disperz.
* Avoid concomitant use of strong CYP3A4/PgP inhibitors. If concomitant use of moderate CYP3A4/PgP inhibitors (e.g., amprenavir, fosamprenavir, aprepitant, erythromycin, fluconazole, verapamil, diltiazem) is required:
  * Reduce Affinitor tablet or Disperz dose by 50%. Administer every other day if dose reduction is required for patients receiving the lowest available strength, and maintain trough concentration 5–15 ng/mL.
  * Assess everolimus trough concentrations approximately 2 weeks after dose reduction.
  * When the moderate inhibitor is discontinued, resume the Afinitor dose that was used before starting the inhibitor 2–3 days after discontinuation. Assess everolimus trough concentrations approximately 2 weeks later.
* Avoid the concomitant use of strong CYP3A4/PgP inducers. If concomitant use of strong inducers of CYP3A4 is required (no alternatives available), double the dose of Afinitor to 9 mg/m^2 once daily. Round to the nearest strength of Afinitor tablets or Disperz.
  * Assess everolimus trough concentration 2 weeks after doubling dose, and adjust dose as necessary to maintain a trough concentration of 5–15 ng/mL.
  * If the strong CYP3A4/PgP inducer is discontinued, return the Afinitor tablet or Afinitor Disperz dose to that used before starting the stong CYP3A4/PgP inducer. Assess everolimus trough concentrations approximately 2 weeks later.
* If dose reduction is required for patients receiving the lowest available strength, administer every other day.
* Once a stable dose is attained, monitor trough concentrations every 3–6 months in patients with changing body surface area, or every 6–12 months in patients with stable BSA for the duration of treatment.
* Temporarily interrupt or permanently discontinue Afinitor tablets or Disperz for severe or intolerable adverse reactions. See package insert for dose modifications for toxicity.
  * If dose reduction required when reinitiating therapy, reduce dose by approximately 50%.
  * If the patient is receiving the lowest available strength, administer every other day.
* Teach patients to AVOID grapefruit, grapefruit juice, and any other nutritional supplements that inhibit cytochrome P450 or PgP activity.

Drug Preparation:
* Afinitor Oral, tablets available in 2.5-mg, 5-mg, 7.5-mg, and 10-mg tablets with no score.
* Afinitor Disperz (tablets for oral suspension): 2-mg, 3-mg, 5-mg tablets for oral suspension, no score.

Drug Administration:

- Do not combine the 2 dosage forms (Afinitor tablets and Afinitor Disperz). Use one dosage form or the other.
- Tablets: Orally, once daily at the same time of day, either consistently with or without food. The patient should swallow tablet whole with a glass of water, and tablets should not be crushed or chewed.
- Afinitor Disperz (Afinitor tablets for oral suspension) for patients with SEGA and TSC, in conjunction with therapeutic drug monitoring.
  - Wear gloves to avoid contact with everolimus when preparing suspension.
    Using an oral syringe:
  - Place prescribed dose of Afinitor Disperz into a 10-mL syringe. DO NOT exceed a total of 10 mg per syringe. Use an additional syringe if higher doses are required. Do not break or crush tablets.
  - Draw about 5 mL of water and 4 mL of air into the syringe. Place the filled syringe into a container (tip up) for 3 minutes, until the Afinitor Disperz tablets are in suspension. Gently invert the syringe 5 times immediately prior to administration.
  - After administration of the prepared suspension, draw 5 mL of water and 4 mL of air into the same syringe, swirling the contents to suspend the remaining particles. Administer the entire contents of the syringe.
    Using a small drinking glass:
  - Place the prescribed dose of Afinitor Disperz into a small drinking glass (maximum 100 mL), containing 25 mL of water. Do not exceed a total of 10 mg per syringe. Use an additional glass if higher doses are required. Do not break or crush tablets.
  - Allow 3 minutes for suspension to occur. Stir the contents gently with a spoon, immediately prior to drinking.
  - After administration of the prepared suspension, add 25 mL of water and stir with the same spoon to re-suspend remaining particles; administer the entire contents of the glass.
  - Disperse tablet completely in glass of water (~30 mL) by gently stirring immediately before drinking dose; rinse glass with same volume of water, and swallow the rinse completely to ensure that the entire dose is taken. Anyone who prepares the suspension for another person should wear gloves to avoid possible contact with the medicine. Take the suspension at about the same time each day, with or without food.
  - Administer immediately after preparation; discard if not used within 60 minutes.
  - Administer suspension orally, once daily at the same time every day, consistently with or without food.
- Monitor renal function, blood glucose, lipids, and hematologic parameters baseline and periodically during therapy.
- Drug is contraindicated in patients who are hypersensitive to the drug or other mTOR inhibitors (e.g., rapamycin derivative).
- Hypersensitivity reactions may include anaphylaxis, dyspnea, flushing, chest pain, or angioedema.

Drug Interactions:
- Everolimus is a substrate of CYP3A, and also is a substrate and moderate inhibitor of P-glycoprotein multidrug efflux pump. It is also a competitive inhibitor of CYP3A4 and a mixed inhibitor of CYP2D6.

HR+ BC, RCC, TSC:
- Coadministration with strong CYP3A4 inhibitors (e.g., ketoconazole, itraconazole, voriconazole, clarithromycin, nafazodone, saquinavir, telithromycin, ritonavir, indinavir, nelfinavir, voriconazole): AVOID.
- Coadministration with moderate CYP3A4 and/or PgP inhibitors (e.g., amprenavir, fosamprenavir, aprepitant, erythromycin, fluconazole, verapamil, diltiazem): AVOID; if unavoidable, see dosage and assessment after dose changes in Dosage section. If the interacting drug is discontinued, a washout period of 2–3 days should occcur before the everolimus dose is increased to the dose prior to initiation of the moderate CYP3A4 and/or PgP inhibitor.
- Coadministration with strong CYP3A4 inducer (e.g., phenytoin, carbamazepine, rifampin, rifabutin, rifapentine, phenobarbital): AVOID; if unavoidable, see dosage and assessment after dose, in Dosage section.
- Grapefruit and grapefruit juice: AVOID; do not take while receiving everolimus.
- St. John's wort can increase the metabolism of everolimus and thus lower drug serum levels; do not use together.
- Inhibitors of P-glycoprotein may decrease the efflux of everolimus from intestinal cells and increase everolimus blood concentrations, so it should be avoided (e.g., ketoconazole, quinidine, erythromycin, verapamil, probenecid, cimetidine). Do NOT coadminister.
- Everolimus is a competitive inhibitor of CYP3A4 and of CYP2D6 microsomal pathways, so that drugs metabolized via these pathways may have higher serum levels; if the drug has a narrow therapeutic window, monitor for side effects or decrease dose of interacting drug.

Lab Effects/Interference:
- Increased creatinine, urinary protein, blood glucose, lipids (hyperlipidemia, hypertriglyceridemia).
- Decreased hemoglobin, lymphocytes, platelets, neutrophils.

Special Considerations:
- Most common adverse reactions (incidence ≥ 30%) include:
  - HR+ BC, advanced PNET, advanced RCC: stomatitis, infections, rash, fatigue, diarrhea, edema, abdominal pain, nausea, fever, asthenia, cough, headache, decreased appetite.
  - Renal angiomyolipoma with TSC: stomatitis.
  - SEGA with TSC: stomatitis, URI.
- *Warnings and Precautions:*
  - Noninfectious pneumonitis: Noninfectious pneumonitis is a class effect of rapamycin derivatives and may occur in up to 19% of patients (up to 4% grade 3, 0.2% grade 4); monitor patients for clinical symptoms and consider noninfectious

pneumonitis in the differential (e.g., hypoxia, pleural effusion, cough, dyspnea when other causes have been excluded). Pneumonitis has been reported even when patient is receiving a reduced dose of everolimus. Teach patient to report any new or worsening respiratory symptoms right away. If symptoms occur:

- Few or no symptoms but with radiological changes suggestive of noninfectious pneumonitis: continue everolimus therapy without dose alteration.
- Moderate symptoms: consider dose interruption until symptoms improve; consider corticosteroid therapy if needed. When symptoms improve, may introduce everolimus at 50% lower than the previous daily dose.
- Grade 3: interrupt drug until resolution to ≤ grade 1; corticosteroids may be indicated. When this occurs, may reintroduce everolimus at 50% lower than the previous daily dose, depending upon the individual clinical circumstances.
- Grade 4: discontinue everolimus. Corticosteroids may be needed to manage clinical symptoms.
- Infections: Everolimus is immunosuppressive, and patients may be at increased risk for developing bacterial, fungal, viral, or protoloan infections, including opportunistic infections, localized, and systemic infections (e.g., pneumonia, mycobaterial infections).
  - Invasive fungal infections such as aspergillosis or candidiasis, and viral infections (including reactivation of hepatitis B virus) have been reported, and some severe infections have been fatal.
  - Patients should complete treatment of preexisting invasive fungal infections prior to starting everolimus.
  - Monitor patients closely for signs/symptoms and treat promptly with appropriate antimicrobials. If an invasive systemic fungal infection is diagnosed, interruption or discontinuation of everolimus should be considered, and the infection treated with antifungal therapy.
- Oral ulceration: mouth ulcers, stomatits, and oral mucositis are common (incidence 44%–78% across clinical trials). Grade 3 or 4 stomatitis occurred in 4–9% of patients.
  - Teach patient to use sytematic oral rinsing and topical treatments (excluding alcohol, hydrogen peroxide, iodine or thyme-containing mouthrinses, which can harm the mucosa).
  - Do not use antifungal agents unless an oral fungal infection has been diagnosed.
- Renal failure: renal failure, including acute renal failure, has occurred and some cases have been fatal. Monitor renal function tests (BUN, urinary protein, or serum creatinine) baseline and periodically during treatment; patients with additional risk factors should be assessed more frequently.
- Impaired wound healing: increased risk of wound-related complications, such as wound dehiscence, wound infection, incisional hernia, lymphocele, seroma, which may require surgical intervention. Monitor patient closely, and use caution in the peri-operative period.
- Geriatric patients: in HR+ BC patients, the incidence of death from any cause within 28 days of the last everolimus dose was 6% in patients age 65 or older, compared to 2% in those younger than age 65. 33% of patients age ≥ 65 permanently

discontinued the drug due to adverse reactions, compared to 17% in patients < 65 years of age. Monitor elderly patients closely and ensure appropriate dose reductions are made for adverse effects.

- Hyperglycemia, hyperlipidemia, and hypertriglyceridemia have been reported. Assess fasting glucose, lipid profile prior to starting everolimus, and discuss appropriate medical therapy with physician or NP/PA prior to patient starting everolimus. Monitor fasting glucose and lipids during therapy, and more closely if the patient is receiving other drugs that may incease blood glucose or lipids.
- Rarely, hypersensitivity reactions to everolimus have occurred; assess for, and teach patient to report/seek emergency care: anaphylaxis, dyspnea, flushing, chest pain, angioedema, and stop drug if these occur.
- Teach patients to AVOID any live vaccinations (e.g., intranasal influenza, measles, mumps, rubella, oral polio, BCG, yellow fever, varicella, and TY21a typhoid) or close contact with people who have received them while the patient is receiving everolimus therapy. The timing of routine vaccinations in pediatric patients with SEGA should be planned prior to starting everolimus therapy.
- Drug can cause embryofetal toxicity. Teach women of reproductive potential to use effective contraception to avoid pregnancy during therapy and for up to 8 weeks after therapy ends.
- If drug is used during pregnancy or if the patient should become pregnant while on the drug, apprise the woman of the potential harm to the fetus.
- Nursing mothers: a decision should be made to discontinue the nursing or to discontinue the drug, taking into account the importance of the drug to the mother's health.

Potential Toxicities/Side Effects and the Nursing Process

I.   POTENTIAL FOR INFECTION related to IMMUNOSUPPRESSION

Defining Characteristics: Everolimus is immunosuppressive and increases risk for opportunistic infections. Infections may be localized or systemic and include pneumonia, other bacterial infections, and invasive fungal infections (e.g., aspergillosis, candidiasis). Incidence is approximately 37%, with 7% grade 3 and 3% grade 4. Cough occurs in 30% of patients, pyrexia in 20%, and dyspnea in 24%. In addition, some patients may experience neutropenia (14%).

Nursing Implications: Assess baseline WBC, lymphocyte, and neutrophil counts, and monitor frequently during therapy. Assess skin integrity, potential for infection, and teach patient measures to prevent infection (e.g., keeping skin intact, avoiding sources of infection, good hand-washing). Teach patient to report any signs/symptoms of infection (e.g., redness, heat, exudate on skin, temperature ≥ 100.4°F, cough, sputum production, dysuria). Assess for signs/symptoms of infection during therapy and at each visit. If a patient develops an infection, discuss with physician or midlevel practitioner interrupting or discontinuing drug, and beginning appropriate antimicrobial treatment.

If the patient is receiving therapy for a preexisting invasive fungal infection, the patient should complete therapy before starting therapy with everolimus. If during everolimus therapy a diagnosis of systemic fungal infection is made, discontinue everolimus and treat with appropriate antifungal therapy.

II.   POTENTIAL ALTERATION IN NUTRITION, LESS THAN BODY REQUIREMENTS, related to STOMATITIS, HYPERGLYCEMIA, HYPERTRIGLYCERIDEMIA, HYPOPHOSPHATEMIA, INCREASED SERUM CREATININE, ANOREXIA, NAUSEA, VOMITING, DIARRHEA

Defining Characteristics: In clinical studies, oral mucositis (e.g., stomatitis, mouth ulcers) affected 44% of patients (compared with 7% placebo) with advanced RCC, and 86% of SEGA patients. In general, this is grade 1 or 2. 6% of PNET developed grade 3–4. Hyperglycemia, hypercholesteremia, and hypophosphatemia have been reported. mTOR is involved in insulin signaling, which possibly explains the hypertriglyceridemia and hyperglycemia. Drug can also increase serum creatinine. Anorexia occurs in 25% of patients. Diarrhea occurs in about 30% of patients, nausea in 26%, and vomiting in 20%.

Nursing Implications: Assess baseline oral mucosa, nutritional status, and appetite. Assess fasting serum triglycerides, cholesterol, phosphate, glucose, BUN, and serum creatinine baseline and during treatment with the drug. Teach the patient to report signs/ symptoms of hyperglycemia (polyuria, polydipsia, polyphagia). Discuss with physician correction of lipids, triglycerides, and glucose if baseline tests are abnormal, prior to beginning everolimus therapy. Assess oral mucosa prior to drug administration, as well as ability to eat and drink at each visit; instruct patient to self-assess and report changes, including the appearance of white patches (candida), pain, and inability to eat or drink. Teach patient oral hygiene measures and self assessment and to avoid alcohol- or peroxide-containing mouthwashes. Antifungal agents should not be used unless fungal infection has been diagnosed. If oral mucositis is painful, or candida is present, discuss prescription of topical analgesics and anti-candidiasis oral treatment. Discuss appropriate antiemetics (e.g., prochlorperazine) and antidiarrheal (e.g., loperamide) medicines if patient develops these symptoms. Teach patient to notify physician/ nurse if oral ulcers occur, if excessive thirst occurs, or any increase in volume or frequency of urination occurs. In addition, call nurse or physician for diarrhea, nausea, or vomiting that does not resolve within 24 hours with recommended over-the-counter medicines. Notify physician of any abnormalities, and discuss implications and management.

III.   ALTERATION IN SKIN INTEGRITY, POTENTIAL, related to RASH

Defining Characteristics: Rash has been reported in 29% of patients. In addition, pruritus was reported in 14% and dry skin in 13% of patients on clinical trials.

Nursing Implications: Assess patient skin integrity, including nails baseline and regularly during treatment. Teach patient self-assessment and local comfort measures, including the use of water-based emollients. Teach patient to report skin changes and, if self-care is ineffective, to discuss plan with physician, especially if severe.

IV. ALTERATION IN COMFORT AND ACTIVITY TOLERANCE, POTENTIAL, related to ASTHENIA, ANEMIA

Defining Characteristics: Asthenia, weakness (affects 33% vs 23%), fatigue 31%, and anemia (92% overall, with 12% grade 3 and 1% grade 4, compared to placebo all grades 79% and 5% grade 3). Headache affects 19%.

Nursing Implications: Assess baseline CBC, Hgb, comfort, and activity tolerance, and reassess during treatment, asking patient to identify what activities now unable to do, sleep habits, and also state of mind. Discuss alternating rest and activity periods and also possibility of other family members or friends assisting with energy-consuming responsibilities to increase energy reserve. Teach patient to report increasing fatigue, signs of severe anemia (shortness of breath, chest pain/angina, headaches). Monitor hemoglobin/hematocrit; discuss transfusion with physician if signs/symptoms develop or hematocrit falls < 25 mg/dL. Teach patient about diet high in iron.

Drug: gefitinib (Iressa)

Class: Tyrosine Kinase Inhibitor of EGFR.

Mechanism of Action: Reversibly inhibits kinase activity in EGFR unmutated (wild-type) and some EGFR mutated (exon 19 deletion or exon 21 point mutation L858R) cancer cells. It also inhibits insulin-like growth factor (IGF) and platelet-derived growth factor (PDGF) signaling.

Metabolism: After oral dosing, peak plasma level occurs 3–7 hours after dosing, and is not influenced by food intake. It is extensively distributed throughout the body, and is 90% protein bound. Drug is a substrate for membrane transport P-glycoprotein (P-gp) but this does not influence drug absorption. Gefitinib is extensively metabolized by the liver, predominantly by CYP3A4. Elimination half-life is 48 hours after IV administration, and steady state is reached in 10 days. Drug and its metabolites are excreted in feces (86%) and to a lesser degree, urine (< 4%). Drug exposure (AUC) is increased by 40% in patients with mild hepatic impairment, 263% if moderate impairment, and 166% in patients with severe impairment. If the patient has a CYP2D6 poor metabolizer phenotype, the patient is at risk for increased gefitinib AUC, and patient should be monitored closely for toxicity. Coadministration with a strong CYP3A4 inducer (e.g., rifampin) reduced gefitinib AUC by 83% while coadministration of a CYP3A4 inhibitor (e.g., itraconazole), increased mean gefitinib AUC by 80%. Drugs affecting gastric pH (e.g., sodium bicarbonate, pH above 5.0) decreased the gefitinib AUC by 47%.

Indication: First-line treatment of metastatic NSCLC that has the following EGFR mutations: exon 19 deletion or exon 21 (L858R) substitution.

Dosage/Range: 250 mg PO once daily without regard to food intake. Withhold drug for up to 14 days for (NCI CTCAE)
• Acute or worsening pulmonary symptoms (e.g., dyspnea, cough, fever).
• Grade 2 or higher increases in AST and/or ALT.
• Grade 3 or higher diarrhea.
• Severe or worsening ocular disorders (e.g., keratitis).
• Grade 3 or higher skin reactions.

Permanently discontinue drug for
• Confirmed interstitial lung disease (ILD).
• Severe hepatic impairment.
• GI perforation.
• Persistent ulcerative keratitis.

Drug Preparation: None. Drug tablets should be stored at room temperature 68°F–77°F (20°C–25°C). If the patient has difficulty swallowing, the tablet should be placed in 4–8 ounces of water, and stirred for about 15 minutes until it dissolves.

Drug Administration:
• Teach patient (1) to take tablet once daily with or without food, OR if taking the dissolved tablet in water, or if difficult or unable to swallow the tablet, (2) have the patient immediately drink the solution containing the dissolved tablet or administer the dose through a nasogastric (NG) tube. Rinse the container used to dissolve the tablet with an additional 4–8 ounces of water and have the patient drink it immediately or administer it through the NG tube. The patient should be taught not to take a missed dose within 12 hours of the next dose.
• Assess ALT and AST baseline and frequently during therapy.
• Assess for changes, and teach patient to report visual changes right away.

Drug Interactions:
• CYP3A4 inducers: will increase gefitinib metabolism and decrease the gefitinib plasma concentration. If patient must take a strong CYP3A4 inducer (e.g., rifampicin, phenytoin, or tricyclic antidepressants) concomitantly, the gefitinib dose should be increased to 500 mg daily.
• CYP3A4 inhibitors: will decrease gefitinib metabolism and increase the gefitinib plasma concentration. If the patient must take a strong inhibitor (e.g., ketoconazole, itraconazole) concomitantly, monitor patients closely for adverse reactions.
• Drugs affecting gastric pH: Drugs increasing gastric pH (e.g., proton pump inhibitors [PPIs], histamine H_2-receptor antagonists, antacids) may decrease gefitinib plasma concentration. Avoid concomitant administration of PPIs. If a PPI is required, the patient should be taught to administer gefitinib 12 hours after the last dose or 12 hours before the next dose of the PPI. If an H_2-receptor antagonist or antacid is required, the patient should take gefitinib 6 hours after or before an H_2-receptor antagonist or antacid.

- Warfarin: increased risk for bleeding. Monitor INR or prothrombin time closely and teach patient to report any bleeding right away.

Lab Effects/Interference:
- Increased AST, ALT
- Proteinuria

Special Considerations:
- Most common adverse reactions occurring in > 20% of patients, and greater than than placebo were skin reactions and diarrhea. Drug should be interrupted for up to 14 days for NCI CTCAE grade 3 or higher diarrhea, or grade 3 or higher skin reactions. Drug should be resumed when toxicity fully resolves or improves to Grade 1.
- Warnings and precautions:
  - ILD: hold drug for worsening pulmonary symptoms (e.g., dyspnea, cough, fever), and discontinue drug if ILD confirmed.
  - Hepatotoxicity: monitor during therapy; hold drug for grade 2 hepatotoxicity (increased ALT, AST, or bilirubin), and discontinue if severe.
  - GI perforation: occurs rarely (0.1%); discontinue drug if it occurs.
  - Severe or persistent diarrhea: Incidence of grade 3/4 toxicity 3%. Hold drug for up to 14 days for grade 3 or higher diarrhea.
  - Ocular disorders (e.g., keratitis, corneal erosion, aberrant eyelash growth, conjunctivitis, dry eye) may occur. Incidence of conjunctivitis, blepharitis, and dry eye was 6%. Rarely (0.1%), drug should be interrupted for severe or worsening ocular disorders.
  - Bullous and exfoliative skin disorders (e.g., toxic epidermal necrolysis, Stevens Johnson syndrome, erythema multiforme) have rarely occurred (0.08%). Interrupt or discontinue drug for severe blistering or exfoliating skin disorders.
  - Embryo-fetal toxicity: drug is fetotoxic. Teach women to use effective contraception during drug therapy and for 2 weeks after last dose. Nursing women should discontinue breastfeeding, or discontinue the drug.
- Nutritional impact symptoms may occur: diarrhea (29%), decreased appetite (17%), vomiting (14%), and stomatitis (7%).

Potential Toxicities/Side Effects and the Nursing Process

I.   ALTERATION IN SKIN INTEGRITY related to RASH

Defining Characteristics: Forty-seven percent of all patients developed skin reactions, which included acne-like rash, dermatitis, drug eruption, erythema, folliculitis, maculopapular rash, and xeroderma. Of these 2% experienced a grade 3 or 4 reaction. Five percent of patients experienced nail disorders, including onycholysis and paronychia.

Nursing Implications: Assess skin integrity of face, neck, arms, and upper trunk baseline and regularly during treatment. Teach patient that rash may occur, its usual course, and self-care measures for comfort. Emphasize the need to keep skin with rash clean to prevent infection, and to continue taking gefitinib until told to stop by nurse or physician. Teach patient that skin may become dry, and to use skin emollients or moisturizers. Assess body image intactness, and if rash develops, its threat to body image. Encourage patient to verbalize feelings, provide emotional support, and individualize care plan based on patient response. For rash management, refer to the introduction in *Chapter 4*. Teach all patients to (1) use a water-based emollient frequently during the day to prevent dryness, (2) stay hydrated, (3) avoid sun exposure and wear SPF 30 (zinc-based). Do not use anti-acne medications. Tetracycline analogues provide anti-inflammatory benefit. **Grade 1/mild rash** (localized, does not interfere with ADLs, and is not infected): Goal is to preserve skin integrity, minimize discomfort, and prevent infection. Key patient teaching includes (1) use a mild soap with active ingredients that reduce skin drying, such as pyrithione zinc (Head & Shoulders); (2) consider applying aloe gel to red, tender areas; (3) report distressing tenderness, as pramoxine (lidocaine topical anesthetic) may help; (4) keep fingernails clean and trimmed; and (5) apply zinc ointment to anal mucosa after washing. **Management: maintain current drug dose, observe or give topical hydrocortisone 1% or 2.5%, or clindamycin 1%** gel (anti-inflammatory benefit), reassess in 2 weeks. **Grade 2/moderate rash** (generalized, mild symptoms, and minimal effect on ADLs, no infection): Goal is to prevent infection and promote comfort. Continue EGFRI dose; use topicals (hydrocortisone 2.5% or clindamycin 1% gel) and consider adding doxycycline 100 mg PO twice daily or minocycline 100 mg PO twice daily (gives antimicrobial and anti-inflammatory effect) and reassess after 2 weeks. **Grade 3–4 or severe rash** (generalized, severe, has significant impact on ADLs, and increased risk of infection): The goal is to prevent infection or identify infection early to minimize complications, and to promote effective coping. Drug should be held for severe rash, CTCAE grade 3 (papules and/or pustules covering > 30% BSA, which may be associated with symptoms of pruritis or tenderness; limiting self care ADL; associated with local superinfection with oral antibiotics indicated) or higher, for up to 14 days. Teach patient to interrupt drug as ordered. Treat rash with topicals (hydrocortisone 2.5%, or clindamycin 1% gel), doxycycline 100 mg PO bid or minocycline 100 mg PO bid, and methylprednisolone (Medrol dose pack); reassess after 2 weeks. (Lacouture et al., 2011; Lynch et al., 2007). If rash appears infected (exudate, vesicular formation, different appearance), obtain C+S, treat empirically until sensitivity received, and/or discuss with provider obtaining dermatology consult.

Teach patient to report any peeling or blistering of skin as bullous and exfoliative skin disorders, such as Stevens Johnson syndrome, may rarely occur; drug should be discontinued in these patients.

Teach patients that nail disorders may occur, and to report them.

II.   ALTERATION IN ELIMINATION PATTERN related to DIARRHEA

Defining Characteristics: Diarrhea was reported in 29% of patients in clinical studies, and was severe in 3%. Diarrhea may occur within 14 days of starting gefitinib, is usually mild to moderate, and well managed with anti-diarrheal medications like loperamide (Shah, 2005). Proteinuria occurred in 35% of patients, and was grade 3/4 in 4.7% (AstaZeneca, 2015).

Nursing Implications: Assess bowel elimination pattern baseline, and regularly during therapy. Teach patient to report diarrhea; teach patient self-care strategies to manage diarrhea such as dietary modification and self-administration of loperamide; teach patient to minimize potential complications such as dehydration and electrolyte depletion. Identify patients at risk for dehydration and follow closely, such as patients with renal insufficiency, diabetes, CHF, or the elderly. If diarrhea does not resolve or is CTCAE grade 3 or higher (grade 3 is an increase of 7 or more stools/day over baseline; incontinence; hospitalization indicated; severe ostomy output compared to baseline; limiting self-care ADL), drug should be interrupted for up to 14 days (Astra-Zeneca, 2015). Discuss with provider lab assessment, fluid and electrolyte replacement, hydration, and further management. If diarrhea is refractory or difficult to manage, this will increase the patient's risk for dehydration and risk for acute renal failure, especially if elderly or if the patient has pre-existing renal disease.

Drug: human papillomavirus bivalent (types 16 and 18) vaccine, recombinant suspension for intramuscular injection (Cervarix)

Class: Vaccine.

Mechanism of Action: Drug is prepared by using recombinant techniques to assemble L1 proteins, which are then assembled into virus-like particles. The adsorbed virus-like particles of each HPV subtype are then combined into the vaccine. It is thought the vaccine efficacy is related to the immune response to the L1 virus-like particles, mediated by the development of IgG neutralizing antibodies against HPV-L1 proteins in the viral caprotein coat surrounding the virus.

Indication: Indicated for the prevention of cervical cancer, cervical intraepithelial neoplasia (CIN) grade 2 or worse, adenocarcinoma in situ, and cervial intraepithelial neoplasia (CIN) grade 1.

Dosage/Range:
- Three doses (0.5 mL each) IM at 0, 1, and 6 months.

Drug Preparation/Administration:
- Available as single-dose prefilled syringes containing a 0.5-mL suspension for injection. Tip caps of the prefilled syringes may contain natural rubber latex, which may cause allergic reactions in latex-sensitive individuals. Do not use TIP-LOK prefilled syringe in latex-sensitive patients.
- Shake syringe well before withdrawal and use. Visually inspect the solution for particulate matter or discoloration, and discard if either is found. It should appear homogeneous, turbid, and white.

- Aseptically remove cap of prefilled TIP-LOK syringe and attach a sterile needle. Prepare site with alcohol swab, and administer IM in the deltoid region of the arm. Do NOT administer IV, intradermally, or subcutaneously.
- Observe the patient for 15 minutes after administration; patient should be sitting down, as syncope may occur.

Drug Interactions:
- Do not mix with any other vaccine in the same syringe or vial.

Lab Effects/Interference:
- Unknown.

Special Considerations:
- Vaccine is FDA-approved for use in females aged 9 through 25 years.
- Limitations of use: vaccine does not provide protection against disease due to all HPV types, and it has not been demonstrated to provide protection against disease from vaccine and nonvaccine HPV types to which a woman has previously been exposed through sexual activity.
- Drug is contraindicated if patient develops severe allergic reaction to the vaccine (anaphylaxis).
- Vaccine may cause syncope, which can result in the patient falling and becoming injured.
  - Patient should be observed for 15 minutes postinjection.
  - Syncope has been associated with tonic-clonic movement and other seizure-like activity. If this occurs, place the patient in a supine or Trendelenburg position to restore cerebral perfusion. Seizure-like activity is usually transient and resolves with supine positioning.
- Most common local adverse reactions in > 20% of patients are pain, redness, swelling at injection site.
- Most common general adverse effects in > 20% of patients are fatigue, headache, myalgia, gastrointestinal symptoms, and arthralgia.
- Safety has not been established in pregnant women. Register women who receive the vaccine while pregnant in the pregnancy registry by calling 1-888-452-9622.
- Immunocompromised patients may have a reduced immune response to the vaccine.

Potential Toxicities/Side Effects and the Nursing Process

I.   ALTERATION IN COMFORT related to INJECTION-SITE DISCOMFORT, FEVER

Defining Characteristics: 92% developed pain, 48% redness, and 44% swelling at the injection site. Fatigue affected 55%, headache, 53%, fever (> 99.5°F) 13%, and rash about 10%. GI symptoms (nausea, vomiting, diarrhea, and/or abdominal pain) affected 28% of patients. Myalgia affected 49%, arthralgia 21%, and urticaria 7% of patients.

Nursing Implications: Teach patient that this may occur, and teach local strategies to minimize this, such as distraction, warm compresses.

Drug: human papillomavirus quadrivalent (types 6, 11, 16, and 18) vaccine, recombinant suspension for intramuscular injection (Gardasil)

Class: Vaccine.

Mechanism of Action: Drug is prepared by using recombinant techniques. Animal studies suggest that the efficacy of L1 VLP vaccines is related to the development of the humoral immune response. The exact mechanism of protection is unknown.

Indication: Indicated in girls and women 9–26 years of age for the prevention of the following diseases caused by HPV types included in the vaccine:
- Cervical, vulvar, vaginal, and anal cancer caused by HPV types 16, 18
- Genital warts (condyloma acuminata) caused by HPV types 6, 11
- Precancerous or dysplastic lesions caused by HPV types 6, 11, 16, 18 (cervical intraepithelial neoplasia (CIN) grade 2–3 and cervical adenocarcinoma in situ; cervical intraepithelial neoplasia (CIN) grade 1; vulvar intraepithelial neoplasia (VIN) grades 2 and 3; vaginal intraepithelial neoplasia (VaIN) grades 2 and 3; anal intraepithelial neoplasia (AIN) grades 1, 2, and 3).

Indicated in boys and men 9–26 years of age for the prevention of the following diseases caused by HPV types included in the vaccine:
- Anal cancer caused by HPV types 16, 18
- Genital warts (condyloma acuminata) caused by HPV types 6, 11
- Precancerous or dysplastic lesions caused by HPV types 6, 11, 16, 18: anal intraepithelial neoplasia (AIN) grades 1, 2, and 3.

Dosage/Range:
- Three doses (0.5 mL each) IM at 0, 2, and 6 months.

Drug Preparation/Administration:
- For IM use only.
- Available as 0.5-mL suspension for injection as a single-dose vial, and prefilled syringes containing a 0.5-mL suspension for injection.
- Shake well before use. Thoroughly agitate immediately before use to maintain vaccine suspension. Do not dilute or mix with other vaccines. After thorough agitation, vaccine is a white, cloudy liquid. Visually inspect the solution for particulate matter or discoloration, and discard if either is found.
- *Single dose vial:* aseptically withdraw the 0.5-mL dose using a sterile needle and syringe and use promptly.
- *Prefilled syringe:* shake well before use; attach a sterile needle by twisting in a clockwise direction until needle fits securely on the syringe.
- Prepare site with alcohol swab, and administer IM in the deltoid region of the upper arm or in the higher anterolateral area of the thigh.
- Observe the patient for 15 minutes after administration; patient should be sitting down, as syncope may occur.

Drug Interactions:
* Gardasil may be administered concomitantly (in a separate injection site) with RECOMBIVAX HB [hepatitis B vaccine (recombinant)].
* Gardasil may be administered concomitantly (in a separate injection site) with Menactra [Meningococcal (Groups A, C, Y, W-135) Polysaccharide Diptheria Toxoid Conjugate Vaccine] and Adacel [Tetanus Toxoid, Reduced Diptheria Toxoid and Acellular Pertussis Vaccine Adsorbed (Tdap)].

Lab Effects/Interference:
* Unknown.

Special Considerations:
* Vaccine is FDA-approved for use in females and males aged 9–26 years.
* *Limitations of use:*
  * Vaccine does not eliminate the necessity for women to continue to undergo recommended cervical cancer screening.
  * Recipients of vaccine should not discontinue anal cancer screening if recommended by a healthcare professional.
  * Vaccine does not provide protection against diseases due to HPV types not contained in the vaccine.
  * Vaccine has not been demonstrated to provide protection against disease from vaccine and nonvaccine HPV types to which a person has previously been exposed through sexual activity.
  * Vaccine is not intended to be used for treatment of active external genital lesions; cervical, vulvar, vaginal, and anal cancers; CIN, VIN, VaIN, or AIN.
  * Not all vulvar, vaginal, and anal cancers are caused by HPV, and vaccine protects only against those vulvar, vaginal, and anal cancers caused by HPV 16 and 18.
  * Vaccine does not protect against genital diseases not caused by HPV.
  * Vaccination may not result in protection in all recipients.
  * Vaccine has not been demonstrated to prevent HPV-related CIN 2/3 or worse in women older than 26 years or age.
* Drug is contraindicated if patient has hypersensitivity, including severe allergic reactions to yeast, a vaccine component, or to a prior Gardasil dose.
* If the patient has an allergic reaction, institute appropriate medical treatment as ordered. Supervision must be readily available in case of anaphylaxis, which has been reported following Gardasil administration.
* Vaccine may cause syncope, which can result in the patient falling and becoming injured.
  * Patient should be observed for 15 minutes postinjection.
  * Syncope has been associated with tonic-clonic movement and other seizure-like activity. If this occurs, place the patient in a supine or Trendelenburg position to restore cerebral perfusion. Seizure-like activity is usually transient and resolves with supine positioning.
* Adverse reactions include headache, fever, nausea, and dizziness; and local injection-site reactions (pain, swelling, erythema, pruritus, and bruising).

- Safety has not been established in pregnant women. Register women who receive the vaccine while pregnant in the pregnancy registry by calling 1-877-888-4231. Safety has not been established in children below the age of 9 years.
- Immunocompromised individuals may have a diminished response to the vaccine.

Potential Toxicities/Side Effects and the Nursing Process

I. ALTERATION IN COMFORT related to INJECTION-SITE DISCOMFORT, HEADACHE, PYREXIA

Defining Characteristics: 83.9% developed pain, 24.7% redness, and 25.4% swelling at the injection site. Pyrexia occurred in 13% girls/women, and 8.3 boys/men. Headache occurred in 12.3% of boys/men.

Nursing Implications: Teach patient that these may occur, and teach local strategies to minimize discomfort, such as, warm compresses for injection-site discomfort. Teach patients to monitor temperature, and to report fever that does not go away, or other discomfort that does not resolve.

Drug: ^{90}Y ibritumomab tiuxetan (Zevalin)

Class: Monoclonal antibody chelated to radioisotope ^{90}Y yttrium.

Mechanism of Action: Ibritumomab tiuxetan is a monoclonal antibody that targets the cell surface antigen CD20, which is found on the surface of normal and malignant B-cell - lymphocytes. The CD20 antigen is also present (expressed) on more than 90% of B-cell non-Hodgkin's lymphoma (NHL) cells, but fortunately is not found on normal bone marrow stem cells, pre-B cells, or other normal tissues. The complex is made up of a murine anti-CD20 monoclonal antibody conjugate to the linker chelator tiuxetan, which then securely chelates the radioisotope ^{90}Y yttrium. The complex attaches to the CD20 receptor, and then the radioisotope delivers high beta energy waves to the malignant cell, causing cell death. The isotope delivers high energy with a short half-life of 64 hours. It appears that if the malignant cells are pretreated with an anti-CD20 antibody (e.g., Rituximab), this clears malignant and normal B lymphocytes from the blood, and ^{90}Y ibritumomab tiuxetan is better able to target the lymphoma B-lymphocytes.

Metabolism: ^{90}Y yttrium has a half-life of 64 hours, and effective half-life in the blood of 28 hours, median biologic half-life of 47 hours, and median area under the curve (AUC) of 25 hours (Wiseman et al., 1996).

Indication: CD20 directed radiotherapeutic antibody administered as part of the Zevalin therapeutic regimen indicated for treatment of patients with
- Relapsed or refractory, low-grade or follicular B-cell non-Hodgkin's lymphoma (NHL).
- Previously untreated follicular NHL who achieve a partial or complete response to first-line chemotherapy.

Dosage/Range:
- Biodistribution is determined prior to dosing determination and administration.
- Day 1: administer rituximab 250 mg/m² intravenously.
- Day 7, 8, or 9: administer rituximab 250 mg/m² IV infusion.
  - If platelets ≥ 150,000/mm³: within 4 hrs after rituximab infusion, administer 0.4 mCi/kg (14.8 MBq per kg) Y-90 Zevalin, intravenously.
  - If platelets ≥ 100,000 but ≤ 149,000/mm³ in relapsed or refractory patients: within 4 hrs after rituximab infusion, administer 0.3 mCi/kg (11.1 MBq per kg) Y-90 Zevalin, intravenously.
- Initiate Zevalin therapeutic regimen following recovery of platelet counts to ≥ 150/000/mm³ at least 6 weeks and no more than 12 weeks, following the last dose of first-line chemotherapy.
- Do not treat patients with platelet counts < 100,000/mm³.
- No contraindications, but drug should not be given to patients with altered biodistribution of Y-90 Zevalin, and patients with ≥ 25% lymphoma marrow involvement or impaired bone marrow reserve.
- Administer rituximab/Zevalin only in facilities where immediate access to resuscitative measures is available.

Drug Preparation/Procedure for determining radiochemical purity and radiation dosimetry:
- Zevalin available as 3.2 mg per 2 mL in a single-use vial.
- See package insert.

Drug Administration:
- Assess CBC/differential and platelet count. Assess medication profile for drug(s) that interfere with platelet function or coagulation. Assess platelet count more frequently in these patients.
- Day 1: administer rituximab 250 mg/m² intravenously.
  - Premedicate with oral acetaminophen 650 mg and diphenhyramine 50 mg before rituximab infusion.
  - Administer rituximab at an initial rate of 50 mg/hr, and if no infusion reaction, escalate the infusion rate in 50-mg/hr increments every 30 min to a maximum of 400 mg/hr. Do not mix or dilute rituximab with other drugs.
  - Immediately stop the rituxmab for serious infusion reactions, and discontinue Zevalin therapeutic regimen.
  - Temporarily slow or interrupt the rituximab infusion for less severed infusion reactions; if symptoms improve, continue the infusion at one-half the previous rate.
- Day 7, 8, or 9:
  - Premedicate with oral acetaminophen 650 mg and diphenhyramine 50 mg before rituximab infusion.
  - Administer rituximab at initial rate of 50 mg/hr; and if no infusion reaction, escalate the infusion rate in 50 mg/hr increments every 30 min to a maximum of 400 mg/hr. Do not mix or dilute rituximab with other drugs.
  - Administer Y-90 Zevalin injection through a free flowing IV line within 4 hrs after rituximab infusion finishes. Use a 0.22 micron low-protein-binding in-line filter

between the syringe and the infusion port. After infusion, flush the line with at least 10 mL of normal saline.

- **If platelet count $\geq$ 150,000/mm³,** administer Y-90 Zevalin over 10 min as an IV injection at a dose of 0.4 mCi/kg (14.8 MBq per kg) actual body weight.
- **If platelet count $\geq$ 100,000/mm³ but < 149,000/mm³,** in relapsed or refractory patients, Y-90 Zevalin over 10 min as an IV injection at a dose of 0.3 mCi/kg (11.1 MBq per kg) actual body weight.
- Do NOT administer more than 32 mCi/kg (1184 MBq) Y-90 Zevalin dose regardless of the patient's body weight.
- Monitor patient closely for extravasation during Y-90 injection. Immediately stop infusion and restart in another limb if signs/symptoms of extravasation occur.

Drug Interactions:
- Increased bone marrow suppression if combined with other myelosuppressive drugs, or drugs interfering with blood clotting.
- Monitor patients receiving medications that interfere with platelet function or coagulation more frequently for thrombocytopenia.

Lab Effects/Interference:
- Decreased WBC and neutrophil, platelet count, and Hgb/HCT.

Special Considerations:
Warnings and Precautions:

- Rituximab, alone or with Y-90 Zevalin, can cause severe, including fatal, infusion reactions. Typically, these are seen during the first rituximab infusion (onset 30–120 minutes).
  - Signs and symptoms of a severe reaction can include urticaria, hypotension, angioedema, hypoxia, bronchospasm, pulmonary infiltrates, ARDS, MI, ventricular fibrillation, and cardiogenic shock. Immediately discontinue rituximab and Y-90 Zevalin for severe infusion reactions.
  - Less severe reactions: temporarily slow or interrupt the rituximab infusion. Ensure resuscitation resources are immediately available in infusion area.
- Prolonged and severe cytopenias are most common severe adverse reactions. Onset is delayed and duration prolonged, sometimes > 12 weeks after infusion. May be complicated by hemorrhage and severe infection.
  - Incidence of severe thrombocytopenia and neutropenia greater in patients with baseline mildly thrombocytopenic counts (e.g., $\geq$ 100,000/mm³ but $\leq$ 149,000/mm³).
  - Do NOT administer Zevalin therapeutic regimen to patients with $\geq$ 25% lymphoma marrow involvement and impaired bone marrow reserve.
  - Monitor CBC/differential and platelet counts weekly until levels recur, or as clinically indicated. Monitor patients for cytopenias and their complications (e.g., febrile neutropenia, hemorrhage) for up to 3 months after Zevalin therapeutic regimen is given. Avoid using drugs that interfere with platelet function or coagulation after Zevalin therapeutic regimen.

- Severe cutaneous and mucocutaneous reactions: Erythema multiforme, Stevens-Johnson syndrome, toxic epidermal necrolysis, bullous dermatitis, and exfoliative dermatitis, sometimes fatal, have been reported. May occur a few days to 4 months after administration of the Zevalin therapeutic regimen. Discontinue Zevalin therapeutic regimen in patients experiencing a severe cutaneous or mucocutaneous reaction.
- Altered biodistribution: 1.3% of patients recorded in a post-marketing registry had altered biodistribution.
- Risk of secondary malignancy: Myelodysplastic syndrome (MDS) and/or acute myelogenous leukemia (AML) were reported in 5.2% of patients with relapsed or refractory NHL enrolled in clinical studies. Median time to diagnosis was 1.9 years after Zevalin therapeutic regimen administration. Incidence in patients who received Zevalin therapeutic regimen after first line chemotherapy was 12.7% compared to 6.8% in the control arm.
- Do not administer live viral vaccines after Zevalin therapeutic regimen is given.
- Use radionucleotide precautions during and after radiolabeling Zevalin with Y-90.
- Y-90 Zevalin can cause fetal harm. Teach women of reproductive potential to use effective contraception to avoid pregnancy for a minimum of 12 months. If Zevalin therapeutic regimen is administered during pregnancy, the patient should be apprised of the potential hazard to the fetus.
- Because IgG is excreted in human milk, nursing mothers should make a decision whether to discontinue nursing or not receive the Zevalin therapeutic regimen, taking into account the importance of the drug to the mother's health.
- After treatment, there is rapid reduction in malignant and normal B-cell lymphocytes, with circulating B cells undetectable for the first 12 weeks, followed by recovery of normal B cells starting in the sixth month after therapy.
- Common adverse events ($\geq$ 10%): cytopenias, fatigue, nasopharyngitis, nausea, abdominal pain, asthenia, cough, diarrhea, and pyrexia.

Potential Toxicities/Side Effects and the Nursing Process

I.   POTENTIAL FOR INJURY related to ANAPHYLAXIS

Defining Characteristics: Rare but potentially life-threatening reaction may occur. Mouse antibodies are used that are foreign and may stimulate anaphylaxis. Rare, fatal anaphylactic reactions have occurred within 24 hours of rituximab dose. Of the reactions, 80% occur during the first rituximab infusion, and within 30–120 minutes of the infusion. Severe infusion reactions include pulmonary infiltrates, acute respiratory distress syndrome, myocardial infarction, ventricular fibrillation, and cardiogenic shock.

Nursing Implications: Assess baseline T, VS. Administer premedications prior to rituximab as ordered, usually acetaminophen and diphenhydramine. Initiate infusion at 50 mg/hr, and increase in 50 mg/hr increments q 30 min to a maximum of 400 mg/hr. If patient develops discomfort, slow infusion; stop infusion if reaction is severe. Once symptoms have improved, resume rate at 50% of previous rate. Have emergency equipment and medications nearby, including epinephrine and corticosteroids. Assess patient for signs/symptoms, including generalized flushing and urticaria leading to pallor, cyanosis, bronchospasm, hypotension, unconsciousness. Teach patient to report signs/ symptoms, including sense of doom, tickle in throat. If signs/symptoms occur, stop infusion immediately, assess VS, notify physician. Physician may prescribe epinephrine 0.3 mL (1:1,000) subcutaneous if hypotensive. Oxygen, antihistamines, corticosteroids may also be used.

II. POTENTIAL FOR INFECTION, BLEEDING, AND FATIGUE related to BONE MARROW SUPPRESSION

Defining Characteristics: Neutropenia common, with 77% incidence, and 25–32% of patients experiencing grade 4 neutropenia, with a median nadir of 900–1100/mm^3; Thrombocytopenia incidence 95% with median platelet nadir of 49,500/mm^3; Anemia incidence 61% with median nadir for red blood cells 9.9 g/dL hemoglobin. Nadir occurred around 7–9 weeks after treatment, and duration of cytopenias was 22–35 days. Chills and fever were common, affecting 27.5% and 21.6% of patients in one study. There appears to be increased hematologic toxicity in patients with bone marrow involvement by tumor, as expected. Rare fatal cerebral hemorrhage, severe infections.

Nursing Implications: Drug contraindicated in patients with > 25% bone marrow hypocellular bone marrow, or history of failed stem cell collection. Assess baseline CBC, platelet count, and monitor closely during and after therapy at least weekly for the first 12 weeks after treatment. Assess risk for increased hematologic toxicity, e.g., whether bone marrow involvement by tumor. Teach patient that blood counts will fall and potential signs/symptoms of infection, bleeding, and fatigue. Teach patient self-care measures, including self-assessment for signs/symptoms of infection, bleeding, and anemia; self-care strategies to minimize risk for infection (e.g., avoiding crowds and proximity to people with colds), bleeding (e.g., avoid aspirin-containing OTC medicines), and fatigue (e.g., alternating rest and activity periods), and what/where to report fever, bleeding, signs/symptoms of infection. Most studies show that few patients developed severe infections, and there were few if any deaths from treatment-related infections. Transfuse red blood cells and platelets as ordered.

III. ALTERATION IN COMFORT related to ASTHENIA, NAUSEA, ABDOMINAL PAIN, HEADACHE

Defining Characteristics: Asthenia commonly affects 21.6%, nausea (grades 1 or 2) 21.6%, and abdominal pain and headache 9.8%. Nausea, vomiting, diarrhea, increased cough, dizziness, arthralgia, anxiety may occur.

Nursing Implications: Assess baseline comfort and energy level. Teach patient that these side effects may occur, and strategies to manage them. If the symptom persists or is unresolved, teach patient to report it, and discuss with physician other management strategies.

IV.   POTENTIAL FOR INJURY related to RADIATION EXPOSURE

Defining Characteristics: ^{90}Y Zevalin is a beta-emitter so that patients should protect others from exposure to their body secretions (saliva, stool, blood, urine).

Nursing Implications: Teach patient importance of specific radiation precautions, beginning at the start of treatment, and continuing for 1 week after treatment is completed: use condom during sexual intercourse, refrain from deep kissing; avoid transfer of body fluids; wash hands thoroughly after using the toilet; and continue effective contraception for 12 months following completion of treatment.

Drug: ibrutinib (Imbruvica)

Class: Bruton's tyrosine kinase (BTK) inhibitor.

Mechanism of Action: Inhibits BTK, an important nonreceptor tyrosine kinase that signals messages through the B-cell lymphocyte antigen receptor (BCR), as well as cytokine receptor pathways. BCR signaling is essential for B-cell development and survival. BCR is believed to be oncogenic in mantle cell lymphoma (MCL) and chronic lymphocytic leukema (CLL), and BTK regulates cell proliferation and cell survival (Hendriks et al., 2014). BCR is composed of immunogobulins that recognize foreign antigens; when bound to the antigen, pathways are activated for B-cell lymphocyte trafficking, chemotaxis, and survival (Pharmacyclics, Inc., 2014). BTK is a key mediator regulating B-lymphocyte apoptosis, adhesion, cell migration, and homing (Pharmacyclics, Inc., 2014). Ibrutinib blocks BCR, resulting in inhibition of malignant B-cell lymphocyte proliferation, cell migration, adhesion to the microenvironment, and survival.

Metabolism: Drug is absorbed with median maximal plasma concentrations (T_{max}) reached in 1–2 hours. If taken with food, drug exposure is twofold greater compared to a fasting state. Drug is 97.3% reversibly bound to plasma proteins. Ibrutinib is metabolized by P450 microenzymes in the liver, CYP3A4 and, to a lesser degree, CYP2D6 into a few metabolites, including the active metabolite, PCI-45227. Ibrutinib affinity for BTK active sites is 15 times that of the active metabolite. Ibrutinib half-life is 4–6 hours. The drug is excreted mainly as metabolites in the stool (80%), with < 10% excreted in the urine. Moderate hepatic impairment increases drug exposure 6 times (Child-Pugh Class B).

Indication: Ibrutinib is FDA-approved for treatment of patients with:
- Mantle cell lymphoma (MCL), who have received at least one prior therapy. Accelerated approval was based on overall response rate and data on improved survival or symptom control have not been shown.
- Chronic lymphocytic leukemia (CLL), who have received at least one prior therapy.
- CLL with 17p deletion.
- Waldenstrom's macroglobulinemia (WM)

Dosage/Range:
- Mantle cell lymphoma (MCL): 560 mg (four 140-mg capsules) orally once daily.
- Chronic lymphocytic leukemia (CLL) and Waldenstrom's macroglobulinemia (WM): 420 mg (three 140-mg capsules) orally once daily.

Dose Modifications:
- Drug should be interrupted for grade ≥3 or higher nonhematologic toxicity, grade ≥3 neutropenia with infection or fever, or grade 4 hematologic toxicity.
- When toxicity has resolved to grade 1 or baseline/recovery, restart ibrutinib at the starting dose.
- If toxicity recurs, after recovery, reduce dose by one capsule; a second dose reduction by 140 mg may be considered as needed. See package insert for specific doses for each indication.
- If toxicity persists or recurs after two dose reductions, discontinue drug.
- Avoid concommitant administration with strong or moderate CYP3A4 inhibitors. If strong CYP3A4 inhibitors (e.g., antifungals, antibiotics) must be used short-term, consider interrupting ibrutinib for the duration. Chronic use of concommitant strong CYP3A4 inhibitors (e.g., boceprevir, indinavir, nefazodone, nelfinavir, ritonavir, saquinavir, telaprevir) is not recommended. If a moderate CYP3A4 inhibitor (e.g., amprenavir, aprepitant, atazanavir, ciprofloxacin, crizotinib, darunavir, diltiazem, erythromycin, fluconazole, fosamprevir, grapefruit products, imatinib, verapamil, Seville oranges) must be used, **decrease ibruitinib dose to 140 mg daily.** Monitor patients receiving concommitant strong or moderate CYP3A4 inhibitors closely for toxicity.
- For patients with mild liver impairment (Child-Pugh class A), recommended dose is 140 mg (1 capsule). Do not administer drug to patients with moderate or severe hepatic impairment.

Drug Preparation/Administration:
- Available in 140-mg capsules.
- Teach patient to take capsule whole, not to open or chew capsule, and to take with water. Drug should be taken at about the same time each day.
- If a dose is missed, it can be taken when remembered on the same day, then resume normal schedule; do not make up a missed dose.

Drug Interactions:
- CYP3A Inhibitors: increase the serum ibritinib levels, increasing toxicity. Do not coadminister strong inhibitors, and reduce ibritinib dose to 140 mg if coadministered with a moderately strong inhibitor. See Dose Modifications.
- CYP3A Inducers: decrease ibritinib serum levels and reduce efficacy; avoid strong CYP3A inducers (e.g., St. John's wort).
- Antiplatelet or anticoagulant therapy: increased risk of bleeding; monitor patients closely, as well as appropriate labs.

Lab Effects/Interference:
- Neutropenia, thrombocytopenia, anemia.
- Increased serum creatinine, uric acid.

Special Considerations:

*   Most common side effects (incidence $\geq$ 25%) in patients with B-cell malignancies (MCL, CLL, WM) were thrombocytopenia, diarrhea, neutropenia, anemia, fatigue, musculoskeletal pain, bruising, nausea, URI, and rash.
*   Bleeding: 5–6% of patients in studies had grade $\geq$ 3 bleeding events (e.g., subdural hematoma, GI bleed, hematuria). Overall bleeding, including bruising, was 48% of MCL patients receiving ibritinib at 560 mg daily, and 63% of CLL patients receiving 420 mg daily. Consider benefit of withholding ibrutinib 3–7 days prior to and after surgery based on type of surgery and risk of bleeding.
*   Tumor lysis syndrome (TLS) may occur. Monitor patients closely for TLS if at risk, and implement medical orders to reduce the risk (e.g., hydration, medication to reduce uric acid).
*   Infection may occur and may be fatal. Grade $\geq$ 3 infection occurred in 25% of MCL and 35% of CLL patients. Monitor patients closely for infection and treat with antimicrobials as indicated.
*   Myelosuppression is common, and grade $\geq$3 cytopenias requiring treatment occurred in 41% of MCL patients and 35% of CLL patients. Incidences were: MCL patients: Neutropenia (29%), thrombocytopenia (17%), anemia (9%); CLL patients: netropenia (27%), thrombocytopenia (10%). Monitor blood counts baseline and monthly.
*   Renal toxicity may occur, with treatment required for increased creatinine up to 1.5 X ULN (incidence 67% in MCL patients, 23% in CLL patients). Creatinine increases 1.5–3 × ULN occurred in 9% patients with MCL, and 4% of patients with CLL. Teach patients to stay well-hydrated and monitor serum creatinine baseline and periodically during therapy.
*   Second primary malignancies have been described in 5% of MCL and 10% of CLL patients treated with ibritinib (skin cancers and other carcinomas).
*   Embryo-fetal toxicity: Teach women of childbearing potential to use effective contraception to avoid pregnancy. If pregnancy occurs while taking the drug, advise patient of potential hazards to fetus.

Potential Toxicities/Side Effects and the Nursing Process

I.   POTENTIAL FOR INFECTION AND BLEEDING related to BONE MARROW DEPRESSION

Defining Characteristics: Neutropenia occurred in 47% of MCL patients (29% grade $\geq$ 3), thrombocytopenia in 57% of patients (17% grade $\geq$3), and decreased hemoglobin in 41% of patients, (29% grade $\geq$ 3). Neutropenia occurred in 54% of CLL patients (27% grade $\geq$ 3), thrombocytopenia in 71% (10% grade $\geq$ 3), and decreased hemoglobin in 44%. Grade $\geq$ 3 infections occurred in 25% of MCL and 35% of CLL patients. Bleeding events, including bruising, occurred in 48% of MCL and 63% of CLL patients receiving recommended doses of ibrutinib. Rarely, grade $\geq$ 3 bleeding occurred. Hemorrhage risk may be increased in patients receiving antiplatelet or anticoagulant therapies.

Nursing Implications: Assess baseline CBC, including WBC and differential and platelet count prior to dosing, and at least monthly. Teach patient self-assessment of signs/symptoms of infection (e.g., T > 100.4°F, dysuria, productive cough) and bleeding (including bruising), and instruct patient to report them right away. Teach patient self-care measures to minimize risk of infection and bleeding, including avoidance of crowds, people with colds, OTC aspirin-containing medications. Discuss dose interruption and modification for grade 3 toxicity with physician. Assess for fever or infection frequently, and discuss need for emergent evaluation and treatment promptly if signs or symptoms of infection are identified.

II.   ALTERATION IN NUTRITION, POTENTIAL, LESS THAN BODY REQUIREMENTS, related to DIARRHEA, NAUSEA, VOMITING, CONSTIPATION

Defining Characteristics: Diarhhea affects 51–63% of patients, nausea 21–31%, constipation 23–25%, vomiting 19–23%, stomatitis 21%, and decreased appetite 21%.

Nursing Implications: Assess baseline nutritional status and bowel elimination status. If patient develops nausea and/or vomiting, teach patient to self-administer antiemetics 1 hour prior to each dose, and to call if nausea/vomiting persist.

Discuss with physician more effective antiemetic regimen if nausea/vomiting persist. Encourage small, frequent intake of cool, bland foods as tolerated if nausea develops. Refer to dietitian as needed for meal planning. Teach patient to report diarrhea that does not respond to OTC antidiarrheal medication. Teach self-care measures of diet modification and oral fluids to 2–3 L during the waking hours. If constipation occurs, teach patient self-care measures to prevent constipation. Assess appetite, and condition of oral mucosa; teach patient self-assessment and systemic oral hygiene after meals and at bedtime.

III.   ALTERATION IN COMFORT related to PAIN, HEADACHE, FATIGUE, ARTHRALGIA, AND FATIGUE

Defining Characteristics: Fatigue affected 41% of patients, peripheral edema 35%, musculoskeletal pain 37% of patients, arthralgias 11% of patients, and abdominal pain affected 24% of patients.

Nursing Implications: Teach patient that these events may occur and to report them, and teach patient strategies to conserve energy. Assess baseline comfort, and monitor closely during treatment. Develop plan to assure comfort depending on symptoms reported. Discuss ineffective strategies with physician.

Drug: idelalisib (Zydelig)

Class: Kinase inhibitor; first-in-class PI3K-delta kinase inhibitor (phosphatidylinositol 3-kinase), a kinase that is expressed by normal and malignant B-cells.

Mechanism of Action: PI3K-delta kinase is found in normal and malignant B lymphocytes. Idelalisib inhibits a number of signaling pathways, including that of the B-cell receptor (BCR), CXCR4, and CXCR5, which help the B-lymphocytes navigate to lymph nodes and bone marrow. Idelalisib inhibits chemotaxis and adhesion. Fiorcari et al. (2013) found that idelalisib inhibited chronic lymphocytic leukemia (CLL) cell adhesion to the endothelial and bone marrow stromal cells that is integrin-mediated. This prevents cell proliferation and results in apoptosis.

Metabolism: After oral administration in a fasting state, T_{max} (median) was seen at 1.5 hours; when administered with a high-fat meal, the idelalisib AUC increased 1.4-fold. However, drug may be given without regard to food. Drug is highly protein bound (> 84%). Drug is metabolized into its principal metabolite GS-563117 in the liver by aldehyde oxidase and CYP3A, with minor metabolism by UGT1A4. The metabolite is not active against PI3K-delta. Terminal elimination half-life is 8.2 hours. Approximately 78% of the drug is excreted in the feces and 14% in the urine. Drug dose does not require modification if renal dysfunction, but patients with hepatic dysfunction require close monitoring and dose modification for toxicity.

Indication:
- For the treatment of:
  - Relapsed CLL, in combination with rituximab, in patients for whom rituximab alone would be considered appropriate therapy due to other comorbidities.
  - Relapsed follicular B-cell non-Hodgkin lymphoma (FL), in patients who have received at least 2 prior systemic therapies.
  - Relapsed small lymphocytic lymphoma (SLL), in patients who have received at least 2 prior systemic therapies.
- Contraindicated in patients with a history of serious allergic reactions, including anaphylaxis and toxic epidermal necrolysis.

Dosage/Range:
- 150 mg orally, twice daily.
- Idelalisib should be continued until disease progression or unacceptable toxicity.

Dose Modification:
- **Pneumonitis:** Discontinue idelalisib for any severity of symptomatic pneumonitis.
- **ALT/AST elevation:**
  - > 3–5 × ULN: Maintain dose; monitor ALT/AST at least weekly until ≤ 1 × ULN.
  - > 5–20 × ULN: Hold drug; monitor at least weekly until ALT/AST is ≤ 1 × ULN; then may resume idelalisib at 100 mg bid.
  - > 20 × ULN: Permanently discontinue idelalisib.
- **Bilirubin elevation:**
  - > 1.5–3 × ULN: Maintain dose; monitor bilirubin at least weekly until ≤ 1 × ULN.
  - > 3–10 × ULN: Hold drug; monitor at least weekly until bilirubin is ≤ 1 × ULN; then may resume idelalisib at 100 mg bid.
  - >10 × ULN: Permanently discontinue idelalisib.

- **Diarrhea:**
  - Moderate (increase of 4–6 stools/day over baseline): Maintain dose; monitor patient at least weekly until resolved.
  - Severe or requiring hospitalization (increase of ≥ 7 stools/day over baseline): Hold drug; monitor patient at least weekly until resolved; then may resume idelalisib at 100 mg bid.
  - Life-threatening: Permanently discontinue idelalisib.
- **Neutropenia:**
  - ANC 1.0 to < 1.5 Gi/L: Maintain idelalisib dose.
  - ANC 0.5 to < 1.0 Gi/L: Maintain idelalisib dose; monitor ANC at least weekly.
  - ANC < 0.5 Gi/L: Interrupt idelalisib; monitor ANC at least weekly until ANC ≥ 0.5 Gi/L; then may resume idelalisib at 100 mg bid.
- **Thrombocytopenia:**
  - Platelets 50 to < 75 Gi/L: Maintain idelalisib dose.
  - Platelets 25 to < 50 Gi/L: Maintain idelalisib dose; monitor platelet count at least weekly.
  - Platelets < 25 Gi/L: Interrupt idelalisib; monitor platelet count at least weekly until platelet count ≥ 25 Gi/L; then may resume idelalisib at 100 mg bid.
- **For other severe or life-threatening toxicities** related to idelalisib, hold drug until toxicity is resolved; then if resuming the drug, dose should be reduced to 100 mg bid. If severe or life-threatening idelalisib-related toxicity recurs, idelalisib should be permanently discontinued.

Drug Preparation:
- Drug is available in 150-mg and 100-mg tablets.
- Drug is FDA-approved with a Risk Evaluation and Mitigation Strategy (REMS) that includes a communication plan to ensure that healthcare providers likely to prescribe Zydelig are fully informed about the risks shown in the black boxed warning (FDA, 2014).

Drug Administration:
- Teach patient to take idelalisib with or without food, to swallow the table whole, and to take at about the same time of day each day.
  - If a dose is missed by < 6 hours, the patient should take the missed dose right away and then the next dose as usual.
  - If a dose is missed by > 6 hours, the patient should skip the missed dose and take the next dose at the usual time.
- Teach female patients of childbearing potential to use effective contraception to avoid pregnancy while taking the drug, and for at least 1 month after last dose of idelalisib.
- Assess CBC/differential and platelet counts baseline and at least every 2 weeks for the first 3 months of therapy, and at least weekly in patients with ANC < 1.0 Gi/L.
- Assess ALT and AST every 2 weeks for the first 3 months of treatment, then every 4 weeks for the next 3 months, then every 1–3 months thereafter. If AST or ALT rises above 3 × ULN, monitor ALT/AST weekly until resolved. Hold idelalisib if AST or ALT is > 5 × ULN, and continue to monitor AST, ALT, and total bilirubin weekly until the abnormality is resolved.
- Assess for signs/symptoms of serious toxicity: diarrhea, cough, dyspnea, hypoxia, new or worsening abdominal pain, chills, fever, nausea/vomiting, rash, allergic reaction, signs/symptoms of infection or bleeding.
- Discuss need for dose modification with physician based on symptoms or laboratory data as needed.

Drug Interactions:
- CYP3A inducers: avoid coadministration with strong CYP3A inducers (e.g., rifampin, phenytoin, carbamazepine, St. John's wort), as this may lower serum level of idelalisib (e.g., 75% reduction in idelalisib AUC) and negate drug effectiveness.
- CYP3A inhibitors: may increase drug serum level and increase toxicity. If patient is taking a strong CYP3A inhibitor with idelalisib, assess patient for signs/symptoms of idelalisib toxicity; dose should be modified accordingly.
- CYP3A substrates: idelalisib is a strong CYP3A inhibitor: avoid coadministration of CYP3A substrates, as this may increase the sensitive substrate serum level fivefold.

Lab Effects/Interference:
- Neutropenia, thrombocytopenia.
- Elevated ALT, AST, bilirubin.
- Hypertriglyceridemia.
- Hyperglycemia.

Special Considerations:
- Drug was approved in FL and SLL through an FDA accelerated approval program based on overall response rate; an improvement in survival or disease-related symptoms has not been established. Continued approval may be contingent upon verification of clinical benefit in confirmatory trials (Gilead Sciences, Inc, 2014).
- Black Boxed Warnings:
  - Hepatotoxicity: fatal and/or serious hepatotoxicity occurred in 14% of patients in clinical trials.
    - Elevations > 5 × ULN have occurred, usually during the first 12 weeks of treatment, and were reversible with dose interruption. When drug was resumed at a lower dose, 26% had recurrent AST/ALT elevations.
    - Monitor hepatic function prior to and during treatment every 2 weeks for first 3 months, every 4 weeks for the next 3 months, then every 1–3 months. Interrupt and then dose-reduce or discontinue drug.
    - See Dose Modifications for monitoring frequency with abnormal values.
    - Avoid coadministration of other potentially hepatotoxic drugs.
    - Teach patient to report right away yellowing of skin or conjunctiva, easy bruising, abdominal pain, or bleeding.
  - Diarrhea or colitis: fatal and/or serious diarrhea or colitis occurred in 14% of idelalisib-treated patients in clinical trials.
    - Review patient medication profile and avoid concurrent use of drugs that cause diarrhea. Idelalisib-related diarrhea does not respond well to anti-motility agents.
    - In clinical trials, diarrhea resolved in 1 week a month after idelalisib was stopped. In some cases, corticosteroids were required.
    - Teach patient to report immediately an increase in the number of stools/day by 6 or more.
  - Pneumonitis: fatal and serious pneumonitis may occur.
    - Monitor patient for pulmonary symptoms (e.g., cough, dyspnea, hypoxia; bilateral interstitial infiltrates); or ≥ 5% decrease in oxygen saturation.

- If these occur, interrupt drug until the etiology is determined. If pneumonitis is confirmed, idelalisib therapy should be discontinued and the patient treated with corticosteroids.
- Teach patient to report immediately any new or worsening respiratory symptoms (e.g., cough, dyspnea).
  - Intestinal perforation: fatal and serious intestinal perforation can occur.
  - This may occur during moderate or severe diarrhea.
  - Teach patient to report immediately new or worsening abdominal pain, chills, fever, nausea/vomiting, and to seek medical care right away.
  - Idelalisib should be permanently discontinued if intestinal obstruction occurs.
- Warnings:
  - Severe cutanous reactions may occur (e.g., grade ≥ 3 cutaneous reactions, such as dermatitis exfoliative, rash, rash erythematous, rash generalized, rash macular, rash macula-papular, rash papular, rash pruritus, exfoliative rash). Monitor patient closely, and discontinue drug if a severe cutaneous reaction occurs.
  - Anaphylaxis: monitor patient for severe allergic reactions and anaphylaxis; discontinue idelalisib if it occurs and provide emergency supportive care. Teach patient to seek emergency medical care right away if patient has difficulty breathing, feels faint, chest pain, or other symptoms of an anaphylactic or serious allergic reaction.
  - Neutropenia: grade 3 or 4 neutropenia occurred in 31% of patients in clinical trials. Monitor blood counts at least every 2 weeks for the first 3 months, then at least weekly in patients with an ANC < 1.0 Gi/T. Teach patient to report any signs or symptoms of infection right away.
  - Embryo-fetal toxicity: advise women of reproductive potential to use effective contraception to prevent pregnancy while taking idelalisib, and for 1 month after the last drug dose. If the drug is used during pregnancy, or if the patient becomes pregnant while taking the drug, the patient should be apprised of the potential risk to the fetus.
- Patients age 65 and older with indolent NHL or CLL had a higher incidence of serious adverse reactions and a higher incidence of death compared to younger patients. Monitor patients age 65 and older closely during therapy.
- Most common adverse effects (incidence ≥ 20%) are diarrhea, pyrexia, fatigue, nausea, cough, pneumonitis, abdominal pain, chills, and rash.
- Women should not breastfeed while receiving idelalisib; the patient should decide to stop nursing or stop taking the drug, taking into account the importance of the drug to the mother's health.

Potential Toxicities/Side Effects and the Nursing Process

I.   POTENTIAL FOR INFECTION AND BLEEDING related to BONE MARROW SUPPRESSION

Defining Characteristics: Neutropenia was common, with 31% of patients having treatment-emergent grade 3 or 4 neutropenia. Infections included pneumonia (23–25%) and sepsis (up to 8%). Pyrexia occurred in 37% of patients and was grade 3–4 in 5%; cough occurred in 19%, and chills in 16%. Thrombocytopenia occurred in 16% (7% grade 3–4), and anemia occurred in 32% with 11% of patients having grade 3–4.

Nursing Implications: Assess CBC/differential and platelet counts baseline and at least every 2 weeks for the first 3 months of therapy as ordered during therapy. Assess CBC/differential weekly in patients with ANC < 1.0 Gi/L. Assess skin integrity, potential for infection, and teach patient measures to prevent infection (e.g., keeping skin intact, avoiding sources of infection, good hand-washing). Teach patient to report any signs/symptoms of infection (e.g., redness, heat, exudate on skin, temperature ≥ 100.4°F, cough, sputum production, dysuria). Assess for signs/symptoms of infection during therapy and at each visit. If a patient develops an infection, discuss with physician or midlevel practitioner interrupting or discontinuing drug, and beginning appropriate antimicrobial treatment. Teach the patient that thrombocytopenia may occur, to avoid situations that could increase bleeding, and to report any signs or symptoms of bleeding right away. Review medication profile, and discuss discontinuance of aspirin or NSAIDs with patient and physician or NP/PA. Follow HGB/HCT and assess patient's tolerance, fatigue, other symptoms, and need for supportive measures.

II.   POTENTIAL ALTERATION IN NUTRITION, LESS THAN BODY REQUIREMENTS, related to NAUSEA, VOMITING, DIARRHEA, HEPATOTOXICITY, RARE INTESTINAL PERFORATION

Defining Characteristics: In clinical studies, nausea occurred in 25–43% of patients (grade 3–4 in 0–1%), vomiting in 13–29% (0–1% grade 3–4), diarrhea in 21–47% (2–14% grade 3–4), constipation in 23%, decreased appetite in 15%, and hypokalemia in 12%. Diarrhea can be fatal and severe diarrhea occurred in 14% of patients. Hypertriglyceridemia, hyperglycemia, and increases in AST and ALT occurred in > 30% of patients. Fatal and serious intestinal perforation can occur.

Nursing Implications: Assess baseline nutritional, and elimination status, and appetite. Assess serum chemistries including glucose, triglycerides, and hepatic function, baseline and during therapy as ordered. Assess patient tolerance of chemotherapy and need for premedication with antiemetics. Teach the patient to report nausea and/or vomiting that is not relieved by prescribed antiemetics. Teach patient that diarrhea or constipation may occur, dietary modifications for each problem, and to call nurse or physician for diarrhea, nausea, or vomiting that does not resolve within 24 hours with recommended over-the-counter or prescription medicines. If patient develops severe diarrhea or colitis, teach patient to stop the drug and to notify physician right away. Drug dose should be interrupted, and then reduced, or drug discontinued per physician. Teach patient to call physician and be prepared to seek emergency care right away if the patient develops severe abdominal pain, with or without fever, as intestinal perforation may occur.

Drug: imatinib mesylate (Gleevec)

Class: Kinase Inhibitor (tyrosine kinase inhibitor).

Mechanism of Action: Inhibits abnormal tyrosine kinase created by the Philadelphia chromosome (Bcr-Abl) in chronic myelocytic leukemia (CML), thus preventing cell proliferation and causing apoptosis in Bcr-Abl positive cell lines (nonreceptor tyrosine kinase inhibitor). Drug also inhibits receptor tyrosine kinases for platelet-derived growth factor (PDGF). Inhibits c-Kit receptor called stem cell factor receptor (SCFR) tyrosine kinases as well, which has resulted in marked responses in GIST (gastrointestinal stromal tumors). 15–85% of GISTs have Kit mutations that result in constitutively active kinases; imatinib mesylate selectively inhibits this mutated tyrosine kinase.

Metabolism: Well absorbed after oral administration with 98% bioavailability and C_{max} in 2–4 hours after dosing. Elimination half-life of imatinib is 18 hours, and 40 hours for primary active metabolite N-desmethyl derivative. Drug is 95% protein-bound. It is metabolized via CYP3A4 hepatic cytochrome P450 enzyme system, with 81% of the dose eliminated in 7 days, primarily via fecal route (68%) and, to a lesser degree, uriinary (13%). 25% of drug dose is excreted unchanged in feces and urine.

Indication: Treatment of
- Newly diagnosed adult and pediatric patients with Philadelphia chromosome chronic myeloid leukemia (Ph+ CML) in chronic phase.
- Ph+ CML in blast crisis (BC), accelerated phase (AP), or in chronic phase (CP) after failure of interferon alpha therapy.
- Adult patients with relapsed or refractory Ph+ acute lymphoblastic leukemia (Ph+ ALL).
- Pediatric patients with newly diagnosed Ph+ ALL in combination with chemotherapy.
- Adult patients with myelodysplastic/myeloproliferative diseases (MDS/MPD) associated with PDGFR gene rearrangements.
- Adult patients with aggressive systemic mastocytosis (ASM), without the D816V c-Kit mutation or c-Kit mutational status is unknown.
- Adult patients with hypereosinophilic syndrome (HES) and/or chronic eosinophilic leukemia (CEL) who have FIP1L1-PDGFRα fusion kinase (mutational analysis or FISH demonstration of CHIC2 allele deletion), as well as those who do not, or it is unknown.
- Adult patients with unresectable, recurrent, and/or metastatic dermatofibrosarcoma protuberans (DFSP).
- Patients with Kit (CD117)-positive unresectable and/or metastatic malignant gastrointestinal stromal tumors (GIST).
- Adjuvant treatment of adult patients following resection of Kit (CD117)-positive GIST.

Dosage/Range:
- Ph+ CML
  - Adults, CP: 400 mg/day PO as a single dose.
  - Adults, AP or BC: 600 mg/day.
  - Adult patients with Ph+ CML CP, AP, and BC: consider dose escalation if no severe adverse drug reaction, no severe nonleukemia-related neutropenia or thrombocytopenia, when (1) disease has progressed, (2) failure to achieve a satisfactory hematologic response after at least 3 months of treatment, (3) failure to achieve a cytogenetic response after 6–12 months of treatment, or (4) loss of a previously achieved hematologic or cytogenetic response.
    - CP: increase dose from 400 mg/day to 600 mg/day.
    - AC, BC: increase dose from 600 mg/day to 800 mg/day (givn as 400 mg twice daily).
  - Pediatrics, CP: 340 mg/m^2/day (not to exceed 600 mg).

- Ph+ALL
  - Adults with Ph+ ALL: 600 mg/day.
  - Pediatric patients with Ph+ ALL: 340 mg/m^2/day (not to exceed 600 mg/day).
- Adults with MDS/MPD: 400 mg/day.
- Adults with ASM: 100 mg/day or 400 mg/day.
- Adults with HES/CEL: 100 mg/day or 400 mg/day.
- Adults with DFSP: 800 mg/day.
- Adults with metastatic and/or unresectable (CD117+) GIST: 400 mg/day; may increase dose up to 800 mg/day (400 mg twice daily) if needed (e.g., showing clear signs of symptoms of disease progression, with no severe adverse drug reactions).
- Adults receiving adjuvant therapy × 36 mo for (CD117+) GIST: 400 mg/day.
- Hepatic impairment: patients with mild or moderate impairment do not require a dose adjustment. Patients with severe hepatic impairment require a 25% decrease in the recommended dose.
- Renal impairment: reduced dose in moderate renal impairment.
  - CrCl = 20–39 mL/min: 50 % reduced starting dose, with future doses increased as tolerated; doses > 600 mg/day are not recommended.
  - Mild renal impairment (CrCl = 40–59): doses > 400 mg/day are not recommended.
  - Severe renal impairment: use with extreme caution; a dose of 100 mg/day has been used (see package insert).
- Concomitant strong CYP3A4 inducers (e.g., dexamethasone, phenytoin, carbamazepine, rifampin, rifabutin, rifampacin, phenobarbital): avoid. If must coadminister, increase the dose of imatinib by at least 50%, and carefully monitor clinical response.

Dose modifications for nonhematologic toxicity (see package insert May 2014):
- Elevations in bilirubin > 3 × IULN (institutional upper limit of normal) or in liver transaminases > 5 × IULN, hold drug until bilirubin has returned to < 1.5 × IULN, and transaminase levels to < 2.5 × ULN. In adults, resume at a reduced daily dose (e.g., 400 mg reduced to 300 mg, 600-mg dose reduced to 400 mg, and 800-mg dose reduced to 600 mg daily). In children, daily doses can be reduced under the same circumstances from 340 mg/m^2/day to 260 mg/m^2/day.
- If a severe nonhematologic reaction occurs (e.g., severe hepatotoxicity or severe fluid retention), hold drug until event resolves. Resume drug as appropriate, depending upon severity of reaction.

Drug modifications for hematologic toxicity (see package insert, May 2014):
- Chronic phase CML at initial dose of 400 mg/day, MDS/MPD, ASM and HES/CEL (starting dose 400 mg) or GIST at initial dose of 400 mg/day: ANC < 1,000/mm^3 and/or platelets < 50,000/mm^3: stop drug until ANC ≥ 1,500/mm^3 and/or platelets ≥ 75,000/mm^3 and then resume at usual 400 mg dose; if recurrence of ANC < 1,000/mm^3, and/or platelets < 50,000/mm^3, hold until recovered, and reduce dose to 300 mg daily.
- Ph+ CML: Accelerated phase and blast crisis (starting dose 600 mg), and Ph+ ALL (starting dose 600 mg): ANC < 500/mm^3 and/or platelets < 10,000/mm^3: determine if related to leukemia by bone marrow aspirate/biopsy; if unrelated to leukemia, reduce dose to 400 mg daily; if cytopenia persists 2 weeks, reduce again to 300 mg daily; if cytopenia

persists 4 weeks and is still unrelated to leukemia, stop imatinib until ANC $\geq 1,000/mm^3$ and platelets $\geq 20/mm^3$, and then resume at 300 mg/day.
- Pediatric newly diagnosed chronic phase CML (starting dose 340 mmg/m^2): ANC $< 1,000/mm^3$ and/or platelets $< 50,000/mm^3$: stop drug until ANC $\geq 1,500/mm^3$ and/or platelets $\geq 75,000/mm^3$ and then resume at previous dose before adverse reaction; if recurrence of ANC $< 1,000/mm^3$, and/or platelets $< 50,000/mm^3$, hold until recovered (ANC $\geq 1,500/mm^3$ and/or platelets $\geq 75,000/mm^3$), then resume at reduced dose of 260 mg/m^2.
- DFSP, ASM associated with eosinophilia (starting dose 100 mg/day), HES/CEL with FIP1L1-PDGFRα fusion kinase (starting dose 100 mg/day): see package insert.

Drug Preparation/Administration:
- Available in scored 100-mg and 400-mg tablets.
- Administer dose orally, once daily (unless the total dose is 800 mg, which is given as 400 mg twice daily), with a meal and a large glass of water.
- In children with CML and Ph+ ALL, the daily dose can be split into two: one portion dosed in the morning and one in the evening, or it can be given as a once-daily dose. There is no experience with imatinib in children < 1 year old.
- Drug can be dissolved in water or apple juice if the patient has difficulty swallowing. Dissolve tablet in a glass of water: use 50 mL for a 100-mg tablet, and 200 mL for the 400-mg tablet; stir with a spoon, and administer immediately after drug dissolves.
- Doses of 800 mg and above: use 400-mg tablets to reduce exposure to iron
- Assess CBC/differential weekly for first month, biweekly for the second month, then as clinically indicated, or periodically, e.g., every 2–3 months. Assess LFTs baseline, then monthly or as clinically indicated.
- Teach patients if they miss a dose, take the dose as soon as possible unless it is almost time for their next dose, in which case they should not take It. Do not take a double dose. Take tablet(s) with a meal and a large glass of water. Teach patients to avoid grapefruit and grapefruit juice.

Drug Interactions:
- *CYP3A4 inhibitors* (ketoconazole, itraconazole, clarithromycin, atazanavir, indinavir, nefazodone, nelfinavir, ritonavir, saquinavir, telithromycin, voriconazole; grapefruit or grapefruit juice) may increase imatinib plasma concentrations; do not coadminister.
- *CYP3A4 inducers* (dexamethasone, phenytoin, carbamazepine, rifampin, phenobarbital; also oxcarbamazepine, fosphenytoin, primidone; St. John's wort) may increase metabolism of imatinib, so imatinib serum levels are reduced. Avoid concomitant use, and find alternative agents. Use together cautiously; when used with dexamethasone, phenytoin, carbamazepine, phenobarbital, rifabutin or rifampin, or other strong inducers, increase imatinib dose by 50%. Doses up to 1200 mg/day (600 mg bid) have been given to patients receiving concomitant strong CYP3A4 inducers. Do not take St. John's wort if taking imatinib.
- *CYP3A4 substrates* with a narrow therapeutic window (e.g., simvastatin, alfentanil, cyclosporine, diergotamine, ergotamine, fentanyl, pimozide, quinidine, sirolimus, tacrolimus; as well as triazolo-benzodiazepines, dihydropyridine calcium channel

blockers, certain HMG-CoA reductase inhibitors) increased serum levels of substrate. For example, imatinib decreases simvastatin metabolism with simvastatin serum levels **increased** 2–3.5 times. Do not administer together, as drug has a narrow therapeutic window. If necessary to coadminister, monitor patient closely for toxicity, and reduce dose of substrate as needed.

- *Other CYP3A4 substrates:* eletriptan (Relpax). Do not administer eletriptan within 72 hours of imatinib. Monitor vital signs closely.
- Warfarin: do not give together with imatinib, as imatinib inhibits warfarin metabolism by CYP2C9 and CYP3A4 enzymes. Use low molecular heparin or standard heparin instead.
- Acetaminophen: systemic exposure expected to increase when coadministered with imatinib mesylate.
- Imatinib mesylate inhibits CYP2D6; when coadministering imatinib with drugs that are a substrate of CYP2D6 having a narrow therapeutic window, use caution and monitor patients closely for toxicity.

Lab Effects/Interference:
- Neutropenia, thrombocytopenia.
- Elevated hepatic transaminases (SGOT/AST, SGPT/ALT), bilirubin, serum creatinine.
- Decreased thyroid function tests (e.g., TSH) in patients who have had thyroidectomy.

Special Considerations:
- Drug is teratogenetic. Women should avoid pregnancy or breastfeeding while taking the drug.
- Fluid retention and edema: drug often causes edema that may be severe in some patients. There is increased risk in patients at higher drug doses and in the elderly (< 65 years). Weigh patients regularly and manage unexpected rapid weight gain by drug interruption and diuretics. Pleural effusion, pericardial effusion, pulmonary edema, and ascites have been reported.
- Drug is associated with neutropenia, thrombocytopenia, and anemia. Blood counts should be checked weekly for the first month, biweekly for the second month, and then periodically thereafter (e.g., every 2–3 months). Patients with accelerated phase CML or blast crisis require closer monitoring. Manage bone marrow depression with dose reduction or dose interruption, and rarely, drug discontinuation. See package insert.
- Severe CHF and left ventricular dysfunction have been reported. Monitor patients carefully if they have cardiac disease, cardiac risk factors, or history of renal failure. Discuss with physician evaluation of patient with signs/symptoms of cardiac or renal failure.
- Hypereosinophilic cardiac toxicity: Patients at risk are those with HES/CEL, and in patients with MDS/MPD or ASM associated with high eosinophil levels. Assess ECHO and serum troponin levels. See package insert for management.
- Dermatologic toxicities: bullous dermatologic reactions (e.g., Stevens-Johnson syndrome, erythema multiforme) have been reported. Assess any rash, and if bullous, discuss drug interruption and confirmation of dermatology diagnosis.

- Hypothyroidism in patients taking levothyroxin replacement after thyroidectomy; monitor TSH levels in these patients.
- Grade 3–4 hemorrhage has been reported in clinical studies in patients newly diagnosed with CML and GIST. GI tumors may be the source of GI bleeds in patients with GIST. Monitor patients for GI symptoms at the start of therapy. Rare reports, including fatalities, of GI perforation have been made.
- GI irritation: patient should take imatinib with food and a large glass of water.
- Severe hepatotoxicity can occur.
  - Cases of liver failure or injury requiring liver transplants have been reported in both short-term and long-term use of imatinib.
  - See Dosage for initial and dose reductions if hepatic impairment.
  - Liver function tests (LFTs) should be monitored baseline and monthly or as clinically indicated.
- Because patients are treated for many years, consider potential long-term toxicities (e.g., liver, kidney, cardiac), as well as immunosuppression.
- Drug is embryo-fetal toxicity: Women of childbearing potential should be taught to use highly effective contraception to avoid pregnancy. If the drug is used during pregnancy or if the patient becomes pregnant while taking the drug, the patient should be apprised of the potential hazard to the fetus.
- Nursing mothers should decide whether to discontinue nursing or discontinue the drug, taking into consideration importance of imatinib to the mother's health.
- Growth retardation has been reported in children and preadolescents receiving imatinib mesylate. The long term effects of prolonged treatment with this drug are unknown. Close monitoring of growth in children is recommended.
- Tumor lysis syndrome may occur in patients with CML, GIST, ALL, and eosinophilic leukemia receiving imatinib mesylate, and it may be fatal. Patients at risk are those with a high proliferative rate or high tumor burden prior to treatment. Monitor these patients closely, and discuss TLS prophylaxis with physician. Correct clinically significant dehydration and treat high uric acid levels before starting imatinib mesylate.
- Most common adverse reactions with an incidence of ≥ 30% were edema, nausea, vomiting, muscle cramps, musculoskeletal pain, diarrhea, rash, fatigue, and abdominal pain.
- Teach patients that they may experience dizziness, blurred vision, or somnolence while taking imatinib and should use caution when driving a car or operating machinery.

Potential Toxicities/Side Effects and the Nursing Process

I. POTENTIAL FOR INFECTION AND BLEEDING related to BONE MARROW DEPRESSION

Defining Characteristics: Neutropenia and thrombocytopenia were common, especially in patients who received higher doses, and in patients with advanced stages of disease (blast crisis and accelerated phase). Median duration of neutropenia was 2–3 weeks, and thrombocytopenia from 3–4 weeks. Dose needs to be held and reduced as noted in Dose Modifications or in package insert. Fever affected 14% (chronic phase) to 38% (accelerated phase) of patients. Hemorrhage (CNS and GI) was treated in 13% (chronic phase) to 48% (accelerated phase) of patients.

Nursing Implications: Assess baseline CBC, including WBC and differential and platelet count prior to dosing, as well as at least weekly during first month of treatment, at least every other week for the second month of treatment, and then as clinically indicated and ordered. Discuss dose interruption and reduction as above for neutropenia and thrombocytopenia (hold for ANC < 500, platelets < 50,000). Teach patient self-assessment of signs/symptoms of infection (e.g., T ≥ 100.4°F, dysuria, productive cough) and bleeding (including epistaxis and development of petechiae), and instruct patient to report them right away. Teach patient self-care measures to minimize risk of infection and bleeding, including avoidance of OTC aspirin-containing medications.

II.   POTENTIAL ALTERATION IN CIRCULATION related to CONGESTIVE HEART FAILURE

Defining Characteristics: The Abelson tyrosine kinase (ABL) protein is necessary for the general health and maintenance of cardiac muscles, especially the mitochondria (Kerkela et al., 2006). Although rare (0.7%) Kerkela et al. reported that 10 patients developed CHF between 1–14 months after starting the drug; although patients had an average LVEF of 56%, on repeat testing, the average LVEF was 25%. Patients with hypereosinophilic infiltration of the myocardium are at risk of cardiogenic shock and left ventricular dysfunction, and it is reversible with systemic steroids, circulatory support strategies, and holding the drug.

Nursing Implications: Patients at risk (e.g., advanced age, cardiac comorbidities) should have determination of their LVEF baseline and periodically while receiving the drug. Assess baseline cardiac status, history, and risk for development of CHF. Closely monitor patient while receiving imatinib mesylate, especially if patient has history of hypertension or is on cardiac medications. Teach patient to report any dyspnea, SOB, chest pain, or heart palpitations, or any unusual feeling. If any abnormalities occur, teach patient to stop drug and to call the physician or nurse immediately.

III.   ALTERATION IN FLUID AND ELECTROLYTE BALANCE related to FLUID RETENTION, EDEMA, AND HYPOKALEMIA

Defining Characteristics: Fluid retention is common (52% chronic phase and 67% accelerated phase patients), especially in the elderly, and primarily reflects periorbital and lower extremity edema. However, pleural effusions, ascites, rapid weight gain, and pulmonary edema may develop, and in some cases, may be life-threatening (e.g., pleural effusion, congestive heart failure, renal failure, pericardial effusion, and anasarca). Hypokalemia was reported to occur in 2–12% of patients.

Nursing Implications: Assess baseline parameters of weight, presence of edema, pulmonary function, and monitor closely during therapy. Teach patient to monitor weight daily at home, and to report weight gain of 2 pounds in 1 week, development of edema, or dyspnea. Teach the patient comfort measures for periorbital edema, such as ice packs, and self-administration of diuretics as ordered. Discuss with physician drug dose modification or interruption if severe fluid retention occurs.

IV. ALTERATION IN NUTRITION, POTENTIAL, LESS THAN BODY REQUIREMENTS, related to NAUSEA, VOMITING, DIARRHEA, HEPATOTOXICITY

Defining Characteristics: Nausea affected 68% of patients with accelerated phase, and 55% with chronic phase; vomiting affected 54% and 28%, respectively. Diarrhea affected 54%, while constipation affected 13%. Dyspepsia affected about 19%.

Nursing Implications: Teach patient to self-administer antiemetics 1 hour prior to each dose, and to call if nausea/vomiting develop. Discuss with physician more effective antiemetic regimen if nausea/vomiting develop. Encourage small, frequent intake of cool, bland foods as tolerated if nausea develops. Refer to dietitian as needed for meal planning. Assess bowel-elimination pattern baseline and at each visit. Teach patient to report diarrhea or constipation that does not respond to antidiarrheal or anticonstipation medications. Teach dietary modifications as appropriate. Monitor LFTs baseline and periodically during therapy. Hold therapy if LFTs become abnormal (see Special Considerations).

V. ALTERATION IN COMFORT related to MUSCLE CRAMPS, MUSCULOSKELETAL (BONE) PAIN, HEADACHE, FATIGUE, ARTHRALGIA, AND ABDOMINAL PAIN

Defining Characteristics: Muscle cramps are common, affecting 25–46% of patients. Musculoskeletal pain affects 27–37% of patients, headache 24–29% of patients, fatigue 33% of patients, rash 32% of patients, and arthralgias 26% of patients. In clinical studies, abdominal pain affected 20% of patients with chronic phase, and 26% of patients in blast crisis.

Nursing Implications: Teach patient that these events may occur and to report them. Assess baseline comfort, and monitor closely during treatment. Develop plan to assure comfort, depending on symptoms reported. For cramps, suggest drinking tonic water and taking calcium gluconate, and if ineffective, discuss with physician the prescription of quinine; for the management of bone pain, suggest NSAIDs as appropriate (Ault et al., 2007). Discuss ineffective strategies with physician, and revise plan as needed.

VI. ALTERATION IN SKIN INTEGRITY related to RASH

Defining Characteristics: Rash may occur. In clinical studies, 32% of patients with accelerated phase, and 36% of patients in chronic phase CML reported rash. Ten percent of patients complained of pruritus.

Nursing Implications: Teach patient that rash may occur and to report it. Assess patient skin integrity, baseline and regularly, during treatment. Teach patient local comfort measures. Teach patient self-application of topical steroids to rash or, if prescribed, systemic steroids (Ault, 2007). Discuss rash and management plan with physician, especially if severe.

Drug: ipilimumab (Yervoy)

Class: Immune checkpoint inhibitor. Human cytotoxic T-lymphocyte antigen-4 (CTLA-4) blocking antibody; IgG1 human monoclonal antibody.

Mechanism of Action: Ipilimumab is a negative regulator of T-cell activation. CTLA-4 is an antigen that is expressed on human activated T-lymphocytes that is important in regulating the body's immune response; it has an affinity for B7 costimulatory molecules, which determine how the T-lymphocyte will interact with antigen-presenting cells. T-lymphocytes are important in immune surveillance to distinguish between self and non–self-antigens. CTLA-4 downregulates (turns off) T-lymphocytes after the invading antigen has been removed so that the immune system does not injure normal tissue. Ipilimumab is a fully human monoclonal antibody that binds to CTLA-4 and blocks its interaction with ligands CD80/CD86. This augments T-cell activation and proliferation. Ipilimumab's effect on malignant melanoma cells is indirect, probably via T-cell mediated antitumor activity.

Metabolism: When given IV every 3 weeks, steady state is achieved after the third dose. The terminal half-life is 14.7 days. Systemic clearance was increased with increasing body weight, but this did not require dose adjustments. Patients with renal or hepatic impairment did not require dose adjustments. Lab testing of pregnant animals showed that there was a higher incidence of abortion, stillbirth, premature delivery, and infant mortality when given in the third trimester.

Indication: Treatment of patients with unresectable or metastatic melanoma.

Dosage/Range:
- 3 mg/kg IV infusion over 90 minutes, every 3 weeks × 4 doses over no more than 16 weeks.
- Permanently discontinue for severe adverse reactions.

Dose Modifications:
- Moderate to severe side effects: hold drug and anticipate MD/NP/PA will order systemic corticosteroids.
- Drug should be held for **moderate immune-mediated adverse reactions or symptomatic endocrinopathy**.
  - If complete or partial resolution of adverse effects (grade 0–1), improvement to mild severity, or return to baseline, and patient is receiving < 7.5 mg of prednisone or equivalent per day, resume drug at the recommended 3 mg/kg IV dose every 3 weeks until all 4 doses have been administered or 16 weeks, whichever comes first.
  - Administer systemic high-dose corticosteroids for severe, persistent, or recurring immune-mediated reactions.

- Drug should be permanently discontinued for any of the following:
  - Persistent moderate adverse reactions, or inability to reduce corticosteroid to 7.5 mg prednisone or equivalent per day.
  - Failure to complete full treatment in 16 weeks from administration of first dose.
  - Severe adverse reactions or life-threatening adverse reactions, including any of the following:
    - Colitis with abdominal pain, fever, ileus, peritoneal signs, 7 or more stools per day over baseline, stool incontinence, need for IV hydration > 24 hr, GI hemorrhage, or GI perforation.
    - Significantly abnormal LFTs: AST or ALT > 5 times ULN, or total bilirubin > 3 times ULN.
    - Stevens-Johnson syndrome, toxic epidermal necrolysis, or rash complicated by full thickness dermal ulceration, or necrotic bullous or hemorrhagic manifestations.
    - Severe motor or sensory neuropathy, Guillain-Barre syndrome, or myasthenia gravis.
    - Severe immune-mediated reactions involving any organ system (e.g., nephritis, pneumonitis, pancreatitis, noninfectious myocarditis); institute systemic high-dose corticosteroid therapy.
    - Immune-mediated ocular disease that is unresponsive to topical immunosuppressive therapy.

Drug Preparation:
- Available in 50-mg/10-mL (5-mg/mL) and 200-mg/40 mL (5-mg/mL) vials.
- Allow drug vial to come to room temperature over 5 min prior to mixing. Inspect and discard if any particulate matter or discoloration is found.
- Withdraw the ordered amount, and aseptically add to either 0.9% sodium chloride injection USP or 5% dextrose injection, USP to create a final concentration of 1 mg/mL–2 mg/mL.
- Mix solution by gently inverting bag. Do not shake.
- Drug may be stored under refrigeration (2–8°C, 36–46°F) or at room temperature (20–25°C, 68–77°F) for ≤ 24 hr.

Drug Administration:
- Assess LFTs, thyroid function tests, and clinical chemistries prior to each dose.
- Administer IV over 90 min via sterile, non-pyrogenic, low-protein binding in-line filter (e.g., 0.22 micron). Flush IV line with 0.9% sodium chloride injection USP or 5% dextrose injection, USP after administration to ensure all drug is administered. Do not mix ipilimumab with any other medicines (with or as an infusion with).
- IV infusion may be associated with infusion reactions, such as chest pain, flushed/red face, and back pain. Stop infusion and assess response. Administer ordered antihistamines (H1 and H2) and corticosteroid.

Drug Interactions:
- Vemurafenib: concurrent administration has resulted in increased grade 3 rise in transaminases, with or without increased bilirubin.

Lab Effects/Interference:
- Elevated LFTs (must distinguish between liver metastases and immune hepatitis).
- Alterations in cortisol, ACTH, testosterone, TSH, free T4 levels.

Special Considerations:
- Increased T-lymphocyte activation and resulting inflammation are responsible for the major toxicities: dermatitis, enterocolitis, and hypophysitis (rare). Rarely, inflammation of the eyes (uveitis), pituitary, thyroid, kidneys (nephritis), lungs (alveolitis), adrenal glands can occur, as can aseptic meningitis and arthritis. Grade 3–4 events are largely reversible with high-dose steroids therapy (Weber, 2007).
- Warnings and Precautions:
  - Permanently discontinue drug for severe immune-mediated reactions.
  - Hold dose for moderate immune-mediated adverse effects until return to baseline, improvement to mild severity, or complete resolution, and patient is receiving < 7.5 mg prednisone or equivalent per day. Administer high-dose corticosteroids for severe, persistent, or recurring immune-mediated reactions.
  - Immune-mediated enterocolitis: Monitor patient for signs/symptoms; see problem 1.
  - Immune-mediated hepatitis: evaluate LFTs before each dose of ipilimumab.
  - Immune-mediated endocrinopathies: monitor thyroid function tests and clinical chemistries prior to each dose. Evaluate at each visit for signs/symptoms of endocrinopathy. Discuss hormone replacement therapy as needed with physician.
- The Immune Mediated Adverse Reaction Management Guide, as well as a Nursing Immune-Mediated Adverse Reaction Checklist are available as part of the Yervoy Risk Evaluation and Mitigation Strategy (REMS), available online at www.YERVOY.com/hcp/rems.
- Assess patient at each visit for signs and symptoms of toxicity. The Yervoy Nursing Immune-Mediated Adverse Reaction Checklist is an excellent tool that was developed as part of Yervoy REMS:
  - Entercolitis (diarrhea, abdominal pain, mucus or blood in stool, fever).
  - Bowel perforation (peritoneal signs, ileus).
  - Hepatitis.
  - Dermatitis (generalized exfoliative full thickness dermal ulceration, ulcerative or bullous dermatitis, skin necrosis, Stevens-Johnson syndrome, or Toxic Epidermal Necrolysis).
  - Neuropathy (motor and sensory, unilateral or bilateral weakness; sensory alterations, paresthesias; severe if interferes with ability to perform ADLs).
  - Endocrine function (hypophysitis, adrenal insufficiency/adrenal crisis, hyper- or hypothyroidism; be alert for signs/symptoms: fatigue, headache, changes in mental status, abdominal pain, unusual bowel habits, hypotension) and discuss need for replacement hormone(s) as needed with physician or midlevel practitioner.
- Wolchok et al. (2011) found that ipilimumab (10 mg/kg) plus dacarbazine (DTIC) significantly improved OS in first-line metatastic melanoma compared to DTIC alone. Median OS was 11.2 months for the ipilimumab group compared to 9.1 months ($p < 0.0009$) in the DTIC alone group. However, PFS was slightly longer in the ipilimumab group (2.8 months vs 2.6 months, $p < 0.006$). The best overall RR was higher in

the ipilimumab arm (15.2%) vs DTIC alone arm (13.3%); and duration of response was longer in the ipilimumab arm (19.3 months vs 8.1 months in DTIC arm). Grade 3–4 events (e.g., diarrhea, rash, elevated ALT) occurred more commonly in the ipilimumab arm (56.3% vs 27.5% in the DTIC alone arm). There were no reports of intestinal perforation or hypophysitis.

- May take up to 3 months after drug is stopped to see a response. Patients may have short-term progression followed by delayed regression with a prolonged duration of clinical response or stable disease (Weber, 2007).
- Concurrent administration of budesonide to prevent diarrhea was ineffective (Weber et al., 2008).
- Women of reproductive potential should use effective birth control measures, and avoid pregancy.
- Nursing mothers should decide whether to discontinue nursing or to discontinue the drug, taking into account the importance of the drug to the mother's health. IgG1 is known to cross the placental barrier, and it is not known if it the drug is excreted in human milk.
- As part of REMS, patients should be given the provided wallet card stating the patient is receiving ipilimumab so that if the patient needs to go to the emergency room, physicians there will know that the patient may be experiencing immune-mediated side effects.

Potential Toxicities/Side Effects and the Nursing Process [see chapter introduction for additional information]

I.   ALTERATION IN ELIMINATION, POTENTIAL, related to DIARRHEA, ENTEROCOLITIS

Defining Characteristics: Incidence of diarrhea is 32% with 5% grade 3–5; colitis affected 8% of patients, with 5% being grade 3–5. Uncontrolled diarrhea may progress to enterocolitis. Rarely, enterocolitis can result in bowel perforation. In the drug studies ($n = 511$), 1% developed intestinal perforation, 0.8% died as a result of complications, and 5% of patients were hospitalized for severe enterocolitis. The median time to onset of grade 2 enterocolitis was 6.3 weeks (range 0.3–18.9 weeks), and to grade 3–5 severe enterocolitis was 7.4 weeks (range 1.6–13.4 weeks). 85% of patients with grade 3–5 enterocolitis were treated with high-dose corticosteroids (≥ 40 mg prednisone equivalent per day), with a median dose of 80 mg/day for a median duration of treatment of 2.3 weeks (ranging up to 13.9 weeks), followed by a corticosteroid taper. For patients studied who had moderate grade 2 enterocolitis, 46% were not treated with high-dose corticosteroids, 29% were treated with < 40 mg prednisone/equivalent/day for a median duration of 5.1 weeks. 25% were treated with high-dose corticosteroids for a median duration of 10 days prior to taper. Infliximab was administered to 8% of patients with moderate, severe, or life-threatening immune-mediated enterocolitis if the patient did not have an adequate response to high-dose corticosteroids. In most patients, symptoms resolved. O'Day et al. (2011) tested a GI management protocol and found that if followed, there was resolution of diarrhea/colitis during ipilimumab treatment: Grade 1 diarrhea: Treat symptomatically without immunosuppressives, unless diarrhea continued for more than 5 days; Grade 2: Treat symptomatically, and if persists for 3–5 days or worsens, treat with corticosteroids; Grade 3 or higher: Treat with systemic high-dose corticosteroids. Median time to resolution to a lower grade was 1 week, and median time to resolution was 2 weeks.

Nursing Interventions: Assess patient's baseline bowel elimination status, and history of bowel dysfunction, such as colitis. Ask about any changes in normal bowel habits or changes from baseline, or last visit: diarrhea, abdominal pain, blood or mucus in stool with/without fever, peritoneal signs consistent with bowel perforation, ileus. Teach patient that diarrhea may occur, to report diarrhea > 4 stools over baseline/day, loose stools, and blood or mucus in the stool. Review the patient's medication profile to identify any bowel medications, and to teach patient to avoid stool softeners and laxatives. Teach patient to take loperamide (or recommended antidiarrheal medication) after the first loose stool if it occurs, and to report right away if diarrhea does not resolve in 24 hours, or if the patient has nausea and/or vomiting and cannot take fluids. MODERATE diarrhea or enterocolitis is defined as diarrhea up to 4–6 stools over baseline/24 hours, abdominal pain, mucus, or blood in stool (grade 1 is < 4 stools over baseline, grade 2 is 4–6 stools over baseline ± abdominal pain, mucus or blood in stool). Moderate enterocolitis is generally treated with loperamide, and the stool tested to ensure another cause is not ignored. Ipilimumab is resumed if symptoms have improved to mild (< 4 stools/day) or resolved completely. If symptoms continue for more than 1 week, expect systemic corticosteroids (e.g., 0.5 mg/kg/day prednisone/equivalent) to be started and continued until improvement or resolution. The corticosteroids should be tapered. Ipilimumab can be resumed when symptoms have improved to at least mild severity and the steroid dose is 7.5 mg prednisone or equivalent, or less. SEVERE, life-threatening, or fatal immune-mediated enterocolitis (grade 3–5) is defined as having diarrhea (7 or more stools over baseline/24 hours), fever, ileus, peritoneal signs. Bowel perforation must be ruled out, and if present, corticosteroids are not started. Expect endoscopy and colonoscopy to be performed, with biopsies, for a definitive diagnosis. If enterocolitis is found, high-dose IV corticosteroids (1–2 mg/kg/day of prednisone or equivalent) are initiated. Once symptoms have resolved, patient should resume nutrition with a progressive low-fat, low-fiber diet. IV corticosteroids can be converted to oral, and the patient discharged home on an oral steroid. The corticosteroid taper should be done over at least 1 month (Weber, 2007). If symptoms do not resolve, the patient should be continually evaluated for evidence of gastrointestinal perforation or peritonitis. Repeat endoscopy should be considered, as should alternative immunosuppressive therapy. If the patient is refractory to high-dose parenteral steroids, infliximab (Remicade, a chimeric MAb targeting TNF-a) as a single dose may be prescribed (Beck et al., 2006). This requires TB testing, as it can reactivate dormant TB. Teach patient to go to the ED or call 911 if severe abdominal pain, with or without vomiting and constipation, occurs, as the patient needs to be evaluated for bowel perforation right away, although this is a rare event. If bowel perforation occurs, anticipate and prepare patient for immediate surgical intervention. Teach patient not to take any OTC medications or dietary supplements until discussing it first with nurse or physician.

II.   ALTERATION IN SKIN INTEGRITY, POTENTIAL, related to DERMATITIS

Defining Characteristics: Dermatitis is a common side effect, often associated with pruritus. Biopsy may show T-lymphocyte infiltrates. In clinical studies, pruritus occurred in

31% of patients, and rash in 29% of patients (2% severe grade 3–5). Severe (grades 3–5) dermatitis appeared in 2.5% of all study patients (e.g., as Stevens-Johnson syndrome, toxic epidermal necrolysis, or rash complicated by full thickness dermal ulceration, or necrotic, bullous, or hemorrhagic manifestations). One patient died of toxic epidermal necrolysis. 12% of patients had moderate (grade 2) dermatitis. Median time to onset of moderate, severe, or life-threatening dermatitis was 3.1 weeks (range up to 17.3 weeks from initiation of ipilimumab). 54% of patients with severe dermatitis received high-dose corticosteroids (median dose 60 mg of prednisone/equivalent) for a median of 14.9 weeks followed by steroid taper. Time to resolution ranged up to 15.6 weeks. Less than half of the patients with moderate dermatitis received high-dose corticosteroids (median dose 60 mg/day prednisone/equivalent, for a median of 2.1 weeks. 11% were treated with topical corticosteroids only, while 49% had neither topic nor systemic steroids. 70% of patients had complete resolution of symptoms, 11% improved to grade 1, and 19% had no improvement.

Nursing Interventions: Assess baseline skin integrity and presence of abnormalities, and monitor during therapy. Teach patient that dermatitis may occur. Moderate dermatitis is defined as diffuse, covering 50% or less of skin surface. If this occurs, ipilimumab dose is held, and topical or systemic corticosteroids administered if there is no improvement of symptoms within 1 week. If symptoms resolve or improve to mild (localized) symptoms, and systemic steroid dose is 7.5 mg prednisone equivalent or less, ipilimumab can be resumed. Severe or life threatening dermatitis is defined as Stevens-Johnson syndrome, toxic epidermal necrolysis, or rash complicated by full thickness dermal ulceration, or necrotic, bullous, or hemorrhagic manifestations. Ipilimumab must be permanently discontinued, and high-dose corticosteroids (1–2 mg/kg/day) started immediately. When the dermatitis is controlled, the corticosteroid should be tapered over at least 1 month. Other symptom management agents that may be used are antipruritic medications such as diphenhydramine and hydroxyzine.

III. ALTERATION IN NUTRITION related to IMMUNE HEPATITIS

Defining Characteristics: Uncommon, but may occur characterized by increasing LFTs. Rarely, severe, and fatal liver inflammation can occur.

Nursing Interventions: Assess LFTs and signs and symptoms of hepatitis baseline and prior to each drug dose. If increasing LFTs (AST, ALT, total bilirubin), check labs every 3 days until stable or decreasing and then weekly per physician's order. Hold drug if moderate elevation in LFTs (AST or ALT > 2.5 times but 1.5 times but 5 times ULN, total bilirubin > 3 times ULN), or failure to complete full treatment course within 16 weeks from administration of first dose. Anticipate that the physician will rule out any infectious or malignant cause. If LFTs continue to rise and immune hepatitis suspected, systemic high-dose corticosteroids (1–2 mg/kg/day prednisone equivalent) should be started, with increased frequency of LFT monitoring until resolution. Once LFTs show sustained improvement or resolve to baseline, the corticosteroid dose should be tapered over at least 1 month. If symptoms do not resolve, consider alternative immunosuppressive therapy, such as mycophenolate mofetil, tacrolimus, or infliximab (Weber, 2007).

IV.   POTENTIAL FOR SENSORY/PERCEPTUAL ALTERATIONS related to NEUROPATHY, GUILLAIN-BARRE SYNDROME, MYASTHENIA GRAVIS

Defining Characteristics: Neurological side effects are rare. A number of cases of Guillain-Barré, one fatal, one case of severe (grade 3) peripheral motor neuropathy, and a case of myasthenia gravis have been reported.

Nursing Interventions: Assess baseline neurological status, and symptoms of motor or sensory neuropathy such as unilateral or bilateral weakness, sensory alterations, or paresthesias, and monitor for these, as well as patient's ability to perform ADLs prior to each dose. Teach patient to report any changes in sensation, perception, or in ability to perform ADLs. Ipilimumab should be held for moderate neuropathy (not interfering with ADLs) but must be permanently discontinued when peripheral neuropathy becomes severe (patient cannot perform ADLs). The drug should also be discontinued if new onset or worsening of severe motor or sensory neuropathy, Guillain-Barré syndrome or myasthenia gravis or failure to complete the full treatment course within 16 weeks from date of first dose. Anticipate that medications appropriate to the type of neurological condition will be instituted; high-dose corticosteroid therapy (1–2 mg/kg/day prednisone/equivalent) should also be considered.

V.   ALTERATION IN BODY FUNCTION AND METABOLISM related to IMMUNE-MEDIATED ENDOCRINOPATHIES, e.g., HYPOPHYSITIS (inflammation leading to hypopituitarism)

Defining Characteristics: Uncommon but significant because symptoms are vague initially (e.g., fatigue, headaches, low TSH, and serum cortisol levels), and if untreated, dysfunction of the hypophysis (such as pituitary enlargement) is far-reaching (e.g., severe headaches, severe fatigue, memory loss, loss of libido) (Blansfield et al., 2005). In clinical studies, 1.8% of patients developed grade 3–4 immune-mediated endocrinopathy (requiring hospitalization, urgent medical interventions, or interfering with patient's ability to perform ADLs). Patients all had hypopituitarism; in addition, some had adrenal insufficiency, hypogonadism, and hypothyroidism. 2.3% of patients had moderate endocrinopathy requiring hormone replacement or medical intervention (grade 2), and conditions included hypothyroidism, adrenal insufficiency, hypopituitarism; one patient had hyperthyroidism, and one had Cushing's syndrome. Median time to onset for moderate to severe immune-mediated endocrinopathy was 11 weeks, with a range up to 19.3 weeks after the first ipilimumab dose.

Nursing Interventions: Monitor TST and clinical chemistries baseline and prior to each ipilimumab dose. Assess baseline activity and comfort levels and at each visit. Teach patient to report onset of worsening fatigue, headaches, changes in mental status, abdominal pain, unusual bowel habits, dizziness (hypotension), or new onset non-specific symptoms. If hypophysitis is suspected, discuss evaluation with physician or NP/PA: MRI to compare size of pituitary baseline, cortisol, ACTH, TSH, and free T4 levels. If the diagnosis of hypophysitis is confirmed, teach patient about, and administer ordered high-dose steroids and hormonal replacement as needed (e.g., thyroid hormone, testosterone for male patients). Expect that most patients will continue on low-dose hydrocortisone to protect the pituitary gland (Blansfield et al., 2005). Ipilimumab should be held for moderate immune-mediated reactions or any symptomatic endocrinopathy until complete resolution or the patient is stable on hormone replacement therapy. Some patients require systemic corticosteroids (1–2 mg/kg/day prednisone/equivalent, as well as hormone-replacement therapy. Ipilimumab should be permanently discontinued if unable to reduce corticosteroid dose to 7.5 mg prednisone/equivalent per day, or failure to complete full treatment course in 16 weeks from first ipilimumab dose.

Drug: lapatinib ditosylate (Tykerb)

Class: Kinase inhibitor (tyrosine); EGFR1 and EGFR2 inhibitor.

Mechanism of Action: Drug inhibits tyrosine kinases of both human epidermal growth factor receptor (EGFR or) HER-1 and (EGFR-2 or) HER-2-neu, leading to arrest of cell growth and/or apoptosis in tumor cells that depend upon ErbB1 and ErbB2 cell signaling. Normally, HER-2 dimerizes with other members of the HER family, including HER-1. The message is then sent repeatedly via the tyrosine kinases to the cell nucleus telling the cell to divide. In 20% of patients with breast cancer, HER-2-neu is overexpressed, leading to increased cell proliferation, invasiveness, and conferring a poor prognosis associated with reduced survival. By blockading the tyrosine kinases, the message for repeated cell division is halted. Crosses the blood brain barrier.

Metabolism: After oral ingestion, drug undergoes incomplete and variable absorption. Initial serum concentration identifiable in 15 minutes (median). Peak concentrations achieved in 4 hours, with steady state reached in 6–7 days of single daily dosing. Dividing the dose results in a twofold higher exposure at steady state. When given with food, systemic exposure is increased threefold higher (low-fat diet) or fourfold higher (high-fat diet). Drug is highly protein-bound (> 99%). Drug is a substrate for the transporter proteins, breast cancer-resistance protein, and P-glycoprotein, and yet, lapatinib is also able to inhibit these efflux transporters. Drug is extensively metabolized by the CYP3A4 and CYP3A5 microenzyme system. Terminal half-life of the drug is 14.2 hours and with daily dosing is 24 hours. Drug is eliminated by the liver (P450 system) with about 27% recoverable from feces and less than 2% from the urine. Drug is not dialyzable due to high protein binding.

Indications: Drug is indicated in combination with:
- Capecitabine, for the treatment of patients with advanced or metastatic breast cancer whose tumors overexpress HER-2 and have received prior therapy, including an anthracycline, a taxane, and trastuzumab. (Limitation of use: Patients should have disease progression on trastuzumab prior to initiation of lapatinib/capecitabine treatment.)
- Letrozole, for the treatment of postmenopausal women with hormone receptor-positive, HER-2+ metastatic breast cancer that overexpresses the HER-2 receptor for whom hormonal therapy is indicated.
- Lapatinib in combination with an aromatase inhibitor has not been compared to a trastuzumab-containing chemotherapy regimen for the treatment of metastatic breast cancer.

Dosage/Range:
- Advanced or metastatic breast cancer: 1,250 mg orally (5 tablets) once daily days 1–21 continuously, in combination with capecitabine, 2,000 mg/m^2/day PO bid on days 1–14, administered orally in 2 doses approximately 12 hours apart, repeated every 21 days.
- Hormone receptor-positive, HER-2+ metastatic breast cancer: 1,500 mg PO (6 tablets) once daily, continuously in combination with letrozole (e.g., 2.5 mg once daily).
- Lapatinib should be taken at least 1 hour before or 1 hour after a meal. The dose should be taken all at once, not divided.

Dose-modify for:
- *Decrease in LVEF:* Discontinue drug in patients with a decreased LVEF that is grade 2 or higher (NCI CTCAE v3), and in patients with an LVEF that drops below the institution's LLN (ILLN). Wait a minimum of 2 weeks, and if the LVEF returns to normal and the patient is asymptomatic, drug may be restarted at a reduced dose of 1,000 mg/day in combination with capecitabine and a dose of 1,250 mg/day in combination with letrozole.
- *Preexisting severe hepatic impairment:* Reduce dose, as systemic exposure to lapatinib (AUC) increased 14% in patients with moderate and 63% in patients with severe preexisting hepatic dysfunction. Thus, patients with severe hepatic impairment (Child-Pugh Class C) should be reduced as follows:
  - HER-2+ metastatic BC indication: to 750 mg/day (from 1,250 mg/day).
  - Hormone receptor-positive, HER-2+ BC indication: to 1,000 mg/day (from 1,500 mg/day), as this predicts a normal AUC; however, there are no clinical data to support this.
  - Discontinue and do not restart drug if patient develops severe changes in liver function tests while receiving lapatinib.
- *Diarrhea:* Interrupt lapatinib for NCI CTCAE grade 3 or grade 1 or 2 with complicating features (e.g., moderate-to-severe abdominal cramping, grade 2 or higher nausea and/ or vomiting, decreased performance status, fever, sepsis, neutropenia, frank bleeding, or dehydration).
  - Lapatinib can be reintroduced at a lower dose (e.g., 1,000 mg/day reduced from 1,250 mg/day, 1,250 mg/day reduced from 1,500 mg/day) when diarrhea resolves to grade 1 or less.
  - Permanently discontinue drug for grade 4 diarrhea.
- Drug Interactions: *Strong CYP3A4 inhibitors*: If avoidance of the drug is not possible, reduce lapatinib dose to 500 mg orally per day, and when interacting drug discontinued, allow 1 week washout period before adjusting lapatinib dose up to 1,250 mg/day. Teach patients NOT to drink grapefruit juice or eat grapefruit to avoid increased serum lapatinib levels.
- Drug Interactions: *Strong CYP3A4 inducers*: If unavoidable, and must give both together, gradually titrate dose of lapatinib up to 4,500 mg/day (from 1,250 mg in HER-2+ metastatic BC) or to 5,500 mg/day (from 1,500 mg in hormone receptor-positive HER-2 BC) based on tolerability; if interacting drug is discontinued, resume 1,250-mg/day dose.
- *Other toxicities*: Discontinue or interrupt drug if patient develops grade 2 or higher toxicities (NCI CTCAE). Resume at 1,250 mg/day or 1,500 mg/day when improvement to grade 1 or less; for recurrent toxicity, restart at a lower dose of 1,000 mg/day (in combination with capecitabine) or 1,250 mg/day in combination with letrozole.
- Drug is contraindicated in patients with known hypersensitivity such as anaphylaxis to the drug or any of its components.

Drug Preparation:
• Oral. Available in 250-mg tablets.

Drug Administration:
• Give lapatinib in a single dose 1 hour before or 1 hour after a meal;
• Capecitabine is given in two divided doses about 12 hours apart with food or within 30 minutes of a meal.
• Letrozole is given in a single dose without regard to food or meals. Do not divide dose.
• Assess baseline LVEF (ECHO or MUGA) results prior to starting lapatinib, and periodically during therapy.
• Assess LFTs baseline and every 4–6 weeks during treatment.
• Assess serum potassium and magnesium, and plan repletion for hypokalemia or hypomagnesemia before lapatinib administration.

Drug Interactions:
• Capecitabine: additive benefits.
• Drugs metabolized by the CYP3A4 and CYP2C8 microenzyme system: lapatinib inhibits CYP3A4 and CYP2C8 (e.g., midazolam, paclitaxel, digoxin); monitor for toxicity of drug coadministered with lapatinib, especially if narrow therapeutic window. If necessary, dose of concomitant drug may need to be reduced.
• Lapatinib inhibits p-glycoprotein (transport system); if given with drugs that are substrates of p-glycoprotein, assess for toxicity resulting from increased substrate concentration, especially if there is a narrow therapeutic window.
• Midazolam (CYP3A4 substrate): increased AUC midazolam 45% when given PO, and 22% when given IV.
• Paclitaxel (CYP2C8 and P-gp substrate): paclitaxel AUC increased 23% (24-hour exposure).
• Digoxin (p-gp substrate): increased digoxin AUC 2.8-fold. Monitor baseline digoxin serum level prior to starting lapatinib, and throughout coadministration. If serum digoxin level is >1.2 ng, digoxin dose should be reduced by half.
• Inhibitors of CYP3A4 (atazanavir, clarithromycin, grapefruit or grapefruit juice, indinavir, itraconazole, ketoconazole, nelfinavir, nefazodone, ritonavir, saquinavir, telithromycin, voriconazole): do not coadminister.
• Inducers of CYP3A4 (carbamazepine, dexamethasone, phenobarbital, phenytoin, rifabutin, rifampin, rifapentine, St. John's wort): do not coadminister.
• Solubility of lapatinib is pH-dependent, but coadministration with proton-pump inhibitor esomeprazole did not reduce lapatinib steady-state level significantly.

Lab Effects/Interference:
• Increased BR, AST, ALT.
• QT/QTc prolongation.
• Decreased WBC, ANC, platelet count when coadministered with capecitabine.

Special Considerations:
Warnings and Precautions:
• Decreased LVEF: 57% of patients in clinical trials had a decrease in LVEF in first 12 weeks of treatment. Assess LVEF in all patients before starting lapatinib to ensure

patient's baseline is within institutional normal limits. Continue to evaluate during therapy to ensure that LVEF does not decline below ILLN.

- Hepatotoxicity can occur (ALT or AST > 3 × ULN and total bilirubin > 2 ULN), occurring days to months after start of therapy, and may be fatal.
  - Monitor LFTs baseline and every 4–6 weeks during treatment, and as clinically indicated. Discontinue and do not restart lapatinib if patients experience severe changes in LFTs.
  - If patient has severe preexisting hepatic impairment, dose-reduce drug. Discontinue and do not restart lapatinib if patients experience severe hepatotoxicity.
- Diarrhea: may be severe, and deaths have been reported. Diarrhea in 50% of patients occurs during 6 days of beginning therapy.
  - Diarrhea ususally lasts 4–5 days, and is low-grade. Grade 3–4 occurs in < 10% and < 1% of patients, respectively.
  - Key to management is early identification: teach patients to report any change in bowel patterns immediately and to take antidiarrheal agent (e.g., loperamide) after the first unformed stool.
  - Severe diarrhea may require oral or IV fluid and electrolyte replacement, antbiotic therapy (e.g., fluoroquinolones, especially if diarrhea persists > 24 hrs, there is fever, or grade 3–4 neutropenia), as well as interruption or discontinuation of lapatinib therapy.
- Drug has been associated with interstitial lung disease and pneumonitis due to EGFR blockade (EGF is necessary for repair of injured lung tissue). Discontinue lapatinib if patients experience grade 3 or greater pulmonary symptoms.
- Lapatinib may prolong the QT interval in some patients.
  - Consider EKG and electrolyte monitoring, especially in patients who have or may develop prolongation of the QTc (patients with hypokalemia, hypomagnesemia, congenital long QT syndrome, taking antiarrhythmic medications or other drugs that lead to QT prolongation, and cumulative high-dose anthracycline therapy).
  - Ensure that hypomagnesemia or hypokalemia is corrected prior to lapatinib administration.
  - Drug can cause fetal harm. Teach women of childbearing potential to use effective contraception to avoid pregnancy. If the drug is used in pregnancy, or if the patient becomes pregnant while on the drug, the patient should be apprised of the potential hazard to the fetus.
- The most common side effects (> 20%):
  - Lapatinib together with capecitabine were diarrhea, nausea, vomiting, palmar-plantar erythrodysesthesia, rash, and fatigue.
  - Lapatinib together with letrozole: diarrhea, rash, nausea, fatigue.

Potential Toxicities/Side Effects and the Nursing Process

I.   ALTERATION IN CIRCULATION, POTENTIAL, related to LEFT VENTRICULAR DYSFUNCTION, QT PROLONGATION, EPISTAXIS

Defining Characteristics: Rarely, patients may develop a decrease in left ventricular ejection fraction (LVEF) to below the institutional lower limit of normal (ILLN). Sixty percent of the time this occurs within the first 9 weeks of treatment. QT prolongation may occur; administer with caution in patients with prolonged or who may develop prolonged QTc (those having hypokalemia, hypomagnesemia, or taking other drugs that prolong the QTc, cumulative high-dose anthracycline therapy). Bleeding may occur, primarily epistaxis (11% incidence).

Nursing Implications: Assess baseline and periodic LVEF tests, as well as assess patients for any signs or symptoms of congestive heart failure. Identify patients at risk for further decrease in LVEF or development of prolonged QTc. Correct electrolyte abnormalities (e.g., magnesium, potassium) before starting lapatinib, and monitor periodically during therapy. If LVEF falls below ILLN, the drug should be stopped for at least 2 weeks until the LVEF is above the ILLN. Discuss any abnormalities with physician or NP. Teach patient bleeding may occur and to come to ED/notify physician/NP right away if bleeding (e.g., epistaxis) does not resolve in 15 minutes with local pressure and cooling.

II. ALTERATION IN NUTRITION, LESS THAN BODY REQUIREMENTS, related to DIARRHEA, NAUSEA, VOMITING, STOMATITIS, DYSPEPSIA, INCREASED LFTs

Defining Characteristics: Diarrhea occurs in 65% of patients, 13% grade 3, and 1% grade 4, compared to patients receiving capecitabine alone (40% with 10% grade 3). If diarrhea precedes or occurs during nadir when coadministered with capecitabine, the patient is at risk for sepsis. Diarrhea generally occurs early, often within 6 days of starting the drug; it lasts 4–5 days, and is generally mild. Nausea occurs in 44% with 2% grade 3, whereas vomiting affected 26% of patients, with 2% grade 3. Capecitabine primary side effects include diarrhea, nausea, and vomiting. Stomatitis affected 14% and dyspepsia 11%. In combination with capecitabine, which causes some elevation of LFTs, BR was elevated in 45% of patients (4% grade 3), AST in 49% of patients, and ALT in 37% of patients. 1% of patients may develop severe hepatotoxicity, which was fatal in some instances.

Nursing Implications: Assess nutritional status, bowel elimination pattern, and appetite, including LFTs, at baseline and repeated periodically during treatment. Teach patient to report right away any change in bowel elimination pattern. Teach patient to take loperamide. Teach patient to report any change in bowel elimination patterns right away. Teach patient to be proactive, and to take antidiarrheal agents (e.g., loperamide) after the first unformed stool, if it occurs. Severe diarrhea requires aggressive support as needed with oral or IV hydration, electrolyte replacement, antibiotics (e.g., fluoroquinolones, especially if diarrhea persists beyond 24 hrs, the patient is febrile, or has grade 3 or 4 neutropenia). Drug should be interrupted (or discontinued) until diarrhea resolves. LFTs should be repeated every 4–6 weeks during treatment. Inform patient these side effects may occur. Teach self-administration of antinausea and antidiarrheal medications (e.g., loperamide) according to protocol and to notify provider if symptoms persist so that the dose can be interrupted per protocol. Teach the patient dietary modification if nausea and vomiting or diarrhea occur (e.g., for diarrhea, BRAT diet: bananas, rice, applesauce, and toast) and to increase oral fluids to prevent dehydration. Consult dietitian to see patient for dietary counseling for anorexia. Discuss any abnormalities with physician or NP.

III.   ALTERATION IN COMFORT related to PALMAR-PLANTAR ERYTHRODYSESTHESIA (PPE), RASH, FATIGUE

Defining Characteristics: PPE is a dose-limiting side effect of capecitabine. The incidence is 53% with 12% grade 3. Acneform rash is characteristic of EGFRIs and is usually mild to moderate. A rash occurred in 28% of patients and dry skin in 10%. Fatigue is common.

Nursing Implications: Assess patient's baseline comfort, and teach that these symptoms may occur. Assess skin integrity (especially sun-exposed skin and palms of hands, soles of feet) baseline and during therapy. Teach symptom management strategies to minimize discomfort. Teach patient to notify nurse or physician if fatigue or rash is severe, or does not resolve with local management. Discuss dose interruption or delay with physician or NP.

Teach patient about PPE: This side effect may occur, and instruct patient to stop drug and call physician/nurse immediately should it occur. If patient has pain, expect dose interruption, with dose reduction if this is the second or subsequent episode at current dose. Teach patient self-assessment of soles of feet and palms of hands daily for erythema, pain, and dry desquamation and to report pain right away. Teach patients to avoid hot showers, whirlpools, paraffin treatments of nails, vigorous repetitive movements of hands and feet, as well as other body areas; avoid tight-fitting shoes and clothes. Teach patients to take cool showers and keep skin surfaces intact and soft with skin emollients. Studies ongoing establishing evidence base for prophylaxis or treatment: vitamin B_6, urea moisturizers, nicotine patch.

Teach patient about EGFRI rash: (Refer also to the Introduction to *Chapter 5.*) Do not use anti-acne medications. Tetracycline analogues provide an anti-inflammatory benefit. Teach all patients to (1) use a water-based emollient frequently during the day to prevent dryness, (2) stay hydrated, (3) avoid sun exposure and wear SPF 30 (zinc-based). **For grade 1 or mild rash (localized, does not interfere with ADLs, and is not infected):** The goal is to preserve skin integrity, minimize discomfort, and prevent infection. Key patient teaching includes to (1) use a mild soap with active ingredients that reduce skin drying such as pyrithione zinc (Head & Shoulders), (2) consider aloe gel for red, tender areas, (3) report distressing tenderness as pramoxine (lidocaine topical anesthetic may help), (4) keep fingernails clean and trimmed, and (5) apply zinc ointment to rectal mucosa after washing. Management: maintain current drug dose; observe or give topical hydrocortisone 1% or 2.5% or clindamycin 1% gel (anti-inflammatory benefit); reassess in 2 weeks. **For grade 2 or moderate rash (generalized, with mild symptoms, and minimal effect on ADLs, and is not infected):** The goal is to prevent infection and promote comfort. Continue EGFRI dose; use topicals (hydrocortisone 2.5% or clindamycin 1% gel) or consider pimecrolimus cream (immunomodulator) and add doxycycline 100 mg PO twice daily or minocycline 100 mg PO twice daily (give antimicrobial and anti-inflammatory effect) and reassess after 2 weeks. **For grade 3–4 or severe rash (generalized, severe, has a significant impact on ADLs, and increased risk of infection):** The goal is to prevent infection or identify it early to minimize complications and maximize patient coping with side effects. Hold drug until rash improves, and treat rash with topicals (hydrocortisone 2.5% or clindamycin 1% gel or pimecrolimus cream, doxycycline 100 mg PO twice daily or minocycline 100 mg PO twice daily, and methylprednisolone, Medrol dose pack); reassess after 2 weeks, and interrupt or discontinue drug if rash worsens (Lynch et al., 2007). If rash appears infected (exudate, vesicular formation, different appearance), obtain C+S, treat empirically until sensitivity received, and/or obtain dermatology consult. Discuss dose modification with a physician.

Drug: lenalidomide (Revlimid)

Class: Immunomodulator with antiangiogenic and antineoplastic properties.

Mechanism of Action: Drug is an analogue of thalidomide with immunomodulatory, antiangiogenic, and antineoplastic properties. Drug inhibits proliferation and induces apoptosis of some hematopoietic tumor cells, including multiple myeloma (MM), mantle cell lymphoma (MCL), and del (5q) myelodysplastic syndrome (MDS) cells. Drug modulates the immune system (is immunomodulatory) by activating T-lymphocytes and natural killer (NK) cells, increasing the numbers of NK T-cells, and inhibiting pro-inflammatory cytokines (e.g., TNF-α and IL-6). Lenalidomide is synergistic with dexamethasone in inhibiting cell proliferation and inducing apoptosis in MM cells.

Metabolism: Rapidly absorbed after oral administration, with maximal plasma concentrations occurring 0.5–6 hours after dose in patients with MM or MDS. Taking the drug with a high-fat meal decreased the AUC about 20% and decreased C_{max} 50% in healthy subjects. However, the studies establishing efficacy and safety did not specify, so the drug can be taken without regard to food intake. Drug exposure (AUC) in MM and MDS patients with normal or mildly impaired renal function (CrCl $\geq$ 60 mL/min) was about 60% higher than in young, healthy male subjects. Drug has approximately 30% protein binding. Drug is primarily excreted by the kidneys, with 90% of a radioactive dose excreted in the urine within 10 days; 4% is excreted in the feces. About 82% of the drug is excreted in the urine as lenalidomide within 24 hours. The mean half-life of the drug is 3 hours in healthy subjects and 3–5 hours in patients with MM, MCL, and MDS.

Dosage/Range:
- MM: 25 mg once daily orally with water days 1–21 of repeated 28-day cycles, together with dexamethasone 40 mg once daily on days 1–4, 9–12, and 17–20 of each 28-day cycle for the first 4 cycles of therapy; then 40 mg/day PO on days 1–4 every 28 days. Starting dose for renal impairment shown below. Treatment is continued or modified based upon clinical and laboratory findings. See package insert for dose modification guidelines.
- MDS: 10 mg once daily orally. Starting dose for renal impairment shown below. Treatment is continued or modified based upon clinical and laboratory findings. **See package insert for dose modification guidelines**.
- MCL: 25 mg once daily orally on days 1–21 of repeated 28-day cycles. Starting dose for renal impairment shown below. Treatment is continued until disease progression or unacceptable toxicity. See package insert for dose modification guidelines.
- After initiation of lenalidomide, subsequent dose modification is based on individual patient treatment tolerance, as shown in package insert.

- Renal impairment: adjust starting dose in patients with moderate or severe renal impairment and on dialysis.
  - Moderate renal impairment (CrCl 30–60 mL/min): MM,MCL = 10 mg every 24 hr; MDS = 5 mg every 24 hr
  - Severe renal impairment (CrCl < 30 mL/min, not requiring dialysis): MM, MCL = 15 mg every 48 hr; MDS = 2.5 mg every 24 hr
  - End-stage renal disease (CrCl < 30 mL/min, requiring dialysis): MM, MCL = 5 mg once daily, administer after dialysis on dialysis days; MDS = 2.5 mg once daily; administer after dialysis on dialysis days.
- Lenalidomide (Revlimid) is not indicated and not recommended for the treatment of patients with chronic lymphocytic leukemia (CLL) outside of controlled clinical trials. Serious cardiac adverse reactions have occurred in this setting.

Drug Preparation:
- Oral available in 2.5-, 5-, 10-, 15-, 20-, and 25-mg capsules. Available only under a restricted distribution program called REVLIMID Risk Evaluation and Mitigation Strategy (REMS) program. Prescribers and pharmacists must be registered with the program.
- Patients must meet all the conditions of the REVLIMID REMS program, and read, agree, and comply with all of the REMS requirements.
- Pregnancy test results must be verified by the prescriber and the pharmacist prior to dispensing the prescription, as drug cannot be given to a pregnant woman.

Drug Administration:
- Oral, at the same time each day, with or without food. Capsules should be swallowed whole with water, and they should not be opened, broken, or chewed.
- Check to make sure that pregnancy tests are negative prior to, monthly, and for four weeks after drug is stopped.
- Assess that the patient is using contraception. See Nursing Problem IV.

Drug Interactions:
- Digoxin: lenalidomide may increase C_{max} and AUC of digoxin; closely monitor digoxin plasma levels.
- Erythropoietin-stimulating agents or estrogen-containing therapies: may increase risk of venous thromboembolism. Use together cautiously in MM patients taking lenalidomide and dexamethasone.
- Additive antitumor effect when combined with dexamethasone in the treatment of multiple myeloma.

Lab Effects/Interference:
- Decreased neutrophil, lymphocyte, platelet, and red blood cell counts.
- Decreased potassium, magnesium, sodium, phosphate, and calcium.
- Increased alanine aminotransferase.

Special Considerations:

- Drug is indicated for the treatment of patients with (1) MM, in combination with dexamethasone, after at least one prior therapy; (2) transfusion-dependent anemia due to low- or intermediate-risk MDS associated with a deletion 5q cytogenetic abnormality, with or without additional cytogenetic abnormalities; (3) MCL, whose disease has relapsed or progressed after two prior therapies, one of which included bortezomib.
- Lenalidomide (Revlimid) is not indicated and not recommended for the treatment of patients with CLL, outside of controlled clinical trials.
- Drug is embryo-fetal toxic and may cause birth defects or embryo-fetal death. Pregnancy must be excluded before treatment starts. Prevent pregnancy during treatment by the use of two reliable methods of contraception. ABSOLUTE CONTRAINDICATION IS PREGNANCY. Two pregnancy tests must be routinely negative prior to beginning therapy in women of childbearing age, one within 10–14 days and the second within 24 hours before prescribing lenalidomide. Pregnancy tests should be continued weekly during the first month, then monthly in women with regular menstrual cycles, or every 2 weeks in women with irregular menstrual cycles. Contraception is mandatory in women and in men, as the drug is found in semen. Nursing mothers should discontinue nursing or discontinue use of the drug. See Nursing Problem IV.
- Drug is associated with significant neutropenia and thrombocytopenia. In patients with deletion5q MDS, 80% of patients required a dose delay/reduction during the major study for the indication. Monitor CBC/differential (1) for MDS patients: weekly for the first 8 weeks, and then at least monthly; (2) for MM patients: every 2 weeks for first 12 weeks, then monthly; (3) for MCL patients: weekly for first cycle (28 days), every 2 weeks during cycles 2–4, then monthly. Based on CBC/differential, discuss dose modifications as indicated in Revlimid package insert, with physician.
- Venous thromboembolism (VTE) has occurred in patients with MM (with dexamethasone, incidence is 9.3%), MDS, and MCL (incidence 4%). Drug significantly increases the risk of deep vein thrombosis (DVT) and pulmonary embolism (PE) in patients with multiple myeloma treated with lenalidomide and dexamethasone. It is not known whether the risk of VTE is reduced by prophylactic anticoagulation or antiplatelet therapy. The physician should decide whether or not to prescribe prophylactic measures after making a careful assessment of the individual patient's underlying risk factors.
- Second primary cancers occurred at a greater frequency in controlled trials of MM patients receiving lenalidomide compared to controls (e.g., acute myelogenous leukemia and B-cell lymphoma).
- Drug is largely excreted unchanged by the kidneys; use cautiously in patients with renal impairment, and dose-reduce per package insert (see Dose Modifications).
- Elderly MM patients receiving lenalidomide and dexamethasone have a higher risk of developing DVT, PE, atrial fibrillation, and renal failure following use of lenalidomide.
- Drug may cause tumor lysis syndrome (TLS) in patients with large tumor burdens prior to treatment that lyse quickly when lenalidomide is given, and it may be fatal. Discuss TLS prophylaxis with physician and closely monitor patients.
- Allergic reactions can occur, including angioedema, Stevens-Johnson syndrome, and toxic epidermal necrolysis, and they can be fatal. Discontinue drug immediately if

reactions are suspected, or if rash is grade 4. DO NOT resume lenalidomide if these reactions are verified. Drug is contraindicated in these patients. Consider lenalidomide interruption or discontinuation for grade 2–3 skin rash.

- Tumor flare reaction, characterized by lymph node swelling, low-grade fever, pain, and rash, have occurred when the drug was studied in patients with CLL (for which the drug is NOT indicated) or lymphoma. In MCL studies, the incidence was 10%, and was grade 1–2, generally occurring during the first cycle. Tumor flare reactions may mimic tumor progression. If needed, corticosteroids, NSAIDs, and/or narcotic analgesics may be considered. If a patient has a grade 3 or 4 reaction, hold lenalidomide until it resolves to ≤ grade 1. Monitor patients with MCL for tumor flare reactions.
- Hepatotoxicity, including hepatic failure, has occurred and some cases have been fatal. Monitor LFTs and stop drug upon elevation of liver enzymes; drug can be resumed after liver enzymes return to baseline, and consider dose reduction.
- Patients must not donate blood during lenalidomide treatment and for 1 month following last drug dose, as the blood may be given to a pregnant female whose fetus would then be exposed to lenalidomide. Men taking thalidomide must not donate sperm.
- Most common side effects in patients with MM: fatigue, neutropenia, constipation, diarrhea, muscle cramp, anemia, pyrexia, peripheral edema, nausea, back pain, URI, dyspnea, dizziness, thrombocytopenia, tremor, rash.
- Most common side effects in patients with MDS: thrombocytopenia, neutropenia, diarrhea, pruritus, rash, fatigue, constipation, nausea, nasopharyngitis, arthralgia, pyrexia, back pain, peripheral edema, cough, dizziness, headache, muscle cramp, dyspnea, pharyngitis, epistaxis.
- Most common side effects in patients with MCL: neutropenia, thrombocytopenia, fatigue, diarrhea, anemia, nausea, cough, pyrexia, rash, dyspnea, pruritus, constipation, peripheral edema, leukopenia.

Potential Toxicities/Side Effects and the Nursing Process

I.   POTENTIAL FOR INFECTION AND BLEEDING related to BONE MARROW
      SUPPRESSION

Defining Characteristics: Significant neutropenia and thrombocytopenia may occur, requiring dose adjustments. In MDS patients, neutropenia occurred in 61.5% of patients, thrombocytopenia in 61.5%, and anemia in 11.5%. Grade 3 or 4 hematologic toxicity was seen in 80% of patients enrolled in the MDS study, and 48% developed grade 3–4 neutropenia. In this study, the median time to onset of neutropenia was 42 days, and median time to recovery was 17 days. In this study, 54% of patients developed grade 3–4 thrombocytopenia, with a median time to onset of 28 days, and median time to recovery was 22 days. In MM patient clinical trials (taking lenalidomide and dexamethasone), incidence of neutropenia was 42.2% (grade 3–4 in 33.4% of patients), thrombocytopenia 21.5% (with 12.2% grade 3–4), and anemia 31.4% (with 9.9% grade 3–4). The incidence in MCL patients was: neutropenia, 49%, thrombocytopenia 36%, and anemia 31%.

Nursing Implications: Assess baseline CBC, WBC, differential, and platelet count prior to lenalidomide, then (1) for MDS patients: weekly for the first 8 weeks of treatment, then monthly; (2) for MM patients: every 2 weeks for first 12 weeks, then monthly; (3) for MCL patients: weekly for first cycle (28 days), every 2 weeks during cycles 2–4, then monthly. Based on CBC/differential, discuss dose modifications as indicated in Revlimid package insert, with physician. Assess for signs/symptoms of infection or bleeding. Teach patient the signs/symptoms of infection or bleeding, and to report these immediately, and teach patient self-care measures to minimize risk of infection and bleeding. This includes avoidance of crowds, proximity to people with infections, and OTC aspirin-containing medications (except if used for thromboprophylaxis). Discuss need for blood product support with physician or NP/PA. Drug should be used in combination with another agent that does not cause bone marrow suppression, like bortezomib (Velcade), rather than chemotherapy.

II. ALTERATION IN COMFORT related to ITCHING, RASH, FATIGUE, LIGHT-HEADEDNESS, AND LEG CRAMPS

Defining Characteristics: Patients may develop itching (7.6% MM/dexamethasone patients, 41.9% MDS patients, 17% MCL patients); rash (21.2% MM/dexamethasone patients, 35.8% MDS patients, 22% MCL patients); and dry skin (9.3% MM/dexamethasone patients and 14.2% MDS patients). In addition, 31.1%–43.9% of patients experience fatigue; 16%–26.3% peripheral edema, 8%–21.6% arthralgias; 13%–25.8% back pain; and 18.2%–33.4% muscle cramps or 13% muscle spasms. About 19.6%–23.2% of patients reported dizziness or headache.

Nursing Implications: Assess patient's baseline comfort, and teach patient that these symptoms may occur. Assess skin integrity baseline and during therapy. Teach symptom management strategies to minimize discomfort. Teach patient to notify nurse or physician if fatigue, rash, itching, or leg cramps are severe, or do not resolve with local management. Teach patient to change position slowly and to report severe dizziness. Teach patient to report leg cramps or new onset of shortness of breath or chest pain right away, and evaluate for DVT or PE.

III. ALTERATION IN NUTRITION, LESS THAN BODY REQUIREMENTS, related to DIARRHEA, CONSTIPATION OR NAUSEA, ELECTROLYTE DISTURBANCE

Defining Characteristics: In clinical studies, diarrhea occurred in 38.5% of MM/dexamethasone patients, 48.6% of MDS patients, and 31% of MCL patients. Constipation occurred in 40.5%, 23.6%, and 16% of patients respectively. Nausea affected 26.1%, 23.6%, and 30% of patients, while vomiting affected 12.2%, 10.1% and 12%, respectively. 15.3% of MM patients receiving lenalidomide/dexamethasone had dysgeusia.

Nursing Implications: Assess baseline nutrition, electrolytes, and bowel elimination pattern. Teach patient that diarrhea, constipation, nausea, and less commonly vomiting, may occur. Teach patient self-care strategies to minimize symptoms and to report them if they do not resolve. Teach patient self-administration of antiemetics or antidiarrheals as prescribed, and to notify provider if diarrhea persists. Teach patient dietary modification if diarrhea, constipation, nausea, or vomiting occur (e.g., the BRAT diet for diarrhea: bananas, rice, applesauce, and toast), and to increase oral fluids to prevent dehydration. Assess electrolytes baseline, as needed if patient develops diarrhea or vomiting, and periodically during treatment. Assess patient taste changes, and suggest dietary modifications if dysgeusia occurs.

IV.   KNOWLEDGE DEFICIT, POTENTIAL, related to PATIENT INSTRUCTIONS (Revlimid REMS), CONTRACEPTION, AND PREGNANCY TESTING

Defining Characteristics: Drug is fetotoxic. Patients must be able to understand the risk to the fetus, comply with REMS requirements, and be able to safeguard the drug in the home.

Nursing Implications: Assess patient's ability to understand rationale, importance of pregnancy testing in women of childbearing age, and to avoid pregnancy 4 weeks prior to drug prescription, and during treatment, treatment holidays, and for 4 weeks following drug discontinuance. Assess the understanding and ability of patients with childbearing potential to comply with contraception requirement and other self-care strategies and agree to the following:

- Female patients: (1) avoiding pregnancy for at least 4 weeks before beginning lenalidomide therapy, during therapy, during dose interruptions, and for at least 4 weeks after completing therapy; (2) committing to either continuous abstinence from heterosexual intercourse or to use 2 methods of reliable birth control beginning 4 weeks prior to starting lenalidomide therapy, during therapy, during dose interruptions, and continuing for 4 weeks following discontinuance of lenalidomide; (3) complying with pregnancy testing 10–14 days and within 24 hours prior to starting lenalidomide; then weekly during first month and monthly thereafter in women with regular menstrual cycles, or every 2 weeks in women with irregular menstrual cycles; and (4) having two negative pregnancy tests before the drug is prescribed.
- Male patients: (1) must always use a latex condom during any sexual contact with females of childbearing potential, as drug is present in the semen; (2) must continue contraception for 28 days after stopping the drug, even if the man has had a successful vasectomy; (3) must not donate sperm.
- Teach patient to notify the physician immediately under the following conditions:
  - Female patient becomes pregnant, thinks she might be pregnant, thinks birth control has failed, stops birth control, misses her menses, or has unusual menstrual bleeding. If so, she must stop taking the drug and notify the physician immediately;
  - Male patient has unprotected sex with a woman who can become pregnant, or if he thinks his sexual partner may be pregnant.
- Patients must not donate blood during treatment with lenalidomide and for 1 month following drug discontinuation.

- Assess ability of patient to keep drug/drug supply out of the reach of children and pets, and NEVER to share drug with anyone else, even if they have similar symptoms. Discuss any concerns with the physician.

Drug: lenvatinib (Lenvima)

Class: Multi-kinase inhibitor (antiangiogenic).

Mechanism of Action: Lenvatinib is a receptor kinase inhibitor of vascular endothelial growth factor: VEGFR1 (FLT1), VEGFR2 (KDR), and VEGFR3 (FLT4). The drug also inhibits fibroblast growth factor (FGF) 1–4, platelet-derived-growth factor receptor alpha (PDGF-α), KIT, and RET. This blockade has been shown to interrupt angiogenesis, tumor growth, and cancer progression.

Metabolism: Following oral administration, peak plasma concentration (T_{max}) occurs 1–4 hours after dosing; when given with food, there is a delay in rate of absorption and T_{max} of 2–4 hours. The drug is highly protein bound (98–99%), and is metabolized by CYP3A enzymes (primarily CYP3A4 and aldehyde oxidase). The terminal elimination half-life of lenvatinib is approximately 28 hours.

Indication: Treatment of patients with locally recurrent or metastatic, progressive, radio-active iodine–refractory differentiated thyroid cancer (DTC).

Dosage/Range:
- 24 mg orally, once daily until disease progression or unacceptable toxicity.
- Severe renal or hepatic impairment: reduce dose to 14 mg once daily.

Dose Modifications:
- *Hypertension (HTN):* Hold drug for grade 4 HTN that persists despite antihypertensive therapy; resume when HTN is controlled at ≤ grade 2 at a reduced dose; discontinue drug for life-threatening HTN.
- *Cardiac dysfunction or hemorrhage:* Withhold drug for grade 3 event until resolved to grade 0–1 or baseline, then resume at a reduced dose or discontinue based on severity and persistence of toxicity. Discontinue drug for grade 4 events.
- *Arterial thrombotic event (ATE):* Discontinue lenvatinib.
- *Renal failure and impairment, or hepatotoxicity:* Withhold drug for grade 3–4 renal failure/impairment or hepatotoxicity until resolved to grade 0–1 or baseline; then resume at a reduced dose or discontinue lenvatinib based on severity and persistence of toxicity. Discontinue drug for hepatic failure.
- *Proteinuria*: Withhold drug for proteinuria (≥ 2 g/24 hr); resume at a reduced dose* when urinary protein < 2 g/24 hr. Discontinue lenvatinib for nephrotic syndrome.
- *Gastrointestinal (GI) perforation or fistula formation:* Discontinue drug for GI perforation or life-threatening fistula.
- *QT prolongation:* Withhold drug for grade 3 or greater QT-interval prolongation; resume at a reduced dose* when QT-interval prolongation resolves to grade 0 or 1, or baseline.

- *Reversible posterior leukoencephalopathy syndrome (RPLS):* Withhold drug until RPLS is fully resolved; then resume at a reduced dose or discontinue drug based on severity and persistence of neurologic symptoms.
- **Recommended dose modifications for persistent and intolerable grade 2 or grade 3 adverse events, or grade 4 laboratory abnormalities (medically manage nausea, vomiting, or diarrhea before interruption or dose reduction):*
  - First occurrence: Interrupt until resolved to grade 0–1 or baseline, then reduce dose to 20 mg (two 10-mg capsules orally once daily).
  - Second occurrence: Interrupt until resolved to grade 0–1 or baseline, then reduce dose to 14 mg (one 10-mg capsule and one 4-mg capsule orally once daily).
  - Third occurrence: Interrupt until resolved to grade 0–1 or baseline, then reduce dose to 10 mg (one 10-mg capsule orally once daily).

Drug Preparation: Available as 4-mg and 10-mg capsules. Keep at room temperature and out of the reach of children and pets.

Drug Administration:
- Assess BP baseline prior to treatment, then after 1 week, then every 2 weeks for the first 2 months, then at least monthly thereafter. Discuss HTN management prior to the patient starting therapy when BP control is documented, or if HTN occurs during therapy.
- Assess patient for signs and symptoms of cardiac dysfunction, ATE, development of neurologic symptom(s), and bleeding. Teach patient to report SOB, chest pain, bleeding, or any abnormality right away.
- Assess renal function tests and LFTs at baseline before starting therapy, then every 2 weeks for the first 2 months, then at least monthly during therapy.
- Assess serum electrolytes at baseline and during treatment, and correct any abnormalities. If the patient has congenital long QT syndrome, CHF, or bradyarrhythmia, or is taking drugs known to prolong the QT interval, monitor the ECG at baseline and during therapy for QT-interval prolongation.
- Assess patient urine dipstick for protein before starting therapy, then periodically during therapy. If dipstick is 2+ or higher, the patient should stop lenvatinib and the provider should evaluate a 24-hour urine sample for protein.
- Assess serum calcium at baseline and at least monthly for hypocalcemia; discuss dose interruption and calcium replacement with the provider if it occurs.
- Assess thyroid-stimulating hormone (TSH) at baseline and monthly; discuss thyroid replacement adjustment with the provider if TSH is elevated.
- Teach females of reproductive potential to use effective contraception during therapy and for at least 2 weeks after stopping the drug. Women should discontinue breastfeeding while taking the drug.
- Teach the patient to self-administer the ordered dose (e.g., 24 mg as two 10-mg capsules and one 4-mg capsule) orally once daily with or without food. Teach the patient to take the medication at the same time every day; if a dose is missed and cannot be taken within 12 hours, skip that dose, and take the next dose at the usual time.

Drug Interactions:
- No dose adjustment is recommended if coadministered with CYP3A, P-glycoprotein, and breast cancer resistance protein (BCRP) inhibitors, or with CYP3A or P-glycoprotein inducers.

Lab Effects/Interference:
- Increased serum creatinine, ALT, AST, or lipase
- Decreased serum calcium or potassium
- Decreased platelet count
- Abnormal TSH
- Prolonged QT interval on ECG

Special Considerations:
- Most common adverse reactions were HTN, fatigue, diarrhea, arthralgia/myalgia, decreased appetite, decreased weight, nausea, stomatitis, headache, vomiting, proteinuria, palmar–plantar erythrodysesthesia (PPE) syndrome, abdominal pain, and dysphonia.
- Most common serious adverse reactions were pneumonia (4%), HTN (3%), and dehydration (3%).
- A dose reduction was necessary for 68% of patients due to adverse reactions.

Warnings and Precautions:
- HTN: BP should be effectively managed before treatment with lenvatinib. The drug should be held for patients with grade 3 HTN despite optimal antihypertensive therapy. It should be discontinued for life-threatening HTN.
- Cardiac failure as evidenced by decreased ejection fraction, cardiac failure, or pulmonary edema occurred in 7% of patients. Withhold the drug for grade 3 dysfunction until resolved to grade 0–1 or baseline; resume at a reduced dose or discontinue drug.
- ATE occurred in 5% of patients, with 3% having grade 3 or higher ATE. Discontinue the drug if ATE occurs. Lenvatinib was not studied in patients who had an ATE within the preceding 6 months.
- Hepatotoxicity may occur. Monitor LFTs at baseline prior to starting therapy, then every 2 weeks for the first 2 months, then at least monthly during therapy. Withhold the drug if grade 3 or higher hepatotoxicity develops; resume the drug when it resolves to grade 0–1 or baseline at a reduced dose, or else discontinue drug.
- Proteinuria occurred in 34% of patients in clinical trials. Monitor urine dipstick at baseline prior to starting the drug, then periodically during treatment. If urine dipstick is 2+ or greater, evaluate a 24-hour urine sample for protein. Withhold the drug if urine protein excretion ≥ 2 g/24 hr, and resume at a reduced dose when proteinuria < 2 g/24 hr. Discontinue the drug if nephritic syndrome develops.
- Renal failure and impairment occurred in 14% of patients compared to 2% in the placebo group, and was primarily related to dehydration and hypovolemia related to diarrhea and vomiting. Withhold the drug for grade 3 or higher renal failure/impairment until resolved to grade 0–1 or baseline; then resume at a reduced dose, or else discontinue the drug.

- GI perforation or fistula formation may occur rarely; discontinue lenvatinib for GI perforation or life-threatening fistula.
- QT prolongation occurred in 9% of patients in study 1 compared to 2% in the placebo group. Assess serum electrolytes and correct any abnormalities; assess and monitor ECG and QT intervals in patients with congenital long QT syndrome, CHF, or bradyarrhythmias, or who are taking drugs that prolong the QT interval (Class Ia and III antiarrhythmics). Withhold the drug for grade 3 or higher QT-interval prolongation; resume the drug when resolved to grade 0–1 or baseline, at a reduced dose.
- Grade 3 or higher hypocalcemia occurred in 9% of patients in study 1 compared to 2% in the placebo group, and responded most often to drug interruption and calcium replacement. Monitor serum calcium at baseline and at least monthly during therapy. Interrupt therapy and adjust the dose based on the severity, ECG changes, and persistence of hypocalcemia.
- RPLS may occur rarely; this diagnosis should be confirmed by MRI. If confirmed, lenvatinib should be stopped until the RPLS is fully resolved; the drug may then be resumed at a reduced dose or discontinued based on the severity and persistence of the neurologic symptoms.
- Hemorrhagic events occurred in 35% of patients in study 1 compared to 18% in the placebo group; grade 3–5 events were similar in the two groups. Epistaxis was most common, but discontinuation of the drug was rare (1%) in the study. Withhold lenvatinib for grade 3 hemorrhage until resolved to grade 0–1, and then either resume the drug at a reduced dose or discontinue it.
- TSH suppression is impaired by lenvatinib; monitor TSH levels monthly and discuss with provider any adjustment of thyroid replacement medication as needed.
- Lenvatinib is embryo-fetal toxic; teach female patients of reproductive age to use effective contraception during lenvatinib therapy and for 2 weeks after therapy is completed.

Potential Toxicities/Side Effects and the Nursing Process

I.   POTENTIAL ALTERATION IN CIRCULATION related to HYPERTENSION, HEMORRHAGE, CARDIAC DYSFUNCTION, AND ARTERIAL THROMBOEMBOLIC EVENTS

Defining Characteristics: Lenvatinib increases the incidence of hypertension—a class effect of all angiogenesis inhibitors that is believed to be caused by the influence of VEGF on nitric oxide and blood vessel dilation, which is now blocked. HTN occurred in 73% of patients (all grades) and was severe (grade 3) in 44%; fewer than 1% of patients had grade 4 HTN. Less commonly, cardiac dysfunction (decreased left or right ventricular function, cardiac failure, or pulmonary edema) occurred in 7% (compared to 2% in the placebo group), and ATE in 5% (2% in the placebo group). Hemorrhagic events occurred in 35% of patients (18% in the placebo group), most commonly epistaxis.

Nursing Implications: Assess baseline BP prior to, then after 1 week, then every 2 weeks for the first 2 months, then at least monthly during treatment. Discuss antihypertensive therapy with the provider as needed. Teach the patient about drug administration, potential side effects, and self-care measures if prescribed antihypertensive medication, such as angiotensin-converting enzyme inhibitors, beta blockers, diuretics, and calcium-channel blockers. Lenvatinib should be temporarily suspended in patients with severe hypertension until BP can be controlled with medical management. The drug should be withheld for grade 3 HTN despite optimal antihypertensive therapy, and resumed at a reduced dose when HTN is well controlled. It should be permanently discontinued if the patient develops hypertensive crisis (diastolic blood pressure > 120 mm Hg) or life-threatening HTN. Monitor the patient for signs and symptoms of cardiac decompensation (e.g., dyspnea, pedal edema); discuss the need for ECHO with the provider if signs and symptoms are found. Teach the patient to report the following conditions immediately and go to ED: severe chest pain or pressure; pain in the arms, back, neck, or jaw; shortness of breath; numbness or weakness on one body side; trouble talking; sudden severe headache; or sudden visual changes. Teach the patient that epistaxis may occur, and to report immediately/come to the emergency room for severe and persistent nose bleeds; vomiting blood; red or black stools; coughing up blood or clots; and heavy or new-onset vaginal bleeding in women.

II.   ALTERATION IN NUTRITION, POTENTIAL, related to NAUSEA, VOMITING, OR DIARRHEA

Defining Characteristics: Diarrhea occurred in 67% of patients and was of grade 3–4 severity in 9%. Nausea occurred in 47%, stomatitis in 41%, vomiting in 36%, constipation in 31%, oral pain in 25%, dry mouth in 17%, and dyspepsia in 13%. Dysgeusia occurred in 18%. Weight was decreased in 51%, and appetite decreased in 54% of patients receiving lenvatinib.

Nursing Implications: Assess nutritional status at baseline and at each visit. Teach the patient that these side effects may occur, and teach self-management strategies such as use of antidiarrheals and antinausea medications, dietary modifications; teach the patient to report any symptoms that do not improve. Discuss prescription medication with the provider if the patient experiences refractory symptoms. Teach the patient tips to increase appetite (e.g., small, frequent meals; use of spices). Offer the services of a dietitian as appropriate.

III.   ALTERATION IN RENAL FUNCTION related to NEPHROTIC SYNDROME, POTENTIAL

Defining Characteristics: Renal impairment occurred in 14% of patients compared to 2% of patients receiving placebo, and was related to dehydration/hypovolemia due to diarrhea and vomiting. Proteinuria occurred in 34% of patients.

Nursing Implications: Assess baseline renal function and presence of protein in urine (1+ or greater by dipstick), and monitor prior to each treatment. Discuss any abnormalities with the physician. Patients with 2+ or higher proteinuria by urine dipstick should stop the drug, and be asked to collect a 24-hour urine sample for protein analysis. The drug should be held for proteinuria ≥ 2 g/24 hr, and resume when proteinuria < 2 g/24 hr. Monitor patients closely if they develop moderate to severe proteinuria until improved or resolved. The drug should be discontinued if the patient develops nephrotic syndrome.

IV.　ALTERATION IN COMFORT related to FATGUE, ARTHRALGIA/MYALGIA, HEADACHE, PALMAR–PLANTAR ERYTHRODYSESTHESIA, AND RASH

Defining Characteristics: Fatigue is common, occurring in 67% of patients, as are arthralgias and myalgias, occurring in 62% of patients. Headache occurred in 38%, palmar–plantar erythrodysesthesia in 32% (but was grade 3 in only 3.4%), rash in 21%, and peripheral edema in 21%. Alopecia was not common, occurring in 12% of patients.

Nursing Implications: Teach the patient that fatigue is common, and offer strategies to manage it, such as alternating rest and activity. Teach the patient that arthralgias and myalgias may occur, and offer strategies to manage them (e.g., acetaminophen or ibuprofen, frequent rest periods, application of heat, massage). Teach the patient that palmar–plantar erythrodysesthesia (PPE) syndrome may occur and should be reported. Assess baseline skin integrity, including the soles of the feet and the palms of the hands. Teach the patient to self-assess all skin areas, and to report rash, as well as redness, swelling, and/or pain anywhere, but particularly on the soles of the feet and the palms of the hands. Teach the patient to avoid activities that increase blood flow in the hands and feet, such as hot showers and baths, and to take tepid showers to reduce the likelihood and severity of hand–foot syndrome. Teach the patient to avoid constrictive clothing and repetitive movements that can irritate the opposing skin. Teach the patient to use skin emollients to prevent skin from drying and cracking starting on day 1 of therapy, followed by wearing cotton gloves or socks to keep the emollient close to the skin until absorbed. Teach the patient to elevate the hands and feet when sitting or lying down; apply ice packs or cool compresses indirectly to the hands or feet for up to 20 minutes; gently pat the skin dry after bathing or washing; and avoid contact with laundry detergents or cleaning products with strong chemicals. Teach the patient to call if pain develops, or if the area (palms of hands, soles of feet, areas of pressure) becomes swollen, and discuss management with the provider.

Drug: nilotinib (Tasigna)

Class: Kinase Inhibitor [Bcr-Abl kinase inhibitor, 2nd generation].

Mechanism of Action: Philadelphia chromosome–positive chronic myelogenous leukemia (Ph+ CML) is caused by a reciprocal mutation involving two chromosomes in the bone marrow (genetic material is exchanged between chromosomes 9 and 22), creating the Philadelphia chromosome. This mutation creates the fusion gene BCR-ABL on chromosome 22, which codes for a Bcr-Abl fusion protein; the ABL gene expresses a membrane tyrosine kinase, while the BCR gene is an oncogene. Thus, the tyrosine kinase is always "turned on" continually stimulating cell division and resulting in CML. Bcr-Abl causes cell proliferation, decreased adhesion/increased migration, inhibition of apoptosis, degradation of regulatory proteins, and prevention of DNA repair. The Bcr portion of the Bcr-Abl fusion protein is a protein kinase that turns on cell proliferation signals that create the excessive production of white blood cells (leukemia); however, the binding site is sometimes blocked (inactive) and sometimes active and able to bind to ATP. When a patient progresses on imatinib, it is because Bcr-Abl is reactivated through a number of processes, such as amplification of Bcr-Abl gene expression, or over 30 point mutations in the Bcr-Abl kinase domain so that the drug cannot bind (Deininger et al., 2005). Nilotinib is a designer drug that is highly specific for and binds very tightly to the ATP binding site of ABL (more selective and 30 times more potent an inhibitor than imatinib mesylate). The drug is active against 32 of the 33 most common Bcr-Abl mutations causing imatinib resistance. The drug also inhibits the KIT and PDGFR-A proteins found in patients with GIST.

Metabolism: The drug is metabolized via the cytochrome P450 microenzyme system in the liver (CYP3A4). A high-fat diet greatly increases drug bioavailability (82%), and thus, the drug must be given on an empty stomach. Peak concentrations reached 3 hours after drug administration. Serum protein binding is 98%. Elimination half-life with daily dosing is 17 hours, and steady state is reached by day 8. Metabolism occurs by oxidation and hydroxylation. Metabolites are not pharmacologically active. More than 90% of administered dose is eliminated within 7 days primarily via the feces. Age, weight, gender, and ethnicity do not significantly affect pharmacokinetics.

Indication: FDA-indicated for the treatment of
- Adult patients with newly diagnosed Ph+ CML in chronic phase (CP). Ongoing and further data will be required to determine long-term outcome.
- Adult patients with Ph+CML-CP and accelerated phase (AP) who are resistant to or intolerant to prior therapy that included imatinib. The effectiveness of nilotinib is based on hematologic and cytogenic response rates.

Dosage/Range:
- Nilotinib should be taken twice daily at approximately 12-hour intervals and MUST be taken on an empty stomach. No food should be eaten for at least 2 hours **before** the dose and for at least 1 hour **after** the dose is taken. Capsule must be taken whole.
- Newly diagnosed Ph+ CML in chronic phase (CP): 300 mg PO twice daily.
- Resistant or intolerant Ph+ CML (accelerated [AP]) or CP: 400 mg orally twice daily.
- An ECG should be repeated 7 days after any dose adjustment.
- Dose adjustment may be required for hematologic and nonhematologic toxicities, and drug interactions (see below).
- Lower starting dose recommended in patients with hepatic impairment (at baseline, see below).

- If clinically indicated, nilotinib may be given in combination with: hematopoietic growth factors (e.g., erythropoietin or G-CSF), hydroxyurea, or anagrelide.
- Nilotinib is contraindicated in patients with hypokalemia, hypomagnesemia, or long QT syndrome.

Dosage Modifications:
- QTc > 480 ms on ECG:
  - Withhold nilotinib, assess serum electrolyte level, and if serum potassium and magnesium are < LLN, replete.
  - Review concomitant medications taken, and reinforce taking medication on empty stomach.
  - Resume drug within 2 weeks at prior dose if QTc returns to < 450 msec and to within 20 msec of baseline.
  - If QTc is between 450 msec and 480 msec after 2 weeks, reduce dose to 400 mg PO once daily.
  - If following dose reduction to 400 mg PO once daily, QTc returns to > 480 msec, nilotinib should be permanently discontinued.
  - An ECG should be repeated 7 days after any dose adjustment.
- Neutropenia and Thrombocytopenia
  - For newly diagnosed Ph+ CML in CP at 300 mg twice daily, and resistant or intolerant Ph+ CML in CP or AP at 400 mg twice daily:
    - If ANC < 1.0×10^9/L and/or platelet count < 50×10^9/L: Stop nilotinib and monitor blood counts;
    - Resume within 2 weeks at prior dose if ANC > 1.0×10^9/L and platelets > 50×10^9/L;
    - If blood counts remain low for > 2 weeks, reduce the dose to 400 mg once daily.
- Selected nonhematologic lab abnormalities
  - Elevated serum lipase or amylase ≥ grade 3: withhold nilotinib, and monitor serum lipase or amylase; resume at 400 mg once daily if serum lipase or amylase returns to ≤ grade 1. Assess serum lipase levels monthly or as clinically indicated.
  - Elevated bilirubin ≥ grade 3: withhold nilotinib and monitor bilirubin; resume at 400 mg once daily if serum bilirubin returns to ≤ grade 1. Assess serum bilirubin levels monthly or as clinically indicated.
  - Elevated hepatic transminases ≥ grade 3: withhold nilotinib and monitor hepatic transaminases; resume at 400 mg once daily if hepatic transaminases return to ≤ grade 1.
- If other clinically significant moderate or severe non-hematologic toxicity develops, hold drug, and resume at 400 mg once daily when resolved. If clinically appropriate, consider escalating dose back to 300 mg (newly diagnosed Ph+ CML in CP) or 400 mg (resistant or intolerant Ph+ CML in CP and Ph+ CML in AP) twice daily.
- Hepatic impairment (at baseline): consider alternative therapies, and if must administer nilotinib, reduce dose:
  - Newly diagnosed Ph+ CML in CP at 300 mg twice daily: mild, moderate, or severe hepatic impairment. Initial dose should be 200 mg twice daily followed by dose escalation to 300 mg twice daily based on tolerability.

- Resistant or intolerant Ph+ CML in CP or AP at 400 mg twice daily.
  - Mild (Child-Pugh Class A) or Moderate (Child-Pugh Class B): Initial dose of 300 mg twice daily, followed by dose escalation to 400 mg twice daily based on tolerability.
  - Severe (Child-Pugh Class C): Initial dose should be 200 mg twice daily, followed by a sequential dose escalation to 300 mg twice daily, and then to 400 mg twice daily based on tolerability.
- Concomitant *Strong CYP 3A4 Inhibitors*:
  - If must take interacting drug, interrupt nilotinib; if must be coadministered, dose-reduce to 300 mg once daily (resistant or intolerant Ph+ CML) or to 200 mg once daily (newly diagnosed Ph+ CML in CP).
  - If the strong CYP3A4 inhibitor is discontinued, a washout period should be allowed before nilotinib is adjusted upward to the indicated dose. Monitor patient closely for prolonged QTc interval.
- Concomitant *Strong CYP 3A4 Inducers*: Do not coadminister, as increasing nilotinib dose will not compensate for loss of drug exposure.

Drug Preparation/Administration:
- Oral.
- Available in 150-mg and 200-mg hard capsules.
- Assess patient's medication profile for possible interacting drugs. Teach patients NOT to eat grapefruit, drink grapefruit juice, or take St. John's wort, as these will affect nilotinib serum levels
- Administer capsules whole on an empty stomach (2 hours after eating any food, and after taking nilotinib, wait at least 1 hour before eating any food) with a glass of water. Drink only water for 1 hour after drug administration. This is a critical point of patient education.
- If the patient is unable to swallow capsules, the contents of each capsule may be dispersed in one teaspoon (NO MORE than this) of applesauce (pureed apple), and taken immediately (within 15 min) and not stored for future use.
- If a dose is missed, the patient should NOT make up the dose but rather resume taking the next prescribed daily dose.
- Therapy is continued until disease progression or unacceptable toxicity.
- Lab monitoring: **CBC/differential** baseline, then every 2 weeks for the first 2 months, and then monthly; ECG to monitor **QTc** baseline, 7 days after first dose, and then periodically, as well as after any dose adjustments; monitor QTc closely in patients with liver impairment or receiving strong CYP3A4 inhibitors; **electrolytes:** baseline and correct prior to starting drug, especially serum magnesium and potassium; monitor magnesium, potassium, calcium, phosphorus, sodium; monitor **serum lipase and glucose** baseline and monthly or as clinically indicated, especially in patients with a history of pancreatitis who require close monitoring; monitor **LFTs** baseline and monthly or as clinically indicated.

Drug Interactions:
- Nilotinib is a competitive inhibitor of CYP3A4, CYP2C8, CYP2C9, CYP2D6, and UGT1A1 in vitro, potentially increasing the concentrations of drugs eliminated by these

enzymes; studies suggest nilotinib may induce CYP2B6, CYP2C8, and CYP2C9, and decrease the concentrations of drugs eliminated by these enzymes (e.g., single dose of nilotinib given with midazolam, a CYP3A4 substrate, increased midazolam exposure by 30%). A single dose of nilotinib given to healthy subjects did not change the pharmacokinetics and pharmacodynamics of warfarin, a CYP2C9 substrate. Use caution when nilotinib is given with substrates for these enzymes have a narrow therapeutic index.
- Nilotinib inhibits human P-glycoprotein. If nilotinib is given with drugs that are substrates of p-gp, increased concentrations of the substrate are likely, and the patient should be monitored closely. In addition, nilotinib is a substrate of P-gp. If nilotinib is administered with drugs that inhibit p-gp, increased concentrations of nilotinib are likely, and should be coadministered very cautiously.
- *CYP3A4 (strong) inhibitors* (e.g., atazanavir, clarithromycin, grapefruit or grapefruit juice, indinavir, itraconazole, ketoconazole, nefazodone, nelfinavir, ritonavir, saquinavir, telithromycin, voriconazole) may increase nilotinib plasma concentrations; do not coadminister. If administration of an interacting drug is necessary, interrupt nilotinib therapy; if continued coadministration is necessary, consider nilotinib dose reduction and monitor patient closely for prolongation of the QT interval. Ketoconazole in healthy subjects at 400 mg once daily × 6 days, increase nilotinib AUC threefold. Teach patient to avoid grapefruit or grapefruit juice.
- *CYP3A4 (strong) inducers* (e.g., carbamazepine, dexamethasone, phenytoin, phenobarbital, rifabutin, rifampicin, rifapentin, St. John's wort) may increase metabolism of nilotinib so that nilotinib serum levels are reduced. For example, rifampicin at 600 mg daily × 12 days reduces nilotinib AUC by approximately 80%; avoid concurrent use. Teach patient not to take St. John's wort if taking nilotinib.
- Drugs that affect gastric pH: Nilotinib's solubility is pH-dependent, with decreased solubility at higher pH. Drugs such as proton pump inhibitors that may increase gastric pH, may decrease nilotinib solubility and reduce its bioavailability. Do not use together if possible, and if they must be coadministered, use caution. If an H_2 blocker or antacid is necessary, separate doses between it and nilotinib by at least several hours.
- Drugs prolonging QTc (e.g., antiarrhythmic drugs such as amiodarone, disopyramide, procainamide, quinidine, and sotalol; chloroquine, clarithromycin, haloperidol, methadone, moxifloxacin, and pimozide): do not use together, as will increase risk of prolonged QTc and sudden death. If treatment with any of these agents is required, interrupt nilotinib therapy. If interruption is not possible, monitor patient closely for prolongation of QT interval.
- Drugs that inhibit drug transport systems: nilotinib is a substrate of the efflux transporter P-glycoprotein (P-gp). If nilotinib is administered with a drug that inhibits P-gp, increased serum levels of nilotinib will likely result; use together cautiously.

Lab Effects/Interference:
- Increased LFTs—AST, ALT, alkaline phosphatase, BR (total)—transient.
- Increased serum creatinine, BUN, lipase (transient), glucose, amylase, CPK, LDH (uncommon), parathyroid hormone.

- Decreased serum calcium, magnesium, phosphate, potassium, sodium.
- Decreased neutrophils, platelet count, red blood cell count.
- QTc prolongation.

Special Considerations:
- Imatinib is successful in treating patients with Ph+ CML (CP, AP, and blast phases) and inducing a complete cytogenic response in 80% of patients; however, 10% will develop resistance by amplification, mutations, additional chromosomal mutations (Ault, 2007). Nilotinib can induce major cytogenetic response in 52% of patients after 6 months in imatinib-resistant or intolerant patients.
- Patient teaching about self-administration on an empty stomach is critical to prevent increased toxicity, and to avoid interacting drugs.
- Grade 3–4 thrombocytopenia, neutropenia, and anemia can occur. Assess CBC baseline and every 2 weeks for the first 2 months, then monthly. Hold dose to reverse myelosupresion, and may require a dose reduction.
- Drug prolongs QTc interval (ventricular repolarization), and sudden deaths have been reported. Prolongation of the QT interval can result in torsades de pointes, a type of ventricular tachycardia that can cause syncope, seizure, and/or death. See the Introduction to *Chapter 5* for full discussion of QT prolongation and sudden death. Patients must have an ECG as follows: before starting the drug, 7 days after starting the drug, with any dose changes, and regularly during nilotinib therapy. Do not give drug to patients with hypokalemia, hypomagnesemia, or long QT syndrome.
  - Before starting nilotinib therapy, assess electrolytes, calcium, and magnesium levels, and correct hypokalemia and/or hypomagnesemia before starting nilotinib. Monitor electrolytes throughout nilotinib therapy.
  - Significant prolongation of QT interval can occur when nilotinib is taken with (1) food (inappropriately), (2) strong CYP3A4 inhibitors, and/or (3) medicinal products known to prolong the QT interval. DO NOT take nilotinib with food or these interacting drugs.
- Nilotinib is contraindicated in patients with:
  - Long QT syndrome.
  - Hypokalemia and/or hypomagnesemia.
- Sudden deaths have been reported rarely in 0.3% of patients; ventricular repolarizatin abnormalities may have contributed.
- Cardiac and vascular events have occurred, including arterial vascular occlusive events, ischemic heart disease-related events, and ischemic cerebrovascular events. Teach patients to seek immediate medical attention if they develop acute signs or symptoms of cardiovascular events. Assess patients for signs/symptoms of cardiovascular events.
- Hepatotoxicity: nilotinib may cause elevations in LFTs. Monitor bilirubin, AST/ALT, alkaline phosphatase; assess baseline, monthly, or as clinically indicated during treatment. Nilotinib exposure is increased and a dose reduction is recommended in patients with impaired hepatic function, and their QT interval (on ECG) should be followed closely for evidence of prolongation.
- Electrolyte abnormalities: Nilotinib can cause hypophosphatemia, hypokalemia, hyperkalemia, hypocalcemia, and hyponatremia. Correct electrolyte abnormalities prior to starting nilotinib therapy, and monitor closely during therapy.

- Drug interactions: avoid CYP3A4 inhibitors or antiarrhythmic drugs (e.g., amiodarone, disopyramide, procainamide, quinidine, sotalol) and other drugs that may prolong QT interval (e.g., chloroquine, clarithromycin, haloperidol, methadone, moxifloxacin, pimozide). Should coadministration of any of these drugs be medically necessary, interrupt nilotinib therapy. If this is not possible, monitor patients for prolongation of QT interval.
- Food effects: nilotinib bioavailability is increased with food, so nilotinib MUST NOT be taken with food; rather, teach patients no food should be consumed for at least 2 hours before and 1 hour after the dose is taken. Teach patients also to avoid grapefruit and grapefruit juice, and other foods known to inhibit CYP3A4 (e.g., noni juice, pomegranate juice). Teach patient to tell nurse or physician before taking ANY over-the-counter medicine, vitamin, or mineral; be sure to tell nurse or physician all medications that patient is taking and whether he or she has had any trouble digesting lactose in the past.
- TLS can occur in patients with resistant or intolerant CML who have malignant disease progression with high WBC and/or dehydration. Assess, discuss TLS prophylaxis (e.g., hydration, uric acid correction) with physician prior to starting nilotinib therapy, and monitor these patients.
- Nilotinib can cause hypophosphatemia, hypokalemia, hyperkalemia, hypocalcemia, and hyponatremia.
- Pancreatitis and elevated serum lipase: Nilotinib can increase serum lipase. Use drug cautiously in patients with history of pancreatitis, and monitor serum lipase baseline, at least monthly, as clinically indicated, and follow closely. If elevated serum lipase is accompanied by abdominal symptoms, interrupt nilotinib dose and consider appropriate diagnostics to exclude pancreatitis.
- Teach women of childbearing age to use effective contraception while receiving the drug, as fetal harm can occur. If the drug is used during pregnancy, or if the patient becomes pregnant while taking the drug, the patient should be apprised of the potential hazard to the fetus. Mothers should not breastfeed; a decision should be made whether to discontinue nursing or to discontinue nilotinib, taking into consideration the importance of the drug to the mother's health.
- Lab monitoring summary:
  - **CBC/differential** baseline and then every 2 weeks for the first 2 months and then monthly;
  - ECG to monitor **QTc** baseline, 7 days after first dose, and then periodically, as well as after any dose adjustments; monitor QTc closely in patients with liver impairment or receiving strong CYP3A4 inhibitors;
  - **Electrolytes:** baseline and correct prior to starting drug, especially magnesium and potassium; monitor magnesium, potassium, calcium, phosphorus, sodium;
  - **Serum lipase and glucose:** baseline and monthly or as clinically indicated, especially in patients with a history of pancreatitis who require close monitoring;
  - **LFTs** baseline and monthly or as clinically indicated.
- Patients who have had a total gastrectomy should be followed more closely, as nilotinib exposure is reduced in these patients. Discuss with physician whether dose increase is appropriate.
- Most common nonhematologic adverse reactions in all patient groups, occurring in 20% or more patients, were: nausea, rash, headache, fatigue, pruritus, vomiting, diarrhea, cough,

constipation, arthralgia, nasopharyngitis, pyrexia, and night sweats. Hematologic adverse reactions include myelosuppression: thrombocytopenia, neutropenia, and anemia.

Potential Toxicities/Side Effects and the Nursing Process

I.   POTENTIAL FOR INFECTION AND BLEEDING related to NEUTROPENIA AND THROMBOCYTOPENIA

Defining Characteristics: Grade 3–4 neutropenia occurred in 28% of patients in chronic phase and 37% of patients with accelerated phase; thrombocytopenia in 28–37% of patients; anemia in 8–23% of patients. Febrile neutropenia occurred in < 10% of patients with accelerated phase CML. Sepsis can occur. Common infections were folliculitis, URI, herpes, candidiasis, pneumonia, UTI, and gastroenteritis.

Nursing Implications: Assess baseline CBC, WBC, differential, and platelet count before initiating therapy, then every two weeks for the first 8 weeks of treatment, and then monthly. Assess for signs/symptoms of infection or bleeding. Teach patient the signs/symptoms of infection or bleeding and to report these immediately, and teach patient self-care measures to minimize risk of infection and bleeding. This includes avoidance of crowds, proximity to people with infections, and OTC aspirin-containing medications. Discuss need for blood product support or growth factors with physician or NP.

II.   ALTERATION IN CIRCULATION, POTENTIAL, related to QTc PROLONGATION

Defining Characteristics: Patients may develop QT prolongation on EKG. Do NOT administer to patients with prolonged or who may develop prolonged QTc (hypokalemia, hypomagnesemia, other drugs that prolong the QTc). Prolonged QTc in the setting of low magnesium and hypokalemia sets the stage for torsades de pointes, with ventricular tachycardia, fibrillation, and sudden cardiac death possible.

Nursing Implications: Assess baseline QTc interval. Identify patients at risk for development of prolonged QTc (congenital long QTc) syndrome, prolonged QTc > 450 msec, taking antiarrhythmics or other drugs that can prolong the QTc interval (hypokalemia, hypomagnesemia, concomitant CYP3A4 strong inhibitors). Correct electrolyte abnormalities (e.g., magnesium, potassium) before starting nilotinib, and monitor periodically during therapy. Hypokalemia and hypomagnesemia in the setting of prolonged QTc may lead to torsades de pointes, ventricular fibrillation, and sudden cardiac death. QTc must be assessed baseline, seven days after drug initiation, and periodically after that, as well as after any dosage adjustments. Teach patient to correctly take nilotinib on an empty stomach to avoid increased drug serum levels, and to avoid any drugs that may interact with nilotinib, until discussion with the physician, NP, PA, or nurse. Teach patient to report feeling lightheaded, faint, or an irregular heartbeat right away. Patients with hepatic impairment should have a dose reduction to avoid increased serum levels of nilotinib. See Introduction to *Chapter 5* for more complete discussion on determining the QTc interval.

III.   ALTERATION IN SKIN INTEGRITY related to RASH, PRURITUS, EDEMA

Defining Characteristics: Rash may occur. In clinical studies, 33% of patients reported rash (2% grade 3–4); 29% of patients complained of pruritus. Peripheral edema occurred in 11% of patients.

Nursing Implications: Teach patient that rash may occur and to report it. Assess patient skin integrity baseline and regularly during treatment. Teach patient local comfort measures. Teach patient self-application of topical steroids to rash or, if prescribed, systemic steroids (Ault, 2007). Discuss rash and management plan with physician, especially if severe. Teach patient to report any weight increase, swelling of the ankles, feet, or face, and any difficulty breathing or shortness of breath.

IV.   POTENTIAL ALTERATION IN NUTRITION related to NAUSEA, DIARRHEA, VOMITING, CONSTIPATION, HEPATOTOXICITY, PANCREATITIS

Defining Characteristics: Nausea affected 31% of patients (1% grade 3–4), and vomiting affected 21% (< 1% grade 3–4). Diarrhea affected 22% (3% grade 3–4), whereas constipation affected 20%. Hepatotoxicity characterized by transient and reversible increase in LFTs. Grade 3–4 lipase increased in 15–17% of patients and glucose in 11% of patients. The largest increase in bilirubin was found in patients with (TA)7 (TA)7 genotype (UGT1A1*28).

Nursing Implications: Teach patient to self-administer antiemetic 1 hour before each dose if needed and to call if nausea/vomiting develop/persist. Discuss with physician more effective antiemetic regimen if nausea/vomiting develop despite antiemetics. Encourage small, frequent intake of cool, bland foods as tolerated if nausea develops. Refer to dietitian as needed for meal planning. Assess bowel elimination pattern baseline and at each visit. Teach patient to report diarrhea or constipation that does not respond to antidiarrheal or anticonstipation medications. Teach dietary modifications as appropriate. Monitor LFTs, serum, lipase, and glucose baseline and periodically during therapy. Discuss abnormalities with physician. Teach patient to report any abdominal pain with nausea or vomiting.

V.   POTENTIAL ALTERATION IN COMFORT related to HEADACHE, FATIGUE, ARTHRALGIA, MYALGIA

Defining Characteristics: In clinical studies, headache affected 30% of patients (3% grade 3–4). Arthralgias affected 18% of patients (2% grade 3–4) and myalgias 14% (2% grade 3–4). Bone pain and muscle spasms affected 11% of patients.

Nursing Implications: Teach patient that these events may occur and to report them. Assess baseline comfort, and monitor closely during treatment. Develop plan to assure comfort depending on symptoms reported. If appropriate, suggest analgesics, the application of heat or cold, for control of myalgias and arthralgias. Discuss ineffective strategies with physician, and revise plan as needed.

Drug: nivolumab (Opdivo) injection

Class: Immune checkpoint inhibitor. Human programmed death 1 (PD-1)–blocking antibody; humanized monoclonal antibody against PD-1.

Mechanism of Action: One of the ways cancer evades the immune system is by taking advantage of the body's process to turn down activated T lymphocytes after an immune response, which is intended to protect the body's organs from autoimmune injury. The programmed cell death 1 (PD-1) receptor is found on T lymphocytes, especially if they have been exposed to an antigen for a long time. It is activated by its ligand, PD-L1 (also known as B7-H1 or CD274), which is often found in the tumor microenvironment (Hamid et al., 2013). PD-1 also has another ligand, PD-L2 (also known as B7-DC or CD273), which is preferentially expressed by antigen-presenting cells. When the ligands PD-L1 and PD-L2 bind to the PD-1 receptor on T lymphocytes, T-cell proliferation and cytokine production are turned off (Bristol-Myers Squibb Co., 2015). Some tumors upregulate PD-1 ligands—a phenomenon that contributes to loss of immune surveillance. Monoclonal antibody drugs (MAbs) that block the ligand PD-L1 from binding to its receptor PD-1 prevent activated T lymphocytes from being turned down/off so that these cells can continue to attack cancer cells. See the chapter introduction for *Immunotherapy*. Because it blocks this immune checkpoint inhibitor, nivolumab has less immune toxicity than ipilimumab, which blocks the inhibitory receptor cytotoxic T-lymphocyte–associated antigen 4 (CTLA-4). However, immune-related toxicity may occur, although it is less common.

Metabolism: Steady-state drug concentrations are reached by week 12 when nivolumab is administered at 3 mg/kg every 2 weeks; its elimination half-life is 26.7 days. Clearance increases as body weight increases, so the dose is weight based. Renal impairment and mild hepatic impairment do not affect clearance, but the drug was not studied in patients with moderate or severe hepatic impairment.

Indication:
- Unresectable or metastatic melanoma and disease progression following ipilimumab therapy, and if the patient is positive for the *BRAF V600* mutation, a BRAF inhibitor. Accelerated approval was granted based on the tumor response rate and durability of response, which may require verification and description of clinical benefit in confirmatory trials.
- Metastatic squamous NSCLC with progression during or after platinum-based chemotherapy.

Dosage/Range:
- 3 mg/kg IV infusion over 60 minutes every 2 weeks, until disease progression or unacceptable toxicity.

Dose Modifications:
- Withhold the drug for grade 2 pneumonitis; grade 2 or 3 colitis; AST or ALT > 3–5 × ULN; serum creatinine > 1.5–6 × ULN or > 1.5 × baseline value.
- Resume drug when reaction resolves to grade 0–1.
- Permanently discontinue the drug for any life-threatening or grade 4 adverse reaction; grade 3 or 4 pneumonitis; grade 4 colitis; AST or ALT > 5 × ULN or total bilirubin

> 3 × ULN; creatinine > 6 × ULN; any severe or grade 3 treatment-related adverse event; inability to reduce corticosteroid dose to ≤ 10 mg of prednisone or equivalent per day within 12 weeks; persistent grade 2–3 treatment-related adverse reactions that do not recover to grade 1 or resolve within 12 weeks after last dose of nivolumab.

Drug Preparation: Available as 40 mg/4 mL and 100 mg/10 mL solutions in single-use vials.
- Visually inspect drug for particulate matter or discoloration (should be opalescent, colorless to pale yellow) and discard if any is found.
- *Preparation*: Withdraw the required drug volume and transfer it to an IV container; dilute with either 0.9% sodium chloride USP or 5% dextrose injection USP, to prepare an infusion with a final concentration 1–10 mg/mL. Mix the diluted solution by inversion, and *do not shake*. Discard any partially used or empty vials.
- *Storage*: As the drug does not contain a preservative, store at room temperature for no more than 4 hours from the time of preparation (includes room-temperature storage of infusion in the IV container **and time for administration of the infusion**). Under refrigeration (2–8°C [36–46°F]), nivolumab infusion is stable for up to 24 hours from time of preparation. *Do not freeze.*

Drug Administration:
- Administer as an infusion over 60 minutes through an IV line containing a sterile, non-pyrogenic, low-protein-binding in-line filter (pore size, 0.2–1.2 micrometer).
- Do not administer other drugs through the same line.
- Flush the IV line at the end of the infusion.

Drug Interactions: Studies have not been conducted.

Lab Effects/Interference:
- Decreased serum sodium, potassium, magnesium, and calcium
- Decreased lymphocyte, red cell, and platelet counts
- Increased creatinine, calcium, potassium, AST, ALT, and alkaline phosphatase

Special Considerations:
- Most common adverse effects (≥ 20% of patients): (1) with melanoma—rash; (2) with advanced squamous NSCLC—fatigue, dyspnea, musculoskeletal pain, decreased appetite, cough, nausea, constipation.
- Immune-mediated adverse reactions are possible. If suspected, exclude other causes.
  - Based on the severity of the reaction, withhold nivolumab and administer high-dose corticosteroid, and as appropriate, administer hormone-replacement therapy.
  - Upon improvement to grade 0–1, begin corticosteroid taper and continue for at least 1 month. Consider restarting nivolumab after the taper is completed if reasonable, but recognize that the drug may require permanent discontinuation.
- Immune-mediated adverse reactions:
  - Pneumonitis: In all clinical trials, incidence was 2.2–6%, with median time to onset of 2.2–3.3 months. Monitor patients for signs and symptoms of pneumonitis. See "Potential Toxicities/Side Effects and the Nursing Process."
  - Colitis: In trial 1, incidence of diarrhea or colitis was 21% compared to 18% of patients receiving chemotherapy alone. Immune-mediated colitis occurred in 0.9–2.2% of patients

in trials 1 and 2. Time to onset was 2.5–6.7 months in trials 1 and 3. Monitor patients for immune-mediated colitis. See "Potential Toxicities/Side Effects and the Nursing Process."
- Hepatitis: Monitor LFTs during treatment and hold the drug for grade 2 hepatotoxicity; discontinue the drug at higher grades.
- Nephritis and renal dysfunction: Monitor serum creatinine baseline and periodically during treatment.
- Hypothyroidism and hyperthyroidism: Monitor thyroid function at baseline and periodically during therapy. If hypothyroidism occurs, the patient should receive hormone replacement therapy. If hyperthyroidism occurs, discuss medical management with the physician/NP/PA. The drug dose does not require modification.
- Other immune-mediated adverse reactions may occur, including after the drug is discontinued. These reactions are uncommon, but include adrenal insufficiency, uveitis, pancreatitis, autoimmune neuropathy, and vasculitis. Consider corticosteroid therapy based on the severity of the reaction.
- In animal models, PD-1 signaling inhibition increases the severity of some infections (e.g., TB) (Bristol-Myers Squibb Co., 2015).
- Nivolumab can cause fetal harm. Teach women of reproductive age to use effective contraception to avoid pregnancy during treatment and for 5 months following the last dose. Women should not breastfeed while receiving the drug.

Potential Toxicities/Side Effects and the Nursing Process

I. ALTERATION IN NUTRITION, POTENTIAL, LESS THAN BODY REQUIREMENTS, related to DECREASED APPETITE, NAUSEA, CONSTIPATION, VOMITING, OR DIARRHEA

Defining Characteristics: Approximately one-third of patients (35%) had decreased appetite. Nausea affected 29%, vomiting 19%, constipation 24%, and diarrhea 18%.

Nursing Implications: Assess nutritional and bowel-elimination patterns, appetite, and presence of nausea and/or vomiting at baseline and at each visit. Teach that diarrhea, constipation, nausea, vomiting, and decreased appetite may occur, and to report them. Assess nutrition impact symptoms and discuss their management with the physician. Teach the patient to self-administer antidiarrheal or antiemetic medication, if needed, and to report symptoms that do not improve. In addition, teach patients to report immediately any diarrhea, blood in stool or black stools, and severe stomach pain or tenderness so that the potential for colitis may be evaluated.

II. ALTERATION IN COMFORT related to FATIGUE, ASTHENIA, MUSCULOSKELETAL PAIN, OR ARTHRALGIA

Defining Characteristics: Fatigue was common in clinical trials, affecting 50% of patients (7% grade 3–4), while asthenia affected 19%, arthralgia occurred in 13%, and musculoskeletal pain in 36%.

Nursing Implications: Teach the patient that these events may occur and to report them. Assess baseline comfort and self-care strategies to maintain comfort. Monitor closely during treatment. Develop a plan to assure comfort, depending on the symptoms reported, and assess its efficacy and revise the plan if needed at each visit.

III. ALTERATION IN SKIN INTEGRITY, POTENTIAL, related to RASH, PRURITUS, OR EDEMA

Defining Characteristics: Pruritus affected 11% of patients in clinical trials, and rash affected 16%. Peripheral edema occurred in 17%.

Nursing Implications: Teach the patient that rash, pruritus, and peripheral edema may occur and to report them. Assess the patient's skin integrity and determine the presence of edema, both at baseline and regularly during therapy.

IV. POTENTIAL ALTERATION IN OXYGENATION related to PNEUMONITIS

Defining Characteristics: In all clinical trials, incidence was 2.2–6%, occurring with median time of onset of 2.2–3.3 months.

Nursing Implications: Teach the patient to report new or worsening cough, chest pain, or shortness of breath. Monitor the patient for signs and symptoms of pneumonitis. Discuss findings with the physician/NP/PA. Expect that after exclusion of other diagnoses, the patient will be evaluated with imaging and pulmonary and infectious disease consultation if respiratory status changes occur.
- Grade 1 (x-ray changes only): Consider holding nivolumab, and monitor every 2–3 days. Reassess at least every 3 weeks, and if improved, resume nivolumab. If the patient's condition worsens, treat as it as grade 2 or 3/4.
- Grade 2 or higher: Withhold the drug until resolution for moderate (grade 2) or higher severity, and permanently discontinue it for severe (grade 3) or life-threatening (grade 4) pneumonitis. Administer corticosteroids at a dose of 1–2 mg/kg/day (prednisone or equivalent) for grade ≥ 2, followed by a taper. Monitor daily. Consult pulmonary and infectious disease specialists, and consider bronchoscopy and lung biopsy. If the patient improves and returns to baseline, taper steroids over at least 1 month. For grade 2 pneumonitis, after the taper is completed, consider resuming nivolumab. If pneumonitis persists or worsens after 2 days, add non-corticosteroid immunosuppressive medication.

V. POTENTIAL ALTERATION IN ELIMINATION AND COMFORT related to COLITIS

Defining Characteristics: In trial 1, the incidence of diarrhea or colitis in patients receiving nivolumab was 21% compared to 18% of patients receiving chemotherapy alone. Immune-mediated colitis occurred in 0.9–2.2% of patients in trials 1 and 3. Time to onset was 2.5–6.7 months in trials 1 and 3. Approximately one-third of patients (35%)

had decreased appetite. Nausea affected 29%, vomiting 19%, constipation 24%, and diarrhea 18%. Grade 1 is defined as symptoms of colitis with fewer than 4 stools over baseline. Grade 2 is symptoms of diarrhea (4–6 stools per day over baseline), abdominal pain, blood in stools, requiring IV fluids for less than 24 hours, and not interfering with ADLs. Grade 3/4 is 7 or more stools per day over baseline with incontinence, interfering with ADLs, and symptoms of severe abdominal pain, requiring medical intervention including IV fluids for 24 hours or longer; this life-threatening condition may include perforation.

Nursing Implications: Teach the patient to report signs and symptoms of colitis (diarrhea, blood in stools or tarry stools, severe abdominal pain). Monitor the patient for immune-mediated colitis, and administer corticosteroids as ordered.

- *Grade 1*: Continue nivolumab.
- *Grade 2*: Hold nivolumab as ordered. If colitis symptoms persist for more than 5 days, or recur, expect a corticosteroid to be ordered at a dose of 0.5–1 mg/kg/day (prednisone or equivalent). Once the patient is improved, and after corticosteroid taper over at least 1 month if used, nivolumab can be resumed. If symptoms worsen or persist for longer than 3–5 days with oral steroids, treat as grade 3/4.
- *Grade 3/4:* Administer corticosteroids 1–2 mg/kg/day (prednisone or equivalent) for grades 3/4, followed by a taper.
- *Grade 3:* Hold nivolumab until the patient is at grade 1, then taper the steroids over at least 1 month. If symptoms persist or worsen or are grade 4, permanently discontinue nivolumab. If the patient's condition is improved from persistent grade 3 or grade 4, continue steroids until the patient is at grade 1, then taper over at least 1 month. Lower GI endoscopy should be considered if needed.

VI. POTENTIAL ALTERATION IN NUTRTION related to HEPATITIS

Defining Characteristics: Immune-mediated hepatitis and abnormal LFTs may occur. Incidence for hepatitis in trial 1 was 1.1%. Increases in AST occurred in 16–28% of patients, increased alkaline phosphatase in 14–22%, increased ALT in 12–16%, and increased total bilirubin in 1.7–9%. Time to onset was 86–113 days. Signs and symptoms of hepatitis include elevated transaminases and total bilirubin, icterus, severe nausea and vomiting, right-sided abdominal pain, drowsiness, dark urine, increased bruisability or bleeding, and anorexia.

Nursing Implications: Assess LFTs at baseline and monitor regularly during therapy. Evaluate the patient for right-sided abdominal pain, drowsiness, dark urine, increased bruising or bleeding, and loss of appetite. Teach the patient to report any yellowing of the skin or whites of the eyes, as well as severe nausea or vomiting. Expect the following orders if abnormal LFTs occur:

- *Grade 1*: AST or AST > ULN to 3.0 × ULN and/or total bilirubin > ULN to 1.5 × ULN: Continue nivolumab and closely monitor LFTs.
- *Grade 2*: AST or ALT > 3.0 to < 5 × ULN and/or total bilirubin > 1.5 to ≤ 3 × ULN: Hold nivolumab and assess LFTs every 3 days; administer 1–2 mg/kg/day prednisone equivalents. If LFTs improve to grade 1 or baseline, resume nivolumab; if steroids were administered, taper them over at least 1 month before resuming nivolumab. Monitor LFTs routinely.

- *Grade 3/4*: AST or ALT > 5 × ULN and/or total bilirubin > 3 × ULN: Permanently discontinue nivolumab, and increase LFT monitoring to every 1–2 days. Consult GI specialist and administer corticosteroids 1–2 mg/kg/day (prednisone or equivalent). When the patient has improved to grade 0–1, taper steroids over at least 1 month. If lab abnormalities persist for more than 3–5 days, worsen, or rebound, add non-corticosteroid immunosuppressive medication.

VII. POTENTIAL ALTERATION IN URINE ELIMINATION related to IMMUNE-MEDIATED NEPHRITIS AND RENAL DYSFUNCTION

Defining Characteristics: Immune-related nephritis or renal dysfunction can occur as evidenced by increased serum creatinine (incidence 13–22%), with the incidence of grade 2–3 immune-mediated nephritis or renal dysfunction being 0.7–0.9%.

Nursing Implications: Assess the patient's baseline renal function, and monitor closely during therapy. Teach the patient to report signs and symptoms such as a decrease in the amount of urine, blood in urine, ankle swelling, loss of appetite.

- *Grades 2 (moderate) to 3 (severe):* Hold nivolumab and administer corticosteroids (prednisone or equivalent of 0.5–1 mg/kg/day, then taper over at least 1 month). If patient worsens or there is no improvement, increase dose to 1–2 mg/kg/day. If there is no improvement or worsening occurs, permanently discontinue nivolumab.
- *Grade 4*: Give corticosteroids 1–2 mg/kg/day (prednisone or equivalent), then taper and permanently discontinue drug.

VIII. POTENTIAL ALTERATION IN ENDOCRINE FUNCTION related to HYPOTHYROIDISM, HYPERTHYROIDISM, OR ADRENAL CRISIS

Defining Characteristics: Incidence of grade 1–2 hypothyroidism in clinical trials was 4.3–8%; incidence of grade 1–2 hyperthyroidism was 1.7–3%. Median onset of hypothyroidism was 2.5–4.1 months; median onset of hyperthyroidism was 1.6–5.2 months.

Nursing Implications: Monitor thyroid function at baseline and periodically during therapy. Teach the patient to report signs and symptoms such as headaches that do not go away, extreme tiredness, weight gain or loss, changes in mood or behavior, dizziness or fainting, hair loss, feeling cold, constipation, and deep and/or hoarse voice. Discuss and teach the patient about ordered hormone replacement therapy for hypothyroidism, or medical management of hyperthyroidism. Expect the following medical management:

- *Asymptomatic endocrinopathy* (TSH < 0.5 × LLN or TSH > 2 × ULN, or consistently out of range in 2 subsequent assessments; include free T_4 at subsequent cycles as clinically indicated): Continue nivolumab; consider endocrine consult.
- *Symptomatic endocrinopathy:* Continue nivolumab for hypothyroidism or hyperthyroidism, but hold drug for other endocrinopathies with abnormal lab/pituitary scan. Monitor endocrine function, and consider pituitary scan if not already done; repeat lab tests in 1–3 weeks, and MRI in 1 month if symptoms persist but lab tests and pituitary scan are within

normal limits. Consider endocrine consult, and start hormone replacement if the patient is symptomatic with abnormal lab tests and pituitary scan.

- *Suspicion of adrenal crisis:* Hold nivolumab, rule out sepsis, obtain an endocrine consult, administer stress-dose of IV steroids with mineralocorticoid activity, and give IV hydration.

Drug: obinutuzumab injection (Gazyva)

Class: IgG$_1$ monoclonal antibody (humanized) targeted at the CD$_{20}$ molecule on B-cell lymphocyte membranes.

Mechanism of Action: Mab binds to the CD$_{20}$ antigen on pre B- and mature B-lymphocytes, and lyses the B-lymphocytes directly through activation of intracellular death pathways, activation of the complement cascade, and indirectly through engagement of immune effector cells (e.g., antibody-dependent cellular cytotoxicity and antibody-dependent cellular phagocytosis).

Metabolism: Half-life approximately 28.4 days.

Indication: Obinutuzumab (Gazyva) is indicated in combination with chlorambucil for the treatment of patients with previously untreated CLL.

Dosage/Range:
- Premedicate with a glucocorticoid (e.g., IV 20 mg dexamethasone, or 80 mg methylprednisolone), acetaminophen (650 mg–1,000 mg), and antihistamine (e.g., diphenhydramine 50 mg). Hydrocortisone is not used, as it is not effective in reducing the rate of infusion reactions.
- Treatment is in combination with chlorambucil, for 6 cycles (28-day).
  - 100 mg day 1, cycle 1 with all premedications.
  - 900 mg on day 2, cycle 1 with all premedications.
  - 1,000 mg on day 8 and 15 of cycle 1 with acetaminophen premedication; if prior infusion reaction (> grade 1), acetaminophen and antihistamine; if prior grade 3 infusion reaction or lymphocyte count > 25 × 10^9 /L prior to treatment, give IV dexamethasone (20 mg) or methylprednisolone (80 mg).
  - 1,000 mg on day 1 of cycles 2–6: with acetaminophen premedication; if prior infusion reaction (> grade 1), acetaminophen and antihistamine; if prior grade 3 infusion reaction or lymphocyte count > 25 × 10^9 /L prior to treatment, give IV dexamethasone (20 mg) or methylprednisolone (80 mg).
- Premedication for microbial prophylaxis: Neutropenic patients should receive antiviral and antifungal prophylaxis.
- Consider treatment interruption for infection, grade 3–4 cytopenia, or ≥ grade 2 nonhematologic toxicity.

Drug Preparation:
- Available in 1,000 mg/40 mL (25 mg/mL) single-use vials.
- Inspect vial for any particulate matter, discoloration; do not use if found.

- Aseptically dilute into a 0.9% sodium chloride PVC or non-PVC polyolefin infusion bag. **Do not use** other diluents (e.g., dextrose 5%).
  - Cycle 1, day 1 (100 mg) and day 2 (900 mg): withdraw 40 mL Gazyva from vial. Dilute 4 mL (100 mg) into a 100-mL 0.9% sodium chloride infusion bag for immediate administration. Dilute the remaining 36 mL (900 mg) into a 250-mL 0.9% sodium chloride infusion bag at the same time for use on day 2 and store at 2°–8°C (36°–46°F) for up to 24 hrs. After allowing the diluted bag to come to room temperature, use immediately. CLEARLY label each infusion bag.
  - Cycle 1, days 8 and 15, and day 1, cycles 2–6: withdraw 40 mL of Gazyva solution (1,000 mg) from the vial and dilute in 250-mL 0.9% sodium chloride infusion bag. Gently rotate bag to mix, but do not shake or freeze. Use diluted infusion immediately, or within 24 hours when refrigerated at 2°–8°C (36°–46°F).
- Administer at a final concentration of 0.4–4 mg/mL.

Drug Administration:
- Administer IV infusion only, never IVP or IVB. Do not mix with other drugs.
- Drug is administered in combination with chlorambucil.
- Administer premedication as above. If the patient has a high tumor burden, and/or high number of circulating lymphocytes ($> 25 \times 10^9$/L), premedicate with antihyperuricemics (e.g., allopurinol), starting 12–24 hrs before initiating obinutuzumab (Gazyva) therapy. Also, ensure adequate hydration to prevent TLS.
- Cycle 1, day 1: Administer IV at 25 mg/hr over 4 hours; do not increase infusion rate.
- Cycle 1, day 2: Administer at 50 mg/hr. The infusion rate can be escalated in increments of 50 mg/hr every 30 min to a maximum rate of 400 mg/hr.
- Cycle 1, days 8 and 15; cycles 2–6, day 1: Start infusion at 100 mg/hr, and increase infusion rate by 100-mg/hr increments every 30 min to a maximum rate of 400 mg/hr.
- If a planned dose is missed, administer it when possible and change schedule accordingly. For example, if a patient does not complete the day 1, cycle 1 dose, may proceed to the day 2, cycle 1 dose.
- Infusion reactions:
  - Grade 4 (life-threatening): Stop infusion, and permanently discontinue obinutuzumab.
  - Grade 3 (severe): Interrupt and manage symptoms. When resolved, consider resuming obinutuzumab at no more than half the previous infusion rate. If the patient does not have further infusion reactions, escalate the infusion rate per cycle day as above. If the patient again has a grade 3 infusion reaction when rechallenged, stop infusion and permanently discontinue.
  - Grade 1–2 (mild-moderate): reduce infusion rate or interrupt infusion, and manage symptoms. When symptoms resolve, continue or resume infusion. If the patient has no further infusion reaction, escalate infusion rate per treatment cycle as above.

Drug Interactions:
- No formal studies have been done.

Lab Effects/Interference:
- Neutropenia, lymphopenia, leukopenia, thrombocytopenia.
- Increased serum potassium, creatinine, AST, ALT, alkaline phosphatase.
- Decreased serum calcium, sodium, albumin, potassium.

Special Considerations:
- Drug may cause hepatitis B reactivation, which rarely may result in fulminant hepatitis, hepatic failure, and death.
- Drug may lead to progressive multifocal leukoencephalopathy (PML), which may be fatal.
- Infusion reactions occurred in 69% of patients during the infusion of the first 1,000 mg of drug infused, but reactions can also occur with later infusions, as well as within 24 hours of the infusion. When premedication was required and the initial dose divided into two days, in clinical trials, the incidence of infusion reactions decreased to 47%. Monitor patients closely during infusions. Symptoms include hypotension, tachycardia, dyspnea, respiratory symptoms (e.g., bronchospasm, laryngeal and throat irritation, wheezing, laryngeal edema), as well as nausea, vomiting, diarrhea, hypertension, flushing, headache, fever, and chills). Premedicate patients with acetaminophen, antihistamine, and glucocorticoid agents, and reactions as needed with glucocorticoids, epinephrine, bronchodilators, and/or oxygen. Stop the drug and permanently discontinue if patient develops anaphylaxis, or any other life-threatening symptoms. For grade 3 reactions, interrupt drug until symptoms resolve. For grades 1–2, interrupt or slow infusion rate (see Drug Administration).
- TLS: Rapid lymphocyte lysis can cause TLS within 12–24 hours of Iinitial drug infusion, characterized by acute renal failure, hyperkalemia, hyperuricemia, and/or hyperphosphatemia. Patients with high tumor burden and/or high circulating lymphocyte counts (> 25 × 10⁹/L) are at high risk and should receive TLS prophylaxis prior to receiving first drug infusion (e.g., antihyperurecemic agent, allopurinol) hydration beginning 12–24 hours before dose. If TLS occurs, correct electrolyte abnormalities, monitor renal function, ensure hydration and fluid balance, and provide supportive care as needed.
- Drug is immunosuppressive, especially in combination with chlorambucil, and may result in serious bacterial, fungal, and new/reactivated viral infections during or after therapy with obinutuzumab. Do not give drug to patients with an active infection, and closely monitor patients with a history of recurring or chronic infections.
  - 34% of patients develop grade 3 or 4 neutropenia; they should be monitored closely for infection and treated promptly when suspected. Neutropenia can occur late, 28 days or more after treatment completed, and can be prolonged, lasting > 28 days. Neutropenic patients should receive antimicrobial prophylaxis throughout treatment, and antiviral and antifungal prophylaxis should be considered.
  - 11% of patients receiving the combination with chlorambucil developed grade 3–4 thrombocytopenia; 5% developd an acute thrombocytopenia occuring within 24 hours after the obinutuzumab infusion. Fatal hemorrhage has also occurred during cycle 1. Monitor patients closely for thrombocytopenia, especially during cycle 1. Monitor platelet counts of patients with grade 3–4 thrombocytopenia more frequently until resolution, and consider subsequent dose delays of obinutuzumab and chlorambucil or dose-reduce chlorambucil.
- Do not immunize patients with live or attenuated viral vaccines during treatment until B-lymphocytes have recovered.
- Drug may cause worsening of preexisting cardiac conditions.

- Drug can cause reactivation of hepatitis B. All patients should be screened for HBV infection (measuring HBsAg and anti-HBc) before starting obinutuzumab therapy. If patient shows evidence of hepatitis B infection, consult with a hepatitis expert about monitoring and consideration for HBV antiviral therapy. Monitor all patients with current or prior HBV infection closely (clinical and laboratory) for signs of hepatitis and HBV reactivation (e.g., increased transaminase levels, bilirubin) during and after completion of treatment. If a patient does experience HBV reactivation, discontinue obinutuzumab and concomitant chemotherapy.
- Drug can rarely cause JC (John Cunningham) virus infection called progressive multifocal leukoencephalopathy (PML). The infection occurs in the brain white matter, damaging cells that make myelin (neuronal insulation). While many people carry the JC virus, it is only virulent if immunosuppressed, and then can be fatal. Consider JC in the differential of any patient with new onset or changes in neurological status. Consider evaluation by a neurologist, brain MRI, and LP. Discontinue obinutuzumab, and consider cessation of chlorambucil if the patient develops PML. Teach patients to report any new neurologic symptoms such as confusion, dizziness, loss of balance, difficulty talking or walking, or vision problems right away.
- The most common side effects were infusion reactions, neutropenia, thrombocytopenia, anemia, fever, cough, and musculoskeletal disorders.

Potential Toxicities/Side Effects and the Nursing Process

I.   POTENTIAL FOR INFECTION related to NEUTROPENIA, IMMUNOSUPPRESSION AND THROMBOCYTOPENIA

Defining Characteristics: Obinutuzumab in combination with chlorambucil resulted in 40% incidence of neutropenia in clinical trials, 34% grade 3–4; this increases risk for infections. The incidence of infections was 38%, 9% grade 3–4. Cough occurs in 10% of patients, as does pyrexia. Thrombocytopenia occurred in 15% of patients, 11% grade 3–4. Anemia occurred in 12% of patients; HBV reactivation can occur in patients who are hepatitis B surface antigen (HBsAg) positive, as well as in patients who are HBsAg negative but hepatitis B core antibody (anti-HBc) positive. Rarely, acute thrombocytopenia can occur within 24 hours of the infusion.

Nursing Implications: Assess baseline WBC, lymphocyte, and neutrophil counts, platelet count, and hemoglobin, and monitor frequently during therapy, especially if the patient develops neutropenia or thrombocytopenia. Assess skin integrity, potential for infection, and teach patient measures to prevent infection (e.g., keeping skin intact, avoiding sources of infection, good hand-washing), bleeding, or worsening fatigue. Teach patient to report any signs/symptoms of infection (e.g., redness, heat, exudate on skin, temperature ≥ 100.4°F, cough, sputum production, dysuria), or bleeding. Assess for signs/symptoms of infection during therapy and at each visit, as well as for bleeding and fatigue. If a patient develops an infection, discuss with physician or midlevel practitioner interrupting or discontinuing drug and beginning appropriate antimicrobial treatment. Neutropenic patients should receive antimicrobial prophylaxis throughout treatment, and antiviral and antifungal prophylaxis should be considered. All patients should be screened for HBV infection (measuring HBsAg and anti-HBc) before starting obinutuzumab therapy. Closely monitor all patients with current or prior HBV infection (clinical and laboratory) for signs of hepatitis and HBV reactivation (e.g., increased transminase levels, bilirubin) during and after completion of treatment.

II. POTENTIAL FOR INJURY related to INFUSION REACTION

Defining Characteristics: Obinutuzumab can cause infusion reactions, so premedication is required. The infusion reaction is characterized by hypotension, tachycardia, dyspnea, bronchospasm, laryngeal edema, wheezing, nausea, vomiting, diarrhea, hypertension, flushing, headache, fever, chills. The risk for severe infusion reaction may be increased in patients with preexisting cardiac or pulmonary conditions.

Nursing Implications: Ensure patient receives premedication with acetaminophen, diphenhydramine or equivalent, and glucocorticoid (dexamethasone or prednisolone). See Drug Administration. Begin infusion using slow infusion rate as in Administration section. Assess for signs/symptoms of infusion reaction, and be prepared to stop infusion. Recall signs/symptoms of anaphylaxis; if these occur, stop drug immediately, notify physician, and assess patient's vital signs. Subjective symptoms are generalized itching, nausea, chest tightness, crampy abdominal pain, difficulty speaking, anxiety, agitation, sense of impending doom, uneasiness, desire to urinate/defecate, dizziness, and chills. Objective signs are flushed appearance; angioedema of face, neck, eyelids, hands, and feet; localized or generalized urticaria; respiratory distress with or without wheezing; hypotension; and cyanosis. Review standing orders or nursing procedures for patient management of anaphylaxis and be prepared to stop drug immediately, notify physician, monitor VS, and administer ordered medications, which may include epinephrine 1:1,000 glucocorticoids, bronchodilator, oxygen, and diphenhydramine. Teach patient to report any unusual symptoms. STOP the infusion for ALL infusion reactions. For severe reactions, institute medical management urgently, such as for angina or other signs/symptoms of myocardial insufficiency. Drug is permanently discontinued for anaphylaxis. If initial reaction is grade 3, interrupt infusion until reaction resolves. For grade 1, 2, interrupt infusion or slow infusion rate, and manage symptoms per physician or mid-level practitioner. Teach patient to report any signs and symptoms of infusion reaction within 24 hours of the infusion (e.g., fever, chills, rash, breathing problems). Closely monitor patients with preexisting cardiac or pulmonary conditions during drug infusion and postinfusion period, as these patients may have more severe reactions. Discuss with physician/mid-level practitioner withholding antihypertensive treatment 12 hours prior to the infusion, during the infusion, and for 1 hour after administration to reduce the risk of hypotension.

Drug: ofatumumab (Arzerra)

Class: IgG_1 monoclonal antibody (fully human) targeted at the CD_{20} molecule on B-cell lymphocyte membranes.

Mechanism of Action: Drug is a CD20-directed cytolytic monoclonal antibody. Drug binds specifically to both the small and large extracellular loop epitope on the CD_{20}

molecule and is released very slowly from the site. An epitope is a location on the antigen that can elicit an immune response. The CD_{20} molecule is expressed on normal B lymphocytes (B-lymphocyte lineage from pre-B to mature B-lymphocyte) and on B-cells in CLL patients. The Fab portion of ofatumumab binds to the CD_{20}, and the Fc portion calls in immune effector cells to kill the B-lymphocytes. Drug has stronger complement-dependent cytotoxicity than rituximab, is more effective in killing tumor cells with lower expression of CD_{20} cells, and is able to kill CD_{20} cells resistant to rituximab.

Metabolism: Ofatumumab is eliminated via target-independent and B-cell–mediated routes. As the B-lymphocytes are killed, the clearance of the drug is slower, so the infusions are scheduled every 4 weeks following 8 weekly infusions. The mean $t_{1/2}$ between infusion 4 and 12 was approximately 14 days (range 2.3–61.5 days). Although volume of distribution and clearance increase with increased body weight, this is not clinically significant.

Indications: For the treatment of
* In combination with chlorambucil, previously untreated patients with CLL for whom fludarabine-based therapy is considered inappropriate.
* Patients with CLL refractory to fludarabine and alemtuzumab.

Dosage/Range:
* Premedicate 30 min to 2 hours prior to each dose of ofatumumab with oral acetaminophen 1,000 mg (or equivalent), oral or IV antihistamine (cetirizine 10 mg or equivalent), and IV corticosteroid (prednisolone 100 mg or equivalent).
* CLL previously untreated, in combination with chlorambucil: 300 mg on cycle 1, day 1, followed by 1,000 mg on cycle 1, day 8, by IV infusion. 1,000-mg IV Infusion on day 1 of subsequent 28-day cycles for a minimum of 3 cycles until best response or a maximum of 12.
* CLL refractory to fludarabine and alemtuzumab: 12 doses as follows:
  * Dose 1: 300-mg initial dose infused at 12 mL/hr (3.6 mg/hr), followed 1 week later by
  * Doses 2–8: 2,000 mg weekly for 7 doses, followed 4 weeks later by
  * Doses 9–12: 2,000 mg every 4 weeks for 4 doses.

Drug Preparation:
* Available as 100-mg/5-mL and 1,000-mg/50-mL single-use vials. Do not shake product. Inspect parenteral drug products for particulate matter and discoloration before administration. Drug should be a clear to opalescent, colorless solution. If discolored or cloudy, or if there are foreign particulates, do not use.
* For the 300-mg dose:
  * Withdraw and discard 15 mL from a 1,000-mL polyolefin bag of 0.9% sodium chloride injection, USP.
  * Withdraw 5 mL from each of 3 100-mg vials of ofatumumab and add to the IV bag. Mix diluted solution by gentle inversion.
* For the 1,000-mg dose:
  * Withdraw and discard 50 mL from a 1,000-mL polyolefin bag of 0.9% sodium chloride injection, USP.
  * Withdraw 50 mL from 1 single-use 1,000-mg vial of ofatumumab and add to the IV bag. Mix diluted solution by gentle inversion.

- For the 2,000-mg dose:
  - Withdraw and discard 100 mL from a 1,000-mL polyolefin bag of 0.9% sodium chloride injection, USP.
  - Withdraw 50 mL from 2 single-use 1,000-mg vials of ofatumumab and add to the IV bag. Mix diluted solution by gentle inversion.
- Store diluted solution at 2–8°C (36–46°F). No incompatibilities between ofatumumab and polyvinylchloride or polyolefin bags and administration sets have been seen.
- START infusion within 12 hours of drug preparation, and discard the prepared solution after 24 hours.

Administration:
- Dilute and administer as an IV infusion; do not administer as an IV push or bolus, or as a subcutaneous injection.
- Premedicate before each infusion. The infusion environment should permit adequate patient monitoring and treatment of infusion reactions.
- Do not mix drug with, or administer as an infusion with, other medicines.
- Administer using an infusion pump and an administration set.
- Flush the IV line with 0.9% sodium chloride injection USP before and after each dose.
- Start infusion within 12 hours of preparation. Discard prepared solution after 24 hours.
- The following infusion rates should be used after the patient has received premedication:
  - Previously untreated CLL:
    - Premedication (or equivalents): acetaminophen 1,000-mg PO, diphenhydramine 50 mg or certirizine 10-mg PO or IV, IV corticosteroid (e.g., prednisilone 50 mg), 30–120 min prior to infusion. If the patient did not have a grade 3 or higher infusion-related adverse event during the first 2 infusions, the dose of corticosteroid may be reduced or omitted for subsequent infusions.
    - Cycle 1, day 1 (300-mg dose): Start infusion at 3.6 mg/hr (12 mL/hr) (median duration of infusion 5.2 hr).
    - Cycle 1, day 8, and cycles 2–12 (1,000-mg doses): Start infusion at 25 mg/hr (25 mL/hr); if prior ≥ grade 3 infusion-related toxicity, start at 12 mg/hr. Median infusion duration for cycle 1, day 8 is 4.4 hrs., and for cycles 2–12 is 4.2–4.4 hrs.
    - If no infusion-related toxicity, increase the infusion rate every 30 min to a maximal rate of 400 mL/hr.

Infusion Rates for Ofatumumab (Arzerra package insert, April 2014):

Interval After Start of Infusion (min)	Cycle 1, Day 1 (mL/hr)	Cycle 1, Day 8, and Cycles 2–12 (mL/hr)
0–30	12	25
31–60	25	50
61–90	50	100
91–120	100	200

(continued)

Infusion Rates for Ofatumumab (Arzerra package insert, April 2014):   *(Continued)*

Interval After Start of Infusion (min)	Cycle 1, Day 1 (mL/hr)	Cycle 1, Day 8, and Cycles 2–12 (mL/hr)
121–150	200	400
151–180	300	400
>180	400	400

- Refractory CLL:
  - Premedication (or equivalent): acetaminophen 1,000-mg PO, diphenhydramine 50 mg or certirizine 10-mg PO or IV, IV corticosteroid (prednisilone 100 mg), 30–120 min prior to infusion. DO NOT reduce corticosteroid dose for doses 1, 2, and 9.
  - Corticosteroid dose may be reduced for doses 3–8, and 10–12 as follows: (1) *Doses 3–8:* Corticosteroid may be reduced or omitted with subsequent infusions if a grade 3 or higher infusion reaction DID NOT occur with the preceding dose; and (2) *Doses 10–12:* Administer prednisolone 50–100 mg or equivalent if a grade 3 or higher infusion reaction DID NOT occur with dose 9.
  - In the absence of infusional toxicity, the rate is increased every 30 minutes.
  - **Dose 1** (300-mg dose): Initiate infusion at a rate of 3.6 mg/hr (12 mL/hr); then increase rate to 25 mL/hr for 30 min; then increase rate to 50 mL/min for 30 min; then increase rate to 100 mL/hr for 30 min; then increase rate to 200 mL/hr for the remainder of the infusion, followed 1 week later by dose 2. Median duration of infusion for dose 1 is 6.8 hrs.
  - **Dose 2** (2,000-mg dose): Initiate infusion at a rate of 24 mg/hr (12 mL/hr), then titrate per table below. Median duration of infusion is 6.8 hrs.
  - **Doses 3–8** (2,000-mg doses): Begin infusion at a rate of 25 mL/hr (50 mg/hr) for 30 min; then increase rate to 50 mL/hr for 30 min; then increase rate to 100 mL/min for 30 min; then increase rate to 200 mL/hr for 30 min; then increase rate to 400 mL/hr for the remainder of the infusion. Doses 3–8 given every week, followed 4 weeks later by **doses 9–12**, which are given every 4 weeks. Median infusion duration doses 3–12 are 4.2–4.4 hrs.
  - Monitor patient closely during infusion, and interrupt infusion if infusion reaction occurs.

Infusion Rates for Ofatumumab in Refractory CLL (Arzerra package insert, April 2014)

Interval After Infusion Start (min)	Dose 1 (mL/hr)	Dose 2 (mL/hr)	Dose 3–12 (mL/hr)
0–30	12	12	25
31–60	25	25	50
61–90	50	50	100
91–120	100	100	200
> 120	200	200	400

- Interrupt infusion for all infusion reactions regardless of severity; if the infusion reaction resolves or remains ≤ grade 2, resume infusion with the following modifications based on the initial grade of the infusion reaction:
  - Grade 1–2: infuse at 50% (one-half) of the previous infusion rate.
  - Grade 3 or 4: infuse at infusion rate of 12 mL/hr.
  - Anaphylaxis: permanently discontinue drug. Consider drug discontinuance if the severity of the infusion reaction does not resolve to ≤ grade 2, despite clinical intervention.
  - After resuming the infusion, the rate may be increased according to the table based on patient tolerance (rate increased every 30 min).

Drug Interactions:
- No studies have been performed; unknown.

Lab Effects/Interference:
- Decreased neutrophil, platelet, red blood cell count.

Special Considerations:
- Ofatumumab can cause infusion reactions; 44% occurred during the initial infusion, 29% on the second-day infusion, and less frequently during subsequent infusions. The infusion reaction is characterized by bronchospasm, dyspnea, laryngeal edema, pulmonary edema, flushing, hypertension, hypotension, syncope, cardiac ischemia/infarction, back pain, abdominal pain, pyrexia, rash, urticaria, and angioedema. STOP the infusion with all infusion reactions. For severe reactions, institute emergency medical management urgently, such as for angina or other signs/symptoms of myocardial insufficiency. The risk for infusion reaction may be increased in patients with moderate to severe COPD. All patients should receive premedication with acetaminophen, antihistamine, and corticosteroid.
- Neutropenia and thrombocytopenia are side effects and can be prolonged (> 1 week) and severe. In clinical trials, the incidence of grade 3–4 neutropenia was 42% (18% grade 4) and sometimes lasted for > 2 weeks. CBC/platelets should be assessed baseline and regularly during therapy, with more frequent blood tests in patients who have grade 3–4 cytopenias.
- Progressive multifocal leukoencephalopathy (PML) can occur, so any patient with a new onset of, or changes in preexisting, neurologic signs or symptoms should be evaluated for PML, including a neurology consult, brain MRI, and LP exam. Ofatumumab should be discontinued if PML is suspected. Teach patients to report any new neurologic symptoms such as confusion, dizziness, loss of balance, difficulty talking or walking, or vision problems right away.
- Reactivation of hepatitis B can occur with monoclonal antibody therapy against CD20, including fulminant hepatitis and death. Screen ALL patients for HBV infection prior to starting the drug (hepatitis B surface antigen (HBsAg) and hepatitis B core antibody positive (anti-HBc). Carriers of hepatitis B should be monitored closely for signs/symptoms of active HBV infection during ofatumumab therapy and for 6–12 months following the last dose of therapy. Ofatumumab must be discontinued in patients who develop viral hepatitis or reactivation of HPV and should then be treated with appropriate antiviral

therapy. The reintroduction of ofatumumab after HPV therapy has not been studied. Teach patients at risk for HBV to report increasing fatigue and yellow discoloration of skin or eyes.

* Obstruction of the small intestines can occur, and patients should have a diagnostic workup to rule this out if symptoms (e.g., abdominal pain, nausea) develop.
* Immunizations: Live vaccines should NOT be administered to patients receiving ofatumumab, and the ability of the patient to generate an immune response to any vaccine is unknown following administration of ofatumumab.
* Drug has not been studied in patients with renal or hepatic impairment; use cautiously in these patients.
* TLS: Rapid lymphocyte lysis can cause TLS within 12–24 hours of initial drug infusion, characterized by acute renal failure, hyperkalemia, hyperuricemia, and/or hyperphosphatemia. Patients with high tumor burden and/or high circulating lymphocyte counts ($> 25 \times 10^9$/L) are at high risk and should receive TLS prophylaxis prior to receiving first drug infusion (e.g., antihyperuricemic agent such as allopurinol, hydration beginning 12–24 hours before dose. If TLS occurs, correct electrolyte abnormalities, monitor renal function and ensure hydration and fluid balance, and provide supportive care as needed.
* Drug may cause fetal harm. Teach women of childbearing age to use effective contraception to avoid pregnancy. Caution should be used if a mother nurses her baby. Published data suggest that neonatal and infant consumption of breastmilk does not result in substantial absorption of maternal antibodies into circulation. However, the local GI and limited systemic exposure of ofatumumab effects are not known.
* Most common side effects (10% or greater incidence) were (1) previously untreated CLL: infusion reactions, neutropenia; (2) refractory CLL: neutropenia, followed by pneumonia, pyrexia, cough, diarrhea, anemia, fatigue, dyspnea, rash, nausea, bronchitis, and URI. The most common serious adverse reactions in patients who received 2,000 mg of ofatumumab were infections (pneumonia and sepsis), neutropenia, and pyrexia. Infections were bacterial, viral, and fungal, affecting 70% of patients. 29% had grade 3 or higher infections, and 12% were fatal. This was less than the incidence (17%) of fatal infections in the group of patients receiving fludarabine and alemtuzumab.

Potential Toxicities/Side Effects and the Nursing Process

I.   POTENTIAL FOR INJURY related to HYPERSENSITIVITY AND INFUSION REACTION

Defining Characteristics: Ofatumumab can cause infusion reactions, so premedication is required. There is a decrease over time in frequency; 44% occurred during the initial infusion, 29% on the second-day infusion, and less frequently during subsequent infusions. The infusion reaction is characterized by bronchospasm, dyspnea, laryngeal edema, pulmonary edema, flushing, hypertension, hypotension, syncope, cardiac ischemia/infarction, back pain, abdominal pain, pyrexia, rash, urticaria, and angioedema. The risk for infusion reaction may be increased in patients with moderate to severe COPD.

Nursing Implications: Ensure patient receives premedication with acetaminophen, diphenhydramine or equivalent, and corticosteroid (prednisolone or equivalent). See Dosage/Range. Begin infusion using slow infusion rate table. Recall signs/symptoms of anaphylaxis, and if these occur, stop drug immediately, notify physician, and assess patient's vital signs. Subjective symptoms are generalized itching, nausea, chest tightness, crampy abdominal pain, difficulty speaking, anxiety, agitation, sense of impending doom, uneasiness, desire to urinate/defecate, dizziness, and chills. Objective signs are flushed appearance; angioedema of face, neck, eyelids, hands, and feet; localized or generalized urticaria; respiratory distress with or without wheezing; hypotension; and cyanosis. Review standing orders or nursing procedures for patient management of anaphylaxis and be prepared to stop drug immediately, notify physician, monitor VS, and administer ordered medications, which may include epinephrine 1:1,000, hydrocortisone sodium succinate, oxygen, and diphenhydramine. Teach patient to report any unusual symptoms. STOP the infusion for ALL infusion reactions. For severe reactions, institute medical management urgently, such as for angina or other signs/symptoms of myocardial insufficiency. If initial reaction is grades 1, 2, or 3, after resolution or if reaction remains ≤ grade 2, resume at one-half the previous infusion rate (for grades 1, 2) or at 12 ml /hr (grade 3). After resuming the infusion, the infusion rate may be increased according to the infusion rate table (every 30 minutes as long as asymptomatic). Teach patient to report any signs and symptoms of infusion reaction within 24 hours of the infusion (e.g., fever, chills, rash, breathing problems).

II. POTENTIAL FOR INFECTION AND BLEEDING related to NEUTROPENIA AND THROMBOCYTOPENIA

Defining Characteristics: Neutropenia and thrombocytopenia are side effects and can be prolonged (> 1 week) and be severe. In clinical trials, the incidence of grade 3–4 neutropenia was 42% (18% grade 4), and sometimes lasted for > 2 weeks. The incidence of infection is 80% (bacterial, viral, and fungal), primarily pneumonia and sepsis. Twelve percent of patients die from their infections. Pyrexia occurs in 20% of patients. Drug may also reactivate HBV infection, so carriers must be monitored closely.

Nursing Implications: Assess CBC and differential/platelets baseline and regularly during therapy, with more frequent blood testing in patients who have grade 3–4 cytopenias. Assess hepatitis B viral screening findings for high-risk individuals and ensure the results are negative before starting drug. Teach patient to report fever and signs/symptoms of infection or bleeding right away. Assess medication profile and OTC medications taken. Teach patient to avoid OTC medications containing NSAIDs or aspirin. Teach patient to talk to nurse or physician before beginning any OTC medications. Monitor before each treatment, during therapy, and more often as needed. Assess risk for infection and integrity of skin and mucous membranes, pulmonary status, and ability to clear secretions, as well as history of past infections, baseline and prior to each treatment. Teach patient to self-administer prophylactic antibiotics, antiviral, and antifungal agents as ordered by physician. Ensure that patient has coverage or can purchase antimicrobial medications if ordered. Teach patient to self-administer oral antifungal agent if ordered for oral candidiasis if it develops. Teach patient to self-assess for signs/symptoms of infection and to call provider immediately or come to the emergency room if temperature > 100.4°F, shaking, chills, rash, productive cough, burning on urination, or any signs/symptoms of infection or bleeding. Teach self-care strategies to minimize risk of infection and bleeding, including avoidance of OTC aspirin-containing medications. Closely monitor hepatitis B carriers for clinical and laboratory signs of active HBV during therapy and for 6–12 months after the last infusion of ofatumumab. Discontinue the drug in patients who develop viral hepatitis or reactivation of viral hepatitis and implement antiviral therapy.

Drug: olaparib (Lynparza)

Class: Poly (ADP-ribose) polymerase (PARP) inhibitor.

Mechanism of Action: Drug inhibits PARP enzymes PARP 1, 2, and 3, which play important roles in DNA transcription, cell-cycle regulation, and DNA repair. This results in disruption of cancer cell processes and cell death, especially in *BRCA*-mutated tumor cells.

Metabolism: Rapid absorption after oral dosing, with peak plasma concentrations occurring 1–3 hours after the patient takes the dose. Taking the drug with a high-fat meal slows the rate of absorption but does not significantly change the extent of absorption. Olaparib is approximately 82% protein bound, and is extensively metabolized by (primarily) CYP3A4. Its terminal plasma half-life is 11.9 ± 4.8 hours, with 15% of the drug being excreted in urine and 6% in feces.

Indication: Accelerated approval as monotherapy for treatment of patients with deleterious or suspected deleterious germline *BRCA* mutation (as detected by an FDA-approved test) advanced ovarian cancer who have received three or more prior lines of chemotherapy. Approval was based on the objective response rate and duration of response; continued approval may be contingent upon verification of clinical benefit in confirmatory trials.

Dosage/Range:
- 400 mg orally (eight 50-mg capsules), taken twice daily (total daily dose of 800 mg), until disease progression or unacceptable toxicity occurs.
- Dose modifications to manage toxicity:
  - Interrupt dose or reduce dose to 200 mg (four 50-mg capsules) twice daily (total 400 mg daily dose).
  - If further dose reduction is necessary, reduce to 100 mg (two 50-mg capsules) taken twice daily (total daily dose of 200 mg).
  - Concomitant CYP3A inhibitors: Avoid use, but if necessary, reduce olaparib dose to 150 mg (three 50-mg capsules) taken twice daily (strong inhibitor) or 200 mg (four 50-mg capsules) taken twice daily (moderate inhibitor).

Drug Preparation: Available as a 50-mg hard capsule. Store at room temperature and keep out of the reach of children and pets.

Drug Administration:
- Teach the patient self-administration: Swallow capsule whole; do not chew, dissolve, or open capsule; do not take capsules that are misshapen or show evidence of leakage.
- If a dose is missed, teach the patient to omit it and to take the next dose at its scheduled time.
- Assess CBC/differential at baseline and monthly thereafter. The drug should not be started until resolution of myelosuppression from prior therapy occurs (grade 0–1).
- If prolonged myelosuppression occurs, interrupt the drug and monitor CBC/differential weekly until recovery. If recovery (grade 0–1) has not occurred by 4 weeks, refer the patient to a hematologist for evaluation, including bone marrow analysis and cytogenetic study. The drug should be discontinued if MDS/AML is confirmed.

Drug Interactions:
- CYP3A inhibitors may increase olaparib serum levels: *Avoid coadministration* with **strong inhibitors** (e.g., itraconazole, telithromycin, clarithromycin, ketoconazole, voriconazole, nefazodone, posaconazole, ritonovir, lopinavir/ritonavir, indinavir, saquinavir, nelfinavir, boceprevir, telaprevir) and **moderate inhibitors** (e.g., amprenavir, aprepitant, atazanavir, ciprofloxacin, crizotinib, darunavir/ritonavir, diltiazem, erythromycin, fluconazole, fosamprenavir, imatinib, verapamil). See the dose modification if the drug must be coadministered with olaparib. Teach the patient to avoid grapefruit and Seville oranges while taking olaparib, as these foods may also increase olaparib serum levels and toxicity.
- CYP3A4 inducers may decrease olaparib serum levels: *Avoid* concomitant administration of **strong inducers** (e.g., rifampicin, phenytoin, carbamazepine, St. John's wort), as this may decrease the serum level of olaparib by as much as 87%. Avoid coadministration with **moderate inducers** (e.g., bosentan, efavirenz, etravirine, modafinil, nafcillin) but if it is unavoidable, assess for decreased olaparib efficacy.
- Anticancer drugs: Potentiation and prolongation of myelosuppression.

Lab Effects/Interference:
- Increased: serum creatinine, MCV
- Decreased: hemoglobin, lymphocyte count, ANC, platelet count

Special Considerations:
- Most common adverse reactions in 20% or more of patients in clinical trials: anemia, nausea, fatigue/asthenia, vomiting, diarrhea, dysgeusia, dyspepsia, headache, decreased appetite, nasopharyngitis/pharyngitis/URI, cough, arthralgia/musculoskeletal pain, myalgia, back pain, dermatitis/rash, abdominal pain/discomfort.
- Warnings and precautions:
  - Myelodysplastic syndrome (MDS)/AML: May occur and be fatal. Incidence in a one-arm study and in a RCT was 2%. MDS/AML was diagnosed in patients receiving the drug for less than 6 months to more than 2 years. All patients had prior chemotherapy with platinum agents and/or other DNA-damaging agents. Most cases were fatal. Monitor baseline CBC/differential at baseline before beginning therapy and at least monthly. Discontinue the drug if MDS/AML is confirmed.

- Pneumonitis may occur and be fatal. If the patient presents with new or worsening respiratory symptoms (e.g., dyspnea, fever, cough, wheezing) or abnormality is seen on x-ray, interrupt the olaparib therapy and discuss further evaluation with the provider. Discontinue the drug if pneumonitis is confirmed.
- Embryo-fetal toxicity: Teach women of reproductive potential to use effective contraception during therapy and for 1 month after the drug is discontinued, and to avoid pregnancy.
- Nursing mothers should discontinue breastfeeding or discontinue the drug.

Potential Toxicities/Side Effects and the Nursing Process

I.   POTENTIAL FOR BLEEDING, INFECTION, ANEMIA, AND FATIGUE related to BONE MARROW SUPPRESSION

Defining Characteristics: In clinical trials, 25–32% of patients experienced neutropenia (7–8% grade 3/4), 26–30% thrombocytopenia (3% grades 3/4), 56% lymphopenia, 25–34% anemia, and 57–85% an elevation in mean corpuscular volume. In addition, 26–43% of patients developed nasopharyngitis or URI. Anemia was common (90%), with 15% of cases being grade 3/4. Fatigue/asthenia occurred in 66% of patients and was severe (grade 3/4) in 8%.

Nursing Implications: Evaluate CBC/differential, hemoglobin/hematocrit, MCV, and platelets at baseline and then monthly. Discuss any abnormalities with the physician/NP/PA. The drug should not be started until resolution of myelosuppression from prior therapy has occurred (grade 0–1). Assess for signs and symptoms of infection, bleeding, and fatigue. Teach the patient about signs and symptoms of infection and bleeding, and to report them immediately. Teach the patient self-care measures to minimize the risk of infection and bleeding, including avoidance of OTC aspirin-containing medications. Teach the patient self-assessment of fatigue, and to alternate rest and activity as needed. If prolonged myelosuppression occurs, interrupt the drug and monitor CBC/differential weekly until recovery. If recovery (grade 0–1) has not occurred by 4 weeks, refer the patient to a hematologist for evaluation, including bone marrow analysis and cytogenetic study. The drug should be discontinued if MDS/AML is confirmed.

II.   ALTERATION IN NUTRITION, POTENTIAL, related to NAUSEA, VOMITING, OR DIARRHEA

Defining Characteristics: Nausea was common in clinical trials (65–75%), as was vomiting (32–43%), diarrhea (28–31%), dyspepsia (25%), decreased appetite (22–25%), and dysgeusia (21%).

Nursing Implications: Assess the patient's nutritional status at baseline and at each visit. Teach the patient that these side effects may occur, and teach self-management strategies such as use of antidiarrheals, antinausea medications, and dietary modifications, and to report any symptoms that do not improve. Discuss prescription medications with the provider if there is a need to manage refractory symptoms. Teach the patient tips to increase appetite (e.g., small, frequent meals, use of spices). Offer the services of a dietitian as appropriate.

III. ALTERATION IN COMFORT related to ARTHRALGIA/MYALGIA, HEADACHE, OR BACKACHE

Defining Characteristics: In clinical trials, arthralgias and musculoskeletal pain occurred in 21–32% of patients (4% grade 3/4), myalgia in 22–25%, back pain in 25%, and headache in 25%.

Nursing Implications: Assess the patient's baseline level of comfort. Teach the patient that these side effects may occur, and teach self-management strategies. Teach the patient to report symptoms that do not improve. If this occurs, discuss with the physician/NP/PA prescription medication for refractory symptoms.

Drug: palbociclib (Ibrance)

Class: Kinase inhibitor; cyclin-dependent kinase (CDK) inhibitor.

Mechanism of Action: Palbociclib inhibits CDK 4 and 6, which stops the cell cycle from proceeding from the G_1 phase to the S phase; thus cell proliferation is halted in ER-positive breast cancer cells. When combined with antiestrogens, palbociclib increased growth arrest and inhibition of ER-positive tumor growth to a greater extent than occurred with either drug alone.

Metabolism: After oral administration, the peak plasma concentration (C_{max}) is reached in 6–12 hours; however, oral bioavailability is 46% (after a dose of 125 mg). Steady state is reached within 8 days. C_{max} is increased by administration of the drug with food. Palbociclib binds to human plasma proteins (about 85%), and undergoes hepatic metabolism, primarily by CYP3A and SULT2A1 (sulfotransferase 2A1) pathways. Almost all of a dose (91.6%) is excreted in 15 days, with 74.1% recovered in the feces and 17.5% in the urine, primarily as metabolites.

Indication: In combination with letrozole, as initial endocrine-based therapy for the treatment of postmenopausal women with ER-positive, *HER-2*–negative advanced breast cancer. FDA-accelerated approval was based on PFS. Continued approval may be contingent on verification and description of clinical benefit in a confirmatory trial.

Dosage/Range:
- With food, in combination with letrozole 2.5 mg once daily, given continuously throughout the 28-day cycle.
- Starting dose: 125 mg orally, once daily with food, for 21 days, followed by 7 days off treatment (28-day cycle).

Dose Modifications:
- First dose reduction to a dose of 100 mg/day; second dose reduction to a dose of 75 mg/day.

- Neutropenia: Grade 3 (ANC < 1,000–500/mm^3): No dose adjustment (unless associated with lymphopenia and opportunistic infection), and consider repeating CBC/ANC 1 week later; withhold initiation of next cycle until recovery to grade ≤ 2 (≥1,000/mm^3). Grade 3 ANC (ANC < 1,000–500/mm^3 + fever (≥38.5°C and/or infection: Withhold palbociclib and initiation of next cycle until recovery to grade ≤ 2 (≥1,000/mm^3) and resume at next lower dose. Grade 4: Withhold palbociclib and begin next cycle once recovery to grade ≤ 2 at the next lower dose.
- Non-hematologic toxicity: Grade 1 or 2: No dose adjustment needed. Grade ≥ 3 (if persisting despite medical therapy): Withhold until symptoms resolve to grade ≤ 1; or grade ≤ 2 if not considered a safety risk for the patient; resume palbociclib at the next lower dose.
- If the drug must be coadministered with a strong CYP3A inhibitor, decrease the palbociclib dose to 75 mg. If the strong inhibitor is discontinued, increase the palbociclib dose to that used prior to adding the strong CYP3A inhibitor once 3–5 half-lives of the inhibitor have passed.
- See the manufacturer's prescribing information for letrozole.

Drug Preparation: Oral. Available as 125-mg, 100-mg, and 75-mg capsules. Store at room temperature, and keep out of the reach of children and pets.

Drug Administration:
- Monitor CBC/ANC prior to start of palbociclib therapy and at the beginning of each cycle, as well as on day 14 of the first two cycles, and as clinically indicated.
- Teach the patient to take the drug at approximately the same time each day. If a dose is missed or vomited, the patient should not take an additional dose, but rather resume dosing at the next scheduled time.
- Teach the patient to swallow the capsule whole; not to chew, crush, or open the capsule; and not to take the capsule if it is broken or cracked.

Drug Interactions:
- CYP3A inhibitors: Increase plasma concentrations of palbociclib (e.g., itraconazole increases C$_{max}$ by 34% and AUC by 87%). Avoid concurrent use with strong CYP3A inhibitors; if such use cannot be avoided, decrease the palbociclib dose.
- CYP3A4 inducers: Decrease plasma concentration of palbociclib (e.g., rifampin decreases C$_{max}$ by 70% and by AUC 85%). Avoid concurrent use with strong and moderate inducers.
- CYP3A substrates: For example, concomitant use of midazolam and palbociclib, increased the midazolam C$_{max}$ by 37%, and AUC by 61%. If the substrate is sensitive and has a narrow therapeutic window, consider dose reduction of the substrate.
- Gastric pH-elevating medications: If the patient is fasting, a proton pump inhibitor (PPI) given concomitantly reduces C$_{max}$ by 80% and AUC by 62%. If the PPI is given to a patient who is eating, there is no significant interaction.

Lab Effects/Interference: Decreased ANC, WBC, lymphocyte count, hemoglobin, and platelet count.

Special Considerations:
- Most common adverse reactions (≥10%): neutropenia, leucopenia, anemia, thrombocytopenia, URI, fatigue/asthenia, nausea, vomiting, stomatitis, decreased appetite, diarrhea, peripheral neuropathy, and epistaxis.

- Warnings and precautions:
  - Neutropenia: Monitor CBC/ANC at baseline and prior to each cycle, as well as on day 14 of the first two cycles. In study 1, 57% of patients had grade 3 neutropenia and 5% had grade 4; the median time to the first episode of any neutropenia was 15 days (range, 13–117 days). Median duration of neutropenia grade ≥ 3 was 7 days. Interrupt the dose, reduce the dose, or delay it if the patient develops grade 3 or 4 neutropenia.
  - Infections: Monitor the patient closely and give medical treatment promptly. Teach the patient to report fever or chills immediately.
  - Pulmonary embolism (PE): In study 1, PE occurred in 5% of patients compared to no cases in those receiving letrozole alone. Monitor the patient closely for signs and symptoms of PE. Teach the patient to report such signs and symptoms immediately, and to seek emergency medical care if any of the following occur: new-onset SOB; sudden, sharp chest pain that may worsen with a deep breath; rapid heart rate; rapid breathing rate.
  - Embryo-fetal toxicity: Palbociclib can cause fetal harm. Teach women of reproductive potential to use effective contraception to avoid pregnancy.
  - Alopecia occurs in 22% of patients (grade 1, 21%; grade 2, 1%).

Potential Toxicities/Side Effects and the Nursing Process

I. POTENTIAL FOR BLEEDING, INFECTION, AND FATIGUE related to BONE MARROW SUPPRESSION

Defining Characteristics: In clinical study 1, 75% of patients developed neutropenia (all grades), with 48% having grade 3 and 6% having grade 4. Thirty-five percent developed anemia, and 17% developed thrombocytopenia. Infections occurred in 31% of patients. Fatigue and asthenia developed in 41% and 13% of patients, respectively.

Nursing Implications: Evaluate CBC/differential, hemoglobin/hematocrit, and platelets at baseline and prior to each 28-day cycle, and on day 14 of the first two cycles. Discuss any abnormalities with the physician/NP/PA. Assess for signs and symptoms of infection, bleeding, and fatigue. Teach the patient about the signs and symptoms of infection and bleeding, and to report them immediately. Teach the patient self-care measures to minimize the risk of infection and bleeding, including avoidance of OTC aspirin-containing medications. Teach the patient self-assessment of fatigue, and to alternate rest and activity as needed. Discuss dose modification for grade 3 or higher neutropenia.

II. ALTERATION IN NUTRITION, POTENTIAL, related to NAUSEA, VOMITING, DIARRHEA, OR STOMATITIS

Defining Characteristics: Stomatitis (aphthous stomatitis, cheilitis, glossitis, glossodynia, mouth ulceration, mucosal inflammation) occurred in 25% of patients. Nausea affected 25%, and vomiting 15%. Diarrhea affected 12% and was severe (grade 3) in 4%.

Nursing Implications: Assess the patient's nutritional status at baseline and at each visit. Assess the oral mucosa for intactness and oral health habits. Teach the patient that these side effects may occur, and teach self-management strategies such as systematic oral cleansing and oral assessment, use of antidiarrheals and antinausea medications, and dietary modifications, and to report any symptoms that do not improve. Discuss prescription medication with the provider if necessary to manage refractory symptoms. Teach the patient tips to increase appetite (e.g., small, frequent meals, use of spices). Offer the services of a dietitian as appropriate.

Drug: panitumumab (Vectibix)

Class: IgG$_2$ human monoclonal antibody targeted against epidermal growth factor receptor (EGFR).

Mechanism of Action: Drug is a human IgG$_2$ monoclonal antibody. It blocks growth factor (ligand, such as epidermal growth factor and transforming growth factor-alpha) from binding to EGFR, thus preventing dimerization and initiation of cell signaling via receptor tyrosine kinase phosphorylation; thus, the message telling the cell to divide does not occur. The drug competes with natural ligands but has a higher affinity for the EGFR than the ligands. In addition to cell growth inhibition, there is induction of apoptosis, and decreased matrix metalloproteinase and vascular endothelial growth factor production. This decreases angiogenesis. Drug is effective only if *KRAS/RAS* genes are normal (called wild-type, WT). If *KRAS/RAS* genes are mutated, the gene turns itself on and sets up an independent signaling cascade bringing a message to the nucleus telling the cell to divide regardless of whether EGFR is blocked by panitumumab.

Metabolism: Steady-state reached by third infusion. Elimination half-life is approximately 7.5 days.

Indication: Treatment of patients with wild-type *KRAS* (exon 2) metastatic colorectal cancer (mCRC) as determined by an FDA-approved test for this use.

- In combination with FOLFOX for first-line treatment.
- As monotherapy following disease progression after prior treatment with fluoropyrimidine, oxaliplatin, and irinotecan chemotherapy-containing regimens.
- Not indicated for the treatment of patients with *KRAS* mutant positive mCRC or for whom *KRAS* status is unknown.

Dosage/Range:
- 6 mg/kg IV over 1 hour every 14 days. If first infusion is well-tolerated, subsequent infusions can be given over 30–60 minutes. Doses > 1,000 mg should infuse over 90 minutes.
- Infusion reactions: reduce infusion rate by 50% for mild reactions; terminate infusion for severe reactions. Depending upon the severity and/or persistence of the reaction, permanently discontinue panitumumab. Medical resources for the treatment of severe infusion reactions should be in the infusion area.

* Dermatologic toxicities:
  * Upon first occurrence of a grade 3 dermatologic reaction, withhold 1–2 doses of panitumumab. If the reaction improves to < grade 3, reinitiate panitumumab at the original dose.
  * Upon second occurrence of a grade 3 dermatologic reaction, withhold 1–2 doses of panitumumab. If the reaction improves to < grade 3, reinitiate panitumumab at 80% of the original dose.
  * Upon third occurrence of a grade 3 dermatologic reaction, withhold 1–2 doses of panitumumab. If the reaction improves to < grade 3, reinitiate panitumumab at 60% of the original dose.
  * Upon the fourth occurrence of a grade 3 dermatologic reaction, permanently discontinue panitumumab.
  * Permanently discontinue panitumumab after the occurrence of a grade 4 dermatologic reaction or for a grade 3 dermatologic reaction that does not recover after withholding 1–2 doses.

Drug Preparation:
* Available as single use (20-mg/mL vials): 100 mg/5mL, 200 mg/10 mL, 400 mg/20mL.
* Inspect drug (should be colorless; do not administer if solution is discolored).
* Do not shake; withdraw ordered dose (6mg/kg).
* Dilute to a total volume of 100 mL with 0.9% sodium chloride injection, USP; doses > 1,000 mg should be diluted to 150 mL 0.9% sodium chloride injection, USP. Final concentration should be ≤ 10 mg/mL. Mix diluted solution by gentle inversion.
* Use the diluted infusion solution within 6 hrs. of preparation if stored at room temperture, or within 24 hours of dilution if stored at 2–8°C (36–46°F). DO NOT FREEZE. Discard any unused portion remaining in the vial.

Drug Administration:
* Administer IV infusion using low-protein binding 0.2-µm or 0.22-µm inline filter using infusion pump over 60 minutes (90 minutes for dose > 1,000 mg).
* Infuse doses of ≤ 1,000 mg over 60 minutes though a peripheral IV line or indwelling IV catheter. If infusion tolerated, administer subsequent infusions over 30–60 minutes. Administer doses > 1,000 mg over 90 minutes.
* Do NOT administer panitumumab by IV push or bolus.
* Flush line before and after panitumumab infusion with 0.9% sodium chloride injection, USP. Do not mix with other drug products or IV solutions.
* Reduce the infusion rate by 50% if patient experiences a mild or moderate (grade 1–2) infusion reaction for the remainder of the infusion.
* Stop and discontinue drug for severe reactions, or persistent reactions, for example, grade 3–4 infusion reactions (symptomatic bronchospasm or anaphylaxis).
* Post-marketing reports indicate that severe infusion reactions occur in 1% of patients and may be fatal.
* Hold drug for severe or intolerable skin toxicity; may resume at 50% dose if toxicity improves.

Drug Interactions:
- IFL: Severe diarrhea (1 fatality). DO NOT COADMINISTER.

Lab Effects/Interference:
- Decreased magnesium 6 weeks after beginning therapy.
- Decreased calcium in some patients.

Special Considerations:
- Panitumumab is not indicated for use in patients with *KRAS* mutation or if mutational status is unknown. Patients with *KRAS* gene mutation in codon 12 or 13 have not shown a treatment benefit, so drug is not recommended in these patients. In fact, increased tumor progression, increased mortality, or lack of benefit was seen in *K-RAS* mutant mCRC (Amgen, 2014). Signal transduction through the EGFR results in activation of wild-type KRAS protein. However, in cells with activating *KRAS* (somatic) mutations, the mutant KRAS protein is continually active and appears independent of EGFR regulation. *K-RAS* tumor status must be determined before using the drug.
- Dermatologic toxicities were reported in 90% of patients and were severe in 16% of patients receiving monotherapy in Study 1. Clinical manifestations included dermatitis cuneiform, pruritus, erythema, rash, skin exfoliation, paronychia, dry skin, and skin fissures. Teach patient to avoid sun exposure, and to use SPF and hat protection if going outside. Closely monitor the patient with rash for the development of inflammatory or infectious sequelae. Life-threatening and fatal infections, including necrotizing fasciitis, abcesses, bullous mucocutaneous skin disease, and sepsis have occurred. Rare cases of Stevens-Johnson syndrome and toxic epidermal necrolysis have been reported post-marketing. Follow dose modifications for grade 3 and grade 4. Hold drug or discontinue drug for dermatologic or soft-tissue toxicity, associated with severe or life-threatening inflammatory or infectious complications.
- Severe infusion reactions occurred in 1% of patients (NCI grade 3–4), and 4% experienced infusion reactions in Study 1. Infusion reactions characterized by anaphylactoid reactions, bronchospasm, and hypotension can occur after panitumumab infusion. Fatal infusion reactions have occurred post-marketing. Terminate the infusion for severe infusion reactions and provide emergency medical care.
- Interstitial lung disease, a class effect, may occur in 1% of patients, but caution should be used when treating patients with a history of interstitial pneumonitis, pulmonary fibrosis, as after the first fatality, these patients were excluded from clinical trials. Permanently discontinue panitumumab if ILD is confirmed. If the patient has a history of interstitial pneumonitis or pulmonary fibrosis, or evidence of interstitial pneumonitis or pulmonary fibrosis, risk versus benefit must be carefully considered.
- Severe diarrhea and dehydration, leading to acute renal failure and other complications, have occurred when panitumumab is administered with chemotherapy.
- Increased mortality and toxicity with panitumumab when added to bevacizumab and chemotherapy so this combination should NOT be used:
  - In an interim analysis of an open-label, multicenter, randomized clinical trial in the first-line setting in patients with mCRC, patients receiving panitumumab, bevacizumab, and chemotherapy had decreased OS and a higher rate of grade 3–5 adverse effects (87% vs 72%).

- Grade 3–4 adverse reactions included rash/cuneiform dermatitis (26% vs 1%); diarrhea (23% vs 12%); dehydration (16% vs 5%); and hydration (16% vs 5%); occurred primarily in patients with diarrhea and hypokalemia (10% vs 4%); stomatitis/mucositis (4% vs < 1%); and hypomagnesemia (4% vs 0).
- Grade 3–5 pulmonary embolism occurred in more patients receiving panitumumab (7% vs 3%), and was fatal in < 1%.
- Patients randomized to receive panitumumab, bevacizumab, and chemotherapy received lower dose intensities for each of the chemotherapy drugs due to adverse events over the first 24 weeks of study, compared to patients receiving bevacizumab and chemotherapy alone.
- Drug may cause grade 3–4 hypomagnesemia in 2% of patients. Hypomagnesemia occurred ≥ 6 weeks after starting panitumumab. Some patients had both hypomagnesemia and hypocalcemia. Assess electrolytes baseline and periodically during and for 8 weeks after the completion of panitumumab therapy. Replete electrolytes as needed.
- Photosensitivity: sunlight exposure can exacerbate dermatolotic toxicity; teach patients to wear sunscreen, hats, and limit sun exposure while receiving panitumumab.
- Keratitis and ulcerative keratitis are risk factors for corneal perforation, and have been reported with panitumumab use. Monitor patient for evidence of keratitis or ulcerative keratitis, and interrupt or discontinue drug for acute or worsening keratitis.
- Tumor should be assessed for EGFR protein expression, using laboratories with demonstrated proficiency.
- Patient should use effective birth control measures to avoid pregnancy. Physicans are encouraged to enroll pregnant patients in Amgen's Pregnancy Surveillance Program (1-800-772-6436). Mothers should not breastfeed while receiving the drug; a decision should be made to discontinue nursing or discontinue the drug, taking into account the importance of the drug to the mother's health.
- Compared with best supportive care (BSC), panitumumab significantly improved PFS, but there was no significant difference in overall survival (OS) between groups.
- Most common adverse reactions (≥ 20%) were skin toxicities (e.g., erythema, dermatitis caneiform, pruritus, exfoliation, rash, fissures), paronychia, hypomagnesemia, fatigue, abdominal pain, nausea, and diarrhea and constipation.

Potential Toxicities/Side Effects and the Nursing Process

I.   POTENTIAL ALTERATION IN BODY IMAGE, SKIN INTEGRITY, COMFORT related to SKIN RASH, PARONYCHIA, SKIN FISSURES, PRURITUS

Defining Characteristics: Drug inhibits epidermal growth factor receptor, so major toxicity is manifested in the skin with 90% of patients experiencing some type of skin toxicity. Most patients develop a mild-to-moderate acnelike rash that is self-limiting. Sixteen percent report a grade 3–4 rash. Rash is a sterile, suppurative rash with multiple follicular or pustular lesions that appear during the first 2 weeks of therapy on the face, upper chest, and back, but in some cases, extended to the arms. Rash resolves when treatment is stopped, without scar formation. Pruritus affects 57%, dry skin 10%, acneform dermatitis 57%, skin desquamation 25%, erythema 65%, paronychia 25%, macular rash 22%, skin fissures 20%, stomatitis 7%, oral mucositis 6%. Fissures can become infected; infection can be treated with topical clindamycin, or oral antibiotics. However, severe dermatologic toxicities result in infectious complications including sepsis, death, and abscesses requiring incision and drainage. Eye-related toxicities occurred in 15% of patients (conjunctivitis 4%, hyperemia 3%, lacrimation 2%, eyelid irritation 1%), median time to most severe toxicity 15 days from starting drug; median time to solution was 84 days. Exposure to UV light exacerbates intensity and severity of rash.

Nursing Implications: Teach patient that rash most likely will occur due to mechanism of drug action. Assess baseline skin integrity on areas of face, neck, and trunk; assess baseline comfort and satisfaction with body image, and monitor at each treatment. Teach patient to report any distress and assess extent of rash. For severe rash (grade 3–4 or intolerable), hold drug for up to one month until it resolves to grade 2 or less; if it does not, discontinue drug. When rash resolves to grade 2 and the patient is symptomatically improved and no more than two doses have been held, resume drug at 50% of the original dose. If skin toxicity recurs, discontinue drug. If skin appears to be infected (exudate, vesicle formation, abnormal appearance), obtain C+S and discuss empiric treatment with physician. For rash, fissure, and paronychia management, refer to the introduction to *Chapter 5*. Teach all patients to (1) use a water-based emollient frequently during the day to prevent dryness, (2) stay hydrated, (3) avoid sun exposure and wear SPF 30 (zinc-based). Do not use anti-acne medications. Tetracycline analogues provide anti-inflammatory benefit. **Grade 1 or mild rash (localized, does not interfere with ADLs, and is not infected):** The goal is to preserve skin integrity, minimize discomfort, and prevent infection. Key patient teaching includes (1) use a mild soap with active ingredients that reduce skin drying such as pyrithione zinc (Head & Shoulders), (2) consider aloe gel for red, tender areas, (3) report distressing tenderness, as pramoxine (lidocaine topical anesthetic) may help, (4) keep fingernails clean and trimmed, and (5) apply zinc ointment to rectal mucosa after washing. Management: maintain current drug dose, observe or give topical hydrocortisone 1% or 2.5% or clindamycin 1% gel (anti-inflammatory benefit) with or without oral doxycycline or minocycline 100 mg BID; reassess in 2 weeks. **For grade 2 or moderate rash that is generalized, mild symptoms, and has minimal effect on ADLs, and no infection:** The goal is to prevent infection and promote comfort. Continue EGFRI dose; use topicals (hydrocortisone 2.5% or clindamycin 1% gel) and add doxycycline or minocycline 100 mg PO twice daily (give antimicrobial and anti-inflammatory effect) and reassess after 2 weeks. **For grade 3–4 or severe rash (generalized, severe, has a significant impact on ADLs, and increased risk of infection):** The goal is to prevent infection or to identify it early to minimize complications and to promote effective coping. Dose-reduce EGFRI drug based on manufacturer's recommendation, and treat rash with topicals (hydrocortisone 2.5% or clindamycin 1% gel, doxycycline 100 mg PO twice daily or minocycline 100 mg PO twice daily, and consider systemic hydrocorticosteroids; reassess after 2 weeks, and interrupt or discontinue drug if rash worsens (Lynch et al., 2007). If rash appears infected (exudate, vesicular formation, different appearance), obtain C+S, treat empirically until sensitivity received, and/or obtain dermatology consult. The STEPP study (Lacouture, 2010) showed that preventive therapy in patients receiving panitumumab, of daily moisturizer, sunscreen, topical hydrocortisone and oral doxycycline 100 mg bid (or minocycline 100 mg daily), reduced the incidence of grade 2 or higher rash compared to patients who received only moisturizer and sunblock, when starting panitumumab therapy.

II. ALTERATION IN NUTRITION, LESS THAN BODY REQUIREMENTS, related to NAUSEA, VOMITING, DIARRHEA, STOMATITIS, CONSTIPATION, ANOREXIA, ABDOMINAL PAIN

Defining Characteristics: Incidence of mild-to-moderate digestive symptoms include nausea (23%), diarrhea (21%), abdominal pain (25%), vomiting (19%), constipation (21%), stomatitis (7%), hypomagnesia (39%), and oral mucositis (6%) in patients in clinical trials.

Nursing Implications: Assess baseline weight and nutritional status. Inform patient that these symptoms may occur, and to report them. Administer antiemetic and other symptom management medications as ordered. Teach patient self-administration of these medications at home. Monitor serum electrolytes (magnesium, calcium) prior to each dose, and replete magnesium as needed. Teach patient dietary modifications to address symptoms such as anorexia (small, frequent high-calorie, high-protein foods, stimulants as permitted by protocol); constipation (high-fiber, high-fluid, high-roughage foods, stool softeners); diarrhea (bananas, rice, applesauce, and toast); nausea (avoid food preparation odors by cooking in zipped plastic bag, or having someone else cook; choose cool, soft, nonspicy, or fatty foods). Teach patient to report any symptoms that do not resolve or improve on the plan. Assess efficacy of intervention, and revise plan as needed. Dehydration is a worrisome complication of diarrhea; teach patient to call right away if diarrhea persists, and/or is unable to drink fluids (e.g., 8 oz every hour while awake).

III. POTENTIAL FOR ALTERATION IN COMFORT related to FATIGUE, DYSPNEA, PERIPHERAL EDEMA, PYREXIA, ARTHRALGIA

Defining Characteristics: In clinical trials, the following symptoms were reported in patients with advanced colorectal cancer: fatigue (51%), cough (18%), dyspnea (14%), peripheral edema (14%), pyrexia (14%), arthralgia (14%), back pain (12%), headache (12%), dizziness (11%), insomnia (11%).

Nursing Implications: Assess patient comfort level, self-care measures baseline and periodically during therapy. Teach patient that these symptoms may arise, either from the drug and/or the treatment. Develop a plan for symptom management, assess efficacy, and revise as needed. Assess level of fatigue and teach energy-conserving strategies, baseline and prior to each treatment. Inform patient that fatigue may occur due to anemia, and teach energy-conserving strategies such as alternating rest and activity periods.

IV. ALTERATION IN ELECTROLYTE BALANCE related to HYPOMAGNESEMIA, POTENTIAL

Defining Characteristics: Magnesium wasting appears related to EGFR inhibition in the renal tubular epithelial cells so that excreted magnesium is not resorbed in the distal convoluted tubules. This leads to initial magnesium wasting, followed by losses of calcium and potassium. Hypomagnesemia occurs in about 38% of patients receiving the drug and is severe in 2–4% of patients. It begins within days to months of receiving the drug, and there is much interpatient variability. There appears to be a direct relationship between duration of EGFRI MAb treatment and severe hypomagnesemia (Fakih, 2007). Symptoms of grade 3–4 hypomagnesemia include fatigue, cramps, and somnolence.

Nursing Implications: Assess baseline electrolyte balance prior to initial treatment and prior to each successive weekly treatment. Grade of hypomagnesemia: Grade 1 is a serum level of < LLN–1.2 mg/dL, grade 2 is 0.9–1.2 mg/dL, grade 3 is 0.7–0.9 mg/dL, and grade 4 is ≤ 0.7 mg/dL. Replete magnesium, calcium, and potassium as needed. Oral magnesium may be ineffective and may result in diarrhea (Tejpar et al., 2007). Magnesium repletion regimens include weekly IV replacement of 4 g magnesium sulfate for grade 2. For grade 3–4, patients may be symptomatic and magnesium replacement may involve once- to twice-weekly IV infusions of 6–10 grams. Provide support for patients as magnesium replacement infusions require lengthy time in clinic, as an 8-g infusion requires 4 hours. Post-IV replacement with every other day serum magnesium monitoring is important until the patient develops a steady state (Fakih, 2007). Continue to monitor after drug has been discontinued (half-life of the drug and time drug persists (e.g., 8 weeks)). Magnesium replacement in IV hydration starting when a patient has grade 1 hypomagnesemia may be effective in preventing worsening hypomagnesemia. For patients who have refractory grade 4 hypomagnesemia, a stop-and-go approach has been effective where EGFRI MAb is held for 4–8 weeks until the magnesium corrects; it is reported that grade 4 hypomagnesemia does not recur when cetuximab is then reintroduced (Fakih, 2007).

Drug: panobinostat capsules (Farydak)

Class: Histone deacetylase (HDAC) inhibitor.

Mechanism of Action: Inhibits HDAC enzyme activity so acetyl groups are not removed from some proteins surrounding DNA. As a result, there is increased acetylation of histone proteins, which relax the DNA helix and permit transcription of genes, such as tumor suppressor genes, that are otherwise turned off by tight coiling of the DNA strands. The drug causes tumor cells to die (cell-cycle arrest and apoptosis). It is more cytotoxic to tumor cells compared to normal cells.

Metabolism: Panobinostat is 21% bioavailable after oral dosing, and reaches its peak concentration about 2 hours after it is taken. The drug is extensively metabolized, primarily through CYP3A, but with minor contributions via the CYP2D6 and CYP2C19 pathways. Its terminal half-life is 37 hours, and metabolites are excreted in the urine and feces. In one study, hepatic impairment increased AUC (mild, by 43%, and moderate, by 105%) in patients receiving panobinostat compared to patients with normal hepatic function.

Indication: For the treatment of patients with multiple myeloma, who have received at least two prior regimens, including bortezomib and an immunomodulatory agent, in combination with bortezomib and dexamethasone. The drug's accelerated approval was based on PFS; continued approval may require verification and description of clinical benefit in confirmatory trials (Novartis, 2015).

Dosage/Range:
- 20 mg orally, once every other day for 3 doses per week (days 1, 3, 5, 8, 10, 12) in weeks 1 and 2 of each 21-day cycle, for 8 cycles.
- Consider continuing treatment for an additional 8 cycles (9–16) if the patient shows clinical benefit, unless unresolved severe or medically significant toxicity occurs.
- Cycles 1–8: Recommended bortezomib dose is 1.3 mg/m^2 on days 1, 4, 8, and 11; dexamethasone dose is 20 mg orally on a full stomach on days 1, 2; 4, 5; 8, 9; and 11, 12 of the 21-day cycle.
- Cycles 9–16: Panobinostat on days 1, 3, 5, 8, 10, 12 of the 21-day cycle; bortezomib on days 1 and 8; and dexamethasone on days 1, 2 and 8, 9 of the 21-day cycle.
- Reduce starting dose to 15 mg in patients with mild hepatic impairment, and to 10 mg in patients with moderate impairment; monitor patients frequently so dose can be further adjusted for toxicity. Do not use the drug in patients with severe hepatotoxicity.
- If the patient is taking concomitant strong CYP3A inhibitors (e.g., boceprevir, clarithromycin, conivaptan, indinavir, itraconazole, ketoconazole, lopinavir/ritonavir), reduce the starting dose to 10 mg.

Dose Modifications:
- Dose and/or schedule modification may be needed to manage toxicity. Manage toxicity by treatment interruption and/or dose reductions. If dose reduction is needed, reduce the panobinostat dose in increments of 5 mg. If dosing is less than 10 mg given 3 times/week, discontinue the drug. Keep the same treatment regimen (3-week treatment cycle) when reducing the dose.
- Thrombocytopenia:
  - **Plt < 50 × 10^9/L (grade 3):** Maintain panobinostat and bortezomib doses and monitor platelet counts at least weekly.
  - **Plt < 50 × 10^9/L (grade 3) with bleeding:** Interrupt panobinostat until Plt ≥ 50 × 10^9/L, monitor platelet counts at least weekly, and then restart at a reduced dose. See the package insert for bortezomib dosing.
  - **Plt < 25 × 10^9/L (grade 4):** Interrupt panobinostat, monitor platelet counts at least weekly until Plt ≥ 50 × 10^9/L, and then restart at a reduced dose. See the package insert for bortezomib dosing.
  - Severe thrombocytopenia: Consider platelet transfusions.
  - Discontinue the drug if thrombocytopenia does not improve despite dose modification or if repeated transfusions are required.
- Neutropenia:
  - **ANC 0.75–1.0 × 10^9/L (grade 3):** Maintain panobinostat and bortezomib doses.
  - **ANC 0.5–0.75 × 10^9/L (grade 3; 2 or more occurrences):** Interrupt panobinostat dose until ANC ≥ 1.0 × 10^9/L, then restart at the same dose; maintain the bortezomib dose.
  - **ANC < 1.0 × 10^9/L (grade 3 with febrile neutropenia any grade):** Interrupt panobinostat until febrile neutropenia resolves, and ANC ≥ 1.0 × 10^9/L, then restart at a reduced dose. See the package insert for bortezomib dosing.

- **ANC < 0.5 × 10⁹/L (grade 4):** Interrupt panobinostat until ANC $\geq$ 1.0 × 10⁹/L, then restart at a reduced dose. See the package insert for bortezomib dosing.
- Grade 3 or grade 4: Consider dose reduction and/or growth factors (e.g., G-CSF).
- Discontinue panobinostat if neutropenia does not improve with dose modification or C-GSFs, or in case of severe infection.
- Anemia (Hgb < 8 g/dL): Interrupt panobinostat until Hgb $\geq$ 10 g/dL, then restart at a reduced dose.
- Diarrhea:
  - **Moderate** (4–6 stools/day): Interrupt panobinostat until the diarrhea is resolved, then restart it at the same dose. Consider interrupting bortezomib and then restarting it at the same dose.
  - **Severe** ($\geq$ 7 stools/day, requiring IV fluids or hospitalization, grade 3): Interrupt panobinostat until the diarrhea is resolved, then restart it at a reduced dose. Interrupt bortezomib and then restart it at a reduced dose when the diarrhea is resolved.
  - **Life-threatening:** Permanently discontinue both panobinostat and bortezomib.
  - Start antidiarrheal medicine (e.g., loperamide) at the first sign of abdominal cramping, loose stools, or onset of diarrhea.
- Nausea or vomiting:
  - **Severe nausea (grade 3 or 4):** Interrupt panobinostat until the nausea is resolved, then restart it at a reduced dose.
  - **Severe/life-threatening vomiting (grade 3/4):** Interrupt panobinostat until the vomiting is resolved, then restart it at a reduced dose.
  - Consider and administer prophylactic antiemetics if needed.
- Grade 3/4 adverse drug reactions other than hematologic or GI: Grade 2 recurrence and grade 3/4: Omit the dose until recovery to grade 0–1, then restart panobinostat at a reduced dose. Grade 3 or 4 toxicity recurrence: Further reduce the dose once the adverse effect has resolved to grade 0–1.

Drug Preparation: Available as 10-mg, 15-mg, and 20-mg capsules.

Drug Administration:
- Assess CBC/ANC before the patient starts treatment; verify baseline platelet count is $\geq$ 100 × 10⁹/L, and ANC $\geq$ 1.5 × 10⁹/L. Monitor CBC weekly or more often as clinically indicated.
- Assess ECG prior to the start of therapy, and repeat during therapy as clinically indicated. Verify QTc is less than 450 msec prior to starting panobinostat therapy. If the QTc increases to 480 msec or longer, therapy should be interrupted. Correct any electrolyte abnormalities. If QT prolongation does not resolve permanently, the drug should be permanently discontinued. In the clinical trial, ECGs were monitored at baseline, and then before each cycle for the first 8 cycles.
- Assess serum electrolytes, including potassium and magnesium, at baseline, and then monitor them during therapy. Correct abnormal electrolyte levels before treatment. During the clinical trial, monitoring was performed prior the start of each cycle, at day 11 of cycles 1–8, and at the start of each cycle for cycles 9–16.
- Teach the patient about the medication schedule—that is, on which days to take panobinostat and dexamethasone, and when to come into the clinic for bortezomib.

• Teach the patient to take the drug orally on the scheduled day at about the same time, with or without food. The patient should swallow the capsule whole with a cup of water; he or she should not open, crush, or chew the capsule. If the patient misses a dose, it can be taken up to 12 hours after the specified dose time. If vomiting occurs, the patient should *not* repeat the dose, but rather take the next scheduled dose at the planned time.

Drug Interactions:
• Panobinostat is a CYP3A substrate, and it inhibits CYP2D6. It is also a P-glycoprotein (P-gp) transporter system substrate.
• Strong CYP3A4 inhibitors: Increase serum level of panobinostat; avoid concomitant use, or decrease the panobinostat dose. Teach the patient to avoid star fruit, pomegranate juice, and grapefruit or grapefruit juice. Reduce the dose of panobinostat to 10 mg if coadministered with a strong CYP3A inhibitor (e.g., boceprevir, clarithromycin, conivaptan, indinivir, itraconazole, ketoconazole, lopinavir/ritonavir, nefazodone, nelfinavir, posaconazole, ritonavir, saquinavir, telaprevir, telithromycin, voriconazole).
• Strong CYP3A4 inducers: Decrease serum level of panobinostat by as much as 70%; avoid concomitant use.
• CYP2D6 substrates: Panobinostat may increase the C_{max} and AUC of sensitive substrates by 80% and 60%, respectively (e.g., atomoxetine, desipramine, dextromethorphan, metoprolol, nebivolol, perphenazine, tolterodine, venlafaxine); it may have the same effect on CYP2D6 substrates with a narrow therapeutic window (e.g., thioridazine, pimozide). Avoid coadministration. If panobinostat and a CYP2D6 substrate must be coadministered, monitor the patient closely for toxicity.
• Drugs that prolong the QT interval (e.g., antiarrhythmic medicines such as amiodarone, disopyramide, procainamide, quinidine, and sotalol; other drugs such as chloroquine, halofantrine, clarithromycin, methadone, moxifloxacin, bepridil, and pimozide): If antiemetic agents that prolong the QT interval are used (e.g., dolasetron, ondansetron, tropisetron), monitor the ECG and QTc frequently.

Lab Effects/Interference:
• Decreased serum phosphate, potassium, and sodium
• Increased serum creatinine
• Thrombocytopenia, lymphopenia, leucopenia, neutropenia, and anemia
• Prolonged QTc interval

Special Considerations:
• Most common adverse effects occurring in 20% or more of patients in clinical trials: diarrhea, fatigue, nausea, vomiting, peripheral edema, decreased appetite, and pyrexia.
• Warnings and precautions:
  • Severe diarrhea occurred in 25% of patients. Monitor and begin antidiarrheal therapy at the first sign of diarrhea, interrupt the drug, and then reduce the dose or discontinue the drug. See the dose modification section.
  • Myelosuppression may be severe, with grade 3–4 thrombocytopenia observed in 67% of patients receiving panobinostat compared to 31% of control patients; severe

neutropenia occurred in 34% (compared to 11% of controls). Assess the patient's baseline CBC, and then monitor it weekly during treatment, and more frequently in the elderly.

- Severe and fatal cardiac ischemic events, severe arrhythmias, and ECG changes may occur; arrhythmias may be exacerbated by electrolyte abnormalities.
  - Obtain an ECG and measure electrolytes at baseline and periodically during treatment. Replete electrolytes promptly. Do not start therapy in patients with a QTc interval > 450 msec or with clinically significant baseline ST-segment T-wave abnormalities.
  - If the QTc interval ≥ 480 msec, the drug should be interrupted and electrolyte abnormalities corrected. If the QTc prolongation does not resolve, discontinue the drug.
  - The drug should not be given to patients who have had a recent MI or have unstable angina.
- Hemorrhage can occur (GI, pulmonary) with thrombocytopenia; monitor the platelet count and give transfusions as needed.
- Localized and systemic infections (e.g., pneumonia; bacterial, invasive fungal, and viral infections) may occur.
- Hepatotoxicity: Monitor hepatic enzymes at baseline and during treatment; adjust the drug dose as needed if LFTs become abnormal.
- The drug can cause fetal harm: Teach females of reproductive potential to use effective contraception to avoid pregnancy during and for at least 1 month after last drug dose. Teach sexually active men to use condoms while on treatment and for 3 months after the last drug dose.

Potential Toxicities/Side Effects and the Nursing Process

I.   ALTERATION IN PATTERN related to DIARRHEA

Defining Characteristics: Diarrhea occurred in 68% of patients (compared to 48% in the control arm), and was severe in 25%. Diarrhea can occur at any time during treatment.

Nursing Implications: Assess the patient's bowel elimination pattern at baseline and then regularly during therapy. Review the patient's medication profile, and teach the patient not to take stool softeners or laxative medications while receiving panobinostat. Assess and monitor patient hydration and electrolyte status (e.g., serum potassium, magnesium, phosphate) at baseline and then at least weekly during therapy. Discuss measures to correct dehydration and electrolyte disturbances with the provider, and implement steps to rehydrate the patient and correct electrolyte abnormalities as soon as possible. Ensure the patient has antidiarrheal medication (e.g., loperamide) on hand prior to starting panobinostat capsules and understands the self-administration directions, including use at the first sign of abdominal cramping, loose stools, or onset of diarrhea. Teach the patient to increase oral fluids to one glass every hour while awake as tolerated, and to make dietary modifications to lessen diarrhea. Teach the patient to stop the drug and call the nurse or provider at the onset of moderate diarrhea (4–6 stools/day), as the drug should be interrupted in such a case; the dose should be reduced if severe diarrhea occurs.

II. POTENTIAL FOR BLEEDING, INFECTION, AND FATIGUE related to THROMBOCYTOPENIA, NEUTROPENIA, AND ANEMIA

Defining Characteristics: Bone marrow suppression may be severe. Thrombocytopenia occurs in 97% of patients, and neutropenia in 75%. In clinical trial of patients with relapsed multiple myeloma, grade 3/4 thrombocytopenia occurred in 67% of patients compared to 31% in the control group, and required dose interruption or reduction in 31% of patients. In addition, nearly one-third (33%) required platelet transfusion. Severe thrombocytopenia can lead to life-threatening hemorrhage. Grade 3/4 hemorrhage occurred in 4% of patients receiving panobinostat.

Neutropenia was severe in 34% of patients compared to 11% of the control group, and 13% of patients had growth factor support. Severe infections occurred in 31% of patients; in some cases, they resulted in death.

Fatigue was common, affecting 60% of patients, and was severe in 25% of patients. Anemia occurred in 62% of patients, and was grade 3/4 in severity in 18%.

Patients with mild and moderate hepatic impairment should have their doses reduced, and the drug should not be used in patients with severe impairment.

Nursing Implications: Assess the patient's baseline WBC, ANC, platelet, and Hgb/Hct; monitor these values at least weekly during treatment, and more frequently if needed in patients older than age 65. Discuss dose modifications based on the CBC/ANC results with the provider. Ensure that the patient does not have an active infection when beginning panobinostat treatment. Assess the patient for signs and symptoms of bleeding and/or infection. If the patient develops an infection, discuss urgent treatment with the provider, to consist of anti-infectives, as well as interruption or discontinuance of panobinostat. Teach the patient to report bleeding, increased bruising, dizziness or weakness, sweats or chills, flu-like symptoms, shortness of breath, blood in sputum, increased severe fatigue, and development of any sores or areas of inflammation on the skin.

Assess the patient's activity level and fatigue at baseline, and monitor them during therapy. Teach the patient to report increasing fatigue, and review strategies to reduce fatigue, such as alternating rest and activity periods and engaging in gentle exercises. Assess the patient's sleep quality and rest while taking dexamethasone, as this agent can cause insomnia.

III. ALTERATION IN OXYGENATION, REDUCED, related to CARDIAC ISCHEMIC EVENTS, ARRYTHMIAS, AND ECG CHANGES

Defining Characteristics: Arrhythmias occurred in 12% of patients compared to 5% in the control arm of the clinical study, while cardiac ischemic events occurred in 4% of patients. This drug is not recommended in patients with a history of a recent MI or unstable angina.

Abnormalities noted on ECG included ST-segment depression, T-wave abnormalities, and prolonged QT interval. Electrolyte abnormalities may exacerbate cardiac arrhythmias. Electrolyte disturbances seen in the clinical trial included hypokalemia (52%), hypophosphatemia (63%), hyponatremia (49%), and hypocalcemia (67%).

Nursing Interventions: Assess the patient's ECG and serum electrolytes at baseline before therapy begins, and then periodically during treatment. QTc must be less than 450 msec prior to the patient beginning the drug, and the drug should be interrupted if the QTc increases to 480 msec or longer during treatment. If QTc prolongation does not resolve with correction of electrolytes, permanently discontinue panobinostat. The drug also should not be given if the ECG shows significant baseline ST-segment or T-wave abnormalities. Discuss prompt repletion of electrolytes once an abnormality is detected. In the clinical trial, ECGs were performed at baseline and prior to the start of each cycle for the first 8 cycles. Serum electrolytes were assessed at baseline and prior to the start of each cycle, at day 11 of cycles 1–8, and at the start of each of cycles 9–16.

Drug: pazopanib (Votrient)

Class: Kinase inhibitor (multi-tyrosine kinase inhibitor).

Mechanism of Action: Drug is a multi-tyrosine kinase inhibitor of vascular endothelial growth factor receptor (VEGFR-1, VEGFR-2, VEGFR-3), platelet-derived growth factor receptor (α, β), fibroblast growth factor receptor (FGFR)-1 and -3, cytokine receptor (Kit), interleukin-2 receptor inducible T-cell kinase (Itk), leukocyte-specific protein tyrosine kinase (Lck), and transmembrane glycoprotein receptor tyrosine kinase (c-Fms).

Metabolism: After oral administration, pazopanib is well absorbed with peak concentrations reached 2 –4 hours after the dose. If tablet is crushed, the area under the curve (AUC) is increased by 46% with increased bioavailability and rate of absorption. Drug should not be crushed. Drug systemic exposure is increased when pazopanib is taken with food, so should be dosed at least 1 hour before or 2 hours after a meal. Drug is highly bound to plasma proteins. Pazopanib is probably a substrate for P-glycoprotein (Pgp). It is primarily metabolized by the liver microenzyme CYP3A4, with a minor contribution by CYP1A2 and CYP2C8. Drug has a half-life of 30.9 hours after drug administration, and it is eliminated primarily via feces and to a lesser degree the kidney (< 4%). Drug clearance from the body is reduced 50% if the patient has moderate hepatic impairment, so a maximum drug dose should be 200 mg PO once daily in these patients.

Indication:
- Treatment of patients with
  - Advanced renal cell carcinoma.
  - Advanced soft-tissue sarcoma, who have received prior chemotherapy.

* The efficacy of the drug in the treatment of patients with adipocytic soft-tissue sarcoma or gastrointestinal stromal tumors (GIST) has not been demonstrated.
* Safety and effectiveness in pediatric patients has not been established, and the drug is not indicated for use in pediatric patients.

Dosage/Range:
* 800 mg PO once daily without food (at least 1 hour prior to or 2 hours after a meal). Do not exceed the 800-mg dose.
* Baseline moderate hepatic impairment: 200 mg orally once daily without food (as above).
* Do not administer to patients with preexisting severe hepatic impairment (total bilirubin > 3 × ULN with any level of ALT).

Dose Modifications:
* RCC: initial dose reduction should be to 400 mg, and additional dose decrease or increase should be in 200-mg increments, based on individual tolerability.
* In soft-tissue sarcoma (STS), a decrease or increase should be in 200-mg increments, based on individual tolerability.
* Hepatic impairment:
  * Mild impairment: no dose adjustment.
  * Moderate hepatic impairment: consider alternatives to pazopanib; if unavailable, reduce dose to 200 mg PO once daily.
  * Drug should not be used in patients with severe hepatic impairment (total bilirubin > 3 × ULN and any level of ALT).
  * Patients with isolated ALT elevations between 3 × ULN and 8 × ULN may be continued on pazopanib with weekly monitoring of LFTs until ALT returns to grade 1 or baseline.
  * Patients with isolated ALT elevations of > 8 × ULN should have dose interrupted until ALT returns to grade 1 or baseline. If the potential benefit for reinitiating treatment outweighs the risk for hepatotoxicity, then reintroduce drug at a reduced dose of no more than 400 mg once daily, and assess LFTs weekly for 8 weeks. Following reintroduction of pazopanib, if ALT elevations > 3 × ULN recur, then pazopanib should be permanently discontinued.
  * If ALT elevations > 3 × ULN occur concurrently with bilirubin elevations > 2 × ULN, pazopanib should be permanently discontinued. Patients should be monitored until resolution. Drug is a UGT1A1 inhibitor: mild, indirect (unconjugated) hyperbilirubinemia may occur in patients with Gilbert's Sydrome. Patients with only a mild indirect hyperbilirubinemia, known as Gilbert's Syndrome, and elevation in ALT > 3 × ULN should be managed as outlined for isolated ALT elevations.
* Patient taking concomitant strong *CYP3A4 inhibitor*: reduce dose of pazopanib to 400 mg PO once daily; if toxicity develops, further reduce dose of pazopanib if adverse effects occur.
* Patients taking strong *CYP3A4 inducers*: do not use together; if must use CYP3A4 inducer (e.g., rifampin), pazopanib should not be used in these patients.
* Refractory HTN: if despite antihypertensive therapy and dose reduction, HTN is severe and persistent, discontinue pazopanib.

Drug Preparation:
- Pazopanib is available as 200-mg tablets. The drug should be stored at room temperature (59–86°F; 15–30°C) and kept out of reach of children or pets.

Drug Administration:
- Administer full dose orally on an empty stomach (at least 1 hour prior to or 2 hours after a meal). Teach patient that drug should NOT be crushed or chewed, as this increases the bioavailability and systemic exposure (and toxicity). If a dose is missed, it should not be taken if it is less than 12 hours until the next dose.
- Teach patient to avoid grapefruit and grapefruit juice.
- Interrupt drug 7 days prior to scheduled surgery.
- Assess LFTs baseline before starting pazopanib and at weeks 3, 5, 7, and 9; thereafter at months 3 and 4, then regularly as clinically indicated.

Drug Interactions:
- CYP3A4 inhibitors increase pazopanib serum level and risk for toxicity.
  - Avoid concurrent administration with strong CYP3A4 inhibitors (e.g., ketoconazole, ritonavir, clarithromycin, grapefruit juice).
  - If must coadminister, reduce dose of pazopanib.
- CYP3A4 inducers decrease pazopanib serum level and effectiveness;
  - Avoid concurrent administration of strong inducers such as rifampin.
  - If this is not avoidable and chronic dosing of a strong inducer is necessary, do not administer pazopanib.
- Other drugs with a narrow therapeutic window that are metabolized by CYP3A4, CYP2D6, or CYP2C8: do not coadminister, as this will inhibit the other drug's metabolism and increase risk of adverse events.
- Simvastatin: concurrent administration increases risk of ALT elevations. Use dose modification if ALT is elevated or an alternative to pazopanib.
- Chemotherapy: increased toxicity. Drug is not approved for combination therapy. However, clinical trials combining pazopanib with pemetrexed and lapatinib resulted in fatal toxicities (pulmonary hemorrhage, GI hemorrhage, sudden death). Do not combine drug with chemotherapy.

Lab Effects/Interference:
- Increased serum transaminase levels, bilirubin, alkaline phosphatase: assess liver chemistries baseline and follow closely during therapy. Interrupt as needed with dose reduction for moderate hepatic toxicity or drug discontinuance for severe hepatotoxicity.
- Hypothyroidism with increased TSH in 27% of patients; monitor thyroid function tests baseline and prior to therapy.
- Proteinuria (9%): assess baseline and during therapy.
- Serum magnesium decreased: 26%, assess and replete. Increased potassium (16%); decreased albumin (34%) and sodium (31%).
- Lipase increased (27% in some studies).

- Glucose: elevated in 41%, decreased in 17%.
- Leukopenia (44%), lymphocytopenia (43%), thrombocytopenia (36%), neutropenia (33%).
- EKG: QT prolongation (≥ 500 msec); assess baseline EKG and repeat during therapy as needed; correct any serum magnesium and potassium abnormalities.

Special Considerations:
- Severe and fatal hepatotoxicity has been observed; monitor hepatic function and interrupt, reduce, or discontinue drug as recommended.
  - Transaminase elevations occur early in treatment course (92.5% occurred in first 18 weeks).
  - Assess liver chemistry baseline prior to starting treatment, then at weeks 3, 5, 7, and 9; then at months 3 and 4, and as clinically indicated.
  - If the patient has isolated ALT elevations between 3 × ULN and 8 × ULN, continue therapy with weekly monitoring of liver function until ALT returns to grade 1 or baseline. Concomitant use of pazopanib and simvastatin increases the risk of ALT elevations and should be used cautiously if at all, with very close monitoring.
  - Interrupt therapy if the ALT is > 8 × ULN until the ALT returns to grade 1 or baseline; if the benefit outweighs the risk of resuming therapy, reintroduce the dose at 400 mg PO once daily and assess liver function tests at least weekly for 8 weeks. If the ALT becomes elevated > 3 × ULN after pazopanib is reintroduced, permanently discontinue pazopanib.
  - If the ALT elevation > 3 × ULN occurs at the same time as the bilirubin is elevated > 2 × ULN, pazopanib should be permanently discontinued. Continue to monitor patient until resolution.
  - Pazopanib is a UGT1A1 inhibitor; mild, indirect (unconjugated) hyperbilirubinemia may occur if the patient has Gilbert's syndrome. Patients with only a mild indirect hyperbilirubinemia (Gilbert's syndrome) and elevations in ALT > 3 × ULN should be managed as isolated ALT elevation.
- Prolongation of QT interval (> 500 msec) occurs rarely (2%) with torsades de pointes (atypical ventricular tachycardia that can change to ventricular fibrillation and sudden death) occurring < 1%.
  - Use pazopanib cautiously in patients with a history of QT prolongation, in patients taking antiarrythmic drugs or other medications that can prolong the QT interval such as methadone, and those with relevant preexisting cardiac disease.
  - Assess ECG baseline and correct serum abnormalities of magnesium and potassium prior to administering pazopanib. Monitor QTc intervals (ECG) and electrolytes (magnesium, calcium, potassium) periodically during therapy. Electrolytes should be maintained WNL during pazopanib therapy.
- Cardiac events have occurred rarely (0.6%), such as decreased LVEF and CHF, and is likely exacerbated by uncontrolled hypertension.
  - BP should be monitored and managed promptly using antihypertensive therapy and dose modification (interruption and reinitiation at a reduced dose based on clinical judgment).

- Monitor patients carefully for clinical signs or symptoms of CHF. Baseline and periodic evaluation of LVEF is recommended in patients at risk for cardiac dysfunction, including those who have received previous anthracycline exposure.
- In clinical trials, HTN may have exacerbated cardiac dysfunction. BP should be monitored and managed promptly using combination antihypertensive agents and dose modification (interruption and reinitiation at a reduced dose based on clinical judgment.
- As with other VEGFR inhibitors, there are class effects:
  - Hemorrhage: Hemorrhagic events may occur (all grades 16%, grades 3–5 in 2%, and death in 0.9%). Most common hemorrhagic events were hematuria (4%), epistaxis (2%), hemoptysis (2%), and rectal hemorrhage (2%). Do not administer the drug to patients with a history of hemoptysis, cerebral hemorrhage, or clinically significant GI hemorrhage in the prior 6 months, as the drug has not been studied in this population.
  - Arterial thrombotic events: MI, angina, ischemic stroke, and transient ischemic attack have occurred (all grades in 3%, grades 3–5 in 2%, fatal events in 0.3%). Use caution in patients who are at risk for these events, and do not use the drug in patients who have had an event within the previous 6 months, as the drug has not been studied in this population.
  - Venous thrombotic events: Venous thrombosis, fatal pulmonary embolus (PE) have occurred. Monitor patients for signs and symptoms of VTE and PE.
  - Reversible posterior leukoencephalopathy syndrome (RPLS) has been reported, and may be fatal. Monitor for signs/symptoms including headache, seizure, lethargy, confusion, blindness, and other visual and neurological disturbances. Patients may also have mild to moderate hypertension. MRI should be done to rule out RPLS. If the patient develops RPLS, the drug should be discontinued.
  - GI perforation and fistula formation occur rarely (0.9%). Fatal fistula occurred in two patients (0.3%). Assess and monitor patients for signs and symptoms of GI perforation or fistula. Do not administer the drug in patients with a history of hemoptysis, cerebral or clinically significant GI hemorrhage in the past 6 months.
  - Hypertension (SBP > 150 mm Hg, or DBP > 100 mm Hg): BP should be well controlled prior to the patient starting pazopanib. Incidence of HTN was 40%, with grade 3–4% in 7%. HTN occurs early in the course of treatment (40% by day 9, and 90% in the first 18 weeks). If HTN is persistent despite antihypertensive therapy, dose-reduce pazopanib. If despite antihypertensive therapy AND dose reduction, HTN is severe and persistent, discontinue pazopanib. If hypertensive crisis develops, discontinue pazopanib.
  - Delayed wound healing: Stop pazopanib therapy at least 7 days prior to scheduled surgery and resume after the surgical wound has fully healed. Discontinue drug if wound dehiscence develops.
  - Proteinuria: Occurs in 9% of patients (all), with < 1% grades 3 and 4. Assess baseline urinalysis and monitor during treatment for proteinuria. If indicated, follow up with a 24-hour urine protein. Interrupt pazopanib therapy and dose-reduce for 24-hour urine protein ≥ 3 grams/24 hr; discontinue for repeat episodes despite dose reductions.

- Hypothyroidism: has been reported in 7% of patients. Assess baseline thyroid function tests and monitor as needed. Diagnosis made on simultaneous rise of TSH and decline of T4.
- Thrombotic microangiopathy (TMA), including thrombocytopenic purpura (TTP), and hemolytic uremic syndrome (HUS) have been reported when pazopanib is used as monotherapy, in combination with bevacizumab, and in combination with topotecan; drug is not indicated for these combinations. Monitor for signs/symptoms of TMA and permanently discontinue pazopanib if patient develops TMA.
- Drug should not be given concommitantly with chemotherapy, as there is increased toxicity and mortality.
- Serious infections: Have occurred with or without neutropenia. Monitor patient for signs/symptoms of infection, and teach patient to report signs and symptoms. Consider drug interruption or discontinuance for serious infections.
- Pregnancy: In animal studies, drug is teratogenic, embryotoxic, fetotoxic, and abortifacient. Women of childbearing potential should be counseled to use effective birth control measures to avoid becoming pregnant. If the drug is used during pregnancy, or if the patient becomes pregnant while using the drug, the patient should be apprised of the potential hazard to the fetus. Mothers who are nursing should make a decision either to stop nursing or to discontinue pazopanib, taking into account the importance of the drug to the mother's health.
- Most common side effects (incidence ≥ 20%): (1) in patients with RCC: diarrhea, HTN, hair color changes (depigmentation), nausea, anorexia, and vomiting, (2) advanced STS: fatigue, diarrhea, nausea, decreased weight, HTN, decreased appetite, hair color changes (depigmentation), vomiting, tumor pain, dysgeusia, headache, musculoskeletal pain, myalgia, GI pain, and dyspnea.

Potential Toxicities/Side Effects and the Nursing Process

I. POTENTIAL ALTERATION IN CIRCULATION related to HYPERTENSION, CARDIAC ISCHEMIA, OR MYOCARDIAL INFARCTION

Defining Characteristics: Hypertension (SBP ≥ 150, DBP ≥100 mm Hg) occurred in 47% of patients studied and occurred early in the course of treatment (40% by day 9, and 90% occurred during the first 18 weeks). In general, it is easily controlled with antihypertensive drugs. Grade 3 HTN was reported in 4–7% of patients. Arterial embolic events occurred in 3% of patients and were severe in 2.3% of patients.

Nursing Implications: Assess baseline blood pressure, and again after starting the drug, within 1 week; and frequently thereafter to ensure BP is controlled. If the BP is slightly elevated, assess weekly and discuss antihypertensive therapy with physician or NP. HTN should be well-controlled prior to initiating pazopanib. Increased BP should be promptly treated with standard antihypertensive agents, and dose reduction or interruption of pazopanib. Pazopanib should be discontinued if hypertensive crisis occurs, or if HTN is severe despite antihypertensive therapy and dose reduction. If a patient develops cardiac ischemia and/or infarction while receiving the drug, discuss drug discontinuance with the physician. The drug should not be used in patients with a history of cardiac ischemia (angina), ischemic stroke, or TIA. If the patient is at risk for these events, monitor the patient closely during therapy.

II.   ALTERATION IN NUTRITION, LESS THAN BODY REQUIREMENTS, related to DIARRHEA, NAUSEA, ANOREXIA, VOMITING, CONSTIPATION

Defining Characteristics: Diarrhea occurs in 52% of patients, nausea 26%, vomiting 21%, anorexia 22%, and dysgeusia 8%. Weight loss occurred in 9% of patients. Elevation of liver function test AST occurs in 53% of patients, while elevation in BR occurred in 36%. Hepatotoxicity may be severe and is potentially fatal. Glucose is increased in 41%, phosphorus decreased in 34%, sodium decreased in 31%, magnesium decreased in 26%, and glucose decreased in 17%.

Nursing Implications: Assess nutrition status, weight, bowel elimination status, serum chemistries including liver function tests baseline and periodically during treatment. AST and BR must be assessed at least once every 4 weeks for the first 4 months of treatment or as clinically indicated. Continue assessments periodically after this time during therapy. Teach patient to report any changes that suggest liver toxicity right away: yellowing of skin or whites of eyes, dark urine, tiredness, nausea or vomiting, loss of appetite, pain on the right side of abdomen, easy bruisability. Teach patient self-care strategies to manage diarrhea, such as about dietary modifications (BRAT diet: bananas, rice, applesauce, and toast), and to avoid raw fruits, vegetables, whole grain breads and cereals, and seeds. Teach about soluble fiber, which absorbs fluid: applesauce, bananas, canned fruit, orange sections, boiled potatoes, white rice, products made with white flour, oatmeal, cream of rice, cream of wheat, and farina. Teach to increase oral fluids to 8–10 glasses of nonalcoholic fluids a day to prevent dehydration. Teach to increase dose-dense calories and fluid in the diet and strategies to increase appetite. Teach patient how to manage nausea, vomiting, and diarrhea by self-administration of OTC medications or prescribed medications, dietary modifications, and increased hydration. Involve nutritionist as needed to minimize symptoms. Teach patient to report symptoms that do not improve or that persist despite interventions. Teach patient signs of hyperglycemia and to report increased thirst, increased voiding, and increased hunger so that blood sugar can be evaluated.

III.   ALTERATION IN CIRCULATION related to HEMORRHAGE, POTENTIAL

Defining Characteristics: Hemorrhage occurred in 16% of patients.

Nursing Implications: Teach patient to report any episodes of bleeding right away, such as hemoptysis. Drug is not indicated for patients with a history of hemoptysis, cerebral hemorrhage, or clinically significant GI hemorrhage within the prior 6 months. If bleeding occurs, have patient evaluated by the physician or nurse practitioner.

IV. ALTERATION IN BODY IMAGE, POTENTIAL, related to HAIR COLOR CHANGES, HAND-FOOT SYNDROME, SKIN DEPIGMENTATION, ALOPECIA

Defining Characteristics: Hair color changes occur in 38% of patients, alopecia in 8%, palmar-plantar erythrodysesthesia (hand-foot syndrome, acral erythema) in 6%, rash in 8%, and skin depigmentation in 3% of patients.

Nursing Implications: Assess baseline skin integrity, including soles of feet and palms of hands, hair color and intactness, and teach patient that these symptoms may occur. If the patient develops calluses on the feet, suggest applying topical exfoliating agents such as Kerasal (over the counter) or Keralac (prescription) on the calluses ONLY. Teach patient to self-assess all skin areas and to report rash, as well as redness, swelling, and/or pain anywhere, particularly the soles of feet and the palms of hands. Teach patient to avoid activities that increase blood flow in the hands and feet, such as hot showers and baths, and to take tepid showers to reduce likelihood and severity of hand-foot syndrome. Teach patient to avoid constrictive clothing and repetitive movements that can irritate the opposing skin. Teach patient to use skin emollients to prevent skin from drying and cracking. Discuss dose modification with physician or NP if patient has pain or desquamation. Assess effect of hair color changes or hair loss. Encourage patient to verbalize feelings and provide emotional support. If needed, involve social worker in supportive counseling. Encourage patient to use scarves or hats as appropriate and to attend supportive educational sessions such as Look Good . . . Feel Better (ACS).

V. POTENTIAL FOR INFECTION AND BLEEDING related to NEUTROPENIA AND THROMBOCYTOPENIA

Defining Characteristics: Neutropenia occurred in 34% and thrombocytopenia in 32% of patients in clinical trials.

Nursing Implications: Assess baseline blood counts and platelets. Teach patient to report fever and signs/symptoms of infection or bleeding right away. Assess medication profile and OTC medications taken. Teach patient to avoid OTC medications containing NSAIDs or aspirin. Teach patient to talk to nurse or physician before beginning any OTC medications.

Drug: pembrolizumab (Keytruda, MK3475)

Class: Immune checkpoint inhibitor. Human programmed death-1 (PD-1)-blocking antibody; humanized monoclonal antibody against PD-1.

Mechanism of Action: One of the ways cancer evades the immune system is by taking advantage of the body's process to turn down activated T-lymphocytes after an immune response to protect the body's organs from autoimmune injury. The programmed cell death 1 (PD-1) receptor is found on T-lymphocytes, especially if they have been exposed to an antigen for a long time. It is activated by its ligand, PD-L1 (also known as B7-H1 or CD274), which is often found in the tumor microenvironment (Hamid et al., 2013). PD-1 also has another ligand, PD-L2 (also known as B7-DC or CD273), which is preferentially expressed by antigen-presenting cells. When the ligands PD-L1 and PD-L2 bind to the PD-1 receptor on T-lymphocytes, it turns off T-cell proliferation and cytokine production (Merck & Co., 2014). Some tumors upregulate PD-1 ligands. Monoclonal antibody drugs (MAbs) that block the ligand PD-L1 from binding to its receptor PD-1 prevent activated T-lymphocytes from being turned down/off so they can continue to attack cancer cells. See chapter introduction on *Immunotherapy*. By blocking this immune checkpoint inhibitor, pembrolizumab has less immune toxicity than others, such as ipilimumab, which blocks the inhibitory receptor cytotoxic T-lymphocyte-associated antigen 4 (CTLA-4). However, immune-related toxicity may occur, although it is uncommon.

Indication: Treatment of patients with unresectable or metastatic melanoma and disease progression following ipilimumab, and if BRAF V600 mutation-positive, a BRAF inhibitor. The indication is an accelerated approval, based on tumor response rate and durability of response. Survival benefit or disease-related symptom improvement has not yet been established. Continued approval may be contingent upon verification and description of clinical benefit in the confirmatory trials (Merck & Co., 2014).

Dosage/Range:
- 2 mg/kg IV infusion over 30 minutes every 3 weeks until disease progression or unacceptable toxicity. Dilute pembrolizumab injection (solution) or reconstituted lyophilized powder prior to IV administration.
- Hold drug for the following grades or higher: pneumonitis-2, colitis-2, nephritis-2, hyperthyroidism-3, any severe or grade 3 adverse reaction, AST or ALT > 3 × ULN or total bilirubin > 1.5 × ULN, symptomatic hypophysitis. See Special Considerations.
- Resume drug when adverse reaction improves to grade 0–1.
- Permanently discontinue drug in the following cases: any life-threatening adverse reaction; grade 3–4 pneumonitis; grade 3–4 nephritis; persistent grade 2–3 reactions that do not improve to grade 0–1 within 12 weeks of last drug dose; any severe/grade 3 reaction that recurs; AST or ALT > 5 × ULN or total bilirubin > 3 × ULN; if patient has liver metastasis and starts drug treatment with grade 2 AST or ALT; if AST or ALT increases by ≥ 50% relative to baseline and lasts for at least 1 week.

Drug Preparation:
- Pembrolizumab is available as a 50-mg lyophilized powder in a single-use vial for reconstitution, and as a 100 mg/4 mL (25 mg/mL) solution in a single-use vial.
- To reconstitute 50-mg lyophilized powder:
  - Add 2.3 mL sterile water for injection, USP by injecting the water along the walls of the vial (not directly into the lyophilized powder), resulting in a concentration of 25 mg/mL.
  - Swirl the vial contents slowly and gently. Allow up to 5 minutes for the bubbles to clear.
  - *Do not shake the vial.*
- To prepare IV solution:
  - Visually inspect the solution for particulate matter or discoloration. The solution should be clear to slightly opalescent, colorless to slightly yellow. If visible particles are seen, discard the vial.
  - Dilute pembrolizumab injection (solution) or reconstituted lyophilized powder prior to IV administration.

- Aseptically withdraw the ordered volume from the vial(s) and transfer to an IV bag containing 0.9% sodium chloride injection, USP.
- Mix the solution together by gentle inversion, resulting in a final concentration of 1–10 mg/mL. Discard any unused drug left in the vial.
- Storage of reconstituted and diluted solutions:
  - Store reconstituted and diluted solution from the pembrolizumab 50-mg vial either
    - At room temperature for no more than 6 hours from time of reconstitution until time the infusion finishes (including room-temperature storage of reconstituted vials, storage of infusion solution in the IV bag, and duration of infusion) **or**
    - Under refrigeration at 2–8°C (36–46°F) for no more than 24 hours from the time of reconstitution. If refrigerated, all the diluted solution to come to room temperature prior to administration.
  - Store the diluted solution from the pembrolizumab 100 mg/4 mL vial either
    - At room temperature ≤ 6 hours from the time of dilution (including room-temperature storage of the infusion solution in the IV bag and duration of infusion), **or**
    - Under refrigeration at 2–8°C (36–46°F) for no more than 24 hours from the time of dilution. If refrigerated, allow the diluted solution to come to room temperature prior to administration.
  - Do not freeze.

Drug Administration:
- Administer infusion solution IV over 30 minutes through an IV line containing a sterile, non-pyrogenic, low-protein-binding 0.2 micron to 0.5 micron in-line or add-on filter.
- Do not coadminister with other drug(s) through the same line.

Drug Interactions:
- Unknown. No formal studies have been conducted.

Lab Effects/Interference:
- Anemia, hypocalcemia, hyponatremia, hypoalbuminemia.
- Hyperglycemia, hypertriglyceridemia, increased aspartate aminotransferase.

Special Considerations:
- FDA granted accelerated approval, based on a study of 173 patients with advanced melanoma refractory to ipilimumab, and found a response rate of 26% lasting 1.4–8.5 months or longer (Robert et al., 2014).
  - In one study, response rate did not differ significantly between patients who had received prior ipilimumab treatment and those who had not (Hamid et al., 2013).
  - Most responses seen within the first 12 weeks of treatment.
- Common adverse events (≥ 20% of patients) were fatigue, cough, nausea, pruritus, rash, decreased appetite, constipation, arthralgia, and diarrhea.
- Warnings and Precautions:
  - Immune-related pneumonitis: occurred in 2.9% of patients with 1.9% grade 2 and 0.2% grade 3; median time to onset was 5 months with a median duration of 4.9 months. Some patients required high-dose systemic corticosteroids, followed by a taper. Most patients had a complete resolution of pneumonitis. Monitor patients for signs and symptoms of pneumonitis, evaluate any suspicious symptoms promptly

with imaging, hold drug and administer high-dose corticosteroids/taper to patients with grade 2 or higher pneumonitis. Permanently discontinue pembrolizumab in patients with grade 3 or 4 pneumonitis.

- Immune-related colitis: occurred in 1% of patients (grade 2 in 0.2% and grade 3 in 0.5%); median time to onset was 6.5 months with a median duration of 2.6 months. Monitor patients for signs and symptoms of colitis, hold drug for grade 2 or higher and administer high-dose corticosteroids/taper, and permanently discontinue drug for grade 4 colitis.

- Immune-related hepatitis: occurred in 0.5% of patients. Monitor LFTs and administer high-dose corticosteroids/taper for grade 2 or higher hepatitis, and hold or discontinue drug based on severity of changes in liver enzymes.

- Immune-related hypophysitis: occurred in 0.5% of patients. Monitor for signs and symptoms of hypophysitis, hold drug and give high-dose corticosteroids/taper for grade 2 or higher. Hold or discontinue drug for grade 3, and permanently discontinue for grade 4 hypophysitis.

- Renal failure and immune-mediated nephritis: occurred in 0.7% of patients. Monitor renal function, hold drug and give high-dose corticosteroids/taper for grade 2 or higher nephritis. Permanently discontinue drug for grade 3 and 4 nephritis.

- Immune-mediated hyperthyroidism and hypothyroidism: occurred in 1.2% and 8.3% of patients respectively. Monitor thyroid function studies baseline, during treatment, and monitor for signs and symptoms of hypo- and hyperthyroidism. Hold drug and give high-dose corticosteroids/taper for grade 3 hyperthyroidism; discontinue drug for grade 4. Hypothyroidism should be treated as needed with thyroid replacement therapy without treatment interruption or steroids.

- Other immune-mediated adverse reactions occurred in < 1% of patients and included exfoliative dermatitis, uveitis, arthritis, myositis, pancreatitis, hemolytic anemia, partial seizures, myasthenic syndrome, optic neuritis, rhabdomyolysis, and adrenal insufficiency. Evaluate; if severe, interrupt drug and give corticosteroids. When resolved to grade 1 or less, start corticosteroid taper and continue for > 1 month. Permanently discontinue drug for any severe or grade 3 immune-mediated adverse reaction.

- Drug causes embryo-fetal toxicity as PD-1/PDL-1 signaling pathways maintain maternal immune tolerance to fetal tissue. Teach women of reproductive potential to use highly effective contraception to avoid pregnancy during treatment and for 4 months after treatment has ended.

Potential Toxicities/Side Effects and the Nursing Process

I.   ALTERATION IN NUTRITION, POTENTIAL, LESS THAN BODY
      REQUIREMENTS, related to DIARRHEA, NAUSEA, DECREASED APPETITE

Defining Characteristics: Diarrhea affected 20%, nausea 30%, decreased appetite 26%, vomiting 16%, constipation 21%, and abdominal pain 12%. There were no grade 3+ reactions. AST was elevated in 24% of patients; hyperglycemia occurred in 40%, hypoalbuminemia in 34%, and hypertriglyceridemia in 25%.

Nursing Implications: Assess nutritional and bowel-elimination patterns, appetite, and presence of nausea and/or vomiting baseline and at each visit. Teach that diarrhea, constipation, nausea, vomiting, and decreased appetite may occur, and to report them. Assess nutrition impact symptoms and discuss management with physician. Teach patient to self-administer antidiarrheal or antiemetic medication, if needed, and to report symptoms that do not improve. Monitor LFTs, glucose, albumin, triglycerides baseline and periodically during therapy as ordered.

II. ALTERATION IN COMFORT related to FATIGUE, ASTHENIA, MYALGIA, HEADACHE, PYREXIA, CHILLS, AND ABDOMINAL PAIN

Defining Characteristics: Fatigue was common, affecting 47% (7% grade 3–4); arthralgia occurred in 20%, myalgia in 14%, headache in 16%, pyrexia in 11%, chills in 14%, and anemia (laboratory) in 55%.

Nursing Implications: Teach patient that these events may occur and to report them. Assess baseline comfort and hemoglobin/hematocrit, and monitor closely during treatment. Develop plan to assure comfort, depending on symptoms reported, and assess efficacy and revise plan if needed at each visit.

III. ALTERATION IN SKIN INTEGRITY, POTENTIAL, related to RASH, PRURITUS, AND VITILIGO

Defining Characteristics: Pruritis affected 30%, rash affected 29%, and vitiligo 11%. Peripheral edema occurred in 17% and was grade 3+ in 1%.

Nursing Implications: Teach patient that rash, pruritus, vitiligo, and peripheral edema may occur and to report it. Assess patient skin integrity and presence of edema, baseline and regularly, during treatment. Teach strategies to patient to maintain skin integrity and evaluate response.

Drug: pertuzumab (Perjeta)

Class: HER-2/neu receptor dimerization inhibitor (HDI). Specifically, it is a recombinant humanized monoclonal antibody that inhibits human epidermal growth factor receptor dimerization, the first of its class. It is a HER-2 receptor antagonist.

Mechanism of Action: In order for a growth signal to be sent to the cell nucleus, a growth factor (ligand) attaches to the human epidermal growth factor receptor, or HER. The growth factor receptor now needs to dimerize or pair with another growth factor receptor to activate the receptor tyrosine kinase; for example, HER-2 receptor needs to dimerize or pair with another HER receptor, such as HER-1 (EGFR), HER-3, or HER-4. Pertuzumab is an IgG_1 monoclonal antibody that binds to the dimerization domain of HER (subdomain II) so the binding of the antibody directly inhibits the ability of HER-2 to dimerize with other HER proteins and no other proteins can bind to it to activate the receptor. This disrupts the activation of downstream effectors so that the growth signal is not sent, notably the mitogen-activated protein kinase (MAP kinase) and phosphoinositide

3-kinase (P13K) pathways, which control cell growth and survival. This leads to cell growth arrest and apoptosis (programmed cell death). In addition, pertuzumab mediates ADCC. Drug blocks a different HER-2 receptor location from that of trastuzumab so drugs can be given together to maximize blockade of HER signaling. This leads to greater antitumor activity than either agent alone (Baselga et al., 2012). Drug is a recombinant, humanized monoclonal antibody.

Metabolism: Steady state concentration of pertuzumab is reached after the first maintenance dose following loading dose. Median drug half-life is 18 days. Pertuzumab exposure in patients with mild and moderate renal impairment was similar to patients with normal renal function.

Indication:
- In combination with trastuzumab and docetaxel for the treatment of patients with HER-2-positive MBC who have not received prior anti-HER-2 therapy or chemotherapy for metastatic disease.
- In combination with trastuzumab and docetaxel for the neoadjuvant treatment of patients with HER2-positive, locally advanced, inflammatory, or early stage breast cancer (either > 2 cm in diameter or node-positive) as part of a complete treatment regimen for early breast cancer. This indication is based on improvement in pathological CR rate. No data are available showing improvement in event-free survival or overall survival.

Dosage/Range: Initial loading dose: 840-mg IV infusion as a 60-minute infusion, followed every 3 weeks thereafter by a 420-mg IV infusion over 30–60 minutes.
- *HER-2 positive metastatic breast cancer (MBC):* pertuzumab IV infusion every 3 weeks, in combination with trastuzumab and docetaxel.
- *Neoadjuvant treatment of breast cancer in HER2-positive patients with locally advanced, inflammatory, or early stage breast cancer:* pertuzumab IV infusion preoperatively every 3 weeks for 3–6 cycles, as part of one of the following treatment regimes for early breast cancer:
  - Four preoperative cycles of pertuzumab in combination with trastuzumab and docetaxel, followed by 3 post-operative cycles of fluorouracil, epirubicin, and cyclophosphamide (FEC), as given in Study 2 in package insert.
  - Three preoperative cycles of FEC alone, followed by 3 preoperative cycles of pertuzumab in combination with docetaxel and trastuzumab, as given in Study 3 in package insert.
  - Six preoperative cycles of pertuzumab in combination with docetaxel, carboplatin, and trastuzumab (TCH) (escalation of docetaxel above 75 mg/m^2 is not recommended), as given in Study 3 in package insert.
  - FOLLOWING SURGERY, patients should continue to receive trastuzumab to complete 1 year of treatment. There is insufficient evidence to recommend continued use of pertuzumab for > 6 cycles for early breast cancer. There is insufficient evidence to recommend concommitant administration of an anthracycline with pertuzumab, and no safety data to support sequential use of doxorubicin with pertuzumab.
- When pertuzumab, trastuzumab, and docetaxel are given, drugs should be given sequentially, with docetaxel administered **after** pertuzumab and trastuzumab. An observation

period of 30–60 minutes is recommended after each pertuzumab infusion and before starting the subsequent infusion of trastuzumab or docetaxel.

- *Dose Modification:*
    - For delayed or missed doses, if the time between two sequential infusions is < 6 weeks, administer the 420-mg dose of pertuzumab; do not wait for the next planned dose. If the time between two sequential infusions is 6 weeks or more, the initial dose of pertuzumab 840 mg should be readministered as a 60-minute IV infusion, followed every 3 weeks thereafter by a dose of 420-mg IV infusion over 30–60 minutes.
    - Pertuzumab should be discontinued if trastuzumab is discontinued. Dose reductions of pertuzumab are not recommended. See docetaxel prescribing information for docetaxel dose modifications.
    - LVEF: Hold pertuzumab and trastuzumab dosing for at least 3 weeks for either:
        - A drop in LVEF to < 45%, or
        - LVEF of 45% to 49% with a 10% or greater absolute decrease below pretreatment values.
        - Pertuzumab may be resumed if LVEF has recovered to > 49%, or to 45–49% associated with less than a 10% absolute decrease below pretreatment values.
        - If after a repeat assessment within approximately 3 weeks, the LVEF has not improved or has declined further, pertuzumab and trastuzumab should be discontinued, unless the benefits for the individual patient are deemed to outweigh the risks.
    - Infusion-related reactions: slow or interrupt infusion if patient develops an infusion-related reaction.
    - Hypersensitivity reactions/anaphylaxis: discontinue infusion immediately.
- Use in HER-2-positive patients only. Patients on study had to have evidence of HER-2 overexpression defined by 3^+ IHC or FISH amplification ratio ≥ 2.0.
- Drug is contraindicated in patients with known hypersensitivity to pertuzumab or to any of its excipients.
- When combined with trastuzumab, the recommended initial dose of trastuzumab is 8 mg/kg given as a 90-min IV infusion, followed every 3 weeks thereafter by a dose of 6 mg/kg IV infusion over 30–90 min.
- When combined with docetaxel for the treatment of MBC, the recommended initial dose of docetaxel is 75 mg/m^2 administered as an IV infusion; the dose can be escalated to 100 mg/m^2 by IV infusion every 3 weeks if initial dose is tolerated well.

Drug Preparation:
- Available as a single-use vial of 420 mg/14 mL (30 mg/mL). Use 0.9% sodium chloride injection bags ONLY. Do not use D5W.
- After inspecting vial to ensure no particulates or discoloration, aseptically withdraw appropriate volume of drug and dilute in 250 mL 0.9% sodium chloride injection PVC or non-PVC polyolefin infusion bag. Mix solution by gentle inversion, but do not shake. Administer immediately after preparation.
- Drug containing infusion bag can be stored at 2–8°C (36-46°F) for up to 24 hr.
- Dilute with 0.9% sodium chloride injection only. DO NOT use dextrose (5%) solution.

Drug Administration:
- Assess pregnancy status prior to first dose, as drug is embryo-fetotoxic.
- Assess findings of ECHO or MUGA scan for LVEF, baseline and at least every 3 months during treatment.
- Initial: IV infusion over 60 min (loading dose) then subsequent: IV infusion over 30–60 min (maintenance doses) every 3 weeks. Do NOT give IVB or IVP. Reduce infusion rate or interrupt if infusion reaction occurs. Permanently discontinue for severe reactions.
- Observe patients closely for 60 min after the first infusion, and 30 minutes after subsequent infusions, and before administering trastuzumab or docetaxel. If a significant infusion reaction occurs, stop the infusion and administer HSR medications as ordered. Monitor patient closely until complete resolution of signs and symptoms. Consider permanent drug discontinuance in patients with severe infusion reactions. Incidence of hypersensitivity/anaphylaxis was 10.8% in pertuzumab group compared to 9.1% in control group, with grade 3–4 HSR 2% in the pertuzumab group and 2.5% in the placebo group.

Drug Interactions:
- No drug-drug interactions observed between pertuzumab and trastuzumab, or between pertuzumab and docetaxel.

Lab Effects/Interference:
- Neutropenia, anemia when given with docetaxel and trastuzumab.

Special Considerations:
- FDA approval based on results of the CLinical Evaluation Of Pertuzumab And TRAstuzumab (CLEOPATRA) clinical trial demonstrating that the addition of pertuzumab significantly increased PFS compared to trastuzumab and docetaxel alone (18.5 vs 12.4 mo, $p < 0.001$). Overall survival data will not be mature until 2014, but trend favors pertuzumab. Addition of pertuzumab did not increase toxicity: febrile neutropenia (48.9% vs 45.8% in control), grade 3 or higher diarrhea (7.9% vs 5%), but no increase in left ventricular systolic dysfunction (1.2% vs 2.8%) (Baselga et al., 2012).
- Drug is embryo-fetal toxic. Women of childbearing age should use effective contraception to prevent pregnancy. Teach patient to contact provider immediately if pregnancy is suspected while receiving the drug. If drug is administered during pregnancy, provider should contact Genentech Adverse Event Line (1-888-835-2555), and pregnant women should enroll in MotHER Pregnancy Registry (1-800-690-6720).
- Infusion reactions occurred during or on the same day as pertuzumab infusion in 13% of patients, compared to 9.8% of control patients who received trastuzumab and docetaxel alone. Pertuzumab was given one day prior to trastuzumab in the study. Most common reactions during the first treatment were pyrexia, chills, fatigue, headache, asthenia, hypersensitivity, and vomiting. Less than 1% of reactions were grade 3–4. During the second cycle, when all drugs were administered on the same day, most common infusion reactions were fatigue, dysgeusia, hypersensitivity, myalgia, and vomiting.

• Cardiomyopathy: pertuzumab can result in subclinical and clinical heart failure, manifesting as CHF, and decreased LVEF. Evaluate cardiac function prior to and during treatment. Discontinue pertuzumab treatment for a confirmed clinically significant decrease in LVEF.

• Overall, the most common toxicities were diarrhea, alopecia, neutropenia, nausea, fatigue, rash, and peripheral neuropathy.

Potential Toxicities/Side Effects and the Nursing Process

I. POTENTIAL FOR INJURY related to HYPERSENSITIVITY/ANAPHYLAXIS AND INFUSION REACTION

Defining Characteristics: When pertuzumab was administered alone on a separate day in Study 1, the incidence of infusion reactions was 13% (compared to 9.8% in the placebo group) with < 1% grade 3 or 4. Most commonly, infusion reaction was characterized by pyrexia, chills, fatigue, headache, asthenia, hypersensitivity, and vomiting. In the second cycle, when all drugs were given on the same day, the most common infusion reactions were fatigue, dysgeusia, hypersensitivity, myalgia, and vomiting.

Incidence of hypersensitivity/anaphylaxis was 10.8% in pertuzumab group compared to 9.1% in control group, with grade 3–4 HSR 2% in the pertuzumab group and 2.5% in the placebo group. In Study 3, overall frequency of hypersensitivity/anaphylaxis was highest in the pertuzumab + TCH group (13.2%), of which 2.6% were grade 3–4.

Nursing Implications: Assess baseline VS and mental status prior to drug administration and periodically during infusion, as needed. Remain with patient during first 15 minutes of first infusions, and observe patient for 30–60 minutes depending upon cycle after drug has finished infusing. Recall signs/symptoms of anaphylaxis; if these occur, stop drug immediately, notify physician, and assess patient's vital signs. Subjective symptoms are generalized itching, nausea, chest tightness, crampy abdominal pain, difficulty speaking, anxiety, agitation, sense of impending doom, uneasiness, desire to urinate/defecate, dizziness, and chills. Objective signs are flushed appearance; angioedema of face, neck, eyelids, hands, and feet; localized or generalized urticaria; respiratory distress with or without wheezing; hypotension; and cyanosis. Review standing physician orders or nursing procedures for patient management of anaphylaxis, and be prepared to stop drug immediately and change IV to a plain NS solution to keep vein patent, notify physician, keep airway patent, monitor VS, and administer ordered medications, which may include epinephrine 1:1,000 IM in the thigh, IV hydrocortisone sodium succinate, and IV diphenhydramine. Teach patient to report any unusual symptoms. Patient should be observed for 1 hour after the initial treatment, 30 minutes after subsequent treatments, and before trastuzumab and docetaxel are administered. Slow infusion or interrupt the drug if patient develops an infusion reaction, and administer ordered medications. Discontinue the drug if the patient has a serious hypersensitivity reaction, and provide emergency intervention and medications as ordered.

II.   POTENTIAL FOR INFECTION related to NEUTROPENIA

Defining Characteristics: Neutropenia occurred in 53% of patients compared to 50% in the control group without pertuzumab. Grade 3–4: 49% vs 46%. Febrile neutropenia occurred in 13.8% compared to 7.6% in controls. Pyrexia occurred in 18.7% of patients, similar to controls.

Nursing Implications: Assess baseline blood counts, WBC, and differential. Teach patient to report fever and signs/symptoms of infection right away (e.g., T $\geq$ 100.4°F, dysuria, productive cough). Assess medication profile and OTC medications taken. Teach patient to avoid OTC medications containing NSAIDs or aspirin. Teach patient to talk to nurse or physician before starting any OTC medications.

III.   POTENTIAL ALTERATION IN NUTRITION related to DIARRHEA, NAUSEA, VOMITING, CONSTIPATION, STOMATITIS, DECREASED APPETITE, DYSGEUSIA

Defining Characteristics: In Study 1 of patients with MBC, diarrhea was most common, affecting 66.7% of patients (grade 3–4 7.9%); compared to 46% in control group without pertuzumab (5% grade 3–4), and ranging in severity from grades 1–3. Nausea and vomiting affected 42% and 24% patients respectively, similar to the control group. Constipation affected 15%, significantly less than the control (25%). Stomatitis occurred in 19% compared to 15% in control group. Decreased appetite affected 29% vs 26% in control, and dysgeusia occurred in 18% of patients (16% in control group).

Nursing Implications: Assess bowel elimination patterns and nutritional status, baseline and prior to each treatment. Teach patient self-care strategies depending upon symptom: to take antidiarrheal medications if diarrhea, to take antiemetic medication as ordered if nausea/vomiting; if constipation, to take fiber supplements or laxatives as needed. To decrease symptoms, teach patient dietary modifications, which might include high fiber, high fluids for constipation, BRAT diet for diarrhea unless it is persistent, and then modify with more protein; avoid fatty and spicy foods if nausea/vomiting. Teach patient to report any symptoms that do not resolve or improve with the established plan. Teach patient strategies to increase appetite (use small plate with small portions of food; take antiemetic pill prior to eating if needed; use small frequent feedings of high-protein, high-calorie foods, including bedtime snack if tolerated; if dysgeusia, based on sensory change, use plastic utensils if metallic taste, and use spices such as Crazy Jane salt).

IV.   ACTIVITY INTOLERANCE, POTENTIAL, related to FATIGUE, ASTHENIA, HEADACHE

Defining Characteristics: Fatigue occurs commonly in patients with advanced cancer who were studied. Fatigue occurred in 38% of patients similar to control group. Asthenia occurred in 26%, less than the control group of 30%. Headache occurred in 21% of patients, and anemia 23% compared to 19% in control group.

Nursing Implications: Assess baseline activity and energy level, and teach patient that this symptom may occur. Assess patient's activity patterns, and suggest ways to conserve energy. Teach patient that headache may occur, and to use self-care measures, such as taking acetaminophen, finding a quiet place without bright light to rest until the headache resolves. Monitor HGB/HCT.

V.   ALTERATION IN BODY IMAGE, POTENTIAL, related to ALOPECIA, SKIN CHANGES

Defining Characteristics: Alopecia occurs in 61% of patients receiving docetaxel, trastuzumab, and pertuzumab, same as the control group without pertuzumab. Skin changes included rash (33.7% vs 24% in control), nail disorder (same as control, 23%), pruritus (14% vs 10%), and dry skin (10.6% vs 4.3%).

Nursing Implications: Assess baseline skin integrity and skin moisture. Teach patient that skin changes, including alopecia, may occur. Encourage patient to obtain a wig (cranial prosthesis) prior to starting therapy. Assess effect of hair loss on patient's body image, as well as skin changes. Encourage patient to verbalize feelings and provide emotional support. If needed, involve social worker in supportive counseling. Encourage patient to use scarves or hats as appropriate and to attend supportive educational sessions such as ACS Look Good . . . Feel Better program. Teach patient to assess for skin and nail changes, to use skin emollients, and to report nail changes. Discuss management of nail changes with nurse practitioner or physician.

Drug: pomalidomide (Pomalyst)

Class: Immunomodulator with antiangiogic and antineoplastic properties.

Mechanism of Action: Third-generation thalidomide analogue that is an immunomodulatory agent with antineoplastic activity. Drug has been shown to inhibit proliferation and cause apoptosis of hematopoietic tumor cells, and to have activity in lenalidomide-resistant multiple myeloma (MM) cell lines. It is synergistic with dexamethasone to bring about tumor cell apoptosis. Pomalidomide enhances T-cell and natural killer (NK) cell-mediated immunity and inhibits production of pro-inflammatory cytokines (TNF-α and IL-6). Drug also has antiangiogenic activity.

Metabolism: After oral administration, C_{max} occurs at 2 and 3 hours after dosing. Drug is distributed in the semen at a concentration of 67% of plasma level 4 hours post dose. In healthy subjects, drug binds to plasma proteins 12–44%. Drug is primarily metabolized in the liver by CYP1A2 and CYP3A4, and to a lesser degree by CYP2C19 and CYP2D6. Median plasma half-life is 9.5 hours in healthy subjects, and 7.5 hours in patients with multiple myeloma. Drug is excreted primarily in the urine (73%, 2% unchanged), and feces (15%, 8% unchanged drug). Drug is a substrate for P-glycoprotein (P-gp).

Indication: The treatment of patients with multiple myeloma (MM) who have received at least two prior therapies, including lenalidomide and bortezomib, and have disease progression on or within 60 days of completing last therapy. Clinical benefit has not been verified.

Dosage/Range:
- 4 mg orally, daily on days 1–21 of repeated 28-day cycles until disease progression. Pomalidomide may be given in combination with dexamethasone.

Dose Modifications:
- Neutropenia (ANC < 500 cells/mm³, or febrile neutropenia (fever ≥ 38.5° C and ANC < 1,000 cells/mm³)): interrupt pomalidomide; follow CBC weekly and resume drug at 3 mg daily when ANC ≥ 500 cells/mm³; for each subsequent decrease to ANC < 500 cells/mm³, interrupt drug then resume at a reduced dose 1 mg less than previous dose, once ANC returns to ANC ≥ 500 cells/mm³.
- Thrombocytopenia (platelets < 25,000 cells/mm³): interrupt pomalidomide, follow CBC weekly, resume drug at 3 mg daily once platelets return to > 50,000 cells/mm³; for each subsequent drop in platelets < 25,000 cells/mm³, interrupt drug then resume at a reduced dose 1 mg less than previous dose, once platelet count returns to > 50,000 cells/mm³.
- Other grade 3 or 4 toxicities: interrupt drug, then restart treatment at 1 mg less than the previous dose when toxicity has resolved to ≤ grade 2 at physician's discretion.
- If toxicities occur after dose reductions to 1 mg daily, discontinue pomalidomide.
- To initiate a new cycle of pomalidomide, the neutrophil count must be at least 500 cells/mm³, and the platelet count must be at least 50,000 cells/mm³.
- Dose adjustment for strong CYP1A2 inhibitors in the presence of strong CYP3A4 and P-gp inhibitors: avoid coadministration of strong CYP1A2 inhibitors. If medically necessary to coadminister strong CYP1A2 inhibitors in the presence of strong CYP3A4 and P-gp inhibitors, reduce pomalidomide dose by 50%.

Drug Preparation:
- Drug is available only through a restricted distribution program called POMALYST Risk Evaluation Mitigation Strategy (REMS). Prescribers and pharmacists must be certified with the program and patients must sign an agreement and comply with requirements.
- Drug is available as capsules in 1-mg, 2-mg, 3-mg, and 4-mg strengths.

Drug Administration:
- Teach patient to take pomalidomide on an empty stomach, without food, at least 2 hours before or 2 hours after a meal. Drug capsule can be taken with water and should not be broken, chewed, or opened.
- Drug is a teratogen that can cause severe birth defects or fetal death.
- Women of reproductive potential must:
  - Have two negative pregnancy tests before starting the drug (the first performed within 10–14 days, and the second, within 24 hours prior to prescribing pomalidomide therapy), then weekly during the first month, then monthly thereafter in women who have regular menstrual cycles, or every two weeks if irregular menstrual cycles.
  - Commit either to abstain continuously from heterosexual intercourse or to use two forms of reliable birth control beginning four weeks prior to starting therapy, during

therapy, during dose interruptions, and continuing for four weeks after stopping pomalidomide treatment.
- Men must always use a latex or synthetic condom during any sexual contact with females of reproductive potential while taking pomalidomide, and for up to 28 days after stopping the drug, even if they have had a successful vasectomy. Drug is present in semen.
- Pomalidomide is excreted primarily in the urine. Do not administer to patients with serum creatinine > 3.0 mg/dL.
- Pomalidomide is metabolized in the liver. Avoid pomalidomide in patients with serum bilirubin > 2.0 mg/dL.
- Consider VTE prophylaxis based on individual patient's underlying risk factors.

Drug Interactions:
- Pomalidomide is primarily metabolized by CYP1A2 and CYP3A; pomalidomide is also a substrate for P-glycoprotein (P-gp).
- Drugs that may increase pomalidomide plasma concentrations:
  - CYP1A2 inhibitors (strong): pomalidomide plasma concentrations may be increased when drug is coadministered with a strong CYP1A2 inhibitor (e.g., fluvoxamine) in the presence of a strong CYP3A4/5 and P-gp inhibitor (e.g., ketoconazole). Ketoconazole in the absence of a CYP1A2 inhibitor does not increase pomalidomide serum levels.
    - Thus, AVOID coadministration of strong CYP1A2 inhibitors (e.g., ciprofloxacin and fluvoxamine) unless medically necessary; and if necessary to coadminister, pomalidomide dose must be reduced.
    - If a CYP1A2 inhibitor without coadministration of a CYP3A4 and P-gp inhibitor is given, monitor patient closely for toxicity, and reduce pomalidomide dose as needed.
- Drugs/substances that may reduce pomalidomide plasma concentrations:
  - Smoking: may reduce pomalidomide serum level due to CYP1A2 induction and reduce efficacy; teach patients that smoking may reduce drug's effectiveness.
  - CYP1A2 inducers: have not been studied, and may reduce pomalidomide serum level. Dexamethasone, a weak CYP3A4 inducer, in combination with pomalidomide, did not change the pharmacokinetics of pomalidomide.

Lab Effects/Interference:
- Neutropenia, thrombocytopenia, anemia.
- Hyperglycemia, hypercalcemia.
- Hyponatremia, hypocalcemia, hypokalemia.
- Increased serum creatinine.

Special Considerations:
- Venous thromboembolic events (VTE): deep vein thrombosis (DVT) and pulmonary embolism (PE) may occur; in clinical trials, prophylactic antithrombotic measures (aspirin, warfarin, heparin, or clopidogrel) were used, which should be considered based on patient risk review. Incidence of DVT or PE was 3%.

- Neutropenia occurs in 50% of patients with an incidence of 43% grade 3–4; anemia and thrombocytopenia also occur. Patients should have CBC/differential and platelet counts monitored weekly for the first 8 weeks, then monthly. Dose interruption and modification are used to manage toxicity.
- Drug can cause dizziness (18%) and confusion (12%). Teach patient to avoid driving and operating heavy machinery until the patient knows the drug's effects, and to avoid any other concurrent medications that can cause dizziness.
- If the patient had a serious hypersensitivity reaction (HSR) to thalidomide or lenalidomide, the patient may be at higher risk for HSR with pomalidomide.
- Neuropathy occurred in 18% of patients, with 9% having peripheral neuropathy. No grade 3 or higher neuropathy was seen in clinical trials.
- Tumor Lysis Syndrome (TLS) may occur. Patients at risk are those with a high tumor burden before initial treatment; discuss TLS prophylaxis with physician, and monitor patient closely.
- Most common adverse reactions were fatigue, asthenia, neutropenia, anemia, constipation, nausea, diarrhea, dyspnea, URIs, back pain, pyrexia.
- Patients must not donate blood during treatment with pomalidomide or for one month after discontinuing the drug, as the blood may be given to a pregnant patient whose fetus must not be exposed to the drug.
- Men should be counseled not to donate sperm, as drug is distributed in semen.
- Drug is contraindicated during pregnancy. If the patient becomes pregnant while taking the drug, the patient should be apprised of the potential hazard to the fetus. Nursing mothers should discontinue the drug or stop nursing.
- POMALYST REMS Program: drug is available only under this program, which includes:
  - Prescribers must be certified with the POMALYST REMS program by enrolling and complying with the REMS requirements.
  - Patients must sign a patient-prescriber agreement form and comply with the REMS requirements (e.g., female patients of reproductive potential who are not pregnant must comply with the pregnancy testing and contraception requirements, and males must comply with the contraception requirements).
  - Pharmacists must be certified with the POMALYST REMS program, must only dispense to patients who are authorized to receive pomalidomide, and must comply with REMS requirements.
  - Further information is available from www.celgeneriskmanagement.com or at 1-888-423-5436.

Potential Toxicities/Side Effects and the Nursing Process

I.   POTENTIAL FOR INFECTION, BLEEDING, FATIGUE related to BONE MARROW SUPPRESSION

Defining Characteristics: Neutropenia occurred in 50% of patients and was grade 3–4 in 43%; febrile neutropenia occurred in 3% of patients. Thrombocytopenia occurred in 25%

(was grade 3–4 in 22%). Anemia occurred in 38% of patients (was grade 3–4 in 22%). Fever occurred in 19%, chills in 9%; pneumonia was reported in 23% of patients, URIs in 32%, and UTIs in 8%. Epistaxis was reported in 15% of patients. Fatigue and asthenia occurred in 55% of patients.

Nursing Implications: Assess baseline CBC, WBC, differential, and platelet count baseline and weekly for the first 8 weeks, then monthly. Hold drug if ANC < 500 cells/mm^3 or platelets < 50,000 cells/mm^3 and dose-modify when ANC and/or platelet count recovers (see dosing section). Assess for signs/symptoms of infection or bleeding. Teach patient the signs/symptoms of infection (e.g., T > 100.4°F, productive cough, dysuria, dyspnea) or bleeding (e.g., epistaxis, pink urine, after brushing teeth), and to report these immediately. Teach patient self-care measures to minimize risk of infection and bleeding. This includes avoidance of crowds, proximity to people with infections, and OTC aspirin-containing medications (except 325 mg PO aspirin daily as DVT prophylaxis), and NSAIDs. Discuss any abnormalities with physician or NP/PA. Teach patient strategies to manage fatigue, and conserve energy, such as altering rest and activity, organizing chores, engaging in gentle exercise.

II. ALTERATION IN NUTRITION, LESS THAN BODY REQUIREMENTS, related to DIARRHEA, CONSTIPATION, NAUSEA, VOMITING, DECREASED APPETITE, WEIGHT LOSS

Defining Characteristics: Nutrition impact symptoms may occur. Constipation occurred in 36% of patients in clinical trials, diarrhea in 34%, nausea 36%, vomiting 14%, decreased appetite 22%, and weight loss 14%. Hyperglycemia occurred in 12%, hyponatremia 10%, hypercalcemia 21%, hypocalcemia 6%, and hypokalemia 10%.

Nursing Implications: Assess baseline nutritional status, including weight and serum lab values (e.g., electrolytes and glucose). Assess bowel elimination pattern, energy level/activity, and appetite. Teach patient that symptoms may occur and to report them. Teach patient self-care management strategies for diarrhea, constipation, nausea, vomiting, and to report if symptom(s) do not resolve. Teach dietary modifications based on symptoms, such as the BRAT diet for diarrhea (bananas, rice, applesauce, and toast), and to increase oral fluids to prevent dehydration. Involve dietitian as needed and available.

III. ALTERATION IN COMFORT related to BACK PAIN, MUSCULOSKELETAL CHEST PAIN, MUSCLE SPASMS, ARTHRALGIA, MUSCULOSKELETAL PAIN, PERIPHERAL EDEMA, RAS

Defining Characteristics: In clinical trials, symptoms occurred with the following incidences: peripheral edema (23%), back pain (32%), musculoskeletal pain (22%), muscle spasms (19%), arthralgia (16%), musculoskeletal pain (11%), rash (22%).

Nursing Implications: Assess patient's baseline comfort, as bone involvement by multiple myeloma may increase discomfort. Teach patient that these symptoms may occur, and to report them. Teach patient self-management strategies and to report them if ineffective, including use of warmth/heat and cold, as tolerated and preferred. Discuss analgesics with physician/NP/PA, recommendations for the patient, and need for prescription analgesics. Teach patient to report rash, and to have it evaluated to rule out allergic reaction.

IV.   POTENTIAL FOR SENSORY/PERCEPTUAL ALTERATIONS related to NEUROLOGIC TOXICITY

Defining Characteristics: In clinical trials, neuropathy occurred in 18% of patients, peripheral neuropathy in 9% of patients, dizziness in 20%, headache in 13%, tremor in 9%.

Nursing Implications: Assess patient's ability to understand rationale and importance of pregnancy testing in women of childbearing age prior to drug prescription, as well as during treatment, treatment holidays, and for four weeks following drug discontinuance. Assess the understanding and the ability of patients with childbearing potential to comply with contraception requirements and other self-care strategies.

Drug: ponatinib (Iclusig)

Class: Kinase inhibitor (multiple).

Mechanism of Action: Drug inhibits tyrosine kinase activity of ABL, BCR-ABL, as well as mutant forms; also inhibits VEGFR, PDGFR, FGFR, KIT, RET, TIE2, and FLT3 kinases.

Metabolism: Peak concentrations are achieved within 6 hours after oral dosing, and they are not influenced by food intake. Aqueous solubility of ponatinib is pH-dependent, with lower solubility in higher pH environments. Drug is highly protein-bound (> 99%) to plasma proteins. Drug is metabolized by CYP3A4 and to a lesser degree CYP2C8, CYP2D6, and CYP3A5, as well as by esterases and/or amidases. Mean terminal half-life is about 24 hours, and primary excretion is via the feces (87%).

Indication: The treatment of adult patients with:
- T3151-positive CML chronic phase (CP), accelerated phase (AP), or blast phase (BP) of T3151-positive Philadelphia chromosome positive (Ph⁺) acute lymphoblastic leukemia (Ph⁺ ALL).
- CML-CP, CML-AP, or CML-BP, or Ph⁺ALL adult patients for whom no other tyrosine kinase inhibitor (TKI) therapy is indicated.
- Indication based on response rate only.

Dosage/Range: See REMS letter for new labeling and safety information (Dec. 2013) available at http://www.iclusigrems.com/factsheet.pdf. The optimal dose is not known, as

59% of patients required a dose reduction to 30 mg or 15 mg once daily during the course of therapy.
- Recommended dose: 45 mg orally once daily with or without food. Consider reducing the dose of ponatinib for chronic phase (CP) CML and accelerated (AP) CML patients who have achieved a major cytogenetic response.
- Patients with hepatic impairment: 30 mg PO once daily.
- Consider discontinuing ponatinib if response has not occurred by 3 months (90 days).

Dose Modifications:
Myelosuppression: ANC < 1.0×10^9/L and thrombocytopenia (platelets < 50×10^9/L that are unrelated to leukemia).
- First occurrence: interrupt ponatinib and resume initial dose of 45 mg daily after recovery of ANC ≥ 1,500 cells/mm³ and platelets ≥ 75,000 cells/mm³.
- Second occurrence: interrupt ponatinib and resume at 30 mg daily after recovery of ANC ≥ 1,500 cells/mm³ and platelets ≥ 75,000 cells/mm³.
- Third occurrence: interrupt ponatinib and resume at 15 mg daily after recovery of ANC ≥ 1,500 cells/mm³ and platelets ≥ 75,000 cells/mm³.
Hepatotoxicity:
- Elevated liver transaminases > 3 × ULN (grade 2 or higher): *if occurs at 45-mg dose:* interrupt dose, monitor LFTs, resume at 30-mg dose after recovery to < 3 × ULN (≤ grade 1); *if occurs at 30-mg dose:* interrupt drug and resume at 15 mg after recovery to ≤ grade 1; *if occurs at 15-mg dose,* discontinue ponatinib.
- Elevation of AST or ALT ≥ 3 × ULN concurrent with elevation in bilirubin > 2 × ULN and alkaline phosphatase < 2 × ULN: discontinue ponatinib.
Pancreatitis and elevated lipase:
- Asymptomatic grade 1 or 2 elevation of serum lipase: consider interruption or dose reduction of ponatinib.
- Asymptomatic grade 3 or 4 elevation of lipase (> 2 × ULN) or asymptomatic radiologic pancreatitis (grade 2 pancreatitis): *if occurs at 45-mg dose:* interrupt dose, and resume at 30 mg after recovery to ≤ grade 1 (< 1.5 × ULN); *if occurs at 30 mg dose:* interrupt drug and resume at 15 mg after recovery to ≤ grade 1; *if occurs at 15-mg dose,* discontinue ponatinib.
- Symptomatic grade 3 pancreatitis: *if occurs at 45-mg dose*, interrupt drug, and resume at 30 mg after complete resolution of symptoms and recovery of lipase elevations to ≤ grade 1; *if occurs at 30-mg dose*, interrupt drug and resume at 15- mg dose after complete resolution and after recovery of lipase elevation to ≤ grade 1; *if occurs at 15-mg dose,* discontinue ponatinib.
- Grade 4 pancreatitis: discontinue ponatinib.
Use with strong CYP3A4 inhibitors: reduce dose to 30 mg orally, once a day.
Ischemic reaction: interrupt and do not restart drug if a serious ischemic reaction occurs, unless potential benefit outweighs the risk of recurrent ischemia and the patient has no other treatment options.

Drug Preparation:
- Available in 15-mg and 45-mg capsules.

Drug Administration:
- Assess lab tests baseline and:
  - CBC/differential every 2 weeks for 3 months, then monthly and as clinically indicated.
  - Serum lipase baseline and monthly during therapy.
  - LFTs at least monthly; more frequently if patient has history of pancreatitis or alchohol abuse.
- Monitor patient for fluid retention; discuss drug interruption, reduction, or discontinuance with physician if fluid retention found.
- Monitor patient's BP, and discuss management of HTN with physician.
- Teach patient to take ponatinib with or without food, and to swallow the capsule whole. Teach patients not to crush or dissolve tablets, and not to take two doses at the same time to make up for a missed dose.
- Teach patient that ponatinib contains 121 mg of lactose monhydrate in a 45-mg daily dose.
- Assess risk for tumor lysis syndrome (TLS) and ensure adequate hydration, correction of uric acid levels prior to initial dose; highest risk in patients with advanced disease and high tumor burden (e.g., CML-AP, CML-BP, Ph+ ALL).
- Temporarily interrupt therapy at least one week prior to major surgery, as drug may interfere with wound healing; resume when wound has healed (based on clinical judgment).

Drug Interactions:
- Drug is a substrate of CYP3A4/5 and to a lesser extent CYP2C8 and CYP2D6. Drug also inhibits the P-glycoprotein (P-gp), ATP-binding G2 (ABCG2, also known as BCRP), and bile salt export pump (BSEP) transporter systems.
- Strong CYP3A4 inhibitors (e.g., ketoconazole): increased ponatinib serum concentration with increased risk of drug toxicity; avoid concomitant administration; if must give together, reduce ponatinib drug dose.
- Strong CYP3A4 inducers (e.g., rifampin): decreased ponatinib serum concentration, with decreased drug effect; avoid concomitant administration unless potential benefit outweighs risk of possible ponatinib underexposure, and monitor for reduced effectiveness.
- pH modifying drugs (e.g., proton pump inhibitors, H2 blockers, antacids): may reduce ponatinib bioavailability; avoid if possible; if must coadminister, assess for signs of decreased ponatinib effectiveness.
- Drugs that are substrates of the P-gp (e.g., aliskiren, ambrisentan, colchicine, dabigatran, etexilate, digoxin, everolimus, fexofenadine, imatinib, lapatinib, maraviroc, nilotinib, posaconazole, ranolazine, saxagliptin, sirolimus, sitagliptin, tolvaptan, topotecan) or ABCG2 (e.g., methotrexate, mitoxantrone, imatinib, irinotecan, lapatinib, rosuvastatin, sulfasalazine, topotecan) transport system: have not been studied so concomitant administration should be avoided.

Lab Effects/Interference:
- Neutropenia, thrombocytopenia, anemia.
- Increased serum lipase, amylase.

- Increased or decreased glucose; decreased phosphorus; increased or decreased calcium; increased or decreased sodium; increased or decreased potassium; decreased bicarbonate; increased calcium; increased creatinine.
- Increased triglycerides.
- Increased LFTs, alkaline phosphatase, decreased albumin.

Special Considerations:
- Monitor CBC, differential, platelet count every two weeks for three months and then monthly as clinically indicated. Interrupt drug for ANC < 1,000 cells/mm^3 or thrombocytopenia < 50,000 cells/mm^3; monitor LFTs baseline then at least monthly; monitor lipase every two weeks for the first two months, then monthly or as clinically indicated.
- Severe myelosuppression (grade 3–4) occurred in 48% of patients, especially patients with CML-AP, CML-BP, and Ph+ ALL, compared to patients with CML-CP. Adjust drug dose as recommended.
- Vascular occlusion: Drug can cause arterial (in at least 20% of patients) and venous (in 5% of patients) thrombosis and occlusions have occurred in at least 27% of ponatinib-treated patients in phase 1–2 trials, including fatal MI, stroke, stenosis of larger arterial vessels of the brain, severe peripheral vascular disease, and the need for urgent revascularization procedures. Drug can cause recurrent or multisite vascular occlusion. Most common VTE were DVT, PE, superficial thrombophlebitis, and retinal vein thrombosis.
  - Patients with and without cardiovascular risk factors, including patients < 50 years old, experienced these events. Overall, 20% of ponatinib-treated patients had an arterial occlusion and thrombus event of any grade. Events more frequent with increasing age and in patients with prior history of ischemia, HTN, diabetes, or hyperlipidemia.
  - Fatal and life-threatening vascular occlusion has occurred within 2 weeks of starting drug, and in patients receiving as little as 15 mg/day.
  - Median time to first vascular occlusion event was 5 months.
  - Monitor for evidence of thromboembolism, vascular occlusion, and arterial thrombotic events; interrupt or stop ponatinib immediately for vascular occlusionsor arterial thrombotic events. A benefit-risk consideration should guide a decision to restart ponatinib.
- CHF occurred in 8% of patients and was serious or fatal in 5%. Monitor patients for signs/symptoms of new or worsening heart failure or LV dysfunction; if it occurs, interrupt ponatinib and treat appropriately; if serious, discontinue ponatinib.
- Hepatotoxicity: hepatotoxicity, liver failure, and death have occurred in ponatinib-treated patients. Ponatinib may cause elevated ALT, AST, or both. Monitor hepatic function baseline, then at least monthly or as clinically indicated. Interrupt ponatinib if hepatotoxicity is suspected, dose-reduce or discontinue drug as clinically indicated.
- Cardiac arrhythmias may occur: symptomatic bradyarrhythmias that may require a pacemaker, supraventricular tachyarrhythmias (5%, atrial fibrillation most common). Teach

patient to report immediately palpitations and dizziness, or slow heartbeat along with fainting, dizziness, or chest pain.

- HTN occurred in 67% of patients requiring treatment (SBP ≥ 140 mmHg, or DBP ≥ 90 mm Hg on at least one occasion), with 2% experiencing symptomatic HTN (confusion, headache, chest pain, or SOB). Monitor and manage HTN to normalize BP; interrupt, dose-reduce, or stop ponatinib if HTN not medically controlled.

- Pancreatitis: clinical pancreatitis occurred in 6% of patients; lipase elevation requiring treatment occurred in 41% of patients. If patients with elevated lipase develop abdominal pain/symptoms, stop drug and evaluate for pancreatitis. Monitor serum lipase every 2 weeks for the first 2 months and then monthly thereafter, or as clinically indicated. Consider additional monitoring in patients with a history of pancreatitis or alcohol abuse. Interrupt or dose-reduce as needed. Do not consider resuming ponatinib until complete resolution of symptoms and serum lipase is < 1.5 × ULN.

- Neuropathy: peripheral neuropathy occurred in 13% of patients (2% grade 3–4) characterized by paresthesia, hypoesthesia, hyperesthesia. Cranial neuropathy developed in 1% of patients (< 1% grade 3–4). Neuropathy occurred during the first month of therapy in 31%. Monitor for symptoms of neuropathy (e.g., hypoesthesia, hyperesthesia, paresthesia, discomfort, burning sensation, neuropathic pain, or weakness). Consider drug interruption and evaluation of suspected neuropathy.

- Ocular toxicity: ocular toxicities leading to blindness or blurred vision have occurred. Retinal toxicities (3% incidence): macular edema, retinal vein occlusion, retinal hemorrhage. 13% of patients developed conjunctival or corneal irritation, dry eye, or eye pain. 6% developed visual blurring. Other toxicities reported: cataracts, glaucoma, iritis, iridocyclitis, and ulcerative keratitis. Perform comprehensive eye exam at baseline, then periodically during treatment.

- Hemorrhage occurred in 24% of patients (serious in 5%); most hemorrhagic events occurred in patients with grade 4 thrombocytopenia. Interrupt drug for serious or severe hemorrhage and evaluate.

- Fluid retention can occur and is serious in 3% of patients. Most commonly, peripheral edema occurred in 16%, pleural effusion in 7%, and pericardial effusions in 3%. Once case of brain edema was fatal. Monitor for fluid retention, manage patients clinically, and interrupt, dose-modify, or discontinue drug as clinically indicated.

- Compromised wound healing and GI perforation: interrupt drug at least 1 week prior to major surgery. Serious GI perforation (fistula) has occurred 38 days post-cholecystectomy.

- Tumor lysis syndrome (TLS) rarely occurred in patients with advanced disease (AP-CML, BP-CML, or Ph+ ALL). Hyperuricemia occurred in 7% of patients (majority CP-CML). In patients with advanced disease, ensure patient has adequate hydration and treat high uric acid prior to starting ponatinib.

- Embryo-fetal toxicity: Advise women of reproductive potential to use effective contraception to avoid pregnancy. If drug is used during pregnancy, or if the patient becomes pregnant while taking the drug, apprise the patient that the drug can cause fetal harm.

- Most common (≥ 20%) side effects were HTN, rash, abdominal pain, fatigue, headache, dry skin, constipation, arthralgia, nausea, and pyrexia. Hematologic adverse effects included thrombocytopenia, anemia, neutropenia, lymphopenia, and leukopenia.

• Patient teaching key points: Teach patients to contact their physician right away for symptoms suggestive of (1) a blood clot (e.g., chest pain, SOB, weakness on one side of the body, speech problems, leg pain, or swelling); (2) CHF or arrythmias (e.g., SOB, chest pain, palpitations, dizziness, or fainting); (3) hepatotoxicity (e.g., yellowing of the eyes or skin, "tea-colored" urine, drowsiness); (4) new or worsening of existing HTN (e.g., headache, dizziness, chest pain, SOB); (5) pancreatitis (e.g., new onset or worsening nausea, vomiting, abdominal pain, or discomfort); (6) neuropathy (e.g., decreased sensation (hypoesthesia), increased sensation (hyperesthesia), "pins and needles" sensation in fingertips/toes, which progresses in a stocking-glove pattern (paresthesias), discomfort, burning, neuropathic pain, or weakness; (7) ocular toxicity (e.g., blurred vision, dry eye, eye pain); (8) hemorrhage (e.g., unusual bleeding or easy bruising); (9) fluid retention (e.g., leg swelling, abdominal swelling, weight gain, SOB); (10) low blood counts (e.g., fever, signs/symptoms of infection). Teach patients to notify their doctor if they are planning to have a surgical procedure or had recent surgery, as drug may interfere with wound healing. Teach female patients of reproductive potential to use effective contraception to avoid pregnancy, as drug can cause embryo-fetal toxicity.

Potential Toxicities/Side Effects and the Nursing Process

I. POTENTIAL FOR INFECTION, BLEEDING, AND FATIGUE, related to BONE MARROW SUPPRESSION

Defining Characteristics: Myelosuppression is common in all patients. Grade 3–4 thrombocytopenia occurred in 36–57% of patients, and grades 3–4 neutropenia occurred in 24–63% of patients. Febrile neutropenia occurred rarely (1–25%, depending upon state of disease). Sepsis occurred in 1–22% (highest in patients with Ph+ ALL). Most common infections were pneumonia (3–13%), UTI (7–12%), URIs (1–11%), nasopharyngitis (0–12%), and cellulitis (0–11%). Anemia occurred in 9–55% of patients. Fatigue and asthenia occurred in 3–39% of patients.

Nursing Implications: Monitor CBC differential, platelet count every two weeks for first three months, then monthly or as clinically indicated. Teach patients to report signs/symptoms of infection (e.g., fever > 100.4°F, sore throat, sputum production, difficulty breathing, dysuria) or bleeding. Teach patients to avoid OTC aspirin, NSAIDs, preparations containing aspirin or NSAIDs, or other drugs that increase the risk of bleeding. Teach patient energy conservation strategies, organization of activities to reduce fatigue, and gentle exercises.

II. ALTERATION IN NUTRITION, POTENTIAL, related to NAUSEA, VOMITING, DIARRHEA, CONSTIPATION, MUCOSITIS, RARE GI HEMORRHAGE, HEPATOTOXICITY

Defining Characteristics: Constipation occurs in 2–47% of patients, diarrhea in 1–26% of patients, nausea 1–32%, vomiting 2–24% of patients, oral mucositis in 1–23%. GI hemorrhage occurred in 11-21% of patients, decreased appetite 8–31%, and 8–31% weight loss. LFTs are abnormal in many patients: increased AST (41%), ALT (53%), bilirubin (19%), increased alkaline phosphatase (37%), decreased albumin (28%). Other laboratory abnormalities: increased glucose (58%), decreased phosphorus (57%), decreased calcium (52%), increased lipase (41%), decreased sodium (29%), decreased glucose (24%), potassium decreased (16%), potassium increased (15%), sodium increased (10%), bicarbonate decreased (11%), increased creatinine (7%), increased calcium (5%), triglycerides (3%), increased amylase (3%).

Nursing Implications: Assess nutritional status baseline and at each visit. Assess laboratory results, especially LFTs (baseline and at least monthly). Monitor lipase every two weeks for the first two months, then monthly or as clinically indicated. Discuss abnormalities with physician, NP, or PA, and understand dose interruption or modification based on prescribing information. Teach patient that nutritional impact symptoms may occur and to report them. Discuss with patient self-care management strategies to manage nausea, vomiting, diarrhea, and mucositis if they occur. Teach patient systematic oral cleansing after meals and at bedtime and to report any sores or pain. Discuss dietary modifications as needed. If patient develops persistent diarrhea, discuss with physician, NP/PA; lab assessment of serum potassium and need for repletion, as well as hydration. Discuss pharmacologic management of symptoms as needed. Teach patient to report right away or to call 911 for severe abdominal pain or GI bleeding.

III.   POTENTIAL ALTERATIONS IN CIRCULATION related to HTN, HEMORRHAGE, CHF, ARTERIAL, AND VENOUS THROMBOEMBOLISM

Defining Characteristics: HTN is a class-related effect of antiangiogenesis agents. Treatment emergent HTN occurred in 67% of ponatinib-treated patients. 2% in clinical trials had symptomatic HTN, such as hypertensive crisis. Patients may require urgent clinical intervention for HTN-associated confusion, headache, chest pain, shortness of breath. Of patients with baseline BP WNL (SBP < 140, DBP < 90 mm Hg), 78% developed treatment-emergent HTN: 49% had Stage 1 (SBP ≥, or DBP ≥ 90 mm Hg), 29% developed Stage 2 HTN (SBP ≥ 160 mm Hg, or DBP ≥ 100 mm Hg). Of patients with Stage 1 HTN at baseline, 61% developed Stage 2 HTN.

Arterial occlusion and thrombosis occurred in at least 20% of patients, and some experienced more than one type. Patients have required revascularization procedures. Cardiac vascular occlusion, such as MI, and coronary artery occlusion occurred in 12%, with or without CHF. Cerebrovascular occlusion, including fatal stroke, occurred in 6%; drug can cause stenosis over multiple segments in major arterial vessels supplying the brain (e.g., carotid, vertebral, middle cerebral arteries). Peripheral arterial occlusive events occurred in 8%, and included fatal mesenteric artery occlusion and life-threatening peripheral artery disease. Patients have developed digital or distal extremity necrosis, requiring amputation. Venous thromboembolism (VTE) occurred in 5% of ponatinib-treated patients and included DVT, PE, superficial thrombophlebitis, and retinal vein thrombosis.

Fatal and serious heart failure or left ventricular dysfunction occurred in 5% of patients. Rarely, arrhythmias may occur: bradycardia (occurred in 1% of patients, e.g., complete heart block requiring pacemaker, sick sinus syndrome, atrial fibrillation with bradycardia and pauses) or supraventricular tachyarrhythmias (occurred in 5%, atrial fibrillation was the most common, with other patients developing atrial flutter, supraventricular tachycardia, or atrial tachycardia). Hemorrhage occurs in about 2–11% of patients, most commonly in patients with grade 3–4 thrombocytopenia.

Nursing Implications: Assess baseline BP, cardiac status, and risk for bleeding baseline and during treatment. Assess BP frequently if elevated, and teach patient to monitor at home as appropriate. If BP elevated, the patient should receive antihypertensive therapy, and if difficult to control, the drug should be stopped until the BP is well controlled. If BP is not able to be medically controlled, ponatinib should be interrupted, dose-reduced, or stopped. Monitor patients for signs/symptoms of heart failure, and discuss treatment with physician, including interruption of ponatinib. If heart failure is serious, drug discontinuation must be considered. Teach patient to report right away (1) severe headaches, (2) light-headedness, dizziness or fainting, (3) changes in vision or eye pain, (4) changes in breathing, (5) chest discomfort, (6) onset of chest pain, (7) pain in the leg or leg swelling, (8) weakness on one side of the body, (9) speech problems, (10) changes in skin color of temperature of fingers or toes, and (11) palpitations, dizziness. Anticipate performing ECG if patient reports chest pain, new onset SOB, or symptoms suggesting fast or slow heartbeat. Discuss treatment emergently with physician or NP/PA.

IV.   ALTERATION IN ACTIVITY AND COMFORT related to FLUID RETENTION, HEADACHE, FEVER, PAIN, DYSPHONIA, RASH

Defining Characteristics: Fluid retention occurred in 23% of patients receiving ponatinib and was serious in 3% of patients (e.g., brain edema that was fatal, pericardial effusion, pleural effusion, ascites). The most common fluid retention events were peripheral edema (16%), pleural effusion (7%), and pericardial effusion (3%). Rash occurred in 34–54% of patients, arthralgias in 1–26%, myalgias in 0–22%, pain in 1–15%, and muscle spasms in 0–13% of patients. Headache occurred in 3–39% of patients.

Nursing Implications: Assess patient weight, skin turgor, baseline and at each visit for evidence of peripheral edema, and teach patients to self-assess for the development of swelling of feet or hands, or any changes in breathing and to report findings. If peripheral edema develops, teach patient to do daily weight tracking and to report any increases. Teach patient to report any changes in breathing right away. Discuss drug interruption, dose reduction, or discontinuance. Assess skin integrity and presence of rash baseline, and at each visit; teach patient that rash may occur and to report it. Assess rash and discuss management with physician, NP, or PA. Teach patient that arthralgias, myalgias, headache, or other symptoms may occur, and discuss self-care strategies to manage them. If they persist, discuss pharmacologic management with physician, NP, or PA.

Drug: ramucirumab injection (Cyramza)

Class: Recombinant human, IgG_1 monoclonal antibody targeted against vascular endothelial growth factor receptor 2 (VEGFR2); angiogenesis inhibitor.

Mechanism of Action: Binds to the VEGF receptor 2 (VEGFR2), as opposed to bevacizumab, which targets the ligand VEGF. Thus, it prevents binding of the ligand VEGF to the receptor, prevents VEGF receptor activation, and subsequent proliferation and migration of endothelial cells to form tumor blood vessels (angiogenesis).

Metabolism: Unknown.

Indication: Ramucirumab is indicated as a single agent for the treatment of patients with advanced or metastatic gastric or gastro-esophageal junction adenocarcinoma with disease progression on or after prior fluoropyrimidine- or platinum-containing chemotherapy.

Dosage/Range: 8 mg/kg IV every 2 weeks, as an IV infusion over 60 minutes. Continue drug until disease progression or unacceptable toxicity.

Dose Modifications:
- Infusion reactions: Grade 1–2: reduce infusion rate by 50%; grade 3–4: permanently discontinue drug.
- Hypertension (HTN): Interrupt drug for severe HTN until controlled with antihypertensive therapy. Permanently discontinue drug for severe HTN that cannot be controlled with antihypertensive therapy.
- Proteinuria: Assess dipstick/urinalysis before each treatment and if 2+ or greater protein, assess 24-hour urine protein.
  - Interrupt drug for urine protein level ≥ 2 g/24 hr. When urine protein < 2 g/24 hr, reinitiate drug at a reduced dose of 6 mg/kg for gastric and mCRC patients (8 mg/kg for NSCLC patients) every 2 weeks. If protein level ≥ 2 g/24 hr happens again, interrupt drug, and when urine protein is < 2 g/24 hr, reinitiate drug at a further reduced dose of 5 mg/kg for gastric patients (6 mg/kg for NSCLC patients) every 2 weeks.
  - Permanently discontinue drug if urine protein level > 3 g/24 hr or if patient develops nephrotic syndrome.
- Wound healing complications: Interrupt drug prior to scheduled surgery and until the surgical wound is fully healed.
- Arterial thrombotic events, GI perforation, or grade 3–4 bleeding: Permanently discontinue drug.

Drug Preparation:
- Available in 100-mg/10mL or 500-mg/50 mL in a concentration of 10-mg/m, as single-dose vials.
- Inspect vials and ensure no particulate matter or discoloration prior to use.
- Calculate dose and aseptically withdraw ordered amount. Further dilute in 0.9% sodium chloride to make a final volume of 250 mL. Do not use dextrose solutions. Gently invert

to mix, and do not shake or freeze. Do not dilute with other solutions or add anything or coinfuse with electrolytes or medications.

* Store diluted infusion bag at 2–8°C (36–46°F) for up to 24 hours, or 4 hours at room temperature (below 25°C [77°F]).
* Discard any unused drug in the vial.

Drug Administration:
* Assess BP and urine for protein (1+ or greater by dipstick/urinalysis), and monitor prior to each treatment. Discuss any abnormalities with the physician. Patients with 2+ or higher proteinuria by urine dipstick/urinalysis should be asked to collect a 24-hour urine sample for protein. Drug should be held for proteinuria ≥ 2 g/24 h, and resume when proteinuria < 2 g/24 h. Monitor patients closely if moderate to severe proteinuria until improved or resolved. Drug should be discontinued if the patient develops nephrotic syndrome or urine protein > 3 g/24 hours.
* Visually inspect infusion bag for particulate matter and discoloration; if found, discard solution.
* Premedicate with an IV histamine H1 antagonist (e.g., diphenhydramine). If the patient has had a prior grade 1–2 infusion reaction, add dexamethasone and acetaminophen to the premedications given.
* Infuse drug over 60 minutes via an infusion pump, through a separate line. Do not give IVP or IVB.
* Use of a protein-sparing 0.22 micron filter is recommended.
* Flush with sterile 0.9% sodium chloride for injection at the end of the infusion.

Drug Interactions:
* No studies have been done. Ramucirumab is incompatible with dextrose solutions.

Lab Effects/Interference:
* Serum hyponatremia; urine proteinemia.
* Anemia.

Special Considerations:
* Ramucirumab was FDA-approved through a Priority Review program. In the phase III REGARD trial, patients receiving the drug had a median overall survival of 5.2 mo vs patients in the placebo plus Best Supportive Care (BSC) group of 3.8 mo (p = 0.0473), and treatment with ramucirumab correlated with an increase in median progression-free survival (p < 0.0001). While 6-mo survival was 42% in the ramucirumab group and 32% in the placebo-plus-BSC group, 12 mo survival was 18% in the ramucirumab group vs 12% in placebo-plus-BSC group (Fuchs et al., 2014).
* Infusion reactions occurred in 16% of patients across clinical trials, before premedication became standard. The infusion reactions generally occurred during or after a first or second infusion. Symptoms included rigors/tremors, back pain/spasms, chest pain/tightness, chills, flushing, dyspnea, wheezing, hypoxia, paresthesia. Rarely, in severe cases, bronchospasm, supraventricular tachycardia, and hypotension occurred. Always premedicate patients, and monitor patients during infusion. Ensure that resuscitation

equipment and oxygen are nearby. Permanently discontinue ramucirumab if grade 3 or 4 infusion reactions occur.

- Patients with Child-Pugh Class B or C cirrhosis: New or worsening encephalopathy, ascites, or hepatorenal syndromes. Risk vs potential benefit should be discussed with the patient, and ramucirumab given only if potential benefits outweigh risks.
- Most common adverse effects:
  - As a single agent (≥ 1% incidence and ≥ 2% higher than placebo): HTN, diarrhea.
  - Together with paclitaxel (≥ 30% incidence): fatigue, neutropenia, diarrhea, epistaxis.
  - Together with docetaxel (≥ 30% incidence): neutropenia, fatigue/asthenia, stomatitis/mucosal inflammation.
  - Together with FOLFIRI (≥ 30% incidence): diarrhea, neutropenia, decreased appetite, epistaxis, stomatitis.
- Ramucirumab was associated with increased risk of side effects due to antiangiogenic class.
  - Hemorrhage, which may be severe and fatal. Incidence in one gastric cancer study was 3.4% versus 2.6% in the placebo-controlled arm. In the NSCLC trial, the incidence was 2.4% for the ramucirumab group compared to 2.3% in the control group. Teach patients to report bleeding or lightheadedness right away. Drug should be permanently discontinued in patients with severe bleeding.
  - Arterial embolic events (ATE) (including MI, cardiac arrest, CVA, cerebral ischemia) occurred in 1.7% of patients in clinical trials: ramucirumab should be permanently discontinued in patients who experience a severe ATE.
  - HTN: Incidence was 8% vs 3% in placebo patients. Control HTN prior to starting ramucirumab; monitor BP baseline and at least every 2 weeks during treatment. Interrupt drug for severe HTN until medically controlled. Permanently discontinue drug if medically significant HTN cannot be controlled with antihypertensive therapy, or if patient develops hypertensive crisis or hypertensive encephalopathy. Teach patient to report severe headache, lightheadedness, or neurologic symptoms right away.
  - GI perforations: Incidence was 0.7%. Permanently discontinue drug if this occurs. Teach patients to report severe diarrhea, vomiting, or severe abdominal pain right away and to come to the emergency department for evaluation.
  - Impaired wound healing: Drug has not been studied in patients with serious or non-healing wounds. Hold drug prior to surgery, and resume drug based on clinical judgment of adequate wound healing. Stop drug if a patient develops wound healing complications while receiving the drug, and resume when wound is fully healed. Teach patient not to undergo surgery without first discussing the risk of impaired wound healing with their healthcare provider.
  - Proteinuria: Occurred in 8% of patients receiving ramucirumab compared to 3% of patients receiving placebo. See Drug Modification and Administration. Drug should be held for proteinuria ≥ 2 g/24 h, and resume when proteinuria < 2 g/24 h. Drug should be discontinued if the patient develops nephrotic syndrome or urine protein > 3 g/24 hours.
- Warnings:
  - Hemorrhage: Increased risk of hemorrhage and GI hemorrhage, which may be severe and fatal. The drug should be permanently discontinued if severe bleeding occurs.

- GI perforation: Permanently discontinue the drug if it occurs.
- Impaired wound healing: Hold the drug prior to surgery, and discontinue it if the patient develops wound healing complications.
- Reversible posterior leukoencephalopathy syndrome (RPLS): May rarely (< 0.1%) occur. If RPLS is suspected, the diagnosis should be confirmed with MRI and the drug discontinued. In many cases, symptoms resolve or improve quickly. However, some patients may have ongoing neurologic problems or may die.
- Monitor thyroid function during therapy. In the mCRC patient study, 2.6% of patients receiving ramucirumab plus FOLFIRI developed hypothyroidism compared to 0.9% of patients receiving FOLFIRI alone.
- Counsel women of childbearing age to use highly effective contraception to avoid pregnancy during and for 3 months following last treatment dose. Antiangiogenic agents are teratogenic and fetotoxic. Drug may also impair fertility. Nursing mothers should decide between nursing and receiving the drug.

Potential Toxicities/Side Effects and the Nursing Process

I. POTENTIAL FOR INJURY related to INFUSION REACTION

Defining Characteristics: Incidence in clinical trials occurred prior to standardly prescribing premedications, and was 16%, including 2 severe events. Most infusion reactions occur during or after first or second drug infusion.

Nursing Implications: Ensure patient receives premedication with diphenhydramine as ordered, and if prior grade 1–2 infusion reactions, also administer dexamethasone and acetaminophen as ordered. Assess baseline VS and mental status prior to drug administration, at 15 minutes and periodically during infusion, as needed. Remain with patient during first 15 minutes of infusions. Signs and symptoms included rigors/tremors, back pain/spasms, chest pain/tightness, chills, flushing, dyspnea, wheezing, hypoxia, paresthesia. Rarely, in severe cases, bronchospasm, supraventricular tachycardia, and hypotension occurred. Recall signs/symptoms of infusion reactions; if these occur, stop drug immediately, notify physician, and assess patient's vital signs. If the infusion reaction is grade 1 or 2, infusion rate should be reduced by 50%. Drug should be permanently discontinued for grade 3–4. Review standing physician orders or nursing procedures for patient management of infusion reaction, and be prepared to stop drug immediately and change IV to a plain NS solution to keep vein patent; notify physician. Ensure oxygen and resuscitation equipment is nearby in infusion area. If severe, keep patent airway, monitor VS, and administer ordered medications, which may include epinephrine 1:1,000 IM in the thigh, IV hydrocortisone sodium succinate, and IV diphenhydramine. Teach patient to report any unusual symptoms.

II. POTENTIAL ALTERATION IN CIRCULATION related to HYPERTENSION

Defining Characteristics: Hypertension occurred in 8–16% of patients (8% grade 3–4) in clinical trials.

Nursing Implications: Assess baseline BP prior to administering first dose of ramucirumab, and at least every 2 weeks during treatment. If the patient has a history of hypertension, monitor BP more closely, although hypertension develops over time rather than during the drug infusion. Blood pressure should continue to be monitored after patient has stopped the drug. Teach patient drug administration, potential side effects, and self-care measures if prescribed antihypertensive medication, such as angiotensin-converting enzyme inhibitors, beta-blockers, diuretics, and calcium channel blockers. Ramucirumab should be temporarily suspended in patients with severe hypertension until BP can be controlled with medical management. Drug should be permanently discontinued if HTN cannot be controlled with antihypertensive therapy, the patient develops hypertensive crisis (diastolic blood pressure > 120 mm Hg), or develops hypertensive encephalopathy.

III.   ALTERATION IN NUTRITION, POTENTIAL, related to DIARRHEA, RARE RISK GI PERFORATION

Defining Characteristics: Diarrhea occurs in 14% of patients and was grade 3–4 in 1% of patients.

Nursing Implications: Assess baseline nutritional status and bowel elimination status. Teach patient that diarrhea may occur, and much more rarely, bowel perforation. Discuss with patient self-care strategies to manage diarrhea if it occurs. Teach patient that GI perforation may rarely occur, and to report and go to the emergency room right away if severe diarrhea, vomiting, and/or severe pain in the abdomen occurs.

Drug: regorafenib (Stivarga)

Class: Kinase inhibitor (multi-kinase inhibitor).

Mechanism of Action: Drug inhibits multiple receptor tyrosine kinases, and the serine/threonine-specific Raf kinase. This theoretically blocks angiogenesis and tumor microenvironment maintenance (inhibiting VEGFR2-TIE2, VEGFR3, PDGFR) and tumor cell proliferation (inhibiting RET, KIT, BRAF). KIT and PDGFR-α are important kinases that drive GastroIntestinal Stromal Tumor (GIST).

Metabolism: After oral dosing of 160 mg, peak plasma level is reached in a median of 4 hours. Tablets are 69% bioavailable compared to 83% when given as an oral solution. A high-fat meal increases the drug's mean AUC by 48% compared to the fasted state, while taken with a low-fat meal the AUC increases only 36%. Drug is highly protein-bound to plasma proteins (99.5%). Regorafenib is metabolized by CYP3A4 and UGT1A9 into the active metabolites M-2 and M-5, which are also highly protein-bound. The mean elimination half-life of regorafenib is 28 hours; the half-life of M-2 is 25 hours; and the half-life of M-5 is 51 hours. The drug is primarily excreted in the feces (71%), and less so in the urine (19%), with 90% of the drug eliminated in 12 days.

Indication: Treatment of patients with

- Metastatic CRC (mCRC), previously treated with fluoropyrimidine-, oxaliplatin-, and irinotecan-based chemotherapy, an anti-VEGF therapy, and if *KRAS*-wild type, an anti-EGFR therapy.
- Locally advanced unresectable or metastatic gastrointestinal stromal tumor (GIST), previously treated with imatinim mesylate and sunitinib maleate.

Dosage/Range:

- 160 mg (four 40-mg tablets) orally once daily, for the first 21 days of a 28-day cycle.
- Do not begin regorafenib unless BP is adequately controlled.

Dose Modifications:

- Dose-reduce drug to 120 mg for:
  - First occurrence of grade 2 Hand-Foot Skin Reaction (HFSR), palmar-plantar erythrodysesthesia, PPE, of any duration.
  - After recovery of any grade 3 or 4 adverse reaction.
  - Grade 3 AST/ALT elevation; resume only if the potential benefit outweighs the risk of hepatotoxicity.
- Interrupt drug for:
  - NCI CTCAE grade 2 HFSR that is recurrent or does not improve within 7 days despite dose reduction; grade 3 HFSR: interrupt drug for a minimum of 7 days.
  - Symptomatic grade 2 HTN.
  - Any grade 3 or 4 adverse reaction.
- Dose-reduce regorafenib to 120 mg.
  - First occurrence of grade 2 HFSR of any duration.
  - After recovery of any grade 3 or 4 adverse reaction.
  - Grade 3 ALT/AST elevation; resume only if the potential benefit outweights the risk of hepatotoxicity.
- Dose-reduce regorafenib to 80 mg:
  - For any recurrence of grade 2 HFSR at the 120-mg dose.
  - After recovery of any grade 3 or 4 adverse reaction at the 120-mg dose (except hepatotoxicity).
- Discontinue drug permanently for:
  - Failure to tolerate 80-mg dose.
  - Any occurrence of AST or ALT > 20 × ULN.
  - Any occurrence of AST or ALT > 3 × ULN with concurrent bilirubin > 2 × ULN.
  - Reoccurrence of AST or ALT > 5 × ULN, despite dose reduction to 120 mg.
  - For any grade 4 adverse reaction; only resume if the potential benefit outweighs the risks.
- Stop drug before surgery, and resume after wound healing. Discontinue drug for wound dehiscence.
- HTN: temporarily or permanently discontinue drug for severe or uncontrolled HTN.
- Hold drug for new or acute cardiac ischemia/infarction and resume only after resolution of acute ischemic events.
- Discontinue drug if reversible posterior leukoencephalopathy syndrome (RPLS) occurs.
- Discontinue drug if GI perforation or fistulae develop.

Drug Preparation:
- None, oral. Available in 40-mg film-coated tablets. Tablets should be kept in the bottle, not put into daily or weekly pill boxes, and any remaining tablets should be discarded 28 days after opening the bottle. The bottle should be kept tightly closed.

Drug Administration:
- Teach the patient to take with a low-fat breakfast (food), and at the same time every day.
- Example: 2 slices white toast with 1 T low-fat margarine and 1 T jelly, 8 oz skim milk (319 calories and 8.2 g fat); or 1 c cereal, 8 oz skim milk, 1 slice toast with jam, apple juice, and 1 cup of coffee or tea (520 calories, 2 g fat).
- Inform patients to take any missed doses on the same day, as soon as they remember, and that they must not take two doses on the same day to make up for a dose missed on the previous day.
- Monitor BP weekly for the first 6 weeks of treatment, then every cycle, or more frequently, as indicated.

Drug Interactions:
- Strong CYP3A4 inducers (e.g., carbamazepine, phenytoin, phenobarbital, rifampin, St. John's wort): decreased serum levels of regorafenib but increased mean exposure of M-5 metabolite; avoid concomitant use.
- Strong CYP3A4 inhibitors (e.g., clarithromycin, grapefruit or grapefruit juice, itraconazole, ketoconazole, posaconazole, telithromycin, voriconazole): increased mean regorafenib serum level, and decreased exposure of metabolites M-2 and M-5. Avoid concomitant administration.

Lab Effects:
- Increased AST (65%), ALT (45%), bilirubin (45%).
- Anemia (79%), thrombocytopenia (41%), lymphopenia (54%), neutropenia (3%).
- Hypocalcemia (59%), hypokalemia (26%), hyponatremia (30%), hypophosphatemia (57%).
- Increased INR (24%), lipase (46%), amylase (26%).

Special Considerations:
- Severe and sometimes fatal hepatotoxicity occurred in clinical trials. Liver biopsies, when done, showed hepatocyte necrosis with lymphocyte infiltration. In Study 1, all the patients who developed liver failure had liver metastases.
  - Monitor LFTs baseline prior to starting therapy, and at least every two weeks for the first two months of treatment. Monitor LFTs monthly thereafter or more frequently as indicated.
  - If the patient develops increased LFTs, monitor LFTs weekly until improved to < 3 × ULN or baseline.
  - Temporarily hold and then dose-reduce or permanently discontinue regorafenib, depending upon severity and persistence.
- Hemorrhage may rarely occur; discontinue drug if severe hemorrhage occurs. Incidence overall was 21% in Study 1 and 11% in Study 2 (vs 8% and 3% in placebo arm). Permanently discontinue drug in patients with severe or life-threatening hemorrhage. Monitor INR levels more frequently in patients receiving warfarin, as INR may become excessively elevated.

- Dermatological toxicity: Increased incidence of toxicity in skin and subcutaneous tissues occurred (72%–78% vs 24% in Studies 1 and 2), including HFSR, and severe rash requiring dose modification.
  - HFSR incidence 45%–67%, appearing first cycle of treatment.
  - Incidence of grade 3 HFSR was 17%–22%, grade 3 rash 6–7%; Stevens-Johnson syndrome occurred in 0.2%, erythema multiforme in 0.2%, and toxic epidermal necrolysis in 0.1%.
  - Hold drug, reduce the dose, or permanently discontinue drug depending upon severity and persistence of dermatologic toxicity.
- HTN: Incidence was 30%–59% in Studies 1 and 2. Hypertensive crisis occurred in 0.25% across all clinical trials. Onset of HTN was within the first cycle of therapy.
  - Do not start regorafenib therapy until BP is well-controlled.
  - Monitor BP weekly for the first 6 weeks of treatment, then every cycle, or more frequently as indicated.
  - Temporarily or permanently withhold drug for severe or uncontrolled HTN.
- Cardiac ischemia and infarction occurred more frequently than in placebo (1.2% vs 0.4%, Study 1). Hold drug in patients that develop new or acute onset cardiac ischemia or infarction. Resume regorafenib only after resolution of acute cardiac ischemic events if the potential benefits outweigh the risks of further cardiac ischemia.
- Reversible posterior leukoencephalopathy syndrome (RPLS) may occur. It is a syndrome of subcortical vasogenic edema, diagnosed by MRI. If a patient presents with seizures, headache, visual disturbances, confusion, or altered mental function, discuss patient evaluation for RPLS with physician. Drug should be discontinued if the diagnosis of RPLS is confirmed.
- GI perforation or fistula occurred in 0.6% of patients across all clinical trials. Permanently discontinue drug if either of these events occur.
- Wound-healing complications: no studies have been conducted, but VEGFR inhibitors can impair wound healing. Stop drug at least 2 weeks prior to scheduled surgery. Resumption of drug after surgery should be based on adequate wound healing. Discontinue the drug if wound dehiscence occurs.
- Drug is embryo-fetal toxic. Counsel women of childbearing potential and men to avoid pregnancy, and to use highly effective contraception during therapy and for two months after drug is discontinued. If the drug is used in pregnancy, or if the patient becomes pregnant while receiving the drug, the patient should be apprised of the potential hazard to the fetus. Nursing mothers should make a decision to discontinue nursing or to discontinue the drug, taking into account the importance of the drug to the patient's health.
- Most common side effects (≥ 20%) are asthenia/fatigue, hand-foot skin reaction (HFSR), diarrhea, decreased appetite/food intake, HTN, mucositis, dysphonia, infection, pain, decreased weight, GI and abdominal pain, rash, fever, nausea.
- In the CORRECT study, patients with advanced mCRC who had progressed on all other standard therapies were randomized to receive regorafenib or placebo. Those in the regorafenib arm had improved OS (6.4 mo vs 5 mo control). Disease control rate was 44% compared to 15% in the placebo group. Drug appears to be more effective in stabilizing disease and delaying progression than marked tumor shrinkage (Grothey et al., 2012).

- In the GRID study, patients with advanced GIST who had progressed after imatinib and sunitinib therapy had significantly greater PFS (60% at 3 mo, 38% at 6 mo, compared to 11% and 0% in the control arm). Disease control for patients in the regorafenib arm was 4.8 mo compared to 0.9 mo (p < 0.001) in the control arm (Demetri et al., 2012).

Potential Toxicities/Side Effects and the Nursing Process

I.   ALTERATION IN NUTRITION, POTENTIAL, related to NAUSEA, VOMITING, DIARRHEA, MUCOSITIS, HYPOTHYROIDISM, HEPATOTOXICITY, POSSIBLE GI PERFORATION OR FISTULA

Defining Characteristics: Diarrhea occurs in 47% of patients, mucositis in 40%, nausea 20%, and vomiting 17% of patients. Hypothyroidism affects 18%, and decreased appetite and food intake 31%. Weight loss occurred in 14% of patients. LFTs are abnormal in many patients: Increased AST (65%), ALT (45%), bilirubin (45%), and INR is increased in 14% of patients. Hypokalemia occurs in 26% of patients. GI perforation or fistula is rare (0.6–2.1%).

Nursing Implications: Assess baseline nutritional status, lab findings especially LFTs (transaminases and bilirubin) and serum potassium. LFTs should be assessed at least every two weeks during the first two months of treatment, then monthly or more frequently as needed. Discuss abnormalities with physician, NP, or PA, and understand dose interruption or modifications per prescribing information (see Dose Modifications above). Teach patient that nutritional impact symptoms may occur and to report them. Discuss with patient self-care strategies to manage nausea, vomiting, diarrhea, and mucositis if they occur. Teach patient systematic oral cleansing after meals and at bedtime, and to report any sores or pain. Discuss dietary modifications to minimize symptoms experienced. If patient has diarrhea that persists, discuss with physician, NP, or PA the need for lab testing of serum potassium, as well as replacement therapy and hydration. If symptoms persist, discuss pharmacological management with physician, NP, or PA. Although rare, GI perforation or fistula may occur. Teach patient to come to the emergency room and to report severe pain in the abdomen, swelling in the abdomen, and high fever right away.

II.   POTENTIAL ALTERATION IN CIRCULATION related to HYPERTENSION, HEMORRHAGE, CHF

Defining Characteristics: HTN is a class-related side effect of antiangiogenesis agents. As the kidney is made up of many capillaries, there may be protein leakage (proteinuria). HTN occurs in 59% of patients, and is grade 3 or higher in 28%. Proteinuria occurs in 60% of patients. Hemorrhage occurs in about 11% of patients and is severe in 4%, affecting respiratory, GI, and genitourinary tracts. Rarely, patients receiving regorafenib had increased risk of myocardial ischemia and MI (1.2% vs 0.04% in controls).

Nursing Implications: Assess baseline BP, cardiac status, and risk for bleeding baseline and during treatment. Patient should have BP assessed weekly for the first 6 weeks, then checked regularly. If elevated, the patient should receive antihypertensives, and the drug should be stopped until the BP is well controlled. Assess urine protein, and if 2+ or greater, discuss obtaining 24-hour urine for protein with provider. Usually drug is held for urine protein > 2 g/24 hours, and resumed after the urine protein is less than that. Teach patient to report severe headaches, light-headedness, or changes in vision. Teach patient to report any changes in breathing, chest discomfort, or the onset of chest pain. Discuss with provider need for ECG, and be prepared to obtain the ECG. Hold drug in patients who develop new or acute onset cardiac ischemia or infarction. Assess platelet count, and INR in patients receiving warfarin. Teach patient to report any signs/symptoms of bleeding. Monitor INR levels closely in patients receiving warfarin, and dose based on INR per physician, NP, or PA. Regorafenib should be discontinued in patients with severe hemorrhage.

III.   ALTERATION IN SKIN INTEGRITY AND COMFORT related to HAND-FOOT SKIN REACTION (HFSR), RASH

Defining Characteristics: Drug causes skin and subcutaneous tissue reactions including HFSR, also known as palmar-plantar erythrodysesthesia (PPE), and severe rash, which require dose modifications. The incidence of HFSR in clinical trials was 45%, with grade 3–4 HFSR occurring in 17–21% of patients in clinical trials. Rash affected 26% of patients, in which 6% were grade 3 or 4. HFSR may involve palms of hands, soles of feet, and other areas that are exposed to friction, such as knees when chronically rubbing together (e.g., in a wheelchair) Most cases appeared during the first treatment cycle, and patients often present with painful blisters, which over weeks to months are replaced by thick, hyperkeratotic areas similar to calluses (Lacouture, 2011). Rash may be severe, and rarely erythema multiforme, Stevens-Johnson syndrome, and toxic epidermal necrolysis have occurred.

Nursing Implications: Assess baseline skin integrity, including soles of feet and palms of hands, and teach patient that these symptoms may occur and to report them. If patient has calluses, they should be trimmed or removed. Teach patient to (1) self-assess for erythema, swelling, blisters, and pain on skin surfaces, and to report them; (2) avoid activities that increase blood flow to the hands and feet, such as hot showers and baths, and to take tepid baths and showers; (3) avoid constrictive clothing and repetitive movements that can irritate the opposing skin; (4) use skin emollients to prevent skin from drying and cracking starting on day 1 of therapy, and to use lotion and therapeutic socks (available from the drug manufacturer) until the lotion is absorbed; (5) elevate hands and feet when sitting down and to apply cool compresses to hands or feet if swollen; (6) gently pat skin dry after bathing and use mild soap. Assess grade of HFSR and teach patient to stop using drug and to call provider if pain is felt, as this may mean drug therapy should be interrupted. See Dose Modifications.

IV.   POTENTIAL FOR INFECTION related to LYMPHOPENIA

Defining Characteristics: Lymphopenia occurred in 54% of patients in clinical trials, and neutropenia in 3%. Infection occurred in 31% of patients, was grade 3 or higher in 9% of patients, and fever occurred in 28% of patients.

Nursing Implications: Assess patient's CBC/differential baseline and during treatment. Teach patient strategies to avoid infection and self-assessment for signs/symptoms of infection, as well as to report signs/symptoms of infection (e.g., T > 100.4°F, productive cough, dysuria, dyspnea). Assess patient for presence of intact mucous membranes and skin, as these are portals for infection.

V.   ALTERATION IN ACTIVITY AND COMFORT related to ASTHENIA, HEADACHE, FEVER, PAIN, DYSPHONIA

Defining Characteristics: Asthenia/fatigue occurred in some patients during clinical trials, and was grade 3 or higher in some patients. Pain occurred in some and fever in others. Anemia occurred in some patients, and was grade 3 or higher in a few patients. Headache occurred in some and dysphonia in some patients.

Nursing Implications: Teach patient that these symptoms may occur and how to manage them, such as alternating rest and activity, energy- conserving measures, gentle exercise. If symptoms persist, discuss prescription pharmacologic management with physician, NP, or PA.

Drug: rituximab (Rituxan)

Class: Monoclonal antibody (anti-CD20 antibody).

Mechanism of Action: Anti-CD20 antibody that is genetically engineered (chimeric monoclonal antibody, or part mouse/part human) directed against the CD20 antigen found on the surface of normal and malignant B-cell lymphocytes. The CD20 antigen is also present (expressed) on more than 90% of B-cell non-Hodgkin's lymphoma (NHL) cells, but fortunately is not found on normal bone marrow stem cells, pre-B cells, normal plasma cells, or other normal tissues. A section of the rituximab (Fab domain), CD20 binds to the CD20 antigen on B lymphocytes; another section of the rituximab (Fc domain) calls together other immune effectors, resulting in lysis of the B lymphocyte.

Metabolism: Serum and half-life of drug vary with dose and sequence, and at 375 mg/m^2, the median serum half-life was 76.3 hours after the first infusion, as compared to 205 hours after the fourth infusion. Drug was detected in patient serum up to 3–6 months after completion of treatment.

Indications: The treatment of patients with
• **NHL:** (1) relapsed or refractory, low-grade or follicular, CD-20 positive, B-cell NHL as a single agent; (2) previously untreated follicular, CD-20 positive, B-cell NHL in combination with first-line chemotherapy and, in patients achieving a complete or partial response to rituximab in combination with chemotherapy, as single-agent maintenance therapy; (3) nonprogressing (including stable disease), low-grade, CD-20 positive B-cell NHL as a single agent after first-line CVP chemotherapy; (4) previously untreated diffuse large

B-cell, CD-20 positive NHL, in combination with CHOP or other anthracycline-based chemotherapy regimens.
- **CLL** in combination with fludarabine and cyclophosphamide (FC) for the treatment of patients with previously untreated or treated CD20-positive CLL.
- **RA,** in adult patients with moderately-to-severely active rheumatoid arthritis (RA) who have had an inadequate response to one or more TNF antagonist therapies.
- **Granulomatosis with Polyangiitis (GPA) (Wegener's Granulomatosis, (WG)),** in adult patients in combination with glucocorticoids for the treatment of GPA (WG) and microscopic polyangiitis (MPA).
- **Rituximab** is not recommended for use in patients with severe, active infections.

Dosage/Range:
- Premedications:
  - Premedicate before each infusion with acetaminophen and an antihistamine. For patients receiving rituximab infusion over 90 minutes, administer glucocorticoid prior to infusion.
  - For RA (rheumatoid arthritis) patients, methylprednisolone 100 mg IV or its equivalent is recommended 30 minutes prior to each infusion.
  - Pneumocystis jiroveci pneumonia (PCP) and antiherpetic viral prophylaxis is recommended for patients with CLL during treatment and for up to 12 months following treatment, as appropriate.
  - Pneumocystis jiroveci pneumonia (PCP) prophylaxis is recommended for patients with GPA and MPA during treatment and for 6 months following last rituximab infusion.

NHL: 375 mg/m^2 IV infusion:
- Relapsed or refractory, low-grade or follicular, CD20-positive, B-cell NHL.
  - 375 mg/m^2 given as IV infusion weekly for 4 or 8 doses.
  - Retreatment for relapsed or refractory, low-grade or follicular, CD-20 positive B-cell NHL: Administer once weekly for 4 doses in responding patients who develop progressive disease after previous rituximab therapy.
- Previously untreated, follicular, CD20-positive, B-cell NHL.
  - 375 mg/m^2 IV infusion day 1 of each cycle of chemotherapy for up to 8 doses.
  - If complete or partial response, start rituximab maintenance therapy 8 weeks following completion of rituximab in combination with chemotherapy. Administer rituximab as a single agent every 8 weeks for 12 doses.
- Nonprogressing, low-grade, CD20-positive, B-cell NHL after first-line CVP chemotherapy.
  - Following completion of 6–8 cycles of CVP chemotherapy, administer rituximab 375 mg/m^2 IV infusion, once weekly for 4 doses every 6 months for up to 16 doses.
- Diffuse large B-cell NHL (DLBCL) in combination with chemotherapy.
  - 375 mg/m^2 IV infusion day 1 of each cycle of chemotherapy for up to 8 infusions.

Chronic lymphocytic leukemia (CLL): If patient is > 70 years of age, there is no benefit in adding rituximab to (FC).
- 375 mg/m^2 initially on the day prior to the start of FC chemotherapy, then 500 mg/m^2 IV on day 1 of cycles 2–6 administered every 28 days. Patient should also receive PCP

and antiherpetic viral prophylaxis during treatment and for up to 12 months following treatment, as needed.
- PCP and antiherpetic viral prophylaxis is recommended during treatment and for up to 12 months following treatment as needed.

As a component of Zevalin (ibritumomab tiuxetan) therapeutic regimen:
- Rituximab 250 mg/m² IV within 4 hours prior to the administration of Indium-111-(In-111-) Zevalin, and within 4 hours prior to the administration of Yttrium-90-(Y-90-) Zevalin.
- Administer rituximab and In-111-Zevalin 7-9 days prior to rituximab and Y-90-Zevalin. Refer to Zevalin package insert for full prescribing information regarding Zevalin therapeutic regimen.

Rheumatoid arthritis: Administer rituximab as two 1,000-mg **(NOT per meter squared)** IV infusions separated by 2 weeks (one course);
- Administer glucocorticoids (methylprednisolone 100 mg IV or equivalent) 30 minutes prior to each infusion to reduce incidence and severity of infusion reactions.
- Subsequent courses should be administered every 24 weeks or based on clinical evaluation, but not sooner than every 16 weeks.
- Rituximab is given in combination with methotrexate.
- Rituximab should not be used in RA patients who have not had an adequate response to one or more TNF antagonists.

Granulomatosis with polyangiitis (GPA, Wegener's granulomatosis or WG) and Microscopic Polyangiitis (MPA):
- 375 mg/m² IV once weekly for 4 weeks, together with glucocorticoid.
- Methylprednisolone 1,000 mg IV per day for 1–3 days, followed by oral prednisone 1 mg/kg/day (not to exceed 80 mg/day and tapered per clinical need) are recommended to treat severe vasculitis symptoms; this regimen should begin within 14 days prior to or with the initiation of rituximab and may continue during and after the 4-week course of rituximab treatment.
- PCP and antiherpetic viral prophylaxis is recommended during treatment and for at least 6 months following the last rituximab treatment.
- There is limited data on the safety and efficacy of subsequent courses of rituximab in patients with GPA and MPA.

Drug Preparation:
- Do not mix with or dilute with other drugs.
- Store at 2–8°C (36–46°F) and protect vials from direct sunlight.
- Available as 100-mg (10-mL) and 500-mg (50-mL) single-use preservative-free vials.
- Inspect for particulate matter and discoloration prior to administration. Do not use vial if particulates or discoloration is present.
- Aseptically withdraw the ordered dose and dilute to a final concentration of 1–4 mg/mL in an infusion bag of either 0.9% sodium chloride USP or 5% dextrose. Gently invert to mix, and inspect for presence of any particulate matter or discoloration. Discard any unused drug left in the vial.
- Drug is stable in infusion solution at 2–8°C (36–46°F) for 24 hours and at room temperature for another 24 hours.

Administration:
- DO NOT GIVE AS AN INTRAVENOUS PUSH OR BOLUS.
- Premedicate before each infusion with acetaminophen and an antihistamine.
- **First infusion**: Initiate infusion at a rate of 50 mg/hr; if no infusion-related problems occur, increase the infusion rate in 50-mg/hr increments every 30 minutes to a maximum of 400 mg/hr. If infusion reaction occurs, slow or stop the infusion depending on severity. If not severe, may continue the infusion at half the previous rate (minimum 50% rate reduction) once symptoms resolve. Discontinue drug if infusion reaction is severe.
- **Subsequent infusions**:
  - Standard infusion: If the first infusion is well tolerated, administer at initial rate of 100 mg/hr, and increase by 100-mg/hr increments every 30 minutes, to a maximum of 400 mg/hr as tolerated.
  - For *previously untreated NHL and DLBCL patients:* If patient did not experience a grade 3–4 infusion-related reaction during cycle 1, a 90-minute infusion can be administered in cycle 2 with a glucocorticoid-containing chemotherapy regimen. Most of the CD20 lymphocytes have been lysed in the first treatment, so the risk of cytokine release syndrome is minimal (Swan et al., 2011).
    - Initiate at a rate of 20% of the total dose given in the first 30 minutes, with the remaining 80% of the total dose given over the next 60 minutes.
    - If the 90-minute infusion is well tolerated in cycle 2, the same rate can be used when giving the remainder of the treatment regimen (through cycle 6 or 8).
    - Do not use the 90 min infusion for patients who have clinically significant cardiovascular disease or who have circulating lymphocyte counts > 5,000/mm^3 before cycle 2.
  - Administer glucocorticoid component of chemotherapy prior to rituximab infusion.
  - Interrupt the infusion or slow the rate if an infusion reaction occurs. Continue the infusion at one-half the previous rate upon symptom improvement.
  - Fatal infusion reactions have rarely occurred within 24 hours of rituximab dose, characterized by hypoxemia, pulmonary infiltrates, ARDS, MI, VF, and shock. Eighty percent of the fatal reactions occurred with the first infusion.

Drug Interactions:
- Renal toxicity when rituximab used in combination with cisplatin. Combination not indicated.

Lab Effects/Interference:
- Decreased lymphocyte count (B cells); decreased IgM and IgG serum levels.
- Hypophosphatemia and hyperuricemia.

Special Considerations:
- *Infusion reactions:* Although infusion reactions are common (fever, chills) during the first infusion, severe infusion reactions can also occur and some cases are fatal. Appropriate emergency medical support to manage severe infusion reactions must be available.
  - Severe reactions typically occurred during the first infusion with onset 30–120 minutes, but they can occur within 24 hours.

- Signs/symptoms include involving urticaria, hypotension, angioedema, broncho-spasm, hypoxia, pulmonary infiltrates, acute respiratory distress syndrome, myocardial infarction, ventricular fibrillation, cardiogenic shock, anaphylactoid events, and death.
- Patients should be premedicated with an antihistamine and acetaminophen prior to drug administration (RA patients should receive methylprednisolone 100 mg IV or equivalent 30 minutes prior to dose).
- STOP infusion for severe reactions and institute emergency medical management (e.g., glucocorticoids, epinephrine, oxygen, bronchodilators, saline) for infusion reactions as needed.
- Depending upon severity of reaction and required interventions, temporarily or permanently discontinue rituximab.
  - For mild-to-moderate infusion reactions, once symptoms have resolved, rituximab may be resumed at 50% of the previous rate. Closely monitor patients who have pre-existing cardiac or pulmonary conditions, those who have had prior cardiopulmonary side effects, and those with high numbers ($\geq 25,000/m^3$) of circulating tumor cells. Infusion reaction is a cytokine release reaction related to the cytokines released when the tumor cells are rapidly lysed by rituximab. The higher the number of circulating tumor cells, the higher the risk of an infusion reaction or cytokine release syndrome.
  - Emergency medications should be readily available: epinephrine, antihistamines, and corticosteroids.
- Severe mucocutaneous reactions may occur, some resulting in death.
  - Reactions include paraneoplastic pemphigus, Stevens-Johnson syndrome, lichenoid dermatitis, vesiculobullous dermatitis, and toxic epidermal necrolysis.
  - Onset can be as early as the first day of therapy to 13 weeks following rituximab dose.
  - Drug should be stopped if a reaction develops; a skin biopsy should be performed.
  - If the patient has a severe mucocutaneous reaction, the drug should be discontinued.
- Hepatitis B (HPV) reactivation can occur in hematologic patients treated with rituximab, usually about 4 months after the first rituximab dose, and about 1 month after the last dose.
  - Reactivation can result in fulminant hepatitis, hepatic failure, or death.
  - All patients at high risk for HPV should be screened for HPV prior to starting rituximab therapy.
  - Carriers of hepatitis B should be closely monitored for clinical and laboratory signs of active HPV infection for several months following rituximab therapy.
  - Patients who develop viral hepatitis should have rituximab discontinued, along with any concomitant chemotherapy, and start appropriate treatment, including antiviral therapy.
  - It is unknown whether rituximab can be safely resumed in these patients.
- Progressive multifocal leukoencephalopathy (PML) can occur following rituximab therapy, usually within 12 months of the last rituximab infusion, and can be fatal.
  - PML is caused by the JC virus, and the disease occurs in patients who have been immunosuppressed, such as patients with hematologic malignancies who received chemotherapy along with rituximab or as part of a stem cell transplant, or with auto-immune disease in patients who had prior or concurrent immunosuppressive therapy.

- Most cases of PML were diagnosed within 12 months of their last rituximab dose. If a patient receiving rituximab has a new-onset neurologic problem, consider PML in the differential, with evaluation by a neurologist, along with brain MRI and lumbar puncture.
  - Rituximab should be discontinued, and the discontinuation or reduction of any concomitant chemotherapy or immunosuppressive therapy in the patient who develops PML should be considered.
- Tumor lysis syndrome (TLS) may occur within 12–24 hours after the first infusion of rituximab for NHL, with acute renal failure, hyperkalemia, hypocalcemia, hyperuricemia, or hyperphosphatemia.
  - Patients at risk for TLS are those with a high number of circulating tumor cells ($\geq 25,000/mm^3$), high tumor burden, and high LDH.
  - Prepare patients at risk prior to rituximab with aggressive IV hydration and antihyperuricemic therapy, correct electrolyte abnormalities, monitor renal function and fluid balance, and administer supportive care, including dialysis, if needed.
- Serious infections can occur during and up to 1 year after the last rituximab-based therapy, including potentially fatal bacterial, fungal, and new or reactivated viral infections (e.g., CMV, herpes simplex, parvovirus B19, varicella zoster, West Nile, hepatitis B and C).
  - If a patient develops a severe infection, discontinue rituximab and begin appropriate antimicrobial therapy.
  - Drug should NOT be administered to patients with severe active infections.
- Cardiac arrythmias and angina can occur and be life-threatening.
  - Patients who develop clinically significant arrythmias should receive cardiac monitoring during and after all subsequent infusions of the drug.
  - Patients with a history of arrhythmias and angina should be cardiac monitored during infusion and immediately postinfusion for evidence of recurrence of these problems.
  - Rituximab should be discontinued if serious or life-threatening cardiac arrhythmias occur.
- Severe renal toxicity can occur in patients with NHL after rituximab therapy, including renal toxicity in patients who develop TLS.
  - Patients should be monitored closely for signs of renal failure
  - Discontinue rituximab in patients with a rising serum creatinine or oliguria.
- Bowel obstruction and perforation can occur rarely in NHL patients receiving rituximab and chemotherapy and sometimes result in death.
  - Typically, abdominal pain, bowel obstruction, and perforation occurred 6 days (range 1–77) after rituximab dosing.
  - Patients with abdominal pain should have a thorough diagnostic evaluation to rule out obstruction or perforation.
- Monitor CBC, platelet count regularly during therapy.
- Live vaccines should not be administered to patients receiving rituximab.
  - Patients with RA receiving rituximab should follow current immunization guidelines for non-live vaccines at least 4 weeks prior to a course of rituximab.
  - In studies, patients receiving rituximab and MTX had lower antibody titers to many immunizations but had similar responses to patients receiving MTX alone for tetanus toxoid and *Candida* skin test (delayed hypersensitivity).

Laboratory monitoring:
- **Malignancies:**
  - Patients receiving monotherapy should have a CBC and platelet count prior to each rituximab infusion.
  - During treatment with rituximab and chemotherapy, CBC and platelets should be monitored with weekly to monthly intervals or more frequently if cytopenias develop.
- **RA, WG, or MPA:** Patients should have a CBC and platelet count at 2- to 4-month intervals during rituximab therapy.
  - Cytopenias that develop during rituximab therapy can last months beyond the treatment period.
  - Concomitant use of biologic agents and DMARDS other than Methotrexate: limited safety data in RA patients with peripheral B-cell depletion following treatment with rituximab; observe patients closely for signs of infection. Concomitant immunosuppressants other than corticosteroids have not been studied in WG or MPA patients exhibiting peripheral B-cell depletion following treatment with rituximab.
- The use of rituximab is not recommended for patients with RA who have not had prior inadequate response to TNF antagonists.
- Retreatment in patients with GPA, WG, and MPA: there are limited data; safety and efficacy have not been established.
- Pregnancy: there are limited human data. Birth control practices during and for 12 months following therapy should be used by individuals of childbearing potential. B-cell lymphopenia occurred in infants exposed in utero.
- Nursing mothers: caution should be used when administering rituximab to a nursing mother.
- Most common adverse reactions:
  - Non-Hodgkin's Lymphoma (NHL) ($\geq$ 25%): Infusion reactions, fever, lymphopenia, chills, infection, and asthenia; CLL, infusion reactions, neutropenia.
  - RA ($\geq$ 10%): URI, nasopharyngitis, UTI, bronchitis; other less-frequent reactions: infusion reactions, serious infections, cardiovascular events.
  - GPA and MPA ($\geq$15%): infections, nausea, diarrhea, headache, muscle spasms, anemia, peripheral edema; other less frequent: infusion reactions.

Potential Toxicities/Side Effects and the Nursing Process

I.   POTENTIAL FOR INJURY related to INFUSION-RELATED REACTIONS

Defining Characteristics: Infusion-related reactions occurred within 30 minutes to 2 hours of the beginning of the first infusion. Fever and chills/rigors affect most patients during the initial infusion. Other infusion-related symptoms include: nausea; urticaria; fatigue; headache; pruritus; bronchospasm; dyspnea; sensation of swelling of tongue, throat; hypotension; flushing; and pain at disease site. Infusion-related reactions generally resolve with slowing or interrupting the drug infusion, and/or symptomatic treatment (IV saline, acetaminophen, diphenhydramine). Premedications often reduce the severity and/or occurrence of these reactions. In patients who receive retreatment after having completed at least one course of drug therapy, reactions that were reported include: fever, chills, asthenia, pruritus, and infusion-related events (fever, chills, pain, and throat irritation). The incidence of abdominal pain, anemia, dyspnea, hypotension, and neutropenia is higher in patients with bulky tumors > 10 cm. Infusion reaction is more likely during or after initial treatment, as it is related to the release of cytokines from the lysed CD20-positive cells. In successive treatments, fewer CD20 cells remain to be lysed, so there is significantly less cytokine release.

Nursing Implications: Discuss with physician or NP/PA the use of premedications, such as acetaminophen and an antihistamine before drug therapy. Ensure that medications necessary for the management of severe infusion reactions are readily available (e.g., epinephrine, antihistamines, corticosteroids). Assess baseline VS and monitor frequently during the infusion. Follow infusion rate guide (see Drug Administration section) for first and subsequent infusions. Slow or stop the infusion if severe infusion-related reactions occur. Monitor VS, and notify physician. Be prepared to provide emergency support as necessary (including IV saline, epinephrine, antihistamines, bronchodilators). If/when symptoms resolve, resume the infusion at 50% of the rate of the previous infusion, as directed by the physician.

II.   ALTERATION IN ELIMINATION, RENAL, related to TUMOR LYSIS SYNDROME

Defining Characteristics: Patients with high tumor burden receiving rituximab for the first time are at risk for rapid tumor lysis. Tumor lysis syndrome (TLS) occurs as a result of rapid release of intracellular contents into the bloodstream. The risk of TLS appears higher in patients with a high number of circulating lymphocytes, e.g., > 25,000/mm^3.

Nursing Implications: For first infusion, expect patient orders to include: Hydration at 150 mL/hr with or without alkalinization, oral allopurinol, strict monitoring of I/O, daily weight, and body balance determination. Monitor baseline and daily BUN, creatinine, potassium, phosphorus, uric acid, and calcium. Monitor for renal, cardiac, neuromuscular signs/symptoms, hyperkalemia, hyperphosphatemia, hypomagnesemia, hypocalcemia, and elevated uric acid.

III.   POTENTIAL FOR INFECTION related to LYMPHOPENIA AND BONE MARROW DEPRESSION

Defining Characteristics: B-cell lymphocytes are reduced in some patients, together with a decrease in immunoglobulins in some patients. Bacterial infections that occurred in these patients were not associated with neutropenia, and some were severe, involving sepsis due to *Listeria, Staphylococcus*, and polymicrobials; posttreatment infections included rare sepsis, and viral infections (herpes simplex and herpes zoster). Leukopenia occurs in some patients, thrombocytopenia in some, and neutropenia in some others. Serious bone marrow suppression was uncommon and may occur up to 30 days following treatment. These include severe neutropenia, thrombocytopenia, and severe anemia. Rarely, transient aplastic anemia or hemolytic anemia may occur. Incidence of neutropenia, anemia, and abdominal pain was higher, as was the severity, in patients with bulky tumors > 10 cm. Limited data is available about safety of biologic agents and DMARDS (other than methotrexate) in RA, as rituximab will deplete peripheral B-cells. Post-marketing reports have noted prolonged rare pancytopenia, marrow hypoplasia, grade 3–4 prolonged or late onset neutropenia.

Nursing Implications: Monitor CBC, platelets baseline and regularly during treatment. If the patient develops cytopenia, monitor more frequently. Assess for signs/symptoms of infection, bleeding, fatigue, and chest pain prior to each treatment. Teach patient to self-assess for these, including taking temperature, and instruct to report them immediately. Transfuse red cells and platelets as ordered. Observe patients with RA who are also taking DMARDS (other than methotrexate) closely for signs of infection.

IV.   LOSS OF SKIN INTEGRITY, POTENTIAL, related to SEVERE MUCOCUTANEOUS REACTIONS

Defining Characteristics: Severe skin reactions have occurred rarely and, in some cases, ended in death of patient. Skin abnormalities include paraneoplastic pemphigus (uncommon autoimmune disorder, may be related to underlying malignancy), Stevens-Johnson syndrome (may be caused by HSV or other infectious disorder), lichenoid dermatitis, vesiculobullous dermatitis, and toxic epidermal necrolysis. Onset is 1–13 weeks following rituximab exposure.

Nursing Implications: Assess baseline skin and mucous membrane integrity. Teach patient that rarely skin and mucous membrane reactions may occur, and to report any changes right away. Manufacturer recommends stopping rituximab therapy and obtaining skin biopsy to determine cause. Discuss with physician. Teach the patient local care strategies depending upon symptoms.

V.   ALTERATION IN COMFORT related to ASTHENIA, HEADACHE, NAUSEA, VOMITING, PRURITUS, MYALGIA, AND DIZZINESS

Defining Characteristics: From single-agent Rituxan studies for relapsed or refractory, low-grade or follicular NHL, there was some incidence of asthenia. Headache, nausea, pruritus, vomiting, myalgia, and dizziness may also occur.

Nursing Implications: Assess baseline comfort prior to each infusion, and tolerance of past infusion. Discuss strategies to manage symptoms. If symptoms are severe, discuss management with physician.

Drug: romidepsin for injection (Istodax)

Class: Histone deacetylase (HDAC) inhibitor.

Mechanism of Action: Romidepsin catalyzes the removal of acetyl groups from acetylated lysine residues in histones, resulting in the modulation of gene expression.

HDACs also deacetylate nonhistone protein transcription factors. Romidepsin causes acetylated histones to accumulate, and induces cell cycle arrest and apoptosis in some cancer cell lines. The antineoplastic mechanism has not been fully characterized.

Metabolism: The drug is highly protein-bound after IV injection (92–94%). It undergoes extensive metabolism in the liver, primarily by the CYP3A4 system, with minor metabolism by CYP3A5, CYP1A1, CYP2B6, and CYP2C19. The terminal half-life is about 3 hours, and there is no accumulated drug with repeated dosing. Mild hepatic impairment does not affect pharmacokinetics, but moderate and severe liver impairment have not been studied. Patients with mild, moderate, or severe renal impairment did not have changes in pharmacokinetics, but patients with end-stage renal impairment have not been studied.

Indication: FDA-approved for the treatment of:
- Cutaneous T-cell lymphoma (CTCL) in patients who have received at least one prior systemic treatment.
- Peripheral T-cell lymphoma (PTCL) in patients who have received at least one prior therapy.

Dosage/Range:
- 14 mg/m^2 IV infusion over 4 hours on days 1, 8, 15 of a 28-day cycle. Repeat cycles every 28 days as long as patient continues to derive benefit and tolerates the drug.
- Discontinue or interrupt with or without dose reduction to 10 mg/m^2 to manage treatment side effects.

Dose Modifications:
- **Nonhematologic toxicities** (excluding alopecia):
  - Grade 2–3: Delay drug until toxicity improves to ≤ grade 1 or baseline; then restart at 14 mg/m^2.
  - If grade 3 toxicity recurs, delay until toxicity improves to ≤ grade 1 or baseline, then permanently dose-reduce to 10 mg/m^2.
  - Grade 4 toxicity: Delay until toxicity improves to ≤ grade 1 or baseline, then permanently dose-reduce to 10 mg/m^2.
  - Discontinue drug if grade 3–4 toxicities recur after dose reduction.
- **Hematologic toxicities:**
  - Grade 3–4 neutropenia or thrombocytopenia: Delay until cytopenia returns to ANC ≥ 1.5 × 10^9/L and/or platelet count returns to ≥ 75 × 10^9/L or baseline; then resume at 14 mg/m^2.
  - Grade 4 febrile (≥ 38.5°C) neutropenia or thrombocytopenia that requires platelet transfusion: Delay until cytopenia returns to ≤ grade 1 or baseline; then permanently dose-reduce to 10 mg/m^2.
- Patients with moderate or severe hepatic impairment or with end-stage renal disease should be treated with caution.

Drug Preparation/Administration:
- Use recommended practices for the safe handling of hazardous drugs.
- Drug is supplied as a kit with (1) sterile, lyophilized powder in a single-use vial containing 10 mg romidepsin and 20 mg of bulking agent, povidone, USP, and

(2) one sterile vial containing 2 mL of diluent (80% propylene glycol, USP, and 20% dehydrated alcohol, USP).

• Reconstitute with supplied diluent, and further dilute with 0.9% sodium chloride injection, USP, before IV infusion.

• Each 10-mL single-use vial is reconstituted with 2 mL of supplied diluent.

• Aseptically withdraw 2 mL from supplied diluents vial, and slowly inject it into the romidepsin for injection vial. Swirl until contents are completely dissolved. The reconstituted solution contains romidepsin 5 mg/mL. The reconstituted solution is chemically stable for at least 8 hours at room temperature.

• Calculate volume of ordered dose, and extract romidepsin from the vial(s), using aseptic technique. Further dilute romidepsin in 500 mL 0.9% sodium chloride injection, USP.

• Infuse IV over 4 hours.

• Solution is chemically stable for at least 24 hours stored at room temperature, but it should be administered as soon after dilution as possible. Diluted solution is compatible with polyvinyl chloride (PVC), ethylene vinyl acetate (EVA), polyethylene (PE) infusion bags, as well as glass bottles.

• Visually inspect for particulate matter and discoloration prior to administration.

Drug Interactions:

• Coumadin/Coumadin derivatives: romidepsin may cause prolongation of PT and elevation of INR. Monitor PT and INR closely in patients receiving this combination.

• Romidepsin is metabolized by CYP3A4. Strong CYP3A4 inhibitors may increase the serum level of romidepsin. Drugs that are strong inhibitors of the CYP3A4 enzyme include atazanavir, clarithromycin, indinavir, itraconazole, ketoconazole, nefazodone, nelfinavir, ritonavir, saquinavir, telithromycin, and voriconazole. Avoid combination if possible, but if romidepsin is initially coadministered with a strong CYP3A4 inhibitor, monitor the patient closely for romidepsin side effects, and follow dose modifications for toxicity.

• Drugs that induce the CYP3A4 enzymes (e.g., carbamazepine dexamethasone, phenobarbital, phenytoin, rifampin, rifabutin, rifapentine) may decrease the serum level of romidepsin and should be avoided if possible. Coadministration with rifampin increased romidepsin exposure by 80%, AUC and C_{max} by 60%, possibly by rifampin inhibition of an unknown hepatic intake process. Patients should NOT take rifampin together with romidepsin. St. John's wort should also not be taken with romidepsin.

• Drugs that inhibit drug transport systems: romidepsin is a substrate of the efflux transporter P-glycoprotein (P-gp) so that drugs that inhibit P-glycoprotein may result in increased serum levels of romidepsin when coadministered. If they are coadministered, caution should be exercised.

Lab Effects/Interference:

• Hypomagnesemia, hypokalemia, hypocalcemi, hypoalbuminemia, hyponatremia, hypophosphatemia.

• Hyperglycemia, hypermagnesemia, hyperuricemia, hyperbilirubinemia.

• Anemia, thrombocytopenia, neutropenia, lymphopenia.

• Increased AST, ALT.

• ECG ST-T wave changes, QTc prolongation.

Special Considerations:
- Thrombocytopenia, neutropenia, lymphopenia, and anemia can occur; monitor CBC/platelets/ANC baseline, prior to each cycle, and during treatment as indicated.
- Drug can prolong the QT interval (time of ventricular contraction and relaxation) with risk of ventricular arrythmias.
- If serum magnesium and potassium are low, this increases the risk for torsades de pointes, a type of ventricular tachycardia that can deteriorate into ventricular fibrillation.
- **Prior to romidepsin administration, ensure that serum magnesium and potassium are WNL.**
- Patients at risk have: congenital long QT syndrome; significant history of cardiovascular disease; or are taking medications that can significantly prolong the QT interval such as amiodarone, chlorpromazine, methadone.
- Patients at risk should have cardiovascular monitoring precautions, such as ECG and electrolytes baseline and during treatment.
- Drug may cause fetal harm, so pregnancy should be avoided; if romidepsin is used during pregnancy, or if the patient becomes pregnancy during therapy, the patient should be apprised of potential harm to the fetus.
- Nursing mothers: a decision should be made whether to discontinue nursing or discontinue the drug, taking into account importance of the drug to the mother's health.
- The most common adverse reactions are neutropenia, lymphopenia, thrombocyteopenia, infections, nausea, fatigue, vomiting, anorexia, anemia, and ECG T-wave changes.
- Serious and sometimes fatal infections have been reported during treatment and within 30 days after treatment with romidepsin. Risk is highest in patients who have a history of extensive or intensive chemotherapy.
- Tumor lysis syndrome (TLS) has been reported during treatment (1–2% incidence); anticipate possible TLS in patients with advanced stage disease and/or high tumor burden, discuss TLS precautions with physician, and monitor closely.

Potential Toxicities/Side Effects and the Nursing Process

I. POTENTIAL FOR INFECTION, BLEEDING, AND FATIGUE related to NEUTROPENIA, THROMBOCYTOPENIA, AND ANEMIA

Defining Characteristics: The highest incidence of anemia was 72% (16% grade 3–4), thrombocytopenia 65% (14% grade 3–4), and neutropenia 57% (27% grade 3–4). Infections occurred in up to 54% of patients, with pyrexia (23%). Serious and sometimes fatal infections, including pneumonia and sepsis, have been reported in clinical trials. These infections can occur during or within 30 days after treatment, and risk may be higher in patients who have had extensive or intensive chemotherapy.

Nursing Implications: Monitor CBC, platelet count; assess at baseline, prior to each treatment, and periodically as indicated. Ensure that dose modifications are performed as indicated in dosage section. Assess for signs and symptoms of infection, bleeding, fatigue, and anemia. Teach patients to self-assess for signs and symptoms of infection, bleeding, and anemia and to call their nurse or physician right away if they occur, or to go to the emergency room. Ensure that the patient has a thermometer at home and that the patient and a family member can read the number and verbally repeat to call if the temperature is 100.4°F or higher. In addition, patients should be taught to report cough, shortness of breath, significant fatigue, chest pain, burning with urination, flulike symptoms, muscle aches, or worsening skin problems. Assess patient medication profile and any over-the-counter medications such as those containing aspirin or NSAIDs that would increase the risk of bleeding. Instruct patient to avoid these drugs and not to begin any over-the-counter medications without first discussing with nurse or physician. Teach patient to alternate rest and activity periods if feeling fatigued and to organize shopping and chores in a way to minimize energy expenditures.

II. POTENTIAL ALTERATION IN CIRCULATION related to CHANGES IN ECG T-WAVE/ST-SEGMENT AND QTc PROLONGATION, HYPOTENSION

Defining Characteristics: ECG ST and T-wave changes occurred in up to 63% of patients. Prolongation of the QTc interval occurred and in rare instances led to drug discontinuation. Ventricular and supraventricular arrhythmias also were reported. Hypotension may occur in up to 23% of patients. Low serum potassium and magnesium increase the risk of arrhythmia in patients with prolonged QTc intervals.

Nursing Implications: Do baseline assessment of cardiac status, including drug profile and possible drugs that may prolong the QT interval. If a patient has risk factors (such as congenital long QT sysndrome, significant cardiovascular disease, or taking antiarrhythmic medications), ensure that baseline ECG with QTc interval has been done and that it is done periodically during treatment. Assess baseline electrolytes, especially serum potassium and magnesium, and ensure levels are WNL before administering romidepsin. Identify patients at risk for developing QTc prolongation, such as patients on antiarrhythmic agents and patients with hypomagnesemia or hypokalemia. Replete magnesium and potassium as ordered.

III. ALTERATION IN NUTRITION, LESS THAN BODY REQUIREMENTS, related to NAUSEA, DIARRHEA, ANOREXIA, DEHYDRATION, VOMITING, DYSGEUSIA, HYPERGLYCEMIA, HYPOALBUMINEMIA

Defining Characteristics: In clinical trials, these side effects occurred with the following frequency: nausea 56%–86% (6% grade 3–4), vomiting 34%–52% (5%–10% grade 3–4), anorexia 23%–54% (< 1%–4% grade 3–4), diarrhea 20%–36%, dysgeusia 15%–40%, constipation 12%–40%, hyperglycemia 2%–51%, hypoalbuminemia < 1%–48%.

Nursing Implications: Assess weight, bowel elimination status, baseline nutritional status, and glucose level along with other labs, and monitor during therapy. Teach patient that symptoms can occur and ways to minimize these effects, such as self-administration of antinausea, anticonstipation, and antidiarrheal medications and to report symptoms that do not resolve with established plan. Assess for taste disturbances, and teach dietary modifications to minimize impact. Teach patient to identify nutritionally dense (high calories and protein in the smallest amount) foods and to keep them handy in the refrigerator. Teach patient to eat small, frequent meals and to have a bedtime snack. Teach patient that goal is to take in at least 2 quarts of fluid a day and to try to drink a glass of fluid every hour while awake. Closely monitor those patients at risk for dehydration (e.g., elderly patients). Teach patient signs and symptoms of hyperglycemia (e.g., excessive thirst, frequent urination) and to report them. Discuss any abnormalities with a physician.

Drug: siltuximab (Sylvant)

Class: Interleukin-6 (IL-6) antagonist, chimeric monoclonal antibody.

Mechanism of Action: Drug is a chimeric mAb that binds human Interleukin-6 (IL-6), thus preventing IL-6 from binding to its IL-6 receptors. IL-6 is a cytokine produced by various cells (e.g., T- and B-lymphocytes, monocytes, fibroblasts, endothelial cells). IL-6 normally induces immunoglobulin secretion. A dysregulated, overproduction of IL-6 from activated B-lymphocytes in affected lymph nodes is believed to cause multicentric Castleman's disease (MCD) with its systemic manifestations (e.g., enlarged lymph nodes, fever, weakness, fatigue, night sweats, weight loss, nausea, vomiting, loss of appetite, nerve damage, and increased risk of infection). Treatment with siltuximab in a clinical trial resulted in significant tumor and symptomatic responses (Wong et al., 2013).

Metabolism: Following IV administration, C_{max} occurred near the end of the infusion. With every 3-week dosing, steady state is reached by the 6th infusion. Mean terminal half-life (t1/2) after the first infusion is 20.6 days (range 14.2–29.7 days). There was no difference in clearance in patients with preexisting mild, moderate, and severe renal impairment compared to normal patients, nor any difference in patients with mild or moderate hepatic impairment compared to patients with normal hepatic function. Patients with end-stage renal disease or severe hepatic dysfunction (Child-Pugh Class C) were not studied.

Indication: Drug approved for the treatment of patients with multicentric Castleman's disease (MCD) who are human deficiency virus- (HIV-) negative and human herpes virus-8- (HHV-8-) negative.
- MCD, a rare blood disorder similar to lymphoma, affects about 1,100–1,300 Americans. It is a serious, chronic disease characterized by an abnormal overgrowth of lymphocytes in lymph nodes and in lymphoid tissue such as the liver and spleen, which become enlarged. The cause is unknown, but it is associated with an overproduction of IL-6. Disease symptoms include fever, night sweats, weight loss, weakness, fatigue, and a weakened immune system leading to infection. Infection, multi-organ system failure, and malignancies, including malignant lymphoma, are common causes of death in MCD.
- Drug has not been studied in patients who are HIV-positive or HHV-8 positive because drug does not bind to virally produced IL-6 in a nonclinical study.
- MCD2001 was the clinical trial leading to FDA priority review and approval, which showed that of 79 patients with symptomatic MCD randomized to best supportive care

(BSC) alone or the combination BSC/siltuximab, 34% of patients receiving the combination had a durable tumor and symptomatic response persisting for a minimum of 18 weeks without treatment failure, compared to zero in the BSC arm (p = 0.0012). 61% of anemic patients had an increase in hemoglobin of 1.5 g/dL in the combination group vs zero in the BSC group (p < 0.05).

Dosage/Range:
- 11 mg/kg administered as a 1 hr IV infusion every 3 weeks, until treatment failure.
- Assess CBC/differential, platelet count prior to each dose for the first 12 months, then every 3 cycles therafter.
- Prior to first siltuximab dose, labs must be: ANC ≥ 1.0×10^9/L, platelet count ≥ 75×10^9/L, Hgb < 17 g/dL.
- Prior to subsequent siltuximab doses, labs must be: ANC ≥ 1.0×10^9/L, platelet count ≥ 50×10^9/L, Hgb < 17 g/dL.
- DO NOT administer drug to patients with severe infections until the infection resolves.
- Discontinue drug in patients with severe infusion-related reactions, anaphylaxis, severe allergic reactions, or cytokine release syndromes. Do not reinstitute treatment in patients who have had a severe hypersensitivity reaction to siltuximab or any of its excipients.
- Drug is contraindicated.

Drug Preparation:
- Available in 100 mg and 400 mg of lyophilized powder in a single-use vial. Obtain 250-mL infusion bags of 5% dextrose in water, made of polyvinyl chloride (PVC) with Di (2-cthylhcxyl), phthalate (DEIIP), or Polyolefin (PO), as well as IV administration sets lined with PVC with DEHP or polyurethane (PU), containing a 0.2 micron inline polyethersulfone (PES) filter.
- Calculate dosage required, total volume or reconstituted drug needed, and number of vials.
- Using a 21-gauge 1-1/2 inch needle, aseptically add 5.2 mL sterile water for injection, USP, to the 100-mg vial, or 20 mL of sterile water for injection, USP, to the 400-mg vial. Each vial will have a concentration of 20 mg/mL. Gently swirl the reconstituted vials until completely dissolved; DO NOT shake or swirl vigorously. Dissolving the lyophilized powder should take < 60 min.
- Once reconstituted and prior to further dilution, inspect for particulate matter and discoloration, and do not use if found or if visibly opaque. Further dilute into the infusion bag within 2 hours.
- Aseptically remove the calculated dose volume (that will be added) from a 250-mL bag of sterile dextrose 5% in water that is made of PVC with DEHP or PO; then slowly add the total calculated volume for the ordered dose of reconstituted siltuximab to the 5% dextrose in water infusion bag. Gently invert to mix.
- Drug will be administered by IV infusion over 1 hour, completed within 4 hr of dilution of the reconstituted solution to the infusion bag.

Drug Administration:
- Drug must be diluted in a 250 mL infusion bags of 5% dextrose in water made of polyvinyl chloride (PVC) with Di2-ethylhexyl phthalate (DEHP) or Polyolefin (PO), and administered by IV administration sets lined with PVC with DEHP or polyurethane (PU), containing a 0.2 micron inline polyethersulfone (PES) filter.

- Administer by IV infusion over 1 hr; infusion must be completed within 4 hours of the time the reconstituted solution was placed into the infusion bag.
- Do not infuse concomitantly with other drugs in the same IV line.
- Stop the infusion if the patient has an infusion reaction. Ensure that the infusion setting has resuscitation equipment, emergency medications, and personnel trained in emergency resuscitation.
  - Mild to moderate reaction: if the reaction resolves, may restart drug at a lower infusion rate per MD or NP/PA; consider premedication with antihistamines, acetaminophen, and corticosteroids. Discontinue drug if the patient does not tolerate the infusion with these interventions.
  - Anaphylaxis: stop the infusion, provide immediate medical intervention, and discontinue siltuximab.

Drug Interactions:
- Cytochrome P450 substrates: infection and inflammation, and cytokines (e.g., IL-6) down regulate cytochrome P450 enzymes in the liver. When IL-6 is inhibited, this may restore CYP450 enzyme activity to higher levels leading to increased metabolism of CYP450 substrates (drugs that are metabolized by CYP450 enzymes). When starting or stopping siltuximab for patients being treated with CYP450 substrates with a narrow therapeutic index, perform therapeutic monitoring of effect (e.g., warfarin or drug concentration such as cyclosporine or theophylline), and adjust dose as needed. The effect of siltuximab on CYP450 enzyme activity can persist for several weeks after stopping siltuximab.
- CYP3A4 substrates (e.g., oral contraceptives, lovastatin, atorvastatin): exercise caution when coadministering, as a decrease in effectiveness may occur and is undesireable.

Lab Effects/Interference:
- Decreased C-reactive protein (CRP), platelet count.
- Hypertriglyceridemia, hypercholesteremia, hyperuricemia.

Special Considerations:
- The most common adverse effects (> 10%) were pruritus, increased weight, rash, hyperuricemia, URI.
- *Warnings and Precautions:*
  - Do not administer drug to patients with severe infections until the infection has resolved. Drug may mask signs and symptoms of acute inflammation including suppression of fever, and acute phase reactants such as CRP. Monitor patients receiving siltuximab closely for infections, stop drug, and promptly treat with anti-infective therapy.
  - Do not administer live vaccines because inhibition of IL-6 may interfere with the normal immune response to new antigens.
  - Infusion reactions: see Drug Administration.
  - GI perforation: reported in clinical trials, though not MCD trials. Use drug cautiously in patients at risk for GI perforation. Patients presenting with symptoms suggestive of GI perforation should be evaluated immediately.
- Infants born to pregnant women treated with siltuximab may be at increased risk of infection; caution is advised in the administration of live vaccines to these infants.

Drug should be used during pregnancy only if the potential benefit justifies the potential risk to the fetus. Advise patients of childbearing potential to avoid pregnancy, using contraception during and for 3 months after treatment ends.

• Nursing mothers: a decision should be made whether to discontinue nursing or to discontinue the drug, taking into account the importance of the drug to the mother's health.

Potential Toxicities/Side Effects and the Nursing Process

I.   POTENTIAL FOR INJURY related to HYPERSENSITIVITY/ANAPHYLAXIS AND INFUSION REACTION

Defining Characteristics: Infusion reactions were reported in 4.8% of patients; symptoms were back pain, chest pain or discomfort, nausea, vomiting, flushing, erythema, and palpitations. Anaphlylalxis occurred in one patient of the approximately 750 patients treated with siltuximab.

Nursing Implications: Ensure resuscitation equipment, emergency medicines, and oxygen are located in the infusion area. Assess baseline VS and mental status prior to drug administration, at 15 minutes, and periodically during infusion, as needed. Remain with patient during first 15 minutes of first infusions. Recall signs/symptoms of anaphylaxis; if these occur, stop drug immediately, notify physician, and assess patient's vital signs. Subjective symptoms are generalized itching, nausea, chest tightness, crampy abdominal pain, difficulty speaking, anxiety, agitation, sense of impending doom, uneasiness, desire to urinate/defecate, dizziness, and chills. Objective signs are flushed appearance; angioedema of face, neck, eyelids, hands, and feet; localized or generalized urticaria; respiratory distress with or without wheezing; hypotension; and cyanosis. Review standing physician orders or nursing procedures for patient management of anaphylaxis, and be prepared to stop drug immediately and change IV to a plain NS solution to keep vein patent, notify physician or NP/PA, keep airway patent, monitor VS, and administer ordered medications, which may include epinephrine 1:1,000 IM in the thigh, IV hydrocortisone sodium succinate, and IV diphenhydramine. Teach patient to report any unusual symptoms. Stop infusion if a reaction occurs. For mild-to-moderate infusion reactions (grade 1–2), the drug may be resumed at a decreased infusion rate per MD or NP/PA; also, consider premedication with an antihistamine, acetaminophen, and a corticosteroid for subsequent treatents. Drug should be discontinued in patients who experience anaphylaxis.

II.   POTENTIAL ALTERATION IN SKIN INTEGRITY related to RASH, PRURITUS, EDEMA

Defining Characteristics: Rash and pruritus each affected 28% of patients during the initial 8 infusions. Edema was reported in 26%.

Nursing Implications: Assess baseline skin integrity, and teach patient that rash, pruritus, and edema may occur, and to report It. If it occurs, assess need for intervention and discuss with MD or NP/PA if it persists or worsens.

Drug: sipuleucel-T (Provenge)

Class: Autologous cellular immunotherapy agent.

Mechanism of Action: Sipuleucel-T induces an immune response in the patient directed against PAP, an antigen expressed in most prostate cancers. In the laboratory, the patient's antigen-presenting cells (APCs) are cultured with PSP-GM-CSF so that the APCs can take up and process the recombinant target antigen into small peptides that are then displayed on the APC surface. These pieces of the tumor antigen can then be recognized by the patient's immune system by T-lymphocytes and NK cells, which will then seek and destroy the prostate cancer cells.

Metabolism: Unknown. Neutralizing antibodies to GM-CSF were transient.

Indication: Drug is FDA-approved for the treatment of asymptomatic or minimally symptomatic metastatic castrate-resistant (hormone refractory) prostate cancer.

Dosage/Range: Recommended course is 3 complete doses at 2-week intervals.
- Each dose of sipuleucel-T contains a minimum of 50 million autologous CD54⁺ (antigen presenting cells that carry a piece of the patient's prostate cancer [antigen] to present to the immune system to stimulate it to attack the patient's prostate cancer), activated with PAP-GM-CSF, suspended in 250 mL of lactated Ringer's injection, USP, in a sealed, patient-specific infusion bag. The bag may also contain other immune cells that have been leukophoresed.
- Each infusion is preceded by a leukapheresis procedure approximately 3 days prior.

Drug Preparation:
- Drug is shipped directly to the patient's physician, who will infuse the drug.
- Sipuleucel-T will arrive in a cardboard shipping box with the drug inside a special insulated polyurethane container. Verify the product and patient-specific label on the top of the insulated container. Do NOT remove the container from the box or open the lid until the patient is ready to receive the infusion.
- Do NOT infuse the drug until confirmation of product release has been received from Dendreon, the manufacturer. They will send a Cell Product Disposition Form containing patient identifiers, expiration date and time, and the disposition status (approved for infusion or rejected) to the infusion site.
- Infusion must begin prior to the expiration date and time indicated on the Cell Product Disposition Form and product label. DO NOT initiate infusion of expired drug. Once the infusion bag is removed from the insulated container, it should remain at room temperature for no more than 3 hours. DO NOT return the infusion bag to the shipping container.
- Once the patient is prepared for infusion, and the Cell Product Disposition Form and product label have been received, remove the sipuleucel-T infusion bag from the insulated container and inspect for signs of leakage. Contents will be slightly cloudy, with a cream-to-pink color. Gently mix and resuspend the contents of the bag, inspecting for clumps and clots, which can be gently dispersed by manual mixing. DO NOT administer if the bag leaks or if clumps remain in the bag.
- Prior to the infusion, match the patient's identity with the patient identifiers on the Cell Product Disposition Form and the infusion bag.

- Sipuleucel-T is to be used for autologous use only.
- Sipuleucel-T is not routinely tested for transmission of infectious diseases and may transmit disease to healthcare professionals. Use universal precautions.

Drug Administration:
- Confirm patient identity (must be same patient leukophoresed that is receiving the drug).
- Inspect the infusion bag; do not administer if there are leaks or clumps that cannot be dissolved.
- Check that the infusion time is prior to the expiration date and time on the Cell Product Disposition Form and product label. Do not use expired sipuleucel-T.
- Administer premedication (acetaminophen and antihistamine such as diphenhydramine).
- Do NOT use a cell filter, and infuse over 60 minutes.
- If the patient has an acute infusion reaction, interrupt or slow the infusion depending upon severity, and discuss further management with physician/NP/PA. If the infusion is interrupted, and then is reinitiated, make sure that the infusion bag has not been standing at room temperature for more than 3 hours. Closely monitor patient, especially those patients with cardiac or pulmonary conditions.
- Observe the patient for 30 minutes after completion of the infusion.

Drug Interactions:
- Unknown, as no studies have been performed. Concomitant use of chemotherapy and immunosuppressive medications with sipuleucel-T has not been studied.

Lab Effects/Interference:
- Anemia.

Special Considerations:
- Drug is indicated solely for AUTOLOGOUS use.
- Acute infusion reactions have been observed. This may require stopping the infusion or slowing it down, depending upon the severity of the reaction. Closely monitor patients with preexisting cardiac or pulmonary problems.
- Use universal precautions when handling the drug. Sipuleucel-T is not routinely tested for transmissible infectious diseases and may transmit disease to healthcare providers handling the product.
- Concomitant use of chemotherapy and immunosuppressive medications with sipuleucel-T have not been studied and is not recommended.
- In two clinical studies, patients receiving sipuleucel-T had significantly longer overall survival (25.8/25.9 months vs 21.7/21.4 months, $p = .032$, $p = .010$).
- The most common side effects are chills, fatigue, fever, back pain, nausea, joint ache, and headache. Suspected adverse reactions can be reported to the FDA at www.fda.gov/medwatch.
- Severe adverse events were reported in 24% of patients, compared to 25% in the control group. These included infusion reactions, cerebrovascular events, and single-case reports of eosinophilia, rhabdomyolysis, myasthenia gravis, myositis, and tumor flare.
- Side effects of leukophoresis 3 days prior to the therapy included citrate toxicity (14%), oral paresthesia (12%), paresthesia (11%), and fatigue (8%).

Potential Toxicities/Side Effects and the Nursing Process

I. POTENTIAL FOR INJURY related to HYPERSENSITIVITY AND INFUSION REACTION

Defining Characteristics: Sipuleucel-T can cause acute infusion reactions within 1 day of infusion. In clinical trials, the incidence was 71%, and of these, 95% were mild or moderate, characterized by chills, fever, and fatigue that resolved within 2 days. Severe or grade 3 reactions occurred in 3.5% of patients and included chills, fever, fatigue, asthenia, dyspnea, hypoxia, bronchospasm, dizziness, headache, HTN, muscle ache, nausea, and vomiting. The incidence of severe reactions was greatest after the second infusion (2.1%) compared to infusion 1 (0.8%). Rarely patients were admitted for management of acute infusion reactions. There were no grade 4 or 5 reactions.

Nursing Implications: Ensure patient identifiers are closely checked. Ensure patient receives premedication with acetaminophen, diphenhydramine, or equivalent. Begin infusion slowly; then speed up to complete within 1 hour. Closely monitor patients with cardiac or pulmonary conditions. Have physician or NP nearby in case of reaction. Recall signs/symptoms of anaphylaxis/infusion reaction, and if these occur, stop drug immediately, notify physician, and assess patient's vital signs. Subjective symptoms are generalized itching, nausea, chest tightness, crampy abdominal pain, difficulty speaking, anxiety, agitation, sense of impending doom, uneasiness, desire to urinate/defecate, dizziness, and chills. Objective signs are flushed appearance; angioedema of face, neck, eyelids, hands, and feet; localized or generalized urticaria; respiratory distress with or without wheezing; hypotension; and cyanosis. Review standing orders or nursing procedures for patient management of anaphylaxis and be prepared to stop drug immediately, notify physician, monitor VS, and administer ordered medications, which may include epinephrine 1:1,000, hydrocortisone sodium succinate, oxygen, and diphenhydramine. Teach patient to report any unusual symptoms. If the patient develops an acute infusion reaction, if severe, stop the reaction; if mild or moderate, discuss with physician or nurse practitioner whether the infusion should be slowed down or interrupted. If severe, institute medical management urgently, such as for angina or other signs/symptoms of myocardial insufficiency. Teach patient to report any signs and symptoms of infusion reaction within 24 hours of the infusion (e.g., fever, chills, rash, breathing problems).

II. ALTERATION IN COMFORT related to CHILLS, FATIGUE, FEVER, BACK PAIN, NAUSEA, JOINT ACHE, HEADACHE

Defining Characteristics: In clinical trials there were chills (53%), fatigue (41%), fever (31%), back pain (29%), nausea (21%), joint ache (19%), headache (18%). Most patients have one or more of these side effects, and in 67% of patients, they are mild or moderate. Back pain and chills were severe in about 2% of patients.

Nursing Implications: Assess baseline comfort level and teach patient that these side effects may occur. Teach self-management for comfort and teach patient to call if symptomatic treatment does not resolve issue in 1–2 days. Discuss with physician or nurse practitioner prescription medication to improve comfort for symptoms that do not respond to conservative management.

Drug: sonidegib (Odomzo)

Class: Hedgehog pathway inhibitor.

Mechanism of Action: The Hedgehog pathway is vital during embryogenesis. In the embryo the Hedgehog pathway is responsible for cell proliferation and cell differentiation into specialized cells and organs, as well as tissue migration to the correct anatomical position within the developing embryo. For example, this pathway is critical to ensuring that the spinal cord ends up in the correct place, that the developing fetus has five fingers on each hand, five toes on each foot, and that the anatomical part is heading in the correct direction (tissue polarity). The Hedgehog pathway also plays a role in cell differentiation, stem cell maintenance, and wound healing in the adult. The Hedgehog gene codes for the sonic hedgehog (SHH) protein, which will bind to a specific cell membrane receptor complex to turn on signal transduction leading to cell proliferation. The receptor complex on the cell membrane is made up of two proteins: patched (PTCH) 1 that binds the ligand SHH, and smoothened (SMO), which turns on the actual signal transduction to activate the target genes controlling cell proliferation. Normally this pathway is almost shut down after the fetus is formed. If the PTCH1 gene becomes mutated, then the PTCH1 protein cannot bind to SMO, releasing SMO to send unlimited messages to the target genes so that unregulated cell proliferation occurs along with angiogenesis. Mutations in PTCH1, PTCH2, SMO, and another gene can occur in basal cell carcinoma (BCC). UV exposure mutates PTCH1, and is thought to be responsible for 70% of BCCs (von Gorlin syndrome). Another 10–20% of BCCs appear to be due to mutations in SMO, leading to unregulated signaling to the genes responsible for cell proliferation. Thus in BCC, the Hedgehog pathway becomes turned on without regulation, resulting in malignant transformation and growth. Hedgehog signaling from the tumor to the stroma (surrounding tissue that stimulates tumor growth) increases tumorigenesis (Gupta et al., 2010). Sonidegib binds to and inhibits SMO, the transmembrane protein that is necessary for activation of Hedgehog signal transduction. By inactivating SMO, the pathway is turned off.

Metabolism: After oral administration, < 10% of the dose is absorbed, and in fasting conditions, the median time to peak concentration (Tmax) was 2–4 hours. Steady state is achieved in about 4 months after starting the drug. A high fat meal increases exposure to sonidegib (AUC, Cmax). Drug is highly bound to human plasma proteins. Elimination half-life ($t_{1/2}$) is about 28 days. Drug is primarily metabolized by CYP3A and the drug and metabolites are eliminated via the hepatic route. Of the absorbed dose, 70% is excreted in the feces, and 30% in the urine. Mild hepatic dysfunction and mild or moderate renal impairment did not affect drug exposure. In a cross study comparison, AUC appears to be 1.7 fold higher in Japanese healthy subjects compared to Western (Whites and Blacks) subjects.

Indication: Treatment of adult patients with locally advanced basal cell carcinoma that has recurred following surgery or RT, or those who are not candidates for surgery or RT.

Dosage/Range: 200 mg PO once daily taken on an empty stomach, at least 1 hour before or 2 hours after a meal. Continue drug until disease progression or unacceptable toxicity.
* Interrupt sonidegib for
  * Severe or intolerable musculoskeletal adverse reactions.
  * First occurrence of serum CK elevation between 2.5-10 X ULN.
  * Recurrent serum CK elevation between 2.5-5 X ULN.
* Resume sonidegib at 200 mg when signs/symptoms resolve.
* Permanently discontinue drug for
  * Serum CK elevation > 2.5 X ULN with worsening renal function.
  * Serum CK elevation > 10 X ULN.
  * Recurrent serum CK elevation > 5 X ULN.
  * Recurrent severe or intolerable musculoskeletal adverse reactions.

Drug Preparation: Available as a 200 mg capsule.

Drug Administration:
* Verify that female patients of reproductive potential are not pregnant. Teach patient to use effective contraception during therapy and for 20 months following last dose.
* Teach male patients to use condoms with a pregnant partner or a female partner of reproductive potential during treatment and for at least 8 months after last dose, to prevent semen exposure that may contain the drug.
* Assess serum creatine kinase (CK) and renal function tests prior to starting drug in all patients.
* Teach patient how to take drug (1) take on an empty stomach, 1 hour before or 2 hours after a meal, and (2) if a dose is missed, resume dosing with the next scheduled dose.

Drug Interactions:
* CYP3A inhibitors: can increase sonidegib peak serum concentration; do not give concomitantly with strong (e.g., saquinavir, telithromycin, ketoconazole, itraconazole, voriconazole, posaconazole, nefazodone) or moderate (e.g., atanzavir, diltiazem, fluconazole) inhibitor. If a moderate CYP3A inhibitor must be coadministered,, administer the moderate CYP3A4 inhibitor for < 14 days and monitor closely for adverse reactions, especially in the musculoskeleton.
* CYP3A4 inducers: may decrease sonidegib peak serum levels (e.g., carbamazepine, efavirenz, modafinil, phenobarbital, phenytoin, rifabutin, rifampin, St. John's Wort). Avoid concomitant administration of strong or moderate CYP3A4 inducers.
* Acid reducing agents: concomitant administration of PPIs or H_2- may decrease the mean sonidegib steady-state AUC by 34%.

Lab Effects/Interference:
* Increased serum creatinine, serum creatine kinase (CK), glucose, lipase, AST, ALT, amylase
* Anemia, lymphopenia

Special Considerations:
- Most common adverse reactions occurring in >/=10% of patients were muscle spasms, alopecia, dysgeusia, fatigue, nausea, musculoskeletal pain, diarrhea, decreased weight, decreased appetite, myalgia, abdominal pain, headache, pain, vomiting, pruritis.
- Warnings and precautions
  - Teach patients not to donate blood or blood products during treatment and for at least 20 months after the last dose.
  - Musculoskeletal adverse reactions: obtain serum CK and creatinine levels prior to starting therapy, periodically during therapy, and as clinically indicated. Interrupt drug temporarily if severe.
    - Muscle spasms most frequent (54%), followed by musculoskeletal pain (32%), and myalgia (19%).
    - Serum CK is monitored as rhabdomyolysis may occur, defined as serum CK > 10 X baseline value with concurrent 1.5 X or greater increase in serum creatinine above baseline value.
    - Assess serum creatinine and CK levels at least weekly in patients with musculoskeletal adverse reactions with concurrent serum CK elevations > 2.5 X ULN until resolution of clinical signs and symptoms.
    - Teach patient to report any unexplained muscle pain, tenderness, or weakness during treatment or after drug has been discontinued, right away.
  - Embryo-fetal toxicity: Drug can cause severe birth defects or embryo-fetal death. Ensure female patients of reproductive potential are not pregnant when starting the drug, and use effective contraception during and after drug therapy (20 months). Ensure male patients with female partners use condoms during therapy and for 8 months after last dose to prevent drug exposure to the female via semen.
- Alopecia occurs in 53% of patients. Fatigue occurs in 41%, headache in 15%, and itching in 10%.
- Nutritional impact symptoms may occur: Dysgeusia occurs in 46% of patients, nausea in 39%, diarrhea in 32%, decreased weight in 30%, decreased appetite in 23%, and vomiting in 11% of patients.

Potential Toxicities/Side Effects and the Nursing Process

I.   ALTERATION IN SEXUALITY/REPRODUCTION related to POTENTIAL TERATOGENICITY

Defining Characteristics: Drug is teratogenic, embryotoxic, and fetotoxic, causing embryo-fetal death and severe birth defects. Drug may be excreted in the semen. Drug can also be passed through blood transfusions to pregnant patients. In clinical studies 2/14 premenopausal women receiving either a 200 mg or 800 mg daily dose developed amenorrhea that lasted for at least 18 months.

Nursing Implications: Assess reproductive status, sexual activity, and birth control measures used for both men and women. Teach male patients to use condoms with spermicide, even after vasectomy, during sexual intercourse with female partners while receiving therapy and for at least 8 months after the last dose. Ensure that women have had a negative pregnancy test within 7 days of starting the drug. Teach women to use highly effective contraception measures that have < 1% risk of failure prior to starting therapy, and to continue using it for at least 20 months after last dose of sonidegib. Teach female patients to notify their providers immediately if they become pregnant while taking the drug or within 20 months after the last drug dose, and male patients to notify provider if his female partner becomes pregnant while taking sonidegib or within 8 months of the last drug dose. Nursing mothers should either discontinue sonidegib or discontinue nursing. Teach patients not to donate blood while taking sonidegib and for 20 months after the last drug dose.

II. ALTERATION IN COMFORT related to MUSCULOSKELETAL ADVERSE EFFECTS

Defining Characteristics: Musculoskeletal adverse reactions are common. Muscle spasms occur in 54% of patients, and are grade 3 in 3%. Musculoskeletal pain affects 32%, and myalgia 19% of patients. Elevation in serum creatine kinase (CK) may occur, and rhabdomyolysis defined as serum CK increase > 10X baseline value with a concurrent increase of 1.5 X or greater increase in serum creatinine above baseline, occurs rarely (0.2%). Musculoskeletal pain and myalgia usually preceded increase in serum CK values. The median time to onset of grade 2 or higher serum CK elevations was 12.9 weeks, and median time to resolution to </− grade 1 was 12 days. Medical intervention was necessary in 29% of patients (magnesium supplementation, muscle relaxants, analgesics, or opioids) including 5% who required IV hydration or hospitalization. Incidence of increased serum creatinine was 92% but remained in the normal range in 76% of patients. Increased CK occurred in 61% and was grade 3–4 in 8%.

Nursing Implications: Teach patient that musculoskeletal adverse events may occur, and to report right away any new or unexplained muscle pain, tenderness, or weakness during treatment or that persists after discontinuing sonidegib. Discuss with provider need for magnesium, muscle relaxants, and/or analgesics, and teach patient self-care strategies. Assess baseline serum CK and creatinine levels before initial dose of sonidegib, during treatment, and if patient reports muscle symptoms. If patient has musculoskeletal adverse reactions and concurrent serum CK elevations > 2.5 X ULN, assess serum creatinine and CK levels at least weekly. Discuss with provider temporary dose interruption or discontinuation based on severity of musculoskeletal symptoms and CK elevations.

III. POTENTIAL ALTERATION IN NUTRITION related to DYSGEUSIA, NAUSEA, DIARRHEA, DECREASED APPETITE, WEIGHT LOSS, VOMITING

Defining Characteristics: Nutritional impact symptoms may occur. Incidence of dysgeusia was 46%, nausea 39%, diarrhea 32%, and vomiting 11%. Decreased weight occurred in 30% of patients, and decreased appetite in 23%. Hyperglycemia occurred in 51%.

Nursing Implications: Assess nutritional status, weight, and bowel elimination status pattern baseline and at each visit. Teach patient self-care measures: to take OTC anti-diarrheal medication as needed; to take antinausea medicine as prescribed; to modify diet if diarrhea (foods to decrease motility, fluids to reverse dehydration); high-calorie, high-protein foods frequently in small amounts if decreased taste, appetite and/or weight loss; taste stimulation strategies for altered taste. Teach patient to report any symptoms that do not resolve or improve with the established plan. To increase appetite, encourage patients to use a small plate, small portions, and not to fill the plate with food; take antiemetic 30 minutes prior to eating if nausea, and to eat small, frequent meals. Arrange dietary consultation if available and needed. Note trends in weight and discuss with provider if significant.

IV.   ACTIVITY INTOLERANCE, POTENTIAL, related to FATIGUE, ASTHENIA, HEADACHE, ABDOMINAL PAIN

Defining Characteristics: Fatigue occurs in 41% of patients, abdominal pain in 18%, headache in 15%, and pain in 14%.

Nursing Implications: Assess baseline activity and energy level, and teach patient this symptom may occur. Assess patient's activity patterns, and suggest ways to conserve energy.

V.   ALTERATION IN BODY IMAGE, POTENTIAL, related to ALOPECIA, PRURITIS

Defining Characteristics: Alopecia occurs in 53% of patients, and pruritis in 10%.

Nursing Implications: Assess baseline skin itching, and hair distribution on scalp. Teach patient that alopecia may occur. Encourage patient to get a wig (cranial prosthesis) prior to starting therapy as appropriate. Assess effect of hair loss on patient's body image. Encourage patient to verbalize feelings and provide emotional support. If needed, involve social worker in supportive counseling. Encourage patient to use scarves and hats as appropriate and to attend supportive educational sessions such as ACS Look Good Feel Better programs if available. Teach patient self-care strategies for pruritis, and to report it if it persists. Teach patient not to scratch because it may impair skin integrity.

Drug: sorafenib (Nexavar)

Class: Multiple targeted tyrosine kinase inhibitor, antiangiogenesis agent.

Mechanism of Action: Drug inhibits a number of tyrosine kinases, including Raf kinase, an enzyme in the RAS pathway (RAS is mutated in about 20–30% of solid tumors), as well as receptor tyrosine kinases VEGFR-2 and PDGFR-b, thus preventing cell proliferation and angiogenesis. First, sorafenib inhibits the signaling cascade in the RAS pathway, blocking uncontrolled cell growth from either excessive stimulation of the RAS pathway, or through mutations of RAS and RAF proteins. In addition, sorafenib inhibits angiogenesis by preventing the message from vascular endothelial growth factor (VEGF), telling endothelial cells to proliferate and migrate, from reaching the cell nucleus (signal transduction), and angiogenesis is prevented. It also inhibits the message that would be sent to the cell nucleus when the ligand platelet-derived growth factor (PDGF) attaches to its receptor PDGFR-b; PDGF is necessary for pericytes around the blood vessels to provide external structure during angiogenesis, and when they are not available, angiogenesis is stopped (Onyx, 2005).

Metabolism: After oral administration, mean relative bioavailability is 38–49%, peak plasma levels in 3 hours, and mean elimination half-life of 25–48 hours. Steady state plasma concentrations reached in 7 days with multiple doses. When drug is given with a high-fat meal, bioavailability is reduced 29% compared to that in a fasted state. Drug is highly protein-bound (99.5%). Drug is metabolized by liver P450 microenzyme system, mediated by CYP3A4, with glucuronidation mediated by UGT1A9. There are eight metabolites of the drug. Following oral dose, 96% of the drug was recovered in 14 days, with 77% of the dose excreted in the feces, and 19% in the urine.

Indication: Indicated for the treatment of patients with
- Advanced renal cell cancer (RCC).
- Unresectable hepatocellular carcinoma (HCC).
- Differentiated thyroid carcinoma (DTC), which is locally recurrent, metastatic, or progressive, and refractory to radioactive iodine.

Dosage/Range:
- For patients with advanced renal cell cancer (RCC), (2) unresectable hepatocellular carcinoma (HCC), and (3) differentiated thyroid carcinoma (DTC), which is locally recurrent, metastatic, or progressive, and refractory to radioactive iodine:
  - 400 mg (two 200-mg tablets) PO bid (total daily dose of 800 mg) taken 1 hour before or 2 hours after a meal, until patient is no longer clinically benefiting from drug, or toxicity is unacceptable.
  - When dose reduction is indicated, reduce to a single 400-mg PO dose daily; if further reduction needed, change to 400-mg PO every other day.

Dose Reductions:
- Skin toxicity HCC or RCC:
  - Grade 1: numbness, dysesthesia, paresthesia, tingling, painless swelling, erythema or discomfort of hands or feet that does not disrupt patient's normal activities: continue treatment and consider topical treatment for symptomatic relief.
  - Grade 2: painful erythema and swelling of hands or feet and/or discomfort affecting ADLs: (1) first occurrence: continue sorafenib, consider topical therapy for symptomatic relief; (2) no improvement within 7 days or second or third occurrence: interrupt sorafenib until toxicity resolves to grade 0–1, then resume sorafenib at a reduced dose by one dose level (e.g., 400 mg daily or 400 mg every other day).

- Grade 3: moist desquamation, ulceration, blistering or severe pain in hands or feet, or severe discomfort, cannot do ADLs or work: (1) first or second occurrence: interrupt sorafenib until toxicity resolves to grade 0–1, then resume sorafenib, dose decreased by one dose level; (2) third occurrence: discontinue sorafenib.

Dose Reductions DTC:

- First dose reduction: 600-mg daily dose taken 400 mg and 200 mg 12 hours apart (either dose can come first).
- Second dose reduction: 400-mg daily dose taken as 200 mg twice daily.
- Third dose reduction: 200 mg once daily.
- Reduce for dermatologic toxicity in DTC:
    - Grade 1: numbness, dysesthesia, paresthesia, tingling, painless swelling, erythema or discomfort of hands or feet that does not disrupt patient's normal activities: continue treatment with sorafenib.
    - Grade 2: painful erythema and swelling of hands or feet and/or discomfort affecting ADLs: (1) First occurrence: decrease sorafenib dose to 600 mg daily; if no improvement within 7 days at reduced dose or if it is the second occurrence, interrupt sorafenib until resolved or improved to grade 1; (2) if sorafenib is resumed, decrease dose as above (dose reductions DTC); (3) if the third occurrence, interrupt sorafenib until resolved or improved to grade 1. If sorafenib is resumed, decrease dose as above (dose reductions DTC); (4) if it is the fourth occurrence, permanently discontinue sorafenib.
    - Grade 3: moist desquamation, ulceration, blistering or severe pain in hands or feet, or severe discomfort, cannot do ADLs or work: (1) first occurrence: interrupt sorafenib until toxicity resolves to grade 0–1, then resume sorafenib, dose decreased by one dose level; (2) second occurrence: interrupt sorafenib until toxicity resolves to grade 0–1, then resume sorafenib, dose decreased by two dose levels; (3) third occurrence: permanently discontinue sorafenib.
    - After improvement of grade 2 or 3 dermatologic toxicity to grade 0–1 after at least 28 days of treatment at the reduced dose, the next sorafenib dose may be increased one dose level from the reduced dose.
- No dose reduction for renal dysfunction (mild, moderate, or severe [not requiring dialysis]).
- Hepatic dysfunction: no dose modification necessary for mild or moderate impairment, but patients with severe impairment have not been studied.
- Drug is contraindicated in patients with hypersensitivity to drug or components, and in combination with carboplatin and paclitaxel in patients with squamous cell lung cancer.

Drug Preparation/Administration:

- None, oral. Take without food, at least 1 hour before or 2 hours after a meal.
- Drug is available in 200-mg tablets.
- HTN should be well controlled.
- Drug should be temporarily interrupted prior to a major surgical procedure. Decision when to resume drug is based on clinical judgment of adequate wound healing.

Drug Interactions:

- CYP3A4 inhibitors (e.g., ketoconazole): none.
- CYP isoform-selective substrates (e.g., midazolam, omeprazole, dextromethorphan): none.
- CYP2C9 substrates (e.g., warfarin): monitor INR regularly.

- CYP3A4 inducers (e.g., carbamazepine, dexamethasone, phenobarbital, phenytoin, rifampin, St. John's wort) are expected to increase the metabolism of sorafenib and decrease sorafenib serum concentration. If they must be coadministered, consider an increase in sorafenib dose, and monitor closely for toxicity.
- CYP2B6 and CYP2C8 substrates: sorafenib inhibits the metabolism of these substrates, thus increasing serum levels. Avoid concomitant administration.
- Warfarin: INR may be elevated. Monitor INR and dose warfarin accordingly.

Lab Effects/Interference:
- Increased lipase (41%), amylase (30%).
- Decreased phosphate (45%).
- Lymphopenia (23%), neutropenia (5%), anemia (44%), thrombocytopenia (12%).
- May prolong QTc on ECG.
- Increased bilirubin, transaminases, INR.
- Low TSH.

Special Considerations:
- Drug is well-tolerated with most common side effects being diarrhea, fatigue, infection, alopecia, hand-foot skin reaction, rash, weight loss, decreased appetite, nausea, GI and abdominal pain, hypertension, and hemorrhage.
- Drug is teratogenic and embryo-fetal toxic. Women of childbearing potential should be advised to avoid pregnancy, or if the patient becomes pregnant while receiving the drug, patient should be apprised of potential hazard to the fetus. Women should not breastfeed while receiving the drug.
- Peripheral sensory neuropathy occurs in 13% of patients.
- Drug should be temporarily interrupted prior to undergoing major surgical procedures, and resumed after the wound has healed.
- Drug may rarely cause gastrointestinal perforation. Patients should be taught to go to the ED immediately if they develop severe abdominal pain, with or without nausea, vomiting, or constipation, and the provider should be notified.
- Sorafenib has been shown to increase overall survival of patients with hepatocellular carcinoma by 44% (SHARP trial; Llovet et al., 2007).
- QT Prolongation: monitor for prolonged QTc intervals in patients with CHF, bradyarrhythmias, drugs known to prolong the QTc (e.g., methadone), and electrolyte abnormalities. Do not use sorafenib for patients with congenital long QT syndrome.
- Risk of cardiac ischemia and/or infarction is higher in the sorafenib-treated patients than those in the placebo group (1.9%–2.9% vs 0%–0.4%).
- Risk of hemorrhage is increased with sorafenib treatment. If bleeding requires medical intervention, consider discontinuing drug. To reduce the risk of bleeding in DTC, prior to treatment with sorafenib, tracheal, bronchial, and esophageal infiltration should be locally treated.
- Sorafenib can cause hypertension. Monitor BP weekly during first 6 weeks of sorafenib therapy. Thereafter, monitor BP and treat HTN according to standard medical practice. If HTN is severe or persistent, consider drug interruption or permanent discontinuance.
- Hand-foot syndrome and rash were the most common sorafenib-related side effects. These were generally grade 1–2 and appeared during first 6 weeks of therapy. Treatment often

includes topical symptomatic relief, temporary treatment interruption, and/or dose modification. If severe or persistent, drug should be permanently discontinued.
- Drug may cause osteonecrosis of the jaw (seen in post-marketing reports).
- Drug-induced hepatitis may occur, characterized by a hepatocellular pattern of liver damage with significant increases in transaminases, which can result in hepatic failure and death. Bilirubin and INR may also increase. Monitor LFTs baseline and regularly during therapy. If transamitnases significantly rise without alternative explanation (e.g., viral hepatitis, or progressive underlying malignancy), discontinue sorafenib.
- Sorafenib can impair thyroid suppression. DTC patients had a baseline TSH < 0.5 mU/L, but on sorafenib therapy, 41% of patients had an elevated TSH compared to 16% receiving placebo. In the study, the median maximal TSH was 1.6 mU/L and 25% had TSH levels > 4.4 mU/L. Monitor TSH levels baseline, then monthly and adjust thyroid replacement medication as needed.
- Drug was studied in chemotherapy-naive patients with NSCLC in combination with carboplatin/paclitaxel, and patients with squamous cell histology had a higher mortality, so drug is contraindicated in this population and also not recommended in patients receiving gemcitabine/cisplatin. Sorafenib is not FDA-approved for treatment of patients with NSCLC.
- Sorafenib is contraindicated in patients with known severe hypersensitivity to sorafenib or its components; it is also contraindicated in combination with carboplatin and paclitaxel in patients with squamous cell lung cancer.

Potential Toxicities/Side Effects and the Nursing Process

I.   POTENTIAL ALTERATION IN CIRCULATION related to HYPERTENSION, CARDIAC ISCHEMIA, MYOCARDIAL INFARCTION OR QT PROLONGATION WITH VENTRICULAR ARRHYTHMIAS

Defining Characteristics: Hypertension occurred in 9–41% of patients studied. Rarely, hypertensive crisis, myocardial ischemia and/or infarction occurred. In the HCC group receiving sorafenib, the incidence of cardiac ischemia/infarction was 2.7% (1.3% in placebo group), and in the RCC group receiving sorafenib, the incidence was 2.9% (0.4% in placebo group). Drug can rarely prolong QT/QTc interval and increase risk of ventricular arrhythmias, including torsades de pointes.

Nursing Implications: Review cardiac history. Assess baseline blood pressure, and monitor weekly during the first 6 weeks of treatment. Discuss antihypertensive therapy with physician or NP. If hypertension is severe and refractory to maximal antihypertensive therapy, drug should be interrupted or discontinued. If a patient develops cardiac ischemia and/or infarction while receiving the drug, discuss drug interruption or discontinuance with the physician. If the patient has cardiac ischemia or has had an infarction, discuss the risks and benefits before beginning therapy. Drug should be avoided in patients with congenital long QT interval. Document baseline QTc in patients with CHF, bradyarrhythmias, taking other drugs known to prolong the QT interval such as antiarrhythmics, and patients with electrolyte imbalances, such as magnesium and potassium. Correct hypomagnesemia, hypokalemia and hypocalcemia in the patients and monitor ECG throughout treatment.

II. ALTERATION IN SKIN INTEGRITY AND COMFORT related to HAND-FOOT SYNDROME, RASH, POTENTIAL

Defining Characteristics: Erythema is common. Rash or skin desquamation occurred in 40% of patients, and hand-foot syndrome (acral erythema) in 30% of patients compared to 16% and 7% of patients, respectively, receiving placebo. Hand-foot syndrome is generally grade 1–2, and appears during the first 6 weeks of treatment. Alopecia occurred in 27% of patients, pruritus in 19%, and dry skin in 11%. Areas of hyperkeratosis may occur on the soles of the feet, forming calluses (Wood, 2006). Rarely, folliculitis, eczema, erythema multiforme occurs. There have been reports of severe dermatologic toxicity (e.g., Stevens-Johnson syndrome (SJS) and toxic epidermal necrolysis (TEN)), which may be life-threatening.

Nursing Implications: Assess baseline skin integrity, including soles of feet and palms of hands, and teach patient that these symptoms may occur. If the patient develops calluses on the feet, suggest applying topical exfoliating agents such as Kerasal (over the counter) or Keralac (prescription) on the calluses ONLY. Teach patient to self-assess all skin areas, and to report rash, as well as redness, swelling, and/or pain anywhere, particularly the soles of feet and palms of hands. Teach patient to avoid activities that increase blood flow in the hands and feet, such as hot showers and baths, and to take tepid showers to reduce likelihood and severity of hand-foot syndrome. Teach patient to avoid constrictive clothing and repetitive movements that can irritate the opposing skin. Teach patient to use skin emollients to prevent skin from drying and cracking starting on day 1 of therapy, followed by wearing cotton gloves or socks to keep the emollient close to the skin until absorbed. Teach patient to elevate hands and feet when sitting or lying down; apply ice packs or cool compresses indirectly to hands or feet for up to 20 minutes; gently pat skin dry after bathing or washing; and avoid contact with laundry detergents or cleaning products with strong chemicals.

After assessment, discuss dose modification with physician or NP if grade 2 (PAIN) or 3, as follows (per manufacturer):

Grade 1: Numbness, dysesthesia, paresthesia, tingling, painless swelling, erythema, or discomfort of the hands or feet that does not disrupt ADLs; no change, use topical therapy for symptomatic relief.

Grade 2: Painful erythema and swelling of the hands or feet and/or discomfort affecting ADLs: First occurrence, continue therapy and use local symptomatic treatment; if no improvement within 7 days, or second or third occurrence, interrupt therapy until grade 0–1, then resume with dose reduction by one dose level, either 400 mg daily or every other day; if fourth occurrence, discontinue drug.

Grade 3: Moist desquamation, ulceration, blistering or severe pain of the hands or feet, or severe discomfort that causes the patient to be unable to work or do ADLs: first or second occurrence, interrupt until toxicity resolves to grade 0–1; then decrease dose by one dose level (400 mg daily or every other day); third occurrence: discontinue drug.

Discontinue drug if SJS or TEN are suspected.

III.　ALTERATION IN NUTRITION, LESS THAN BODY REQUIREMENTS, related to DIARRHEA, NAUSEA, ANOREXIA, VOMITING, CONSTIPATION

Defining Characteristics: Diarrhea occurs in 43% of patients, constipation 15%, nausea 23%, vomiting 16%, and anorexia 16%.

Nursing Implications: Assess nutrition status, bowel elimination status baseline and periodically during treatment. Involve nutritionist as needed to minimize symptoms, such as BRAT diet for patient with diarrhea (e.g., bananas, rice, applesauce, and toast); increase dose-dense calories and fluid in the diet, and strategies to increase appetite. Teach patient how to manage nausea, vomiting, diarrhea, and constipation, including self-administration of OTC medications or prescribed medications, dietary modifications, and increased hydration. Teach patient to report symptoms that do not improve or that persist despite interventions.

IV.　ALTERATION IN CIRCULATION related to HEMORRHAGE, POTENTIAL

Defining Characteristics: Hemorrhage occurred in 15% of patients as compared to 8% in the placebo arm. In patients with hepatocellular carcinoma, 2.4% of patients bled from esophageal varices (compared to 4% in control group). Incidence of grade 3–4 bleeding was 2% and 0% respectively.

Nursing Implications: Teach patient to report any episodes of bleeding right away. If bleeding requires medical intervention, discuss drug discontinuation with the physician.

V.　POTENTIAL FOR INFECTION AND BLEEDING related to NEUTROPENIA AND THROMBOCYTOPENIA

Defining Characteristics: Neutropenia occurred in 5% of patients, anemia in 44% of patients, and thrombocytopenia in 12% of patients in clinical trials.

Nursing Implications: Assess baseline blood counts and platelets. Teach patient to report fever, and signs/symptoms of infection or bleeding right away. Assess medication profile and OTC medications taken. Teach patient to avoid OTC medications containing NSAIDs or aspirin. Teach patient to talk to nurse or physician before beginning any OTC medications.

Drug: sunitinib malate (Sutent)

Class: Multitargeted tyrosine kinase inhibitor.

Mechanism of Action: Drug has both antitumor and antiangiogenesis activity, and inhibits multiple receptor tyrosine kinases that are involved in tumor growth, angiogenesis, and metastatic cancer progression. It inhibits platelet-derived growth factor receptors (alpha and beta), vascular endothelial growth factor receptors (VEGFR-1, -2, -3), stem cell factor receptor (KIT), fms-like tyrosine kinase-3 (FLT-3), colony-stimulating factor receptor type 1 (CSF-1R), and the glial cell-line–derived neurotrophic factor receptor (RET).

Metabolism: After oral ingestion, maximal plasma concentrations are reached within 6–12 hours, regardless of food intake. Drug and primary metabolite bind to plasma protein 90–95%. Drug is metabolized by the cytochrome P450 enzyme CYP3A4 to produce its primary metabolite, which is then itself metabolized by CYP3A4. Terminal half-life of sunitinib and its primary metabolite are 40–60 hours and 80–110 hours, respectively. Drug is primarily excreted via the feces.

Indication: Drug is FDA-approved for the treatment of patients with
- Gastrointestinal stromal tumor (GIST) after disease progression on imatinib mesylate.
- Advanced renal cell carcinoma (based on response rate and response duration).
- Progressive, well-differentiated pancreatic neuroendocrine tumors (pNET) when disease is unresectable locally advanced or metastatic.

Dosage/Range:
- Gastrointestinal stromal tumor (GIST) or advanced renal cell carcinoma (RCC): 50 mg PO daily for 4 weeks, followed by 2 weeks off, in a 6-week cycle.
- Pancreatic neuroendocrine tumors (pNET): 37.5 mg taken orally once daily, with or without food, continuously. Max dose for pNET patients studied is 50 mg.
- Dose-interrupt or dose-modify in 12.5-mg increments or decrements.
- Dose-interrupt and/or reduce in patients without signs/symptoms of CHF who have an LVEF < 50% and > 20%.
- If coadministration with strong CYP3A4 inhibitors is necessary: Reduce dose sunitinib to a minimum of 37.5 mg (GIST and RCC) or 25 mg (pNET).
- If coadministration with strong CYP3A4 inducer is necessary: Increase sunitinib dose to a maximum of 87.5 mg (GIST and RCC) or 62.5 mg (pNET) daily. If the dose is increased, monitor patient carefully for toxicity.

Drug Preparation/Administration:
- None, oral tablet. Take with or without food.
- Available as 12.5-mg, 25-mg, and 50-mg capsules.
- Laboratory monitoring:
  - CBC with platelet count, serum chemistries, including phosphate and LFTs at the beginning of each treatment cycle.
  - Assess baseline thyroid function, as acquired hypothyroidism may occur.
  - Assess baseline ECHO; if cardiac risk factors, monitor the ECHO periodically, as well as assess for signs/symptoms of CHF.
  - Patient should have a baseline ECG with calculation of QTc interval, and this should be monitored during therapy. Frequency of monitoring should increase if the patient is taking an interacting drug with increased risk of toxicity.

Drug Interactions:
- CYP3A4 inhibitors (e.g., atazanavir, clarithromycin, indinavir, itraconazole, ketoconazole, nelfinavir, nefazodone, ritonavir, saquinavir, telithromycin, voriconazole, grapefruit or

grapefruit juice): Increase plasma level of sunitinib; do not give together, or dose-reduce sunitinib if used concurrently.
- CYP3A4 inducers (e.g., carbamazepine, dexamethasone, phenobarbital, phenytoin, rifabutin, rifampin, rifapentine, St. John's wort): Decrease plasma level of sunitinib by 23–46%; do not give together, or increase dose of sunitinib if given concurrently.

Lab Effects/Interference:
- Decreased lymphocyte (38%), neutrophil (53%), red blood cell (26%), and platelet counts (38%). Elevated serum lipase (25%) and amylase (17%).
- Elevated AST/ALT (39%), alkaline phosphatase (24%), total bilirubin (16%), indirect bilirubin (10%).
- Elevated serum creatinine (12%), uric acid (15%).
- Decreased phosphate (9%), increased or decreased potassium (6%, 12%), increased or decreased sodium (10%, 6%).
- Decreased thyroid function (acquired hypothyroidism).
- QT/QTc prolongation on ECG.

Special Considerations:
- Drug is teratogenic and embryo-fetal toxic. Women of childbearing potential should be advised to avoid pregnancy, or if the patient becomes pregnant while receiving the drug, patient should be apprised of potential hazard to the fetus. Women should not breastfeed while receiving the drug.
- Patient should have CBC with platelet count, serum chemistries, including phosphate and liver function tests at the beginning of each treatment cycle; check baseline thyroid function, as acquired hypothyroidism may occur. In addition, patients should have a baseline ECHO, and if cardiac risk factors, the ECHO should be monitored periodically, as well as assessment for signs/symptoms of CHF. Patient should have a baseline ECG with calculation of QTc interval, and this should be monitored during therapy. Frequency of monitoring should increase if the patient is taking an interacting drug, with increased risk of toxicity.
- Drug has been associated with hepatotoxicity, rarely resulting in liver failure or death. Observe patient for signs/symptoms of liver failure (jaundice, elevated LFTs with encephalopathy, coagulopathy, and/or renal failure). Assess LFTs before starting the drug, during each treatment cycle, and as clinically indicated. Interrupt drug for grade 3–4 hepatotoxicity, and if unresolved, permanently discontinue drug. Drug should NOT be restarted if patient subsequently experiences severe changes in LFTs or has other signs/symptoms of liver failure.
- Drug may cause adrenal insufficiency, so patients who are experiencing stress (e.g., surgery, trauma, severe infection) should be monitored closely.
- Drug may cause bleeding, hypertension, and reduction of left ventricular ejection fraction with increased risk of CHF.
- Sunitinib should be discontinued in the presence of clinical manifestations of CHF.
- In patients without clinical evidence of CHF but a decrease in LVEF to < 50% but > 20% below baseline, the dose should be interrupted or reduced.

- The patient should be monitored for signs/symptoms of CHF during treatment.
- Baseline and periodic evaluations of LVEF should be performed during therapy, and in patients without cardiac history, a baseline evaluation of LVEF should be considered.
- Drug may prolong QTc interval (drug interval for depolarization and repolarization of the heart).
  - It is dose-dependent, and torsades de pointes or ventricular tachycardia has occurred in < 0.1% of patients.
  - Use drug cautiously in patients at risk for prolonged QT intervals (patients with a history of QT prolongation, who are taking antiarrhythmics, with a preexisting cardiac disease, bradycardia, or electrolyte disturbance).
  - Monitor patient electrolytes and ECG baseline and during treatment, and replete electrolytes to normal values (especially potassium and magnesium).
  - If the patient is also receiving concomitant treatment with a strong CYP3A4 inhibitor that can increase sunitinib plasma concentrations, consider dose reduction of sunitinib and use caution.
- 2% of patients receiving sunitinib developed DVT.
- Patients with brain metastases receiving the drug may rarely develop seizures.
- Patients on sunitinib may rarely develop pancreatitis (1%); if this occurs, the drug should be discontinued.
- Hemorrhagic events may occur, involving the GI or respiratory systems, urinary tract, brain, and tumor. The incidence of bleeding in clinical trials was 30% compared to 8% with IFN-α. Rarely, GI perforation has occurred.
- Therapy should be temporarily interrupted in patients undergoing major surgical procedures due to risk of delayed wound healing. Ensure complete wound healing prior to resuming drug after major surgery; discuss with physician.
- Osteonecrosis of the jaw may rarely occur with sunitinib therapy. Consider completing preventive dentistry prior to starting drug. Avoid invasive dental procedures, especially in patients receiving IV bisphosphonates.
- Tumor lysis syndrome has occurred, especially in newly diagnosed patients with high tumor burden; monitor patients closely and if at risk, prophylax with hydration, correction of uric acid, and monitoring of renal and electrolytes.
- Thyroid dysfunction may occur.
  - Assess baseline thyroid function prior to starting sunitinib; as needed, patients should receive medical management of thyroid dysfunction prior to starting sunitinib.
  - Assess patients for signs/symptoms of hyperthyroidism, hypothyroidism, and thyroiditis during sunitinib therapy; if identified, patients should have laboratory monitoring and management of thyroid dysfunction.
- Dermatologic toxicities: severe cutaneous reactions have been reported (e.g., erythema multiforme (EM), toxic epidermal necrolysis (TEN), Stevens-Johnson syndrome (SJS)) and may be fatal.
  - If signs/symptoms of EM, SJS, or TEN occur (eg., progressive skin rash, blisters, or mucosal lesions), discontinue sunitinib.

- If a diagnosis of EM, SJS, or TEN is confirmed, sunitinib must not be restarted.
- Necrotizing fasciitis has been reported and may be fatal. Sites included the perineum and some were secondary to fistula formation. Discontinue sunitinib if necrotizing fasciitis occurs.
- Proteinuria and nephrotic syndrome have been reported. Assess urinalysis for protein baseline and periodically during treatment, with a 24-hour urine collection for protein if proteinuria occurs.
  - Interrupt sunitinib and dose reduce for 24-hour urine protein ≥ 3 grams.
  - Discontinue sunitinib in patients with nephrotic syndrome or repeat episodes of urine protein ≥ 3 grams depite dose reductions.
  - The safety of continued sunitinib therapy in patients with moderate to severe proteinuria is unknown.
- Most common adverse reactions (≥ 20%) are fatigue, asthenia, fever, diarrhea, nausea, mucositis/stomatitis, vomiting, dyspepsia, abdominal pain, constipation, hypertension, peripheral edema, rash, hand-foot syndrome, skin discoloration, dry skin, hair color changes, altered taste, headache, back pain, arthralgia, extremity pain, cough, dyspnea, anorexia, and bleeding.
- There are no randomized trials of sunitinib demonstrating clinical benefit, such as increased survival or improvement in disease-related symptoms in renal cell carcinoma.

Potential Toxicities/Side Effects and the Nursing Process

I.   ALTERATION IN CIRCULATION, POTENTIAL, related to LEFT VENTRICULAR DYSFUNCTION, HEMORRHAGE

Defining Characteristics: Fifteen percent of patients had a decrease in left ventricular ejection fraction (LVEF) to below the lower limit of normal (LLN). Some patients (18–37%) developed bleeding events: epistaxis was most common. Less commonly, patients experienced rectal, gingival, upper GI, genital, wound bleeding, and tumor hemorrhage (NSCLC, squamous histology). Rarely, patients on clinical trials had myocardial ischemia, and one patient experienced a fatal myocardial infarction while on treatment. Rarely, GI complications including GI perforation have occurred in patients with intra-abdominal malignancies treated with sunitinib.

Nursing Implications: Assess baseline and periodic LVEF tests, as well as assess patients for any signs or symptoms of congestive heart failure. Ensure patient has a baseline determination of LVEF and that patients with cardiac disease have the determination repeated regularly during therapy. Discuss any abnormalities with physician or NP. Patients with CHF prior to starting therapy should begin sunitinib at a reduced dosage. Teach patient to perform daily weights at home and to report a weight gain of 5 lbs. or more, as well as any signs or symptoms of dyspnea or bleeding right away. Teach patient that nosebleeds may occur, and to apply pressure and hold the head down; if nosebleed does not stop within 15 minutes, patient should go to ED and call physician.

II. ALTERATION IN CIRCULATION, POTENTIAL, related to QTc PROLONGATION

Defining Characteristics: Patients may develop QT prolongation on EKG. Do NOT administer to patients with prolonged QTc or who may develop prolonged QTc (hypokalemia, hypomagnesemia, hypocalcemia, other drugs that prolong the QTc). Prolonged QTc in the setting of low magnesium and hypokalemia sets the stage for torsades de pointes, with ventricular tachycardia, fibrillation, and sudden cardiac death possible.

Nursing Implications: Assess patient's drug profile to ensure that the patient is not taking any drugs that may increase the QTc interval. Assess baseline QTc interval. Identify patients at risk for development of prolonged QTc (congenital long QTc) syndrome, prolonged QTc > 450 msec, taking antiarrhythmics or other drugs that can prolong the QTc interval (hypokalemia, hypomagnesemia, concomitant CYP3A4 strong inhibitors). Correct electrolyte abnormalities (e.g., magnesium, calcium, potassium) before starting vandetanib, and monitor periodically during therapy. Hypokalemia, hypocalcemia, and hypomagnesemia in the setting of prolonged QTc may lead to torsades de pointes, ventricular fibrillation, and sudden cardiac death. QTc must be assessed baseline, and periodically during therapy. Following any dose reduction for QT prolongation, or any dose interruptions > 2 weeks, QT assessment should be conducted as previously described. If the patient has diarrhea, serum electrolytes and EKGs will need to be assessed more frequently, and electrolytes repleted. Because of the long half-life of 50–100 hr of sunitinib and its principal metabolite, a prolonged QT interval may take a few weeks to resolve. Serum potassium level should be maintained at 4 mEq/L or higher (within normal range) and serum magnesium and calcium kept WNL. Teach patient to correctly take sunitinib as prescribed, and to avoid any drugs that may interact with it, until discussion with the physician, NP, PA, or nurse. See Introduction to *Chapter 5* for a full discussion of assessing the QT (QTc) interval in patients receiving drugs that may increase the risk of serious complications.

III. POTENTIAL ALTERATION IN CIRCULATION related to HYPERTENSION

Defining Characteristics: Hypertension occurred in 15–28% of patients being studied, compared to 11% receiving placebo. Rarely, hypertensive crisis, myocardial ischemia, and/or infarction occurred. Rarely on clinical trials, patients presented with seizures and radiologic evidence of reversible posterior leukoencephalopathy syndrome RPLS (hypertension, headache, decreased alertness, altered mental functioning, and visual loss). In patients with metastatic RCC, sunitinib-associated hypertension is associated with improved clinical outcomes without HTN-associated adverse events (Rini et al., 2011).

Nursing Implications: Assess baseline blood pressure, and monitor weekly during the first treatment cycle. Discuss antihypertensive therapy with physician or NP. If hypertension is severe (SBP > 200 mm Hg, DBP > 100 mm Hg), or refractory to maximal antihypertensive therapy, drug should be interrupted until BP controlled, or discontinued. If RPLS occurs, the drug should be interrupted.

IV.   ALTERATION IN SKIN INTEGRITY AND COMFORT related to SKIN DISCOLORATION, HAND-FOOT SYNDROME, RASH, DEPIGMENTATION OF HAIR

Defining Characteristics: Rash affected 14% of patients, skin discoloration (yellow color) 30%, and hand-foot syndrome (HFS) 14%. HFS differs from classic chemotherapy induced HFS in that the lesions are localized and hyperkeratotic. Changes may present as painful, symmetrical erythematous and edematous areas on palms and soles, ± paresthesias (Kollmannsberger et al., 2011). Preexisting sole hyperkeratosis may increase risk of developing painful lesions that restrict mobility. Hair-color changes occurred in 7% of patients: when on the drug for 4 weeks, the hair is depigmented (white), while pigment returns on the 2-week break off treatment, giving the hair a zebra-like appearance. Alopecia occurred in 5% of patients.

Nursing Implications: Assess baseline skin integrity, including soles of feet and palms of hands, and teach patient that these symptoms may occur. If patient has hyperkeratotic areas, discuss with physician/midlevel referral to podiatrist for evaluation/potential callus removal. Teach patient to self-assess all skin areas, and to report rash, as well as redness, swelling, and/or pain anywhere, particularly the soles of feet and palms of hands. Teach patient to moisturize skin on soles of feet, palms of hands frequently and to wear thick cotton socks and avoid constrictive footwear, hot water, and excessive friction. Teach to avoid activities that increase blood flow in the hands and feet, such as hot showers and baths, and to take tepid showers to reduce likelihood and severity of hand-foot syndrome. Teach patient to avoid constrictive clothing and repetitive movements that can irritate the opposing skin. Teach patient to use skin emollients to prevent skin from drying and cracking. As needed, discuss with physician/midlevel, prescription of symptomatic medications: topical or systemic analgesics, pregabalin, steroid creams, dermabond (Kollmannsberger et al., 2011). Discuss with physician/midlevel dose modifications if grade 2 (dose interruption, usually for 3 days), and restart at same dose or dose reduction.

V.   ALTERATION IN BOWEL ELIMINATION STATUS related to DIARRHEA, CONSTIPATION

Defining Characteristics: Diarrhea occurs in 40% of patients, constipation 20%. Diarrhea may be irregular, with diarrhea occurring on a few days, alternating with days of normal bowel movements.

Nursing Implications: Assess bowel elimination status, baseline and periodically during treatment. Teach patient how to manage diarrhea including self-administration of OTC medications (e.g., immodium) or prescribed medications; avoidance of stool softeners and some fiber supplements, magnesium-containing antacids; dietary modifications (avoid spicy, fatty foods, caffeine, fruit); and increased hydration. Involve nutritionist as needed to minimize symptoms, such as BRAT diet for patient with diarrhea (i.e., bananas, rice, applesauce, and toast); increase dose-dense calories and fluid in the diet, and strategies to increase appetite. If patient develops constipation, teach self-care strategies to prevent it (stool softeners, increased fluids, fruits, and vegetables). Teach patient to report symptoms that do not improve or that persist despite treatment.

VI. POTENTIAL FOR INFECTION AND BLEEDING related to NEUTROPENIA AND THROMBOCYTOPENIA

Defining Characteristics: Neutropenia occurred in 39–45% of patients, anemia 25–37% of patients, and thrombocytopenia 18–19% of patients in clinical trials.

Nursing Implications: Assess baseline blood counts and platelets. Teach patient to report fever, and signs/symptoms of infection or bleeding right away. Assess medication profile and OTC medications taken. Teach patient to avoid OTC medications containing NSAIDs or aspirin. Teach patient to talk to nurse or physician before beginning any OTC medications.

VII. ALTERATION IN NUTRITION, LESS THAN BODY REQUIREMENTS, related to NAUSEA, STOMATITIS

Defining Characteristics: Patients developed nausea (31%), vomiting (24%), stomatitis (29%), and anorexia (33%). Other changes that may occur are taste changes, dry mouth, indigestion, and anorexia.

Nursing Implications: Assess nutritional status, integrity of oral mucosa baseline and periodically during treatment. Teach patient that these side effects may occur and to report them. Teach patient self-administration of antiemetics prior to administration of drug if nausea or vomiting has occurred. Teach patient other self-care strategies, such as to eat small, frequent meals; avoid foods that are sweet, fried, or fatty; avoid bad smells; and drink small amounts of fluids frequently. Teach patient to report persistent or continued nausea and/or vomiting. Assess efficacy and discuss change in antiemetic drug with physician if regimen ineffective. Teach patient to assess oral mucosa regularly, use oral hygiene regimen such as sodium bicarbonate in water after meals and at bedtime, and report signs/symptoms of stomatitis. Teach patient diet modification to minimize oral discomfort, such as avoiding hot, spicy, or acidic foods; eating small pieces of cool or cold foods; using a straw for drinking liquids.

Drug: temsirolimus (Torisel)

Class: Kinase inhibitor (mTOR inhibitor).

Mechanism of Action: Drug binds to the intracellular protein FKBP-12, and the protein-drug complex inhibits mTOR (mammalian target of rapamycin or FKBP 12) kinase that is responsible for cell division. mTOR is also responsible for sensing the nutrients in the cell's environment and also for organizing actin, trafficking of the membrane, insulin secretion, protein degradation, protein kinase C signaling, and tRNA synthesis. Inhibition of the kinase makes the cell think it is starving and it stops growing (arrests cell growth in

G1 phase of the cell cycle). This reduces the levels of hypoxia-inducible factors (HIF) and VEGF. As more is learned about the function of this pathway, it appears that rapamycin and mTOR inhibitors affect only some of mTOR functioning.

Metabolism: The drug is metabolized by the P450 microenzyme system in the liver (CYP3A4) into five metabolites. Sirolimus is the active metabolite. Metabolites are primarily excreted in the feces (82% within 14 days). Mean half-lives of temsirolimus and sirolimus were 17.3 hours and 54.6 hours, respectively. Patients with baseline bilirubin > 1.5 × ULN have an increased risk of grade 3–4 adverse effects and death.

Indication: For the treatment of advanced renal cell cancer.
• Drug is contraindicated in patients with bilirubin > 1.5 × ULN.

Dosage/Range :
• 25 mg IV over 30–60 minutes weekly until tumor progression or intolerable toxicity. Pretreat with an diphenhydramine as ordered.
• Dose-reduce in patients with mild hepatic impairment (BR > 1–1.5 × ULN or AST > ULN but BR ≤ ULN): Reduce dose to 15 mg/week.
• Concomitant strong CYP3A4 inhibitors: avoid; if must be coadministered, reduce temsirolimus dose to 12.5 mg/week. If the strong inhibitor is discontinued, allow a washout period of one week before adjusting the temsirolimus dose back to dose used before initiation of strong CYP3A4 inhibitor.
• Concomitant strong CYP3A4 inducers: avoid; if must be coadministered, raise temsirolimus dose from 25 mg/week up to 50 mg/week. If the strong inducer is discontinued, return to the temsirolimus dose used prior to starting the strong inducer.

Drug Preparation:
• Temsirolimus is supplied as a Torisel kit containing temsirolimus vial (25 mg/mL) and diluent vial containing 1.8 mL (with overfill).
• Before preparation, store in the refrigerator at 2–8°C (36–46°F) and protect from light.
• During preparation, protect from excessive room light and sunlight. Inspect product for particulate matter and decolorization before administration.
• Do not use bags or tubing containing the plasticizer DEHP [di(2-ethylhexyl) phthalate], which may leach DEHP from the PVC infusion bags or sets into IV solution and be administered into the patient.
• Step 1: Inject 1.8-mL of supplied diluent into vial that together with an overfill of 0.2 mL results in a 10-mg/mL solution.
• Invert vial to mix, and allow air bubbles to subside. This vial is stable for 24 hours at controlled room temperature. ALWAYS combine temsirolimus injection with the supplied diluent BEFORE adding to infusion bag. Direct addition of drug to aqueous solution will result in precipitation of the drug.
• Step 2: Withdraw ordered drug amount from vial [prepared in step 1 (e.g., 2.5 mL for a temsirolimus dose of 25 mg)], and further dilute into an infusion bag containing 250 mL of 0.9% sodium chloride injection. Use an IV container such as glass, polyolefin, or polyethylene. Invert bag or bottle to mix but do not shake, as this will cause foaming. Protect IV bag containing temsirolimus from excessive room light and sunlight.

- Inspect the solution for particulate matter and discoloration prior to administration.
- Drug must be used within 6 hours.
- Drug contains polysorbate 80, which increases the rate of DEHP extraction from PVC.

Drug Administration:
- Check CBC weekly, and chemistries every other week. Hold for ANC < 1,000 cells/mm^3, platelet count < 75,000 cells/mm^3, or grade 3 or higher toxicity (NCI CTCAE). Assess baseline LFTs, as dose is reduced in patients with impaired hepatic function.
- Drug should be stored in bottles (glass, polypropylene) or plastic IV bags (polypropylene, polyolefin) that do not contain DEHP. The drug should be administered through a non-DEHP, non-polyvinylchloride (non-PVC) tubing with appropriate filter. An administration set that does not contain DEHP with an inline filter < 5 microns, such as a polyethylene-lined administration set with an inline polyether sulfone filter with a pore size < 5 microns, should be used. D not use bags or tubing containing the plasticizer DEHP [di(2-ethylhexyl) phthalate], which may leach from the PVC infusion bags or sets into IV solution and be administered into the patient.
- Administer the final diluted drug solution within 6 hrs from the time that temsirolimus is first added to the 0.9% sodium chloride injection, USP.
- Premedicate with 25–50 mg diphenhydramine 30 minutes before temsirolimus dose.
- After premedication, administer temsirolimus IV over 30–60 minutes once a week via an infusion pump if possible.
- Hypersensitivity/infusion reactions (e.g., flushing, chest pain, dyspnea, hypotension, apnea, loss of consciousness, hypersensitivity, anaphylaxis) may occur rarely, and occur very early in the first infusion, but may also occur in subsequent infusions.
  - Monitor patient closely. If a reaction occurs, stop the drug immediately, and keep vein open with a plain IV solution (e.g., 0.9% Sodium Chloride).
  - Have emergency equipment nearby. If stable, observe the patient for 30–60 minutes, depending upon severity of reaction.
  - Physician/NP/PA may decide to resume the drug after the administration of an H1-receptor antagonist (e.g., diphenhydramine) if not already administered and/or H2 receptor antagonist (e.g., IIV famotidine 20 mg or IV ranitidine 50 mg), 30 minutes before resuming the infusion.
  - Resume infusion at a slower rate (e.g., up to 60 minutes).
  - A benefit-risk assessment must be done prior to continuing temsirolimus therapy if severe or life-threatening reaction occurs.
- Teach patient not to eat/drink grapefruit or grapefruit juice, and not to take St.John's wort.

Drug Interactions:
- Strong CYP3A4 inhibitors (e.g., atazanavir, clarithromycin, indinavir, itraconazole, ketoconazole, nelfinavir, nefazodone, ritonavir, saquinavir, telithromycin, voriconazole, grapefruit juice); do not coadminister or reduce temsirolimus dose.
- Strong CYP3A4 inducers (carbamazepine, dexamethasone, phenobarbital, phenytoin, rifabutin, rifampin, rifampacin, St. John's wort): do not coadminister, or consider dose adjustment if medically necessary to coadminister.

- Interactions with drugs metabolized by CYP2D6: no clinically significant effect anticipated.
- Sunitinib: Grade 3–4 dose-limiting toxicities.

Lab Effects/Interference:
- Hyperglycemia, hypertriglyceridemia, hypophosphatemia; elevated AST, alkaline phosphatase, and serum creatinine; decreased potassium.
- Neutropenia, thrombocytopenia, anemia, lymphopenia.

Special Considerations:
- Use with caution, if at all, in patients with hypersensitivity to drug, sirolimus, or polysorbate 80.

Warnings and Precautions:
- Hypersensitivity infusion reactions:
  - May be characterized by flushing, chest pain, dyspnea, hypotension, apnea, loss of consiousness, hypersensitivity, and anaphylaxis.
  - May occur very early in first infusion, but also may occur with subsequent infusions.
  - Monitor patient throughout the infusion; if a severe infusion reaction occurs, interrupt the infusion, and provide appropriate supportive care as ordered.
  - If a patient develops a hypersensitivity reactions (HSR), stop the infusion, and observe the patient for at least 30–60 minutes, depending upon severity of HSR. Physician may order the drug infusion resumed with administration of an H1-receptor antagonist if not previously administered, and/or a H2-receptor antagonist (e.g., IV famotidine 20 mg) approximately 30 minutes prior to restarting the temsirolimus infusion. Resume the infusion at a slower rate (up to 60 minutes).
  - If the patient has a severe or life-threatening reaction, a benefit-risk assessment should be done prior to continuing temsirolimus therapy.
- Hepatic impairment:
  - Patients with baseline bilirubin > 1.5 × ULN had greater toxicity than patients with lower baseline bilirubin, and grade 3 and higher adverse events occurred more frequently in patients with bilirubin > 1.5 × ULN, including death.
  - Dose should be reduced in patients with mild hepatic impairment (see Dosage/Range).
- Hyperglycemia/glucose intolerance, occurs commonly with 89% having at least one episode of elevated serum glucose during clinical trials and 26% of patients reporting hyperglycemia as an adverse event.
  - This may necessitate an increase in the dose of, or initiation, of insulin and/or oral hypoglycemic agent therapy.
  - Monitor serum glucose baseline, and during treatment. Teach patients to report excessive thirst or increased volume or frequency of urination.
- Infections may occur as temsirolimus may be immunosuppressive. Observe patients carefully for occurrence of infections, including opportunistic infections.
- Interstitial lung disease (ILD) may occur, and some cases may be fatal.
  - Patients may be asymptomatic or minimally symptomatic with infiltrates seen on CT or CXR.
  - Symptomatic patients may have dyspnea, cough, hypoxia, fever.

- Teach patient to report any new or worsening respiratory symptoms right away.
- Patient should undergo baseline radiographic assessment by lung CT scan or chest radiograph prior to starting temsirolimus therapy. Follow these assessments periodically even if patient has no clinical respiratory symptoms.
- Patients should be followed closely for clinical respiratory symptoms:
  - If clinically significant symptoms develop, consider holding temsirolimus until after recovery of symptoms and radiologic improvement related to pneumonitis.
  - Discuss medical management with physician or NP/PA. Empiric treatment with corticosteroids and/or antibiotics may be considered.
  - Opportunistic infections such as PJP should be considered in the differential diagnosis, and if the patient requires corticosteroids, PJP prophylaxis should also be considered.
- Hyperlipidemia occurs commonly and may require the initiation of, or increase in dose of, the patient's current lipid-lowering agent. Assess serum triglycerides and cholesterol baseline and during temsirolimus therapy.
- Abnormal wound healing: drug has been associated with abnormal wound healing. Use drug cautiously in perioperative period. Ensure that wound is well healed before giving drug.
- Bowel perforation occurs rarely and may be fatal. Teach patients to report worsening abdominal pain and bloody stools right away and to come to the emergency department for immediate evaluation.
- Renal failure has occurred, and cases of rapidly progressive and sometimes fatal renal failure have been reported.
- Intracerebral hemorrhage: patients with CNS tumors (primary or metastatic) and/or receiving anticoagulation therapy may be at increased risk of intracerebral bleeding during temsirolimus therapy.
- Coadministration with inducers or inhibitors of CYP3A metabolism: avoid coadministration, and if medically necessary to coadminister, adjust temsirolimus dose. Teach patients NOT to eat grapefruit or drink grapefruit juice, and NOT to take St. John's wort.
- Concomitant use of temsirolimus with sunitinib: resulted in dose-limiting toxicities (grade 3–4 erythematous maculopapular rash, gout/cellulitis requiring hospitalization).
- Vaccinations: avoid live vaccines (e.g., intranasal influenza, measles, mumps, rubella, oral polio, BCG, yellow fever, varicella, and TY21a typhoid) during temsirolimus therapy.
- Use in pregnancy:
  - Drug is likely to cause fetal harm. If drug is used in pregnancy, or if the patient becomes pregnant while receiving the drug, the patient should be apprised of the potential hazard to the fetus.
  - Teach women of reproductive potential to use reliable contraception to avoid pregnancy during treatment and for 3 months after last dose.
  - Teach men with partners of childbearing potential to use reliable contraception and to continue this for 3 months after the last temsirolimus dose.
- Elderly patients are more likely to experience diarrhea, edema, and pneumonia.
- Laboratory monitoring: in clinical trials, CBC assessed weekly, and chemistry panels every 2 weeks; monitoring may be more or less frequently at physician's discretion.

Most common (≥ 30%) side effects are rash, asthenia, mucositis, nausea, edema, anorexia.
* Most common lab abnormalities (≥ 30%) were: anemia, hyperglycemia, hyperlipidemia, hypertriglyceridemia, lymphopenia, elevated alkaline phosphatase, elevated serum creatnine, hypophosphatemia, thrombocytopenia, elevated AST, and leukopenia.

Potential Toxicities/Side Effects and the Nursing Process

I.   **POTENTIAL FOR INJURY related to INFUSION-RELATED REACTIONS AND HYPERSENSITIVITY**

Defining Characteristics: The incidence of hypersensitivity is uncommon, as most patients received premedication with diphenhydramine (Chan et al., 2005).

Nursing Implications: Administer premedication with diphenhydramine. Stop the infusion right away if the patient has a reaction; monitor VS and O_2 saturation for at least 30–60 minutes depending on the severity of the reaction. Discuss the addition of an H_2 antagonist 30 minutes prior to resuming the infusion to prevent further hypersensitivity with physician. Ensure that medications necessary for the management of hypersensitivity/anaphylaxis are readily available (e.g., epinephrine, antihistamines, corticosteroids). Assess baseline VS and monitor frequently during the infusion, as specified by the infusion. Be prepared to provide emergency support as necessary (including IV saline, epinephrine, antihistamines, bronchodilators). If/when symptoms resolve, resume the infusion at 50% of the rate of the previous infusion, as directed by the physician.

II.   **POTENTIAL FOR INFECTION AND BLEEDING related to NEUTROPENIA AND THROMBOCYTOPENIA**

Defining Characteristics: Incidence of decreased neutrophils was 19% (grade 3–4 5%), platelets 40% (1%), hemoglobin 94% (20%), and lymphocytes 53% (16%). Grade 3 or 4 neutropenia occurred in 7% of patients, thrombocytopenia in 5%, and anemia in 9% of patients in clinical trials comparing doses 75–250 mg weekly. Drug is immunosuppressive, and thus, patients are at risk for opportunistic infections.

Nursing Implications: Assess baseline blood counts and platelets. Teach patient to report fever, and signs/symptoms of infection or bleeding right away. Assess medication profile and OTC medications taken. Teach patient to avoid OTC medications containing NSAIDs or aspirin. Teach patient to talk to nurse or physician before beginning any OTC medications.

III. **POTENTIAL ALTERATION IN NUTRITION, LESS THAN BODY REQUIREMENTS, related to MUCOSITIS, NAUSEA, ANOREXIA, DIARRHEA, HYPERGLYCEMIA, HYPERTRIGLYCERIDEMIA, BOWEL PERFORATION**

Defining Characteristics: In clinical studies, mucositis affected 70% of patients, nausea 43%, diarrhea 27%, and anorexia 40% of patients. Bowel perforation occurs rarely but may be fatal. Presentation includes fever, abdominal pain, metabolic acidosis, bloody stools, diarrhea, and/or acute abdomen. The incidence of hypercholesterolemia is 87%, triglyceridemia 83%, and hyperglycemia was 89%; in terms of grade 3 and 4 toxicities, hyperglycemia occurred in 17% of patients, hypophosphatemia 13%, and hypertriglyceridemia in 6% of patients. mTOR is involved in insulin signaling, which possibly explains the hypertriglyceridemia and hyperglycemia.

Nursing Implications: Assess serum triglycerides, cholesterol, glucose baseline and during treatment with the drug. Teach the patient to report any new or worsening abdominal pain or bloody stools right away and to come to the emergency department for immediate evaluation. Premedicate with antiemetics. Encourage small, frequent meals of cool, bland foods, and increase fluid intake. Assess oral mucosa prior to drug administration and instruct patient to report changes. Teach patient oral hygiene measures and self-assessment. Teach patient to notify physician/nurse if excessive thirst or any increase in volume or frequency of urination. Notify physician of any abnormalities and discuss implications and management.

IV. ALTERATION IN SKIN INTEGRITY, POTENTIAL, related to RASH

Defining Characteristics: Maculopapular rash is the most common toxicity, affecting 47%; 10% had acne, 14% had a nail disorder, 11% had dry skin, and 19% pruritus.

Nursing Implications: Assess patient skin integrity, including nails baseline and regularly during treatment. Teach patient self-assessment and local comfort measures, including the use of water-based emollients. Teach patient to report skin changes and if self-care ineffective, discuss plan with physician, especially if severe.

V. ALTERATION IN COMFORT AND ACTIVITY TOLERANCE, POTENTIAL, related to ASTHENIA

Defining Characteristics: Asthenia affects 51% of patients in clinical studies, depression 4%, but at the higher dose of 250 mg q week, 5% had grade 3 and 4 depression.

Nursing Implications: Assess baseline comfort, mental status, and activity tolerance, and reassess during treatment, asking patient to identify what activities now unable to do, sleep habits, and also feeling state. Discuss alternating rest and activity periods, and also possibility of other family members or friends assisting with energy-consuming responsibilities to increase energy reserve. Assess baseline alertness, sleep patterns. Assess other drugs taken, especially those with sedating qualities, and alcohol ingestion. Instruct patient to avoid alcohol and to take drug at bedtime. Assess degree of drowsiness and dizziness for safety of patient. If significant, teach measures to ensure safety.

Drug: thalidomide (Thalomid)

Class: Immunomodulatory and antiangiogenic agent.

Mechanism of Action: While the mechanism of action is not fully understood, drug has immunomodulatory, anti-inflammatory, and antiangiogenic properties. Drug probably suppresses excessive TNF-α production and modulates some cell surface adhesion molecules involved in leukocyte migration. In multiple myeloma (MM), drug treatment is accompanied by an increase in the number of circulating natural killer (NK) and T-cell derived cytokines associated with cytotoxic activity. Thalidomide inhibits angiogenesis, possibly by blocking the proliferation of endothelial cells.

Metabolism: Slow absorbtion after oral administration. Mean peak serum level reached at 2–5 hours after drug administration. Drug is not a substrate of the P450 hepatic enzyme system. The mean elimination half-life was 5.5–7.3 hrs. The majority of a radioactive dose is excreted within 48 hrs., primarily in the urine as hydrolic metabolites (91.9%), with minor fecal excretion (< 2% of drug). There is a linear relationship between body weight and estimated thalidomide clearance.

Indication: Drug is indicated for the treatment of patients with:
• Newly diagnosed multiple myeloma (MM) in combination with dexamethasone.
• Acute treatment of cutaneous manifestations of moderate to severe erythema nodosum leprosum (ENL) and maintenance therapy for the prevention and suppression of the cutaneous manifestations of ENL recurrence.
• Drug is not indicated as monotherapy for ENL treatment if the patient has moderate-severe neuritis.

Dosage/Range:
• Drug is only available through a restricted distribution program, the THALOMID Risk Evaluation and Mitigation Strategies (REMS) program. This requires that:
  • Prescribers must be certified with THALOMID REMS program by enrolling and complying with the REMS requirements.
  • Patients must sign a Patient-Provider agreement form and comply with the REMS requirements (e.g., pregnancy testing for females of reproductive potential, and contraception for females and males, see Drug Preparation/Administration).
  • Pharmacies must be certified with THALOMID REMS program, must dispense only to patients who are authorized to receive thalidomide, and comply with REMS requirements.

Multiple myeloma (MM):
• In combination with dexamethasone in 28-day treatment cycles: Thalidomide 200 mg orally once daily with water, preferably at bedtime, at least 1 hour after the evening meal. Give dexamethasone 40 mg orally daily on days 1–4, 9–12, 17–20, every 28 days.
• Patients who develop constipation, somnolence, or peripheral neuropathy or other adverse events, may benefit by either temporarily discontinuing the drug or continuing at a lower dose.
• With abatement of these adverse reactions, the drug may be started at a lower dose or at the previous dose based on clinical judgment.
• Consider thromboprohylaxis based on individual patient's underlying risk factors.

Cutaneous erythema nodosum leprosum (ENL):
• For an episode of ENL: 100–300 mg/day, administered once daily with water, preferably at bedtime, at least 1 hour after the evening meal. Patients weighing < 50 kg should be started at the low end of the dose range.

- Patients with severe ENL reaction, or those who required higher doses to control the reaction: Start at higher doses up to 400 mg/day once daily at bedtime, or in divided doses with water, at least 1 hour after meals.
- Patients with moderate to severe neuritis associated with a severe ENL reaction: corticosteroids may be started concomitant with thalidomide. Steroid usage can be tapered and discontinued when neuritis has improved.
- Thalidomide is not indicated as monotherapy for acute treatment in the presence of moderate-severe neuritis.
- Thalidomide is usually continued until signs and symptoms of active reaction have subsided, usually a period of at least 2 weeks. Patients may be tapered off thalidomide in 50-mg decrements every 2–4 weeks.
- Patients with a documented history of requiring prolonged maintenance treatment to prevent the recurrence of cutaneous ENL, or who flare during tapering, should be maintained on the minimum dose necessary to control the reaction. Tapering off medication should be attempted every 3–6 mo, in decrements of 50 mg every 2–4 weeks.

Drug Preparation/Administration:
- Drug is contraindicated in a pregnant woman or in patients with demonstrated hypersensitivity to the drug or its components.
- Available as 50-mg, 100-mg, 150-mg, and 200-mg capsules.
- Pregnancy must be excluded prior to starting therapy, and female patients with reproductive potential must use two reliable methods of contraception.
  - Females of reproductive potential must avoid pregnancy for at least 4 weeks before beginning thalidomide, during therapy, during dose interruptions, and for at least 4 weeks after completing therapy.
  - Females must commit either to abstain continuously from heterosexual intercourse, or to use two reliable methods of birth control, beginning at least 4 weeks before beginning thalidomide, during therapy, during dose interruptions, and for at least 4 weeks after discontinuance of thalidomide therapy.
  - Two negative pregnancy tests must be obtained prior to initiating therapy. First test should be performed within 10–14 days, and the second test within 24 hours prior to prescribing thalidomide therapy, then weekly during the first month, then monthly thereafter in women with regular menstrual cycles or every 2 weeks in women with irregular menstrual cycles.
- Men must always use a latex or synthetic condom during any sexual contact with females of reproductive potential when taking thalidomide and for up to 28 days after thalidomide discontinuance, even if the man has undergone a successful vasectomy. Drug is present in semen.
- Initiate thalidomide treatment only if ANC is ≥ 750 cells/mm³.
  - CBC/differential should be monitored on an ongoing basis, especially in patients prone to neutropenia, such as HIV-seropositive patients.
  - If ANC < 750 cells/mm³ while on treatment, reevaluate the patient's medication regimen, and if neutropenia persists, consider withholding thalidomide if clinically appropriate.

- Oral, give at bedtime if possible, at least 1 hour after the evening meal.
  - Females of reproductive potential should avoid contact with thalidomide capsules, and capsules should be stored in blister packs until ingestion. If there is skin contact with non-intact capsules or the powder contents, exposed area should be washed with soap and water.
  - Healthcare providers should wear gloves if handling drug capsules to prevent potential cutaneous exposure. If exposed to body fluids from patients receiving thalidomide, exposed area should be washed with soap and water.
- Teach patient that if a dose is missed and it has been < 12 hours since the regular time to take the dose, to take the dose as soon as it is remembered. If it has been > 12 hours, the missed dose should be skipped. The patient should not take 2 doses at the same time.

Drug Interactions:
- Opioids, antihistamines, antipsychotics, antianxiety agents, other CNS depressants including alcohol: increased sedation; avoid coadministration.
- Drugs that cause bradycardia (e.g., calcium channel blockers, beta blockers, alpha/beta-adrenergic blockers, digoxin, cimetidine, famotidine, lithium, tricyclic antidepressants, succinylcholine): possible additive bradycardic effect; use together cautiously.
- Drugs that cause peripheral neuropathy (e.g., bortezomib, amiodarone, cisplatin, docetaxel, paclitaxel, vincristine, disulfiram, phenytoin, metronidazole, alcohol): possible additive effect; use together with caution.
- Hormonal contraceptives increase the risk of thromboembolism. It is unknown if concomitant use of hormonal contraceptives further increases risks for thromboembolism when given with thalidomide.
- Drugs that interfere with hormonal contraceptives (e.g., HIV-protease inhibitors, griseofulvin, modafinil, penicillins, rifampin, rifabutin, phenytoin, carbamazepine, or certain herbal supplements like St. John's wort) when used concomitantly with hormonal contraceptive agents may reduce the effectiveness of contraception up to one month after discontinuation of these concomitant therapies. Women requiring treatment with one or more of these drugs must use 2 OTHER effective or highly effective methods of contraception while taking thalidomide.

Lab Effects/Interference:
- Decreased leukocytes, neutrophils.
- Hyperglycemia.
- Hypocalcemia.
- Increased serum bilirubin.
- HIV RNA levels may be increased in HIV-seropositive patients.

Special Considerations:
- Thalidomide is a powerful teratogen that induces a high frequency of severe and life-threatening birth defects, even after a single dose.
  - Thalidomide is ABSOLUTELY CONTRAINDICATED IN PREGNANCY. Pregnancy tests must be routinely negative prior to beginning therapy in women of childbearing age.

- Reliable contraception is mandatory in men and women. Nursing mothers should discontinue drug or nursing, taking into account the importance of the drug to the mother's health. See above Drug Dosage, Drug /Administration for THALOMID REMS details.
- Further information is available at www.celgeneriskmanagement.com, or at 1-888-423-5436.
- Thalidomide is present in semen. Men taking thalidomide must not donate sperm.
- Women taking hormonal contraception concomitantly with drugs that may reduce effectiveness of contraception MUST use two other effective or highly effective methods of contraception when on thalidomide therapy. See Drug Interactions.
- Thalidomide when used to treat MM increases risk of venous thromboembolism events (VTE) such as DVT and pumonary embolism (PE). This risk is significantly increased when combined with standard chemotherapy agents, including dexamethasone.
- In one controlled trial, the incidence was 22.5% in patients receiving thalidomide plus dexamethasone, compared to 4.9% in patients receiving dexamethasone alone (p = 0.002). Consider thromboprophylaxis based on assessment of individual patient's risk factors. Assess patients for signs/symptoms of VTE, and teach patient to call healthcare provider/get medical care right away for SOB, chest pain, arm or leg swelling.
- Drowsiness and somnolence: teach patients to avoid situations where drowsiness may be a problem, and not to take take other drowsiness-inducing medicines. Teach patients that their ability to perform hazardous tasks, such as driving a car, or operating complex or dangerous machinery, may be impaired (mentally and/or physically) and to avoid these activities. Thalidomide dosage may need to be reduced.
- Dizziness and orthostatic hypotension may occur. Teach patients to sit upright for a few minutes before standing up from a recumbent position.
- Peripheral neuropathy is common, affecting ≥ 10% of patients, and may be irreversible.
  - Peripheral neuropathy generally occurs with chronic use over a period of months but occurrence after relatively short-term use has been reported. Symptoms may occur after thalidomide treatment has been stopped, and resolve slowly if at all.
  - Assess patients for signs/symptoms of peripheral neuropathy (e.g., numbness, tingling or pain in the hands and feet) baseline, at least monthly for the first 3 months, then periodically during thalidomide therapy.
  - Consider electrophysiological testing (measurement of sensory nerve action potential (SNAP) amplitudes) baseline, and every 6 months to identify asymptomatic neuropathy.
  - If symptoms of drug-induced neuropathy develop, discontinue thalidomide immediately to limit further nerve damage, if clinically appropriate. Usually, thalidomide is reinitiated only if neuropathy returns to baseline status.
  - Use medications known to be associated with neuropathy cautiously in patients receiving thalidomide.
- Neutropenia: Thalidomide should be initiated only if ANC is ≥ 750 cells/mm^3, and CBC/differential should be monitored on an ongoing basis, especially in patients who are prone to neutropenia (e.g., HIV-seropositive patients). Reevaluate patient's medication regimen if ANC falls to < 750 cells/mm^3 while on treatment. If neutropenia

persists, consider withholding thalidomide if clinically appropriate. Patients may require dose reduction.

- Increased plasma HIV RNA levels may occur in HIV seropositive patients. Measure viral load baseline, after the first and third months of treatment, and then every 3 months thereafter. Bradycardia in patients receiving thalidomide has been reported. Monitor patients for bradycardia and syncope. Dose reduction or discontinance may be required. Medications known to decrease heart rate should be used cautiously in patients receiving thalidomide.

- Severe dermatological reactions, including Stevens-Johnson syndrome (SJS) and toxic epidermal necrolysis (TEN) have been reported, and may be fatal. Stop thalidomide if rash occurs, and resume thalidomide only after appropriate clinical evaluation. If rash is exfoliative, purpuric, or bullous, or if SJS or TEN is suspected, do not resume thalidomide.

- Seizures, including grand-mal seizures, have been reported post-approval. If a patient has a history of seizures, or other risk factors for developing seizures, monitor the patient closely for clinical changes that could precipitate acute seizure activity.

- Tumor lysis syndrome (TLS) may occur in patients with a high tumor burden before treatment. Identify these patients, and discuss with physician, NP, or PA TLS prophylaxis.

- Hypersensitivity to thalidomide has been reported, characterized by erythematous macular rash, possibly associated with fever, tachycardia, and hypotension; if severe, interrupt thalidomide therapy. If the reaction occurs again after drug is resumed, discontinue thalidomide.

- Risks of certain contraceptive methods: Because some patients receiving thalidomide may develop sudden, severe neutropenia and/or thrombocytopenia, use of an intrauterine device (IUD) or implantable contraceptive may increase the risk of infection or bleeding either at insertion, removal, or during use. Thalidomide treatment in the presence of an underlying malignancy and/or use of an estrogen-containing contraceptive can each increase the risk of VTE. While it is not known if the risks of VTE are additive, the risks should be considered when the patient is selecting contraceptive methods.

- Patients receiving thalidomide should not donate blood during treatment or for one month after the drug has been discontinued, as the blood might be given to a pregnant woman, putting the fetus at risk of exposure to thalidomide.

- Most common side effects when thalidomide is used to treat MM are fatigue, hypocalcemia, edema, constipation, sensory neuropathy, dyspnea, muscle weakness, leukopenia, neutropenia, rash/desquamation, confusion, anorexia, nausea, anxiety/agitation, asthenia, tremor, fever, weight loss, thrombosis/embolism, motor neuropathy, weight gain, dizziness, dry skin.

- Most common side effects when thalidomide is used to treat ENL: somnolence, rash, headache.

- Safety and effectiveness in pediatric patients < 12 years old have not been established.

- In Study 2 of MM patients receiving thalidomine with dexamethasone, patients 65 years of age or older had higher incidences of atrial fibrillation, constipation, fatigue, nausea, hypokalemia, DVT, hyperglycemia, PE, and asthenia compared to patients < 65.

Potential Toxicities/Side Effects and the Nursing Process

I.   ALTERATION IN SEXUALITY/REPRODUCTION related to POTENTIAL TERATOGENICITY

Defining Characteristics: Drug is teratogenic and a single dose can cause birth defects. Drug is distributed in semen.

Nursing Implications: Assess reproductive status, sexual activity, and birth control measures used for both men and women. The THALOMID REMS program requires that prescribers be certified with the program (enrolling and complying with REMS), patients must sign a Patient-Prescriber agreement form and comply with the REMS requirements, and pharmacies must be certified with the THALOMID REMS program, must only dispense to authorized patients, and must comply with REMS requirements. Women of reproductive potential must commit to using two forms of reliable contraception (or abstain continuously from heterosexual sexual intercourse) to avoid pregnancy for four weeks before starting thalidomide, during therapy, during dose interruptions, and for at least four weeks after drug has been discontinued. Two negative pregnancy tests must be verified prior to starting therapy, one 10–14 days before, and one within 24 hours of prescribing thalidomide therapy, then weekly for the first month, then monthly if regular menses, or every two weeks in women with irregular menstrual cycles.

Male patients must commit to always using a latex or synthetic condom during any sexual contact with females of reproductive potential while taking thalidomide, and for up to 28 days after discontinuing the drug. This is regardless of whether the man has had a successful vasectomy. Men should be told not to donate sperm.

Teach women to tell their healthcare provider right away if they have unprotected sex or think that their birth control has failed. If the patient thinks she has become pregnant, she should stop taking thalidomide right away and call her healthcare provider. Teach men to tell their healthcare provider if they have unprotected sexual contact with a female who is or could become pregnant; if their female partner becomes pregnant, they should tell their healthcare provider right away. If the healthcare provider is not available, the patient can call 1-800-332-1088 for medical information. Healthcare providers and patients should report all pregnancies to FDA MedWatch at 1-800-332-1088, and Celgene Corporation at 1-888-423-5436.

II.   ALTERATION IN OXYGENATION, POTENTIAL, related to VENOUS THROMBO EMBOLISM (VTE)

Defining Characteristics: In MM patients, VTE risk is significantly increased when thalidomide is combined with standard chemotherapy agents, including dexamethasone. In one controlled trial, the incidence was 22.5% in patients receiving thalidomide plus dexamethasone, compared to 4.9% in patients receiving dexamethasone alone ($p = 0.002$). In the safety study, DVT occurred in 13% of patients compared to 2% in placebo/dexamethasone group.

Nursing Implications: Assess for signs/symptoms of VTE at each visit. Discuss with physician or NP/PA need for thromboprophylaxis given the individual patient's underlying risk for developing VTE. Teach MM patients taking thalidomide and dexamethsone that there may be an increased risk of blood clots in the veins of the legs and lungs; and the patient should call the healthcare provider or get medical help right away if the patient experiences SOB, chest pain, or arm or leg swelling.

III.   ALTERATION IN SENSORY/PERCEPTUAL PATTERNS related to PERIPHERAL NEUROPATHY, DIZZINESS, SEIZURE

Defining Characteristics: Sensory neuropathy occurs commonly ($\geq$ 10%) and in the safety study in combination with dexamethasone, the incidence was 54% (4% grade 3–4). Motor neuropathy occurred in 22% (8% grade 3–4). Neuropathy is potentially severe and may be irreversible. Neuropathy generally occurs after chronic use over a period of months, but reports after short-term use have been made. Symptoms may occur after thalidomide has been stopped, and may resolve slowly or not at all. Confusion was reported in 28% of MM patients receiving thalidomide and dexamethasone in the safety study 1. Dizziness/ light-headedness occurred in 20% of MM patients. Orthostatic hypotension may occur. Seizures, including grand mal, have been described in post-marketing reports.

Nursing Implications: Assess baseline neurologic status, especially presence of neuropathy. Teach patient to stop drug and report immediately numbness, tingling, pain, or a burning sensation in hands, legs, or feet. Perform assessment for neuropathy at every visit. Patient should have a monthly examination for the first three months of therapy, and regularly after that for signs/symptoms of neuropathy. Manufacturer recommends consideration of electrophysiological testing (measurement of sensory nerve action potential or SNAP amplitudes) baseline and every six months to detect asymptomatic neuropathy. Teach patient to avoid any situation where dizziness might be unsafe, and to avoid taking other medicines that increase dizziness or light-headedness. Teach patient to change position slowly, sitting for a few minutes after moving from a lying position, before standing up. Monitor patients with a history of seizures, or who are at risk of a lowered seizure threshold (e.g., other medications) closely for any changes that could precipitate seizure activity. Teach patient to report any changes.

IV.   ALTERATION IN SENSORY/PERCEPTUAL PATTERNS related to DROWSINESS

Defining Characteristics: Drug has sedative qualities, and drowsiness is a frequent side effect. Tolerance to daytime drowsiness occurs over several weeks of use.

Nursing Implications: Assess baseline alertness, sleep patterns. Assess other drugs taken, especially those with sedating qualities, and alcohol ingestion. Instruct patient to avoid alcohol and to take drug at bedtime. Assess degree of drowsiness and dizziness and safety of patient. If significant, teach measures to ensure safety. Advise patients to avoid driving a car or operating machinery.

V.   ALTERATION IN SKIN INTEGRITY, POTENTIAL, related to RASH, PRURITUS

Defining Characteristics: Pruritic, erythematous macular rash may occur. Incidence was 30% in MM patients (rash/desquamation) and 20.8% in ENL patients. Hypersensitivity has been reported with signs/symptoms of erythematous macular rash, possibly associated with fever, tachycardia, and hypotension. Drug rechallenge often results in immediate reaction of rash, tachycardia, and fever. Rash resolves with drug discontinuation. Serious dermatological reactions can occur, including Stevens-Johnson syndrome (SJS) and toxic epidermal necrolysis (TEN), which can be fatal.

Nursing Implications: Assess patient for rash/desquamation at each visit. Teach patient to self-assess for rash; if rash occurs, patient should stop thalidomide and to call provider for evaluation. If rash is exfoliative, purpuric, or bullous, or if SJS or TEN is suspected, drug should not be resumed. Teach patient that an allergic reaction may occur and if the patient develops a red, itchy rash, fever, a fast heartbeat, or if the patient feels dizzy or faint, to call the healthcare provider or get medical help right away.

VI.   ALTERATION IN ELIMINATION related to CONSTIPATION

Defining Characteristics: Mild constipation occurs commonly, with an incidence of 55% in MM patients (Safety Study 1).

Nursing Implications: Instruct patient to prevent constipation by using stool softeners, mild laxatives if needed (e.g., Milk of Magnesia), and to use bulk (e.g., psyllium). In addition, teach dietary interventions (e.g., increased fiber, fluids of 3 quarts/day), and mild exercise. Instruct patient to report constipation unresponsive to these interventions.

VII.   POTENTIAL FOR INFECTION related to NEUTROPENIA

Defining Characteristics: Neutrophils are decreased in 31% of MM patients (20% grade 3–4) (Safety Study 1).

Nursing Implications: Determine baseline WBC and absolute neutrophil count (ANC). Do not initiate therapy if ANC < 750/mm^3. If on treatment, ANC < 750/mm^3, the patient's medication regimen should be reevaluated, and if neutropenia persists, consideration should be given to withholding the drug. Drug may be reinstituted after neutrophil recovery. WBC and ANC should be monitored in an ongoing fashion in all patients, especially in patients prone to neutropenia, such as HIV-seropositive patients.

Drug: trametinib (Mekinist)

Class: Kinase inhibitor (MEK kinase inhibitor, first in class).

Mechanism of Action: The mitogen-activated extracellular signal regulated kinase 1 (MEK1) and MEK2 proteins are upstream regulators of the ERK (extracellular signal-related kinase) pathway, which promote cell division. Trametinib is a reversible inhibitor of MEK1 and MEK2 activation, as well as their kinase activity. The BRAF pathway includes MEK1 and MEK2, and if there is a BRAF V600E mutation, this turns on the pathway resulting in a continual signal being sent to the cell nucleus calling for cell proliferation. Trametinib turns this pathway off in tumors with the BRAF V600E mutation, such as certain malignant melanoma tumors, and leads to cell death (apoptosis).

Metabolism: After oral dosing, peak plasma level is reached 1.5 hours after the dose (T_{max}). Mean absolute bioavailability is 72%. Administration with a high-fat, high-calorie meal decreased AUC by 24%, C_{max} by 70%, and delayed T_{max} by about 4 hours, compared to when the drug is taken in a fasting state. Drug is 97.4% bound to plasma proteins. Metabolism occurs by deacetylation alone, or with mono-oxygenation, or in combination with glucuronidation. The elimination half-life of the drug is 3.9–4.8 days. Most (> 80%) of the drug and metabolites are excreted in the feces, with < 20% excreted in the urine. Mild hepatic impairment does not affect drug pharmacokinetics, but the drug was not studied in patients with moderate or severe hepatic impairment. Mild or moderate renal impairment does not affect pharmacokinetics, but the drug was not studied in patients with severe renal dysfunction.

Indication:
- As a single agent for the treatment of patients with unresectable or metastatic melanoma with BRAF V600E or V600K mutations as detected by an FDA-approved test. Drug is **not** indicated for patients who have received prior BRAF-inhibitor therapy.
- In combination with dabrafenib for the treatment of patients with unresectable or metastatic melanoma with BRAF V600E or V600K mutations as detected by an FDA-approved test. Indication based on demonstration of a durable response rate, and there are no data showing symptom improvement or survival advantage.

Dosage/Range:
- Presence of BRAF V600E or V600K mutations must be confirmed prior to starting drug.
- Recommended dose:
  - As a single agent, 2 mg orally once daily, taken at least 1 hour before or at least 2 hours after a meal.
  - In combination, 2 mg orally once daily, taken at least 1 hour before or at least 2 hours after a meal, with dabrafenib 150 mg taken twice daily.
- Continue treatment until disease progression or unacceptable toxicity occurs.
- Teach patient not to take a missed dose within 12 hours of the next trametinib dose, and when given in combination with dabrafenib, to take trametinib with either the morning or evening dose of dabrafenib.

Dose Modifications:
- Dose Levels:
  - When trametinib is administered as single agent or in combination: (1) First dose reduction dose is 1.5 mg orally once daily; (2) second reduction dose is 1 mg orally daily; if unable to tolerate1 mg orally, discontinue trametinib.
  - Dabrafenib dose reductions are (1) first dose reduction: 100 mg twice daily; (2) second reduction 75 mg twice daily; (3) third dose reduction is 50 mg twice daily; if unable to tolerate dabrafenib at 50 mg twice daily, discontinue dabrafenib.
- Fever:
  - 101.3°–104°F: no change in trametinib, hold dabrafenib until fever resolves, and resume at same or lower dose level.
  - If fever > 104°F, or fever complicated by rigors, hypotension, dehydration, or renal failure: hold trametinib or both drugs. If combination used until fever resolves, then resume trametinib at same or lower dose and dabrafenib at a lower dose level, or permanently discontinue dabrafenib.
- Cutaneous: Intolerable grade 2 skin toxicity or grade 3 or 4 skin toxicity: Hold trametinib and dabrafenib (if combination) for up to 3 weeks; if improved, resume trametinib (and dabrafenib if combination) at lower dose level; if not improved, discontinue drug(s) permanently.
- Cardiac:
  - Asymptomatic, absolute decrease in LVEF of 10% OR from baseline AND is < institutional LLN from pretreatment value: hold drug up for up to 4 weeks, and if improved to normal LVEF value, resume trametinib dose at a lower dose level; if not improved to normal LEVf, discontinue drug permanently; if combination, do not modify the dabrafenib dose.
  - Symptomatic CHF, or absolute decrease in LVEF > 20% from baseline that is below LLN, permanently discontinue trametinib; if combination therapy, hold dabrafenib, and if LVEF improved, resume at the same dose.
- Venous thrombembolism:
  - Uncomplicated DVT or PE: hold trametinib for up to 3 weeks; if improved to grade 0–1, resume at a lower dose level; if not, permanently discontinue trametinib. Do not modify dabrafenib dose.
  - If life-threatening PE, permanently discontinue trametinib, as well as dabrafenib if combination used.
- Ocular:
  - Grade 2–3 retinal pigment epithelial detachments (RPED): hold drug up to 3 weeks; if improved to grade 0–1 within 3 weeks, resume trametinib at a lower dose; if not, permanently discontinue trametinib. Do not modify dabrafenib if combination used.
  - Retinal vein occlusion: permanently discontinue trametinib; do not modify dabrafenib dose if combination used.
  - Uveitis and iritis: do not modify trametinib dose; if combination used, hold dabrafenib for up to 6 weeks; if improved to grade 0–1, resume at same dose; if not improved, permanently discontinue dabrafenib.
- Pulmonary:
  - ILD/pneumonitis: permanently discontinue trametinib; if combination, do not modify dabrafenib.

- New primary noncutaneous malignancies: if patient is taking combination, permanently discontinue dabrafenib in patients who develop RAS mutation-positive noncutaneous malignancies.
- Other:
  - Intolerable grade 2 or any grade 3 adverse reaction: hold (and dabrafenib if combination) for up to 3 weeks; if improved to grade 0–1, resume each drug at lower dose level; if not improved, permanently discontinue trametinib and dabrafenib (if combination used).
  - First occurrence of grade 4 adverse reaction: hold trametinib and dabrafenib if combination used until adverse reaction improves to grade 0–1; then resume drugs each at a lower dose level, or permanently discontinue drug(s).
  - Recurrent grade 4 adverse reaction, permanently discontinue trametinib and dabrafenib if combination used.

Drug Preparation:
- Drug available in 0.5-mg, 1-mg, and 2-mg tablets.

Administration:
- Assess LVEF findings (ECHO or MUGA scan prior to initiating drug, then one month after initiation, and then at two- to three-month intervals). Hold treatment if absolute LVEF value decreases by 10% from pretreatment values and is < LLN.
- Oral on an empty stomach, taken at least 1 hour before or at least 2 hours after a meal.

Drug Interactions:
- No formal studies have been conducted.
- Drug is not a substrate of CYP enzymes or efflux transporters P-gp or BCRP in vitro.
- Drug is an inhibitor of CYP2C8 in vitro.
- Drug is an inducer of CYP3A4 in vitro, but administration with the sensitive CYP3A4 substrate everolimus did not clinically affect AUC or C_{max} of everolimus.

Lab Effects/Interference:
- Increased AST (60%), increased ALT (39%), increased alkaline phosphatase (24%).
- Hypoalbuminemia (43%), anemia (38%).
- Hyperglycemia when trametinib is combined with dabrafenib.
- Increased LVEF by ECHO or MUGA.

Special Considerations:
- Cardiomyopathy occurred in 7% of patients in clinical trials. Hold treatment if absolute LVEF value decreases by 10% from pretreatment values and is < LLN. Permanently discontinue drug for symptomatic cardiomyopathy or persistent asymptomatic LVEF dysfunction that does not resolve within four weeks.
- Retinal vein occlusion occurred in 0.2% of patients.
  - Retinal vein occlusion may lead to macular edema, decreased visual function, neovascularization, and glaucoma.

- If patient reports loss of vision or other visual disturbances, patient should have an urgent (within 24 hours) ophthalmological evaluation.
- Drug should be discontinued if retinal vein occlusion is found. If trametinib is combined with dabrafenib, do not modify dabrafenib dose.
- Retinal Pigment Epithelial Detachment (RPED) can occur when trametinib is given as a single agent or in combination with dabrafenib.
  - The incidence of RPED is 0.8%. If RPED occurs, it is often bilateral and multifocal in the macular region of the retina. RPED results in decreased visual acuity, which resolves in 3–71 days (median 11.5 days) after trametinib was stopped.
  - Patients who develop visual disturbances should have an ophthalmological evaluation, and trametinib should be held if RPED is identified.
  - If RPED resolves within 3 weeks, resume drug at a lower dose level; if there is no improvement, discontinue trametinib. If used with dabrafenib, do not modify dabrafenib dose.
- ILD occurred in 2% of patients in clinical trials. Time to first presentation was 160 days (range 60–172 days). Hold drug in patients presenting with new or progressive pulmonary signs/symptoms, including cough, dyspnea, hypoxia, pleural effusion, or infiltrates, while pulmonary symptoms are worked up. If ILD is found, discontinue trametinib. If ILD develops in a patient receiving a combination with dabrafenib, do not modify dabrfenib dose.
- Skin toxicity is common (87%, 12% severe) and includes rash, dermatitis, acneiform rash, palmar-plantar erythrodysesthesia syndrome (PPES), and erythema. See Dose Modifications.
- Drug is embryo-fetal toxic.
  - Counsel women and men of reproductive potential to use highly effective contraception during drug therapy and for four months after treatment.
  - If patient is receiving trametinib and dabrafenib, teach patient to use nonhormonal method of contraception, as dabrafenib can make this type of contraceptive ineffective.
  - Teach patient that if pregnancy is suspected, to advise provider right away.
  - Nursing mothers should decide whether to discontinue nursing or discontinue the drug, taking into account the importance of the drug to the mother's health.
  - Drug may impair fertility in female patients.
- Most common side effects were rash, diarrhea, and lymphedema.
- Drug can cause increased transaminases and alkaline phosphatase. Although no dose adjustment is necessary for patients with mild hepatic impairment, the appropriate dose for patients with moderate or severe hepatic impairment has not been established.
- Hypertension occurred in 15% of patients (12% grades 3 or 4), and hemorrhage in 13%.
  - Monitor BP baseline and during treatment.
  - Teach patient to report epistaxis, gingival bleeding, rectal bleeding, vaginal bleeding, bleeding from hemorrhoids, blood in urine, or red conjunctiva.
- FDA approval was based on the METRIC study, which showed that patients who had previously received chemotherapy had significantly improved progression-free survival, as well as overall survival, compared to those receiving chemotherapy (controls).

- When trametinib is combined with dabrafenib:
  - Dabrafenib may cause (1) tumor promotion in patients with BRAF wild-type melanoma, (2) hemolytic anemia in patients with glucose-6-phosphate dehydrogenase deficiency (6GPD).
  - Incidence of basal cell carcinoma was increased (9%) compared to dabrafenib alone; the incidence of cutaneous squamous cell cancer was lower with the combination, as was the incidence of new primary melanomas. Perform dermatologic evaluations prior to starting combination, every 2 months while on therapy, and for up to 6 months after discontinuance of the combination. No dosage adjustments are recommended for patients who develop primary cutaneous malignancies.
  - Noncutaneous malignancies: rare RAS mutation-positive cancers (e.g., pancreatic adenocarcinoma, CRC). Monitor patients closely for signs and symptoms of noncutaneous malignancy, and permanently discontinue dabrafenib in patients who develop RAS-mutation-positive noncutaneous cancers.
  - Increased risk of hemorrhage (16% vs 2% with dabrafenib alone). Incidence is 5%, but it can be fatal (e.g., intracranial). Permanently discontinue trametinib, as well as dabrafenib, if given together for all grade 4 hemorrhage events, as well as grade 3 events that do not improve. Hold trametinib (and dabrafenib if used in combination) for up to 3 weeks for grade 3 hemorrhagic events; if improved, resume at a lower dose level.
  - Increased risk of venous thromboembolism (DVT, PE): 7% vs 0%. Teach patients to seek medical care right away if they develop symptoms of DVT or PE (e.g., shortness of breath, chest pain, arm or leg swelling). Discontinue both drugs if life-threatening PE occurs. Hold trametinib for up to 3 weeks for uncomplicated DVT and PE; if improved, resume trametinib at a lower dose level; do not modify dabrafenib dose.
  - Cardiomyopathy: Incidence of trametinib-related cardiomyopathy in clinical trials was 11% as a single agent and 8% when given with dabrafenib. Assess ECHO or MUGA baseline, then 1 month after drug(s) initiation, then at 2–3 monthly intervals during treatment. Hold trametinib for up to 4 weeks if absolute LVEF value decreases by 10% from baseline and is < LLN. For symptomatic cardiomyopathy or persistent, asymptomatic LV dysfunction that does not resolve within 4 weeks, permanently discontinue trametinib and hold dabrafenib. Resume at the same dose upon cardiac function recovery.
  - Uveitis and iritis: uveitis occurred in 1% of patients, and if it occurs, steroid and mydriatic ophthalmic drops should be used for symptomatic improvement. Monitor patients for uveitis (change in vision, photophobia, eye pain). If diagnosed, hold dabrafenib for up to 6 weeks until it resolves to grade 0–1; if it is not improved, discontinue dabrafenib. Do not modify trametinib dose.
  - Febrile reactions occurred in 71% of patients receiving combination drugs, compared to 26% in patients receiving dabrafenib alone, while 25% had serious febrile reactions (with hypotension, rigors or chills, dehydration, or renal failure) compared to 2% in patients receiving dabrafenib alone. Median time to onset of fever was 30 days, with a median duration of 6 days in patients receiving the combination, compared to 19 days in patients receiving dabrafenib alone. Hold dabrafenib for fever ≥ 101. 3°F; hold trametinib for fever > 104°F. Hold both drugs if the patient has serious febrile

reactions or fever with rigors, chills, hypotension, dehydration, or renal failure, and evaluate for infection. Consider prophylaxis with antipyretics when resuming either drug.

- Skin toxicity can occur with either agent: rash, dermatitis caneiform rash, palmar-plantar erythrodysesthesia syndrome, and erythema (incidence 87% in trametinib-treated patients, compared to 68% receiving dabrafenib. When patients receive both drugs, skin toxicity occurs in 1–225 days (median 37days), with resolution in a median of 33 days. Hold both drugs if patients develop intolerable or severe skin toxicity; resume drugs at a reduced dosage level when skin recovers within 3 weeks.
- Hyperglycemia may occur when both drugs are administered; patient may require an increase in the dose of insulin or oral hypoglycemic agent, or initiation of insulin, or of an oral hypoglycemic agent, if not already taking it. Monitor serum glucose levels, especially in patients with preexisting diabetes or hyperglycemia. Teach patients to report symptoms of hyperglycemia.

Potential Toxicities/Side Effects and the Nursing Process

I. ALTERATION IN CIRCULATION related to CARDIOMYOPATHY

Defining Characteristics: Cardiomyopathy defined as cardiac failure, LV dysfunction, or decreased LVEF, occurred in 7% of patients in clinical trials. When combined with dabrafenib, incidence was 11%. Median time to onset of cardiomyopathy was 63 days (range 16–156 days). Cardiomyopathy resolved in 71% of patients.

Nursing Implications: Assess baseline cardiac function, including pulse, BP. Review history, and identify patients at risk who have CHF, hypertension, coronary artery disease. Patients should have baseline ECHO or gated blood pool scan to determine left ventricular ejection fraction (LVEF), and this should be monitored at least every 2–3 months during therapy and at the conclusion of therapy. Assess for signs and symptoms at each visit: dyspnea, increased cough, paroxysmal nocturnal dyspnea, peripheral edema, S3 gallop, and decrease in left ventricular function when tested. Teach patient to report cough, weight gain, light-headedness, edema of ankles or feet, difficulty breathing, feeling like the heart is pounding or racing, or need to use more pillows at night. Hold treatment if absolute LVEF value decreases by 10% from pretreatment values and is < LLN. Permanently discontinue drug for symptomatic cardiomyopathy or persistent asymptomatic LVEF dysfunction that does not resolve within four weeks.

II. ALTERATION IN SENSORY PERCEPTION, POTENTIAL, related to VISUAL CHANGES

Defining Characteristics: Retinal pigment epithelial detachments (RPED) was rare (incidence 0.8%), but may lead to blindness. RPED led to reduced visual acuity that resolved after a median of 11.5 days (range 3–71 days) after drug interruption. Ocular coherence tomography (OCT) abnormalities were present a month after drug interruption in some cases. Retinal vein occlusion can also rarely occur (0.2% of patients), which may lead to macular edema, decreased visual function, neovascularization, and glaucoma.

Nursing Implications: Teach patient that visual changes may occur rarely but must be reported right away to prevent worsening, as rarely blindness may occur. Patient should immediately report blurred vision, loss of vision, other visual changes, seeing color dots, or seeing a halo (blurred outline around objects). Discuss with physician or NP/PA ophthamologic evaluation baseline. Assess patient for visual changes, and ensure patient has an ophthalmological evaluation at any time new or changed visual disturbances are reported. If patient reports loss of vision or other serious visual disturbances, patient should have an urgent (within 24 hours) ophthalmological evaluation. Drug should be discontinued if retinal vein occlusion is found.

III.   ALTERATION IN SKIN INTEGRITY, POTENTIAL, related to RASH, DERMATITIS, ACNEIFORM RASH, PPES, ERYTHEMA

Defining Characteristics: Skin toxicity is common (87%, 12% severe) and includes rash (57% incidence), dermatitis acneiform (19%), dry skin (11%), pruritus (10%), and paronychia (10%). Six percent of patients required hospitalization, commonly for secondary infection. Median time to onset was 15 days (1–221 days), and median time to resolution was 48 days (1–282 days).

Nursing Implications: Assess baseline skin integrity and dryness. Teach patient that these side effects may occur and to report them. Teach self-care measures based on symptoms that arise. For PPES, teach patient to keep skin moisturized, avoid repetitive hand or foot motions such as jogging, avoid hot water, and use tepid bath water. Teach patient to report erythema, edema, desquamation (peeling), or any changes in sensation. Teach patient to keep nails trimmed and clean. If rash itches at night, suggest patient wear cotton gloves to avoid scratching rash and possibly infecting it. Teach patient management of itching, and to avoid scratching, as secondary infections may require IV antibiotics. If paronyrchia develop, suggest measures to reduce distress, such as steroid tape.

IV.   ALTERATION IN NUTRITION related to DIARRHEA, STOMATITIS

Defining Characteristics: Diarrhea affected 43% of patients (no grade 3–4), and stomatitis 15% (2% grade 3–4).

Nursing Implications: Assess patient for bowel elimination pattern, and status of oral mucosa. Teach patient that these side effects may occur, and to report them. Teach patient to self-assess oral mucosa and to use a systematic oral cleansing after meals and at bedtime. Teach patient to report any pain, or difficulty eating or drinking. If stomatitis worsens, discuss topical treatment with diphenhydramine or lidocaine plus antacid mixture. See Dose Modifications.

Drug: trastuzumab (Herceptin, humanized anti-HER-2 antibody, rhuMAbHER2)

Class: Monoclonal antibody, unconjugated.

Mechanism of Action: Recombinant humanized monoclonal antibody targeted against the human epidermal growth factor receptor 2 (*HER-2*). *HER-2* is an oncogene that is overexpressed in a number of cancers, including 25–30% of breast cancers. The drug binds to HER-2 tightly, thus inhibiting cell signaling and cell proliferation. This monoclonal antibody is believed to act through three different mechanisms: (1) the antagonizing function of the growth-signaling properties of *HER-2*, (2) signaling immune cells to attack and kill malignant cells with this receptor (ADCC), and (3) synergistic and/or additive effects seen with many chemotherapeutic agents. HER-2 signaling appears necessary for repair of cardiac damage; this explains why cardiotoxicity develops when administered following a cardiotoxic agent, such as doxorubicin.

Metabolism: Initial studies using a loading dose of 4 mg/kg followed by a weekly maintenance dose of 2 mg/kg, a mean half-life of 6 days, with a range of 1–32 days was seen. The mean half-life is 16 days (range, 11–23 days) when a loading dose of 8 mg/kg followed by a three-weekly 6 mg/kg dose is used. Steady state is reached between weeks 6 and 37.

Indications:
- Adjuvant treatment of HER-2 overexpressing node positive or node-negative (ER/PR negative or with one high-risk feature) breast cancer: breast cancer.
  - As part of a treatment regimen consisting of doxorubicin, cyclophosphamide, and either paclitaxel or docetaxel.
  - With docetaxel and carboplatin.
  - As a single agent following multi-modality anthracycline-based therapy.
- Treatment of HER-2 overexpressing metastatic breast cancer.
  - In combination with paclitaxel for first-line treatment.
  - As a single agent in patients who have received one or more chemotherapy regimens for metastatic disease.
- HER-2 overexpressing metastatic gastric cancer or gastroesophageal junction adenocarcinoma, in combination with cisplatin and capecitabine or 5-fluorouracil, in patients who have not received prior treatment for metastatic disease.

Dosage/Range:
- **DO NOT substitute Herceptin (trastuzumab) for or with ado-trastuzumab emtansine.**
- Do not administer as an IV push or bolus. Do not mix trastuzumab with other drugs.
- *Adjuvant (for a total of 52 weeks):*
- When given during **and following** paclitaxel, docetaxel, or docetaxel/carboplatin:
  - Initial dose of 4 mg/kg IV infusion over 90 minutes week 1, then at 2 mg/kg as an IV infusion over 30 minutes weekly during chemotherapy for the first 12 weeks (paclitaxel or docetaxel) or 18 weeks (docetaxel/carboplatin).
  - One week following the last weekly dose of trastuzumab, administer trastuzumab at 6 mg/kg as an IV infusion over 30–90 minutes every 3 weeks.

- As a single agent within 3 weeks following completion of multi-modality, anthracycline-based chemotherapy regimens:
  - Initial dose at 8 mg/kg as an IV infusion over 90 minutes.
  - Subsequent doses at 6 mg/kg as an IV infusion over 30–90 minutes every 3 weeks. Extending adjuvant therapy beyond 1 year is not recommended.

Metastatic Treatment for Breast Cancer:
- Administer trastuzumab, alone or in combination with paclitaxel, at an initial dose of 4 mg/kg as a 90-minute infusion, followed by subsequent once-weekly doses of 2 mg/kg as a 30-minute IV infusion, until disease progression.

Metastatic Gastric Cancer:
- Administer trastuzumab at an initial dose of 8 mg/kg as a 90-minute IV infusion, followed by subsequent doses of 6 mg/kg IV infusion over 30–90 minutes every 3 weeks, until disease progression.
- *If infusion reaction occurs*, decrease the rate of infusion for mild or moderate reaction; interrupt the infusion in patients with dyspnea or clinically significant hypotension; discontinue trastuzumab for severe or life-threatening infusion reactions.
- *Assess LVEF baseline* prior to starting trastuzumab therapy, and at regular intervals during treatment.
  - Hold trastuzumbab dose for at least 4 weeks for either (1) ≥ 16% absolute decrease in LVEF from pretreatment value, or (2) LVEF below institutional limits of normal and ≥ 10% absolute decrease in LVEF from pretreatment values.
  - Resume trastuzumab if, within 4–8 weeks, the LVEF returns to normal limits and the absolute decrease from baseline is ≤ 15%.
  - Permanently discontinue trastuzumab for a persistent (> 8 wks) LVEF decline or for suspension of trastuzumab dosing no more than 3 occasions for cardiomyopathy.

Drug Preparation:
- Check drug label to make sure drug being prepared is Herceptin (trastuzumab) and NOT ado-trastuzumab emtansine.
- Drug is available as a lyophilized sterile powder of 440 mg per vial for parenteral administration. Requires refrigeration at 2–8°C (36–46°F). DO NOT FREEZE.
- Reconstitute with 20 mL of bacteriostatic water for injection, USP, containing 1.1% benzyl alcohol, which is supplied with each vial, to make a multidose solution. If the patient is allergic to benzyl alcohol, reconstitute with 20 mL sterile water for injection without preservative to yield a single-use solution. DO NOT SHAKE.
- Using a sterile syringe, slowly inject the 20 mL diluent into the vial, directing the stream into the lyophilized cake.
- Swirl the vial gently to mix; DO NOT SHAKE.
- Slight foaming may occur; allow vial to stand undisturbed for about 5 minutes.
- Inspect for particulate matter or discoloration, and if found, do not use. Solution should be clear to slightly opalescent, colorless to pale yellow, without particles.
- Store reconstituted trastuzumab at 2–8°C (36–46°F); discard unused trastuzumab after 28 days. If reconstituted with sterile water for injection without preservatives, use immediately and discard any unused portion.
- Reconstituted solution contains 21 mg/mL. Further dilute ordered dose in 250 mL of 0.9% sodium chloride injection, USP. DO NOT use dextrose (5%) solution. Gently invert to mix.

- Vial is designed for multiple use, and is stable for 28 days following reconstitution at 2–8°C (36–46°F). If patient is hypersensitive to this bacteriostatic diluent, use 20 mL sterile water for injection without preservatives as a single solution (not multidose).

Drug Administration:
- Administered IV infusion; initial loading dose is administered over 90 minutes, and initial maintenance dose (week 2 or dose 2) is administered over 30–60 minutes. Never give as IV push or bolus.
- Observe patient for 1 hour following completion of initial loading dose, and if well tolerated, observe patient for 30 minutes following completion of initial maintenance dose (week or dose 2). If well tolerated, no further postinfusion observation is needed in subsequent weekly infusions.
- Subsequent maintenance doses are administered over 30 minutes if prior administration was well tolerated without fever or chills.
- Continue to administer over 90 minutes if fever, chills experienced in prior administrations.
- Assess results of ECHO or MUGA for LVEF, baseline then every 3 months and upon completion of trastuzumab therapy.
- If trastuzumab is held for significant LV dysfunction, assess LVEF findings at 4-week intervals.

Drug Interactions:
- Paclitaxel: twofold decrease in trastuzumab clearance in animals and a 1.5-fold increase in trastuzumab serum level in human clinical studies.
- Chemotherapy: increased neutropenia and febrile neutropenia.
- Doxorubicin, anthracyclines: additive cardiotoxicity; DO NOT GIVE CONCURRENTLY.
- Everolimus may circumvent trastuzumab resistance when used concurrently by blocking mTOR, which is downstream of P13K. Hyperactivation of the P13K/AKT pathway appears to be the cause of trastuzumab resistance (Morrow et al., 2010).

Lab Effects/Interference:
- Decreased LVEF; monitor baseline and throughout treatment.
- Decreased absolute neutrophil count when given with chemotherapy.

Special Considerations:
- HER-2 protein overexpression must be determined prior to treatment. Use FDA-approved tests for the specific tumor type (e.g., breast or gastric/GE junction adenocarcinoma) to assess HER-2 protein overexpression and HER-2 gene amplification. Use laboratories with demonstrated proficiency. FISH (tests for HER-2 gene amplification) are more accurate in identifying HER-2 overexpression; in some centers, patient tumors are tested with IHC (measures HER-2 protein overexpression), and if 2+, sent for FISH testing. IHC 3+ demonstrates definite HER-2 overexpression. Discordant lab values (false negatives or positives) occur more commonly in labs doing less than 100 tests per month (24%) compared with a lab doing 100 or more a month (3%) (Paik et al., 2002).
- Trastuzumab is very well-tolerated; given that it is a humanized antibody, no premedication is recommended. Infusion reactions, if they occur, are characterized by fever,

chills, with or without nausea, vomiting, pain (may be at tumor site), headache, dizziness, dyspnea, hypotension, rash, and asthenia.

- Rarely, trastuzumab may cause hypersensitivity/allergic reactions, so emergency equipment should be available during infusions. Post-marketing reports have described serious and fatal infusion reactions characterized by bronchospasm, anaphylaxis, angioedema, hypoxia, and severe hypotension usually during or immediately after initial infusion.
- Severe infusion reactions and pulmonary toxicity can occur within 24 hours of the drug dose. Interrupt treatment for dyspnea or significant hypotension. Discontinue drug if patient develops anaphylaxis, angioedema, interstital pneumonitis, or ARDS.
- There are no data identifying patients who may be retreated with trastuzumab after a severe infusion reaction. Premedication with antihistamines and/or corticosteroids is recommended, and despite this, some patients may again have a severe infusion reaction.
- Drug has been associated with serious and fatal pulmonary toxicity. Dyspnea, interstitial pneumonitis, pulmonary infiltrates, pleural effusions, noncardiogenic pulmonary edema, pulmonary insufficiency and hypoxia, ARDS, and pulmonary fibrosis have been described and may occur following infusion reactions. Symptoms usually occur during or within 24 hours of trastuzumab administration. Risk appears greater in patients with intrinsic lung disease or extensive lung metastases, resulting in dyspnea at rest. Interrupt infusion for dyspnea or clinically significant hypotension. Discontinue drug for anaphylaxis, angioedema, interstitial pneumonitis, or ARDS.
- Phase III clinical trials studied coadministration together with doxorubicin/cyclophosphamide (AC) showed an increased risk of subclinical and clinical cardiomyopathy (CHF and decreased LVEF). DO NOT give trastuzumab concurrently with anthracycline chemotherapy. Left ventricular function should be evaluated prior to and during treatment with trastuzumab therapy.
- Trastuzumab administration can result in subclinical and clinical cardiac failure. The incidence was highest in patients receiving trastuzumab with anthracycline-containing chemotherapy regimens.
- There is a fourfold to sixfold increase in the incidence of symptomatic myocardial dysfunction in patients receiving trastuzumab as a single agent or in combination compared with those not receiving trastuzumab.
- Evaluate LVEF in all patients prior to and during treatment with trastuzumab. If clinically significant decrease in LVEF, discontinue trastuzumab in patients receiving adjuvant therapy and withhold in patients with metastatic disease.
- Withhold trastuzumab for ≥ 16% absolute decrease in LVEF from pretreatment values or an LVEF value < intitutional limits of normal and ≥ 10% absolute decrease in LVEF from pretreatment values.
- Cardiac monitoring: Patient should have a thorough cardiac assessment, including history, physical exam, and LVEF determination (by ECHO of MUGA scan) at the recommended schedule:
  - Baseline LVEF immediately prior to beginning trastuzumab.
  - LVEF meaurements every 3 months during and upon completion of trastuzumab.
  - Repeat LVEF measurements at 4-week intervals if trastuzumab is withheld for significant left ventricular cardiac dysfunction.
  - LVEF measurements every 6 months for at least 2 years following trastuzumab when used in the adjuvant setting.

- Planned assessment of LVEF is intended to prevent the development of clinical cardiomyopathy. In an Italian study, Troponin I was an independent predictor of trastuzumab-induced cardiotoxicity (able to identify patients early who would be at risk for developing trastuzumab-induced cardiotoxicity), as well as those for whom cardiotoxicity would be irreversible (Cardinale et al., 2010).
- Exposure to trastuzumab during pregnancy can result in oligohydramnios (decreased amniotic fluid), and oligohydramnios sequence manifesting as pulmonary hypoplasia, skeletal abnormalities, and neonatal death (Genentech, 2014). Women of childbearing age should use effective contraception.
- Trastuzumab may exacerbate chemotherapy-induced neutropenia (grade 3–4).
- Resistance to trastuzumab develops with the loss of the tumor suppressor protein PTEN and hyperactivation of the P13K/AKT pathway. PTEN is a tumor suppressor that helps to ensure that the cell cycle is controlled and that uncontrolled cell division does not occur. To do this, it suppresses activation of the P13K/AKT/mTOR pathway. Thus, when PTEN is silenced, P13K/AKT is hyperactivated, which can lead to inhibition of apoptosis and resistance to drugs like trastuzumab and cisplatin (Becker, 2008). More recently, microRNA-21 (or miRNA-21) has been identified as the culprit in trastuzumab resistance by turning off the PTEN gene. miRNA are pieces of a gene that control cell behavior by turning certain genes on and off (Rehman et al., 2010). HER-2+ tumor cells with high levels of miRNA became resistant to trastuzumab by turning off the PTEN gene, which led to increased cell proliferation.
- Subcutaneous injection over 5 minutes of a subcutaneous formulation of trastuzumab was non-inferior in terms of pharmacokinetic, efficacy, and safety, when compared to IV administration (Ismael et al., 2012).

Potential Toxicities/Side Effects and the Nursing Process

I.   ALTERATION IN CIRCULATION related to CARDIOMYOPATHY

Defining Characteristics: Trastuzumab administration may result in ventricular dysfunction and congestive heart failure. The risk is significantly greater when given with doxorubicin (28% compared with 7% with AC alone), and thus, trastuzumab should NOT be given with doxorubicin and cyclophosphamide. It should begin after the completion of AC in the adjuvant setting. In addition, there is a theoretical slight increase when given together with paclitaxel, but clinical studies have shown a similar incidence of 2% when trastuzumab is given as monotherapy after adjuvant AC to that of AC followed by paclitaxel. Thus, the two drugs can be given concurrently. The 52-week incidence of trastuzumab-related cardiotoxicity, when given to follow AC concurrent with paclitaxel for 12 weeks and then as a single agent, is about 4%. If allowed to progress, failure may be severe, and the following have been reported: severe cardiac failure, death, and mural thrombosis leading to stroke. Thus, during adjuvant therapy, it is critical that cardiac function be monitored baseline and at least every 3 months. Rare events described following treatment with trastuzumab were vascular thrombosis, pericardial effusion, heart arrest, hypotension, syncope, hemorrhage, shock, and arrhythmia. Risk factors in the NSABP B-31 clinical trial were declining LVEF after completion of AC chemotherapy and increasing age.

Nursing Implications: Assess baseline cardiac function, including apical pulse, BP. Review history, and identify patients at risk who have CHF, hypertension, coronary artery disease. Patients should have baseline ECHO or gated blood pool scan to determine left ventricular ejection fraction (LVEF), and this should be monitored at least every 3 months during adjuvant trastuzumab therapy and at the conclusion of therapy. Repeat LVEF test every 4 weeks if trastuzumab is held for significant changes in LVEF. After completion of adjuvant therapy, assess LVEF every 6 months for at least 2 years. Assess for signs and symptoms at each visit: dyspnea, increased cough, paroxysmal nocturnal dyspnea, peripheral edema, S3 gallop, and decrease in left ventricular function when tested. Teach patient to report cough, weight gain, edema of ankles, difficulty breathing, or need to use more pillows at night. If patient develops a significant decrease in LVEF, the drug should be held for at least 4 weeks and LVEF repeated every 4 weeks for either of the following: (1) ≥ 16% absolute decrease in LVEF from pretreatment values below institutional LLN and (2) ≥ 10% absolute decrease in LVEF from pretreatment values and below LLN. Resume drug if within 4–8 weeks, the LVEF returns to normal limits, and the absolute decrease from baseline is 15% or less. Discontinue drug for a persistent (> 8 weeks) LVEF decline or for suspension of trastuzumab dosing on more than three occasions for cardio-myopathy. LVEF should continue to be monitored every 6 months for at least 2 years following completion of trastuzumab adjuvant therapy.

II.   POTENTIAL FOR INJURY related to HYPERSENSITIVITY, INFUSION RATE

Defining Characteristics: Infusion-related reactions (e.g., fever and/or chills) were reported in about 40% of patients with their first treatment, and 10% with subsequent infusions. Infusion reactions are characterized by a symptom complex of fever and chills, with or without nausea, vomiting, pain (may be at tumor site), headache, dizziness, dyspnea, hypotension, rash, and asthenia. Severe hypersensitivity reactions are rare but have been reported, including post-marketing serious and fatal infusion reactions. Bronchospasm, ana-phylaxis, angioedema, hypoxia, and severe hypotension can occur during or immediately after the infusion but may have an initial improvement followed by rapid clinical deteriora-tion. Severe deterioration may be delayed by hours to days after a serious infusion reaction.

Nursing Implications: Assess VS baseline and frequently during infusion, especially during initial loading dose, and subsequent maintenance infusions. Observe patient for 1 hour following completion of loading dose, and 30 minutes after initial maintenance dose if loading dose was well tolerated. If not well tolerated, continue to monitor for 60 minutes until well tolerated. Notify physician if fever or chills develop and assess need for acetamin-ophen and slowing of infusion. Although severe allergic reactions are uncommon, have emergency equipment available and nearby, and be prepared to provide emergency support if necessary. **Stop drug if patient develops dyspnea,** severe bronchospasm, hypoxia, or severe hypotension. Notify physician/midlevel and be prepared to administer epinephrine, corticosteroids, diphenhydramine, bronchodilators, and oxygen. Discuss permanent dis-continuation of drug for severe infusion reactions. A reaction can occur within 24 hours of the drug dose, and thus, if the patient is symptomatic, consider admitting patient for obser-vation. Discontinue drug for severe and life-threatening infusion reactions. If the patient is to receive the drug again after an infusion reaction during the prior administration, discuss with the physician, and ensure that the patient is premedicated with antihistamines and corticosteroids. Monitor the patient very carefully during the infusion, as despite the premedications, severe infusion reactions can still occur.

III. ALTERATION IN OXYGENATION, POTENTIAL, related to DYSPNEA, PULMONARY COMPLICATIONS

Defining Characteristics: After trastuzumab, patients have rarely developed serious and fatal pulmonary toxicity. Pulmonary events that have been described include dyspnea, interstitial pneumonitis, pulmonary infiltrates, pleural effusions, noncardiogenic pulmonary edema, pulmonary insufficiency, hypoxia, ARDS, and pulmonary fibrosis. These may be complications of infusion reactions.

Nursing Implications: Assess patient's baseline pulmonary status, including history of pulmonary disease, breath sounds, and respiratory rate. Patients at risk for developing pulmonary complications are (1) those with symptomatic intrinsic lung disease, and (2) those patients with extensive tumor involvement of the lungs so that they are dyspneic at rest. Monitor patients closely during the infusion, and teach patient to report any changes in respiratory function or dyspnea right away. If dyspnea or other symptoms are severe, the patient should come to the emergency room right away for evaluation.

IV. ALTERATION IN COMFORT related to PAIN, ASTHENIA

Defining Characteristics: Generalized pain may affect 11% of patients, and asthenia 5%. Abdominal pain may specifically affect 3% of patients.

Nursing Implications: Teach patients to report alterations in comfort, especially pain and dyspnea. Distinguish new onset of symptoms versus those experienced prior to treatment due to malignancy. Discuss intensity of symptoms and need for pharmacologic and nonpharmacologic interventions. Monitor response to intervention between weekly treatments, and need for alternative strategies.

V. POTENTIAL FOR INFECTION related to EXACERBATION OF CHEMOTHERAPY-INDUCED NEUTROPENIA

Defining Characteristics: In patients with metastatic breast cancer, the incidences of grades 3 and 4 neutropenia, and febrile neutropenia were higher in patients receiving trastuzumab in combination with myelosuppressive chemotherapy.

Nursing Implications: For patients with metastatic breast cancer receiving chemotherapy and trastuzumab, monitor CBC, platelet count baseline and prior to each treatment. Assess for signs and symptoms of infection (e.g., T ≥ 100.4°F, dysuria, productive cough). Teach patient self-care measures to prevent or minimize the risk of infection. Teach patient self-assessment for signs and symptoms of infection and to call the provider immediately if they occur.

Drug: tretinoin (Vesanoid, ATRA, all-trans-retinoic acid)

Class: Retinoid.

Mechanism of Action: Induces maturation of acute promyelocytic leukemia (APL) cells, thus decreasing proliferation. In patients who achieve a complete response to this therapy, there is an initial maturation of primitive leukemic cells, and then cells in both the bone marrow and peripheral blood are normal, polyclonal blood cells. The exact mechanism is unknown.

Metabolism: This drug is well absorbed orally into the systemic circulation, with peak concentrations in 1–2 hours. Drug is > 95% protein-bound, primarily to albumin. Oxidative metabolism occurs via the cytochrome P450 enzyme system in the liver. Drug is excreted in the urine (63% in 72 hours) and feces (31% in 6 days).

Indication: Indicated for the induction remission of patients with APL (FAB-M3), characterized by the presence of the t(15:17) translocation and/or presence of the PML/RAR (alpha) gene.

Dosage/Range:
- 45 mg/m^2 per day.

Drug Preparation:
- None: oral.
- Available as 10-mg capsules.
- Protect from light.

Drug Administration:
- Drug is to be used for induction remission only.
- Administer in evenly divided doses until complete remission (CR) is achieved, then for an additional 30 days, or after 90 days of treatment, whichever comes first.

Drug Interactions:
- Drugs that either inhibit or induce the cytochrome P450 hepatic enzyme system potentially will interact with this drug, but there are no data to suggest that these drugs either increase or decrease tretinoin activity.
- Drugs that induce the enzyme system: rifampin, glucocorticoids, phenobarbital, pentobarbital; drugs that inhibit the enzyme system: ketoconazole, cimetidine, erythromycin, verapamil, diltiazem, cyclosporin.
- Antifibrinolytic agents.

Lab Effects/Interference:
- Increased cholesterol and triglyceride levels (60% of patients).
- Increased LFTs (50–60% of patients).

Special Considerations:
- Absorption is enhanced when taken with food.
- Monitor CBC, platelets, coagulation studies, liver function tests, and triglyceride and cholesterol levels frequently during therapy.

Potential Toxicities/Side Effects and the Nursing Process

I.   ALTERATION IN OXYGENATION, POTENTIAL, related to RETINOIC - ACID-APL SYNDROME

Defining Characteristics: Syndrome occurs in approximately 25% of patients and varies in severity, but has resulted in death. Syndrome is characterized by fever, dyspnea, weight gain, pulmonary infiltrates on X-ray, and pleural and/or pericardial effusions. May also be accompanied by impaired myocardial contractility, hypotension, ± leukocytosis, and because of progressive hypoxemia and multisystem organ failure, some patients have died. Usually occurs during first month of treatment, but may follow initial drug dose.

Nursing Implications: Assess VS, pulmonary exam, and weight at each visit. Teach patient to do daily weights, and to report any SOB, fever, weight gain. If this occurs, notify physician and discuss obtaining CXR and focused exam. Discuss chest X-ray findings with physician. Be prepared to give high-dose steroids at the first sign of the syndrome (e.g., dexamethasone 10 mg IV q 12 h × 3 days or until symptom resolution (necessary in 60% of patients). Provide pulmonary and hemodynamic support as necessary. Discuss whether drug should be discontinued based on severity and patient's response to high-dose steroids.

II.   ALTERATION IN COMFORT related to VITAMIN A TOXICITY

Defining Characteristics: Almost all patients experience some toxicity, but they do not usually have to discontinue the drug. Toxicity of high-dose vitamin A includes headache (86%) starting the first week of treatment, but fading after that; fever (83%); skin/mucous membrane dryness (77%); bone pain (77%); nausea/vomiting (57%); rash (54%); mucositis (26%); pruritus (20%); increased sweating (20%); visual disturbances (17%); ocular disorders (17%); skin changes (17%); alopecia (14%); changed visual acuity (6%); visual field defects (3%).

Nursing Implications: Teach patient about possible side effects of high-dose vitamin A as above and to report them if they occur. Teach patient symptom management. Assess severity of symptom(s) and discuss with physician symptom management of fever, headache unresponsive to acetaminophen, nausea/vomiting. If headache is severe in a child, have child evaluated for pseudotumor cerebri.

III.   POTENTIAL FOR INJURY related to PSEUDOTUMOR CEREBRI

Defining Characteristics: Benign intracranial hypertension has occurred in children treated with retinoids. Early signs and symptoms are papilledema, headache, nausea and vomiting, and visual disturbances.

Nursing Implications: Teach patient/parents to report symptoms. Assess patient for symptomatology on regular basis. If headache is severe, discuss with physician analgesics and therapeutic lumbar puncture.

IV.   POTENTIAL DISTURBANCE IN CIRCULATION

Defining Characteristics: The following disturbances may occur: arrhythmia (23%), flushing (23%), hypotension (14%), hypertension (11%), phlebitis (11%), cardiac failure (6%); 3% of patients studied developed cardiac arrest, myocardial infarction, enlarged heart, heart murmur, ischemia, stroke, and other serious disturbances.

Nursing Implications: Assess cardiac status baseline and presence of risk factors (e.g., hypertension). Assess VS at each visit and teach patient in a manner not to induce anxiety to report any symptoms such as chest pain, SOB, heart palpitations, or any changes that occur.

V.   ALTERATION IN NUTRITION, LESS THAN BODY REQUIREMENTS, related to GI DYSFUNCTION

Defining Characteristics: Some problems are related to APL, and together with drug may emerge, such as GI bleeding/hemorrhage, which may occur in up to 34% of patients. Other GI problems include abdominal pain (31%), diarrhea (23%), constipation (17%), dyspepsia (14%), abdominal distention (11%), hepatosplenomegaly (9%), hepatitis (3%), and ulcer (3%).

Nursing Implications: Assess GI status and presence of GI dysfunction baseline. Teach patient to report any GI disturbances or changes in bowel status. If these occur, assess severity and need for symptom management, or discussion/intervention with physician. Monitor liver function studies frequently during therapy.

VI.   SENSORY/PERCEPTUAL ALTERATIONS related to CHANGES IN EAR SENSATION/HEARING

Defining Characteristics: 23% of patients report earache or fullness in ears. Other ear problems that may occur are reversible hearing loss (5%) and irreversible hearing loss (1%).

Nursing Implications: Teach patient that this may occur and to report it if it occurs. Assess severity and need for intervention.

VII.   POTENTIAL FOR INJURY related to CNS, PERIPHERAL NERVOUS SYSTEM CHANGES, AND AFFECT CHANGES

Defining Characteristics: Changes that may occur include dizziness (20%), paresthesias (17%), anxiety (17%), insomnia (14%), depression (14%), confusion (11%), cerebral hemorrhage (9%), agitation (9%), and hallucinations (6%). Rarely, the following may occur: forgetfulness, gait disturbances, convulsions, coma, facial paralysis, tremor, leg weakness, somnolence, slow speech, aphasia, and other CNS changes.

Nursing Implications: Teach patient in a manner that does not cause anxiety to report any changes in affect, sensorium, or functional ability (e.g., to walk, speak). Assess severity of symptom(s) if they arise and potential for injury. If severe, modify patient's environment to minimize risk of injury and discuss medical intervention with physician.

VIII. ALTERED URINARY ELIMINATION, POTENTIAL, related to RENAL CHANGES

Defining Characteristics: Uncommonly, renal insufficiency may occur (11%), dysuria (9%), acute renal failure (3%), urinary frequency (3%), renal tubular necrosis (3%), and enlarged prostate (3%).

Nursing Implications: Assess baseline urinary elimination pattern. Teach patient to report any changes. Monitor BUN/creatinine periodically during therapy and discuss any abnormalities with physician.

Drug: vandetanib (Caprelsa, D6474)

Class: Kinase inhibitor (multiple tyrosine kinase inhibitor, TKI).

Mechanism of Action: Vandetanib is a potent, selective inhibitor of multiple tyrosine kinases; it blocks vascular endothelial growth factor receptor (VEGFR-2), as well as the epidermal growth factor receptor (EGFR-1) tyrosine kinases. This blocks endothelial cell migration, proliferation, survival, and new blood vessel formation during angiogenesis. It inhibits EGFR-dependent cell survival, as well as EGF-stimulated receptor tyrosine kinase phosphorylation in tumor and endothelial cells, as well as VEGF-stimulated tyrosine kinase phosphorylation in endothelial cells. In mouse tumor models, the drug reduced tumor cell-induced angiogenesis, tumor vessel permeability, and inhibited tumor growth and metastasis. It also blocks RET (rearranged during transfection) kinase, protein tyrosine kinase 6 (BRK), TIE2 (receptor tyrosine kinase found on endothelial cells and necessary for tumor angiogenesis, as well as normal vascular development), members of the EPH receptors' kinase family (important role in cell signaling and cancer development), and members of the Src family of tyrosine kinases (may contain oncogenic protein), which may be important in certain tumors. There is no relationship between RET mutations and efficacy with vandetanib.

Metabolism: The median plasma half-life is 19 days following daily dosing. The drug is slowly absorbed, with a peak plasma concentration in a median of 6 hours (range 4–10 hours). Food does not affect absorption. Steady state is achieved in about 3 months. Drug is about 90% protein bound. The drug is metabolized in the liver by enzymes including CYP3A4, forming two major metabolites. 69% of the drug is excreted within 21 days (44% in feces, and 25% in urine), with additional drug being excreted after this time given long half-life.

Indication: Indicated for the treatment of symptomatic or progressive medullary thyroid cancer in patients with unresectable locally advanced or metastatic disease. Use in patients with indolent, asymptomatic, or slowly progressing disease only after careful consideration of the treatment-related risks.

Dosage/Range:
- Prescribers and pharmacies distributing vandetanib must be certified through the Vandetanib Risk Evaluation Mitigation Strategy (REMS) program, a restricted distribution program. To enroll in the Vandetanib REMS program, call 1-800-817-2722 or visit www.vandetanibrems.com. The drug will be dispensed exclusively through Biologics, Inc.'s pharmacy unit, an integrated oncology management company.
- 300 mg once daily orally with or without food.
- Renal impairment: Starting dose should be reduced to 200 mg once daily in patients with moderate (creatinine clearance 30 to 50 mL/min) to severe (creatinine clearance < 30 mL/min) renal impairment; monitor QTc interval closely.
- Do not start drug in patients whose QTc interval is > 450 ms.
- *Dosage Modifications:*
  - When needed, decrease the 300-mg daily dose to 200 mg (two 100-mg tablets), and then if further dose reduction needed, to 100 mg daily.
  - If QTc (corrected QT interval, see Introduction to *Chapter 5* for how to determine this) > 500 ms, interrupt drug dosing until QTc < 450 ms, then resume at reduced dose. Because of the drug's 19-day half-life, adverse reactions, including prolonged QT interval, may not resolve quickly. Monitor appropriately.
  - For grade 3 or greater toxicity, interrupt dosing until toxicity resolves or improves to CTCAE grade 1, then resume at a reduced dose.
- Drug should not be used for/by:
  - Patients with moderate (Child-Pugh Class B) and severe (Child-Pugh Class C) hepatic impairment; there is limited data on patients with a serum bilirubin > 1.5 × ULN, and the safety and efficacy have not been established.
  - Patients with congenital long QT syndrome.
  - Patients with hypocalcemia, hypokalemia, and/or hypomagensemia.
  - Patients with a history of hemoptysis of ≥ 1/2 tsp.

Drug Preparation:
- Oral. Available as 100-mg and 300-mg tablets. Do not crush.
- Only prescribers and pharmacies certified with the restricted distribution program are able to prescribe and dispense vandetanib (Caprelsa).

Drug Administration:
- Assess electrolytes, and replete so that serum calcium, potassium, and magnesium are WNL before vandetanib administration. Monitor periodically during therapy, and correct as needed and ordered.
- Assess TSH baseline, 2–4 weeks, and 8–12 weeks after starting vandetanib, and every 3 months thereafter.
- Teach patient to:
  - Take tablet orally, daily at about the same time, with or without food.
  - If the patient misses a dose, do not take it if less than 12 hours before the next dose.
  - If the patient cannot swallow the tablet whole, disperse the tablet(s) in a glass containing 2 oz. of noncarbonated water, and stir for approximately 10 minutes until well dispersed (will not completely dissolve). To ensure full dose is consumed, add an

additional 4 oz. of noncarbonated water swirl to mix the remaining residues, and have the patient swallow the solution.

- Dispersed drug can be administered through nasogastric or gastrostomy tubes.
- Avoid direct contact of skin or mucous membranes with crushed drug; if this occurs, wash the area thoroughly.
- Monitor ECG (QTc interval), electrolytes (serum potassium, calcium, magnesium), TSH baseline, during week 2–4, then again weeks 8–12 after starting vandetanib therapy.

Drug Interactions:
- Strong CYP3A4 inducers (e.g., dexamethasone, phenytoin, carbamazepine, rifampin, rifabutin, rifapentine, phenobarbital), St. John's wort: may reduce vandetanib levels; DO NOT take together.
- Drugs that prolong QT interval [antiarrhythmic drugs (e.g., amiodarone, disopyramide, procainamide, sotalol, dofetilide); others (chloroquine, clarithromycin, dolasetron, granisetron, haloperidol, methadone, moxifloxacin, pimozide)]: Increase risk of QTc prolongation; avoid concomitant administration.
- Metformin, other drugs transported by the organic cation transporter type 2 (OCT2): increased plasma concentrations of metformin; use together cautiously and monitor for toxicities.
- Digoxin: increased digoxin plasma concentrations: monitor digoxin levels closely, and monitor patients for digoxin toxicity.

Lab Effects/Interference:
- Prolongs QTc interval
- Decreased serum calcium (57%), decreased serum glucose (24%); increased ALT (51%, 2% grade 3–4).
- Bilirubin increased (13%), creatinine increased (16%).
- Decreased: WBC (19%), Hgb (13%), neutrophils (10%), platelets (9%).
- Proteinuria (10%).
- TSH may be increased if the patient develops hypothyroidism; decreased T_4.

Special Considerations:
- QT prolongation and torsades de pointes.
  - Torsades de pointes (a type of ventricular tachycardia), ventricular tachycardia, and sudden death have occurred in patients receiving the drug.
  - Do not start drug in patients whose QTc interval is > 450 ms.
  - Drug should not be prescribed for patients with a history of torsades de pointes, congenital long QT syndrome, bradyarrhythmias, or uncompensated heart failure.
  - Drug exposure is increased in patients with renal impairment; the starting dose should be reduced to 200 mg in patients with moderate to severe renal impairment, and monitor QT interval frequently.
  - Risk of torsades de pointes increased in patients with hypokalemia, hypomagnesemia, and/or hypocalemia.
  - Perform ECG and assess serum potassium, calcium, magnesium, and TSH baseline, at 2–4 weeks, and 8–12 weeks after starting vandetanib, then every 3 months. Monitor electrolytes more frequently if patient develops diarrhea.

- Maintain serum potassium at 4 mEq/L or higher (within normal range) and maintain serum and calcium levels WNL.
- Avoid using vandetanib with drugs that prolong the QT interval, and if medically necessary to coadminister, monitor ECG for QT-interval prolongation more frequently.
- Following any dose reduction for QT prolongation, or any dose interruption > 2 weeks, assess QT interval as described above.
- Stop vandetanib in patients who develop a QTc > 500 ms until the QTc returns to < 450 ms. Resume vandetanib at a reduced dose.
- Drug has not been studied in patients with ventricular arrhythmias or recent myocardial infarction.
- Skin reactions and Stevens-Johnson syndrome: severe skin reactions, including Stevens-Johnson syndrome have occurred. Photosensitivity reactions can occur during therapy and for 4 months after last dose. Permanently discontinue drug for severe skin reactions. Drug is not recommended for patients with moderate (Child-Pugh Class B) or severe (Child-Pugh Class C) hepatic impairment; limited data exists on patients with a serum bilirubin > 1.5 times ULN, and the safety and efficacy have not been established.
- Interstitial lung disease (ILD), resulting in death, has been reported; interrupt drug immediately if patient has unexplained dyspnea, cough, and fever. If ILD is confirmed, permanently discontinue drug, and treat ILD.
- Ischemic cerebrovascular events occurred in 1.3% of patients. Discontinue vandetanib in patients who experience a severe ischemic cerebrovascular event.
- Hemorrhagic events have occurred. Drug should not be prescribed in patients with a recent history of hemoptysis (≥ 1/2 teaspoon).
- Heart failure has been observed in patients receiving the drug; it may not be reversible on stopping the drug, and may be rarely fatal. Monitor for signs/symptoms of heart failure. Drug discontinuance should be considered in patients with heart failure; heart failure may not be reversible when drug is stopped.
- Diarrhea, grade 3 or higher, occurred in 11% of patients. If diarrhea occurs, monitor patient's serum electrolytes and ECGs to reduce risk and enable early detection of QT prolongation resulting from dehydration. Interrupt vandetanib for severe diarrhea; when symptom improves, resume drug at a reduced dose.
- Hypothyroidism: Most patients studied had undergone thyroidectomy. Assess patients for onset of hypothyroidism: assess TSH baseline, then at 2–4 weeks, 8–12 weeks after starting the drug, then every 3 months thereafter. If signs/symptoms of hypothyroidism occur (e.g., fatigue, sluggishness, increased sensitivity to cold, constipation, dry skin, puffy face, hoarse voice, increased serum cholesterol, unexplained weight gain, joint stiffness, muscle weakness, brittle fingernail/hair, depression, heavy menses), assess TSH and discuss with physician or NP/PA, adjustment of thyroid replacement therapy dose as needed.
- Hypertension may occur. Monitor all patients for HTN, and discuss vandetanib dose reduction or interruption for HTN. Vandetanib should not be resumed if HTN is not controlled.
- Reversible posterior leukoencephalopathy syndrome (RPLS), a syndrome of subcortical vasogenic edema diagnosed by brain MRI, may occur.

- If patient presents with seizures, headache, visual disturbances, confusion, or altered mental function, RPLS should be considered in the differential diagnosis.
- Three out of the four patients who developed RPLS while receiving vandetanib also had HTN.
- Discontinue vandetanib in patients who develop RPLS.
- Renal impairment: vandetanib exposure is increased so starting dose must be reduced to 200 mg in patients with moderate to severe renal impairment. Monitor QT interval closely. No information is available for patients with end-stage renal disease who require dialysis.
- Embryo-fetal toxicity: If the drug is used during pregnancy, or if the patient becomes pregnant while receiving the drug, the patient should be apprised of the potential hazard to the fetus. Teach women of childbearing potential to use effective contraception during treatment, and for at least 4 months after the last dose.
- Most common adverse drug reactions (≥ 20%, and with a difference between arms of ≥ 5%) were diarrhea/colitis, rash, acneiform dermatitis, nausea, hypertension, headache, URI, decreased appetite, and abdominal pain;
- Most common lab abnormalities (≥ 20%) were decreased serum calcium and glucose, and increased ALT.

Potential Toxicities/Side Effects and the Nursing Process

I. ALTERATION IN CIRCULATION, POTENTIAL, related to QTc PROLONGATION

Defining Characteristics: Patients may develop QT prolongation on EKG. Do NOT administer to patients with prolonged or who may develop prolonged QTc (hypokalemia, hypomagnesemia, hypocalcemia, other drugs that prolong the QTc). Prolonged QTc in the setting of low magnesium and hypokalemia sets the stage for torsades de pointes, with ventricular tachycardia, fibrillation, and sudden cardiac death possible. Incidence of electrolyte disturbances: decreased calcium 57% (6% grade 3–4), decreased magnesium 7% (< 1%), decreased potassium 6% (1%). 14% had QTc prolonged: 69% had QTc > 450 ms, 7% had QTc > 500 ms. Only physicians certified by the Vandetanib REMS can prescribe, and only certified pharmacies can dispense the drug.

Nursing Implications: Assess patient's drug profile to ensure that the patient is not taking any drugs that may increase the QTc interval. Assess baseline QTc interval. Identify patients at risk for development of prolonged QTc (congenital long QTc) syndrome, prolonged QTc > 450 msec, taking antiarrhythmics or other drugs that can prolong the QTc interval, hypokalemia, hypomagnesemia, concomitant CYP3A4 strong inhibitors. Correct electrolyte abnormalities (e.g., magnesium, calcium, potassium) before starting vandetanib, and monitor periodically during therapy. Hypokalemia, hypocalcemia, and hypomagnesemia in the setting of prolonged QTc may lead to torsades de pointes, ventricular fibrillation, and sudden cardiac death. QTc must be assessed baseline, at 2–4 weeks, and 8–12 weeks after starting vandetanib therapy, then every 3 months thereafter. Following any dose reduction for QT prolongation, or any dose interruptions > 2 weeks, QT assessment should be conducted as previously described. If the patient has diarrhea, serum electrolytes and EKGs will need to be assessed more frequently, and electrolytes repleted. Because of the long half-life of 19 days, a prolonged QT interval may take a few weeks to resolve. Serum potassium level should be maintained at 4 mEq/L or higher (within normal range) and serum magnesium and calcium kept WNL. Teach patient to correctly take vandetanib as prescribed, and to avoid any drugs that may interact with vantedanib, until discussion with the physician, NP, PA, or nurse. Patients with renal impairment should have a dose reduction to avoid increased serum levels of vandetanib. See Introduction to *Chapter 5* for a full discussion of assessing the QT (QTc) interval in patients receiving drugs that may increase the risk of serious complications.

II.   ALTERATION IN CIRCULATION, POTENTIAL, related to BLEEDING AND HYPERTENSION

Defining Characteristics: Like all antiangiogenic agents, vandetanib can cause serious hemorrhagic events and hypertension (HTN).

Nursing Implications: Drug should not be given to patients with a recent history of hemoptysis of ≥ 1/2 tsp. of red blood. Teach patient that bleeding may occur and to come to the emergency department and notify physician or nurse practitioner right away if bleeding (e.g., epistaxis) does not resolve in 15 minutes with local pressure and ice. Ensure that major surgery is planned with adequate time for drug elimination from body (half-life 19 days) and that it is not resumed until after adequate wound healing. Assess patient for hypertension, and if uncontrolled, hypertensive crisis. Assess at each visit, and discuss if needed, medical management of HTN. If not able to be medically controlled, stop drug until HTN well-managed. Drug should be permanently discontinued in patients with severe hemorrhage or uncontrollable hypertension.

III.   POTENTIAL ALTERATION IN SENSORY PERCEPTUAL PATTERNS related to ISCHEMIC CEREBROVASCULAR EVENTS, REVERSIBLE POSTERIOR LEUKOENCEPHALOPATHY SYNDROME (RPLS)

Defining Characteristics: Ischemic cerberovascular events have occurred and are rarely fatal, with incidence 1.3%. RPLS, a syndrome of subcortical vasogenic edema as shown on brain MRI, may also occur rarely and may be more likely in patients with HTN. Blurred vision affected 9% of patients.

Nursing Implications: Assess baseline neurological status. Teach patient to report any changes in behavior, thinking, visual changes, or any new signs or symptoms. If seizure, headache, visual disturbances, confusion, or altered mental function, discuss patient RPLS evaluation with physician or midlevel practitioner. MRI is used to identify RPLS pathology. Drug should be permanently discontinued in patients who have either ischemic cerberovascular events or RPLS. If patient complains of blurred vision, discuss with physician or midlevel practitioner, have evaluation by ophthalmologist, and slit lamp examination. Those studied had corneal opacities (vortex keratopathies), which led to halos and decreased visual acuity. If blurred vision, advise patient not to drive or operate machinery.

IV. POTENTIAL ALTERATION IN SKIN INTEGRITY related to RASH

Defining Characteristics: Rash occurred in 53% of patients, with 5% being grade 3–4. Rash included rash erythematous, generalized, macular, maculo-papular, papular, pruritic, exfoliative, dermatitis, dermatitis bullous, generalized erythema, and eczema. Dermatitis acneiform/acne occurred in 35% of patients, while 15% had dry skin, and 11% pruritus. Rash was usually mild to moderate. Photosensitivity reactions are increased (13%). Severe skin reactions, including Stevens-Johnson syndrome, have been reported; some have been fatal.

Nursing Implications: Assess skin integrity baseline and periodically during therapy. Teach patient that rash may occur, and give general symptom-management strategies to minimize discomfort. Mild-to-moderate skin reactions (rash, dry skin, dermatitis, pruritus, photosensitivity, palmar-plantar erythrodysesthesia syndrome) may require topical and systemic corticosteroids, oral antihistamines, and topical and systemic antibiotics. Advise patient to wear sunscreen and protective clothing when exposed to the sun (during drug treatment and for 4 months following discontinuance). If rash is grade 3, then the drug should be stopped until improvement; when resolved or improved, discuss with physician dose reduction or discontinuance. Teach patient to stop drug and notify nurse or physician if rash begins to peel, is severe, or does not resolve with local management. If rash is severe, treatment may require corticosteroids and vandetanib should be permanently discontinued.

V. POTENTIAL ALTERATION IN OXYGENATION related to INTERSTITIAL LUNG DISEASE (ILD)

Defining Characteristics: ILD or pneumonitis may occur rarely and may result in death. EGFR blockade may be responsible for this, as EGF is necessary to repair injury to the lung tissue. Nonspecific respiratory signs and symptoms are hypoxia, pleural effusion, cough, or dyspnea when infectious, malignant, and other causes have been excluded.

Nursing Implications: Assess patient's respiratory patterns baseline and periodically during treatment. Tell patient to report any new or worsening respiratory symptoms right away. Discuss management plan with physician or midlevel practitioner: imaging to identify ILD changes, and rule out other causes. If symptoms are absent or minimal, and radiological changes are suggestive of ILD, physician may continue vandetanib and closely monitor the patient. If symptoms are moderate, vandetanib therapy is often interrupted until symptoms improve, with or without corticosteroids and antibiotics. If symptoms of ILD are severe, vandetanib should be stopped/permanently discontinued, with corticosteroids and antibiotic therapy instituted.

VI. ALTERATION IN NUTRITION, LESS THAN BODY REQUIREMENTS, related to DIARRHEA, NAUSEA, VOMITING, ANOREXIA, INCREASED LIVER FUNCTION TESTS

Defining Characteristics: Diarrhea occurred in 57% of all patients in study, with 11% being grade 3–4; it is usually well managed with routine antidiarrheal agents. Nausea affected

33% (1% grade 3–4) of patients, and vomiting 15% (1% grade 3–4). 21% of patients had decreased appetite (4% grade 3–4), and 10% experienced weight loss. ALT was elevated in 51% of patients, 2% grade 3–4.

Nursing Implications: Assess nutritional status, bowel elimination pattern, and appetite baseline, and repeat at each visit or telephone call during treatment. Assess LFTs baseline, and ALT every 3 months per physician. Inform patient that these side effects may occur. Teach self-administration of antinausea and antidiarrheal medications (e.g., loperamide) and to notify provider if symptoms persist so that dose can be interrupted and more aggressive antidiarrheal strategies implemented. Since electrolytes can be lost with diarrhea, patient will need recheck of serum electrolytes if diarrhea is persistent or severe. If severe, vandetanib should be interrupted until diarrhea is controlled. When controlled, the vandetanib dose should be reduced when drug is resumed. Teach patient dietary modification if nausea and vomiting or diarrhea occur (e.g., for diarrhea, BRAT diet of bananas, rice, applesauce, and toast) and to increase oral fluids to prevent dehydration. Consult a dietitian to see the patient for dietary counseling for anorexia. Discuss any abnormalities with physician or nurse practitioner.

VII.   ALTERATION IN COMFORT related to HEADACHE, FATIGUE, ABDOMINAL PAIN

Defining Characteristics: Headache affected 26% of patients (1% grade 3–4), fatigue 24% (6% grade 3–4), abdominal pain 21% (3% grade 3–4), asthenia 15% (3% grade 3–4).

Nursing Implications: Assess patient's baseline comfort, and teach that these symptoms may occur. Teach symptom-management strategies to minimize discomfort. Teach patient to notify physician if fatigue or headache becomes severe and does not respond to local therapy.

Drug: vemurafenib (Zelboraf, PLX4032)

Class: Kinase (BRAF) inhibitor. BRAF is a serine-threonine kinase.

Mechanism of Action: 40–60% of patients with malignant melanoma have a mutation in the *BRAF* gene (BRAF V600E), which controls a protein involved in cell signaling. This leads to constitutive activation of downstream signaling via the MAPK pathway (the message for the cell to divide continues to be sent to the cell nucleus via this pathway, even though the cell never received a message to divide from outside the cell). The RAS-RAF pathway is very important in normal cell growth and survival. Mutation of the *BRAF* gene mutation keeps the BRAF protein in an active state causing excessive signaling). Vemurafenib potently inhibits the mutated *BRAF* gene and turns off the MAPK signaling, so the message no longer goes to the cell nucleus. In addition, it allows cells to undergo apoptosis. However, patients ultimately develop resistance to the drug, so it may require concomitant administration with a MEK or AKT inhibitor. Drug may cross the blood–brain barrier.

Metabolism: After oral administration of 960 mg twice daily for 15 days, the T_{max} was 3 hours, with steady state achieved in 15–22 days. Relationship of dosing with food ingestion has not been studied. Drug is highly protein bound (> 99%). The drug is excreted in the feces (94%) and urine (1%). The elimination half-life is 57 hours. Drug clearance in patients with mild to moderate hepatic or renal insufficiency was similar to patients with normal organ function, but clearance in patients with severe dysfunction was not studied. Drug is a substrate of CYP3A4, and both a substrate and inhibitor of the efflux transporter P-glycoprotein (P-gp).

Indication: Drug is indicated for the
- Treatment of patients with unresectable or metastatic melanoma with BRAF V600E mutation as detected by a FDA-approved test.
- Not indicated for the treatment of patients with wild-type BRAF melanoma.

Dosage/Range:
- Confirm the presence of BRAF V600E mutation in tumor specimens prior to initiation of treatment.
- 960 mg PO twice daily, approximately 12 hours apart, with or without a meal. Dose-modify based on toxicity. Doses < 480 mg twice daily are not recommended.

Dose Modifications:
- For new, primary cutaneous malignancies: no dose modifications are necessary.
- For other adverse reactions:
  - Permanently discontinue drug for any of the following:
    - Grade 4 adverse reactions, first appearance (if clinically appropriate), or second appearance.
    - QTc prolongation > 500 ms and increased by > 60 ms from pretreatment values.
  - Withhold vemurafenib for NCI CTCAE (v.4.0) for intolerable grade 2 or higher adverse reactions.
  - Upon recovery to grade 0–1, restart vemurafenib at a reduced dose as follows: (1) 720 mg twice daily for first appearance of intolerable grade 2 or grade 3 adverse reactions; and (2) 480 mg twice daily for the second appearance of intolerable grade 2, or grade 3 adverse reactions, or for the first appearance of grade 4 adverse reaction (if clinically appropriate).
  - Do not dose-reduce to below 480 mg twice daily.

Drug Preparation:
- Oral. Available as 240-mg tablet.

Drug Administration:
- Oral without regard to food ingestion.
- Teach patient to:
  - Swallow whole with a glass of water, and teach patient not to chew or crush tablet. May take with or without food.
  - If a dose is missed, it can be taken up to 4 hours prior to the next dose to maintain the twice daily regimen. Do not take both doses at the same time. Continue treatment until disease progression or unacceptable toxicity.
  - Do not take an additional dose if vomiting occurs, but continue with next scheduled dose.

Drug Interactions:
- Drug is a substrate of CYP3A4.
  - Strong CYP3A4 inhibitors (ketoconazole, itraconazole, clarithromycin, atazanavir, nefazodone, saquinavir, telithromycin, ritonavir, indinivir, nelfinavir, voriconazole) may increase vemurafenib serum level and increase toxicity. Use alternative drug if possible; if not, use together cautiously if at all, and monitor patient closely for vemurafenib toxicity.
  - Strong inducers (phenytoin, carbamazepine, rifampin, rifabutin, rifapentine, phenobarbital) can decrease vemurafenib concentrations; use alternative drug if possible; if not, use together cautiously if at all, and monitor patient closely for vemurafenib effect.
- Drug is a moderate CYP1A2 inhibitor, a weak CYP2D6 inhibitor, and a CYP3A4 inducer.
- CYP2D6 substrate (dextromethorphan): increased AUC (up to 47%); use together cautiously.
- Midazolam (CYP3A4 substrate): decreased midazolam AUC by 39%.
- Effect of vemurafenib on CYP1A2 substrates: concomitant use of vemurafenib with drugs having a narrow therapeutic window that are predominantly metabolized by CYP1A2 is not recommended.
  - If it cannot be avoided, monitor patient closely for toxicities, and consider a dose reduction of the concomitant CYP1A2 substrate.
  - CYP1A2 substrate (caffeine): increased mean AUC of caffeine by 2.6-fold.
- Warfarin: 18% increase in warfarin AUC (CYP2C9 substrate); use together cautiously and monitor patient's INR closely for warfarin dosing.
- Ipilumumab: increased transaminases and bilirubin in the majority of patients receiving vemurafenib and ipilumumab together.
- Vemurafenib is both a substrate of and an inhibitor of the efflux transporter P-glycoprotein (P-gp).

Lab Effects/Interference:
- Increased LFTs (AST, ALT, alkaline phosphatase, bilirubin).
- Increased QTc interval.

Special Considerations:
- Patients must be BRAF-mutation positive (Cobas 4800 BRAF V600 Mutation test is one test to determine this) to benefit from this drug. It may be possible that the drug, if used in patients with BRAF-wild-type genotype, will cause progression of melanoma (Chapman et al., 2011). In addition, the drug will not work in BRAF-wild-type cancers, and may cause secondary tumors in internal organs in addition to the skin (any organ with squamous epithelium).

Warnings and Precautions:
- Cutaneous squamous cell carcinoma, keratocanthoma, and melanoma occurred at a higher incidence in patients receiving drug, as compared to control arm in Trial 1.
  - Incidence of cutaneous squamous cell carcinomas and keratocanthomas occurred in 24% of patients compared to < 1% in the control.
  - Median time to first appearance of cutaneous squamous cell carcinoma was 7–8 weeks; about 33% of patients who developed this on vemurafenib experienced at least one additional occurrence, with median time between occurrences of 6 weeks.

- Risk factors included age ≥ 65, prior skin cancer, and chronic sun exposure.
- Patients should have dermatologic evaluations prior to starting therapy, and every 2 months while on therapy. Manage suspicious skin lesions with excision and dermatopathologic evaluation. Consider dermatologic monitoring for 6 months after last dose of vemurafenib.
- Noncutaneous squamous cell carcinoma (SCC) of the head and neck can occur. Monitor patients closely for this.
- Vemurafenib may promote malignancies associated with activation of RAS through mutation or other mechanisms. Monitor patients closely for signs or symptoms of other malignancies.
- Tumor promotion in BRAF wild-type melanoma: Paradoxical activation of MAP-kinase signaling and increased proliferation of BRAF wild-type cells exposed to BRSAF inhibitors can occur. Ensure drug is only used in patients with tumors having BRAF V600E mutations.
- Serious hypersensitivity reactions may occur, including generalized rash and erythema, hypotension, drug reaction with eosinophilia and systemic symptoms (DRESS syndrome) during and upon reinitiation of vemurafenib treatment. Monitor patients closely, permanently discontinue drug, and manage serious hypersensitivity reactions.
- Severe dermatologic reactions, including Stevens-Johnson syndrome and toxic epidermal necrolysis, have occurred. Drug should be permanently discontinued if severe reactions occur.
- QT prolongation may occur, and may lead to increased risk of ventricular arrhythmia, including torsades de pointes.
  - Patients should have an ECG with QTc measurement and serum electrolytes (especially potassium, magnesium, calcium) baseline, then 15 days after treatment initiation or dose modification for QTc prolongation, then monthly during the first 3 months, then every 3 months or as clinically indicated.
  - DO NOT start vemurafenib in patients with uncorrected electrolyte abnormalities, QTc > 500 ms, or Long QT syndrome, or in patients taking medicines known to prolong the QT interval.
  - If QTc > 500 ms (grade 3), withhold drug and assess/correct electrolyte abnormalities; control cardiac risk factors for QT prolongation. Upon recovery to QTc ≤ 500 ms (grade 2 or less), restart vemurafenib at a reduced dose.
  - Permanently discontinue vemurafenib if the QTc interval remains > 500 ms and increased > 60 ms from pretreatment values after controlling cardiac risk factors for QT prolongation (e.g., electrolyte abnormalities, CHF, and bradyarrhythmias).
- Hepatotoxicity: Abnormal elevations of LFTs can occur. Monitor LFTs baseline, then monthly during treatment, increasing frequency as needed, as drug can cause abnormalities.
- Concurrent administration with ipilumumab: safety and effectiveness not established; in dose finding study, grade 3 increases in transaminases and bilirubin occurred in a majority of patients.
- Photosensitivity: Teach patient to avoid sun exposure, wear protective clothing, and use a broad spectrum UVA/UVB sunscreen and lip balm (SPF ≥ 30) when outdoors, as drug can cause photosensitivity.

- Serious ophthalmologic reactions may occur (uveitis, blurry vision, and photophobia), so teach patient to report any visual changes, and discuss ophthalmologic evaluation with physician or midlevel practitioner.
- Drug can cause fetal harm, and fetal drug levels were 5% of maternal levels.
  - Teach women of childbearing age to use effective contraception during therapy and for at least 2 months after last dose of vemurafenib.
  - If the drug is used in pregnancy or if the patient becomes pregnant while taking the drug, the patient should be apprised of potential hazard to the fetus.
  - Mothers should make a decision to stop nursing or to stop the drug, taking into account the importance of the drug to the mother's health.
- Chapman et al. (2011) demonstrated that there was a significant survival advantage for patients with previously untreated metastatic melanoma receiving vemurafenib compared to those taking dacarbazine (DTIC): at 6 months, 84% of patients were alive compared to 64% in the DTIC group. Response rates were 48% for the vemurafenib group compared to 5% in the DTIC group. Patients receiving vemurafenib had a 74% reduction in risk of progression (or death) compared to patients receiving DTIC ($p < 0.001$). Mean progression-free survival was 5.3 months for the vemurafenib group compared to 1.6 months in the DTIC group. Because the early interim results were so astounding, an independent data and safety monitoring board recommended that patients receiving DTIC cross over to vemurafenib.
- A phase 2 study showed a confirmed response rate of 53% and a median duration of response of 6.7 months (Ribas et al., 2011).
- Most common adverse events ($\geq$ 30%) were:
  - Arthralgia, rash, alopecia, fatigue, photosensitivity reactions, nausea, pruritus, and skin papilloma.
  - Patients who developed cutaneous squamous cell carcinoma had the lesion excised and continued vemurafenib therapy.
- Su et al. (2011) showed that resistance is likely because of reactivation of the RAS/RAF pathway and activation of an alternative pathway. This study supports future studies in which an MEK or AKT inhibitor is added to vemurafenib to combat resistance. Another study comparing combinations of a BRAF inhibitor (GSK436) and an AKT inhibitor (GSK212) showed that the combination was safe with preliminary antitumor activity in patients with advanced melanoma (Infante et al., 2011).
- In trying to understand the increased incidence of squamous cell carcinomas and keratoacanthomas in patients treated with vemurafenib, researchers found that 60% of tumors had a *RAS* mutation, suggesting that perhaps the *BRAF* inhibition activates mutations in RAS. This might be prevented by combining treatment with an MEK inhibitor, as mentioned above.

Potential Toxicities/Side Effects and the Nursing Process

I.   ALTERATION IN COMFORT related to FATIGUE, ARTHALGIA

Defining Characteristics: Fatigue occurred in 38–54%, and arthalgias in 53–67% of patients.

Nursing Implications: Teach patients to report alterations in comfort, especially joint pain and fatigue. Distinguish new onset of symptoms versus those experienced before treatment due to malignancy. Teach patient to manage arthralgias and energy-conserving strategies to manage fatigue.

II. ALTERATION IN SKIN INTEGRITY, POTENTIAL, related to INCREASED RISK FOR ALOPECIA, KERATOACANTHOMA, SQUAMOUS CELL CARCINOMA, NEW MELANOMA, AND PHOTOSENSITIVITY

Defining Characteristics: Alopecia, photosensitivity, and rarely development of keratocanthoma or squamous cell carcinoma may occur. Keratocanthoma is a common low-grade skin tumor thought to originate from the hair follicle. It is often considered a form of squamous cell carcinoma. It is found in sun-exposed skin (e.g., face, forearms, and hands). It is dome-shaped, symmetrical, and surrounded by inflamed skin. There are often keratin scales and debris. It grows rapidly, and if not treated, will eventually necrose and heal with scarring. New primary melanomas may occur. Rash occurs in up to half of patients. Photosensitivity affects 33-49% of patients, and pruritus up to 30%.

Nursing Implications: Patient should have a baseline dermatologic evaluation prior to beginning therapy, then every 2 months while on therapy, and continuing for 6 months after completion of drug therapy. Any suspicious lesion should be excised and biopsied, then treated as per standard of care. Drug dose is not changed Assess patient's skin baseline and at each visit. Teach patient to stop taking the drug and call provider right away if the patient develops a severe skin reaction, such as blisters on the skin, in the mouth, fever, peeling of the skin, or redness or swelling of face, hands or soles of feet. Teach patient to self-assess skin regularly, and advise provider if notice a new wart, sore, or bump that bleeds or does not heal, or a mole that changes in color. Teach patient to use strong UVA/UVB sunblock (SPF 30 or higher), lip balm, and protective clothing or to avoid exposing skin to the sun. Teach to wear a hat to protect the scalp, especially if experiencing alopecia, and to cover exposed skin with a shirt or cover. Teach patient to wear sunglasses to protect the eyes when out in the sun if it cannot be avoided. Teach the patient to report any new skin lesions on sun-exposed body parts, especially if it is growing quickly. Discuss with physician referral to dermatology to obtain an excisional biopsy of the lesion.

III. ALTERATION IN NUTRITION, LESS THAN BODY REQUIREMENTS, related to NAUSEA, DIARRHEA

Defining Characteristics: Nausea occurred in 35–37%, vomiting in 18–26%, diarrhea in 28–29%, and constipation in 12–16% of patients in two clinical trials.

Nursing Implications: Assess weight, bowel elimination status, and baseline nutritional status, and monitor during therapy. Teach patient that symptoms can occur and ways to minimize this effect, such as self-administration of antinausea and antidiarrheal medications per protocol and to report symptoms that do not resolve with established plan. If patient has constipation, teach diet modifications to increase peristalsis, self-administration of cathartics and hydration as needed. Teach patient to identify nutritionally dense (high calories and protein in the smallest amount) foods and to keep them handy in the refrigerator. Teach patient to eat small, frequent meals and to have a bedtime snack. Teach patient that goal is to drink a glass of fluid every hour while awake. Teach patient to call provider if symptoms do not resolve within 24 hours. Monitor closely patients, such as older persons, who are at risk for dehydration. Discuss any abnormalities with a physician.

IV.   ALTERATION IN CIRCULATION, POTENTIAL, related to QTc PROLONGATION

Defining Characteristics: Patients may develop QT prolongation on ECG. In the setting of low electrolyte levels (potassium, magnesium, calcium), this can set the stage for ventricular arrythmias, especially torsades de pointes, which may cause sudden death. Drug is not recommended for patients with uncorrectable electrolyte abnormalities, Long QT syndrome, a QTc > 500 ms, or who are taking medications known to prolong the QT interval (e.g., methadone, haloperidol).

Nursing Implications: Assess patients at risk (cardiac history, medications that may prolong QTc including serotonin antagonists, history of cardiac arrythmias). Assess ECG and serum electrolytes; discuss correction of electrolytes prior to starting drug. Monitor ECG and electrolytes should be at day 15 after drug initiation, then monthly during first 3 months of therapy, then every 3 months during therapy. If the QTc > 500 ms (grade 3) at any time, stop the drug, correct electrolyte abnormalities, and control cardiac risk factors for QT prolongation (e.g., CHF, bradyarrythmias). Once the QTc is < 500 ms, restart the drug at a lower dose. Permanently discontinue drug if after correction of risk factors, the QTc increases again both > 500 ms, and > 60 ms change from pretreatment values. See introduction to *Chapter 5* for a full discussion of assessing the QT (QTc) interval in patients receiving drugs that may increase the risk of serious complications. Teach patient to call provider right away, or go to the emergency room if feeling faint, or have a rapid heartbeat.

Drug: vismodegib (Erivedge)

Class: Hedgehog pathway inhibitor.

Mechanism of Action: The Hedgehog pathway is vital during embryogenesis, and it is a complicated pathway. A simplified version is described. In the embryo, the Hedgehog pathway is responsible for cell proliferation and differentiation into specialized cells, organ formation, and tissue migration to the correct anatomical position within the developing embryo. That way, the fetus develops with the spinal cord in the right place, with five fingers on each hand, five toes on each foot, and the anatomical part heading in the right direction (tissue polarity). The Hedgehog pathway also plays a role in cell differentiation, stem cell maintenance and wound healing in adults. The Hedgehog gene codes for the sonic hedgehog (SHH) protein, which will bind to a specific cell membrane receptor complex to turn on signal transduction leading to cell proliferation. The receptor complex on the cell membrane is made up of two proteins: patched (PTCH) 1 that binds the ligand SHH, and smoothened (SMO), which turns on the actual signal transduction to activate the target genes controlling cell proliferation. Normally this pathway is almost shut down after the fetus is formed. If the PTCH1 gene becomes mutated, then the PTCH1 protein cannot bind to SMO, releasing SMO to send unlimited messages to the target genes so that unregulated cell proliferation occurs along with angiogenesis. Mutations in PTCH1, PTCH2, SMO, and another gene may be mutated in basal cell carcinoma (BCC). UV exposure mutates PTCH1, and is thought to be responsible for 70% of BCCs (von Gorlin syndrome). Another 10–20% of BCCs appear to be due to mutations in SMO, leading to unregulated signaling to the genes responsible for cell proliferation. Thus, in BCC, the Hedgehog pathway becomes turned on without regulation, resulting in malignant transformation. Hedgehog signaling from the tumor to the stroma (surrounding tissue that stimulates tumor growth) increases tumorigenesis (Gupta et al., 2010). Vismodegib binds to and inhibits SMO, the transmembrane protein that is necessary for activation of signal transduction. By inactivating SMO, the pathway is turned off.

Metabolism: The drug is highly permeable but has low solubility in water. After an oral dose, the absolute bioavailability is 31.8%. The drug binds to plasma proteins > 99%. More than 98% of the total circulating drug components are parent drug. Drug is metabolized by oxidation (CYP2C9, CYP3A4/5), glucuronidation, and pyridine ring cleavage. Drug and metabolites are eliminated via the liver with 82% of administered dose found in the feces, and 4.4% in the urine. Elimination half-life is 4 days after continuous daily dosing, and 12 days after a single dose. Drug has not been studied in patients with hepatic or renal impairment.

Indication: The treatment of adults with metastatic basal cell carcinoma, or with locally advanced basal cell carcinoma that has recurred following surgery or who are not candidates for surgery, and who are not candidates for radiation therapy.

Dosage/Range:
- 150-mg capsule PO daily, with or without food until disease progression or unacceptable toxicity.

Drug Preparation:
- None, oral. Available as 150-mg capsules, in a bottle containing 28 capsules. Teach patient to keep bottle at room temperature and out of reach of children and pets.

Drug Administration:
- Verify patient is not pregnant before starting therapy with vismodegib.
- Teach patient to take tablet with or without food, and to swallow capsule whole. Do not open or crush capsules. If a dose is missed, do not make it up. Resume drug with next scheduled dose.

Drug Interactions:
- Vismodegib is a substrate of CYP2C9 and CYP3A4; there appear to be no effects from CYP3A4 inducers or inhibitors on vismodegib serum levels.
- Drugs that inhibit the efflux of P-glycoprotein (P-gp) (clarithromycin, erythromycin, azithromycin): since vismodegib is a substrate of P-gp, these drugs may increase vismodegib serum levels and risk for toxicity; avoid concurrent use.

- Drugs that alter gastric pH (proton pump inhibitors, H_2-receptor antagonists, antacids): may alter vismodegib solubility and reduce bioavailability, thus reducing efficacy; avoid concurrent use.
- Vismodegib is an inhibitor of CYP2C8, CYP2C9, CYP2C19, and the transporter BCRP (breast cancer resistance protein). The significance is unknown.

Lab Effects/Interference:
- Hyponatremia, hypokalemia, azotemia.

Special Considerations:
- Drug is teratogenic, embryotoxic, and fetotoxic in rats. It can cause embryo-fetal death and severe birth defects.
  - Verify patients of childbearing potential are not pregnant before starting vismodegib.
  - Teach women of childbearing potential to use effective contraception during and after treatment.
  - Teach men with partners with childbearing potential to use condoms, as there is potential risk of drug exposure through semen.
  - Teach patients to contact their healthcare provider immediately if they suspect they (or for males, their female partner) may be pregnant.
    - Immediately report exposure during pregnancy (either directly or through seminal fluid) to Genentech Adverse Event Line at 1-888-835-2555.
    - Encourage women who may have been exposed during pregnancy (either directly or through seminal fluid) to participate in the ERIVEDGE pregnancy pharmaco-vigilance program (contact Genentech at the above number).
  - If drug is used during pregnancy, or the patient becomes pregnant while using the drug, the patient should be apprised of the potential hazard to the fetus.
- Nursing mothers should make a decision to discontinue nursing or to discontinue the drug, taking into account the importance of the drug to the mother's health.
- Patients should not donate blood or blood products while receiving the drug and for at least 7 months following the last dose of vismodegib.
- Most common adverse effects ($\geq 10\%$) are muscle spasms, alopecia, dysgeusia, weight loss, fatigue, nausea, diarrhea, decreased appetite, constipation, arthralgias, vomiting, and ageusia.
- Drug is fetotoxic and teratogenic. Females of reproductive age and males should be counseled on pregnancy prevention and planning. If pregnancy occurs, report exposure (either directly or through seminal fluid) immediately to Genentech Adverse Event Line 1-888-835-2555. Encourage patient participation in the ERIVEDGE pregnancy pharmaco-vigilance program. Verify pregnancy status prior to initiating drug.

Potential Toxicities/Side Effects and the Nursing Process

I.   ALTERATION IN SEXUALITY/REPRODUCTION related to POTENTIAL TERATOGENICITY

Defining Characteristics: Drug is teratogenic and fetotoxic, causing embryo-fetal death and severe birth defects. Drug may be excreted in semen. Amenorrhea has been observed in premenopausal women; it is unknown if it is reversible.

Nursing Implications: Assess reproductive status, sexual activity, and birth control measures used for both men and women. Instruct male patients to use condoms with spermicide, even after a vasectomy, during sexual intercourse with female partners while receiving therapy and for 2 months after the last dose when drug has been stopped. Ensure that women have had a negative pregnancy test within 7 days of starting the drug. Teach women to use highly effective contraception measures that have < 1% risk of failure prior to starting therapy, and to continue using it for 7 months after the last dose of vismodegib has been taken. Teach female patients to tell their providers immediately if pregnant (during therapy or for 7 months post-therapy) or if a male patient's female partner becomes pregnant while the patient is taking vismodegib. Exposure to the drug during pregnancy should be reported to Genentech Adverse Event Line (1-888-835-2555). Encourage the patient to participate in the Erivedge pregnancy pharmacovigilance program. Nursing mothers should either discontinue the drug or discontinue nursing.

II. POTENTIAL ALTERATION IN NUTRITION related to NAUSEA, DIARRHEA, CONSTIPATION, VOMITING, DECREASED APPETITE, WEIGHT LOSS, DYSGEUSIA, AGEUSIA

Defining Characteristics: Nausea (incidence 30%), diarrhea (29%), constipation (21%), vomiting (14%), weight loss (45%), decreased appetite (25%), dysgeusia (changes in taste sensation) (55%), and ageusia (inability to taste sweet, sour, bitter, salty) (11%) can occur.

Nursing Implications: Assess nutritional status and bowel elimination pattern baseline and at each visit. Teach patient self-care measures: to take OTC antidiarrheal or constipation medication as needed, to take antinausea medicine as prescribed; to modify diet (e.g., increase fiber and fluids if constipated, foods to slow diarrhea and fluids to reverse dehydration; high-calorie, high-protein foods in small amounts if decreased taste, appetite, and weight loss); and if taste disturbances, use taste stimulants such as Crazy Jane salt and pepper. Teach patient to report any symptoms that do not resolve or improve with the established plan. To increase appetite, encourage patients to use a small plate, take small portions, and not to fill the plate; take antiemetic 30 minutes prior to eating; and to eat small, frequent meals. Arrange dietary consultation if available and needed. Monitor weight at each visit to note trends.

III. ACTIVITY INTOLERANCE, POTENTIAL, related to FATIGUE, ASTHENIA, HEADACHE

Defining Characteristics: Fatigue occurs commonly in patients with advanced cancer who were studied. Fatigue occurred in 40% of patients.

Nursing Implications: Assess baseline activity and energy level, and teach patient that this symptom may occur. Assess patient's activity patterns, and suggest ways to conserve energy.

IV.   ALTERATION IN BODY IMAGE, POTENTIAL, related to ALOPECIA, SKIN CHANGES

Defining Characteristics: Alopecia occurs in 64% of patients receiving vismodegib.

Nursing Implications: Assess baseline skin integrity, and teach patient that alopecia may occur. Encourage patient to obtain a wig (cranial prosthesis) prior to starting therapy. Assess effect of hair loss on patient's body image, as well as skin changes. Encourage patient to verbalize feelings and provide emotional support. If needed, involve social worker in supportive counseling. Encourage patient to use scarves and hats as appropriate and to attend supportive educational sessions such as ACS Look Good . . . Feel Better programs if available.

V.   ALTERATION IN COMFORT related to MUSCLE SPASMS, ARTHRALGIAS

Defining Characteristics: Muscle spasms occurred in 72% of patients, and arthralgias, in 16%.

Nursing Implications: Teach patient that these side effects may occur and to report them. Teach patient to use local measures to reduce discomfort, such as use of heat or cold, acetaminophen. Teach patient to report symptoms that do not respond to self-care strategies, and discuss with provider muscle relaxants and other measures.

Drug: vorinostat (Zolinza, suberoylanilide hydroxamic acid, SAHA)

Class: Histone deacetylase (HDAC) inhibitor.

Mechanism of Action: Histones are proteins that give structure and support to the DNA helix and DNA coils around the histones. Some tumors have excess HDAC, which causes the DNA to stay tightly packed. The DNA cannot be transcribed, and genes are not expressed and thus are silenced, like important tumor-suppressor genes. Vorinostat inhibits the enzymatic activity of histone deacetylases HDAC1, HDAC2, and HDAC3 (class I) and HDAC6 (class II). This results in increased histone acetylation and uncoiling of DNA so that the DNA is open; genes are expressed and can be transcribed for protein synthesis. These proteins are critical in normal cell-cycle regulation. The drug induces cell-cycle arrest and apoptosis in some transformed cells; the mechanism of action of antineoplastic effect has not been fully characterized.

Metabolism: After oral ingestion, the drug becomes 71% protein-bound. It is metabolized via glucuronidation and hydrolysis followed by β-oxidation, resulting in two inactive metabolites. Drug is eliminated primarily through metabolism, with < 1% of drug recoverable in the urine.

Indication: Indicated for the treatment of cutaneous manifestations of cutaneous T-cell lymphoma (CTCL) in patients who have progressive, persistent, or recurrent disease on or after two systemic therapies.

Dosage/Range:
- 400 mg orally once daily with food until disease progression or unacceptable toxicity.
- If intolerant to therapy, reduce dose to 300 mg orally once daily with food. If necessary, reduce the dose further to 300 mg once daily with food for 5 consecutive days and repeated weekly.
- Reduce dose in patients with mild or moderate hepatic impairment (BR 1-3 × ULN or AST > ULN): 300 mg once daily with food. There are no recommendations for patients with severe hepatic dysfunction (BR > 3 × ULN).
- Dose-reduce for thrombocytopenia, anemia.

Drug Preparation/Administration:
- Available in 100-mg gelatin capsules.
- Take with food; do not crush or open capsules.
- Monitor CBC, chemistry tests (electrolytes, glucose, serum creatinine, magnesium) every 2 weeks during first 2 months and then monthly thereafter; EKG with QTc measurement baseline and periodically during treatment.

Drug Interactions:
- Other HDACs (e.g., valproic acid): severe thrombocytopenia, GI bleeding; use together cautiously and monitor platelet count every 2 weeks during first 2 months.
- Coumarin-derivative antigoagulants: prolonged PT and INR. Monitor INR closely and dose accordingly.

Lab Effects/Interference:
- Decreased platelet and red blood cell count.
- Increased serum creatinine (46% of patients) and protein in urine (57% of patients).
- Hyperglycemia, hypokalemia, hyponatremia.
- QT/QTc prolongation, rarely.

Special Considerations:
Warnings:
- Pulmonary embolism (PE) occurred in 5% of patients, and deep vein thrombosis (DVT) has been reported: Monitor for signs and symptoms, especially patients with a history of thromboembolic events, and teach patient to report SOB, chest pain, other symptoms right away or call 911.
- Dose-related thrombocytopenia and anemia; May require dose modification or drug discontinuance. Monitor CBC/differential, platelet count every 2 weeks for the first 2 months, then monthly.
- Nausea, vomiting, diarrhea: patients may require antiemetics, antidiarrheals, and fluid and electrolyte replacement to prevent dehydration. Preexisting nausea, vomiting, and diarrhea should be well controlled before starting vorinostat therapy.
- Hyperglycemia: Monitor blood glucose every 2 weeks during the first 2 months, and then monthly; monitor diabetic patients closely.
- Clinical chemistry abnormalities: Measure and correct abnormal electrolytes, creatinine, magnesium, and calcium baseline. Correct hypokalemia and hypomagnesemia before

beginning vorinostat therapy. Monitor clinical chemistries as above every 2 weeks for the first 2 months, then at least monthly.
- Severe thrombocytopenia and GI bleeding has been reported when HDAC inhibitors are combined (e.g., vorinostat and valproic acid). Monitor platelet counts more frequently.
- Fetal harm can occur if administered to a pregnant woman, as drug crosses the placenta and drug is found in fetal animal plasma levels up to 50% of maternal concentrations.
  - Counsel women of reproductive potential to use effective contraception to avoid pregnancy. If drug is used during pregnancy or the patient becomes pregnant while taking the drug, the patient should be apprised of the potential hazard to the fetus.
  - Nursing mothers should decide whether to discontinue nursing or to discontinue vorinostat, taking into consideration the importance of the drug to the mother's health.
- Use in patients with hepatic impairment. Vorinostat AUC increases 50–66% in patients with hepatic impairment, and the incidence of grade 3–4 thrombocytopenia was increased in patients with mild or moderate hepatic impairment. Reduce dose in these patients.
- Most common side effects (≥ 20%):
  - GI: diarrhea, nausea.
  - Constitutional: fatigue.
  - Hematologic: thrombocytopenia.
  - Nutritional disorders: dysgeusia, anorexia.

Potential Toxicities/Side Effects and the Nursing Process

I.   POTENTIAL FOR BLEEDING AND FATIGUE related to THROMBOCYTOPENIA AND ANEMIA

Defining Characteristics: Thrombocytopenia occurs in 25.6% (5.8% grade 3–4) of patients and anemia in 14% (grade 3–4, 2.3%).

Nursing Implications: Monitor CBC, platelet count baseline and periodically during therapy. Assess for signs and symptoms of bleeding, fatigue, and anemia. Teach patient to self-assess for signs and symptoms of bleeding and anemia and to call if they occur. Assess patient medication profile and any over-the-counter medications, such as those containing aspirin or NSAIDs that would increase the risk of bleeding. Instruct patient to avoid these drugs and not to begin any over-the-counter medications without first discussing with nurse or physician. Teach patient to alternate rest and activity periods if feeling fatigued and to organize shopping and chores in a way to minimize energy expenditures.

II.   ALTERATION IN NUTRITION, LESS THAN BODY REQUIREMENTS, related to NAUSEA, DIARRHEA, ANOREXIA, DEHYDRATION, VOMITING, DYSGEUSIA, HYPERGLYCEMIA

Defining Characteristics: In clinical trials, these side effects occurred with the following frequency: diarrhea (52%), nausea (41%), dysgeusia (28%), anorexia (24%), dry mouth (16%), vomiting (15%), constipation (15%), and anorexia (14%).

Nursing Implications: Assess weight, bowel elimination status, baseline nutritional status, and glucose level, and monitor during therapy. Teach patient that symptoms can occur and ways to minimize this effect, such as self-administration of antinausea and antidiarrheal medications and to report symptoms that do not resolve with established plan. Teach patient to identify nutritionally dense (high calories and protein in the smallest amount) foods and to keep them handy in the refrigerator. Teach patient to eat small, frequent meals and to have a bedtime snack. Teach patient that goal is to take in at least 2 quarts of fluid a day and to try to drink a glass of fluid every hour while awake. Monitor those patients at risk for dehydration closely, such as the elderly. Teach patient signs and symptoms of hyperglycemia (excessive thirst, frequent urination) and to report these. Discuss any abnormalities with a physician.

III. POTENTIAL ALTERATION IN CIRCULATION related to PULMONARY EMBOLISM, QTc PROLONGATION, PERIPHERAL EDEMA

Defining Characteristics: Pulmonary embolism occurred in 4.7% of patients, prolongation of the QTc interval occurred but has not been studied definitively, and peripheral edema occurred in 12% of patients.

Nursing Implications: Do baseline assessment of cardiac status, including the presence of peripheral edema, and ensure that baseline EKG with QTc interval has been done and that it is done periodically during treatment. Identify patients at risk for developing QTc prolongation, such as patients on antiarrhythmic agents and patients with hypomagnesemia or hypokalemia. Check electrolytes and magnesium every 2 weeks during first 2 months of therapy and then monthly after that. Replete magnesium and potassium as ordered, or teach patient about self-administration of medications. Teach patient to report new pain in the back of the leg, a red streak up the leg, or difficulty breathing right away and to come to the emergency department for evaluation.

Drug: ziv-aflibercept (Zaltrap)

Class: Angiogenesis inhibitor: VEGF trap, recombinant fusion protein.

Mechanism of Action: Drug is a soluble decoy receptor that binds to VEGF-A, VEGF-B, and placental growth factor (PIGF) so that the VEGF growth factors cannot bind to their receptors on the endothelial cells. It is made up of portions of the external receptors [extracellular domains of Vascular Endothelial Growth Factor (VEGF) Receptor 1 and 2] for the VEGF ligands, that are fused to the Fc (constant region) of a human IgG1 antibody. The fusion protein attracts VEGFs (VEGF-A, B, PIGF) more strongly than do the tumor VEGF receptors so that VEGF binds to the trap and not to the tumor VEGF receptors. This theoretically inhibits tumor angiogenesis and causes the tumor to regress (shrink). VEGFs have an 800 times stronger affinity to aflibercept than to bevacizumab.

Metabolism: Terminal elimination half-life is 4–7 days. Steady state is reached by the second dose. Patients weighing ≥ 100 kg had a 29% increase in systemic exposure compared to patients weighing 50–100 kg. There are no changes in pharmacokinetics in patients with mild or moderate hepatic dysfunction, or mild, moderate, or severe renal impairment. The drug was not studied in patients with severe liver impairment.

Indication: Drug is indicated for the treatment of patients with metastatic colorectal cancer (mCRC) that is resistant to or has progressed following an oxaliplatin-containing regimen, in combination with 5-fluorouracil, leucovorin, irinotecan (FOLFIRI).

Dosage/Range: 4 mg/kg IV infusion every 2 weeks in combination with 5-fluorouracil, leucovorin, irinotecan (FOLFIRI).

Dose Modifications:
* Temporarily suspend drug for (1) at least 4 weeks before elective surgery; (2) recurrent or severe hypertension until controlled; upon resumption of drug, permanently dose- reduce to 2 mg/kg; (3) proteinuria ≥ 2 g/24 hr and resume drug when urine protein < 2 g/24 hr at a permanently reduced dose of 2 mg/kg. For recurrent proteinuria, suspend drug until proteinuria is < 2 g/24 hr, and then permanently reduce aflibercept dose to 2 mg/kg.
* Discontinue drug for (1) severe hemorrhage, (2) GI perforation, (3) compromised wound healing, (4) fistula formation, (5) hypertensive crisis or hypertensive encephalopathy, (6) arterial thrombotic events, (7) nephrotic syndrome or thrombotic microangiopathy (TMA), (8) reversible posterior leukoencephalopathy syndrome (RPLS).

Drug Preparation/Administration:
* Available in single-use vials: 100 mg/4 mL (25 mg/mL), and as 200 mg/8 mL (25 mg/mL). Inspect vial before use: drug is clear, colorless to pale yellow solution. Do not reenter the vial after initial puncture. Withdraw ordered dose and dilute in 0.9% sodium chloride or 5% dextrose solution for injection USP to achieve a final concentration of 0.6–8 mg/mL. Use polyvinyl chloride (PVC) infusion bags containing bis-(2-ethylhexyl) phthalate (DEHP) or polyolefin infusion bags. Store undiluted drug at 2–8° C (36–46° F) for up to 4 hours. Discard any unused portion left in the infusion bag.
* Assess CBC/differential baseline and before each cycle. Ensure that ANC ≥ 1.5 × 10^9/L. Assess urine dipstick/urinalysis for protein.
* Administer as an IV infusion over 1 hour, through a 0.2 micron polyethersulfone filter (do not use polyvinylidene fluoride (PVDF) or nylon filters), every 2 weeks. Do not administer IV push or bolus. Administer prior to any component of FOLFIRI regimen on the day of treatment. Do not combine aflibercept with other drugs in the same infusion bag or IV line. Administer using an infusion set made of (1) PVC containing DEHP, (2) DEHP-free PVC containing trioctyl-trimellitate (TOTM), (3) polypropylene, (4) polyethylene-lined PVC, or (5) polyurethane.

Drug Interactions:
* None known, but specific studies not done.

Lab Effects/Interference:
* Proteinuria (62% of patients in the VELOUR study).
* Leukopenia, thrombocytopenia, neutropenia.

- Increased serum creatinine.
- Increased AST, ALT.

Special Considerations:

- Drug has angiogenesis inhibitor class (side) effects: hypertension, proteinuria (although the incidence is higher with aflibercept compared to bevacizumab), GI , hemorrhage, and compromised wound healing.
- Hemorrhage can be severe and sometimes fatal. Incidence (all grades) was 38% (3% grade 3–4) in patients receiving aflibercept/FOLFIRI vs 19% (1% grade 3–4) receiving FOLFIRI alone. Monitor patients for signs/symptoms of GI bleeding and other severe bleeding. Do not administer drug to patients with severe hemorrhage, and discontinue the drug if it occurs.
- GI perforation: discontinue drug in patients who develop GI perforation. In clinical studies, incidence was 0.8% compared to 0.2% in the placebo/FOLFIRI arm. Monitor patients for signs/symptoms of GI perforation.
- Compromised wound healing: suspend drug at least 4 weeks prior to elective surgery, and do not resume for at least 4 weeks following major surgery and until the surgical wound is fully healed. Grade 3 impaired wound healing occurred in 0.3% of patients compared to 0 in the placebo/FOLFIRI arm. Minor surgery such as port placement, biopsy, or tooth extraction; drug may be resumed after the surgical wound has fully healed.
- Fistula formation: discontinue drug if fistula develops. Incidence is rare: 1.5% in study arm, compared to 0.5% in placebo/FOLFIRI arm. In patients with mCRC, fistulas were enterovesical, anal, entercutaneous, colovaginal, and intestinal sites.
- Hypertension: monitor BP and treat hypertension. Monitor BP every 2 weeks or more frequently as clincally indicated during therapy. Treat with appropriate antihypertensive agent(s) and continue monitoring BP regularly. Temporarily suspend drug if hypertension is uncontrolled. Discontinue drug if hypertensive crisis or hypertensive encephalopathy develops.
- Arterial thrombotic events (ATE): e.g., TIAs, CVA, angina pectoris, may develop. ATEs were reported in 2.6% of patients treated with aflibercept /FOLFIRI vs 1.7% in patients receiving placebo/FOLFIRI. Discontinue drug if an ATE event occurs.
- Proteinuria, nephrotic syndrome, and thrombotic microangiopathy (TMA) occurred more frequently in patients receiving aflibercept. Proteinuria was reported in 62% of patients receiving aflibercept/FOLFIRI compared to 31% receiving placebo/FOLFIRI. Nephrotic syndrome occurred in 0.5% patients in the aflibercept/FOLFIRI arm. Monitor urine protein by dipstick, and/or urinary protein tinine ratio (UPCR) for the development of, or worsening of proteinuria during aflibercept therapy. If patients have a dipstick of ≥ 2+ for protein, or a UPCR > 1, they should undergo a 24-hr urine collection. Suspend drug if proteinuria ≥ 2 g/24 hr, and resume when proteinuria is < 2 g/24 hr. If recurrent, suspend until proteinuria is < 2 g/24 hr and then permanently reduce the aflibercept dose to 2 mg/kg. Discontinue drug if nephrotic syndrome or thrombotic microangiopathy (TMA) develops.
- Reversible posterior leukoencephalopathy syndrome (RPLS) was reported in 0.5% of patients receiving aflibercept alone or in combination. Confirm diagnosis of RPLS with MRI and discontinue drug if RPLS confirmed. Symptoms usually resolve or improve within days.

- Neutropenia and neutropenic complication (febrile neutropenia) occurred in a higher incidence of patients receiving aflibercept. Grade 3–4 neutropenia occurred in 37% mCRC patients receiving aflibercept/FOLFIRI compared to 30% in patients receiving placebo/FOLFIRI. Grade 3–4 febrile neutropenia occurred in 4% of patients receiving aflibercept/FOLFIRI compared to 2% receiving placebo/FOLFIRI, while grade 3–4 infection/sepsis occurred in 1.5% of patients receiving aflibercept/FOLFIRI compared to 1.2% receiving placebo/FOLFIRI. Monitor CBC/differential baseline and prior to beginning each cycle of aflibercept/FOLFIRI. Delay drug administration until ANC $\geq 1.5 \times 10^9$/L.
- Diarrhea and dehydration may be severe and the incidence of severe diarrhea is increased in patients receiving aflibercept/FOLFIRI (grade 3–4 in 19% vs 8% receiving FOLFIRI alone); ensure that patients are monitored closely, taught to report symptoms, and to remain hydrated. Incidence of diarrhea is increased in patients age 65 or older, compared to those < 65 years old; monitor elderly patients with diarrhea more closely.
- Most common side effects (incidence $\geq$ 20%) were leukopenia, diarrhea, neutropenia, proteinuria, increased AST, stomatitis, fatigue, thrombocytopenia, increased ALT, hypertension, decreased weight, anorexia, epistaxis, abdominal pain, dysphonia, increased serum creatinine, and headache.
- Grade 3–4 drug side effects of aflibercept plus FOLFIRI were diarrhea, asthenia, fatigue, stomatitis, infection, hypertension, GI or abdominal pain, neutropenia or neutropenic complications, and proteinuria.

Potential Toxicities/Side Effects and the Nursing Process

I.   POTENTIAL ALTERATION IN CIRCULATION related to HYPERTENSION, ARTERIAL THROMBOTIC EVENTS (ATE), HEMORRHAGE

Defining Characteristics: Hypertension is a class effect of angiogenesis inhibitors, and it may occur. In general, hypertension was more common (41% of patients) with 20% grade 3 or higher, than with bevacizumab combined with FOLFIRI in the 1st line setting of mCRC (AVIRI study, 28% overall, 10% grade 3 or higher). ATE occurred in 2.6% (grade 3–4, 1.8%) of patients compared to 1.7% (0.7%) in patients receiving placebo plus FOLFIRI. The incidence of bleeding/hemorrhage in study patients was 38% (3% grade 3–4) compared to 19% (1% grade 3–4) in patients receiving placebo/FOLFIRI.

Nursing Implications: Assess baseline BP prior to and during treatment, at least for the first treatment, then prior to each drug infusion. If the patient has a history of hypertension, monitor BP more closely, although hypertension develops over time rather than during the drug infusion. BP monitoring should continue after the patient has stopped the drug. Teach patient potential drug side effects and self-care measures. Discuss prescription of antihypertensive medications as needed. Angiotensin-converting enzyme (ACE) inhibitors or angiotensin II receptor blockers are preferred as they have low interaction potential with angiogenesis inhibitors, help reduce proteinuria, and prevent the expression of plasminogen-activator inhibitor-1 (may be stimulated by angiogenesis inhibitors and increasing risk of thrombosis) [Izzedine et al., 2009; Wang & Lockhart, 2012]. Review patient medical history for history of bleeding, hemorrhage, or ATEs. Assess patient for signs/symptoms of bleeding, or arterial thrombotic events, and teach patient to report/seek emergency care immediately if any bleeding or ATE events occur.

II. POTENTIAL FOR FLUID VOLUME DEFICIT related to DIARRHEA, DEHYDRATION

Defining Characteristics: The incidence of diarrhea and dehydration is increased when aflibercept is added to FOLFIRI. Diarrhea in the combination occurred in 69% of patients (19% grade 3–4) compared to 57% (8% grade 3–4) in patients receiving placebo/FOLFIRI. Dehydration was similarly increased: combination: 9% (4% grade 3–4) versus 3% (1% grade 3–4) in the placebo/FOLFIRI group. Incidence of diarrhea is increased in patients age 65 or older, compared to those < 65 years old.

Nursing Implications: Assess baseline bowel elimination and hydration status. Teach patient that these side effects may occur, and to report uncontrolled diarrhea (persisting > 24 hours despite antidiarrheal medication) or inability to drink 2–3 liters of fluid in 24 hours. Involve caregiver in the discussion, and emphasize need to drink fluids, 8 oz an hour while awake, to maintain hydration status, especially fluids that contain salt or electrolytes. Teach patient to take immodium per irinotecan recommendations (4 mg at first instance of diarrhea, then 2 mg every 2 hours until 12 hours without diarrhea) to prevent uncontrolled diarrhea, and to report severe (persistent, bloody, or with mucus). If the patient is elderly, telephone the patient a day or two following treatment to assess tolerance and status, and to report any difficulties early. Teach patient to self-assess temperature, as (FOLFIRI) nadir may occur while the patient is experiencing diarrhea, leading to sepsis.

III. POTENTIAL FOR INFECTION AND BLEEDING related to NEUTROPENIA, THROMBOCYTOPENIA

Defining Characteristics: Neutropenia and neutropenic complications are more common when aflibercept is added to FOLFIRI than FOLFIRI alone. The incidence of neutropenia was 67% (37% grade 3–4) in the combination group compared to 57% (30% grade 3–4) in the placebo/FOLFIRI group. Febrile neutropenia occurred in 4% of patients receiving the combination, compared to 2% of patients receiving placebo/FOLFIRI. Neutropenic infection/sepsis occurred in 1.5% of patients compared to 1.2% treated with placebo/FOLFIRI. Thrombocytopenia occurred more frequently in the combination arm [48% (3% grade 3–4)] versus 35% (2% grade 3–4) in the placebo/FOLFIRI arm. Epistaxis occurred in 28% patients (0.2% grade 3–4) in the combination arm, compared to 7% in the placebo/FOLFIRI arm.

Nursing Implications: Assess patient baseline and prior to each treatment for risk of infection as well as signs and symptoms of infection and bleeding. Ensure that ANC $\geq 1.5 \times 10^9$/L. Teach patient self-care measures to avoid infection (e.g., avoid crowds, avoid close proximity to people with colds, wash hands frequently, but especially after touching anything that may be unclean), and to self-assess for signs/symptoms of infection (e.g., temperature ≥ 100.4°F, productive cough, pain on urination) and to report these right away. Teach patient and caregiver that diarrhea will increase the risk for infection if the ANC is low, and to contact the nurse or physician immediately with a fever and uncontrolled diarrhea. Teach patient to avoid injury and increased risk for bleeding. Review medication profile and ensure the patient is not taking aspirin or NSAIDs. Teach patient to report signs/symptoms of bleeding right away. Teach patient to apply pressure to the bridge of the nose if epistaxis occurs, and to report a nosebleed that does not resolve in 15–20 minutes.

Today, a number of autoimmune diseases, such as rheumatoid arthritis (RA), are being treated with chemotherapy or biotherapy (here defined by the general term chemotherapy), using drugs that in many cases have traditionally been used to treat cancer. This chapter will focus on treatment of RA. Drug administration and care of the patient receiving the drug often become the responsibility of the oncology infusion nurse, or the generalist nurse on a medical-surgical unit. Although oncology nurses usually have resources to learn about such drugs, generalist nurses lack these resources. It is important to understand the rationale for using these drugs, as well as the drug mechanism of action, potential side effects, and nursing implications to administer the drugs safely, as they are considered hazardous. The Oncology Nursing Society (ONS, 2013) has issued a position statement on the education of the RN who administers and cares for individuals receiving chemotherapy and biotherapy, and this includes the following, which the RN will find in the 2015 ONDH:

- Principles, types, and classifications of chemotherapy and biotherapy.
- Principles of safe preparation, storage, labeling, and disposal of chemotherapeutic and biologic agents.
- Patient preassessment, administration procedures, and post-administration patient care.

Following discussion of why these agents are used to treat RA, this chapter presents nine drugs FDA-indicated for its treatment. Please see *Chapter 1 Introduction* for nursing assessment of the patient prior to chemotherapy administration, and standardized nursing care plan for the management of hypersensitivity reactions/infusion reactions. Please also see *Chapter 1* for a discussion of methotrexate, and *Chapter 4* for a discussion of rituximab and monoclonal antibodies.

Autoimmune diseases represent the third largest major illness group in the United States, and it includes more than 100 distinct diseases (AARDA, 2013). One of the most common autoimmune diseases is RA. While the side effect profile of many of the drugs used to treat autoimmune diseases is similar to those used to treat patients with cancer, the doses are usually lower so the side effects are less frequent or severe. However, certain side effects remain the same: hypersensitivity reactions (HSRs) and secondary infections (Zack, 2012).

The cause of RA is not known, but hormones, environmental factors such as smoking, and heredity may all play a role (RA Fact Sheet, 2008). The disease affects more than a million people and tends to affect women more than men; the peak incidence is between ages 35–50 years (Dewing et al., 2012). The average age of the person with RA is 66.8 years (Helmick et al., 2008). RA is characterized by chronic inflammation of the joint lining with subsequent destruction of the underlying cartilage and bone, orchestrated by a flawed immune system. This leads to disability and increased morbidity.

Normally, the immune system is very powerful in identifying and removing invading microorganisms from the body, and also identifying and removing abnormal or damaged cells like cancer cells. The body is able to identify antigens that are "self" (by recognizing HLA or human leukocyte antigen) and distinguish the antigen from "nonself" (i.e., foreign). Foreign antigens are targeted and neutralized. The immune system does this by directly attacking the invading organism or foreign antigen by macrophages, dendritic cells, and killer T-lymphocytes, and also calling in other immune cells to kill other cells with the same antigen. Once the foreign antigen is located, white blood cells migrate to the area and begin an inflammatory response. Macrophages and dendritic cells can mount fragments of the antigen on the cell surface and become antigen-presenting cells (APCs). They travel to a lymph node to become activated, and then signal more immune cell elements to attack any cell that has this antigen. It also uses inflammatory cytokines such as tumor necrosis factor (TNF-α), a proinflammatory cytokine, and by making an antibody that coats the foreign antigen, attracting more immune cells. Complement proteins work with antibodies to punch holes in the cell membrane of the invading cell with the foreign antigen, killing it. Once the war against the invader is won, the body needs to turn off the immune fight so that normal cells and tissues are not harmed. Because the immune system is so powerful, specialized regulatory T-lymphocytes usually turn off the immune attack once the invading microorganism (e.g., antigen) is neutralized.

However, in RA, the immune system does not recognize antigens on cells lining the joint that belong to self (the body); the immune system makes autoantibodies against the normal cells in the lining of the synovium (joint lining). Once activated, the T-lymphocytes and macrophages invade the synovial lining and cause the proinflammatory cytokine TNF-α and interleukins (IL-1, 2, 6, 8, 10, 17) to be released. This results in inflammation and proliferation of the synovial tissue and cartilage, along with bone destruction. In addition, B-lymphocytes infiltrate the synovium, produce immunoglobulins, and activate synovial fibroblasts that destroy the matrix and tissue of the joint. Unfortunately, the regulatory T-lymphocytes do not shut off the immune response. The inflammation is chronic and leads to a thickened synovium and swollen joints. Over time, the immune elements in the inflamed synovium invade and destroy the underlying joint cartilage and bone, as discussed above. RA usually affects symmetric joints, often the wrist and finger joints, which become warm, edematous, and tender. RA symptoms include morning stiffness, which improves with movement, and it may also include systemic symptoms of anorexia, weakness, low-grade fever, and fatigue (Dewing et al., 2012).

The goal of treatment is medical remission or low disease activity (Singh et al., 2012), using NSAIDs and disease-modifying anti-rheumatic drugs (DMARDs). It has been found that joint damage from RA occurs early, often within the first two years following diagnosis (El-Miedany, 2002). While DMARDs should be started upon diagnosis, they are often delayed. In 2012, the American College of Rheumatology (ACR) guidelines were updated to guide rheumatologists in the management of RA. Recommendations are based on how long the person has had RA, how severe the RA is, and what prior treatments the patient has received. These can be found at http://onlinelibrary.wiley.com/doi/10.1002/acr.21641/pdf for a treatment decision tree and narrative.

NSAIDs, including selective COX-2 inhibitors, help to promote comfort by reducing the production of pro-inflammatory and pain-producing prostaglandins, and salicylates, which are used together with DMARDs (Dewing et al., 2012). In order to reduce the occurrence of adverse effects, medications to protect the stomach should be taken along with, or combined with the NSAID (e.g., proton pump inhibitor, or combination ibuprofen+famotidine, or naproxen+lansoprazole). Low-dose oral glucocorticoids, low-dose delayed-release prednisone, or glucocorticoid injections are sometimes used short-term to help control pain until a DMARD is effective (Dewing et al., 2012).

DMARDs are categorized as non-biologic or biologic. Non-biologic therapies are used first and include hydroxychloroquine, leflunomide, methotrexate, minocycline, and sulfasalazine. Methotrexate is a well-known chemotherapeutic agent that is a folic acid antagonist and is used first line (Wilkie, 2010). Patients receiving methotrexate should have their LFTs assessed baseline, at 1 month, and then every 8–12 weeks to identify any potential liver toxicity. Folic acid 1–2 mg daily should be prescribed with methotrexate to minimize the occurrence of side effects (e.g., stomatitis, nausea, hepatic toxicity, alopecia (Wilkie, 2010).

Biologic DMARDs target either receptors on the B-lymphocytes that help orchestrate inflammation, or pro-inflammatory cytokines that cause inflammation and joint damage. They are classified as non-TNF or anti-TNF. TNF-α is a pro-inflammatory cytokine. Non-TNF biologics are abatacept (Orencia, a fully human monoclonal antibody that binds to CD80/86 on the lymphocyte, blocking activation of T-lymphocytes), rituximab (Rituxan, a monoclonal antibody that depletes circulating B lymphocytes with CD20 on their cell surface), and tocilizumab (Actemra, which binds to IL-6 receptors, blocking pro-inflammatory changes). Anti-TNF biologics are used second line, and include adalimumab (Humira), certolizumab pegol (Cimzia), etanercept (Enbrel), golimumab (Simponi), and infliximab (Remicade). When used, infliximab should be combined with methotrexate to prevent neutralizing antibodies to infliximab (Wilkie, 2010). The anti-TNF agents are significantly immunosuppressive. All patients should be screened for TB before starting anti-TNF therapy. TNF is critical for the formation of granulomas, so when blocking TNF, TB may complicate therapy (Wilkie, 2010). Because of the immunosuppressive action of anti-TNF agents, infections can progress quickly and become severe; patients need to be taught self-assessment of signs/symptoms of infection and to report them right away. The drug should be interrupted as the patient receives anti-infective therapy. Anti-TNF agents may also increase the risk of CHF, malignancy, and very rarely, demyelinating disease (e.g., multiple sclerosis).

The severity of the patient's RA, symptom duration, risks vs. benefits, and co-morbidities help the rheumatologist determine which agents should be used. As a better understanding of the specific immune elements involved in RA emerges, new biological agents will emerge. Tofacitinib (Xeljanz), a Janus kinase inhibitor, is an oral agent recently FDA-approved. It blocks transmission of the message to the white blood cells to turn on inflammation (blocking signaling proteins, which transmit the message). Another agent being studied that targets signaling pathways is fostamatinib (Oskira), which inhibits Syk (spleen tyrosine kinase, located on the cell surface of many immune cells).

Other recommendations for patient care are to encourage patients to do regular aerobic exercise and strengthening exercises to improve and maintain function.

References

Actemra package insert. Genentech Inc., South San Francisco, CA. October 2013. Available at http://www.gene.com/download/pdf/actemra.prescribing.pdf, accessed 4.30.13.

AARDA (American Autoimmune-Related Diseases Association, 2013). Available at https://www.aarda.org/mission_statement.php, accessed 4.28.13.

Arthritis Foundation. (2008). Rheumatoid Arthritis Fact Sheet. Available from http://www.arthritis.org/files/images/advocacy/ambassador-kit/RAFactSheet.pdf, accessed 4.27.13.

Cimzia package insert. UCB Inc., Smyrna GA, Oct 2013. Available at http://cimzia.com.pdf/Prescribing_Information.pdf, accessed 6.10.14.

Dewing KA, Setter SM, Slusher BA. (2012). Osteoarthritis and rheumatoid arthritis 2–12: Pathophysiology, diagnosis, and treatment. Available at http://www.clinicaladvisor.com/osteoarthritis-and-rheumatoid-arthritis-2012-pathophysiology-diagnosis-and-treatment/article/265549/2/, accessed 4.28.13.

El-Meidany Y. (2002). The evolving therapy of rheumatic diseases, the future is now. *Curr Drug Targets Immune Endocr Metabol Disord.* 2(1): 1–11.

Enbrel package insert. Amgen., Thousand Oaks, CA, November 2013, available at http://pi.amgen.com/united_states/enbrel/derm/enbrel_pi.pdf, accessed 9.3.14.

Helmick C, Felson D, Lawrence R, Gabriel S, et al. (2008). Estimates of the prevalence of arthritis and other rheumatic conditions in the United States. *Arthritis & Rheumatism* 58(1), 15–25.

Oncology Nursing Society. (2012). Oncology Nursing Society Position on Education of the RN Who Administers and Cares for the Individual Receiving Chemotherapy and Biotherapy. Available at http://www.ons.org/Publications/Positions/RNed/, accessed 4.25.13.

Orencia package insert. Bristol Myers Squibb, Princeton, NJ, Dec. 2013, available at http://packageinserts.bms.com/pi/pi_orencia.pdf, accessed 6.10.14.

Remicade package insert. Janssen Biotech Inc., Horsham, PA, November 2013, available at http://www.remicade.com/shared/product/remicade/prescribing-information.pdf. accessed 9.3.14.

Simponi package insert. Janssen Biotech Inc., Horsham, PA, January 2014, available at http://www.simponi.com/hcp/interactive-prescribing-information, accessed 9.3.14.

Singh JA, Furst DE, Bharat A, et al. (2012). Update of the 2008 American College of Rheumatology recommendations for the use of disease-modifying antirheumatic drugs and biologic agents in the treatment of rheumatoid arthritis. *Arthritis Care & Research* 64(5): 625–639.

Wilkie WS. (2012). Rheumatoid Arthritis. *Cleveland Clinic Center for Medical Education.* Available at http://www.clevelandclinicmeded.com/medicalpubs/diseasemanagement/rheumatology/rheumatoid–arthritis; accessed 4.24.13.

Xeljanz prescribing information. Pfizer Inc., New York, NY, May 2014. Available at http://labeling.pfizer.com/ShowLabeling.aspx?id=959, accessed 9.3.14.

Zack E. (2012). Chemotherapy and biotherapeutic agents for autoimmune diseases. *Clin J Oncol Nurs* 16(4): E125–E132.

Drug: abatacept (Orencia)

Class: Selective T-cell costimulation modulator.

Mechanism of Action: Abatacept is a soluble fusion protein made up of the extracellular domain of the human cytotoxic T-lymphocyte associated antigen4 (CTLA-4) linked to a modified Fc (constant antibody domain) of the immunoglobulin IgG1. The drug is made using recombinant DNA technology. The drug inhibits T-lymphocyte activation by binding to CD80 and CD86, which blocks interaction with CD28. Blocking this interaction stops the full T-lymphocyte activation, which otherwise causes inflammation and damage to the joint synovium in RA. In addition, the drug decreases T-lymphocyte proliferation, and inhibits the production of TNF-α, interferon gamma and interleukin-2, all pro-inflammatory cytokines. This results in suppressed inflammation and decreased antibody production.

Metabolism: Bioavailability following subcutaneous administration is 78.6%. Pharmacokinetics of IV and subcutaneous administration are similar. Terminal half-life is 13–16 days.

Indication: (1) Adult RA that is moderately to severely active, as monotherapy or concomitantly with DMARDs other than TNF antagonists; (2) juvenile idiopathic arthritis that is moderately to severely active polyarticular juvenile idiopathic arthritis in children 6 years and older, as monotherapy or concomitantly with methotrexate. Drug should NOT be given concomitantly with TNF antagonists.

Dosage/Range:
- Drug can be administered IV or SQ.
- IV for adult RA:
  - weight < 60 kg: 500 mg (2 vials)
  - weight 60–100 kg: 750 mg (3 vials)
  - weight > 100 kg: 1,000 mg (4 vials)
- Subcutaneous for adult RA: Give 125 mg subcutaneously once weekly and may be initiated with or without an IV loading dose.
  - If a loading dose is given, abatacept should be initiated with a single IV loading dose (as above), followed within a day by the first 125-mg subcutaneous injection.
  - Patients transitioning from abatacept IV therapy to subcutaneous administration should administer the first subcutaneous dose instead of the next scheduled IV dose.
- Juvenile ideopathic arthritis:
  - Children weighing < 75 kg should receive 10 mg/kg IV based on weight.
  - Patients weighing ≥ 75 kg should receive drug following adult IV dosing regimen not to exceed a maximum dose of 1,000 mg. Give at 2 and 4 weeks after first infusion, then every 4 weeks.

Drug Preparation:
- Drug is available in a 250-mg lyophilized powder in single-use vials for IV infusion, or 125-mg/mL solution in a single-dose prefilled syringe.
- Aseptically add 10 mL of Sterile Water for Injection USP using only the silicone-free disposable syringe provided with each vial, and an 18- to 21-gauge needle. Silicone syringes may cause development of translucent particles and cannot be used. Direct the stream to the glass wall of the vial. Rotate with gentle swirling motion until completely dissolved. Do not shake or agitate. Vent with a needle to dissipate any foam that may be present. The reconstituted solution contains 25 mg/mL.
- Inspect prepared solution for opacity, discoloration, or particulate matter; do not use if found.

- Further dilute reconstituted drug to 100 mL. From a 100-mL infusion bag or bottle, withdraw a volume of 0.9% Sodium Chloride USP equal to the volume of the reconstituted drug solution required for the dose. Slowly add the reconstituted solution to the infusion bag, using the same silicone-free disposable syringe provided with the vial. Do not shake the bag or bottle. The final concentration depends on the amount of added drug but will not be more than 10 mg/mL.
- Administer using a filter.
- Inspect again for color and presence of particulate matter.

Drug Administration:
- Ensure patient has had a latent TB test, and if positive, patient has begun anti-TB therapy before starting abatacept; patients should also be screened for hepatitis B.
- Juvenile idiopathic arthritis patients should have all necessary immunizations prior to starting abatacept, as drug may blunt effectiveness of immunizations.
- Adult patients: abatacept may be administered either by IV or SQ route.
- *Intravenous Infusion:*
  - Administer as a 30-min IV infusion via a sterile, nonpyrogenic low-protein binding filter (pore size 0.2 μm–1.2 μm). Use a separate IV line and do not mix with other agents.
  - Drug infusion must be completed within 24 hours of reconstitution of abatacept vials. If needed, store the fully diluted solution at room temperature or refrigerated at 2–8°C (36°–46°F).
  - Following initial dose, give at 2 and 4 weeks, then every 4 weeks.
- *Subcutaneous Injection:*
  - 125-mg syringe is not intended for IV infusion. Patient may have an initial IV loading dose, with the first SQ dose within a day of the IV loading dose.
  - Patient may be taught self-administration if appropriate.
  - Syringe contents should be visually inspected for color or particulate matter and not used if present. Color should be clear, colorless to pale yellow.
  - Teach patient to inject the entire 1 mL (125 mg) and to rotate sites, avoiding sites if the skin is tender, bruised, red, or hard.

Drug Interaction:
- TNF antagonists: do not coadminister, as there is an INCREASED RISK OF SERIOUS INFECTION.
- Other biologic DMARDs: do not give concurrently.
- Live vaccines: do not give concurrently or for 3 months after last dose.

Lab Effects/Interference:
- Falsely elevated blood glucose readings on the day of infusion.

Special Considerations:
- Drug can cause serious infections, which may be more frequent in patients with a history of recurrent infections or underlying conditions (e.g., COPD) predisposing them to infection. Stop drug if serious infection develops. Concomitant immunosuppressive drugs increase the risk of serious infection.

- Very rarely, patients may have a hypersensitivity reaction, characterized by hives, facial edema, dyspnea. Emergency equipment and medications should be available where IV infusions are administered. Patients receiving subcutaneous medications should be taught to seek emergency care if this occurs.
- Do not give live vaccines during therapy or for 3 months after therapy ends.
- Drug may blunt the effectiveness of some immunizations.
- Most common side effects are headache, URI, nasopharyngitis, and nausea.
- Pregnancy category C: Women of childbearing potential should be counseled that the drug should be used during pregnancy only if the potential benefit to the mother outweighs the risk.
- Nursing mothers should make a decision to discontinue nursing or discontinue the drug, taking into consideration the importance of the drug to the mother's health.

Potential Toxicities/Side Effects and the Nursing Process

I.   POTENTIAL FOR INFECTION related to IMMUNOSUPPRESSION

Defining Characteristics: Patients receiving abatacept are at increased risk for developing infections. Nasopharyngitis occurred in 12% of patients during clinical trials, and UTIs in 6% of patients.

Nursing Implications: Assess results of patient's latent TB test and HBV testing and discuss any abnormalities with physician/NP/PA. If TB is positive, patient should begin anti TB therapy before beginning abatacept therapy. Assess baseline patient risk for infection (e.g., comorbidities, preexisting infections, any concomitant immunosuppressive drugs). Patient should not receive this drug together with any other biologic DMARD, including anti-TNF agents. Teach patient to self-assess for signs/symptoms of infection (e.g., T > 100.4°F, cough, chest pain, sputum production, dysuria), and to report them right away. Closely monitor patient for signs/symptoms of infection during and after treatment with abatacept, including TB reactivation, even if latent TB test is negative, and teach patient to report any changes (e.g., fever, sweats, chills, cough, SOB, blood in sputum, weight loss). Drug should be discontinued if patient develops a serious infection or sepsis, and appropriate antimicrobial therapy should be instituted right away.

II.   KNOWLEDGE DEFICIT related to SUBCUTANEOUS INJECTION TECHNIQUE

Defining Characteristics: Selected patients may choose to self-inject their abatacept doses.

Nursing Implications: Assess patient or caregiver readiness to learn, and assess learning style and limitations. Review with patient drug administration schedule, and to not administer, and notify physician/nurse if patient develops an infection. Provide Medication Guide and Instructions for Use available from Bristol Myers Squibb, the drug manufacturer. Teach patient how to care for drug (prefilled syringes should be stored in refrigerator at 2–8°C (36–46°F) in the original container until used, and protected from light. Patient should inspect syringe for cloudiness or particles and not use it if these are found. Patient should be careful and protect glass syringe, as it may break. Drug should be kept out of reach of children and pets. Teach patient hand-washing, aseptic technique, subcutaneous injection technique, and how to dispose of syringe/needle. Teach patient to rotate sites and to apply local measures if injection-site reactions occur. Validate patient understanding by having patient describe measures taught, and ideally, by repeating the demonstration of subcutaneous injection technique. Teach patient to develop documentation tool to record site rotation and any site irritation or reaction.

Drug: adalimumab (Humira)

Class: TNF inhibitor, human monoclonal antibody.

Mechanism of Action: Adalimumab binds to TNF-α and blocks its ability to bind to TNF cell surface receptors (p55, p75), thus decreasing the pro-inflammatory and immune action of TNF-α. The drug also lyses surface TNF expressing cells when complement is present, further decreasing TNF effect. This decreases levels of acute phase reactants of inflammation (C-reactive protein) and the proinflammatory cytokine IL-6. Drug decreases leukocyte migration immune response. Elevated TNF levels are found in synovial joint fluid of patients with RA, JIA, PsA, and AS, and they contribute to inflammation and joint destruction.

Metabolism: Following subcutaneous injection, the absolute bioavailability of adalimumab is 64%. Maximum serum concentration is reached in 131 ± 56 hours, and the mean terminal half-life of the drug is approximately 2 weeks (10- to 20-day range). Adalimumab concentrations in the synovial fluid ranged from 31–96%. Methotrexate reduces adalimumab clearance by 29% after single dosing, and 44% after multiple doses.

Indications:
- Rheumatoid Arthritis (RA): to reduce signs and symptoms, induce major clinical response, inhibit progression of structural damage, and improve physical functioning in adults with moderately to severely active RA.
- Juvenile Idiopathic Arthritis (JIA): to reduce signs and symptoms of moderately to severely active polyarticular JIA in children 4 years and older.
- Psoriatic Arthritis (PsA): to reduce signs and symptoms, inhibit progression of structural damage, and improve physical functioning in adults with active PsA.
- Ankylosing Spondylitis (AS): to reduce signs/symptoms in adult patients with active AS.
- Crohn's Disease: to reduce signs/symptoms and induce and maintain clinical remission in adults with moderately to severely active Crohn's disease who have had an inadequate response to conventional therapy, who have lost the response, or who are intolerant to infliximab.
- Ulcerative Colitis (UC): to induce and sustain clinical remission in adults with moderately to severely active UC who have had an inadequate response to immunosuppressants (e.g., corticosteroids, azathioprine, or 6-MP).
- Plaque Psoriasis (Ps): to treat adults with moderate to severe chronic Ps who are candidates for systemic therapy or phototherapy, and when other systemic therapies are medically less appropriate.

Dosage/Range:

- RA, Psoriatic Arthritis (PsA), Ankylosing Spondylitis (AS): 40 mg every other week; some RA patients not receiving methotrexate may benefit from increasing the frequency to 40 mg weekly.
- Juvenile Idiopathic Arthritis (JIA): 15 kg (33 lbs) to < 30 kg (66 lbs): 20 mg every other week; weight ≥ 30 kg (66 lbs): 40 mg every other week.
- Crohn's Disease and Ulcerative Colitis (UC): initial dose day 1: 160 mg (four 40-mg injections in one day or two 40-mg injections per day on two consecutive days); second dose two weeks later (day 15): 80 mg; third dose two weeks later (day 29): begin maintenance dose of 40 mg every other week. Patients with UC only: continue adalimumab only in patients who have shown evidence of clinical remission by 8 weeks (day 57) of therapy.
- Plaque Psoriasis (Ps): 80-mg initial dose, followed by 40 mg every other week, starting one week after initial dose.

Drug Preparation:

- None; drug is available in pre-filled syringes (40 mg/0.8 mL or 20 mg/0.4 mL or pen); also available in single-use glass vial for institutional use.

Drug Administration:

- For subcutaneous injection, rotate sites.
- Do not start drug during an active infection.
- Anaphylaxis or serious allergy can rarely occur.

Drug Interactions:

- Abatacept (Orencia) or anakinra (Kineret) in combination with adalimumab: increased risk of serious infection; do not give concomitantly.
- Live vaccines: do not administer while patient is receiving adalimumab.
- CYP450 enzyme formation may be suppressed by increased levels of cytokines, and once inflammation is suppressed, may change the enzyme formation. Monitor patients taking CYP450 substrate drug with a narrow therapeutic window (e.g., warfarin) closely, or monitor drug concentrations (e.g., cyclosporine or theophylline) closely and adjust dose as needed.

Lab Effects/Interference:

- Rare cytopenias, pancytopenia.
- Rare increases in cholesterol, lipids, and alkaline phosphatase.
- Rare increases in LFTs.

Special Considerations:

- Adalimumab increases the risk for serious infections requiring hospitalization, including TB, bacterial sepsis, invasive fungal infections (e.g., histoplasmosis), and other opportunistic infections. Most patients who developed serious infections were also taking concomitant immunosuppressants, such as methotrexate or corticosteroids. If an infection develops, monitor patient carefully and stop drug if infection becomes serious. Drug should be discontinued if patient develops a serious infection or sepsis.

- If the patient has chronic or recurrent infections, has been exposed to TB, or has a history of opportunistic infection, carefully consider the risks vs. benefits of using adalimumab.
- If the patient develops a systemic illness, consider empiric antifungal therapy for those who reside in or travel to regions where mycoses are endemic.
- All patients should have test for latent TB; if positive, anti-TB treatment should start before beginning adalimumab. Consider anti-TB therapy in patients with a past history of latent or active TB and in whom an adequate course of treatment cannot be confirmed.
  - Cases of TB reactivation and new onset of TB infection have occurred in patients receiving adalimumab who previously received treatment for latent or active TB (e.g., pulmonary and extrapulmonary (disseminated)).
  - Consider anti-TB therapy prior to starting adalimumab in patients who have had latent or active TB but for whom it cannot be confirmed whether they completed an adequate course of TB therapy.
- All patients should be monitored for TB during treatment, even if their latent TB test was negative.
- Hepatitis B reactivation can occur. Monitor HBV carriers during and for several months after therapy. If reactivation occurs, stop drug and begin antiviral therapy.
- Demyelinating disease can be exacerbated; rarely, there may be new onset.
- Cytopenias and pancytopenias may rarely occur; patient should be evaluated and should consider discontinuing drug.
- Heart failure may worsen, or there may be new onset of CHF with adalimumab.
- Lupus-like syndrome may develop; if so, discontinue adalimumab.
- Lymphoma and other malignancies have been reported in children and adolescents receiving adalimumab.
- Post-marketing reports document cases of hepatosplenic T-cell lymphoma, a rare, aggressive, fatal, T-cell lymphoma in young adults with inflammatory bowel disease.
  - Most patients had Crohn's disease or ulcerative colitis, were adolescent or young adults, and had received prior treatment with immunosuppressants azathioprine or 6-mercaptopurine (6-MP) concomitantly with a TNF-blocker.
  - The combination of adalimumab with either azathioprine or 6-MP should be used with caution.
- Anaphylaxis and angioneurotic edema have occurred after adalimumab administration.
  - If anaphylaxis occurs, immediately discontinue the drug and provide emergency interventions as ordered.
  - Reactions reported in clinical trials in adults include allergic rash, anaphylactoid reaction, fixed drug reaction, nonspecific drug reaction, and urticaria.
- Pregnancy category B: Teach women of reproductive potential that the drug should be used in pregnancy only if the potential benefit to the mother outweighs the potential risk to the fetus, as there are no well-controlled studies. If pregnancy occurs, patient should be encouraged to register with the Pregnancy Registry at 1-877-311-8972.
- Most common adverse effects were infections (e.g., URI, sinusitis), injection-site reactions, headache, and rash.

Potential Toxicities/Side Effects and the Nursing Process

I.   POTENTIAL FOR INFECTION related to IMMUNOSUPPRESSION

Defining Characteristics: Patients receiving adalimumab are at increased risk for developing serious infections requiring hospitalization. Although uncommon and occurring in patients receiving multiple immunosuppressant medications (e.g., methotrexate and corticosteroids), opportunistic infections may be disseminated on presentation, such as fulminating fungal infections. In clinical trials, most common infections were URI (17%), sinusitis (14%), pharyngitis (11%), and UTI (8%).

Nursing Implications: Assess results of patient's latent TB and HBV testing and discuss any abnormalities with physician, NP, or PA. If TB test is positive, patient should begin anti-TB therapy before beginning adalimumab therapy. Assess baseline risk for infection (e.g., comorbidities, preexisting infections, concomitant immunosuppressants like methotrexate or corticosteroids). Teach patient to self-assess for signs/symptoms of infection (e.g., T > 100.4°F, cough, chest pain, sputum production, dysuria), and to report them right away. Closely monitor patient for signs/symptoms of infection during and after treatment with adalimumab, including TB reactivation even if latent TB test is negative, and teach patient to report any changes (e.g., fever, sweats, chills; cough; SOB; blood in sputum; weight loss; warm, red, or painful skin or sores on body; diarrhea or stomach pain; burning when urinating; urinating more often than usual; feeling very tired). Drug should be discontinued if patient develops a serious infection or sepsis, and appropriate antimicrobial therapy instituted right away. If the patient is at risk for fungal infection and develops severe systemic illness, discuss with physician, NP, or PA empiric antifungal therapy.

II.   KNOWLEDGE DEFICIT related to SUBCUTANEOUS INJECTION TECHNIQUE

Defining Characteristics: Drug is administered subcutaneously, and appropriate patients (or caregivers) can be taught to administer the drug.

Nursing Implications: Assess patient or caregiver readiness to learn, learning style, and limitations. Review with patient drug administration schedule; tell patient not to administer, and to notify physician/nurse, if patient develops an infection. Provide Medication Guide and Instructions for Use available from AbbVie Inc, the drug manufacturer. Teach patient how to care for drug (should be stored in refrigerator at 2–8°C [36°–46°F] in the original container until used, and it should be protected from light). Patient should inspect syringe for cloudiness or particles and should not use if these are found. Patient should be careful to protect glass syringe, as it may break. Drug should be kept out of reach of children and pets. Teach patient hand-washing, aseptic technique, subcutaneous injection technique, and how to dispose of syringe/needle. Teach patient to rotate sites and to apply local measures if injection-site reactions occur. Validate patient understanding by having patient describe measures taught, and ideally, by returning the demonstration of subcutaneous injection technique. Teach patient to develop documentation tool to record site rotation and any site irritation or reaction.

Drug: certolizumab pegol (Cimzia)

Class: Tumor Necrosis Factor (TNF) blocker (antagonist).

Mechanism of Action: Drug binds to human TNF-α, a key proinflammatory cytokine. By neutralizing TNF-α effect, none of the immune inflammatory molecules are activated, so inflammation is suppressed. The drug does not have an Fc (fragment crystallizable of the antibody) region, so it cannot fix complement, cause antibody-dependent cell-mediated cytotoxicity (ADCC), or cause apoptosis (programmed cell death). Elevated levels of TNF-α are found in Crohn's disease (bowel wall) and RA patients (synovial fluid), and TNF-α plays a central role in disease and progression.

Metabolism: After subcutaneous administration, peak plasma concentrations are found 54–171 hours after injection. Bioavailability is 80%. Terminal half-life is about 14 days. The antibody (Fab portion) is cleaved and excreted primarily in the urine.

Indication: For (1) reducing signs and symptoms of Crohn's disease and maintaining clinical response in adult patients with moderately to severely active disease who have had an inadequate response to conventional therapy; (2) treatment of adult patients with moderately to severely active RA; (3) treatment of adult patients with active psoriatic arthritis; (4) treatment of adults with active ankylosing spondylitis.

Dosage/Range:
- **Crohn's disease:** 400 mg initially (2 subcutaneous injections of 200 mg each), and again at weeks 2 and 4; if response occurs, follow with 400 mg subcutaneously every 4 weeks.
- **RA:** 400 mg initially (2 subcutaneous injections of 200 mg each), and at weeks 2 and 4, followed by 200 mg every other week; for maintenance dosing, 400 mg subcutaneously every 4 weeks can be considered. Certolizumab pegol may be used as monotherapy or be combined with nonbiological DMARDs.
- **Psoriatic arthritis:** 400 mg initially and at weeks 2 and 4, followed by 200 mg every other week for maintenance dosing; 400 mg every 4 weeks can be considered.
- **Alkylosing spondylitis:** 400 mg (given as 2 subcutaneous injections of 200 mg each) initially, and at weeks 2 and 4, followed by 200 mg every other week, or 400 mg every 4 weeks.

Drug Preparation:
- Drug available as:
  - 200-mg lyophilized powder for reconstitution, in a single-use glass vial, to be reconstituted with 1 mL of Sterile Water for Injection, USP; use 20-gauge needle included with vial. Use a new syringe to aspirate the contents of each vial (1 ml = 200 mg certolizumab pegol). Replace 20-gauge needle with a 23-gauge needle for administration.
  - 200-mg/mL solution in a single-use prefilled glass syringe.

- Inspect solution carefully for particulate matter, discoloration prior to administration, and do not use if cloudy or particulate matter found.

Drug Administration:
- Ensure patient has been screened for both active and latent TB (e.g., tuberculin skin test and CXR); if results are positive, ensure that the patient has begun anti-TB therapy prior to starting therapy with certolizumab pegol.
- For subcutaneous injection, rotate injection sites and avoid areas where skin is tender, bruised, red, or hard.
- When administering a 400-mg dose, two injections of 200 mg should be given at separate sites in the thigh or abdomen.
- Teach patient or caregiver to administer certolizumab pegol when appropriate.

Lab Effects/Interference:
- Certolizumab pegol may interfere with APTT tests.

Drug Interactions:
- Biological DMARDs: increased risk of infection; do not use concomitantly.
- Live vaccines: do not give with certolizumab pegol.

Special Considerations:
- Drug increases risk of serious infections leading to hospitalization or death, with highest risk in patients receiving another concomitant immunosuppressive drug like methotrexate or corticosteroids.
    - Opportunistic infections include TB and invasive fungal infections where the patient may present with disseminated disease.
    - Consider empiric antifungal therapy in patients who reside in or travel to regions where mycoses are endemic.
- Do not start drug if patient has an active infection, and discontinue drug if a serious infection develops.
- Patients should be closely monitored for signs/symptoms of infection during and after treatment, including the development of TB in patients who tested negatively for latent TB.
- Prior to initial therapy, patients should be evaluated for active TB and tested for latent infection. If initial TB test is positive, patients should begin anti-TB therapy prior to beginning certolizumab pegol. Monitor all patients for active TB during and after treatment, even if initial latent TB test is negative.
- Drug may lead to reactivation of hepatitis B (HBV).
    - Patients should be tested for hepatitis B infection before starting certolizumab pegol.
    - If the test is positive for hepatitis B surface antigen, discuss whether to proceed with a physician specializing in the treatment of patients with hepatitis B.
    - If the patient is an HBV carrier, closely monitor for signs/symptoms of disease activation during and following treatment.
    - Certolizumab pegol should be stopped if HBV is reactivated, and antiviral therapy should be started.

- Demyelinating disease, both new onset and progression of existing disease, has rarely occurred in patients receiving certolizumab pegol. Carefully consider risks vs. benefit in using drug in patients with demyelinating disease.
- Rarely, cytopenias and pancytopenia have occurred.
- Rarely, serious allergic reactions, including anaphylaxis, may occur.
  - Assess for angioedema, dyspnea, hypotension, rash, serum sickness, and urticaria during infusion.
  - If reaction occurs, discontinue drug and institute appropriate medical interventions as ordered.
- Lupus-like syndrome may rarely occur; if it does, stop certolizumab pegol.
- Lymphoma and other malignancies have been reported in patients receiving TNF blockers.
  - These have been reported in children, adolescents, and young adults. Drug is not indicated for the treatment of pediatric patients.
  - Half of cases were lymphomas (HD and NHL).
  - Most patients were receiving immunosuppressants as well; diagnosis occurred after a median of 30 months of therapy.
  - Hepatosplenic T-cell lymphoma (aggressive, often fatal) has been reported in patients treated with TNF blockers, in adult males with Crohn's disease or ulcerative colitis. Most had drug in combination with immunosuppressants.
  - Periodic skin examinations are recommended for all patients, especially those with risk factors for skin cancer.
- Most common side effects are URI (18%), rash (9%), and UTI (8%).
- Pregnancy category B: Counsel women of reproductive potential that the drug should be used during pregnancy only if the benefit exceeds the potential risk, as there are no well-controlled studies in pregnancy. If pregnancy develops, encourage the patient to register in the Pregnancy Surveillance Program (1-877-311-8972). Nursing mothers should decide whether to stop nursing or stop using the drug.

Potential Toxicities/Side Effects and the Nursing Process

I.   POTENTIAL FOR INFECTION related to IMMUNOSUPPRESSION

Defining Characteristics: Patients receiving certolizumab pegol are at increased risk of developing serious infections requiring hospitalization. Although uncommon and occurring in patients receiving combination immunosuppressant medications (e.g., methotrexate and corticosteroids), opportunistic infections may be disseminated on presentation, such as fulminating fungal infections. In clinical trials, most common infections were URI and UTI.

Nursing Implications: Assess results of patient's latent TB and HBV testing and discuss any abnormalities with physician, NP, or PA. If TB test is positive, patient should begin anti-TB therapy before beginning certolizumab pegol therapy. If HBV is positive, discuss if patient should receive therapy (see above). Assess baseline risk for infection (e.g., comorbidities, preexisting infections, concomitant immunosuppressants like methotrexate or corticosteroids). Teach patient to self-assess for signs/symptoms of infection (e.g., T > 100.4°F, cough, chest pain, sputum production, dysuria), and to report them right away. Closely monitor patient for signs/symptoms of infection during and after treatment with certolizumab pegol, including TB reactivation even if latent TB test is negative; teach patient to report any changes (e.g., fever, sweats, chills, cough, SOB, blood in sputum, weight loss). Drug should be discontinued if patient develops a serious infection or sepsis, and appropriate antimicrobial therapy instituted right away. If the patient is at risk for fungal infection and develops severe systemic illness, discuss with physician, NP, or PA empiric antifungal therapy.

II.   KNOWLEDGE DEFICIT related to SUBCUTANEOUS INJECTION TECHNIQUE

Defining Characteristics: Drug is administered subcutaneously, and appropriate patients (or caregivers) can be taught to administer the drug.

Nursing Implications: Assess patient or caregiver readiness to learn, and assess learning style and limitations. Review with patient drug administration schedule; teach patient not to administer and to notify physician or nurse if patient develops an infection. Provide Medication Guide and Instructions for Use from the drug manufacturer UCB, Inc. Teach patient how to care for drug; it should be stored in refrigerator at 2–8°C (36°–46°F) in the original container until used, and it should be protected from light. Drug must not be frozen. Patient should inspect syringe for cloudiness or particles, and should not use if these are found. Patient should be careful to protect glass syringe, as it may break. Drug should be kept out of reach of children and pets. Teach patient hand-washing, aseptic technique, subcutaneous injection technique, and how to dispose of syringe/needle. Teach patient to rotate sites and to apply local measures if injection-site reactions occur. Validate patient understanding by having patient describe measures taught, and ideally, by returning the demonstration of subcutaneous injection technique. Teach patient that allergic reactions are rare, but to call provider right away or seek emergency care if signs/symptoms of allergic reaction occur (e.g., hives, swollen face, trouble breathing, chest pain). Teach patient to develop documentation tool to record site rotation and any site irritation or reaction.

Drug: etanercept (Enbrel)

Class: TNF Blocker (antagonist).

Mechanism of Action: TNF is a pro-inflammatory cytokine and plays a central role in the inflammatory processes of rheumatoid arthritis (RA), polyarticular juvenile idiopathic arthritis (JIA), psoriatic arthritis (PsA), ankylosing spondylitis (AS), and psoriasis (PsO). Elevated levels of TNF are found in the joints and tissues of these patients. Etanercept prevents TNF from binding to its two TNF receptors (α and β) so TNF is unable to stimulate the pro-inflammatory response. The drug also modulates other immune and biological responses regulated by TNF.

Metabolism: Maximal peak serum level is reached in 69 ± 34 hours after a single dose, and mean drug half-life is 102 ± 30 hours.

Indication: (1) Reducing signs and symptoms, inducing major clinical response, inhibiting the progression of structural damage, and improving physical function in patients with moderately to severely active RA, in combination with methotrexate (MTX) or alone; (2) reducing signs and symptoms of moderately to severely active JIA in patients ages 2 and older; (3) reducing signs and symptoms, inhibiting the progression of structural damage, and improving physical function in patients with PsA, and can be used with MTX in patients who do not respond adequately to MTX alone; (4) reducing signs and symptoms in patients with active AS; (5) treatment of adult patients (18+ years old) with chronic moderate to severe plaque psoriasis (PsO) who are candidates for systemic therapy or phototherapy.

Dosage/Range: By subcutaneous injection:
- Adult RA and PsA: 50 mg once weekly with or without methotrexate.
- AS: 50 mg once weekly.
- PsO: starting dose 50 mg twice weekly for three months, followed by maintenance dose of 50 mg once weekly.
- Polyarticular JIA age 2 and older: weight < 63 kg (138 lbs): 0.8 mg/kg weekly (max 50 mg weekly); weight 63 kg (138 lbs) or more: 50 mg weekly.
- Adult RA, AS, PsA: MTX, glucocorticoids, salicylates, NSAIDs, or analgesics can be continued with etanercept treatment.

Drug Preparation:
- 50 mg single-use prefilled syringe (0.98 mL of a 50-mg/mL drug solution).
- 50-mg single-use prefilled SureClick Autoinjector (0.98 mL of a 50-mg/mL drug solution).
- 25-mg single-use prefilled syringe (0.51 mg of a 50-mg/mL drug solution).
- Allow prefilled syringe or SureClick Autoinjector to reach room temperature (15–30 min); do not remove needle cover. Check to see if the amount of liquid falls between the two purple fill-level indicator lines on the syringe. If there is too little liquid, do not use that syringe.
- 25-mg multiuse vial (25 mg etanercept):
  - Use 1 mL of the supplied Sterile Bacteriostatic Water for Injection USP (0.9% benzyl alcohol), giving a solution of 25 mg etanercept per 1.0 mL.
  - Use the supplied vial adapter to aseptically reconstitute the lyophylized powder, unless multiple doses will be withdrawn; in that case, use a 25-gauge needle to reconstitute and withdraw dose. Label multidose vial (must be used within 14 days).
  - If using the vial adapter, twist the adapter onto the diluent syringe. Then place the vial adapter over the Enbrel vial and insert the vial adapter into the vial stopper. Push down on the plunger to inject the diluent into the Enbrel vial.
  - If using a 25-gauge needle to reconstitute and withdraw the Enbrel dose, inject the diluent very slowly into the Enbrel vial. Normally, some foaming occurs.
  - Keep the diluent syringe in place and gently swirl the contents of the vial; do not shake or vigorously agitate.
  - Drug should dissolve in 10 min. Inspect for cloudiness or particulate matter, and if found, do not use. Withdraw the correct dose of reconstituted drug into the syringe. Some foam or bubbles may be present.

- Remove the syringe from vial adapter or remove the 25-gauge needle from syringe. Place 27-gauge needle to inject drug. Do not filter at any time.

Drug Administration:
- Drug should be given subcutaneously.
- Teach patient or caregiver to inject patient when appropriate and if certain that they will comply with medical follow-up as necessary.
- Children should have recommended immunizations given before starting etanercept.

Drug Interactions:
- Live vaccines: do not give with etanercept.
- Immune-modulating biological products (e.g., anakinra): increased immunosuppression; do not give concomitantly.
- Cyclophosphamide: do not use with etanercept.

Lab Effects/Interference:
- Hypoglycemia in diabetic patients (rare).
- Rare cytopenias.

Special Considerations:
- Drug increases risk of serious infections leading to hospitalization or death, with risk highest in individuals receiving another concomitant immunosuppressive drug like methotrexate or corticosteroids. Opportunistic infections include TB and invasive fungal infections where the patient may present with disseminated disease. Consider empiric antifungal therapy in patients at risk for invasive fungal disease who develop severe systemic illness.
- Do not start drug if patient has an active infection, and discontinue drug if a serious infection develops. Drug is contraindicated in sepsis.
- Patients should be closely monitored for signs/symptoms of infection during and after treatment, including the development of TB in patients who tested negatively for latent TB.
- Prior to initial therapy, patients should be evaluated for active TB and tested for latent TB infection. If initial latent TB test is positive, begin anti-TB therapy prior to beginning etanercept. Monitor all patients for active TB during and after treatment, even if initial latent TB test is negative.
- Drug may lead to reactivation of hepatitis B (HBV). Patients should be tested for HBV infection before starting etanercept. If the test is positive for hepatits B surface antigen, discuss whether to proceed with a physician specializing in the treatment of patients with hepatitis B. If the patient is a HBV carrier, close monitoring for signs/symptoms of disease activation should occur during and following treatment. Etanercept should be stopped if HBV is reactivated, and antiviral therapy should be started.
- Demyelinating disease, both new onset and progression of existing disease, has rarely occurred to patients receiving etanercept. Carefully consider risk vs. benefit in using drug in patients with demyelinating disease.
- CHF—new onset or worsening of existing disease—has occurred rarely in patients receiving etanercept.

- Rarely, pancytopenia (< 0.1%) and very rarely, aplastic anemia (< 0.01%), have occurred.
- Allergic reactions have occurred in < 2% of patients, and anaphylaxis has been reported. Drug should be discontinued if anaphylaxis occurs.
- Stop drug if patient develops lupus-like syndrome or autoimmune hepatitis.
- Lymphoma and other malignancies have been reported.
- Most common side effects are infections and injection-site reactions.
- Pregnancy category B: Counsel women of reproductive potential that drug should be used in pregnancy only if benefit outweighs potential risk. If pregnancy develops, encourage patient to register in Amgen's Pregnancy Surveillance Program (1-800-772-6436). Nursing mothers should decide whether to stop nursing or to discontinue the drug.

Potential Toxicities/Side Effects and the Nursing Process

I.   POTENTIAL FOR INFECTION related to IMMUNOSUPPRESSION

Defining Characteristics: Patients receiving etanercept are at increased risk of developing serious infections requiring hospitalization. Although uncommon and occurring in patients receiving multiple immunosuppressant medications (e.g., methotrexate and corticosteroids), opportunistic infections may be disseminated on presentation, such as fulminating fungal infections. In clinical trials, 50–81% of RA patients developed infections. The most common infections were URI (38–65%), while non-URI infections were 21–54%.

Nursing Implications: Assess results of patient's latent TB test and HBV testing and discuss any abnormalities with physician, NP, or PA. If TB test is positive, patient should begin anti-TB therapy before beginning etanercept therapy. Assess baseline patient risk for infection (e.g., comorbidities, preexisting infections, any concomitant immunosuppressive drugs). Teach patient to self-assess for signs/symptoms of infection (e.g., T >100.4°F, cough, chest pain, sputum production, dysuria), and to report them right away. Closely monitor patient for signs/symptoms of infection during and after treatment with etanercept, including TB reactivation even if latent TB test is negative, and teach patient to report any changes (e.g., fever, sweats, chills, cough, SOB, blood in sputum, weight loss). Drug should be discontinued if patient develops a serious infection or sepsis, and appropriate antimicrobial therapy should be instituted right away. If the patient is at risk for fungal infection and develops severe systemic illness, discuss with physician empiric antifungal therapy.

II.   KNOWLEDGE DEFICIT related to SUBCUTANEOUS INJECTION TECHNIQUE

Defining Characteristics: Drug is administered subcutaneously, and appropriate patients (or caregivers) can be taught to administer the drug.

Nursing Implications: Assess patient or caregiver readiness to learn, and assess learning style and limitations. Review with patient drug administration schedule, and teach patient not to administer and to notify physician/nurse if patient develops an infection. Provide

Medication Guide and Instructions for Use from the drug distributor, Amgen. Teach patient how to care for drug; it should be stored in refrigerator at 2–8°C (36°–46°F) in the original container until used, and it should be protected from light. Drug must not be frozen. Patient should inspect syringe for cloudiness or particles and should not use if these are found. Patient should be careful to protect glass syringe, as it may break. Drug should be kept out of reach of children and pets. Teach patient hand-washing, aseptic technique, subcutaneous injection technique, and how to dispose of syringe/needle. Teach patient to rotate sites, and to apply local measures if injection-site reactions occur. Validate patient understanding by having patient describe measures taught, and ideally, by demonstrating the subcutaneous injection technique. Teach patient that allergic reactions are rare, but to call provider right away or seek emergency care if signs/symptoms of allergic reaction occur (hives, swollen face, trouble breathing, chest pain). Teach patient to develop documentation tool to record site rotation and any site irritation or reaction.

Drug: golimumab (Simponi)

Class: Tumor Necrosis Factor Blocker (antagonist).

Mechanism of Action: Golimumab is a human monoclonal antibody that binds to soluble and transmembrane forms of TNF-α, a pro-inflammatory cytokine that plays a central role in inflammation of arthritic joints. High levels of TNF-α are found in blood, synovium, and joints of patients with RA, psoriatic arthritis (PsA), and ankylosing spondylitis (AS). Thus, golimumab blocks TNF-α so it is unable to bind to its receptors, suppressing joint inflammation and destruction.

Metabolism: Following subcutaneous injection, the absolute bioavailability of golimumab is 53%. Time to maximum serum concentration is 2–6 days, and steady state is reached by week 12. There is limited extravascular distribution. Median terminal half-life is about 2 weeks. Methotrexate combined with golimumab reduces the formation of antigolimumab antibodies, so the combination should be used in patients with RA. In the PsA and AS trials, concomitant methotrexate did not appear to influence clinical efficacy or safety. Combinations of NSAIDs, oral corticosteroids, or sulfasalazine with golimumab does not affect golimumab clearance.

Indications: (1) RA: adult patients with moderately to severely active RA in combination with methotrexate (MTX); (2) PsA: adult patients alone or in combination with MTX; (3) AS: adult patients with active AS; (4) Ulcerative colitis: adult patients with moderately to severely active ulcerative colitis who have demonstrated corticosteroid dependence or who have had an inadequate response to or failed to tolerate oral aminosalicylates, oral corticosteroids, azathioprine, or 6-mercaptopurine (6-MP) for (a) inducing and maintaining clinical response; (b) improving endoscopic appearance of the mucosa during induction; (c) inducing clinical remission; (d) achieving and sustaining clinical remission in induction responders.

Dosage/Range:
- RA: 50-mg subcutaneous injection once a month.
- RA patients should receive methotrexate in combination with golimumab; for patients with PsA or AS, golimumab may be given with or without methotrexate or other non-biologic DMARDs.
- RA, PsA, AS patients: corticosteroids, nonbiologic DMARDs, and/or NSAIDs can be continued during golimumab therapy.
- Ulcerative Colitis (UC): 200 mg initially administered by subcutaneous injection at week 0, followed by 100 mg at week 2, and then maintenance dose of 100 mg every 4 weeks.
- Prior to beginning golimumab and periodically during therapy, patients should be evaluated for active TB and tested for latent infection. In addition, prior to starting drug, patients should be tested for hepatitis B viral infections.

Drug Preparation:
- Drug is available in 50-mg and 100-mg strengths for SQ injection:
- Smartject® autoinjector:
  - Each 50-mg single-dose SmartJect® autoinjector contains a prefilled glass syringe (27-gauge 1/2-inch) providing 50 mg of golimumab per 0.5 mL solution.
  - Each 100-mg single-dose SmartJect® autoinjector contains a prefilled glass syringe (27-gauge 1/2-inch) providing 100 mg of golimumab per 1.0 mL solution.
- Prefilled syringe:
  - Each 50-mg single-dose prefilled glass syringe (27-gauge 1/2-inch) contains 50 mg of golimumab per 0.5 mL of solution. Each 100-mg single-dose prefilled glass syringe (27-gauge 1/2-inch) contains 100 mg of golimumab per 1.0 mL of solution.

Drug Administration:
- Teach patient or caregiver proper aseptic SQ injection technique if/when appropriate.
- Allow the prefilled syringe or autoinjector to sit at room temperature for 30 min. outside the carton prior to SQ administration. Do not warm in any other way.
- Inspect syringe for particles or discoloration, and do not use if present; solution should be clear to slightly opalescent or light yellow.
- Do not use any leftover product in the prefilled syringe or autoinjector.
- The needle cover contains dry natural rubber (latex derivative) on prefilled syringe and prefilled syringe with autoinjector cap, and should not be handled by people with a latex sensitivity.
- When multiple injections are given, give in different sites. Rotate injection sites, avoiding where skin is tender, bruised, red, or hard.

Drug Interactions:
- Methotrexate: increased response with golimumab in RA patients.
- Biologic DMARDs (e.g., abatacept, anakinra): increased risk of serious infection; do not administer concomitantly.
- Live vaccines: do not administer while patient is receiving golimumab.
- CYP450 enzyme formation may be suppressed by increased levels of cytokines (e.g., TNF) during chronic inflammation, and thus may be normalized with golimumab when TNF levels are reduced. Assess INR frequently in patients receiving warfarin, or

closely monitor patient receiving other CYP450 substrates with a narrow therapeutic window.

Lab Effects/Interference:
• Increased ALT, AST.
• Rare pancytopenia, leukopenia, neutropenia, thrombocytopenia; very rare aplastic anemia.

Special Considerations:
• Drug increases risk of serious infections leading to hospitalization or death. Patients at greatest risk are those > 65 years old, those with comorbid conditions, and/or those taking concomitant immunosuppressants, such as corticosteroids or methotrexate. Opportunistic infections include TB, hepatitis B infection, and invasive fungal infections where the patient may present with disseminated disease. Consider empiric antifungal therapy in patients who reside in or travel to regions where mycoses are endemic. Other serious infections included sepsis.
• Do not start the drug if patient has an active infection, and monitor patient closely. If an infection develops, stop drug if the infection becomes serious.
• Patients should be closely monitored for signs/symptoms of infection during and after treatment, including the development of TB in patients who initially tested negative for latent TB.
• Prior to initial therapy, patients should be evaluated for active TB (CXR) and tested for latent infection (e.g., induration ≥ 5mm is a positive TB skin test, even if previously vaccinated with BCG). If initial latent TB test is positive, patient should begin anti-TB therapy prior to beginning golimumab.
  • Test for active and latent TB during and after golimumab therapy, even if initial latent TB test is negative.
  • Treatment of latent TB prior to TNF-blocker therapy has been shown to reduce the risk of TB reactivation during therapy.
  • Consider anti-TB therapy prior to golimumab therapy in patients with a past history of latent or active TB, when it cannot be confirmed that an adequate course of therapy has been completed.
  • Cases of active TB have occurred in patients treated with golimumab during and after treatment for latent TB.
  • Monitor patients for signs and symptoms of TB during golimumab therapy even if the patients tested negative for latent TB infection prior to starting therapy, patients were on treatment for latent TB, or patients were previously treated for TB.
• Drug may lead to reactivation of hepatitis B (HBV). Patients should be tested for HBV infection before starting golimumab. If the test is positive for hepatitis B surface antigen, discuss whether to proceed with a physician specializing in the treatment of patients with hepatitis B. If the patient is an HBV carrier, closely monitor the patient for signs/symptoms of disease activation during and following treatment. Golimumuab should be stopped if HBV is reactivated, and antiviral therapy should be begun.
• CHF, new onset or worsening of existing disease, has occurred rarely.
• Cytopenias and pancytopenia have rarely occurred.
• Serious hypersensitivity reactions, including anaphylaxis, have rarely occurred.

- Lymphoma and other malignancies have been reported in children, adolescent, and young adult patients receiving TNF-blockers who started therapy at or younger than 18 years of age.
  - Median onset was 30 months after starting TNF-blocker therapy, and most patients were receiving concomitant immunosuppressants.
  - Rare post-marketing reports of hepatosplenic T-cell lymphoma in patients receiving TNF-blockers, a rare and aggressive lymphoma, primarily in patients with Crohn's disease who had previously received azathioprine or 6-MP.
- Most common side effects are URI, injection-site reaction, and viral infections. Rarely, psoriasis may occur or worsen in patients with the disease who receive golimumab therapy.
- Pregnancy category B: Counsel women of reproductive potential that drug should be used during pregnancy only if benefit exceeds potential risk to the fetus, as there have been no controlled trials. Infants who were exposed to the drug in utero should not receive live vaccinations for 6 months following the mother's last dose of golimumab. Nursing mothers should decide whether to stop nursing or discontinue the drug.

Potential Toxicities/Side Effects and the Nursing Process

I.   POTENTIAL FOR INFECTION related to IMMUNOSUPPRESSION

Defining Characteristics: Patients receiving golimumab are at increased risk for developing serious infections (e.g., bacterial, viral, fungal) requiring hospitalization. Although uncommon and occurring in patients receiving multiple immunosuppressant medications (e.g., methotrexate and corticosteroids), opportunistic infections may be disseminated on presentation, such as fulminating fungal infections (e.g., histoplasmosis, coccidiodomycosis, candidiasis, aspergillosis, pneumocystosis) or extrapulmonary TB. In clinical trials, most common infections were URI (17%), sinusitis (14%), pharyngitis (11%), and UTI (8%).

Nursing Implications: Assess results of patient's latent TB and HBV testing and discuss any abnormalities with physician, NP, or PA. If TB test is positive (e.g., induration of 5 mm or greater on skin tuberculin test), patient should begin anti-TB therapy before beginning golimumab therapy. Assess baseline risk of infection (e.g., comorbidities, preexisting infections, concomitant immunosuppressants like methotrexate or corticosteroids). Teach patient to self-assess for signs/symptoms of infection (e.g., T > 100.4°F, cough, chest pain, sputum production, dysuria), and to report them right away. Closely monitor patient for signs/symptoms of infection during and after treatment with golimumab, including TB reactivation even if latent TB test is negative, and teach patient to report any changes (e.g., fever, sweats, chills, cough, SOB, blood in sputum, weight loss). Drug should be discontinued if patient develops a serious infection or sepsis, and appropriate antimicrobial therapy instituted right away. If the patient is at risk for fungal infection and develops severe systemic illness, discuss empiric antifungal therapy with physician, NP, or PA.

II.   KNOWLEDGE DEFICIT related to SUBCUTANEOUS INJECTION TECHNIQUE

Defining Characteristics: Drug is administered subcutaneously, and appropriate patients (or caregivers) can be taught to administer the drug.

Nursing Implications: Assess patient or caregiver readiness to learn, and assess learning style and limitations. Review with patient drug administration schedule, and teach not to administer and to notify physician/nurse if patient develops an infection. Provide Patient Instructions for Use available from Janssen Biotech (patient package insert). Teach patient how to care for drug; it should be stored in refrigerator at 2–8°C (36–46°F) in the original container until used, and protected from light. Patient should inspect syringe for cloudiness or particles, and not use if these are found. Patient should be careful to protect glass syringe, as it may break. Teach patient not to use any leftover product remaining in the prefilled syringe/autoinjector. Teach patients with a latex sensitivity not to handle the needle cover on the prefilled syringe/autoinjector, as it contains dry natural rubber (derivative of latex), and to use gloves. Drug should be kept out of reach of children and pets. Teach patient hand-washing, aseptic technique, subcutaneous injection technique, and how to dispose of syringe/needle. Teach patient to rotate sites and to apply local measures if injection-site reactions occur. If multiple injections are needed, teach patient to use separate injection sites. Validate patient understanding by having patient describe measures taught, and ideally, by demonstrating the subcutaneous injection technique. Teach patient to develop documentation tool to record site rotation and any site irritation or reaction.

Drug: infliximab (Remicade)

Class: Tumor Necrosis Factor (TNF) blocker (antagonist).

Mechanism of Action: Chimeric monoclonal antibody targeting TNF. TNF-α is important in initiating the acute phase reaction in systemic inflammation. TNF-α functions to induce pro-inflammatory cytokines (e.g., IL1 and IL6), enhances leukocyte migration, activates neutrophil and eosinophilic functional activity, induces acute phase reactants and other liver proteins, as well as tissue-degrading enzymes produced by cells in the joints (synoviocytes and/or chrondrocytes). Infliximab is a chimeric monoclonal antibody, made up of 25% mouse and 75% human protein, that binds to soluble and transmembrane TNF-α so that TNF-α cannot bind to its receptors. This neutralizes TNF-α effect and reduces inflammation. TNF-α concentrations are elevated in tissues/fluids of patients with rheumatoid arthritis (RA), Crohn's disease, ulcerative colitis (UC), ankylosing spondylitis (AS), psoriatic arthritis (PsA), and plaque psoriasis. The drug reduces inflammatory cell infiltration into tissue, levels of IL-6, and C-reactive protein.

Metabolism: After IV infusion, median terminal half-life of infliximab is 7.7–9.5 days. Development of antibodies to infliximab increases its clearance. Coadministration with methotrexate decreases formation of antibodies to infliximab.

Indication: For the treatment of patients with (1a) Crohn's disease to reduce the signs and symptoms, and induce and maintain clinical remission in adult patients with moderately to severely active disease who have had an inadequate response to conventional therapy; as well as (1b) to reduce the number of draining enterocutaneous and rectovaginal fistulae, and to maintain fistula closure in adult patients with fistulizing disease; (2) pediatric Crohn's disease, to reduce the signs and symptoms, and induce and maintain clinical remission in children aged 6 years old and older, with moderately to severely active disease who have had an inadequate response to conventional therapy; (3) ulcerative colitis (UC), to reduce signs and symptoms, to induce and maintain clinical remission and mucosal healing, and to eliminate corticosteroid use in adult patients with moderately to severely active disease who have had an inadequate response to conventional therapy; (4) pediatric UC, to reduce signs and symptoms, and to induce and maintain clinical remission in children, aged 6 years and older, with moderately to severely active disease who have had an inadequate response to conventional therapy; (5) rheumatoid arthritis (RA) in combination with methotrexate, to reduce signs and symptoms, to inhibit the progression of structural damage, and to improve physical function in patients with moderately to severely active disease; (6) ankylosing spondylitis (AS) to reduce signs and symptoms in patients with active disease; (7) psoriatic arthritis to reduce signs and symptoms of active arthritis and to prevent the progression of structural damage and improve physical functioning; (8) plaque psoriasis, in adult patients with chronic severe (extensive or disabling) disease who are candidates for systemic therapy and when other systemic therapies are medically less appropriate.

Dosage/Range:
- Crohn's disease: 5 mg/kg at 0, 2, and 6 weeks, then every 8 weeks as maintenance therapy. Some adults who respond may benefit from increasing the dose to 10 mg/kg if responsiveness is lost. Patients who do not respond by week 14 are unlikely to respond, and drug should be discontinued.
- Pediatric Crohn's disease: 5 mg/kg at 0, 2, and 6 weeks, then every 8 weeks as maintenance therapy.
- Ulcerative colitis: 5 mg/kg at 0, 2, and 6 weeks, then every 8 weeks as maintenance therapy.
- Pediatric Ulcerative colitis: 5 mg/kg at 0, 2, and 6 weeks, then every 8 weeks as maintenance therapy.
- RA in conjunction with methotrexate, 3 mg/kg at 0, 2, and 6 weeks, then every 8 weeks as maintenance therapy. Some patients may benefit from increasing the dose up to 10 mg/kg or treating as often as every 4 weeks. However, incidence of infection is higher with higher doses.
- AS: 5 mg/kg at 0, 2, and 6 weeks, then every 6 weeks as maintenance therapy.
- Psoriatic arthritis and plaque psoriasis: 5 mg/kg at 0, 2, and 6 weeks, then every 8 weeks as maintenance therapy.
- DO NOT administer doses > 5 mg/kg to patients with moderate-to-severe heart failure.
- Drug is contraindicated in patients who have a severe hypersensitivity reaction to the drug or to murine components.
- Prior to starting infliximab therapy, and during therapy, patient should be evaluated for active TB and tested for latent infection.

Drug Preparation:
- Available as 100 mg of lyophilized infliximab in a 20-mg vial for IV use.
- IV:
  - Calculate the dose, the total volume of reconstituted infliximab solution required, and the number of vials needed. Each vial will contain 100 mg of the infliximab antibody.
  - Reconstitute each vial with 10 mL Sterile Water for Injection USP, using a syringe with a 21-gauge or smaller needle as follows: Remove the flip top from the vial and wipe the top with an alcohol swab. Insert the needle aseptically into the vial through the center of the rubber stopper and direct the stream of sterile water to the glass wall of the vial. Gently swirl the solution by rotating the vial to dissolve the lyophilized powder, but do not shake or use vigorous agitation. Foaming of the solution may occur; allow the reconstituted solution to stand for 5 minutes.
  - Inspect the solution; it should be colorless to light yellow and opalescent, and it may contain a few translucent particles of infliximab, as it is a protein. Do not use if lyophlized cake has not fully dissolved or if opaque particles, discoloration, or other foreign particles are seen.
  - Dilute the total volume of the reconstituted infliximab dose to 250 mL with sterile 0.9% Sodium Chloride Injection, USP by withdrawing a volume equal to the volume of reconstituted drug from the 250 mL bag of 0.9% Sodium Chloride Injection, USP. Slowly add the entire volume of reconstituted drug to the bag or infusion bottle, then gently mix. The resulting infusion concentration should range from 0.4–4 mg/mL.
  - Begin the infliximab infusion within 3 hours of reconstituting and diluting the drug.

Drug Administration:
- Infusion reactions: 20% of patients experienced an infusion reaction in clinical trials; monitor patient closely during the infusion, as anaphylaxis may occur at any time. Discuss with physician, NP, or PA premedications (e.g., antihistamine, acetaminophen, corticosteroid) to reduce the risk.
- Administer IV over a minimum of 2 hours, using an infusion set with a low-protein-binding filter.
  - Mild-moderate infusion reactions: slow or stop infusion; once it resolves, resume at lower infusion rate; and/or administer antihistamines, acetaminophen, and/or corticosteroids.
  - If patient cannot tolerate infusion with these interventions, discontinue drug.
  - If patient has a severe infusion reaction during or after the infusion, infliximab should be discontinued.
  - Severe infusion reactions: manage signs and symptoms as ordered and have emergency equipment readily available.
- Assess baseline TB and HBV screening results. Anti-TB therapy should be started before starting infliximab.
- Drug should be discontinued if patient has a severe infusion-related hypersensitivity reaction.
- Do not give the drug if patient has an active infection, including a clinically important localized infection, or if patient develops lupus-like syndrome.

- Live vaccines should not be given with infliximab. Bring pediatric patients up-to-date with all vaccinations prior to initiating infliximab.
- Use caution when switching between biological DMARDs, as there may be overlapping biological activity with further increased risk of infection.
- Common adverse effects during administration are flulike symptoms, headache, dyspnea, hypotension, transient fever, chills, GI symptoms, skin rash.

Drug Interactions:
- Anakinra (Kineret, abatacept (Orencia), tocilizumab (Actemra), etanercept (Enbrel), or other biological therapies: concurrent use increases risk of neutropenia and serious infections; DO NOT GIVE CONCOMITANTLY.
- Methotrexate and other concomitant medications (e.g., NSAIDs, folic acid, corticosteroids): may decrease the incidence of anti-infliximab antibody production, and increase infliximab concentrations and potential efficacy.
- Immunosuppressants: reduce number of infusion reactions in patients with Crohn's disease; when used baseline, drugs such as corticosteroids, antibiotics (metronidazole or ciprofloxacin) and aminosalicylates do not appear to affect serum infliximab concentrations.
- Cytochrome (CYP) P450 substrates: formation of CYP450 enzymes may be suppressed by increased cytokine levels (TNF-α, IL-1, IL-6, IL-10, IFN) during chronic inflammation; thus, when infliximab is administered, it is likely that CYP450 enzyme levels will normalize; monitor for increased drug interactions.
- Live vaccines: may result in clinical infection; do not give concurrently.
- BCG, other therapeutic infectious agents: can result in clinical infection and dissemination; do not give concurrently.

Lab Effects/Interference:
- Decreased leucocyte, platelet, and red blood cell counts.
- Rare elevation of LFTs.

Special Considerations:
- Due to severe immunosuppression, patients are at increased risk for developing serious infections that require hospitalization and that may be fatal. Patients at risk are those taking concomitant immunosuppressants like methotrexate or corticosteroids. Drug should be discontinued if a serious infection or sepsis develops, and patient should be given appropriate antimicrobial therapy immediately.
- Patients should be tested for latent TB prior to infliximab use; if needed, patients should begin anti-TB medications prior to starting infliximab.
- Opportunistic infections include bacterial, viral, and invasive fungal, and the patient may present with disseminated disease. Consider empiric antifungal therapy in patients at risk for invasive fungal disease who develop severe systemic illness.
- Patients should be closely monitored for signs/symptoms of infection during and after treatment, including TB, even if the patient tested negatively for latent TB.

- Lymphoma and other malignancies, especially in children and adolescents with Crohn's disease or ulcerative colitis. Patients at risk received prior treatment with azathioprine or 6-MP concomitantly with infliximab.
- Melanoma and merkel cell carcinoma have occurred in some patients. All patients should receive baseline and periodic skin examinations, especially those with increased risk factors for skin cancer.
- Drug may lead to reactivation of hepatitis B (HBV). Patients should be tested for HBV infection before starting infliximab. If the test is positive for hepatitis B surface antigen, discuss whether to proceed with a physician specializing in the treatment of patients with hepatitis B. If the patient is an HBV carrier, closely monitor the patient for signs/symptoms of disease activation during and following treatment. Infliximab should be stopped if HBV is reactivated, and antiviral therapy should be begun.
- Severe hepatotoxicity may occur, beginning 2 weeks to > 1 year after starting infliximab. Evaluate all patients with signs/symptoms of liver dysfunction; if jaundice or marked elevation in liver enzymes occur ($\geq 5 \times$ ULN), discontinue infliximab and evaluate patient thoroughly.
- Infliximab has been shown to worsen heart failure. Patients should be advised of the potential risk vs. benefit, and if drug is given, patient should be closely monitored during therapy. Drug should be discontinued if new or worsened symptoms occur.
- Drug may cause leukopenia, neutropenia, thrombocytopenia, and pancytopenia. Infliximab should be discontinued if significant hematology abnormalities occur.
- Hypersensitivity reactions (HSRs) can occur during or within 2 hours of drug infusion (e.g., urticaria, dyspnea, hypotension). Rarely, serum sickness-like reaction can occur and is associated with development of anti-infliximab antibodies (e.g., fever, rash, headache, sore throat, myalgias, polyarthralgias, hand and facial edema, dysphagia). Discontinue drug for severe HSRs and have emergency medications and equipment in the infusion room; treat with acetaminophen, antihistamines, corticosteroids, and/or epinephrine per physician.
- In RA, Crohn's disease, and psoriasis clinical trials, there was a higher incidence of reactions when the drug was readministered after a long treatment break. See prescribing information.
- Rarely, CNS reactions have occurred (e.g., systemic vasculitis, seizures, and CNS demyelinating disorders such as multiple sclerosis). Caution should be used when deciding to use infliximab in patients with preexisting neurological disorders.
- Most common adverse reactions were infections (URI, sinusitis, pharyngitis), infusion-related reactions, headache, and abdominal pain.
- Care should be taken when switching from one biological DMARD to another, as overlapping biological activity may increase risk of infection.
- Do not give live vaccines to patients receiving infliximab, as it has resulted in clinical infections. Caution is advised when giving live vaccines born to women treated with infliximab during pregnancy, as drug crosses the placental barrier and can persist in the serum of infants born to mothers treated with infliximab during pregnancy for up to 6 months.
- All pediatric patients should be brought up-to-date with all vaccinations prior to starting infliximab.

Potential Toxicities/Side Effects and the Nursing Process

I. POTENTIAL FOR INJURY related to INFUSION-RELATED REACTIONS

Defining Characteristics: Infliximab is a chimeric monoclonal antibody with at least 25% murine protein, which increases the risk of HSRs. About 20% of patients in clinical trials had infusion reactions (e.g., flulike symptoms, headache, dyspnea, hypotension, transient fever, chills, GI symptoms, and skin rashes). Although rare, anaphylaxis may occur at any time during the infusion (incidence < 1%). Patients who developed antibodies to infliximab were more likely to have an infusion reaction.

Nursing Implications: Discuss with physician premedications (e.g., acetaminophen plus antihistamine or corticosteroid) prior to drug infusion. Ensure that emergency medications (e.g., epinephrine, antihistamines, corticosteroids) and equipment are readily available if needed for a severe infusion reaction. Assess baseline vital signs and monitor frequently during infusion (see http://www.janssenaccessone.com/pages/remicade/pubs/infusion/infusion.jsp for a template for documentation of infliximab monitoring and infusion). Stop infusion for infusion reactions, assess patient, and discuss next steps with physician, NP, or PA. If severe, in addition, keep vein open with 0.9% normal saline or other IV solution via new tubing (without infliximab in it) and prepare to give emergency support (see *Chapter 1*). Mild-to-moderate infusion reactions may improve after slowing or interrupting the infusion. Once the reaction has been treated and resolves, resume the infusion at a slower rate per physician, NP, or PA. If the patient does not tolerate the infusion after these steps, or if the infusion reaction is severe, infliximab should be discontinued.

II. POTENTIAL FOR INFECTION related to IMMUNOSUPPRESSION

Defining Characteristics: Patients receiving infliximab are at increased risk of developing serious infections (e.g., bacterial, viral, fungal) requiring hospitalization. Although uncommon and occurring in patients receiving multiple immunosuppressant medications (e.g., methotrexate and corticosteroids), opportunistic infections may be disseminated on presentation, such as fulminating fungal infections. In clinical trials, most common infections were URI, which occurred in 32% of patients with RA receiving four or more infliximab infusions, sinusitis (14%), pharyngitis (12%), bronchitis (10%), and UTI (8%).

Nursing Implications: Assess results of patient's latent TB and HBV testing and discuss any abnormalities with physician, NP, or PA. If TB test is positive, patient should begin anti-TB therapy before beginning infliximab therapy. Assess baseline risk of infection (e.g., comorbidities, preexisting infections, concomitant immunosuppressants like methotrexate or corticosteroids). Teach patient to self-assess for signs/symptoms of infection (e.g., T > 100.4°F, cough, chest pain, sputum production, dysuria), and to report them right away. Closely monitor patient for signs/symptoms of infection during and after treatment with infliximab, including TB reactivation, even if latent TB test is negative, and teach patient to report any changes (e.g., fever, sweats, chills, cough, SOB, blood in sputum, weight loss).

Drug should be discontinued if patient develops a serious infection or sepsis, and appropriate antimicrobial therapy should be instituted right away. If the patient is at risk for fungal infection and develops severe systemic illness, discuss empiric antifungal therapy with physician, NP, or PA.

Drug: tocilizumab (Actemra)

Class: Interleukin-6 (IL-6) receptor antagonist.

Mechanism of Action: Drug binds to soluble and membrane-bound IL-6 receptors to inhibit IL-6-mediated signaling to the receptors, thus stopping messages to the cell that drive inflammation. IL-6 is a pro-inflammatory cytokine produced by a number of immune cells, including T and B lymphocytes, monocytes, and fibroblasts. IL-6 participates in T-lymphocyte activation, immunoglobulin secretion, and initiation of hepatic acute phase protein synthesis, and it is produced by synovial and endothelial cells. In RA, IL-6 helps produce joint inflammation. Blockade of IL-6 turns off inflammation.

Metabolism: Steady state is reached after the first infusion. The terminal half-life of the drug is concentration-dependent and is 11–13 days for adults with RA, and 16–23 days in children. Doses > 800 mg per infusion are not recommended.

Indication: For the treatment of (1) adults with moderately to severely active RA who have had an inadequate response to one or more DMARDs; (2) patients 2 years of age and older with active polyarticular juvenile idiopathic arthritis (PJIA); (3) patients with active systemic juvenile idiopathic arthritis (SJIA) 2 years of age and older.

Drug is not recommended for patients with active hepatic disease or hepatic impairment.

Dosage/Range:
- **RA:**
- IV infusion: 4 mg/kg IV infusion over 60 minutes every 4 weeks, followed by an increase to 8 mg/kg every 4 weeks based on clinical response.
    - Drug can be used as monotherapy or concomitantly with methotrexate or other non-biologic DMARDs.
    - Interrupt drug and dose-reduce from 8 mg/kg to 4 mg/kg if neutropenia (ANC < 1,000 cells/mm^3), thrombocytopenia (< 100,000 cells/mm^3), elevated LFTs (see package insert).
    - Do not exceed 800 mg per infusion.
- SQ injection: Patients < 100 kg weight: 162 mg SQ every other week, followed by an increase to every week based on clinical response; patients ≥ 100 kg weight: 162 mg SQ every week.
    - When transitioning from IV to SQ administration, administer the first SQ dose instead of the next scheduled IV dose.
- Management of increased LFTs, neutropenia, thrombocytopenia: Interruption of dose or reduction in frequency from every week to every other week dosing.

- Liver enzymes > 1–3 × ULN: dose modify concomitant DMARD if appropriate; if persistent increases in this range: for patients receiving IV tocilizumab, reduce dose to 4 mg/kg or hold drug until ALT, AST have normalized; for patients receiving SQ tocilizumab, reduce injection frequency to every other week or hold dosing until ALT, AST have normalized. Resume tocilizumab at every other week and increase frequency to every week as clinically appropriate.
- Liver enzymes > 3–5 × ULN (confirm by repeat testing): hold tocilizumab until < 3 × ULN, and follow recommendations for 1–3 × ULN; for persistent increases > 3 × ULN, discontinue tocilizumab.
- ANC > 1,000 cells/mm$_3$: maintain dose.
- ANC 500–1,000 cells/mm$_3$: hold tocilizumab; when ANC > 1,000 cells/mm$_3$: IV: resume at 4 mg/kg and increase to 8 mg/kg as clinically appropriate; SQ, resume at every other week dosing and increase frequency to every week as clinically appropriate.
- ANC < 500 cells/mm$_3$: discontinue tocilizumab.
- Platelets 50,000–100,000 cells/mm$_3$: hold tocilizumab, and when platelets > 100,000 cells/mm$_3$, IV: resume tocilizumab at 4 mg/kg and increase to 8 mg/kg as clinically appropriate; SQ, resume at every other week dosing and increase frequency to every week as clinically appropriate.
- Platelets < 50,000 cells/mm$_3$: discontinue tocilizumab.
- Monitor CBC, LFTs, lipids 4–8 weeks after start of therapy, then every 3 months.

Polyarticular Juvenile Idiopathic Arthritis (PJIA): IV over 60 minutes, every 4 weeks, alone or in combination with methotrexate.

- Patients < 30 kg weight: 10 mg/kg.
- Patients > 30 kg weight: 8 mg/kg.
- Do not change dose based solely on a single-visit body weight measurement, as weight may fluctuate.
- Interrupt if low neutrophil or platelet counts, increased LFTs; consider dose modification if methotrexate also given; see package insert.
- SQ administration is not approved for SJIA

Systemic Juvenile Idiopathic Arthritis (SJIA): IV over 60 minutes once every 2 weeks, alone or in combination with methotrexate.

- Patients < 30 kg weight: 12 mg/kg.
- Patients > 30 kg weight: 8 mg/kg.
- Do not change dose based solely on a single-visit body weight measurement, as weight may fluctuate.
- Interrupt if low neutrophil or platelet counts, increased LFTs; consider dose modification if methotrexate also given; see package insert.
- SQ administration is not approved for SJIA.
- Drug should not be started in patients with an ANC < 2,000 cells/mm^3, platelet count < 100,000 cells/mm^3, or who have ALT or AST ≥ 1.5 × ULN. If ANC < 500 cells/mm^3, drug should be discontinued.

Drug Preparation:
- Available in single-use vials (20 mg/mL): 80 mg/4 mL, 200 mg/10 mL, and 400 mg/ 20 mL.

IV Administration:
- Aseptically prepare IV infusion bag.
- Adult RA and PJIA, SJIA patients weighing > 30 kg: use a 100-mL infusion bag or bottle of 0.9% Sodium Chloride Injection USP.
- PJIA and SJIA patients weighing < 30 kg: use a 50-mL infusion bag or bottle of 0.9% Sodium Chloride Injection USP.
- Preparation:
  - Withdraw volume equal to the volume of tocilizumab required for the patient dose from the IV bag or bottle. [4 mg/kg = 0.2 mL/kg (adult RA); 8 mg/kg (adult RA, SJIA, and PJIA ≥ 30 kg body weight) = 0.4 mL/kg; 10 mg/kg (PJIA < 30 kg of body weight) = 0.5 mL/kg; 12 mg/kg (SJIA (< 30 kg of body weight) = 0.6 mL/kg]
  - Withdraw the amount of tocilizumab for IV infusion from the vial(s). Slowly add tocilizumab for IV infusion from each vial to the infusion bag or bottle; gently invert bag to mix.
  - Fully diluted drug can be stored at 2–8°C (36–46°F) or room temperature for up to 24 hours; protect from light. Allow refrigerated drug to come to room temperature prior to infusion.
- Inspect for particulate matter and discoloration; if found, do not use.
- **SQ administration:** RA patients only. Do not use for IV administration.
- Patient/caregiver can be taught to prepare and administer if/when appropriate. Use Instructions for Use in package insert for teaching tool.
- Inspect for particulate matter, cloudiness, and discoloration; if found, do not use prefilled syringe (PFS).
- Drug should be clear and colorless to pale yellow.

Drug Administration:
- ANC must be > 2,000 cells/mm^3, platelet count > 100,000 cells/mm^3, and ALT/AST ≤ 1.5 × ULN.
- Assess results of latent TB test, and if positive, patient must begin anti-TB therapy prior to starting tocilizumab therapy.
- Patients with PJIA and SJIA should have their immunizations brought up to date before starting drug.
- IV: Administer by IV infusion over 60 minutes in its own IV; do not mix with other drugs. Monitor for infusion reactions.
- SQ: Teach patient to inject the full amount in the syringe (0.9 mL), providing 162 mg tocilizumab, according to the directions in the Instructions for Use.
- Teach patient to rotate sites with each injection, and to avoid moles, scars, and areas that are tender, bruised, red, hard, or not intact.
- Teach patient that if hypersensitivity reactions, including anaphylaxis, occur, to seek immediate medical attention if they have any signs or symptoms (e.g., dyspnea, feeling faint, body rash).

Drug Interactions:
- Biologic DMARDs: increased immunosuppression, increased risk for infection; DO NOT give concomitantly.
- Live vaccines: do not give during tocilizumab therapy.

- Simvastatin (a CYP3A4 and OATP1B1 substrate): simvastatin effect may be reduced.
- Omeprazole (CYP2C19 and CYP3A4 substrate): omeprazole effect may be reduced.
- Dextromethorphan (CYP2D6 and CYP3A4 substrate): dextromethorphan effect may be increased after drug infusion.
- Monitor patients receiving drugs that are CYP substrates closely to determine effect (e.g., patients on warfarin) and monitor INR.

Lab Effects/Interference:
- Neutropenia, thrombocytopenia.
- Increased LFTs.
- Increased total cholesterol, triglycerides, LDL, and HDL cholesterol.

Special Considerations:
- Serious infections may occur, and patients receiving other concomitant immunosuppressant medications are at greatest risk (e.g., methotrexate, corticosteroids); opportunistic infections include invasive fungal infections that may present as disseminated rather than localized disease. Do not administer drug during an active infection, including localized infections. Interrupt drug if a serious infection develops.
- All patients should be tested for latent TB, and if positive, anti-TB therapy should be started prior to beginning tocilizumab therapy. Closely monitor patient during tocilizumab therapy for signs/symptoms of infection, including TB, even if the patients had a negative latent TB test.
- Monitor Absolute Neutrophil Count (ANC), platelet count, serum lipids, and LFTs: baseline. Monitor ANC, platelet count, and ALT and AST levels 4–8 weeks after start of therapy, then every 3 months thereafter in RA patients. Risk of hepatotoxicity (increased LFTs) is greater in patients also receiving methotrexate. Patients with PJIA should have baseline and repeat testing at the time of the second infusion, then every 4–8 weeks; SJIA patients should have these labs tested every 2–4 weeks. Lipids should be monitored every 4–8 weeks.
- Use drug cautiously in patients at risk for GI perforation, as this has rarely occurred.
- Rarely, hypersensitivity reactions (HSRs) have occurred (incidence 0.1–0.2%), including anaphylaxis. If severe HSR occurs, drug should be permanently discontinued and emergency measures instituted.
- Rarely, demyelinating disorders have been reported in RA patients. Use drug cautiously in patients with preexisting or recent onset demyelinating disorders.
- Live vaccines should not be given to patients receiving tocilizumab.
- Malignancies have been reported in patients receiving the drug.
- The drug can cause infusion reactions. Patients did not receive premedication in clinical studies, and during 24 hours surrounding drug administration between 4–20% developed infusion reactions (e.g., rash, nausea, hypotension, dizziness, urticaria, diarrhea, epigastric distress, arthralgia, headache), but only 0.1–0.2% involved anaphylaxis or HSRs requiring treatment discontinuation; these occurred despite premedication.
- Most common side effects are URI, nasopharyngitis, headache, HTN, and increased ALT.
- Pregnancy category C: Counsel women of childbearing age that drug should be used in pregnancy only if benefit exceeds potential risks, as there are no well-controlled

studies. If patient becomes pregnant, encourage her to register with the Pregnancy Registry, 1-877-311-8972. Nursing mothers should stop nursing or discontinue the drug.

Potential Toxicities/Side Effects and the Nursing Process

I. POTENTIAL FOR INFECTION related to IMMUNOSUPPRESSION

Defining Characteristics: Patients receiving tocilizumab are at increased risk of developing serious infections (e.g., bacterial, mycobacterial, viral, fungal, protozoan) leading to hospitalization or death. Although uncommon and often occurring in patients receiving other immunosuppressant medications (e.g., methotrexate, corticosteroids), opportunistic infections may be disseminated on presentation, which in addition to RA predispose the patient to infection. In clinical trials, most common infections were URI (6–8%), nasopharyngitis (4–7%), and bronchitis (3–4%), while serious infections were pneumonia, UTI, cellulitis, herpes zoster, gastroenteritis, diverticulitis, sepsis, and bacterial arthritis. Patients with latent TB may develop activated TB. Viral infections can be reactivated, such as herpes zoster. Signs and symptoms of acute inflammation may be reduced due to suppression of acute phase reactants.

Neutrophils (17% over 12 weeks) and platelets (4% over 12 weeks) may be decreased.

Nursing Implications: Review patient history; drug should not be given to a patient with active infection, including localized infections. Physician should review the risks and benefits of using tocilizumab therapy in patients with chronic or recurrent infections, as well as those who have been exposed to TB, have a history of serious or opportunistic infection, have lived or traveled in areas of endemic TB or other mycoses, or with underlying conditions that may predispose them to infection.

Assess results of patient's latent TB testing and discuss any abnormalities with physician, NP, or PA. If TB test is positive, patient should begin anti-TB therapy before beginning tocilizumab therapy. Anti-TB therapy should also be considered, based on input from a TB specialist, for those patients with a history of latent or active TB where an adequate course of therapy cannot be confirmed, or if the patient tested negative for latent TB but has risk factors.

Assess baseline labs, and verify that ANC > 2,000 cells/mm^3, and platelet count is > 100,000 cells/mm^3. ANC and platelet count should be monitored baseline and every 4–8 weeks. Assess baseline risk for infection (e.g., comorbidities, preexisting infections, concomitant immunosuppressants like methotrexate or corticosteroids). Teach patient to self-assess for signs/symptoms of infection (e.g., T > 100.4°F, cough, chest pain, sputum production, dysuria), and to report them right away. Closely monitor patient for signs/ symptoms of infection during and after treatment with tocilizumab, and teach patient to report any changes. Drug should be interrupted if patient develops a serious infection, opportunistic infection, or sepsis. If a patient develops a new infection while receiving tocilizumab therapy, prompt and comprehensive evaluation of an immunocompromised patient should be done.

II.   POTENTIAL FOR INJURY related to INFUSION-RELATED REACTIONS

Defining Characteristics: Patients can develop infusion reactions during or within 24 hours of tocilizumab administration. Incidence of reactions during the infusion ranged from 4–6%. Reactions within 24 hours after the infusion occurred in 16–20%. Anaphylaxis was reported in < 1% of patients. Symptoms that occurred during the infusion included headache, nausea, and hypotension; reactions occurring during the 24 hours following infusion were rash, urticaria, diarrhea, epigastric discomfort, arthalgia, dizziness, and hypotension. Incidence of HSRs requiring drug discontinuation were < 0.2%.

Nursing Implications: Discuss with physician premedications (e.g., acetaminophen plus antihistamine or corticosteroid) prior to drug infusion. While anaphylaxis is rare, ensure that emergency medications (e.g., epinephrine, antihistamines, corticosteroids) and equipment are readily available if needed. Assess baseline vital signs before and after the infusion, as well as during the infusion if needed. Stop infusion for infusion reactions, assess patient, and discuss next steps with physician, NP, or PA. If severe, in addition, keep vein open with 0.9% Normal Saline or other IV solution via new tubing (without tocilizumab in it) and prepare to give emergency support (see *Chapter 1*).

Drug: tofacitinib citrate (Xeljanz)

Class: Janus Kinase Inhibitor (JAK inhibitor).

Mechanism of Action: JAKs are enzymes within the cell that carry messages from receptors on the cell surface, which have been activated by cytokine or growth factors, to the cell nucleus. JAKs tell the immune system to turn on and to activate other blood cells using phosphorylation, which activates signal transducers and transcription (STATs), which in turn regulate cell activities, as well as turning on genes in the cell's DNA. JAK inhibitors modulate the signaling pathway, thus stopping this message from being sent so that STATs are not activated and the immune system (inflammation) is not turned on. Drug causes dose-dependent decreases in circulating Natural Killer lymphocytes (NK, CD16/56+ cells) with maximal effect in 8–10 weeks after therapy has started. Changes resolve in 2–6 weeks after the drug is discontinued. After treatment with tofacitinib, there is a rapid decrease in serum C-reactive protein (CRP) that takes longer than the drug's half-life to reverse.

Indications: For the treatment of adult patient with moderately to severely active RA who has had an inadequate response or intolerance to methotrexate. It may be used as monotherapy or in combination with methotrexate or other nonbiologic DMARDs. Limitations of use: use of tofacitinib citrate with biologic DMARDs or with potent immunosuppressants (e.g., azathioprine and cyclosporine) is not recommended.

Dosage/Range:
* 5 mg orally twice daily without regard to meals.
    * As monotherapy or in combination with methotrexate (MTX) or other nonbiologic DMARD.

- Do not initiate drug if absolute lymphocyte count < 500 cells/mm^3, ANC < 1,000 cells/mm^3, or if Hgb < 9 g/dL.
- Do not use drug if patient develops a serious infection until the infection is controlled.
- Dose interruption for management of lymphopenia, neutropenia, and anemia.
- If moderate or severe renal impairment, or moderate hepatic impairment: reduce dose to 5 mg orally once daily. Do not use drug in patients with severe hepatic impairment.
- Dose modifications:
  - Lymphocyte count < 500 cells/mm^3 (confirm by repeat testing): discontinue drug.
  - Absolute Neutrophil Count (ANC) 500–1,000 cells/mm^3: interrupt drug until ANC > 1,000 cells/mm^3 and then resume at usual dose; if ANC < 500 cells/mm^3 (repeat testing confirmation), discontinue drug.
  - Hgb: ≤ 2 g/dL decrease and ≥ 9.0 g/dL: maintain dose; if > 2 g/dL decrease or < 8.0 g/dL (confirm by repeat testing), interrupt drug until hemoglobin values have normalized.
- If given with strong CYP3A4 inhibitor (e.g., ketoconazole): reduce dose to 5 mg orally once daily.
- If given with a moderate CYP3A4 inhibitor **and** potent inhibitor of CYP2C19 (e.g., fluconazole): decrease dose to 5 mg orally once daily.
- If given with potent CYP3A4 inducers (e.g., rifampin, St. John's wort): may reduce or nullify clinical response. Do not co administer. Teach patient not to take St. John's wort.

Drug Preparation:
- Available as 5-mg tablets.

Drug Administration:
- Assess lymphocyte and neutrophil count, hemoglobin, LFTs, and lipids baseline and frequently during therapy. Lymphocyte count must be ≥ 500 cells/mm^3, and ANC ≥ 1,000 cells/mm^3 for drug to be given. Hgb should be ≥ 9.0 g/dL.
- Stop drug during active infection, including localized infections.
- Interrupt tocilizumab if a serious infection develops, and do not resume until the infection is controlled.
- Do not give drug to patients with severe hepatic impairment.
- Monitor ANC and Hgb baseline, then after 4–8 weeks of treatment, then every 3 months; lymphocyte counts baseline and every 3 months; monitor LFTs, lipids baseline, then lipids after 4–8 weeks. Assess results of tests for active and latent TB, and viral hepatitis screens.

Drug Interactions:
- Strong CYP 3A4 inhibitors (e.g., ketoconazole): increased tofacitinib serum level (because drug metabolism is reduced); reduce tocilizumab dose if coadministered (see *Chapter 4 Introduction* for a review of CYP3A4).
- Moderate CYP3A4 inhibitors (e.g., fluconazole) and potent CYP2C19 inhibitors: increased tofacitinib serum levels; reduce tocilizumab dose if coadministered.
- Potent CYP3A4 inducers (e.g., rifampin): decreased tofacitinib serum level with decreased tofacitinib activity.

- Immunosuppressive drugs (e.g., azathioprine, tacrolimus, cyclosporine), or other DMARDs: increased risk of infection; DO NOT give concomitantly.

Lab Effects/Interference:
- Initial lymphocytosis at 1 month, followed by a decrease in mean absolute lymphocyte counts below baseline of 10% during 12 months of therapy. Lymphocyte counts < 500 cells/mm^3 were associated with increased risk of serious infection.
- Decreased lymphocyte and neutrophil counts (rare).
- Increased LDL and HDL cholesterol, total cholesterol, triglycerides.
- Increased LFTs.
- Anemia.

Special Considerations:
- Drug should not be given to patients with active, serious infections, including localized infections. Risk vs. benefit should be carefully assessed before starting drug in patients:
  - With chronic or recurrent infection;
  - Who have been exposed to TB;
  - With a history of a serious infection or opportunistic infection;
  - Who have traveled to areas of endemic TB or endemic mycoses, or who have an underlying condition predisposing them to infection.
- Serious infections requiring hospitalization, including TB and bacterial, invasive fungal, and viral opportunistic infections may occur; monitor patient closely.
  - Most common serious infections included pneumonia, cellullitis, herpes zoster, and UTI.
  - Opportunistic infections included myocobacterial infections, cryptococcosis, esophageal candidiasis, pneumocystosis, multidermatomal herpes zolster, cytomegalovirus, and BK virus. Some patients presented with disseminated disease and were often taking concommitant immunomodulating agents, such as MTX or corticosteroids.
  - Drug must not be started in patients with an active, serious infection, including localized infections.
  - Interrupt drug if patient develops a serious infection, an opportunistic infection, or sepsis. Appropriate antimicrobial intervention should occur promptly.
- Prior to beginning therapy, patient should be tested for latent TB; if positive, delay tofacitinib until anti-TB treatment is started.
- Monitor all patients closely for active TB during treatment, even if latent TB test is negative.
- GI perforations have occurred; use cautiously in patients at increased risk, such as those taking NSAIDs, methotrexate, or corticosteroids.
- Do not give live immunizations (vaccines) while patient is receiving tofacitinib.
- Lymphoma and other opportunistic malignancies have occurred in patients treated with tofacitinib.
- Viral reactivation, including herpes have occurred. Patients should be screened for viral hepatitis prior to starting drug.
- Epstein-Barr virus-associated post-transplant lymphoproliferative disorder has been observed at an increased rate in renal transplant patients treated with tofacitinib and concomitant immunosuppressive medications.

- Non-melanoma skin cancer has been reported in patients; perform periodic skin assessment in patients at risk for skin cancer.
- Pregancy category C: Counsel women of reproductive potential that drug should be used in pregnancy only if benefit outweighs potential risk, as there are no well-controlled studies. In laboratory studies, at very high doses, tocilizumab may be fetocidal and teratogenic. If patient becomes pregnant while taking tocilizumab, encourage her to register on the Pfizer Pregnancy Registry at 1-877-311-8972. Nursing mothers should discontinue nursing or stop using tocilizumab.
- Most common side effects during first three months of therapy are URI (4.5%), headache (4.3%), diarrhea (4%), and nasopharyngitis (3.8%).
- Monitor lymphocyte counts baseline and every 3 months thereafter. Monitor ANC and hemoglobin baseline, then after 4–8 weeks of treatment, then every 3 months thereafter. Dose modify based on ANC (see package insert). Assess lipids baseline then after 4–8 weeks of therapy as maximum effects observed within 6 weeks. Patients with lipid elevations should be managed according to clinical guidelines for hyperlipidemia.

Potential Toxicities/Side Effects and the Nursing Process

I.   POTENTIAL FOR INFECTION related to IMMUNOSUPPRESSION

Defining Characteristics: Patients receiving tofacitinib are at increased risk of developing serious infections (e.g., bacterial, mycobacterial, viral, fungal, protzoan). Lymphopenia and neutropenia may occur rarely with lymphocyte counts < 500 cells/mm^3 occurring in 0.04% of patients and ANC < 1,000 cells/mm^3 occurring in 0.07% of patients. There was no association between neutropenia and infection. Latent TB may become reactivated TB (pulmonary or extrapulmonary). Opportunistic infections (OIs) may occur, including invasive fungal infections (e.g., cryptococcus and pneumocystosis) that may be disseminated on presentation (patients were usually taking tofacitinib with concomitant immunomodulating agents such as methotrexate or corticosteroids). Most common OIs were TB, mycobacterial infections, cryptococcus, esophageal candidiasis, pneuomocystosis, and cytomegalovirus. Most common infections are pneumonia, cellulitis, herpes zoster, and UTIs. Tofacitinib can cause viral reactivation; patients who screen tested positive for hepatitis B or C were excluded from studies.

Nursing Implications: Review patient history; drug should not be given to a patient with active infection, including localized infections. Assess results of patient's latent TB testing and discuss any abnormalities with physician, NP, or PA. If TB test is positive, patient should begin anti-TB therapy before beginning tofacitinib therapy. Anti-TB therapy should also be considered for patients with a history of latent or active TB, and an adequate course of therapy cannot be confirmed. Monitor all patients for active TB during treatment, even if initial latent TB test is negative. Physician should discuss risks vs. benefits of tofacitinib in patients with chronic or recurrent infections, exposed to TB, with a history of a serious OI, who have resided or traveled to an area of endemic TB or mycoses, or with underlying conditions besides RA that may predispose them to infection.

If the patient screened positive for hepatitis B or C, discuss with physician whether patient is a candidate for the drug, as tofacitinib may react with hepatitis virus. If the patient is treated with tofacitinib, teach the patient to report immediately increased fatigue, yellow conjunctiva (eyes looking yellow), anorexia, vomiting, clay-colored bowel movements, fever, chills, stomach discomfort, muscle aches, dark urine, or skin rash.

Assess CBC/differential baseline labs and at each visit prior to drug administration, and verify that lymphocyte count is > 500 cells/mm^3 and ANC > 1,000 cells/mm^3. Assess baseline risk for infection (e.g., comorbidities, history of infections). Teach patient to self-assess for signs/symptoms of infection (e.g., T > 100.4°F, cough, chest pain, sputum production, dysuria), stop drug, and report any signs/symptoms immediately. Closely monitor patient for signs/symptoms of infection, including TB, during and after treatment with tofacitinib, and teach patient to report any changes (e.g., fever, sweats, rigors, weight loss, blood in sputum). Drug should be interrupted if patient develops a serious infection, opportunistic infection, or sepsis. If a patient develops a new infection while receiving tofacitinib therapy, prompt and comprehensive evaluation of an immunocompromised patient should be done, and antimicrobial therapy should be given.

Teach patient strategies to manage fatigue and conserve energy, such as alteration of rest and activity, and organizing chores.

Section 2
Symptom Management

Chapter 6
Pain

Pain in the patient with cancer may result from a variety of stimuli. A careful assessment is critical in order to identify the physical causes and psychosocial factors that modulate pain intensity and perception. Pain can be acute or chronic. Acute pain results from stimuli such as surgical procedures, pathologic fractures, and obstruction of a hollow viscus where the stimulus can be removed (e.g., healing, radiation to the bone metastatic site, or resection of obstructing tumor), while chronic pain reflects the more common cancer pain where the stimulus cannot be removed, such as pain resulting from tissue inflammation caused by tumor. Patients often have both acute and chronic components of pain. Acute pain lasts from minutes to months and ceases when the cause of pain is removed (e.g., pain caused by spinal cord compression is removed when the patient undergoes laminectomy or radiotherapy to relieve the compression). This type of pain is often associated with anxiety, and one sees symptoms of sympathetic nervous system arousal (increased heart rate, increased/decreased BP) as well. In contrast, chronic pain lasts from months to years; the cause cannot be removed, and this type of pain is often associated with depression. The long duration of chronic pain dampens sympathetic response, so the patient does not manifest changes in heart rate or BP. Many patients with cancer pain have persistent pain that requires around-the-clock analgesia to prevent pain. In addition, patients can develop breakthrough pain, which may be precipitated by an anticipated event, such as movement, or it just may occur. It is estimated that 64–89% of patients with chronic cancer pain have breakthrough pain, with most episodes lasting 120 minutes or less, and a single patient having four to seven episodes a day (Zeppetella et al., 2000). Less commonly, pain can be intermittent, and this is characteristic of acute pain. Here, short-acting analgesia is given intermittently.

Symptoms often accompanying unrelieved pain are sleeplessness, anorexia (loss of appetite), fatigue, irritability, and fear. In fact, as early as the first century AD, it was recognized that fear of pain was significant. Epictetus (AD 55–135) is reported to have said "It is not death or pain that is to be dreaded, but the fear of pain or death" (Crossley, 2006). Nurses play a critical role in advocating for effective cancer pain management and alleviation of other accompanying symptoms. Fortunately, there are a variety of available analgesic medications, including non-opioid and opioid, adjuvant agents such as antidepressants, as well as nonpharmacologic techniques such as relaxation exercises.

Opioid agents are available in immediate-onset formulations for acute pain, and long-duration agents that allow superior control for chronic pain by avoiding the peaks and valleys of serum drug levels associated with immediate preparations. While analgesics do not remove the source or stimulus for the pain, they decrease or modulate the impulse so that the pain impulse perceived by the patient is reduced or absent, thus decreasing the distress and discomfort perceived by the patient. *Non-opioid* medications are helpful for mild-to-moderate pain, and some, such as acetaminophen, provide added analgesia as well.

Most non-opioid analgesics work peripherally to decrease prostaglandin synthesis (NSAIDs), but some agents may have a central action as well, possibly at the level of the hypothalamus (McEvoy et al., 1992). Pain receptors appear to be sensitized to mechanical and chemical stimulation by prostaglandins, so interruption of prostaglandin synthesis diminishes the painful impulse. For example, bone destruction and pain from metastasis appear to be mediated by prostaglandins, so NSAIDs that inhibit prostaglandin synthesis are first-line analgesics (Foley, 2000). In addition, the anti-inflammatory action of NSAIDs contributes to analgesia. Principal side effects of this class are alteration in hemostasis (aspirin inhibits platelet aggregation, while other salicylates may alter hepatic synthesis of blood coagulation factors); alteration in GI mucosal integrity (aspirin and other NSAIDs can erode GI mucosal surface, causing bleeding or ulceration); and altered renal elimination due to inhibition of renal prostaglandins responsible for renal blood flow and function.

NSAIDs achieve their anti-inflammatory effect by inhibiting the enzyme cyclooxygenase (COX), which is necessary for synthesis of prostaglandins and thromboxanes. There are two isoforms of the enzyme: COX-1, which appears to protect the gastric mucosa and is found in most tissues, including platelets, and COX-2, which is found in brain and kidney tissue, as well as other body tissues at the site of inflammation. NSAIDs traditionally inhibit both COX-1 and COX-2 isoforms, resulting in a high risk of gastric ulceration and perforation.

Adjuvant analgesics play a vital role in cancer pain management. These drugs are indicated for purposes other than analgesia but can be combined with primary analgesics to increase analgesia and/or manage symptoms related to pain or the adverse effects of the opioids. There may be wide variations in patient responses. The major classes used as adjuvant drugs are antidepressant (*Chapter 9*), corticosteroid (*Chapter 1*), anticonvulsant, and specialty drugs for bony metastasis (*Chapter 10*).

The *antidepressants* enhance pain-modulating pathways that are mediated by serotonin and norepinephrine, and interestingly, clomipramine and amitriptyline have been shown to increase morphine levels (Wilkie, 1995). Not only can these agents help reduce the depression associated with chronic pain, but they can also relieve sleep problems, and often offer significant benefit in the management of neuropathic pain (McDonald & Portenoy, 2006). Antidepressant groups that offer benefit include the tricyclic antidepressants, the serotonin-reuptake inhibitors, as well as others such as venlafaxine, bupropion, and duloxetine. Paroxetine (Paxil) has shown benefit in reducing the painful symptoms of peripheral neuropathy in diabetic patients (Sindrup et al., 1990) and itching in patients with advanced cancer (Zycliz, 1996). Duloxetine (Cymbalta) has been shown to significantly reduce painful chemotherapy-induced peripheral neuropathy, and also improved function and quality of life (Smith et al., 2013). In dosing antidepressants, the starting dosage should be low and given at bedtime. The dose should be titrated up slowly to the usually effective range. It is important to allow 1 week between dose titrations to evaluate the benefit of a given dose. Side effects include sedation, orthostatic hypotension, constipation, dry mouth, dizziness and, less commonly, precipitation of acute angle-closure glaucoma, urinary retention, and arrhythmia.

Corticosteroids are useful in both acute and chronic pain management, such as that associated with metastatic bone pain, neuropathic pain, lymphedema, hepatic capsular distension,

MANAGEMENT

and brain metastasis. The dosing is individualized to the etiology of the pain and patient requirements, from low doses to high doses for patients with brain metastasis. It is important to identify patients at risk for peptic ulceration, and then to use corticosteroids cautiously if at all. In addition, patients need to be cautioned not to take concomitant aspirin.

Anticonvulsants may provide analgesia for lancinating, neuropathic pain. Second-generation drugs (gabapentin, pregabalin, and lamotrigine) have largely replaced first-generation drugs (carbamazepine, phenytoin, clonazepam, and valproate).

Specialty drugs for the management of bony metastasis are bisphosphonate pamidronate disodium (Aredia) and zoledronate (Zometa), indicated for use in managing pain related to bony metastases. Pamidronate and zoledronate have been shown to inhibit osteoclast activity and reduce pain from bony metastasis. Treatment is given IV every 4 weeks. Radiopharmaceuticals such as strontium-89 are taken up in bone mineral preferentially, in sites of metastasis. However, the subsequent development of acute leukemia has limited interest in radiopharmaceutical management of pain.

Cancer Pain Management: According to McCaffery (1982), pain is "whatever the patient says it is, occurring where the patient says it is." Use of quantifiable measurement tools is helpful to identify pain intensity (see Figure 6.1) and pain *relief* in response

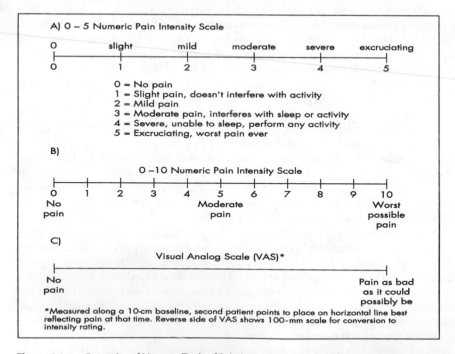

Figure 6.1   Examples of Measure Tools of Pain Intensity

Data from Agency for Healthcare Research and Quality (1992). Acute Pain Management: Operative or medical procedures and trauma, Clinical Practice Guideline No. 1 AHCPR Publication No 92-0032. Rockville, MD. pp116–117.

to intervention. The World Health Organization recommends a two-step approach to cancer pain management, beginning with non-opioids for slight-to-mild pain and adding an opioid as the pain intensity increases. Opioids have different potencies, and when a patient is changed from one opioid to another, it is imperative that equianalgesic dosages be used. Equianalgesic dose tables are based on comparative potencies to morphine (see Table 6.1). Opioids and non-opioids can be combined for additive analgesia. Opioid agonist-antagonists, such as pentazocine (e.g., Talwin), should be used with caution, if at all, since they may cause withdrawal syndrome.

Opioid analgesics are the cornerstone of management of moderate-to-severe cancer pain. These drugs, opiate agonists, attach to specific opiate receptors in the limbic system, thalamus, hypothalamus, spinal cord, and organs such as intestines. This leads to altered pain perception at the spinal cord and higher CNS levels. Because of this action, side effects that may occur include suppressed cough reflex; alterations in consciousness and mood (drowsiness, sedation, euphoria, dysphoria, mental clouding); respiratory depression; nausea/vomiting; constipation; and dependence. A recent study compared sustained-release oral morphine to transdermal fentanyl and oral methadone in cancer pain management (Mercadante et al., 2008). No differences in pain or symptom intensity were found or in adverse effects during titration or chronic treatment. Methadone was significantly less expensive. However, oral methadone requires skill in dosing and management (NCCN, 2013) due to the drug's biphasic half-life when used for chronic pain.

Unfortunately, some patients with cancer pain suffer needlessly because healthcare providers (physicians) underprescribe and (nurses) undermedicate (Marks and Sacher, 1973). Chronic cancer pain requires the patient to self-administer opioids "around-the-clock" rather than "as needed (PRN)" to prevent moderate-to-severe pain. The NCCN (2013) provides an excellent resource for cancer professionals to provide a comprehensive patient pain assessment, including consideration of a patient's cultural and linguistic ability so that patient and family education can be tailored to the patient, and reassessment can be accurate. Key concepts in cancer pain management are tolerance, physical and psychological dependence. Tolerance is the ability to receive larger amounts of a drug without ill effect and to show decreased effect (i.e., pain relief) with continued use of the same drug dose. Tolerance occurs over time, depending on the drug and the route of administration. In addition, tolerance to the respiratory depressant effects of opiates develops over time with chronic usage for prevention of cancer pain. For instance, a patient with severe cancer pain who has been receiving escalating doses over a period of time may require very high doses to finally eliminate or reduce the pain to acceptable levels, as in the case of a patient with head and neck cancer who required 1,200 mg/hour of morphine yet was still ambulatory and able to interact with family and friends. Opiate agonists may cause physical dependence (causing physical signs and symptoms of withdrawal if drug is stopped abruptly after chronic usage) and addiction (psychological dependence). However, addiction is VERY RARE in cancer patients, occurring in less than 0.1% of patients. This is important for healthcare professionals, as under-medication of patients with cancer pain causes the patient to have to "watch the clock" and request pain medication whenever it is due, giving the uninformed healthcare professional the impression the patient is "drug seeking" when, in fact, the patient is not receiving adequate analgesics.

MANAGEMENT

Table 6.1 Equianalgesic Dose Table

Drug / Opioid Agonist	Approximate Equianalgesic Oral Dose	Approximate Equianalgesic Parenteral Dose	Recommended Starting Dose (Adults > 50 kg Body Weight)	
			Oral	Parenteral
Morphine	30 mg q 3–4 h (around-the-clock dosing) 60 mg q 3–4 h (single dose or intermittent dosing)	10 mg q 3–4 h	30 mg q 3–4 h	10 mg q 3–4 h
Codeine	200 mg q 3–4 h	75 mg q 3–4 h	60 mg q 3–4 h	60 mg q 2 h (IM, SQ)
Fentanyl	—	0.1	—	
Hydromorphone (Dilaudid)	7.5 mg q 3–4 h	1.5 mg q 3–4 h	6 mg q 3–4 h	1.5 mg q 3–4 h
Hydrocodone (in Lorcet, Lortab, Vicodin, others)	30 mg q 3–4 h	Not available	10 mg q 3–4 h	Not applicable
Levorphanol (Levo-Dromoran)	4 mg q 6–8 h	2 mg q 6–8 h	4 mg q 6–8 h	2 mg q 6–8 h
Methadone (Dolophine, others)	20 mg q 6–8 h	10 mg q 6–8 h	20 mg q 6–8 h	10 mg q 6–8 h
Oxycodone (Roxicodone, also in Percocet, Percodan, Tylox, others)	15–20 mg q 3–4 h	Not available	10 mg q 3–4 h	Not applicable
Oxymorphone (Numorphan)	10 mg	1 mg q 3–6 h	10 mg q 3–6	1 mg q 3–6 h

Data from AHCPR, Public Health Service, U.S. Department of Health and Human Services. Rockville, MD. AHCPR Publication No. 92-0032; National Comprehensive Cancer Network Clinical Practice Guidelines: Adult Cancer Pain, v.2.2015. Available at http://www.nccn.org/professionals/physician_gls/pdf/pain.pdf, accessed 10.8.15.

Breakthrough pain management continues to be a significant challenge for healthcare professionals. Recognizing the different needs of different patients has led to a variety of formulations, especially of fentanyl, for the treatment of breakthrough pain in opioid-tolerant patients. Fentanyl is available as a transdermal patch delivery of fentanyl (20 times more potent than morphine) and as an immediate-release oral lozenge with mucosal absorption system (Actiq and generic equivalents). Other formulations available are fentanyl buccal tablet (Fentora), fentanyl buccal soluble film (Onsolis), sublingual (Abstral), sublingual spray (Subsys), and as a nasal spray (Lazanda). In addition, in an effort to avoid the pitfalls of the individuals who abuse drugs, OxyContin was reformulated to discourage abuse. In the past, abusers were able to use the controlled-release product to release a large quantity of oxycodone all at once. The reformulated OxyContin has tamper-resistant properties, although it can still be abused. In 2006, more than 4 million people aged 12 and over reported using OxyContin for nonmedical uses at least once in their lifetime, and more than 500,000 were new, nonmedical users (U.S. Substance Abuse and Mental Health Services Administration, 2007, 2008). All long-acting and extended-release opioid analgesics now require an accompanying Risk Evaluation and Mitigation Strategy (REMS) program. Similar to that for ESAs, the REMS includes a patient medication guide and provider educational programs and materials (which include appropriate patient selection and dosing) so that prescribers, pharmacists, and patients will understand their responsibilities for the safe prescription, dispensing, and self-administration of the drug. Some drugs, such as the new fentanyl formulations, require a signed patient educational review. Newer technology is being incorporated into novel formulations to discourage opioid abuse and tampering, such as the oxycodone fomulation Oxecta, which uses Aversion Technology to discourage abuse of the oxycodone for injection (forms a gel that cannot be dissolved) or snorted (irritates the nasal passages). A REMS for transmucosal immediate release fentanyl (TIRF) is required by the FDA to assure standardization between/among products and to ensure informed risk-benefit decisions before starting and during treatment. TIRF medications are indicated only for the management of breakthrough pain in adult cancer patients age 18 and over (age 16 and over for Actiq and generic equivalents) who are already receiving and are tolerant to around-the-clock opioid therapy for cancer-related persistent pain. Opioid-tolerant is defined as taking at least: 60 mg of oral morphine/day, 25 mcg transdermal fentanyl/hr, 30 mg oral oxycodone/day, 8 mg oral hydromorphone/day, 25 mg oral oxymorphone/day, or an equianalgesic dose of another opioid/day for a week or longer. Patients receiving TIRF medications should be screened for, and taught about avoidance of, drugs that are CYP3A4 inhibitors, as the drug interaction may result in an increased fentanyl plasma serum level and increased toxicity (e.g., possibly fatal respiratory depression).

When trying to evaluate an opioid intervention, it is important to recall that this is the century of genomics. It is now clear that there is considerable genetic polymorphism in the cytochrome P450 family of enzymes (Bernard and Bruera, 2000), and that this can influence analgesic effect. For example, Payne (1998) states that 15% of Caucasians lack the enzyme CYP2D6 that is required to metabolize codeine to morphine, so this group will require higher doses to achieve the same effect. As genotyping becomes more a part of designing a plan of care, it is important to remember this. In addition, as nurses have always done, when one opioid is ineffective, care planning with physician colleagues is necessary to make sure that another opioid from a different class is tried.

MANAGEMENT

Non-Opioids: To meet the increasing needs of alternative administration formulations, ketorolac and acetaminophen are available as *parenteral* formulations.

Numerous practice guidelines are available, led by the National Comprehensive Cancer Network (NCCN, 2013). The guidelines give titration recommendations for patients who are either opioid-naïve or opioid-tolerant. Key points include the need for rapid titration of short-acting opioids to manage severe pain, before then determining the optimal analgesic regimen to control the patient's pain. For opioid-tolerant patients with a pain rating of > 4 (on a score of 0–10), calculate the previous 24-hour opioid requirement, convert to IV equivalent, and give 10–20% of the total dose. Other key points in the NCCN guidelines are (1) supplemental doses of analgesics should be administered when a pain from a procedure is anticipated, (2) if a patient is receiving a continuous IV PCA and it must be stopped due to a procedure/transport, administer the prescribed IV bolus dose immediately before the procedure/transport and give a subcutaneous dose equivalent to a 2-hour basal infusion rate, (3) anxiolytics should be given preemptively when feasible, and (4) titrate an opioid with caution in patients with risk factors, such as decreased renal/hepatic function, sleep apnea, or poor performance status.

References

Archimedes Pharma US Inc. Lazanda Prescribing Information. Bedminster, NJ: Archimedes Pharma US Inc., June 2011.

Bernard SA, Bruera E. Drug Interactions in Palliative Care. *J Clin Oncol* 2000; 18(8) 1780–1790.

Cadence Pharmaceuticals, Inc. Ofirmev Prescribing Information. San Diego, CA: Cadence Pharmaceuticals, Inc., November 2010.

Eliot L, Geiser R, Loewen G. Steady State Pharmacokinetic Comparison of a New Once-daily, Extended Release Morphine Formulation (Morphelan) and OxyContin Twice Daily. *J Oncol Pharm Pract* 2001; 71–78.

Epictetus, arranged and translated by Hastings Crossley as part of the Gutenberg Project (released 2006). The Golden Sayings of Epictetus. The Project Gutenberg E Book. Available online at http://www.gutenberg.org/files/871/871-h/871-h.htm, accessed July 2, 2011.

Ferrell BR, Rivera LM. Cancer Pain Education for Patients. *Semin Oncol Nurs* 1997; 13 42–48.

Foley KM. Controlling Cancer Pain. *Hospital Practice* 2000; 35(4) 101–112.

Foley KM. The Treatment of Cancer Pain *N Engl J Med* 1995; 313 84–95.

Food and Drug Administration 2012; Transmucosal Immediate Release Fentanyl Risk Evaluation Mitigation Strategy Access Program: Available at http://www.tirfremaccess.com, accessed June 22, 2012.

Holmes MD, Chen WY, LiL, et al. Aspirin Intake and Survival after Breast Cancer. *J Clin Oncol* 2010; 28(9) 1467–1472.

Horizon Pharma USA Inc. Duexis Prescribing Information. Northbrook, IL: Horizon Pharma USA Inc., April 2011.

Jacox A, Carr DB, Payne R. Management of Cancer Pain. *Clinical Practice Guideline No 9 (AHCPR Pub No 94–0592)*. Rockville, MD: Agency for Health Care Policy & Research USDHHS; 1994.

Jannsen Pharmaceuticals, Inc. Duragesic [package insert]. Titusville, NJ: April 2014.

Kaiko RF, Wallenstein SL, Rogers AG, et al. Opioids in the Elderly. *Med Clin North Am* 1982; 66 1079–1089.

Marks RM, Sacher EJ. Undertreatment of Medical Inpatients with Opioid Analgesics. *Ann Intern Med* 1973; 78 173–181.

McCaffery M. *Nursing. Management of the Patient with Pain.* Philadelphia, PA: JB Lippincott Co.; 1982.

McDonald AA and Portenoy RK. How to Use Antidepressants and Anticonvulsants as Adjuvant Analgesics in the Treatment of Neuropathic Cancer Pain. *Supportive Oncology* 2006; 4(1) 43–52.

Meda Pharmaceuticals, Inc. *Onsolis* [package insert] Somerset, NJ: Meda Pharmaceuticals, Inc.; June 2009.

Mercadante S, Porzio G, Ferrera P, et al. Sustained-Release Oral Morphine Versus Transdermal Fentanyl and Oral Methadone in Cancer Pain Management. *Eur J Pain* published online at DOI 10.1016/j.ejpain.2008.01.013. Accessed June 24, 2008.

National Comprehensive Cancer Center. *Adult Cancer Pain.* v.2.2013. Rockville, MD; NCCN.

Payne R, *Pharmacologic Management of Pain, Section IA3. Berger A, Portenoy RK, Weissman DE, Principles and Practice of Supportive Oncology.* Philadelphia, PA: Lippincott-Raven Publishers; 1998.

ProStraken Inc. Abstral Prescribing Information. Bedminster NJ: ProStraken Inc, January 2011.

Purdue Pharma. Oxycontin Prescribing Information. Stamford, CT: Purdue Pharma LP, November 2010.

Roxane Laboratories. Dear Doctor Letter: Important Safety Information Regarding Morphine Sulfate Oral Solution 100 mg per 5 mL (20 mg/mL). December 2010.

Smith EM, Pang H, Cirrincione C et al. (2013). Effect of duloxetine on pain, function, and quality of life among patients with chemotherapy-induced painful peripheral neuropathy: A randomized clinical trial. *J Am Med Assoc* 309(13) 1359–67.

Tokunaga A, Saika M, Senba E. 5-HT2A Receptor Subtype Is Involved in the Thermal Hyperalgesic Mechanism of Serotonin in the Periphery. *Pain* 1998; 76 349–355.

U.S. Substance Abuse and Mental Health Services Administration, Office of Applied Studies. *Results from the 2006 National Survey on Drug Use and Health: National Findings.* 1007; NSDUH Series H 32, DHHS Publication No (SMA) 07–4293. Rockville, MD.

US Substance Abuse and Mental Health Services Administration. Oxycontin Prescription Drug Abuse: 2008 Revision. *Substance Abuse Treatment Advisory* 2008; 7(1) 1–8.

Wilkie D. Neural Mechanisms of Pain: A Foundation for Cancer Pain Assessment and Management. Maguire DB, Yarbro CH, Ferrell BR, *Cancer Pain Management* 2nd ed. Sudbury, MA: Jones and Bartlett Publishers; 1995; 61–87.

Zeppetella G, O'Doherty CA, Collins S. Prevalence and Characteristics of Breakthrough Pain in Cancer Patients Admitted to a Hospice. *J Pain Symptom Manage* 2000; 20 87–92.

Zycliz Z, Smits C, Krajnik M. Paroxetine for Pruritus in Advanced Cancer. *J Pain Symptom Management* 1996; 16 121–124.

MANAGEMENT

NON-OPIOID ANALGESICS

Drug: acetaminophen (Acephen, Actamin, Anacin-3, Apacet, Anesin, Dapa, Datril, Genapap, Genebs, Gentabs, Halenol, Liquiprin, Meda Cap, Panadol, Panex, Suppap, Tempra, Tenol, Ty Caps, Tylenol)

Class: Miscellaneous analgesic/antipyretic.

Mechanism of Action: Appears to inhibit prostaglandin synthesis centrally, thus preventing sensitization of pain receptors to chemical or mechanical stimulation. Mechanism is similar to salicylates but is not uricosuric. May have weak anti-inflammatory effects in nonrheumatoid conditions (e.g., after oral surgery). Reduces fever by direct effect on hypothalamus; heat is lost through vasodilation and increased peripheral blood flow. Analgesic and antipyretic action similar to aspirin.

Metabolism: Rapidly absorbed from GI tract; 25% serum protein-binding. Elimination half-life is 1–3 hours. Metabolized by the liver and excreted in the urine.

Indication: For the relief of pain and discomfort, and to reduce fever.

Dosage/Range:
- 325–650 mg every 4–6 hours PRN for pain, discomfort. Some individuals may need increased single doses of 1 g.
- Maximum dose in 24 hours: Adults: 10 tablets (3,250 mg) and in children 5 tablets (1,625 mg).

Drug Preparation:
- Ensure seals on tamper-resistant package are intact when opening new package.

Drug Administration:
- Oral, rectal, elixir.

Drug Interactions:
- Hepatotoxicity of acetaminophen may be increased by chronic use of high doses of drugs using hepatic microsomal enzyme system: barbiturates, carbamazepine, rifampin, phenytoin, sulfinpyrazone.
- Alcohol: increased risk of hepatic damage with chronic, excessive use.
- Diflunisal: increased acetaminophen serum level; avoid concurrent use.
- Phenothiazines: possible severe hypothermia may occur when used concomitantly.

Lab Effects/Interference:
- None known.

Special Considerations:
- Elixirs contain alcohol (Tylenol, Valadol).
- Contraindicated in patients with known hypersensitivity; use cautiously, if at all, in patients with hepatic or renal dysfunction.
- Chronic ingestion of large doses of acetaminophen may slightly potentiate effects of coumarin and other anticoagulants.

Potential Toxicities/Side Effects and the Nursing Process

I.   KNOWLEDGE DEFICIT related to SELF-ADMINISTRATION

Defining Characteristics: Fever curve or excessive fever can be masked by self-dosing with acetaminophen.

Nursing Implications: Instruct patient to report temperature over 38.3°C (101°F) or persistent or recurrent fever. Assess other over-the-counter (OTC) medicines the patient may be taking.

II.   POTENTIAL INJURY related to HEPATOTOXICITY

Defining Characteristics: Excessive alcoholic intake and other drugs can increase risk for hepatotoxicity.

Nursing Implications: Assess total acetaminophen dosage/24 hours, taking into account OTC medications. Assess baseline LFTs, especially if the patient has primary hepatoma or liver metastasis. Teach patient to avoid excessive alcohol intake and/or excessive acetaminophen intake.

Drug: acetaminophen injection (Ofirmev)

Class: Miscellaneous analgesic/antipyretic.

Mechanism of Action: Appears to inhibit prostaglandin synthesis centrally, thus preventing sensitization of pain receptors to chemical or mechanical stimulation. Mechanism is similar to salicylates but is not uricosuric. May have weak anti-inflammatory effects in nonrheumatoid conditions (e.g., after oral surgery). Reduces fever by direct effect on hypothalamus; heat is lost through vasodilation and increased peripheral blood flow. Analgesic and antipyretic action similar to aspirin.

Metabolism: C_{max} (maximum concentration) reached at end of 15-minute IV infusion, and is about 70% higher than that achieved with oral administration of the same dose. However, the AUC is similar following oral and IV administration of the same dose. Low binding (10–25%) to plasma proteins. Metabolized by the liver (primarily CYP2E1 microenzyme) and metabolites excreted in the urine (< 5% intact drug). Elimination half-life is 1–3 hours, with > 90% of the administered dose excreted within 24 hours.

Indications: FDA-indicated for the management of mild-to-moderate pain, management of moderate-to-severe pain with adjunctive opioid analgesics, and reduction of fever.

Contraindications: Severe liver impairment, severe active liver disease, or hypersensitivity to drug or its components.

Dosage/Range:
- Adults and adolescents weighing > 50 kg: 1,000 mg every 6 hours or 650 mg every 4 hours to a maximum of 4,000 mg/day. Minimum dosing interval is 4 hours.
- Adults and adolescents weighing < 50 kg: 15 mg/kg every 6 hours or 12.5 mg/kg every 4 hours to a maximum or 75 mg/kg/day. Minimum dosing interval is 4 hours.
- Children > 2 years to 12 years old: 15 mg/kg every 6 hours or 12.5 mg/kg every 4 hours to a maximum of 75 mg/kg/day. Minimum dosing interval is 4 hours.
- Use cautiously in patients with liver impairment or active hepatic disease, alcoholism, chronic malnutrition, severe hypovolemia, or severe renal impairment.

Drug Preparation: Injection for IV infusion: each 100 mL glass vial contains 1,000 mg acetaminophen (10 mg/mL). Inspect the vial for any particulate matter or discoloration, and discard if found. Aseptically, attach a vented intravenous (IV) set into the septum of the 100-mL vial for patients ordered for 1,000-mg dose. Drug can be administered without further dilution.

Do not add any other medications to the vial or infusion device. For doses < 1,000 mg, aseptically withdraw the ordered amount from an intact sealed vial and place in a separate, empty sterile container (e.g., glass bottle, plastic IV container, or syringe) for IV infusion.
- Available in carton of 24 vials. Store at 20–25°C (68–77°F).
- Vial is a single-use, preservative-free vial, and any unused portion must be discarded. Put small-volume pediatric doses up to 60 mL in a syringe and administer over 15 minutes.
- Once vacuum seal of the glass vial has been penetrated, or the contents transferred to another container, administer the dose within 6 hours.
- DO NOT add other medications to IV tubing; e.g., diazepam and chlorpromazine HCl are physically incompatible.

Drug Administration: Administer 1,000-mg dose IV via vented IV set over 15 minutes, ensuring that at the completion of the infusion, the tubing is shut off to prevent inadvertent air embolism.

Drug Interactions:
- Incompatible with diazepam and chlorpromazine HCl.
- Ethanol: Increased risk of hepatotoxicity. Substances that induce or regulate hepatic cytochrome enzyme.
- CYP2E1 may alter the metabolism of acetaminophen and increase its hepatotoxic potential (substrates are acetaminophen, alcohol; inhibitors are disulfiram [Antabuse]; inducers are ethanol and isoniazid [Laniazid]). Ethanol has a complex relationship with acetaminophen: Excess ethanol intake can induce hepatic cytochromes, but it also acts as a competitive inhibitor of acetaminophen metabolism.
- Anticoagulants: Increased INR when administered with chronic administration of oral acetaminophen at 4,000 mg/day; data shows INR increases in some patients who have been stabilized on sodium warfarin; assess INR more frequently and dose warfarin accordingly.

Lab Effects/Interference: May increase LFTs.

Special Considerations:
- Drug is contraindicated in patients with (1) known hypersensitivity to acetaminophen or to any of the excipients in the IV formulation, or (2) with severe hepatic impairment or severe active liver disease. Administration of acetaminophen in doses higher than recommended may result in hepatic injury, including the risk of severe hepatotoxicity and death. Do not exceed the maximum recommended daily dose of acetaminophen.
- Use caution when administering acetaminophen to patients with: (1) hepatic impairment or active hepatic disease, (2) alcoholism, (3) chronic malnutrition, (4) severe hypovolemia, or (5) severe renal impairment (creatinine clearance < 30 mL/min).
- Post-marketing reports indicate that hypersensitivity and anaphylaxis have occurred, characterized by swelling of the face and throat, respiratory distress, urticaria, rash, and pruritus. Discontinue drug immediately if allergic or hypersensitivity reactions occur. DO NOT administer to patients with an allergy to acetaminophen.
- Most common adverse reactions were nausea, vomiting, headache, and insomnia in adult patients; in children, nausea, vomiting, constipation, pruritus, agitation, and atelectasis are most common.
- Overdosage: acute overdosage is dose-dependent and potentially fatal. Sequelae are hepatic necrosis (90% hepatic damage in patients with acetaminophen level > 300 mcg/mL

at 4 hours after ingestion; minimal damage if plasma level < 150 mcg/mL at 4 hours or < 37.5 mcg/mL at 12 hours), renal tubular necrosis, hypoglycemic coma, and thrombocytopenia. Early symptoms of potentially hepatotoxic overdose: nausea, vomiting, diaphoresis, general malaise. Laboratory evidence of hepatotoxicity may not be apparent until 48–72 hours post-ingestion. Antidote is N-acetylcysteine (NAC, e.g., Mucomyst), which should be administered emergently. Poison Control Center 1-800-222-1222.

- Use in special populations:
  - Drug is pregnancy class C: Use drug only if clearly needed (no studies have been done with IV formulation).
  - Nursing mothers: Studies show infant receives about 1–2% of the mother's dose; use drug cautiously, if at all, in nursing mothers.
  - Pediatrics < 2 years old: Has not been studied, and is not recommended.
  - Severe renal impairment (creatinine clearance < 30 mL/min): Consider reduced daily dose given with longer dosing intervals.

Potential Toxicities/Side Effects and the Nursing Process

I.   KNOWLEDGE DEFICIT related to SELF-ADMINISTRATION

Defining Characteristics: Fever curve or excessive fever can be masked by self-dosing with acetaminophen.

Nursing Implications: Instruct patient to report temperature over 38.3°C (101°F) or persistent or recurrent fever. Assess other over-the-counter (OTC) medicines the patient may be taking.

II.   POTENTIAL INJURY related to HEPATOTOXICITY

Defining Characteristics: Excessive alcoholic intake and other drugs can increase risk for hepatotoxicity.

Nursing Implications: Assess total acetaminophen dosage/24 hours, taking into account OTC medications. Assess baseline LFTs, especially if the patient has primary hepatoma or liver metastasis. Teach patient to avoid excessive alcohol intake and/or excessive acetaminophen intake.

Drug: aspirin, acetylsalicylic acid (ASA, Aspergum, Bayer Aspirin, Easprin, Ecotrin, Empirin)

Class: Salicylate.

Mechanism of Action: Inhibits prostaglandin synthesis, peripherally preventing sensitization of pain receptors by mechanical and chemical stimuli. Also has anti-inflammatory effect, producing analgesic and antipyretic effects. Central action via hypothalamus unclear.

MANAGEMENT

Metabolism: Rapidly and well absorbed from GI tract, and distributed throughout the body with high concentrations in liver and kidney. Drug is bound to serum proteins, especially albumin. Metabolized by liver and excreted in urine.

Indication: For the relief of pain and the reduction of fever.

Dosage/Range:
- 325–650 mg PO or PR every 4 hours PRN for pain or fever (maximum 3.9 g/day).

Drug Preparation:
- Keep in closed container, away from heat, to prevent drug decomposition.
- Do not use if strong, vinegar-like odor is present. Do not crush enteric-coated aspirin.

Drug Administration:
- Oral or rectal suppositories. Give oral dose with 240 mL water or milk to decrease gastric irritation.
- Oral solution may be made from effervescent aspirin powders (e.g., Alka-Seltzer); Alka-Seltzer chewable aspirin tablets available.

Drug Interactions:
- Ammonium chloride, ascorbic acid, or methionine (urine acidifiers): Decrease ASA excretion, so increase risk of ASA toxicity.
- Antacids, urinary alkalizers: May increase ASA excretion, so may decrease the ASA effect. Alcohol increases the risk of GI ulceration, bleeding.
- Decreased effect of angiotensin-converting enzyme (ACE) inhibitors. When used together, the effect of anticoagulants may be enhanced (additive hypothrombinemic effect), leading to prolonged bleeding time. DO NOT USE TOGETHER.
- Beta-adrenergic blockers (e.g., propranolol): Possible decrease in antihypertensive effect.
- Corticosteroids: Increase in aspirin excretion with decrease in aspirin effect.
- Methotrexate: Increase in methotrexate serum levels with increased toxicity. DO NOT USE CONCURRENTLY.
- NSAIDs: Decrease in NSAID serum concentration; may have increased incidence of GI side effects. Not recommended to be used together.
- Probenecid, sulfinpyrazone: aspirin (doses ≥ 3 g/day) antagonizes uricosuric drug effect.
- Spirolactone: Aspirin may inhibit diuretic effect.
- Sulfonylureas, exogenous insulin: Aspirin may have hypoglycemic effect and may potentiate these drug actions. Monitor for hypoglycemia.
- Valproic acid: Aspirin displaces drug and decreases its excretion, resulting in increased serum levels and possible valproic acid toxicity.

Lab Effects/Interference:
- Prolonged bleeding time, leukopenia, thrombocytopenia.

Special Considerations:
- Patients receiving myelosuppressive chemotherapy should be cautioned not to take aspirin due to increased risk of bleeding.
- Patients should be instructed to take drug with food or milk.

- Use cautiously in patients with asthma, rhinitis, or nasal polyps (can cause severe bronchospasm).
- Drug is contraindicated in patients with GI ulcer, GI bleeding, hypersensitivity to aspirin, increased bleeding tendencies.
- Use cautiously in patients with liver damage, hypoprothrombinemia, or with vitamin K deficiency.
- Aspirin administration in patients with breast cancer may reduce recurrence and death, as aspirin appears to inhibit metastases. A study showed that women who were alive for at least 1 year after being diagnosed with breast cancer, who took aspirin (1–7 days of aspirin use per week), had a decreased risk of recurrence and death compared to those who did not take aspirin (Holmes et al., 2010).

Potential Toxicities/Side Effects and the Nursing Process

I. ALTERATION IN NUTRITION, LESS THAN BODY REQUIREMENTS, related to GI TOXICITY

Defining Characteristics: Nausea, dyspepsia (5–25% of patients), heartburn, epigastric discomfort, anorexia, and acute, reversible hepatotoxicity may occur. Risk increases with dose. May potentiate peptic ulcer disease.

Nursing Implications: Teach patient self-administration with 8 oz (240 ml) water or milk. If GI distress develops, discuss use of enteric-coated aspirin (e.g., Ecotrin). If patient receiving high doses of aspirin, monitor LFTs. Drug contraindicated in patients with peptic ulcer disease.

II. POTENTIAL FOR BLEEDING related to INHIBITION OF PLATELET AGGREGATION

Defining Characteristics: Aspirin may cause prolongation of bleeding time, leukopenia, thrombocytopenia, purpura, shortened erythrocyte survival time.

Nursing Implications: Teach patient to avoid aspirin and aspirin-containing drugs if receiving myelosuppressive chemotherapy. Review concurrent medications to identify risk for drug interactions. Monitor Hgb, HCT over time; teach patient signs/symptoms of anemia, and instruct to report them (headache, fatigue, chest pain, irritability). Monitor stool guaiacs.

III. INJURY related to MILD SALICYLISM

Defining Characteristics: Administration of large doses of salicylates may cause salicylism, characterized by dizziness, tinnitus, diminished hearing, nausea, vomiting, diarrhea, mental confusion, CNS depression, headache, sweating, and hyperventilation

MANAGEMENT

at serum salicylate concentration 150–300 μg/mL (use in cancer patients usually 100 μg/mL).

Nursing Implications: Teach patient to reduce dose, interrupt dose if signs/symptoms occur. Assess concurrent medications for possible drug interactions.

Drug: choline magnesium trisalicylate (Trilisate)

Class: Choline and magnesium salicylate combination.

Mechanism of Action: Analgesic effect through peripheral and central pathways, decreasing pain perception. Prostaglandin inhibition probably involved in peripheral mechanism. Antipyretic effect via hypothalmic heat regulation center. Does not interfere with platelet aggregation.

Metabolism: Rapidly absorbed from GI tract. Metabolized by the liver and excreted in the urine.

Indication: For the relief of pain, including pain related to osteoarthritis, RA.

Dosage/Range:
- Trilisate 750 mg bid or dose-increase to maximum 3200 mg/day.

Drug Preparation:
- Trilisate liquid 5 mL or Trilisate 500-mg tablet contains ASA equivalent of 650 mg.
- Trilisate 750-mg tablet contains 975 mg ASA.
- Trilisate 1,000-mg tablet contains 1,300 mg ASA.

Drug Administration:
- Oral.

Drug Interactions:
- Antacids, urine alkalinizers: Increase salicylate excretion and decrease drug effect. Do not administer with antacids.
- Ammonium chloride, ascorbic acid, methionine (urine acidifiers): Decrease salicylate excretion, so increased risk of salicylate toxicity.
- Concomitant administration with alcohol, steroids, other NSAIDs may increase GI side effects.
- Corticosteroids: May increase salicylate excretion and decrease trilisate effect.
- Warfarin: May have increased warfarin levels and increased PT; monitor patient closely, and reduce warfarin dosage as needed.

Lab Effects/Interference:
- Free T_4 may be increased with a concurrent decrease in total plasma T_4 (does not affect thyroid function).

Special Considerations:
- Drug does not interfere with platelet aggregation.
- Use cautiously in patients with chronic renal failure, gastritis.

- Contraindicated if known hypersensitivity to salicylates.
- Drug contains magnesium, so periodic evaluation of serum magnesium should be performed.

Potential Toxicities/Side Effects and the Nursing Process

I.   ALTERATION IN NUTRITION, LESS THAN BODY REQUIREMENTS, related to GI TOXICITY

Defining Characteristics: Fewer GI side effects than aspirin. Nausea, dyspepsia (5–25% of patients), heartburn, epigastric discomfort, anorexia, and acute reversible hepatotoxicity may occur. Risk increases with dose. May potentiate peptic ulcer disease.

Nursing Implications: Teach patient self-administration with food, or 8 oz. (240 mL) water or milk. If patient is receiving antacid, administer antacid 2 hours after meals and Trilisate before meals. Assess baseline liver and renal function and monitor if patient is receiving high doses on ongoing basis. Guaiac stool to assess occult blood, as gastric ulceration may occur.

II.   INJURY related to MILD SALICYLISM

Defining Characteristics: Administration of large doses of salicylates may cause salicylism, characterized by dizziness, tinnitus, diminished hearing, nausea, vomiting, diarrhea, mental confusion, CNS depression, headache, sweating, and hyperventilation at serum salicylate concentration 150–300 µg/mL (use in cancer patients usually 100 µg/mL).

Nursing Implications: Teach patient to reduce dose, interrupt dose if signs/symptoms occur. Assess concurrent medications for possible drug interactions.

III.   POTENTIAL ALTERATION IN URINARY ELIMINATION related to RENAL PROSTAGLANDIN INHIBITION

Defining Characteristics: Rarely, elevated serum BUN and creatinine may occur.

Nursing Implications: Assess baseline serum BUN, creatinine, and monitor during therapy.

Drug: clonidine hydrochloride (Duraclon)

Class: Antiadrenergic agent.

Mechanism of Action: Acts centrally to stimulate alpha-2-adrenergic receptors in the CNS, thus inhibiting sympathetic vasomotor centers. When given epidurally, the drug is believed to mimic norepinephrine activity at presynaptic and postjunctional alpha-2-adrenoceptors in the dorsal horn of the spinal cord. Is administered together with opioids for severe cancer pain to maximize analgesia. Clonidine HCl shows best efficacy against neuropathic pain.

Metabolism: Drug is highly lipid-soluble and rapidly distributes into extravascular sites and into the CNS; enters the plasma via the epidural veins, leading to hypotensive effect. Drug is metabolized and excreted in the urine (72% of the administered dose in 96 hours, and 40–50% of that is unchanged drug).

Indication: In combination with opiates for the treatment of severe pain in cancer patients that is not adequately relieved by opioid analgesics alone. Drug may be more effective in patients with neuropathic pain than somatic or visceral pain.

Contraindicated in patients sensitive or allergic to clonidine HCl; epidural administration contraindicated if (1) injection-site infection occurs, (2) patient is receiving anticoagulation, (3) patient has bleeding diathesis, (4) administered above the C4 dermatome, (5) patient has severe cardiac disease or is hemodynamically unstable, or (6) used in obstetrical or postoperative analgesia.

Dosage/Range:
To be administered in combination with opioids via epidural route:
• Initial: Starting dose is 30 µg/hr.
• May be titrated up to 40 µg/hr or down, based on degree of pain relief and extent of side effects.

Drug Preparation:
• Preservative-free preparation.
• Given epidurally in combination with opioid via continuous epidural infusion device.

Drug Interactions:
• CNS depressants (e.g., alcohol, barbiturates): Potentiation of CNS depression.
• Opioid analgesics: May potentiate hypotension due to clonidine.
• Tricyclic antidepressants: May antagonize hypotensive effect of clonidine.
• Beta-blockers: May exacerbate hypertensive symptoms of clonidine withdrawal.
• Epidural local anesthetics: Clonidine may prolong pharmacologic effects of local anesthetic; both motor and sensory blockade.

Lab Effects/Interference:
• None known.

Special Considerations:
• Use cautiously in patients receiving digitalis, calcium channel blockers, and beta-blockers, as there may be additive effects of bradycardia and AV block.
• Severe hypotension may occur during first 2 days of clonidine therapy, especially when drug is infused into the upper thoracic spinal segments—monitor vital signs frequently.
• Do not suddenly withdraw drug, as this may result in nervousness, agitation, headache, tremor, rapid increase in blood pressure; scrupulously maintain drug administration equipment to prevent accidental interruption of drug. Drug dose should be gradually decreased over 2–4 days. If patient is receiving a beta-blocker, the beta-blocker should be discontinued several days before the gradual discontinuation of epidural clonidine. Teach patient NOT to discontinue drug on own.

Potential Toxicities/Side Effects and the Nursing Process

I.   ALTERED TISSUE PERFUSION related to HYPOTENSION

Defining Characteristics: Hypotension usually occurs within the first 4 days after beginning epidural clonidine but may also occur throughout treatment. Increased risk in patients receiving infusion into upper-thoracic spinal segments, in women, and in patients who have low body weight. Hypotension may be accentuated by concurrent opiate administration. Clonidine decreases sympathetic CNS outflow, decreasing peripheral resistance, decreasing renal vascular resistance, and decreasing heart rate and BP.

Nursing Implications: Monitor T, BP, HR frequently, especially during first few days of therapy. Notify physician of significant changes. Expect IV fluids to be given to correct hypotension, and if needed, IV ephedrine. Symptomatic bradycardia can be treated with atropine.

II.   ALTERED TISSUE PERFUSION related to REBOUND HYPERTENSION

Defining Characteristics: Withdrawal symptoms can occur if drug is interrupted or stopped abruptly; characterized by nervousness, agitation, headache, tremor, rapid increase in BP. Increased risk in patients receiving high drug doses, patients receiving beta-blockers, or patients with a history of hypertension. Rarely, this may result in CVA, hypertensive encephalopathy, or death.

Nursing Implications: Scrupulously manage/maintain catheter and pump to prevent interruption in flow; teach patient catheter and pump care and use; instruct patient never to abruptly discontinue medicine; anticipate physician will discontinue beta-blockers prior to gradual taper of drug over 2–4 days when drug is being discontinued.

III.   POTENTIAL FOR INFECTION related to IMPLANTED DEVICE

Defining Characteristics: Implanted epidural catheter may become infected, leading to epidural abscess or meningitis.

Nursing Implications: Scrupulously maintain catheter, using sterile technique; teach patient catheter care and management; monitor for signs/symptoms of infection and teach patient this assessment. If in the hospital, monitor for fever and pain and notify the physician immediately if either occurs. Instruct patient to report fever, pain to the physician immediately if at home.

Drug: gabapentin (Neurontin)

Class: Anticonvulsant.

Mechanism of Action: Not clearly understood. Drug is structurally related to neurotransmitter GABA (gamma-amino-butyric acid), but drug does not bind to GABA receptor

MANAGEMENT

sites. It is unclear whether drug has activity at NMDA receptor sites. Drug has been shown to bind to receptor sites in neocortex and hippocampus.

Metabolism: Bioavailability of drug decreases as dose increases, and drug absorption unaffected by food. Drug half-life is 5–7 hours, and drug excreted unchanged in the urine. Plasma clearance may be reduced in elderly and is reduced in renal insufficiency.

Indication: For the management of patients with post-herpetic neuralgia, and epilepsy.

Dosage/Range:
- Initial titration: 300 mg on day 1, 300 mg bid on day 2, and 300 mg tid on day 3.
- As needed, dose may be titrated up to 400 mg tid, in increments, to a maximum dose of 600 mg tid (1,800 mg total dose per day).
- Dose-reduce in renal insufficiency:

Creatinine Clearance	Drug Dose
30–60 mL/min	300 mg bid
15–30 mL/min	300 mg/day
< 15 mL/min	300 mg every other day

Drug Preparation:
- Oral, take without regard to food intake.
- Take 1 hour before, or 2 hours after, antacid.
- Take initial dose at bedtime to enhance somnolence and minimize dizziness, fatigue, and ataxia.
- Doses should not be separated by > 12 hours (must be tid, e.g., every 8 hours).
- If drug is discontinued or changed to another anticonvulsant, gradually discontinue drug over 1 week.

Drug Interactions:
- Antacids: decrease bioavailability of drug.
- Cimetidine: decreases renal excretion of drug with potential for excess toxicity; monitor patient closely and dose-reduce if both drugs must be given concomitantly.

Lab Effects/Interference:
- Urinary protein test using Ames N-Multistix may be falsely positive.
- Drug may cause leukopenia, anemia, thrombocytopenia.

Special Considerations:
- Dose-reduce in patients with renal insufficiency, and consider dose reduction in the elderly.
- Drug helpful in the management of painful peripheral neuropathies.
- Drug may cause dizziness, fatigue, drowsiness, ataxia, so patient should be taught to avoid activities requiring mental acuity, such as driving, until after full effect of drug is known.

Potential Toxicities/Side Effects and the Nursing Process

I.   SENSORY/PERCEPTUAL ALTERATIONS related to CNS CHANGES

Defining Characteristics: The most common side effects are somnolence, ataxia, dizziness, and fatigue. Less commonly, nystagmus, tremor, nervousness, dysarthria, amnesia, depression, abnormal thought processes, incoordination, headache, confusion, emotional lability, paresthesia, areflexia, anxiety, hostility, syncope, hypesthesia may occur. Seizures have been reported, as have suicidal tendencies. Other sensory side effects that rarely occur are diplopia, abnormal vision, dry eyes, photophobia, ptosis, and hearing loss.

Nursing Implications: Assess baseline neurologic status and document. Instruct patient of general side effects that may occur, and to report them. Assess for suicidal ideation. If significant CNS changes occur, discuss dose reduction or change to an alternative drug with physician. Instruct patient not to drive a car or to do activities that require mental acuity until full effect of drug is known.

II.   ALTERATION IN NUTRITION related to GI TOXICITY

Defining Characteristics: Nausea and vomiting may occur. Less commonly, dyspepsia, dry mouth, constipation, increased or decreased appetite, thirst, stomatitis, taste changes, increased salivation, fecal incontinence may occur

Nursing Implications: Assess patient tolerance of GI side effects. Instruct patient to report side effects. If nausea and vomiting occur, discuss changing to another medication or adding antiemetic agent to regimen if relief of peripheral neuropathy is achieved.

III.   ALTERATION IN SKIN INTEGRITY related to RASH

Defining Characteristics: Rash may occur, as may pruritus, acne, alopecia, hirsutism, herpes simplex, dry skin, and increased sweating.

Nursing Implications: Perform baseline skin assessment, and note any areas that are not intact. Teach patient to self-assess for rash, other changes, and to report them. If rash develops, instruct patient to notify provider immediately. If itch occurs, discuss symptomatic management.

IV.   ALTERATION IN RESPIRATORY PATTERN related to RHINITIS, COUGH

Defining Characteristics: Rhinitis, pharyngitis, coughing, pneumonia, dyspnea may occur. Rarely, epistaxis and apnea have been reported.

Nursing Implications: Assess baseline respiratory pattern, and instruct patient to report any changes. Discuss any significant changes with physician, and discuss management versus change of drug.

MANAGEMENT

V.   ALTERATION IN URINARY ELIMINATION related to URINARY CHANGES

Defining Characteristics: Hematuria, dysuria, frequency, urinary incontinence, cystitis, urinary retention may occur.

Nursing Implications: Assess baseline urinary elimination pattern, and instruct patient of possible side effects and to report them. Discuss symptomatic management, or discuss drug change with physician if changes are significant.

VI.   POTENTIAL FOR SEXUAL DYSFUNCTION related to VAGINAL CHANGES AND IMPOTENCE

Defining Characteristics: Vaginal hemorrhage, amenorrhea, dysmenorrhea, menorrhagia, inability to climax, abnormal ejaculation, and impotence have been reported.

Nursing Implications: Assess baseline sexuality, and instruct patient to report any changes. If changes occur, discuss impact and distress caused, and together with physician and patient, discuss drug alternatives.

VII.   POTENTIAL ALTERATION IN OXYGENATION related to TACHYCARDIA, HYPOTENSION

Defining Characteristics: Rarely, hypertension, vasodilatation, hypotension, angina pectoris, peripheral vascular disease, palpitation, tachycardia, and appearance of a murmur may occur.

Nursing Implications: Assess baseline cardiovascular status, and instruct patient to notify provider if any changes occur. Instruct patient to report palpitations, fast heartbeat, dizziness, or chest pain immediately. If significant changes occur, discuss alternative drug therapy with physician.

Drug: ibuprofen (Advil, Genpril, Haltran, Ibuprin, Midol 200, Nuprin, Rufen; parenteral Caldolor injection)

Class: NSAID.

Mechanism of Action: Peripherally acting analgesic, anti-inflammatory, and antipyretic agent; anti-inflammatory action probably due to prostaglandin synthetase inhibition, but is not well understood.

Metabolism: 80% of oral dose absorbed from GI tract, and absorption rate is slowed by administration with food. Peak serum concentrations with tablet occur in 2 hours; suspension in 1 hour. Highly protein-bound (90–99%) and has a plasma half-life of 2–4 hours. Excreted in urine. The parenteral form has an elimination half-life of 2.22–2.44 hours.

Indications: (1) PO: relief of mild-to-moderate pain, pain from RA and osteoarthritis, treatment of primary dysmenorrhea; (2) IV formulation indicated for the short-term management of mild-to-moderate pain, for management of moderate-to-severe pain as an adjunct to opioid analgesia, and for the reduction of fever. Use lowest dosage for shortest duration to achieve desired effect. Drug may cause serious and potentially fatal cardiovascular thrombotic events, as well as serious and potentially fatal GI reactions.

Dosage/Range:
- Oral: 200–800 mg every 4–8 hours PRN to maximum of 3,200 mg/24 hours.
- IV: Pain: 400 mg–800 mg IV over 30 minutes every 6 hours as needed; fever: 400 mg IV over 30 minutes, followed by 400 mg every 4–6 hours or 100–200 mg every 4 hours as needed.

Drug Preparation:
- Tablets: 200 mg, 300 mg, 400 mg, 600 mg, 800 mg.
- Caplets: 200 mg.
- Oral suspension: 100 mg/5 mL.
- IV: Available as 400 mg/4 mL and 800 mg/8 mL (100 mg/mL). Aseptically add ordered dose to 200 mL (for 800-mg dose) or 100 mL (for 400-mg dose) 0.9% sodium chloride, 5% dextrose injection USP, or lactated Ringer's solution, so final concentration is 4 mg/mL or less. Stable for up to 24 hours at ambient temperature (20–25°C) and room lighting.

Drug Administration:
- Oral.
- IV: Administer over at least 30 minutes. Patients must be well-hydrated before drug is given.

Drug Interactions:
- Oral anticoagulants, thrombolytic agents: Possible increase in PT with increased bleeding; use with caution and monitor patient closely.
- Other NSAIDs, aspirin: Possible increase in GI toxicity; do not administer concomitantly.
- Furosemide, thiazide diuretics: Decreased diuretic effect when administered concomitantly.
- ACE inhibitors: NSAIDs may diminish the antihypertensive effect of ACE inhibitors.

Lab Effects/Interference:
- Slight decrease in Hgb not exceeding 1 g/dL without signs of bleeding; decrease in Hgb > 1 g/dL may be associated with signs of bleeding.
- IV formulation: Elevated hepatic transaminases, which may progress to liver failure.

Special Considerations:
- Contraindicated in patients with known hypersensitivity, asthmatic patients with nasal polyps and other patients who develop bronchospasm or angioedema with aspirin or other NSAIDs, and patients with peptic or duodenal ulcer. IV formulation also contraindicated during the perioperative period in the setting of coronary artery bypass graft (CABG) surgery.

- Use cautiously in patients with cardiac or renal dysfunction.
- NSAIDs may increase the risk of serious cardiovascular thrombotic events, myocardial infarction, and stroke, which can be fatal; risk appears to increase with duration of use.
- Discontinue IV formulation if abnormal LFTs persist or worsen.
- Long-term administration of NSAIDs can lead to papillary necrosis and other renal injury. Use cautiously in patients at risk (e.g., elderly; patients with renal impairment, heart failure, hepatic dysfunction, taking diuretics or ACE inhibitors).
- Fluid retention, edema, CHF can occur with NSAIDs; use cautiously in patients with edema or heart failure.
- Hypertension can occur with NSAIDs; monitor BP during therapy.
- Anaphylactoid reactions can occur with patients receiving NSAIDs. Discontinue drug if this occurs.
- Rarely, drug can cause serious skin reactions, such as epidermal necrolysis, which can be fatal. Discontinue drug if rash or other allergic signs or symptoms occur.

Potential Toxicities/Side Effects and the Nursing Process

I.   ALTERATION IN NUTRITION, LESS THAN BODY REQUIREMENTS, related to GI SIDE EFFECTS

Defining Characteristics: Dyspepsia, heartburn, nausea, vomiting, anorexia, diarrhea, constipation, stomatitis, bloating, epigastric and abdominal pain may occur.

Nursing Implications: Assess history of GI symptoms and history of ulcer disease. Teach patient to take NSAID with meals or milk. Teach patient potential side effects, and instruct to report them. If symptoms are severe, discuss alternative NSAIDs with physician.

II.   POTENTIAL FOR BLEEDING related to INHIBITION OF PLATELET AGGREGATION

Defining Characteristics: Drug can prolong bleeding time and inhibit platelet aggregation. Peptic ulceration and occult GI bleeding can occur and be life-threatening. Increased risk factors: smoking, alcoholism.

Nursing Implications: Assess risk, history of peptic ulcer disease or GI bleeding. Assess baseline Hgb, HCT, and presence/absence of occult bleeding by guaiac of stools. Instruct patient to report signs/symptoms of abdominal pain, black stools, blood per rectum, epistaxis, menorrhagia. If patient is at risk for bleeding, discuss with physician use of misoprostol to protect GI mucosa. Teach patient to avoid concurrent use of aspirin, other NSAIDs.

III.   POTENTIAL SENSORY/PERCEPTUAL ALTERATIONS related to CNS CHANGES

Defining Characteristics: Dizziness, headache, nervousness, fatigue, drowsiness, malaise/light-headedness, anxiety, confusion, mental depression, and emotional lability may occur.

Decreased hearing, visual acuity, changes in color vision, conjunctivitis, diplopia, and cataracts have been reported. In addition, though rare, aseptic meningitis has occurred.

Nursing Implications: Assess baseline neurologic and mental status. Instruct patient to report changes in sensory/perceptual pattern, especially VISUAL CHANGES. If visual changes occur, discuss with physician referral to ophthalmologist as soon as possible. Assess for rare occurrence of aseptic meningitis (fever, coma). Discuss drug continuance with physician for significant symptoms.

IV. ALTERATION IN NUTRITION, LESS THAN BODY REQUIREMENTS, related to HEPATIC TOXICITY

Defining Characteristics: Severe and sometimes fatal hepatotoxicity has occurred. Jaundice and hepatitis occur rarely. Borderline increase in LFTs occurs in 15% of patients, while values increase by three times in 1%.

Nursing Implications: Assess baseline LFTs and monitor periodically during long-term therapy. Instruct patient to report jaundice, abdominal pain. Discuss discontinuance of drug with physician for significant toxicity.

V. ALTERATION IN RENAL ELIMINATION related to INHIBITION OF RENAL PROSTAGLANDINS

Defining Characteristics: Acute renal failure may occur rarely within first few days of treatment in patients with preexisting renal dysfunction. Other signs/symptoms of renal dysfunction that may occur rarely are azotemia, cystitis, hematuria, increased serum BUN and creatinine, and decreased creatinine clearance. Peripheral edema has also been described.

Nursing Implications: Assess baseline renal function. Instruct patient to report any changes in urinary function. Monitor periodic serum BUN, creatinine during chronic therapy.

VI. ALTERATION IN SKIN INTEGRITY related to RASH

Defining Characteristics: Rash (urticaria, vesicles, or erythematous macular) may occur, as may Stevens-Johnson syndrome, flushes, alopecia, rectal itching, and acne.

Nursing Implications: Assess baseline skin integrity and presence of lesions. Teach patient to report abnormalities. Provide symptomatic relief for rashes, pruritus.

VII. POTENTIAL FOR FATIGUE, THROMBOCYTOPENIA, AND INFECTION related to BONE MARROW INJURY

Defining Characteristics: Neutropenia, agranulocytosis, aplastic anemia, hemolytic anemia, and thrombocytopenia may occur *rarely*.

MANAGEMENT

Nursing Implications: Assess baseline CBC, WBC, differential, and platelet count. Discuss abnormalities with physician. Instruct patient to report severe fatigue, infection, bleeding. Monitor lab values periodically during treatment.

Drug: ibuprofen/famotidine (Duexis)

Class: Combination NSAID and histamine H_2-receptor antagonist.

Mechanism of Action: Ibuprofen appears to provide analgesic and antipyretic actions via prostaglandin synthetase inhibition, which can increase the risk of gastrointestinal (GI) ulceration, especially in the setting of gastric acid. Famotidine is a competitive inhibitor of histamine H_2-receptor antagonist, which inhibits gastric secretion, resulting in suppression of both acid concentration and volume of gastric secretion.

Metabolism: Both ibuprofen and famotidine are rapidly absorbed, resulting in maximal ibuprofen serum concentration (C_{max}) in 1.9 hours after oral administration. C_{max} for famotidine is reached about 2 hours after dosing. Ibuprofen is extensively bound to plasma proteins, while 15–20% of famotidine is protein bound. Ibuprofen is eliminated from systemic circulation 2 hours after administration; it is rapidly metabolized and excreted in the urine so that ibuprofen is totally excreted in 24 hours after the last dose. Famotidine has a half-life of 4 hours, and is excreted by renal (65–70%) and metabolic routes.

Indication: (1) Relief of signs and symptoms of RA and osteoarthritis, and 2) reduction in the risk of developing upper GI ulcers (e.g., gastric and/or duodenal ulcers) in patients taking ibuprofen for those indications.

Dosage/Range: Drug tablet contains fixed-dose combination of ibuprofen 800 mg and famotidine 26.6 mg. One tablet orally, three times per day.

Drug Preparation: None. Available in a bottle of 90 tablets.

Drug Administration:
- Oral: Teach patient to swallow drug whole, and not to cut to supply a lower dose. Do not chew, divide, or crush tablet. If a dose is missed, it should be taken as soon as possible. If the next scheduled dose is due, do not take the missed dose but take the next dose on time. Do not take two doses at one time to make up for a missed dose.
- Drug is not recommended in patients with renal creatinine clearance < 50 mL/min as the elimination half-life of famotidine is increased and may exceed 20 hours.

Drug Interactions:
- Warfarin-type anticoagulants: Increased risk of serious GI bleeding.
- Aspirin: Increased risk of GI bleeding, other adverse events.
- Corticosteroids, antiplatelet drugs: Increased risk of GI bleeding.
- ACE-inhibitors and diuretics: Ibuprofen may reduce the effectiveness of these drugs.
- Lithium: Increased lithium levels (by ibuprofen interaction).
- Methotrexate: NSAIDs may decrease tubular secretion of methotrexate in the kidney; also displaces methotrexate from plasma proteins, increasing risk of methotrexate toxicity;

use together cautiously. Selective serotonin reuptake inhibitors (SSRIs): Increased risk of GI bleeding.

- Cholestyramine: Delayed absorption of ibuprofen.

Lab Effects/Interference: Increased LFTs, anemia, abnormal serum creatinine.

Special Considerations:

- FDA approval supported by data showing fewer upper GI ulcers when treated with ibuprofen/famotidine compared to ibuprofen alone (REDUCE-1 and REDUCE-2 studies).
- Contraindicated in patients: (1) with preexisting asthma, urticaria, or allergic reactions after taking aspirin or other NSAIDs; (2) in the perioperative period in the setting of coronary artery bypass graft surgery (CABG); (3) pregnant at 30 weeks gestation or later, as may cause premature closure of the ductus arteriosus in the fetus; or (4) with known hypersensitivity to other H_2-receptor antagonists.
- Two large, controlled clinical trials of a COX-2 selective NSAID for the treatment of pain in the first 10–14 days following CABG surgery found an increased incidence of stroke and MI. Thus drug is contraindicated in these patients.
- Anaphylaxis has been reported; discontinue drug immediately if an anaphylactoid reaction occurs.
- Serious skin reactions can occur (exfoliative dermatitis, Stevens-Johnson syndrome, toxic epidermal necrolysis, which can be fatal): Discontinue drug if rash or other signs of local skin reaction occur.
- Hepatic injury ranging from elevated LFTs to liver failure can occur. Discontinue drug immediately if abnormal LFTs persist or worsen, if clinical signs and symptoms of liver disease develop, or if systemic manifestations occur.
- NSAIDs increase the risk of serious GI adverse reactions, including bleeding, ulceration, and perforation of stomach or intestines, which can be fatal. Reactions can occur at any time without warning symptoms.
- The elderly are at greatest risk.
- Use drug cautiously with the elderly and in patients with:
  - Hypertension, which can occur with NSAID treatment; monitor BP closely during treatment.
  - CHF and edema; fluid retention and edema can occur with NSAID treatment.
  - Risk of bleeding; active and clinically significant bleeding from any source can occur; discontinue drug if active bleeding occur.
  - Renal impairment, heart failure, liver impairment, taking diuretics or ACE inhibitors: Long-term administration of NSAIDs can result in papillary necrosis and other renal injury.
  - Cardiovascular disease or risk factors for cardiovascular risk; thrombotic events, MI, and stroke, which may be fatal, may occur. Risk may increase with duration of use.
- Drug is pregnancy category C and should be used during pregnancy only if the potential benefit justifies the potential risk to the fetus (may cause premature closure of ductus arteriosus). Nursing mothers: Use drug with caution, as it is unknown if drug is excreted in human milk. Most common adverse reactions (> 1% than ibuprofen alone): nausea, diarrhea, constipation, upper abdominal pain, headache.

MANAGEMENT

Potential Toxicities/Side Effects and the Nursing Process

I.   ALTERATION IN NUTRITION, LESS THAN BODY REQUIREMENTS, related to GI SIDE EFFECTS

Defining Characteristics: Dyspepsia, heartburn, nausea, vomiting, anorexia, diarrhea, constipation, stomatitis, bloating, epigastric and abdominal pain may occur.

Nursing Implications: Assess history of GI symptoms and history of ulcer disease. Teach patient to take NSAID with meals or milk. Teach patient potential side effects, and instruct to report them. If symptoms are severe, discuss alternative NSAIDs with physician.

II.   POTENTIAL FOR BLEEDING related to INHIBITION OF PLATELET AGGREGATION

Defining Characteristics: Drug can prolong bleeding time and inhibit platelet aggregation. Peptic ulceration and occult GI bleeding can occur and be life-threatening. Increased risk factors: smoking, alcoholism.

Nursing Implications: Assess risk, history of peptic ulcer disease or GI bleeding. Assess baseline Hgb, HCT, and presence/absence of occult bleeding by guaiac of stools. Instruct patient to report signs/symptoms of abdominal pain, black stools, blood per rectum, epistaxis, menorrhagia. If patient is at risk for bleeding, discuss with physician use of misoprostol to protect GI mucosa. Teach patient to avoid concurrent use of aspirin, other NSAIDs.

III.   POTENTIAL SENSORY/PERCEPTUAL ALTERATIONS related to CNS CHANGES

Defining Characteristics: Dizziness, headache, nervousness, fatigue, drowsiness, malaise/ light-headedness, anxiety, confusion, mental depression, and emotional lability may occur. Decreased hearing, visual acuity, changes in color vision, conjunctivitis, diplopia, and cataracts have been reported. In addition, though rare, aseptic meningitis has occurred.

Nursing Implications: Assess baseline neurologic and mental status. Instruct patient to report changes in sensory/perceptual pattern, especially VISUAL CHANGES. If visual changes occur, discuss with physician referral to ophthalmologist as soon as possible. Assess for rare occurrence of aseptic meningitis (fever, coma). Discuss drug continuance with physician for significant symptoms.

IV.   ALTERATION IN NUTRITION, LESS THAN BODY REQUIREMENTS, related to HEPATIC TOXICITY

Defining Characteristics: Severe and sometimes fatal hepatotoxicity has occurred. Jaundice and hepatitis occur rarely. Borderline increase in LFTs occurs in 15% of patients receiving NSAIDs, while values increase by three times in 1%.

Nursing Implications: Assess baseline LFTs and monitor periodically during long-term therapy. Instruct patient to report jaundice, abdominal pain. Discuss discontinuance of drug with physician for significant toxicity.

V. ALTERATION IN RENAL ELIMINATION related to INHIBITION OF RENAL PROSTAGLANDINS

Defining Characteristics: Acute renal failure may occur rarely within first few days of treatment with NSAIDs in patients with preexisting renal dysfunction. Other signs/symptoms of renal dysfunction that may occur rarely are azotemia, cystitis, hematuria, increased serum BUN and creatinine, and decreased creatinine clearance. Peripheral edema has also been described. Drug should not be used in patients with creatinine clearance < 50 mL/min.

Nursing Implications: Assess baseline renal function. Instruct patient to report any changes in urinary function. Monitor periodic serum BUN, creatinine during chronic therapy.

VI. ALTERATION IN SKIN INTEGRITY related to RASH

Defining Characteristics: Rash (urticaria, vesicles, or erythematous macular) may occur, as may Stevens-Johnson syndrome, flushes, alopecia, rectal itching, and acne.

Nursing Implications: Assess baseline skin integrity and presence of lesions. Teach patient to report abnormalities. Provide symptomatic relief for rashes, pruritus. Discuss drug discontinuance with physician/midlevel if rash develops.

VII. POTENTIAL FOR FATIGUE, THROMBOCYTOPENIA, AND INFECTION related to BONE MARROW INJURY

Defining Characteristics: Neutropenia, agranulocytosis, aplastic anemia, hemolytic anemia, and thrombocytopenia may occur rarely in patients taking NSAIDs.

Nursing Implications: Assess baseline CBC, WBC, differential, and platelet count. Discuss abnormalities with physician. Instruct patient to report severe fatigue, infection, bleeding. Monitor lab reports periodically during treatment.

Drug: indomethacin (Indocin, Indocin SR, Indotech)

Class: NSAID, structurally related to sulindac.

Mechanism of Action: Actions similar to other NSAIDs: anti-inflammatory action, probably by inhibition of prostaglandin synthesis, as well as by inhibiting migration of leukocytes to infection site and stabilization of neutrophils so lysosomal enzymes cannot be released; may also interfere with the production of autoantibodies (mediated by prostaglandins).

Analgesic and antipyretic effects appear to result from inhibition of prostaglandin synthesis. Probably reduces tumor-associated fever by inhibition of synthesis of prostaglandin (PGE_1) in hypothalamus. However, drug has serious side effects, so should not be used routinely as an antipyretic.

Metabolism: Rapidly and completely absorbed from GI tract. When administered with food or antacid (aluminum and magnesium hydroxide), peak plasma drug concentrations may be slightly decreased or delayed. Drug is 99% bound to plasma proteins. Crosses BBB slightly, and placenta freely. Metabolized by liver, undergoes enterohepatic circulation, and is excreted in urine.

Indication: Effective for the treatment in active stages of (1) moderate to severe RA including acute flares; (2) moderate-to-severe anklylosing spondylitis; (3) moderate-to-severe osteoarthritis; (4) acute painful shoulder (bursitis and/or tendinitis); and (5) acute gouty arthritis.

Dosage/Range:
- Capsules: 10 mg, 25 mg, 50 mg, 75 mg, given in 2–4 divided doses.
- Sustained release: 75 mg, given once or bid.
- Oral suspension: 25 mg/5 mL, given in 2–4 divided doses.
- Suppositories: 50 mg, given in 2–4 divided doses.

Drug Preparation:
- Drug is sensitive to light. Store capsules in well-closed containers at temperatures < 40°C (104°F).
- Oral suspension should be stored in tight, light-resistant containers at 30°C (86°F).
- Suppositories should be stored at temperatures < 30°C (86°F).

Drug Administration:
- Give with food or antacid to protect GI mucosa.
- Rectal suppository must remain in rectum for at least 1 hour for maximum absorption.
- Consider reduced dose in patients with renal dysfunction.
- Indocin suspension contains 1% alcohol.

Drug Interactions:
- Indomethacin can displace or be displaced by other protein-bound drugs: oral anticoagulants, hydantoins (e.g., phenytoin), salicylates, sulfonamides, sulfonylureas. Therefore, if taking any of these medications with indomethacin, the patient must be assessed for increased toxicity of each drug.
- Antihypertensive effect of hydralazine, captopril, furosemide, beta-adrenergic blockers, or thiazide diuretics may be decreased.
- NSAIDs: concurrent administration with salicylates does not improve drug effects but increases toxicity (GI, aplastic anemia) so should NOT be given concurrently. Diflunisal may decrease renal excretion of indomethacin and increase risk of GI hemorrhage; AVOID concurrent use.
- Triamterene: may precipitate renal failure. DO NOT USE CONCURRENTLY.
- Digoxin: serum levels may be increased and prolonged, so digoxin levels should be monitored closely.

- Methotrexate, especially HIGH DOSE: increased, prolonged serum methotrexate levels can be fatal; AVOID concurrent use.
- Potassium (K+) supplements, K+ sparing diuretics: indomethacin may increase serum K+ concentrations, especially in the elderly or patients with renal dysfunction. Use with caution and monitor K+ serum levels.
- Lithium: may increase plasma lithium levels; assess patient for lithium toxicity.
- Cyclosporine: possible increased nephrotoxicity; use with caution and monitor renal function.
- Probenecid: increased plasma level and therapeutic effects of indomethacin; decrease indomethacin dose.

Lab Effects/Interference:
- May prolong bleeding time.
- Rarely, hemolytic anemia, leukopenia, thrombocytopenia.

Special Considerations:
- Avoid use or use cautiously in the elderly or in patients with epilepsy, Parkinson's disease, renal dysfunction, mental illness.

Potential Toxicities/Side Effects and the Nursing Process

I. POTENTIAL SENSORY/PERCEPTUAL ALTERATIONS

Defining Characteristics: Dose-related headache occurs in 25–50% of patients (more severe in morning); may be associated with frontal throbbing, vomiting, tinnitus, ataxia, tremor, vertigo, and insomnia. Dizziness, depression, fatigue, and peripheral neuropathy may occur in 3–9% of patients; 1% of patients may have confusion, psychic disturbances, hallucinations, and nightmares. May accentuate epilepsy and Parkinson's disease symptomatology. Blurred vision, corneal and retinal damage, and hearing loss may occur with long-term use.

Nursing Implications: Assess baseline mental and neurologic status. Teach patient to report headache, changes in sensation or perception, and sleep problems. Discuss drug discontinuance with physician if neurologic side effects occur. Patients with visual disturbances or pain, or changes from baseline, should be seen by an ophthalmologist.

II. ALTERATION IN NUTRITION, LESS THAN BODY REQUIREMENTS, related to GI TOXICITY

Defining Characteristics: Nausea, with or without vomiting and indigestion, heartburn, and epigastric pain occur in ~ 10% of patients. Diarrhea, abdominal pain/distress, and constipation may occur in ~ 3%. Other effects occurring in ~ 1% are anorexia, distension, flatulence, gastroenteritis, rectal bleeding, stomatitis. Severe GI bleeding may occur in 1% of patients, as drug decreases platelet aggregation.

Nursing Implications: Teach patient potential side effects and to self-administer drug with food or antacid. Teach patient to avoid OTC aspirin-containing drugs, alcohol, or steroids, all of which can increase GI toxicity and risk for GI bleeding. Instruct patient to report any signs/symptoms of GI bleeding, abdominal pain immediately, and to stop taking the drug. Guaiac stool for occult blood periodically. If drug must be used, and risk of GI ulceration is high, discuss with physician use of misoprostol to protect the GI mucosa.

III. POTENTIAL FOR INFECTION, FATIGUE, BLEEDING related to BONE MARROW INJURY

Defining Characteristics: Although rare (1%), potential toxicities include hemolytic anemia, bone marrow depression (leukopenia, thrombocytopenia), aplastic anemia, thrombocytopenic purpura. Drug inhibits platelet aggregation, but this will reverse to normal within 24 hours of drug discontinuance. May prolong bleeding time, especially in patients with underlying bleeding problems.

Nursing Implications: Assess all medicines the patient is taking and teach patient to avoid OTC aspirin-containing drugs. Teach patient to self-assess and instruct to report signs/ symptoms of bleeding, fatigue, and infection.

IV. POTENTIAL FOR ALTERATION IN ELIMINATION PATTERN related to RENAL DYSFUNCTION

Defining Characteristics: Acute interstitial nephritis with hematuria, proteinuria, nephrotic syndrome may occur in 1% of patients. Patients with renal dysfunction may have worsening of renal function. Increased K+ levels may occur in the elderly or in patients with renal dysfunction. Risk increases with long-term therapy.

Nursing Implications: Assess baseline renal status. Discuss alternate drugs if renal dysfunction. Monitor serum K+, sodium (Na+), especially if receiving other drugs that affect serum K+ level (e.g., amphotericin, diuretics), or in the elderly.

V. POTENTIAL FOR ALTERATION IN CARDIAC OUTPUT related to CARDIAC EFFECTS

Defining Characteristics: CHF, tachycardia, chest pain, arrhythmias, palpitations, hypertension, and edema may occur in < 1% of patients.

Nursing Implications: Assess baseline cardiovascular status and monitor periodically while receiving the drug. Assess efficacy of antihypertensive medication due to possible drug interaction.

VI. POTENTIAL FOR INJURY related to DERMATOLOGIC AND SENSITIVITY REACTIONS

Defining Characteristics: Dermatologic effects occur in < 1% of patients and include pruritus, urticaria, rash, exfoliative dermatitis, and Stevens-Johnson syndrome. Allergic reactions occur in < 1%, characterized by asthma in aspirin-sensitive individuals, dyspnea, fever, acute anaphylaxis.

Nursing Implications: Assess baseline dermatologic, pulmonary status, and continue during drug use. Instruct patient to report any adverse reactions immediately.

Drug: ketorolac tromethamine (Toradol)

Class: NSAID.

Mechanism of Action: Inhibits prostaglandin synthesis peripherally to exert analgesic, anti-inflammatory, and antipyretic activity.

Metabolism: Drug completely absorbed following PO or IM administration of the drug, with peak serum levels in 44 minutes and 50 minutes, respectively. Drug is extensively bound to serum protein (99%). Terminal half-life is 2.4–9.2 hours. Excreted by the kidney.

Indication: For the short-term (< 5 days) treatment of acute pain that requires analgesia at the opioid level, usually in the post-operative setting. Therapy should be initiated with IV formulation, followed by tablets to continue treatment, if necessary. Combined use of oral and IV is not to exceed 5 days.

Contraindications: In patients with (1) recent GI bleed or perforation, history of peptic ulcer disease, or GI bleeding; (2) advanced renal impairment or at risk for renal failure due to volume depletion; (3) nursing mothers; (4) hypersensitivity to the drug, or allergy to aspirin or other NSAIDs; (5) as prophylactic analgesia before surgery or intra-operatively; (6) currently taking aspirin or NSAIDs; (7) for neuraxial (epidural or intrathecal) administration; (8) concomitant use of drug with probenecid.

Dosage/Range:
- Single dose: IM, 60 mg; IV, 30 mg.
- Multiple doses: IM/IV, 30 mg q 6 h (maximum daily dose is 120 mg).
- 50% dose reduction for patients aged ≥ 65 years, renal impaired, or weight < 50 kg.
- Oral: for continuation therapy.
- Patients < 65 years old: 20 mg, × 1, then 10 mg q 4–6 h (max 40 mg/24 hours).
- Patients ≥ 65: 10 mg q 4–6 h (max 40 mg/24 hours).
- MAXIMUM USE OF KETOROLAC IS 5 DAYS.

Drug Preparation:
- Store at controlled room temperature of 15–30°C (59–86°F) and protect from light.

Drug Administration:
- PO, IM, or IV.

Drug Interactions:
- Other salicylates: displace ketorolac from protein binding. DO NOT USE together or dose-reduce ketorolac.
- Anticoagulants: possible increase in bleeding time; use with caution and monitor closely.
- Furosemide: decreased diuretic response; need to increase diuretic dose.

* Probenecid: causes prolonged, increased serum ketorolac levels; use cautiously, and reduce dose.
* Lithium, methotrexate: theoretically increased serum levels, so should be dose-reduced if given with ketorolac.

Lab Effects/Interference:
* None known.

Special Considerations:
* Concurrent use with other NSAIDs NOT recommended due to risk of additive toxicity.
* Contraindicated in persons with hypersensitivity to ketorolac, or patients with asthma, nasal polyps, angioedema, and bronchospastic reaction to aspirin or other NSAIDs; also in patients with active peptic ulcer disease or GI bleeding, and patients with advanced renal insufficiency.

Potential Toxicities/Side Effects and the Nursing Process

I.   ALTERATION IN NUTRITION, LESS THAN BODY REQUIREMENTS, related to GI SIDE EFFECTS

Defining Characteristics: Dyspepsia, heartburn, nausea, vomiting, anorexia, diarrhea, constipation, stomatitis, bloating, epigastric and abdominal pain may occur.

Nursing Implications: Assess history of GI symptoms and history of ulcer disease. Teach patient to take NSAID with meals or milk. Teach patient potential side effects and instruct to report them. If symptoms are severe, discuss alternative NSAIDs with physician.

II.   POTENTIAL FOR BLEEDING related to INHIBITION OF PLATELET AGGREGATION

Defining Characteristics: Drug can prolong bleeding time and inhibit platelet aggregation. Peptic ulceration and occult GI bleeding can occur and be life-threatening. Increased risk factors: smoking, alcoholism.

Nursing Implications: Assess risk, history of peptic ulcer disease or GI bleeding. Assess baseline Hgb, HCT and presence/absence of occult bleeding by guaiac of stools. Instruct patient to report signs/symptoms of abdominal pain, black stools, blood per rectum, epistaxis, menorrhagia. If patient at risk for bleeding, discuss with physician use of misoprostol to protect GI mucosa. Teach patient to avoid concurrent use of aspirin, other NSAIDs.

III.   POTENTIAL SENSORY/PERCEPTUAL ALTERATIONS related to CNS CHANGES

Defining Characteristics: Dizziness, headache, nervousness, fatigue, drowsiness, malaise/light-headedness, anxiety, confusion, mental depression, and emotional lability may occur. Decreased hearing, visual acuity, changes in color vision, conjunctivitis, diplopia, and cataracts have been reported. In addition, though rare, aseptic meningitis has occurred.

Nursing Implications: Assess baseline neurologic and mental status. Instruct patient to report changes in sensory/perceptual pattern, especially VISUAL CHANGES. If visual changes occur, discuss with physician referral to ophthalmologist as soon as possible. Assess for rare occurrence of aseptic meningitis (fever, coma). Discuss drug continuance with physician for significant symptoms.

Equianalgesic Dosing:

Ketorolac	Meperidine		Morphine
IM			
30 or 90 mg	100 mg		12 mg
10 mg	50 mg		6 mg
Ketorolac	Ibuprofen	Aspirin	Acetaminophen
PO			
10 mg	400 mg	650 mg	600 mg

IV. ALTERATION IN NUTRITION, LESS THAN BODY REQUIREMENTS, related to HEPATIC TOXICITY

Defining Characteristics: Severe and sometimes fatal hepatotoxicity has occurred. Jaundice and hepatitis occur rarely. Borderline increase in LFTs occurs in 15% of patients, while values increase by three times in 1%.

Nursing Implications: Assess baseline LFTs and monitor periodically during long-term therapy. Instruct patient to report jaundice, abdominal pain. Discuss discontinuance of drug with physician for significant toxicity.

V. ALTERATION IN RENAL ELIMINATION related to INHIBITION OF RENAL PROSTAGLANDINS

Defining Characteristics: Acute renal failure may occur rarely within first few days of treatment in patients with preexisting renal dysfunction. Other signs/symptoms of renal dysfunction that may occur rarely are azotemia, cystitis, hematuria, increased serum BUN and creatinine, and decreased creatinine clearance. Peripheral edema has also been described.

Nursing Implications: Assess baseline renal function. Teach patient to report any changes in urinary function. Monitor periodic serum BUN, creatinine during chronic therapy.

MANAGEMENT

VI.   ALTERATION IN SKIN INTEGRITY related to RASH

Defining Characteristics: Rash (urticaria, vesicles, or erythematous macular) may occur, as may Stevens-Johnson syndrome, flushes, alopecia, rectal itching, and acne.

Nursing Implications: Assess baseline skin integrity and presence of lesions. Instruct patient to report abnormalities. Provide symptomatic relief for rashes, pruritus.

VII.   POTENTIAL FOR FATIGUE AND INFECTION related to BONE MARROW INJURY

Defining Characteristics: Neutropenia, agranulocytosis, aplastic anemia, hemolytic anemia, and thrombocytopenia may occur rarely.

Nursing Implications: Assess baseline CBC, WBC, differential, and platelet count. Discuss abnormalities with physician. Instruct patient to report severe fatigue, infection, bleeding. Monitor lab values periodically during treatment.

Drug: pregabalin (Lyrica)

Class: Anticonvulsant, analgesic for peripheral neuropathy.

Mechanism of Action: Unknown, but believed to reduce the calcium-dependent release of several neurotransmitters, possibly by modulating the calcium channel function. In neuropathic pain, voltage-gated calcium channels let extra calcium into the neuron ending, which then binds to vesicles containing pain-causing chemicals (neurotransmitters). The vesicles then migrate to the neuronal membrane, and secrete them into the nerve endings. Pregabalin binds with the alpha-2-delta site (axillary subunit of the voltage-gated calcium channel) in CNS tissues (but not cardiac-related, voltage-gated calcium channels).

Metabolism: Well absorbed from GI tract with peak plasma levels in 1.5 hours; bioavailability is > 90% independent of dose. Drug does not bind to plasma proteins. Steady state is reached in 24–48 hours. Drug is not metabolized in the body, and 90% of intact drug is eliminated in the urine. Because of this, drug elimination rate is proportional to the creatinine clearance, so drug dose must be reduced in patients with renal compromise. Drug crosses blood–brain barrier in laboratory animals, so is presumed to do so in humans. The drug has an elimination half-life of 6 hours.

Indications: For (1) neuropathic pain associated with diabetic peripheral neuropathy; (2) postherpetic neuralgia; (3) adjunctive therapy for adult patients with partial onset seizures; (4) fibromyalgia; and (5) neuropathic pain associated with spinal cord injury.

Dosage/Range:
- Diabetic peripheral neuropathy: Begin dosing at 50 mg PO tid, and increase to 100 mg PO tid over 1 week, to goal of 300 mg/day within 1 week, with or without food, in patients with creatinine clearance of > 60 mL/minute. Dose-reduce for patients with creatinine clearance < 60 mL/minute.

- Postherpetic neuralgia: Begin dosing at 75 mg PO bid or 50 mg PO tid with goal 300 mg/day within 1 week; maximum dose of 600 mg/day.
- Adjunctive therapy for adult patients with partial onset seizures: 2–3 divided doses per day, to a maximum of 600 mg/day.
- Fibromyalgia: 2 divided doses per day, goal 300 mg/day within 1 week; maximum of 450 mg/day.
- Neuropathic pain associated with spinal cord injury: 2 divided doses a day, goal 300 mg/day within 1 week. Maximum dose of 600 mg/day.
- Patients with renal impairment: Dose should be reduced 50% if creatinine clearance is 30–60 mL/minute, another 50% if creatinine clearance is 15–30 mL/minute, and a further 50% if < 15 mL/minute (see package insert).
- If patient is being hemodialyzed, see package insert for supplementary doses.

Drug Preparation:
- Available 25-, 50-, 75-, 100-, 150-, 200-, 225-, 300-mg capsules; 20 mg/mL oral solution (16 fl oz).
- Oral; take with food or on an empty stomach.
- Teach patients to keep medication in a safe place, out of reach of children and pets.

Drug Interactions:
- None.

Lab Effects/Interference:
- ↑ Creatine kinase in 2% of patients.
- ↓ Platelets (20% below baseline in 3% of patients).
- EKG changes: PR interval prolongation by 3–6 msec.

Special Considerations:
- As with any antiepileptic drugs, the drug should be withdrawn gradually to minimize the potential of increased seizure frequency in patients with seizure disorders. If discontinued, the drug should be gradually reduced in dose over at least 1 week.
- Abrupt discontinuation of drug may result in insomnia, headache, nausea, and diarrhea (discontinue over a minimum of 1 week).
- Although uncommon, 2% of patients had creatine kinase > 3 times the ULN; patients should be taught to report immediately unexplained muscle pain or tenderness, especially if these muscle symptoms are associated with malaise or fever so that they can be further evaluated, and rhabdomyolysis or myopathy ruled out. Discontinue drug if myopathy is suspected or confirmed, or if patient develops markedly elevated creatine kinase.

Potential Toxicities/Side Effects and the Nursing Process

I.   SENSORY/PERCEPTUAL ALTERATIONS related to CNS CHANGES

Defining Characteristics: The most common side effects are somnolence (22%), dizziness (29%), blurred vision (6%), abnormal thinking (concentration and attention). Somnolence and dizziness start right after the drug is initiated, increase in frequency as the dose is increased, and may persist throughout treatment. Less commonly, ataxia, vertigo, confusion, diplopia, euphoria, incoordination, and amnesia may occur. Increased sleepiness and dizziness if taking concomitant opioids for pain, alcohol, or antianxiety/ sedatives.

Nursing Implications: Assess baseline neurologic status and document. Instruct patient of general side effects that may occur, and to report them as well as any changes that may occur, such as reduced visual acuity. Assess for suicidal ideation. If significant CNS changes occur, discuss dose reduction or change to an alternative drug with physician. Instruct patient not to drive a car or to do activities that require mental acuity until full effect of drug is known. If blurred vision, dizziness, or weakness occurs, teach patient to report this immediately.

II.   ALTERATION IN NUTRITION related to GI TOXICITY

Defining Characteristics: Gastroenteritis and increased appetite with weight gain (7% over baseline over 13 weeks) may occur. Weight gain of diabetic patients averaged 1.6 kg. Less commonly, cholecystitis, cholelithiasis, colitis, dysphagia, esophagitis, gastritis, GI hemorrhage, melena, mouth ulceration, pancreatitis, rectal hemorrhage, and tongue edema may occur. Rarely, aphthous stomatitis may occur.

Nursing Implications: Assess patient tolerance of GI side effects. Instruct patient to report side effects. Discuss symptomatic management depending upon symptoms. If patient is also taking rosiglitazone (Avandia) or pioglitazone (Actos), counsel about increased risk of weight gain.

III.   ALTERATION IN SKIN INTEGRITY related to PRURITUS, EDEMA

Defining Characteristics: Pruritus is common; infrequently, patients may develop alopecia, dry skin, eczema, hirsutism, skin ulcer, urticaria, or vesiculobullous rash. Rarely, patients may develop exfoliative dermatitis. Edema, principally peripheral edema, occurs in 6% of patients, especially in diabetic patients taking thiazolidinedione antidiabetic agents (these drugs in and of themselves can cause fluid retention and weight gain).

Nursing Implications: Perform baseline skin assessment, and note any areas that are not intact, are swollen, or itch. Teach patient to self-assess for itch, swelling, other changes, and to report them. If rash develops, instruct patient to notify provider immediately. If itch occurs, discuss symptomatic management.

IV.   ALTERATION IN COMFORT related to ARTHRALGIA, LEG CRAMPS, MYALGIA, EDEMA, PERIPHERAL EDEMA, ECCHYMOSIS, ABDOMINAL PAIN

Defining Characteristics: Although not common, arthralgias, leg cramps, myalgias, ecchymosis, and abdominal pain can occur.

Nursing Implications: Perform baseline comfort assessment, and teach patient to report these side effects if they occur. Develop a plan for symptomatic relief.

Drug: ziconotide intrathecal infusion (Prialt)

Class: Selective blocker of neuronal N-type calcium channels in the nerves that normally conduct pain signals from the periphery to the spinal cord.

Mechanism of Action: Synthetic equivalent to a naturally occurring conopeptide found in a marine snail (*Conus magus*), which binds to N-type calcium channels on the primary afferent nerves (A-d and C) of the dorsal horn of the spinal cord. Voltage-sensitive calcium channels (VSCC) permit the cell to regulate the amount of calcium entering and leaving the cell; this directly influences membrane excitability, among other cellular processes. Ziconotide appears to block these channels so that pain messages from the periphery do not get passed through to the spinal cord and up the spinal cord where pain perception occurs.

Metabolism: Following 1 hour IT administration of 1–10 µg of drug, total and peak exposure were variable but dose proportional; as a continuous IT infusion, once a quantifiable serum level of drug is identified, the serum level remains constant at least up to 9 months. Drug is 50% bound to human plasma proteins, and CSF volume of distribution is the same as the total CSF volume of 140 mL. Terminal half-life in the CSF is 4.6 hours, and is cleared from the CSF at approximately the human CSF turnover rate of 0.3–0.4 mL/min. Drug passes across the blood–brain barrier into systemic circulation with a serum half-life of 1.3 hours. Drug is cleaved at multiple sites of the peptide; it is degraded via the ubiquitin-protease system in many organs (kidney, liver, lung) into component amino acids. < 1% of intact ziconotide is recovered in the urine.

Indication: For the management of severe chronic pain in adults for whom intrathecal therapy is warranted, and who are intolerant of or refractory to other treatment, such as systemic analgesics, adjunctive therapies, or intrathecal morphine.

Dosage/Range:
- Initial dose no more than 2.4 mcg/day (0.1 mcg/hr) and titrated to patient response.
- Increase dose by up to 2.4 mcg/day (0.1 mcghr) at intervals of no more than 2–3 times/week based on patient response, up to recommended MAXIMUM of 19.2 mcg/day (0.8 mcg/hr) by day 21.
- May use dose increases in increments of less than 2.4 mg/day less frequently than 2–3 times a week.
- With each dosage titration ensure that the pump infusion rate is adjusted correctly (either implanted microinfusion device or external microinfusion device and catheter).
- Available in 1-, 2-, and 5-mL vials (100 mcg/mL) for diluted use; and 20-mL vial (25 mcg/mL) for undiluted use.
- Diluted ziconotide: Use 0.9% sodium chloride injection USP (preservative-free) using aseptic procedures to achieve pump manufacturer's recommended concentration.
- Once the appropriate dose has been established, the 100 mcg/mL formulation may be used undiluted.
- Store unopened vials at 2–8°C (36–46°F) but do not freeze; refrigerate (2–8°C) after preparation, protect from light, and use within 24 hours.
- Initial (naïve) pump priming: Use 2 mL of undiluted 25-mc/mL formulation to rinse the internal surfaces of the pump; repeat twice more for a total of three rinses.

- Initial pump fill: Use undiluted 25 mcg/mL ONLY to fill the naïve pump after priming; begin dosing NO HIGHER than 2.4 mcg/day (0.1 mcg/hr). Initial pump fill loses drug through adsorption on internal device surfaces and by dilution in the residual space in the device—this does not occur with subsequent pump filling. Refill the pump reservoir within 14 days of the initial fill to ensure accurate drug administration.
- Pump refills: Fill the pump at least every 40 days if used diluted; if undiluted drug, fill the pump at least every 60 days. Use the Medtronic refill kit to empty the pump contents prior to refill with new drug. If an implanted pump must be surgically replaced while the patient is receiving the drug, the replacement pump should be primed, and the initial drug replaced in 14 days as above.

Drug Preparation:

Ziconotide IT Infusion	Initial Fill (Expiration)	Refill (Expiration)
25 mcg/mL, undiluted 14 days	14 days	60 days
100 mcg/mL, undiluted N/A	N/A	60 days
100 mcg/mL, diluted N/A	N/A	60 days

Drug Preparation:
- Refer to manufacturer's pump manual for specific instructions. When using an external microinfusion device, and filling it the first time, use a concentration of 5 mcg/mL; dilute drug with 0.9% sodium chloride USP (preservative-free); the flow rate for the external microinfusor usually starts at 0.02 mL/hr to deliver the initial dose rate of 2.4 mcg/day (0.1 mcg/hr).

Drug Administration:
- Continuous IT infusion via Medronic SynchroMed EL (Medtronic Inc.), SynchroMed II Infusion System (Medtronic Inc.), Simms Deltec Cadd Micro (Ardus Medical, Inc.) External Microinfusion Device and Catheter pumps.
- Most patients continue to receive opioids.
- There is no known antidote for the drug; if overdosage, most patients recover within 24 hours after drug withdrawal; if inadvertent IV or epidural injection of drug, support blood pressure by recumbent positioning, and BP support as needed.

Drug Interactions:
- Additive effect when given with opioid medications as drug does not bind to opiate receptors.
- CNS depressant drugs: increased incidence of CNS adverse events (e.g., dizziness, confusion).

Lab Effects/Interference:
- Increased serum creatine kinase levels (40% of patients), which may be associated with muscle weakness; rare renal failure related to rhabdomyolysis and very high CK elevations.

Special Considerations:

- Severe psychiatric symptoms and neurologic impairment may occur during ziconotide IT infusion; patients with a history of psychosis should NOT receive the drug; monitor patients frequently for signs/symptoms of cognitive impairment, hallucinations, or changes in mood or level of consciousness; interrupt or discontinue drug for severe psychiatric or neurologic symptoms/signs.
- Drug can be interrupted or discontinued abruptly without risk of withdrawal syndrome.
- Drug is embryotoxic in animals.
- Use cautiously in elderly patients as incidence of confusion is higher; start at lower dose and titrate more slowly.
- Patients should be taught not to engage in hazardous activity, such as operation of heavy machinery.
- Patients should notify provider IMMEDIATELY for any of the following:
  - Change in mental status such as lethargy, confusion, disorientation, decreased alertness.
  - Change in mood or perception, such as hallucinations (e.g., unusual tactile sensations in oral cavity).
  - Symptoms of depression or suicidal ideation.
  - Nausea, vomiting, seizures, fever, headache, and/or stiff neck, as these may herald developing meningitis.

Potential Toxicities/Side Effects and the Nursing Process

I.   SENSORY/PERCEPTUAL ALTERATIONS related to CNS CHANGES

Defining Characteristics: CNS depression and changes in mental status may occur, including psychiatric symptoms, cognitive impairment, and decreased alertness/unresponsiveness. These are characterized by confusion (33%, with a higher incidence in the elderly), memory impairment (22%), speech disorder (14%), aphasia (12%), abnormal thinking (8%), and amnesia (1%). Psychiatric symptoms are more likely to occur in patients with pretreatment psychiatric disorders, and include hallucinations (12%), paranoid ideation (2%), hostility (2%), delirium (2%), psychosis (1%), and manic reactions (0.4%). Cognitive impairment may be gradual a few weeks after starting therapy. Once dose is interrupted or discontinued, symptoms usually resolve in 2 weeks. Patients may become depressed with suicidal ideation. Other sensory/perceptual alterations include: dizziness (47%), somnolence (22%), abnormal vision (22%), ataxia (16%), abnormal gait (15%), hypertonia (11%), nystagmus (8%), dysesthesia (7%), paresthesia (7%), and vertigo (7%).

Nursing Implications: Assess past medical history for psychiatric and neurologic problems. Assess baseline gait, movement, mental, affective, and neurologic status. Assess medication profile to identify other contributions, i.e., CNS depressants, antiepileptics, neuroleptics, sedatives, diuretics. Teach patient and family that these side effects may

MANAGEMENT

occur, and instruct patient/family to report any changes. Teach patient/family to notify provider IMMEDIATELY for any of the following:

- Change in mental status such as lethargy, confusion, disorientation, decreased alertness.
- Change in mood or perception, such as hallucinations (e.g., unusual tactile sensations in oral cavity).
- Symptoms of depression or suicidal ideation.

Assess patient safety and measures to ensure safety. Discuss any significant changes with physician and need to interrupt/discontinue drug based on severity of symptoms.

OPIOID ANALGESICS

Drug: codeine (as sulfate or phosphate); may be combined with acetaminophen (Phenaphen with Codeine, Tylenol with Codeine, nl Capital and Codeine, Codaphen [Odalan]), or with aspirin (Empirin with Codeine, Soma Compound with Codeine, Fiorinal with Codeine)

Class: Opioid analgesic (opioid agonist).

Mechanism of Action: Resembles morphine but has milder action; binds to opiate receptors in CNS (limbic system, thalamus, striatum, hypothalamus, midbrain, spinal cord), altering pain perception at level of spinal cord and higher centers, as well as the emotional response to pain. Also suppresses cough reflex.

Metabolism: Well absorbed after oral or parenteral administration. Metabolized by liver; excreted in urine, and small amount in feces.

Indication: Relief of mild-to-moderately severe pain, unrelieved by nonopioid analgesic, where the use of an opioid analgesic is appropriate.

Dosage/Range: Mild pain: 30 mg q 4 h (range 15–60 mg), PO, subcutaneous, or IM.

Drug Preparation:
- Store tablets in tight, light-resistant containers at 15–30°C (59–86°F).
- Injection should be protected from light and stored at 15–40°C (59–104°F).
- At home, teach patient to store oral doses in a safe place away from children and pets.

Drug Administration:
- PO, subcutaneous, IM.

Drug Interactions:
- Injection is incompatible with solutions containing aminophylline, ammonium chloride, amobarbital sodium, chlorothiazide sodium, heparin sodium, methicillin sodium, nitrofurantoin, phenobarbital sodium, sodium bicarbonate.
- Alcohol, CNS depressants: additive effects.

Lab Effects/Interference:
• None known.

Special Considerations:
• Parenteral dose is 2/3 oral dose for equianalgesic effect.
• Onset of action after PO or subcutaneous dose is 15–30 minutes, with duration of analgesia 4–6 hours.
• Addition of acetaminophen or aspirin gives additive analgesia.
• Give smallest effective dose to prevent development of tolerance, physical dependency.
• Reduce dose in debilitated patients, or patients receiving other CNS depressants.
• Use with caution in patients with hepatic or renal dysfunction, hypothyroidism, Addison's disease, severe CNS depression, respiratory depression, head injury, elevated intracranial pressure.
• If required, naloxone HCl (Narcan) will reverse opiate toxicity (e.g., respiratory depression). However, it is important that acute withdrawal symptoms be prevented by giving only enough naloxone to reverse respiratory depression and that this be continued for opioid drug half-life.
• Teach patient that opioid analgesics may impair the mental and/or physical ability to drive and use machines, and to avoid these activities until the effect of the drug is known.

Potential Toxicities/Side Effects and the Nursing Process

I.   SENSORY/PERCEPTUAL ALTERATIONS related to CNS DEPRESSION

Defining Characteristics: Drowsiness, sedation, mood changes, euphoria, dysphoria, dizziness, mental clouding may occur. At high doses, may cause seizures. Miosis (papillary constriction) may occur.

Nursing Implications: Assess baseline neurologic status. Use cautiously, if at all, in patients with head injury, increased intracranial pressure, severe CNS depression, acute alcoholism, or who are elderly or debilitated. Assess other concurrent medications. Use with caution in patients receiving other opioids, tranquilizers, hypnotics, monoamine oxidase (MAO) inhibitors, since increasing CNS depressant effects can occur. Monitor neurologic status closely. Teach patient to avoid driving and operating machinery while taking the medicine, and to AVOID concurrent alcohol.

II.   ALTERATION IN OXYGENATION related to RESPIRATORY DEPRESSION

Defining Characteristics: Opiate agonists directly depress respiratory center in brain stem, causing decreased sensitivity and responsiveness to increased pCO_2 (CO_2 tension in serum). Also may depress deep breathing and reflex to sigh. Tolerance to respiratory depressant effects occurs with chronic use.

Nursing Implications: Assess baseline pulmonary status, and monitor periodically during drug use. Use cautiously in patients with bronchial asthma, chronic obstructive pulmonary disease (COPD), respiratory depression, and monitor closely.

III.   ALTERATION IN ELIMINATION related to CONSTIPATION, ILEUS

Defining Characteristics: Opium agonists bind to opiate receptors in bowel, slowing peristalsis, leading to constipation. Untreated constipation may result in bowel perforation.

Nursing Implications: Assess baseline elimination, fluid intake, diet, and exercise patterns. Teach patient about prevention of constipation: goal is to move bowels at least every 2 days by increasing fluid intake to 3 L/day, following a diet high in fiber (beans, vegetables, fruit), and taking moderate exercise. Assess need for bowel softeners, bulk-forming laxatives, and osmotic cathartics, and discuss prescription with physician. Teach patient self-administration of medications.

IV.   ALTERATION IN NUTRITION, LESS THAN BODY REQUIREMENTS, related to GI TOXICITY

Defining Characteristics: Nausea, vomiting, dry mouth may occur. Gastric, biliary, and pancreatic secretions are decreased by opiate agonists; digestion is delayed. Biliary tract muscle tone is increased, and spasm of Oddi's sphincter may occur (morphine > meperidine > codeine).

Nursing Implications: Assess patient tolerance of GI side effects. Teach patient to report side effects. If nausea/vomiting occur, change to another opioid, or premedicate with antiemetic to prevent nausea/vomiting. Assess GI pain, biliary spasm, and consider alternative opioid.

V.   ALTERATION IN CARDIAC OUTPUT related to HYPOTENSION, BRADYCARDIA

Defining Characteristics: Orthostatic hypotension, bradycardia due to cholinergic effect, and peripheral vasodilation may occur with rapid IV dosing. There may be histamine-related flushing, pruritus, diaphoresis with chronic drug usage; tolerance develops to this effect.

Nursing Implications: Assess baseline cardiovascular status. Teach patient to change position slowly and to hold onto stable, nearby structure for support as needed. Be careful when giving IV push opioids, and caution patient to remain in supine position for 15–20 minutes after injection. Monitor cardiovascular status after injection.

VI.   ALTERATION IN URINE ELIMINATION related to URINARY RETENTION

Defining Characteristics: Increased smooth muscle tone in urinary tract and spasm may occur. Bladder tone is increased and may cause urgency. Vesical sphincter tone may be increased, leading to difficulty urinating. Increased risk of urinary retention in patients with prostatic hypertrophy or urethral stricture.

Nursing Implications: Assess baseline urinary elimination pattern. Teach patient to increase fluids to 3 L/day, and encourage voiding every 2–3 hours. Instruct patient to report problems with urination.

VII. KNOWLEDGE DEFICIT related to DRUG ADMINISTRATION, POTENTIAL FOR TOLERANCE, AND DEPENDENCY

Defining Characteristics: Psychological dependence (addiction) occurs rarely in patients taking opioid agonists for cancer pain (< 1%). Physical dependence (precipitation of withdrawal symptoms) occurs with chronic use of the drug for the relief of chronic cancer pain. In addition, tolerance, or less analgesic effect over time with the same drug dose, occurs and requires increased dosage of drug.

Nursing Implications: Assess baseline knowledge of opioid analgesics, and attitude about their use for cancer pain management. Teach patient about proper self-administration, possible side effects, and self-care measures. Suggest patient maintain diary of pain intensity, precipitating and alleviating factors, drug dose and time taken, and relief. Teach patient to self-administer opioid agonists for relief of chronic cancer pain around-the-clock, not PRN, to prevent pain. Explain use of prescribed short-acting opioid for rescue or to manage breakthrough pain. Discuss with physician dose increase or change in frequency of administration if tolerance develops. Teach patient that withdrawal symptoms may occur if chronic, around-the-clock dosing is interrupted. Withdrawal (abstinence) symptoms that may be seen are restlessness, lacrimation, rhinorrhea, yawning, perspiration, gooseflesh, restless sleep, mydriasis in first 24 hours. These are followed by twitching and leg spasm; severe aching of the back, abdomen, and legs; cramping in abdomen and legs; hot/cold flashes; insomnia; nausea/vomiting, diarrhea; severe sneezing; and increased heart rate, BP, and temperature (T), which peak at 36–72 hours. Withdrawal syndrome can be prevented by administration of at least ¼ of previous opioid dose.

VIII. SEXUAL DYSFUNCTION related to IMPOTENCE, ↓ LIBIDO

Defining Characteristics: Opiate agonists may suppress gonadotropin, causing impotence and decreased libido.

Nursing Implications: Assess baseline sexual pattern. Discuss potential toxicity and impact on sexuality. Provide information, emotional support, and referral as needed.

Drug: fentanyl buccal soluble film (Onsolis)

Class: Opioid analgesic (opioid agonist), oral transmucosal fentanyl soluble film.

Mechanism of Action: Fentanyl is a pure opioid agonist that binds to opioid μ-receptors located in the brain, spinal cord, and smooth muscle. Fentanyl is a transmucosal fentanyl product that is formulated as a soluble film that dissolves in 15–30 minutes and is absorbed through the buccal mucosa. The onset of analgesia is at 15 minutes, with significant decrease in pain intensity at 30 minutes in 50% of patients, and duration of action of 60 minutes.

Metabolism: Following an initial rapid absorption from the buccal mucosa, there is a more prolonged absorption if swallowed from the GI tract. The absolute bioavailability is 71%, with 51% of the total dose absorbed from the buccal mucosa and 49% of the dose swallowed with saliva and then slowly absorbed from the GI tract. Of the swallowed fentanyl, 20% does not have first-pass (liver, intestines) elimination and becomes systemically available. If the film is accidently chewed and swallowed, there will be lower peak concentrations and lower bioavailability. Compared to oral transmucosal fentanyl citrate (Actiq), the soluble film has 62% greater maximum plasma concentration and 40% greater systemic exposure (AUC). Fentanyl is metabolized in the liver and in the intestinal mucosa to norfentanyl by the CYP3A4 enzymes. The metabolite is nonactive. Fentanyl is highly lipophilic and is rapidly distributed to the brain, heart, lungs, kidneys, and spleen, with slower redistribution to muscle and fat. Fentanyl is 80–85% protein-bound. More than 90% of fentanyl is excreted as inactive metabolites, with less than 7% excreted in the urine unchanged, and 1% unchanged in the feces. The terminal elimination half-life of the drug is 14 hours.

Indication: Drug is an opioid analgesic indicated for the management of breakthrough pain in patients with cancer, patients 18 years and older, and patients who are already receiving and who are tolerant to opioid therapy for their underlying persistent cancer pain. Tolerance is defined as taking at least 60 mg of oral morphine a day or 25 mcg of fentanyl per hour, or at least 30 mg of oxycodone daily, or at least 8 mg of hydromorphone daily, or an equianalgesic dose of another opioid, for at least 1 week or longer. Patients must remain on around-the-clock opioids while taking fentanyl buccal soluble film (Onsolis).

Dosage/Range:

- To be used in opioid-tolerant patients only (have been receiving 60 mg PO morphine/day, 25 mcg transdermal fentanyl/hr, 30 mg PO oxycodone/day, 8 mg PO hydromorphone/day, 25 mg oxymorphone/day, or an equianalgesic dose of another opioid for 1 week or longer).
- Initial starting dose of 200 mcg of fentanyl buccal soluble film in *all* patients, even if patient has been on another oral transmucosal fentanyl product.
- Titrate using 200-mcg film increments (up to a maximum of four 200-mcg films or a single 1,200-mcg film) to adequate analgesia without intolerable side effects. Start with 200-mcg dose, and if that is inadequate, increase the dose by 200 mcg in each subsequent episode until the patient reaches a dose that relieves pain with tolerable side effects.
- Maximum is one dose per breakthrough pain episode, no more than four doses per day, separated by at least 2 hours.
- Prescribers of Onsolis on an outpatient basis must enroll in the Transmucosal Immediate Release Fentanyl (TIRF) Risk Evaluation and Mitigation Strategy (REMS) Access Program and comply with the REMS requirements to ensure safe use of Onsolis. Their outpatients, pharmacies who dispense, and distributors must enroll in the program. This is not required for inpatient administration, including hospices and long-term care facilities.

Drug Preparation:
- Available in buccal soluble film in 200-mcg, 400-mcg, 600-mcg, 800-mcg, and 1,200-mcg dosage strengths.

Drug Administration:
- Use the tongue to wet the inside of the cheek or rinse the mouth with water to wet the area for placement of the fentanyl soluble film. Open the drug package immediately prior to using it.
- Place the entire film near the tip of a dry finger with the pink side facing up and hold in place. Place the pink side of the film against the inside of the cheek. Press and hold the film in place for 5 seconds, and then the film should stay in place by itself. Do not drink liquids for 5 minutes.
- Do not cut, tear, chew, or swallow the film; do not manipulate with tongue or finger, and do not eat food until the film is dissolved (15–30 minutes).
- When using multiple film strips, do not place on top of each other, but rather in separate places on the buccal mucosa; use both sides of the mouth.
- Teach patient that opioid analgesics may impair the mental and/or physical ability to drive and use machines, and to avoid these activities until the effect of the drug is known.

Drug Interactions:
- Use with CYP3A4 inhibitors may cause potentially fatal respiratory depression. CNS depressants (other opioids, sedatives, hypnotics, general anesthetics, phenothiazines, tranquilizers, skeletal muscle relaxants, sedating antihistamines), potent inhibitors of cytochrome P450 CYP3A4 isoform (erythromycin, ketoconazole, certain protease inhibitors), and alcohol: increased CNS depression, with risk of hypoventilation, hypotension, and profound sedation. Moderate CYP3A4 inhibitors (aprepitant, diltiazem, grapefruit juice, verapamil): may increase fentanyl plasma levels; use together cautiously.
- MAO inhibitors within 14 days: potentiation of opioid, do not give together.
- Monitor patients who stop therapy with, or decrease the dose of, inducers of CYP3A4 (e.g., barbiturates, carbamazepine, efavirenz, glucocorticoids, modafinil, nevirapine, oxcarbazepine, phenobarbital, phenytoin, pioglitazone, rifabutin, rifampin, St. John's wort, or troglitazone) for signs of opioid toxicity.

Lab Effects/Interference:
- None known.

Special Considerations:
- DO NOT substitute for any other fentanyl products.
- Drug is available through a restricted distribution program called Transmucosal Immediate Release Fentanyl Risk Evaluation and Mitigation Strategy (TIRF REMS) Access Program. Outpatients, healthcare professionals who prescribe to outpatients, pharmacies, and distributors are required to enroll in the program. Outpatients must understand the risks and benefits and sign a Patient-Prescriber Agreement. If questions, more information is available at www.TIRFREMSAccess.com.
- Contraindicated in patients who are not opioid-tolerant or who have acute or postoperative pain, including headache/migraine or dental pain; contraindicated for use in

MANAGEMENT

the emergency room; contraindicated for those intolerant or hypersensitive to fentanyl, Onsolis, or its components. Drug should not be used in patients who have received MAO inhibitors within 14 days, or nursing mothers, as fentanyl is excreted in human milk causing potentially fatal respiratory depression, as well as physical dependence and withdrawal when no longer nursing.

- Use with other CNS depressants or CYP3A4 inhibitors may increase depressant effects including hypoventilation, hypotension, and profound sedation. Consider dosage adjustments if needed.
- Drug can impair ability to do dangerous tasks, such as driving a car or operating machinery. Teach patients to avoid these activities until the drug's effect is determined.
- Titrate drug cautiously in patients with chronic obstructive pulmonary disease, or preexisting medical conditions that predispose the person to hypoventilation; administer with EXTREME caution in patients susceptible to intracranial effects of CO_2 retention.
- Use cautiously if at all in patients with hepatic and/or renal dysfunction, chronic pulmonary disease, head injuries with increased intracranial pressure, and bradyarrhythmias. If drug must be used in a pregnant woman, benefit must outweigh potential risk to the fetus.
- Teach patient that drug must be kept out of reach of children and pets, as dose can be LETHAL to children and pets.
- Drug is an opioid and may cause physical dependence and withdrawal if stopped (along with maintenance opioid) abruptly.
- Manufacturer recommends disposal of unused drug: Foil packet should be opened, and fentanyl film dropped into the toilet for each film; then flush the toilet.

Potential Toxicities/Side Effects and the Nursing Process

I.   POTENTIAL ALTERATION IN OXYGENATION related to HYPOVENTILATION

Defining Characteristics: Increased cough and/or dyspnea are rare, but the chief toxicity in naïve patients or if excessive dosing is respiratory depression. Drug may cause bradycardia; thus, use with caution in patients with bradyarrhythmias.

Nursing Implications: Assess baseline pulmonary status. Use with caution in patients with COPD, bradycardia, or renal or hepatic dysfunction, and in the older population. Teach patient to report any pulmonary difficulties immediately. Ensure that patient knows that if respiratory difficulty develops, the drug must be removed from mouth and discarded immediately. Ensure that patient understands how to administer drug safely and to keep drug supply out of reach of children and pets.

II.   SENSORY/PERCEPTUAL ALTERATIONS related to CNS CHANGES

Defining Characteristics: CNS depression and changes in mental status may occur, characterized by somnolence (7%) or dizziness (11%), confusion (8%), depression (8%), anxiety (5%), and insomnia (6%).

Nursing Implications: Assess baseline gait, mental, affective, and neurologic status. Assess medication profile to identify other contributions (i.e., CNS depressants). Instruct patient to report any changes. Assess patient safety and measures to ensure safety. Teach patient not to take alcohol, sleep aids, or tranquilizers, except as ordered by the oncology provider. Teach patient not to operate heavy machinery or to drive until the drug's effect has been determined. Discuss any significant changes with provider.

III. ALTERATION IN COMFORT related to HEADACHE, FATIGUE, ASTHENIA

Defining Characteristics: Headache occurs in about 9% of patients, asthenia (13%), and fatigue (12%).

Nursing Implications: Assess baseline comfort and activity level. Teach patients strategies to minimize fatigue. Teach patient to report symptoms and manage based on severity. Assess impact on patient's quality of life. If severe, discuss alternative strategies with physician.

IV. ALTERATION IN NUTRITION, LESS THAN BODY REQUIREMENTS, related to NAUSEA/VOMITING

Defining Characteristics: Nausea occurred in 21% of patients, vomiting occurred in 21%, and dry mouth in 7% of patients. Dehydration occurred in 13% of patients, anorexia in 8%, and decreased weight in 7%.

Nursing Implications: Assess baseline nutritional status, including electrolyte and fluid balance. Teach patient to take antiemetic agents as prescribed, to drink 8–10 ounces of fluid hourly while awake, and to eat small, frequent, calorie-dense foods. Teach patient to report nausea, vomiting, anorexia, and dehydration. Manage symptomatically. Assess severity and impact on quality of life. Discuss severe or unmanaged symptoms with physician.

V. ALTERATION IN ELIMINATION related to CONSTIPATION OR DIARRHEA

Defining Characteristics: Opium agonists bind to opiate receptors in bowel, slowing peristalsis, leading to constipation. Untreated constipation may result in bowel perforation. Constipation occurred in 11% of patients and diarrhea in 9% of patients.

Nursing Implications: Assess baseline elimination, fluid intake, diet, and exercise patterns. Instruct patient regarding prevention of constipation: goal is to move bowels at least every 2 days by increasing fluids to 3 L/day (drink 8- to 10-ounce glasses of fluid every hour while awake), following a diet high in fiber (beans, vegetables, fruit), and taking moderate exercise. Review bowel regimen, and assess need for additional bowel softeners, bulk-forming laxatives, and osmotic cathartics, and discuss prescription with physician. Teach patient self-administration of medications. However, all patients MUST be started on bowel regimen when receiving an opioid.

MANAGEMENT

Drug: fentanyl buccal tablet (Fentora)

Class: Opioid analgesic (opioid agonist).

Mechanism of Action: Fentanyl is a pure opioid agonist that binds to opioid μ-receptors located in the brain, spinal cord, and smooth muscle. Fentanyl in a buccal tablet is formulated using OraVescent technology so that when the tablet contacts saliva, the resulting reaction releases carbon dioxide and changes the local pH, allowing dissolution and passage of the fentanyl through the buccal membrane. The onset of analgesia is at 15 minutes, with significant decrease in pain intensity at 30 minutes in 50% of patients, and duration of action of 60 minutes.

Metabolism: Approximately 50% of the drug is absorbed through the buccal mucosa. The remaining half of the total dose is absorbed via the GI tract. Absolute bioavailability is 65%. After buccal absorption, there is a steep rise in mean plasma fentanyl concentration, peaking at 46.8 minutes. Drug is highly lipophilic and highly protein-bound (80–85%). Drug is taken up in tissues and eliminated primarily by biotransformation into inactive metabolites in the liver. It is metabolized in the liver primarily and to a lesser extent in the intestinal mucosa to norfentanyl by cytochrome P450 3A4 isoform. In population studies, patients with lower weight have a higher systemic exposure to the drug (men, Japanese subjects). Patients with renal and/or hepatic dysfunction who are receiving high doses of drug may have significantly decreased metabolic elimination of the drug. Four single 100-mcg tablets deliver 12–13% more drug than a single 400-mcg tablet. The dwell time (time tablet takes to disintegrate) does not affect early systemic exposure to fentanyl.

Indication: Indicated for the management of breakthrough pain in patients with cancer 18 years or older, who are already receiving and are tolerant to around-the-clock opioid therapy for persistent cancer pain (taking at least 60 mg of oral morphine a day, or 25 mcg of fentanyl per hour, or at least 30 mg of oxycodone daily, or at least 8 mg of hydromorphone daily, or an equianalgesic dose of another opioid, for at least 1 week or longer).

Dosage/Range:
- Principles: Patients must require and use around-the-clock opioids when taking this drug. Initial dose is 100 mcg. Initiate titration using multiples of 100 mcg of Fentora tablet. Limit patient access to only one strength of Fentora at one time. Individually titrate to a tolerable dose that provides adequate analgesia using single Fentora tablet. No more than 2 doses per breakthrough pain (BTP) episode. Wait at least 4 hours before treating another episode of BTP with Fentora. Place entire tablet in buccal cavity or under tongue; tablet must not be split, crushed, sucked, chewed, or swallowed whole.
  - Starting dose is 100 mcg; redose within a single BTP episode may occur 30 minutes after the start of administration of buccal fentanyl using the same dose strength.
  - Prescription is written: place tablet above a rear molar between the upper cheek and gum; one tablet per BTP episode; may repeat once if pain is not relieved after 30 minutes.
  - Titrate to adequate dose by patient diary and discussion with provider to achieve single tablet strength that provides relief; when doses above 100 mcg needed, patient

should place one 100-mcg tablet on buccal mucosa on each side of the mouth; if this is ineffective, increase dose by placing two 100-mcg tablets on each side of the mouth, for a total of four 100-mcg tablets.
  • Titrating above 400 mcg: increase dose in 200-mcg increments.
• When converting from oral transmucosal fentanyl (Actiq), a dose of buccal tablet is one-half or less than the Actiq dose (e.g., Actiq 200 or 400 mcg = Fentora 100 mcg; Actiq 600 or 800 mcg = Fentora 200 mcg; Actiq 1,200–1,600 mcg =Fentora 400 mcg).
• The goal is to determine necessary dose in a single tablet.
• After an effective dose has been determined, when the patient requires more than four breakthrough pain episodes per day, increase the maintenance (around-the-clock) opioid by an equivalent amount.
• Increase the fentanyl buccal tablet dose when a patient requires more than one dose per breakthrough pain episode.
• Drug is available through a restricted distribution program called Transmucosal Immediate Release Fentanyl Risk Evaluation and Mitigation Strategy (TIRF REMS) Access Program. Outpatients, healthcare professionals who prescribe to outpatients, pharmacies, and distributors are required to enroll in the program.

Drug Preparation/Administration:
• Available in a carton of seven blister cards with four tablets in each card; blister pack is child-resistant and encased in peelable foil.
• Available in 100-, 200-, 400-, 600-, and 800-mcg fentanyl base tablets.
• Open blister pack immediately before use: tear single blister unit from card, bend blister unit, and peel backing to expose the tablet (do not try to push through the backing).
• Remove tablet from blister unit, and place entire tablet in buccal cavity, usually above a rear molar, between the upper cheek and teeth, or place entire tablet under the tongue; patient should NOT try to split the tablet and/or chew, suck, or swallow the tablet, as this results in lower plasma fentanyl levels.
• Leave the tablet against buccal mucosa until it has fully disintegrated (14–25 minutes).
• After 30 minutes, if tablet remnants remain, the patient can swallow them with a drink of water.
• Teach patient to alternate sides of mouth when administering subsequent doses in the buccal cavity.
• Teach patient that opioid analgesics may impair the mental and/or physical ability to drive and use machines, and to avoid these activities until the effect of the drug is known.
• For patients requiring opioid discontinuation, gradually titrate downward, as it is not known at what level the opioid may be discontinued without causing signs/symptoms of abrupt withdrawal.

Drug Interactions:
• CNS depressants (other opioids, sedatives, hypnotics, general anesthetics, phenothiazines, tranquilizers, skeletal muscle relaxants, sedating antihistamines), potent inhibitors of cytochrome P450 CYP3A4 isoform (erythromycin, ketoconazole, certain protease inhibitors), and alcohol: increased CNS depression, with risk of hypoventilation, hypotension, and profound sedation.

- Moderate CYP3A4 inhibitors (aprepitant, diltiazem, grapefruit juice, verapamil): may increase fentanyl plasma levels; use together cautiously.
- MAO inhibitors within 14 days: potentiation of opioid, do not give together.

Lab Effects/Interference:
- None known.

Special Considerations:
- Contraindicated in patients who are not opioid-tolerant, have postoperative pain, who have received MAO inhibitors within 14 days, nursing mothers, as fentanyl is excreted in human milk causing potentially fatal respiratory depression, as well as physical dependence and withdrawal when no longer nursing.
- Use cautiously in patients with hepatic and/or renal dysfunction, chronic pulmonary disease, head injuries with increased intracranial pressure, and bradyarrhythmias. If drug must be used in a pregnant woman, benefit must outweigh potential risk to the fetus.
- Teach patient that drug must be kept out of reach of children and pets, as dose can be LETHAL to children and pets.
- Drug is an opioid and may cause physical dependence and withdrawal if stopped (along with maintenance opioid) abruptly.
- Application-site reactions occur in about 10% of patients (range from paresthesia to irritation to ulceration and bleeding) but rarely cause drug discontinuation.
- Most common ($\geq 10\%$) adverse reactions: nausea, dizziness, vomiting, fatigue, anemia, constipation, peripheral edema, asthenia, dehydration, headache.

Potential Toxicities/Side Effects and the Nursing Process

I.   POTENTIAL ALTERATION IN OXYGENATION related to HYPOVENTILATION

Defining Characteristics: Increased cough and/or dyspnea are rare, but the chief toxicity in naïve patients or if excessive dosing is respiratory depression. Drug may cause bradycardia; thus, use with caution in patients with bradyarrhythmias.

Nursing Implications: Assess baseline pulmonary status. Use with caution in patients with COPD, bradycardia, or renal or hepatic dysfunction, and in the older population. Teach patient to report any pulmonary difficulties immediately. Ensure that patient knows that if respiratory difficulty develops the drug must be removed from mouth and discarded immediately. Ensure that patient understands how to administer drug safely and to keep drug supply out of reach of children and pets.

II.   SENSORY/PERCEPTUAL ALTERATIONS related to CNS CHANGES

Defining Characteristics: CNS depression and changes in mental status may occur, characterized by somnolence (9%) or dizziness (13%), confusion (7%), depression (8%), and insomnia (6%). Rarely, hypoesthesia, lethargy, balance problems, anxiety, disorientation, and hallucinations may occur.

Nursing Implications: Assess baseline gait, mental, affective, and neurologic status. Assess medication profile to identify other contributions (i.e., CNS depressants). Instruct patient to report any changes. Assess patient safety, and measures to ensure safety. Teach patient not to take alcohol, sleep aids, or tranquilizers, except as ordered by the oncology provider. Discuss any significant changes with provider.

III. ALTERATION IN COMFORT related to HEADACHE, PAIN, PERIPHERAL EDEMA

Defining Characteristics: Headache occurs in about 10% of patients, abdominal pain (9%), peripheral edema (12%), asthenia (11%), and fatigue (16%). Back pain (5%) and arthralgia (6%) were reported less commonly.

Nursing Implications: Assess baseline comfort. Assess baseline skin integrity, presence of peripheral edema, and weight. Teach patient to report symptoms and manage based on severity, including elevating legs if peripheral edema present. Assess impact on patient's quality of life. If severe, discuss alternative strategies with physician.

IV. ALTERATION IN NUTRITION, LESS THAN BODY REQUIREMENTS, related to NAUSEA/VOMITING

Defining Characteristics: Nausea occurred in 29% of patients, and vomiting occurred in 20% of patients. Dehydration occurred in 11% of patients, anorexia 8%, and hypokalemia 6%.

Nursing Implications: Assess baseline nutritional status, including electrolyte and fluid balance. Teach patient to take antiemetic agents as prescribed, to drink 8–10 ounces of fluid hourly while awake, and to eat small, frequent, calorie-dense foods. Teach patient to report nausea, vomiting, anorexia, and dehydration. Manage symptomatically. Assess severity and impact on quality of life. Discuss severe or unmanaged symptoms with physician.

V. ALTERATION IN ELIMINATION related to CONSTIPATION OR DIARRHEA

Defining Characteristics: Opium agonists bind to opiate receptors in bowel, slowing peristalsis, leading to constipation. Untreated constipation may result in bowel perforation. Constipation occurred in 12% of patients and diarrhea in 8% of patients.

Nursing Implications: Assess baseline elimination, fluid intake, diet, and exercise patterns. Instruct patient regarding prevention of constipation: goal is to move bowels at least every 2 days by increasing fluids to 3 L/day (drink 8- to 10-ounce glasses of fluid every hour while awake), following a diet high in fiber (beans, vegetables, fruit), and taking moderate exercise. Review bowel regimen, and assess need for additional bowel softeners, bulk-forming laxatives, and osmotic cathartics, and discuss prescription with physician. Teach patient self-administration of medications. However, all patients MUST be started on bowel regimen when receiving an opioid.

MANAGEMENT

Drug: fentanyl citrate oral transmucosal lozenge, oral transmucosal fentanyl citrate (OTFC) [Actiq, generic equivalents]

Class: Opioid analgesic (opioid agonist).

Mechanism of Action: Fentanyl is a pure opioid agonist that binds to opioid μ-receptors located in the brain, spinal cord, and smooth muscle. The oral transmucosal preparation of the drug is a solid formulation of fentanyl citrate placed on a handle so the drug is placed between the cheek and lower gum, with the patient occasionally moving the drug matrix from one side to the other, over a 15-minute period. Sucking the drug dose coats the oral mucosa, through which 25% of the drug is rapidly absorbed, reportedly as fast as IV morphine.

Metabolism: Initial rapid absorption of about 25% of total dose across buccal mucosa, into systemic circulation, and longer prolonged absorption of swallowed fentanyl (75% of dose) from GI tract. One-third of drug escapes first-pass elimination and enters the systemic circulation for a total of 50% of the total dose that is bioavailable. Following absorption, drug is rapidly distributed to brain, heart, lungs, kidneys, and spleen. Plasma binding is 80–85%. The drug is primarily metabolized in the liver, by the CYP3A4 isoenzyme; < 7% of the dose is excreted in the urine. The terminal elimination half-life is approximately 7 hours.

Indication: Management of breakthrough pain (BTP) in cancer patients 16 years of age and older who are already receiving and who are tolerant to around-the-clock opioid therapy for their underlying persistent cancer pain. Tolerance to opioids is defined as taking at least: 60 mg of morphine/day, 25 mcg/hr transdermal fentanyl, 30 mg oral oxycodone/day, 8 mg oral hydromorphone/day, 25 mg oral oxymorphone/day, or an equianalgesic dose of another opioid daily for a week or longer. Limitations: drug can be dispensed only to patients enrolled in the TIRF (Transmucosal Immediate Release Fentanyl) REMS (Risk Evaluation and Mitigation Strategy) Access Program.

Contraindications: Opioid-naïve patients; treatment of acute or postoperative pain, including headache/migraine, dental pain. Life-threatening respiratory depression and death can occur at any dose in opioid nontolerant patients, or when used postoperatively. Also contraindicated in patients allergic to fentanyl, or OTFC components, as anaphylaxis and HSR can occur. Do not administer to patients who have received MAO inhibitors within 14 days, as unpredictable potentiation of the opioid may occur. Do not administer to nursing mothers.

Dosage/Range: *Adult (16 years of age and older)*
- Oral Transmucosal Fentanyl Citrate (OTFC) is available only through a restricted program. OTFC can be dispensed only to patients enrolled in the TIRF REMS Access Program. OTFC can be prescribed, dispensed, and distributed only by physicians, pharmacists, and vendors enrolled in the TIRF REMS Access Program. To obtain a list of qualified pharmacies/distributors, see www.TIRFREMSAccess.com, or call 1-866-822-1483.

- *Initial dose of OTFC is always 200 mcg.* Patient should have an initial supply of six 200 mcg OTFC units. Patient should use all units before increasing to a higher dose to prevent confusion and possible overdose.
  - For example, patient begins using a 200-mcg unit for BTP and sucks the medicine for 15 minutes. If the pain is unrelieved, the patient waits an additional 15 minutes, and then administers a second 200-mcg unit (now 30 minutes after starting initial dosage unit).
  - The patient should take a maximum of two doses of OTFC for any BTP episode. Patient should wait at least four hours before treating another episode of BTP with OTFC. To reduce risk of overdosing, patient should only have one strength of OTFC for any BTP episode.
  - Patients should record their usage of OTFC over several episodes of BTP and share this with their provider to determine if a dosage adjustment is needed.
- *Maintenance dosing:* Once an effective dose is reached, patient should use only one OTFC unit of the appropriate strength per pain episode.
  - If the BTP is not relieved in 15 minutes after completion of the OTFC unit, patient can take only one additional dose using the same strength for that episode 15 minutes later.
  - Once the dose has been determined that relieves BTP with a single dose, the patient should require only four or fewer doses a day.
  - If more than four doses are required, then the ATC (long-acting) opioid dose should be evaluated and likely increased.
- Generally, OTFC dose should be increased only when a single administration of the current BTP dose fails to treat the BTP episode effectively for several consecutive episodes.
- The patient should notify the physician if drug is required more than four times per day, so that the long-acting opioid can be increased.

Drug Preparation:
- Drug is available in dosage strengths of 200, 400, 600, 800, 1,200, and 1,600 mcg. Initial dose is always 200 mcg.
- Drug is on a handle, sealed in a child-resistant foil pouch that requires scissors to open. The drug dose is color-coded.
- Trade name Actiq is manufactured by Cephalon, and generic OTFC lozenges are manufactured by Anesta Corp, Mallinckrodt Inc., and Par Pharmaceutical Companies Inc.

Drug Administration:
- Use scissors to open blister pack immediately before use. Patient should place drug dose unit in the mouth between cheek and lower gum, occasionally moving the drug matrix from one side to the other using the handle. Patient should suck, NOT CHEW, the medication over 15 minutes, as this would result in lower peak concentrations and lower bioavailability.
- If patient has signs of excessive opioid effects before unit is consumed, the dosage unit should be removed from the patient's mouth, disposed of properly, and subsequent doses should be reduced.
- If the patient achieves adequate analgesia or develops excessive side effects, the drug should be removed from the mouth and discarded immediately. The remaining drug is very dangerous if a child or pet ingests it, so maximum precautions must be taken.

MANAGEMENT

- Destroy any medication remaining on the handle by dissolving it under hot water, and place handle out of reach of children and pets. If unable to dispose of remaining drug right away, place in an empty jar, tightly close lid, and place out of reach of children and pets. Dispose of properly as soon as possible.
- Any remaining drug must be disposed of properly. It can be fatal to a child or pet if ingested, so maximum precautions must be taken.
- Keep medication away from patient's eyes, skin, or mucous membranes when not sucking the medication, and the patient should wash hands after discarding unused medication portion.
- At home, teach patient to store oral doses in a safe place away from children and pets.
- Titrate drug cautiously in patients with COPD or preexisting medical conditions predisposing them to respiratory depression and in patients susceptible to intracranial effects of CO_2.
- Teach patient that opioid analgesics may impair the mental and/or physical ability to drive and use machines, and to avoid these activities until the effect of the drug is known.
- If patient requires discontinuance of opioids, a gradual downward titration is recommended to prevent withdrawal symptoms: yawning, sweating, lacrimation, rhinorrhea, anxiety, restlessness, insomnia, dilated pupils, piloerection, chills, tachycardia, hypertension, nausea/vomiting, cramping, abdominal pain, diarrhea, muscle aches and pains.

Drug Interactions:

- CNS depressants (e.g., other opioids, alcohol, sedatives, hypnotics, general anesthetics, phenothiazines, tranquilizers, skeletal muscle relaxants, sedating antihistamines) may increase CNS depression (hypoventilation, hypotension, profound sedation, especially in opioid nontolerant patients). Patients who require concomitant drugs should be monitored for a change in opioid effects. Consider adjusting the dose of OTFC if needed.
- Strong CYP3A4 inhibitors (e.g., ritonavir, ketoconazole, itraconazole, troleandomycin, clarithromycin, nelfinavir, nefazodone) or moderate inhibitors (e.g., amprenavir, aprepitant, diltiazem, erythromycin, fluconazole, fosamprenavir, verapamil), and grapefruit/grapefruit juice: may result in increased fentanyl serum levels, increasing opioid side effects, including fatal respiratory depression; avoid concomitant administration. If required, carefully monitor patient for an extended period of time. If dosage increase is required, do so very conservatively and carefully.
- Strong CYP3A4 inducers: may decrease serum fentanyl levels, and decrease analgesia. Avoid concomitant administration.
- MAO inhibitors, or within 14 days of discontinuation; do not administer OTFC.

Lab Effects/Interference:

- None known.

Special Considerations:

- Once an effective dose is identified, drug provides rapid relief of BTP.
- Patients should be taught to call nurse or physician if taking two of the same strength units within 60 minutes without relief or if taking drug more than four times per day.
- When prescribing, do NOT convert a patient to OTFC from any other fentanyl product on a mcg-per-mcg basis, as OTFC and other fentanyl products are NOT equivalent. There are NO safe conversions; therefore, the initial dose of OTFC should ALWAYS be 200 mcg.

- OTFC is NOT a generic version of fentanyl buccal tablet (Fentora). DO NOT substitute an OTFC prescription for fentanyl buccal tablets (Fentora) under any circumstances. The drugs are NOT equivalent; there are substantial differences in pharmacokinetic profile, rate, and extent of absorption.
- Teach patient that drug must be kept out of reach of children, as dose can be LETHAL to children. This has occurred when a child accidentally played with a parent's OTFC. Patients and their caregivers should be taught to keep both used and unused dosage units out of reach of children and pets. All units should be disposed of immediately after use. Providers and nurses should specifically question patients about children in the home (living there or visiting). Actiq offers an interim safe-storage container, "Actiq Child Safety Kit," obtainable by providers by calling Cephalon Inc. at 1-800-896-5855, or accessing it on the Web at www.actiq.com.
- Administer cautiously to patients with hepatic or renal dysfunction.
- Use cautiously in patients with chronic pulmonary disease (degree of hypoventilation), cardiac conduction disease (bradycardia), and the elderly.
- Use extreme caution when administering OTFC, if at all, to patients with increased intracranial pressure or impaired consciousness, as they are susceptible to intracranial effects of CO_2 retention. Opioids can also make accurate neurological assessment difficult or impossible.
- Respiratory depression is the chief hazard with opioids, such as fentanyl, the opioid in OTFC. This most often occurs in patients who are elderly, have underlying respiratory disorders, or are debilitated; when large doses are prescribed to an opioid-naïve patient; or when opioids are given together with other respiratory depressing drugs. Patients experiencing respiratory depression have a decreased urge to breathe, depressed respiratory rate, a "sighing" pattern of respiration (deep breaths separated by abnormally long pauses). CO_2 retention from this depressed breathing can exacerbate opioid-induced sedation. Patients should be monitored for this. This was not reported in the clinical trials with Actiq.
- Most common adverse effects (occurring $\geq$ 5%): nausea, dizziness, somnolence, vomiting, asthenia, headache, dyspnea, constipation, anxiety, confusion, depression, rash, and insomnia. The most serious adverse effects reported with all opioids are respiratory depression, circulatory depression, hypotension, and shock.
- Each OTFC unit contains about 2 grams of sugar (hydrated dextrates). Diabetic patients should be warned this may affect their blood glucose levels and medication needed to control their diabetes. In addition, dental decay can be accelerated by the sugar content, and may be exacerbated by opioid-induced dry mouth. Post-marketing reports confirmed cases of dental decay. Patients should be told to contact their dentist to ensure they are performing appropriate oral hygiene.

Potential Toxicities/Side Effects and the Nursing Process

I.   ALTERATION IN OXYGENATION related to HYPOVENTILATION

Defining Characteristics: Dyspnea (7–22%) may occur. Patients are also receiving ATC long-acting opioids.

Nursing Implications: Assess baseline pulmonary status. Use with caution in patients with COPD, bradycardia, or renal or hepatic dysfunction, and in the elderly. Teach patient to report any pulmonary difficulties immediately. Ensure that patient knows that if respiratory difficulty develops, the drug must be removed from mouth and discarded immediately; also, the patient must know to suck and not to chew drug. Ensure that patient understands how to handle drug safely to prevent additional absorption of unused drug. Teach patient and family members to call 911 if the patient is very sedated.

II.   SENSORY/PERCEPTUAL ALTERATIONS related to CNS CHANGES

Defining Characteristics: CNS depression and changes in mental status may occur, characterized by somnolence or dizziness (9–16%); abnormal gait, anxiety, confusion, depression, insomnia, hypesthesia, vasodilation (3–10% incidence).

Nursing Implications: Assess baseline gait and mental, affective, and neurologic status. Assess medication profile to identify other contributions, i.e., CNS depressants. Instruct patient to report any changes. Assess patient safety, and take measures to ensure safety. Discuss any significant changes with physician. Teach patient that opioid analgesics may impair the mental and/or physical ability to drive a car or operate machinery, so these activities should be avoided until the drug's full effects are known.

III.   ALTERATION IN SELF-CARE, POTENTIAL, related to LACK OF KNOWLEDGE OF SELF-ADMINISTRATION

Defining Characteristics: Instructions regarding self-administration may be confusing to patients, especially if English is not the patient's native language.

Nursing Implications: Ensure that the patient is taking a long-acting opioid (ATC) and has for at least one week. Teach patient about OTFC, that it is an opioid with very important self-care administration points, and why it is being recommended for the management of BTP in this patient. Review the medication guide that comes with the OTFC with the patient. Ask if children live or visit at home, and emphasize how important it is to keep the drug out of reach of children and pets. Teach patient that fentanyl can be abused, so it should never be shared with other people. Teach patient that all patients start with a 200-mcg dose and the patient should have only one strength of OTFC at home at one time. OTFC doses should be four hours apart, unless the pain is unrelieved by a single dose; in that case, a second dose can be taken 30 minutes after the first. The goal is to need only four doses of BTP medication per day, along with the long-acting ATC opioid; the patient must work with the nurse and doctor to find the right dose. The patient should be given a diary to record pain level, time of BTP dose, activity, and relief achieved. Teach patient to call the nurse or physician if the OTFC with a repeated dose in 15 minutes after the end of the dose (total time 30 minutes) does not control the pain, or if the pain gets worse after taking two doses of BTP OTFC, or if the patient requires more than four BTP medication doses a day. It may be necessary to adjust the dose. Teach patient that opioids may cause constipation, and that the goal is to move bowels at least once every 1–2 days. If nausea and vomiting develop, ensure that patient has a prescription for an antiemetic, along with instructions on how to self-administer.

IV. ALTERATION IN COMFORT related to HEADACHE, FEVER

Defining Characteristics: Headache and asthenia are reported in 4–20% and 15–38% of patients respectively who required OTFC.

Nursing Implications: Assess baseline comfort. Teach patient to report symptoms and manage based on severity. Assess impact on patient's quality of life. If severe, discuss alternative strategies with physician.

V. ALTERATION IN NUTRITION, LESS THAN BODY REQUIREMENTS, related to NAUSEA/VOMITING

Defining Characteristics: Nausea occurs in 24–45% and vomiting in 7–31% of patients.

Nursing Implications: Assess baseline nutritional status. Teach patient to report nausea, vomiting, anorexia, dyspepsia. Manage symptomatically. Teach self-administration of antiemetics 30 minutes prior to drug dose, if possible, and as directed. Assess severity and impact on quality of life. Discuss severe or unmanaged symptoms with physician and revise plan. Ensure that patient is taking adequate fluids to keep hydration status normal.

VI. ALTERATION IN ELIMINATION related to CONSTIPATION OR DIARRHEA

Defining Characteristics: Opium agonists bind to opiate receptors in bowel, slowing peristalsis, leading to constipation. Untreated constipation may result in bowel perforation. In long term treatment, constipation occurred in 20% of patients (any dose).

Nursing Implications: Assess baseline elimination, fluid intake, diet, and exercise patterns. Instruct patient regarding prevention of constipation: goal is to move bowels at least every 2 days by increasing fluids to 3 L/day, following a diet high in fiber (beans, vegetables, fruit), and taking moderate exercise. Assess need for bowel softeners, bulk-forming laxatives, and osmotic cathartics, and discuss prescription with physician. Teach patient self-administration of medications. Patient MUST be started on bowel regimen.

Drug: fentanyl nasal spray (Lazanda)

Class: Opioid analgesic (opioid agonist).

Mechanism of Action: Fentanyl is a pure opioid agonist that binds to opioid μ-receptors located in the brain, spinal cord, and smooth muscle, to achieve analgesia.

MANAGEMENT

Metabolism: Fentanyl nasal spray is absorbed from the nasal mucosa, and the T_{max} (maximal concentration) is achieved from 15–21 minutes after a single dose. Presence of allergic rhinitis does not affect absorption. Bioavailability of drug is 20% higher than when administered in an oral transmucosal formulation. Drug is highly lipophilic, with 80–85% plasma binding. Fentanyl is metabolized by the liver and in the intestinal mucosa to norfentanyl by cytochrome P450 CYP3A4 isoform. Fentanyl is excreted (> 90%) by biotransformation into inactive metabolites. Less than 7% of administered dose is excreted unchanged in the urine, and 1% excreted unchanged in the stool.

Indications: Mangement of breakthrough pain (BTP) in cancer patients aged 18 years and older who are already receiving and who are tolerant to opioid therapy for their underlying persistent cancer pain. Drug is available through a restricted distribution program called Transmucosal Immediate Release Fentanyl Risk Evaluation and Mitigation Strategy (TIRF REMS) Access Program. Outpatients and healthcare professionals who prescribe to outpatients, pharmacies, and distributors are required to enroll in the program.

Contraindications: (1) Opioid NON-tolerant patients; (2) management of acute or postoperative pain, including headache/migraine, or dental pain; (3) intolerance or hypersensitivity to fentanyl or drug's components.

Dosage/Range:
- Opioid-tolerant patients ONLY. Outpatient prescriber, patient, dispensing outpatient pharmacy, and supplier must all be enrolled in and compy with the TIRF REMS Access Program.
- Nasal spray, where each spray delivers 100 mcL of solution containing either 100 mcg or 400 mcg fentanyl base. Supplied in a 5-mL bottle containing 8 sprays.
- Individually titrate to an effective dose, from 100 mcg to 200 mcg, to 400 mcg, and up to a maximum of 800 mcg, with tolerable side effects.
  - Initial dose: 100 mcg. Teach patient to administer one spray in ONE nostril.
  - Do not give another spray for this episode; WAIT AT LEAST 2 HOURS BEFORE USING SPRAY FOR THE NEXT EPISODE.
  - Evaluate whether pain relief was adequate after 30 minutes; if yes, use the same dose for the next pain episode, and this will be the successful and usual dose.
  - If no, for the next pain episode, increase to the next higher dose (e.g., 200 mcg, one 100-mcg spray in EACH nostril). If not effective in 30 minutes, in 2 hours use next higher titration level (e.g., 400 mcg, one 400-mcg spray in ONE nostril). If not effective in 30 minutes, in 2 hours, use final titration level (e.g., 800 mcg, one 400-mcg spray in EACH nostril).
  - Confirm apparent successful dose of drug with a second episode of breakthrough pain, and review experience with physician/midlevel to determine if that dose is appropriate or whether further adjustment is needed.
  - If pain relief at 30 minutes is inadequate following nasal spray, or if breakthrough pain occurs again within 2 hours, use rescue medications as directed by healthcare professional.

Dosage Readjustment:
- If there is a marked change in response or adverse reaction, you may need to readjust dose. If patient has > 4 episodes of breakthrough pain per day, reevaluate dose of the

long-acting opioid used for control of persistent underlying cancer pain. If the dose of the long-acting opioid is increased, reevalute and retitrate the fentanyl nasal spray dose.
- Limit use of fentanyl nasal sprays to treat < 4 episodes of breakthrough pain/day.
- Any dose retitration must be carefully monitored by a healthcare professional.

Drug Preparation: Nasal spray: Each spray delivers 100 mcL of solution, containing either 100 mcg or 400 mcg fentanyl base, supplied in a 5-mL bottle containing 8 sprays. Fentanyl nasal spray bottle MUST be stored out of reach of children and pets, in the specially provided child-resistant container.

Drug Administration:
- Prime the device before use by spraying into the pouch (4 sprays in total), following the instructions for use in the *Medication Guide* provided with the REMS Lazanda pack.
- Insert the nozzle of fentanyl nasal spray bottle 1/2 inch (1 cm) into the nose and point toward the bridge of the nose, tilting the bottle slightly.
- Press down firmly on the finger grips until the patient hears a click, and the number in the counting window advances by one; the fine mist spray is not always felt on the nasal mucosal membrane, so the patient should rely on hearing the audible click and the advancement of the dose counter to confirm a spray has been administered.
- When the 8 doses in the bottle have all been given, the patient should dispose of any remaining drug by aiming the bottle into the provided pouch, and discharge the remaining liquid into the pouch by pressing down on the finger grips a total of 4 times to ensure that any remaining liquid is trapped in the pouch. After the 8 therapeutic sprays have been emitted, the patient will not hear a click and the counter will not advance beyond 8 when spraying the residual into the pouch. Then seal the pouch. Place both the empty bottle and sealed pouch into the child-resistant storage container and discard in the trash.
- Patient should be instructed to wash hands with soap and water immediately after handling the pouch.
- If the pouch is lost, use a pouch from another Lazanda pack to prime and dispose of unused medicine from the current bottle, as well as from the next bottle. If the patient does not have an available empty pouch, teach the patient to call 1-866-435-6775 to order and receive a replacement pouch in the mail.
- Teach patient that opioid analgesics may impair the mental and/or physical ability to drive and use machines, and to avoid these activities until the effect of the drug is known.

Drug Interactions:
- Monitor patients who begin therapy with, or increase the dose of, inhibitors of CYP3A4 for signs of opioid toxicity (e.g., indinavir, nelfinavir, ritonavir, clarithromycin, itraconazole, ketoconazole, nefazodone, saquinavir, telithromycin, aprepitant, diltiazem, erythromycin, fluconazole, grapefruit juice, verapamil, or cimetidine). Coadministration may increase or prolong adverse opioid effects, including potentially fatal respiratory depression.
- Monitor patients who stop therapy with, or decrease the dose of, inducers of CYP3A4 (e.g., barbiturates, carbamazepine, efavirenz, glucocorticoids, modafinil, nevirapine, oxcarbazepine, phenobarbital, phenytoin, pioglitazone, rifabutin, rifampin, St. John's wort, troglitazone) for signs of opioid toxicity. Coadministration of an inducer and

fentanyl can decrease the fentanyl serum level, so when stopping the CYP3A4 inducer, the patient may experience a sudden increase in the fentanyl plasma concentration. Adjust fentanyl nasal spray dose accordingly.
- Agents used to treat allergic rhinitis: Coadministration of a vasoconstrictive nasal decongestant may cause fentanyl nasal spray to be less effective. In addition, if the patient is experiencing an acute episode of rhinitis and the fentanyl dose is titrated, an incorrect titration may occur so that when the allergic rhinitis drug is stopped, the drug dose is too high. DO NOT COADMINISTER.
- MAO inhibitors within 14 days: Potentiation of opioid; do not give together.
- CNS depressants (e.g., other opioids, sedatives or hypnotics, general anesthetics, phenothiazines, tranquilizers, skeletal muscle relaxants, sedating antihistamines, alcohol): May increase risk for CNS depression (e.g., hypotension, hypoventilation, profound sedation); do not coadminister; if must coadminister, consider reducing fentanyl nasal spray dose.

Lab Effects/Interference: Increased alkaline phosphatase.

Special Considerations:
- Lazanda is available only through the restricted Lazanda TIRF REMS program, and healthcare providers who prescribe to outpatients, pharmacies, and distributors are required to enroll in the TIRF REMS Access Program.
- Drug is an opioid and may cause physical dependence and withdrawal if stopped (along with maintenance opioid) abruptly. In addition, it can lead to psychological dependence (addiction) if inappropriately used.
- Use drug cautiously in the elderly, who are more sensitive to opioids.
- Clinically significant respiratory and CNS depression can occur. Monitor patients accordingly.
  - Use cautiously, if at all, in patients with hepatic and/or renal dysfunction, head injuries, increased intracranial pressure, cardiac disease (especially with bradyarrhythmias), and chronic pulmonary disease. If a pregnant woman must use the drug, benefit must outweigh potential risk to the fetus.
  - Titrate fentanyl nasal spray cautiously in patients with COPD or preexisting medical conditions predisposing them to hypoventilation.
  - Administer fentanyl nasal spray with extreme caution in patients susceptible to intracranial effects of CO_2 retention.
- DO NOT convert patients to fentanyl nasal spray from other fentanyl products on a mcg-per-mcg basis, or substitute a fentanyl nasal spray prescription for another fentanyl product, as this may result in a fatal overdose.
- Use with other CNS depressants and potent CYP3A4 inhibitors may increase depressant effects including hypoventilation, hypotension, and profound sedation. Consider dosage adjustments if warranted.
- Fentanyl citrate is not mutagenic but is embryocidal in rats; in addition, it has been shown to impair fertility. DO NOT use drug during labor and delivery, as it may cause respiratory depression in the fetus. Nursing mothers should not use the drug.
- Teach patient that drug must be kept out of reach of children and pets, as dose can be LETHAL to children and pets. Keep drug in the specially provided child-resistant container.

- Most common side effects during titration (frequency > 5%): nausea, vomiting, dizziness.
- Most common side effects during maintenance phase (frequency > 5%): vomiting, nausea, pyrexia, constipation.

Potential Toxicities/Side Effects and the Nursing Process

I. POTENTIAL ALTERATION IN OXYGENATION related to HYPOVENTILATION

Defining Characteristics: Increased cough and/or dyspnea are rare, but the chief toxicity in opioid-naïve patients, or if excessive dosing, is respiratory depression. Drug may cause bradycardia; thus, use with caution in patients with bradyarrhythmias.

Nursing Implications: Assess baseline pulmonary status. Use with caution in patients with COPD, bradycardia, or renal or hepatic dysfunction, and in the older population. Drug is contraindicated in opioid-naïve patients. Teach patient to report any pulmonary difficulties immediately. Ensure that patient knows that if respiratory difficulty develops to call the emergency response system (e.g., 911). Ensure that patient understands how to administer drug safely and to keep drug supply out of reach of children and pets in the specially provided secure container.

II. SENSORY/PERCEPTUAL ALTERATIONS related to CNS CHANGES

Defining Characteristics: CNS depression and changes in mental status may occur, characterized by somnolence (9%) or dizziness (6%), confusion, and headache; dysgeusia may also occur.

Nursing Implications: Assess baseline gait, mental, affective, and neurologic status. Assess medication profile to identify other contributions (i.e., CNS depressants). Instruct patient to report any changes. Assess patient safety, and measures to ensure safety. Teach patient not to take alcohol, sleep aids, or tranquilizers, except as ordered by the oncology provider. Discuss any significant changes with provider. Teach patient that drug may impair the mental and/or physical ability to operate a car or heavy machinery, and to avoid doing so while taking the drug.

III. ALTERATION IN COMFORT related to BACK PAIN, PAIN IN EXTREMITY, ARTHRALGIA

Defining Characteristics: Although uncommon, back pain, extremity pain, and arthralgias may occur.

Nursing Implications: Assess baseline comfort. Teach patient to report symptoms and manage based on severity. Assess impact on patient's quality of life. If severe, discuss alternative strategies with physician.

MANAGEMENT

IV.   ALTERATION IN NUTRITION, LESS THAN BODY REQUIREMENTS, related to NAUSEA/VOMITING

Defining Characteristics: Nausea occurred in 7% of patients during both titration and maintenance. Vomiting occurred in 6% during titration and 10% during maintenance. Dysgeusia, dry mouth, dyspepsia, mouth ulcer, proctalgia rarely occurred.

Nursing Implications: Assess baseline nutritional status, including electrolyte and fluid balance. Teach patient to take antiemetic agents as prescribed, to drink 8–10 ounces of fluid hourly while awake, and to eat small, frequent, calorie-dense foods. Teach patient to report nausea, vomiting, anorexia, and dehydration. Manage symptomatically. Assess severity and impact on quality of life. Discuss severe or unmanaged symptoms with physician.

V.   ALTERATION IN ELIMINATION related to CONSTIPATION

Defining Characteristics: Opium agonists bind to opiate receptors in bowel, slowing peristalsis, leading to constipation. Untreated constipation may result in bowel perforation. Constipation occurred in 6% of patients and diarrhea in 8%.

Nursing Implications: Assess baseline elimination, fluid intake, diet, and exercise patterns. Instruct patient regarding prevention of constipation: goal is to move bowels at least every 2 days by increasing fluids to 3 L/day (drink 8- to 10-ounce glasses of fluid every hour while awake), following a diet high in fiber (beans, vegetables, fruit), and taking moderate exercise. Review bowel regimen, and assess need for additional bowel softeners, bulk-forming laxatives, and osmotic cathartics, and discuss prescription with physician. Teach patient self-administration of medications; however, all patients MUST be started on bowel regimen when receiving an opioid.

Drug: fentanyl sublingual tablets (Abstral)

Class: Opioid analgesic (opioid agonist).

Mechanism of Action: Fentanyl is a pure opioid agonist that binds to opioid μ-receptors located in the brain, spinal cord, and smooth muscle, resulting in analgesia.

Metabolism: Orally administered fentanyl undergoes pronounced hepatic and intestinal first-pass effects. Sublingual tablets are absorbed through the oral mucosa. Bioavailability is 54%. Drug is highly lipophilic, and rapidly distributed to the brain, heart, lungs, spleen, and kidneys, followed by a slower redistribution to muscles and fat. Drug is 80–85% plasma bound; it is primarily metabolized by the liver and intestinal mucosa to norfentanyl by cytochrome P450 3A4 isoform. This metabolite is not pharmacologically active. More than 90% of fentanyl is eliminated by biotransformation into inactive metabolites. Less than 7% of intact drug is excreted in the urine and about 1% is excreted in the feces.

Indication: Indicated for the management of breakthrough pain (BTP) in patients who are at least 18 years old and who are already receiving and are tolerant to opioid therapy for their underlying and persistent cancer pain. A patient who is considered tolerant is taking at least 60 mg oral morphine/day; or at least 25 mcg transdermal fentanyl/hour; 30 mg oral oxycodone/day; 8 mg oral hydromorphone/day; 25 mg oral oxymorphone/day; or an equianalgesic dose of another opioid for a week or longer. Drug is available through a restricted distribution program called Transmucosal Immediate Release Fentanyl Risk Evaluation and Mitigation Strategy (TIRF REMS) Access Program. Outpatients and healthcare professionals who prescribe to outpatients, pharmacies, and distributors are required to enroll in the program.

Contraindications: (1) Opioid nontolerant patients; (2) management of acute or postoperative pain, including headache/migraine, dental pain, or use in the emergency department; (3) intolerance or hypersensitivity to fentanyl, Abstral, or its components.

Dosage/Range: Opioid-tolerant patients ONLY.
- Initial dose: 100 mcg.
- **Individually titrate** to an effective dose, from 100 mcg to 200 mcg, to 400 mcg, to 600 mcg, and up to a maximum of 800 mcg, with tolerable side effects.
- Evaluate whether pain relief was adequate after 30 minutes; if yes, use the same dose for the next pain episode, and this will be the successful and usual dose.
- If not, patient may use a second dose after the 30-minute evaluation period as directed by healthcare provider. No more than 2 doses of fentanyl sublingual tablets should be used to treat an episode of breakthrough pain. Patients must wait at least 2 hours before treating another episode of breakthrough pain with fentanyl sublingual tablets.
- If adequate analgesia was not obtained with the first 100-mcg dose, then continue dose escalation in a stepwise manner over consecutive breakthrough episodes until adequate analgesia with tolerable side effects is achieved.
  - Increase the dose by 100-mcg multiples up to 400 mcg as needed (four 100-mcg tablets, two 200-mcg tablets, or one 400-mcg tablet)
  - If adequate analgesia is not achieved at 400-mcg dose, titrate up to 600 mcg (three 200-mcg tablets or one 600-mcg tablet).
  - If adequate analgesia is not achieved at 600-mcg dose, titrate up to 800 mcg (four 200-mcg tablets or one 800-mcg tablet).
  - If adequate analgesia is not achieved 30 minutes after the dose of sublingual fentanyl, patient may repeat the same dose. No more than two doses of the drug should be used to treat an episode of breakthrough pain.
  - Rescue medication as directed by the healthcare provider can be used if adequate analgesia is not achieved with the two doses of sublingual fentanyl.
  - Patients must be supervised by healthcare professionals during dose titration.
- Maintenance: Once the optimal dose has been identified, instruct patient to use only one sublingual fentanyl tablet of the appropriate strength per dose. If patient does not achieve adequate relief, a second dose may be used after 30 minutes (as directed by healthcare provider). Patients should wait at least 2 hours before treating another episode of breakthrough pain.

- Dosage readjustment: If there is a marked change in response or adverse reaction, it may be necessary to readjust dose. If patient has more than 4 episodes of breakthrough pain per day, reevaluate dose of the long-acting opioid used for control of persistent underlying cancer pain. If the dose of the long-acting opioid is increased, reevalute and retitrate the fentanyl nasal spray dose.
- Limit use of fentanyl sublingual to treat fewer than 4 episodes of breakthrough pain per day once a successful dose is determined.
- When prescribing, do not convert patients on a mcg-per-mcg basis from any other oral transmucosal fentanyl product to Abstral.
- When dispensing, do not substitute with any other fentanyl product.
- Use with CYP3A4 inhibitors may cause fatal respiratory arrest. Assess patient medication profile for CYP3A4 inhibitors and discuss with physician or NP/PA if found.
- If the patient discontinues opioid therapy, consider discontinuing sublingual fentanyl tablets gradually along with other opioids to prevent possible withdrawal effects.

Drug Preparation: Available in 100 mcg (marked 1 on tablet), 200 mcg (marked 2 on tablet), 300 mcg (marked 3 on tablet), 400 mcg (marked 4 on tablet), 600 mcg (marked 6 on tablet), and 800 mcg (marked 8 on tablet) tablets; comes in a blister card with four blister units (each containing a tablet). Store at room temperature in the original blister pack; do not remove to store in a temporary container such as a pill box. Teach patient to store oral doses in a safe place away from children and pets, as dose of tablet may be fatal, and to protect from theft.

Drug Administration:
- Remove one blister unit from card by tearing at perforation, then peel back the foil and gently remove tablet. DO NOT try to push through the foil as it will damage the tablet.
- Teach patient to place tablet(s) on the floor of the mouth directly under the tongue, immediately after removing the tablet(s) from the blister pack. Do not chew, suck, or swallow the tablet. Allow the tablet to completely dissolve under the tongue, and do not drink or eat anything until the tablet is completely dissolved. If the patient has a dry mouth, suggest using a small amount of water to moisten the buccal mucosa before taking the tablet(s).
- Teach patient to keep drug in a safe place away from children and pets.
- Teach patient that opioid analgesics may impair the mental and/or physical ability to drive and use machines, and to avoid these activities until the effect of the drug is known.
- Disposal: Dispose of any unused tablets by removing from blister pack and flushing down toilet.

Drug Interactions:
- Monitor patients who begin therapy with, or increase the dose of, inhibitors of CYP3A4 for signs of opioid toxicity (e.g., indinavir, nelfinavir, ritonavir, clarithromycin, itraconazole, ketoconazole, nefazodone, saquinavir, telithromycin, aprepitant, diltiazem, erythromycin, fluconazole, grapefruit juice, verapamil, or cimetidine). Coadministration may increase or prolong adverse opioid effects, including potentially fatal respiratory depression.
- Monitor patients who stop therapy with, or decrease the dose of, inducers of CYP3A4 (e.g., barbiturates, carbamazepine, efavirenz, glucocorticoids, modafinil, nevirapine, oxcarbazepine, phenobarbital, phenytoin, pioglitazone, rifabutin, rifampin, St. John's wort, troglitazone) for signs of opioid toxicity. Coadministration of an inducer and fentanyl can

decrease the fentanyl serum level, so when stopping the CYP3A4 inducer, the patient may experience a sudden increase in the fentanyl plasma concentration. Adjust fentanyl sublingual tablet dose accordingly.

- CNS depressants (other opioids, sedatives, hypnotics, general anesthetics, phenothiazines, tranquilizers, skeletal muscle relaxants, sedating antihistamines), potent inhibitors of cytochrome P450 CYP3A4 isoform (erythromycin, ketoconazole, certain protease inhibitors), and alcohol: Increased CNS depression, with risk of hypoventilation, hypotension, and profound sedation.
- Moderate CYP3A4 inhibitors (aprepitant, diltiazem, grapefruit juice, verapamil): May increase fentanyl plasma levels; use together cautiously.
- MAO inhibitors with 14 days: Potentiation of opioid, do not give together.

Lab Effects/Interference:
- None known.

Special Considerations:
- Abstral is available only through the restricted Abstral REMS program, and healthcare providers who prescribe to outpatients, pharmacies, and distributors are required to enroll in the program. Further information is available at www.abstralrems.com or by calling 1-888-227-8725.
- DO NOT convert patients to fentanyl sublingual tablets from other fentanyl products on a mcg-per-mcg basis; do not substitute Abstral for any other fentanyl product, as it may result in fatal overdose.
- Drug is an opioid and may cause physical dependence and withdrawal if stopped (along with maintenance opioid) abruptly. In addition, it can lead to psychological dependence (addiction) if inappropriately used.
- Use fentanyl sublingual tablets with extreme caution in patients:
  - With hepatic and/or renal dysfunction, head injuries, increased intracranial pressure, cardiac disease (especially with bradyarrythmias), and chronic pulmonary disease.
  - With chronic obstructive pulmonary disease or preexisting medical conditions predisposing them to hypoventilation.
  - Susceptible to intracranial effects of CO_2 retention.
  - Taking other CNS depressants and potent CYP3A4 inhibitors; they may have increased depressant effects, including hypoventilation, hypotension, and profound sedation. Consider dosage adjustments if warranted.
  - Who are elderly; they are more sensitive to opioids.
  - Who are pregnant: fentanyl citrate is not mutagenic but is embryocidal in rats; in addition, it has been shown to impair fertility. If drug must be given to a pregnant woman, benefit must outweigh potential risk to the fetus.
- DO NOT use drug during labor and delivery, as it may cause respiratory depression in the fetus. Nursing mothers should not take the drug.
- Clinically significant respiratory and CNS depression can occur; monitor patients accordingly.
- Teach patient that drug must be kept out of reach of children and pets, as dose can be LETHAL to children and pets.

- Most common side effects during titration (frequency > 3%): nausea and somnolence.
- Most common side effects during maintenance phase (frequency > 3%): headache, nausea, constipation.

Potential Toxicities/Side Effects and the Nursing Process

I.   POTENTIAL ALTERATION IN OXYGENATION related to HYPOVENTILATION

Defining Characteristics: Increased cough and/or dyspnea are rare, but the chief toxicity in opioid-naïve patients or if excessive dosing is respiratory depression. Drug may cause bradycardia; thus, use with caution in patients with bradyarrhythmias.

Nursing Implications: Assess baseline pulmonary status. Use with caution in patients with COPD, bradycardia, or renal or hepatic dysfunction, and in the older population. Teach patient to report any pulmonary difficulties immediately. Ensure that patient knows that if respiratory difficulty develops, the drug must be removed from mouth and discarded in the toilet immediately. Ensure that patient understands how to administer drug safely and to keep drug supply out of reach of children and pets. If respiratory distress occurs, teach patient to call 911 or the local emergency number.

II.   SENSORY/PERCEPTUAL ALTERATIONS related to CNS CHANGES

Defining Characteristics: CNS depression and changes in mental status may occur, characterized by somnolence (4%) or dizziness (2%), and headache (2%). Less commonly, dysgeusia, attention disturbance, amnesia, hypoesthesia, lethargy, labile affect, confusion, depression, disorientation, dysphoria, insomnia, change in mental status, paranoia, sleep disorder, tremor, parosmia (distortion in sense of smell) may occur.

Nursing Implications: Assess baseline gait, mental, affective, and neurologic status. Assess medication profile to identify other contributions (i.e., CNS depressants). Instruct patient to report any changes. Assess patient safety, and measures to ensure safety. Teach patient not to take alcohol, sleep aids, or tranquilizers, except as ordered by the oncology provider. Discuss any significant changes with provider.

III.   ALTERATION IN NUTRITION, LESS THAN BODY REQUIREMENTS, related to NAUSEA/VOMITING

Defining Characteristics: During the titration phase, nausea occurred in 6% of patients; in the maintenance phase, nausea (6%), stomatitis (2%), constipation (5%), and dry mouth (2%) occurred. Rare: abdominal discomfort, dyspepsia, gingival ulceration, impaired gastric emptying, lip ulceration, tongue disorder, and stomatitis occurred.

Nursing Implications: Assess baseline nutritional status including fluid balance. Teach patient to take antiemetic agents as prescribed if needed, to drink 8–10 ounces of fluid hourly while awake, and to eat small, frequent, calorie-dense foods. Teach patient to report nausea, vomiting, anorexia, and dehydration. Manage symptomatically. Assess severity and impact on quality of life. Discuss severe or unmanaged symptoms with physician.

IV. ALTERATION IN ELIMINATION related to CONSTIPATION

Defining Characteristics: Opium agonists bind to opiate receptors in bowel, slowing peristalsis, leading to constipation. Untreated constipation may result in bowel perforation. Constipation occurred in 5% of patients.

Nursing Implications: Assess baseline elimination, fluid intake, diet, and exercise patterns. Instruct patient regarding prevention of constipation: Goal is to move bowels at least every 2 days by increasing fluids to 3 L/day (drink 8- to 10-ounce glasses of fluid every hour while awake), following a diet high in fiber (beans, vegetables, fruit), and taking moderate exercise. Review bowel regimen, and assess need for additional bowel softeners, bulk-forming laxatives, and osmotic cathartics, and discuss prescription with physician. Teach patient self-administration of medications. However, all patients MUST be started on bowel regimen when receiving an opioid.

Drug: fentanyl sublingual spray (Subsys)

Class: Opioid analgesic (opioid agonist).

Mechanism of Action: Fentanyl is a pure opioid agonist that binds to opioid μ-receptors located in the brain, spinal cord, and smooth muscle, to achieve analgesia.

Metabolism: Following a sublingual spray administration of 400 mcg, the mean bioavailability of fentanyl was 76%. The pharmacokinetics are based on how much of the drug is transmucosally absorbed and how much is swallowed. Peak serum levels achieved in 1.5–2 hours. Patients with mucositis had higher AUC drug levels: grade 1: 73% greater maximum plasma concentration (C_{max}) and systemic exposure compared to patients without mucositis, and patients with grades 2 had 4–7 times greater C_{max}. Primarily metabolized by the liver and intestinal microflora to norfentanyl via CYP3A4 microenzyme system. Drug is highly lipophilic, and is rapidly distributed to the brain, heart, lungs, kidneys, and spleen, then more slowly to the muscles and fat. Drug is 80–85% bound to plasma proteins. More than 90% of drug is eliminated as inactive metabolites, with < 7% excreted in urine, and < 1% in feces, as unchanged drug. Terminal half-life after sublingual spray is 5–12 hours.

Indication: Management of breakthrough pain (BTP) in cancer patients 18 years and older who are already receiving and are tolerant to opioid therapy for their underlying persistent cancer pain. Patient must remain on around-the-clock opioids when taking Subsys. A patient who is considered tolerant is taking at least 60 mg oral morphine/day; or at least 25 mcg transdermal fentanyl/hour; 30 mg oral oxycodone/day; 8 mg oral hydromorphone/day; 25 mg oral oxymorphone/day; or an equianalgesic dose of another opioid for a week or longer. Drug is available through a restricted distribution program called Transmucosal Immediate Release Fentanyl Risk Evaluation and Mitigation Strategy (TIRF REMS) Access Program. Outpatients and healthcare professionals who prescribe to outpatients, pharmacies, and distributors are required to enroll in the program.

MANAGEMENT

Contraindications: (1) Opioid nontolerant patients; (2) management of acute or postoperative pain, including headache/migraine, dental pain; (3) intolerance or hypersensitivity to fentanyl, Subsys, or its components.

Dosage/Range:
- Patients must require around-the-clock opioids when taking fentanyl sublingual spray.
- Initial dose is 100 micrograms (mcg); initial prescription should be for 100-mcg spray only (except if already receiving Actiq).
- Individually titrate to an effective and tolerable dose using a single sublingual spray breakthrough dose per episode.
  - No more than two doses can be taken per breakthrough pain episode.
  - Wait at least 4 hours before treating another episode of breakthrough pain with sublingual fentanyl.
  - Limit consumption to 4 or fewer doses per day once a successful dose is found.
  - See package insert and patient educational material for titration steps.
- If patient already receiving Actiq: start with dosing schedule below, and teach patient to stop using Actiq and to dispose of any remaining units.
  - Current Actiq dose: 200 mcg = initial Subsys dose (mcg) 100-mcg spray
  - Current Actiq dose: 400 mcg = initial Subsys dose (mcg) 100-mcg spray
  - Current Actiq dose: 600 mcg = initial Subsys dose (mcg) 200-mcg spray
  - Current Actiq dose: 800 mcg = initial Subsys dose (mcg) 200-mcg spray
  - Current Actiq dose: 1,200 mcg = initial Subsys dose (mcg) 400-mcg spray
  - Current Actiq dose: 1,600 mcg = initial Subsys dose (mcg) 400-mcg spray
- Do not switch patients on a mcg-per-mcg basis from any other oral transmucosal fentanyl product to Subsys.
- To reduce risk of overdosage during titration, patients should have only one strength of Subsys available at any one time.

Drug Preparation:
- Available in 100-mcg, 200-mcg, 400-mcg, 600-mcg, and 800-mcg dosage strengths.

Drug Interactions:
- CYP 3A4 inhibitors: (strong or moderate): may increase depressant effects, including respiratory depression, hypotension, and profound sedation. Consider dosage adjustments if needed.
- CNS depressants: may increase depressant effects, including respiratory depression, hypotension, and profound sedation. Consider dosage adjustments if needed.

Lab Effects/Interference:
- None known.

Special Considerations:
- Clinically significant respiratory depression can occur. Monitor patients closely.
  - Titrate drug cautiously in patients with COPD, or preexisting medical conditions predisposing them to respiratory depression and in patients susceptible to intracranial effects of CO_2 retention.
  - Administer cautiously to patients with liver or renal dysfunction.

- Teach patient/caregiver to safely store and dispose of drug as appropriate and to keep it away from children and pets, as drug can be fatal to a child.
- Most common adverse effects during treatment (> 5%): vomiting, nausea, constipation, dyspnea, somnolence.
- Teach patient that opioid analgesics may impair the mental and/or physical ability to drive and use machines, and to avoid these activities until the effect of the drug is known.

Potential Toxicities/Side Effects and the Nursing Process

I.   POTENTIAL ALTERATION IN OXYGENATION related to HYPOVENTILATION

Defining Characteristics: Increased cough and/or dyspnea are rare, but the chief toxicity in opioid-naïve patients or if there is excessive dosing is respiratory depression. Drug may cause bradycardia; thus, use with caution in patients with bradyarrhythmias.

Nursing Implications: Assess baseline pulmonary status. Use with caution in patients with COPD, bradycardia, or renal or hepatic dysfunction, and in the older population. Teach patient to report any pulmonary difficulties immediately. Ensure that patient knows that if respiratory difficulty develops, the drug must be removed from mouth and discarded in the toilet immediately. Ensure that patient understands how to administer drug safely and to keep drug supply out of reach of children and pets. If respiratory distress occurs, teach patient to call 911 or the local emergency number.

II.   SENSORY/PERCEPTUAL ALTERATIONS related to CNS CHANGES

Defining Characteristics: CNS depression and changes in mental status may occur, characterized by somnolence (4%) or dizziness (2%), and headache (2%). Less commonly, dysgeusia, attention disturbance, amnesia, hypoesthesia, lethargy, labile affect, confusion, depression, disorientation, dysphoria, insomnia, change in mental status, paranoia, sleep disorder, tremor, parosmia (distortion in sense of smell) may occur.

Nursing Implications: Assess baseline gait, mental, affective, and neurologic status. Assess medication profile to identify other contributions (i.e., CNS depressants). Instruct patient to report any changes. Assess patient safety, and measures to ensure safety. Teach patient not to take alcohol, sleep aids, or tranquilizers, except as ordered by the oncology provider. Discuss any significant changes with provider.

III.   ALTERATION IN NUTRITION, LESS THAN BODY REQUIREMENTS, related to NAUSEA/VOMITING

Defining Characteristics: During the titration phase, nausea occurred in 6% of patients; in the maintenance phase, nausea (6%), stomatitis (2%), constipation (5%), and dry mouth (2%) occurred. Rare: abdominal discomfort, dyspepsia, gingival ulceration, impaired gastric emptying, lip ulceration, tongue disorder, and stomatitis occurred.

Nursing Implications: Assess baseline nutritional status, including fluid balance. Teach patient to take antiemetic agents as prescribed, if needed, to drink 8–10 ounces of fluid hourly while awake, and to eat small, frequent, calorie-dense foods. Teach patient to report nausea, vomiting, anorexia, and dehydration. Manage symptomatically. Assess severity and impact on quality of life. Discuss severe or unmanaged symptoms with physician.

IV.   ALTERATION IN ELIMINATION related to CONSTIPATION

Defining Characteristics: Opium agonists bind to opiate receptors in bowel, slowing peristalsis, leading to constipation. Untreated constipation may result in bowel perforation. Constipation occurred in 5% of patients.

Nursing Implications: Assess baseline elimination, fluid intake, diet, and exercise patterns. Instruct patient regarding prevention of constipation: Goal is to move bowels at least every 2 days by increasing fluids to 3 L/day (drink 8- to 10-ounce glasses of fluid every hour while awake), following a diet high in fiber (beans, vegetables, fruit), and taking moderate exercise. Review bowel regimen; assess need for additional bowel softeners, bulk-forming laxatives, and osmotic cathartics; and discuss prescription with physician. Teach patient self-administration of medications. However, all patients MUST be started on bowel regimen when receiving an opioid.

Drug: fentanyl transdermal system (Duragesic)

Class: Opioid analgesic (opioid agonist).

Mechanism of Action: Strong opioid analgesic; 20–30 times more potent than parenteral morphine when given transdermally to opioid-naïve patients. Drug interacts primarily with opioid μ-receptors, found in the brain, spinal cord, and other tissues, causing analgesia and sedation. Duragesic patches provide continuous-released fentanyl from a transdermal reservoir system at a constant amount per unit time. The drug moves from areas of higher concentration (patch) to areas of lower concentration (skin). Initially, the skin under the patch absorbs the fentanyl, and the drug is concentrated in the upper skin layers. The drug gradually enters the systemic circulation, leveling off 2–24 hours later, and remaining fairly constant for the 72-hour application period.

Metabolism: Primarily metabolized by the liver; 75% of IV dose excreted in urine, 9% in feces, and < 10% as unchanged drug. Peak levels occur 24–72 hours after a single application. Half-life is approximately 17 hours (after system removal, serum fentanyl concentrations fall to 50% in approximately 17 hours; range, 13–22 hours).

Indication: In opioid-tolerant patients, management of pain severe enough to require daily, around-the-clock, long-term opioid treatment, and for which alternative treatment is inadequate. A patient who is considered tolerant is taking at least 60 mg oral morphine/day; or 30 mg oral oxycodone/day; 8 mg oral hydromorphone/day; or an equianalgesic dose of another opioid for a week or longer.

Limitations of use: Because of risks of addiction, abuse, and misuse of opioids, drug is reserved for use in patients for whom alternative treatment options (e.g., nonopioid analgesics or immediate-release opioids) are ineffective, not tolerated, or would be otherwise inadequate to provide sufficient management of pain.

Contraindications: (1) Opioid-intolerant patients; (2) acute or intermittent pain, postoperative pain, mild pain; (3) respiratory compromise, acute or severe asthma; (4) parqalytic ileus; (5) patients with known hypersensitivity to fentanyl or any components of transdermal system, including adhesives.

Dosage/Range:
- Each transdermal system is intended to be worn for 72 hours. Reduce dose in geriatric patients or if patient has persistent fever.
- Do not use in patients with severe hepatic impairment.
- If patient has mild-to-moderate hepatic dysfunction, start with one-half the usual Duragesic dose; monitor closely for sedation and respiratory depression, initially and with every dosage increase.
- Renal impairment: Avoid Duragesic if severe renal impairment; if mild or moderate, start with one-half of the usual Duragesic dose; monitor closely for sedation and respiratory depression, initially and with every dosage increase.
- Initial doses for patients currently receiving opioid analgesics who are tolerant can be calculated from Table 6.2 (which is NOT an equianalgesic table; see package insert):

Alternatively, for adult and pediatric patients taking opioids or doses not listed in Table 6.2, use the following methodology and Table 6.3 (see package insert):

1. Calculate the previous 24-hour analgesic requirement.
2. Convert this amount to the equianalgesic oral morphine dose, using a reliable reference. The following table gives the range for 24-hour oral morphine doses recommended for conversion to each Duragesic dose. Initiate Duragesic treatment using the recommended dose and titrate patients upwards (no more frequently than

Table 6.2   Dose Conversion to Duragesic

Current Analgesic	Daily Dosage (mg/day)	Daily Dosage (mg/day)	Daily Dosage (mg/day)	Daily Dosage (mg/day)
Oral MORPHINE	60–134	135–224	225–314	315–404
IM or IV MORPHINE	10–22	23–37	38–52	53–67
Oral OXYCODONE	30–67	67.5–112	112.5–157	157.5–202
Oral HYDROMORPHONE	8–17	17.1–28	28.1–39	39.1–51
IV HYDROMORPHONE	1.5–3.4	3.5–5.6	5.7–7.9	8–10
Oral METHADONE	20–44	45–74	75–104	105–134
DURAGESIC DOSE	25 mcg/hr	50 mcg/hr	75 mcg/hr	100 mcg/hr

Data from: Jannsen Pharmaceuticals, Inc. Duragesic Package Insert. Titusville, NJ: April 2014.

Table 6.3   Recommended Initial Duragesic Dose Based Upon DAILY ORAL MORPHINE DOSE

Oral 24-Hour Morphine (mg/day)	Duragesic Dose (mcg/hr)
45–134	25
135–224	50
225–314	75
315–404	100
405–494	125
495–584	150
585–674	175
675–764	200
765–854	225
855–944	250
945–1,034	275
1,035–1,124	300

From: Jannsen Pharmaceuticals, Inc. Duragesic Package Insert. Titusville, NJ: April 2014.

3 days after the initial dose and every 6 days thereafter) until effective analgesia is attained.

3. Do not use this table to convert from Duragesic to other therapies as this table is conservative, and will overestimate the dose of the new agent.

Titration and Maintenance of Therapy:
Individually titrate Duragesic to a dose that gives adequate analgesia and minimizes toxicity. This requires continual reevaluation to assess pain control and incidence of adverse reactions, including frequent telephone calls or communication between prescriber or nurse, the patient, and or home-care nurse.

- Dosing interval is 72 hours; do not increase the dose for the first time until at least 3 days after initial Duragesic patch is applied.
- Titrate the dose based on the patient's need for supplemental (short-acting, breakthrough pain (BTP)) medication on days 2 and 3 after application until the next patch is due. It may take up to 6 days for fentanyl levels to reach equilibrium on a new dose. Thus, further titration should wait until two 3-day applications have been made before any further dose increase.
- Base dosage increments on the amount of daily BTP medications needed using the ratio of 45 mg/24 hours or oral morphine to a 12 mcg/hr increase in Duragesic dose.
- Adjust the dose to achieve analgesia and to balance any adverse effects that occur.

Some patients will require a 48-hour change in Duragesic but an increase in Duragesic dose every 3 days, prior to decreasing the interval to 48 hours. This may occur if the patient has persistent fever, and the patch is absorbed after 48 hours. Dosing intervals < every 72 hours has not been studied in children or adolescents.

Drug Preparation:
- Transdermal systems available: 12-mcg/hr, 25-mcg/hr, 50 mcg/hr, 75-mcg/hr, 100-mcg/hr.

Drug Administration:
- Apply to nonirritated and nonirradiated skin; clip hair (not shave) as needed. May cleanse with water only and dry completely if necessary.
  - Apply patch immediately after removal from package, and after removal of the outer protective hard plastic liner.
  - Press firmly into place with palm of hand for 10–20 seconds, making sure contact is complete, especially around edges. Patient wears for 72 hours, then changes patch. Some patients may need to reapply new patches every 48 hours.
  - Short-acting opioids must be continued for at least 24 hours until serum fentanyl level achieved to provide breakthrough pain analgesia and until correct Duragesic dose determined.
  - If adhesion is a problem, the edges may be taped, and if problem persists, patch may be overlaid with a transparent adhesive film dressing.
  - If the patch falls off before 72 hours, it should be properly disposed of and a new patch should be applied in a different skin site.
  - If a patient develops fever, or increased core body temperature due to strenuous exertion, the drug may be more quickly absorbed and the patient at risk for increased toxicity; the patient may need dose reduction.
- Patient/Caregiver Teaching:
  - Wash hands with soap and water after applying the patch to prevent accidental exposure to a child or other person (e.g., if hugging).
  - Store oral doses in a safe place away from children and pets, as accidental ingestion can be fatal.
  - Opioid analgesics may impair the mental and/or physical ability to drive and use machines; avoid these activities until the effect of the drug is known.
  - Heat can increase fentanyl absorption from the patch, this increasing risk of overdosage, which may be fatal. This can occur when the anatomical location is exposed to direct heat source, such as an electric blanket, heat/tanning lamp, hot bath, sauna, hot tub, heated water bed, or while sunbathing.
  - Disposal: at home, patient must fold so adhesive side of system adheres to itself; then flush it down the toilet. In hospital, used patches must be returned to pharmacy for proper disposal.
- Pediatric use: safety and efficacy in pediatric patients < 2 years old has not been established. To guard against accidental ingestion by children, use caution when choosing the application site.

Drug Initiation:
- Assess patient for 24–72 hours, when serum concentrations from the initial patch will peak.
- Discontinue all other around-the-clock medications when Duragesic is initiated.
- It is preferable to underestimate the patient's 24-hour fentanyl requirement and provide rescue medication than to overestimate it and have the patient somnolent.
- Use Dosing Table 6.2.
- Hypotensive effects: monitor BP and pulse during initiation and titration.

MANAGEMENT

Drug Interactions:
- Potentiation of CNS depressant effects, when administered concurrently with other opioids, benzodiazepines, or other CNS depressants.
- Mixed agonist/antgonist and partial opioid analgesics: Do not use together, as they may reduce analgesic effect or precipitate withdrawal symptoms.
- CYP3A4 inhibitors: May result in increased fentanyl plasma concentrations and risk for toxicity. Avoid coadministration.
- CYP3A4 inducer: May decrease fentanyl plasma levels. If they are concomitantly administered, and the CYP3A4 inducer is discontinued, assess for increased fentanyl plasma levels and increased risk for toxicity.
- Monomine oxidase inhibitors (MAOIs): Avoid use with Duragesic in these patients or within 14 days of stopping MAOIs.

Lab Effects/Interference:
- None known.

Special Considerations:
- Serious, life-threatening respiratory depression can occur; observe for respiratory depression during initiation, or following dose increase.
- Use with caution in the following patients, and monitor closely for sedation and respiratory depression:
  - COPD predisposed to hypoventilation
  - Head injuries, brain tumor (very sensitive to effects of CO_2 retention)
  - Cardiac disease (may cause bradyarrhythmias)
  - Hepatic or renal dysfunction
  - Elderly or cachectic, debilitated patients, and those with chronic pulmonary disease
- Interactions with CNS depressants: concomitant use may cause profound sedation, respiratory depression, and death. If must be coadministered, consider dose reduction of one or both drugs.
- Drug may cause fetal harm. Teach women of childbearing potential who become or are planning to become pregnant to talk to their healthcare provider before starting or continuing Duragesic therapy.
- Prolonged use of Duragesic during pregnancy can result in neonatal opioid withdrawal syndrome, which may be life-threatening.
- Nursing mothers should make a decision to stop nursing or to stop Duragesic, taking into account the importance of the drug to the mother's health.
- Most common adverse reactions ($\geq$ 5%) are nausea, vomiting, somnolence, dizziness, insomnia, constipation, hyperhidrosis, fatigue, feeling cold, anorexia, headache, diarrhea.
- Assess each patient's risk for addiction, abuse, or misuse prior to prescribing Duragesic, and monitor patients for the development of these behaviors.

Potential Toxicities/Side Effects and the Nursing Process

I.   ALTERATION IN OXYGENATION related to HYPOVENTILATION, FEVER

Defining Characteristics: Dyspnea, hypoventilation, apnea (3–10% of patients); hemoptysis, pharyngitis, hiccups rare; stertorous breathing, asthma, respiratory dysfunction.

Nursing Implications: Assess baseline pulmonary status. Use with caution in patients with COPD, brain tumors, increased intracranial pressure (ICP), hepatic failure. NEVER exceed 25 mcg/h if patient not tolerant to opioids. Must continue to observe patient for 17 hours after dose removed for signs/symptoms of toxicity—same is true if naloxone HCl (Narcan) required to reverse opioid. Theoretically, a temperature of 39°C (102°F) will increase serum fentanyl by 33% due to drug delivery and skin absorption. If patient develops fever, observe for signs/symptoms of overdosage. Elderly patients (> 60–65 years old) may have reduced ability to clear drug, so start at 25 mcg/hr unless already tolerant of > 135 mg morphine sulfate/24 hours.

II. SENSORY/PERCEPTUAL ALTERATIONS related to CNS CHANGES

Defining Characteristics: CNS depression and changes in mental status may occur, characterized by somnolence, confusion, depression, asthenia (> 10%), dizziness, nervousness, hallucinations, anxiety, depression, euphoria (3–10%), tremors, abnormal coordination, speech disorder, abnormal thinking, dreams. Rare: aphasia, vertigo, stupor, hypotonia, hypertonia, hostility.

Nursing Implications: Assess baseline mental, neurologic status. Dose of other opioids and benzodiazepines should be 50%. Use cautiously in substance abusers.

III. ALTERATION IN CARDIAC OUTPUT related to ARRYTHMIA, ANGINA

Defining Characteristics: Arrhythmia, chest pain may occur; IV fentanyl has caused bradyarrhythmias.

Nursing Implications: Assess baseline cardiac status, and monitor during drug use. Instruct patient to report palpitations, chest pain.

IV. ALTERATION IN NUTRITION, LESS THAN BODY REQUIREMENTS, related to NAUSEA, VOMITING

Defining Characteristics: Nausea, vomiting, anorexia, dyspepsia, rare abdominal distension.

Nursing Implications: Assess baseline nutritional status. Instruct patient to report nausea, vomiting, anorexia, dyspepsia.

V. ALTERATION IN ELIMINATION related to CONSTIPATION, ILEUS

Defining Characteristics: Opium agonists bind to opiate receptors in bowel, slowing peristalsis, leading to constipation. Untreated constipation may result in bowel perforation. Opiate receptors in bowel decrease peristalsis.

Nursing Implications: Assess baseline elimination, fluid intake, diet, and exercise patterns. Instruct patient regarding prevention of constipation: goal is to move bowels at least every

MANAGEMENT

2 days, by increasing fluids to 3 L/day, following a diet high in fiber (beans, vegetables, fruit), and taking moderate exercise. Assess need for bowel softeners, bulk-forming laxatives, and osmotic cathartics, and discuss prescription with physician. Teach patient self-administration of medications. MUST be started on bowel regimen.

VI.   ALTERATION IN CARDIAC OUTPUT related to HYPOTENSION, BRADYCARDIA

Defining Characteristics: Orthostatic hypotension, bradycardia due to cholinergic effect, and peripheral vasodilation may occur with rapid IV dosing. There may be histamine-related flushing, pruritus, diaphoresis with chronic drug usage; tolerance develops to this effect.

Nursing Implications: Assess baseline cardiovascular status. Teach patient to change position slowly and to hold onto stable, nearby structure for support as needed.

Be careful when giving IV push opioids, and caution patient to remain in supine position for 15–20 minutes after injection. Monitor cardiovascular status after injection.

VII.   ALTERATION IN URINE ELIMINATION related to URINARY RETENTION

Defining Characteristics: Increased smooth muscle tone in urinary tract and spasm may occur. Bladder tone is increased, which may cause urgency. Vesical sphincter tone may be increased, leading to difficulty urinating. Increased risk of urinary retention in patients with prostatic hypertrophy or urethral stricture. Rare bladder pain, oliguria, urinary frequency.

Nursing Implications: Assess baseline urinary elimination pattern. Teach patient to increase fluids to 3 L/day, and encourage voiding every 2–3 hours. Instruct patient to report problems with urination.

VIII.   ALTERATION IN SKIN INTEGRITY/COMFORT related to RASH, PRURITUS

Defining Characteristics: Sweating, pruritus, rash; erythema, papules, itching, edema, exfoliative dermatitis, pustules at application site; headache rare.

Nursing Implications: Teach patient proper drug application and to rotate sites.

Drug: hydromorphone (Dilaudid)

Class: Opioid analgesic (opioid agonist).

Mechanism of Action: Hydromorphone is a hydrogented ketone of morphine. Binds to opiate receptors in CNS (limbic system, thalamus, striatum, hypothalamus, midbrain, spinal cord), altering pain perception at level of spinal cord and higher centers, as well as the emotional response to pain. Also suppresses cough reflex.

Metabolism: Well absorbed after oral, rectal, and parenteral administration. Onset of action is 15–30 minutes (more rapid than morphine), with a duration of action of 4–5 hours. Metabolized by liver and excreted in urine.

Indication: For the management of pain in patients where an opioid analgesic is appropriate. Dilaudid-HP (high-potency) is intended for use only in opioid-tolerant patients.

Contraindications: Patients with (1) known hypersensitivity to hydromorphone, (2) respiratory depression in the absence of resuscitative equipment, (3) status asthmaticus, and (4) obstetrical analgesia.

Dosage/Range:
- Use caution in
  - Patients who have not received opiates before and have not developed tolerance.
  - Elderly patients who may require doses lower than 2–4 mg every 4 hours.
- Moderate pain: oral: 1–6 mg q 4–6 h; subcutaneous or IM: 2–4 mg q 4–6 h, 3 mg rectal suppository.
- Severe pain: oral: 4 mg or more q 4 h; subcutaneous or IM: 4 mg or more, then titrate based on patient response and tolerance.
- Moderate hepatic dysfunction: start at lower dose and monitor closely during dose titration.
- Hydromorphone oral liquid: 2.5 mg–10 mg (2.5 mL–10mL, or 1/2 tsp to 2 tsp) of 1 mg/1 mL liquid, every 3–6 hours as directed.
- Hydromorphone tablets: 2mg–4 mg orally, every 4–6 hours as needed for pain.
- Initial dose should be reduced in patients with renal or hepatic impairment.

Drug Preparation:
- Available as hydromorphone oral liquid (1 pint, 473 mL); hydromorphone 2-mg, 4-mg, and 8-mg tablets; and Dilaudid IV: 1-, 2-, and 4-mg/mL ampules; and Dilaudid-HP (high-potency) in 10-mg/mL ampules and vials.
- Store tablets in tight, light-resistant containers at 15–30°C (59–86°F).
- Injection should be protected from light and stored at 15–40°C (59–104°F).

Drug Administration:
- PO (liquid or tablet), subcutaneous, IM, IV. Use highly concentrated injectable solution for patients who are tolerant to opiate agonists.
- At home, teach patient to store oral doses in a safe place away from children and pets.
- Teach patient that opioid analgesics may impair the mental and/or physical ability to drive and use machines, and to avoid these activities until the effect of the drug is known.
- Chronic pain: Requires around-the-clock dosing (with hydromorphone at frequent intervals or preferably with a long-acting opiate), with 5–15% of the total daily hydromorphone dosage every 2 hours as breakthrough pain (BTP) medication.
- Continue to reassess pain after initial dosing to ensure adequate pain control through titration.

MANAGEMENT

Drug Interactions:
• Alcohol, CNS depressants: Additive effects.

Lab Effects/Interference:
• None known.

Special Considerations:
• Parenteral dose is 1/5 oral dose for equianalgesic effect.
• Additive benefit when combined with acetaminophen or aspirin.
• Give smallest effective dose to prevent development of tolerance (e.g., takes more drug to provide the same relief over time), physical dependency (e.g., withdrawal symptoms if drug is stopped abruptly). These are separate and distinct from abuse and addiction.
• Drug can lead to drug abuse and addiction if not used for the relief of pain.
• Reduce dose in debilitated patients or patients receiving other CNS depressants.
• Use with caution in patients with hepatic or renal dysfunction, hypothyroidism, Addison's disease, severe CNS depression, respiratory depression, head injury, elevated ICP.
• Most common adverse reactions are lightheadedness, dizziness, sedation, nausea, vomiting, sweating, flushing, dysphoria, euphoria, dry mouth, pruritus, constipation.
• If required, naloxone HCl will reverse opiate toxicity (e.g., respiratory depression). However, it is important that acute withdrawal symptoms be prevented by giving only enough naloxone to reverse respiratory depression and that this be continued for opioid drug half-life.
• Drug should not be used by nursing mothers, and use is contraindicated during labor and delivery.

Potential Toxicities/Side Effects and the Nursing Process

I.   SENSORY/PERCEPTUAL ALTERATIONS related to CNS DEPRESSION

Defining Characteristics: Drowsiness, sedation, mood changes, euphoria, dysphoria, dizziness, mental clouding may occur. At high doses, may cause seizures. Miosis (papillary constriction) may occur.

Nursing Implications: Assess baseline neurologic status. Use cautiously, if at all, in patients with head injury, increased ICP, severe CNS depression, acute alcoholism, the elderly, and the debilitated. Assess other concurrent medications. Use with caution in patients receiving other opioids, tranquilizers, hypnotics, MAO inhibitors, since increasing CNS depressant effects can occur. Monitor neurologic status closely. Teach patient to avoid driving and operating machinery while taking the medicine, and to AVOID concurrent alcohol.

II.   ALTERATION IN OXYGENATION related to RESPIRATORY DEPRESSION

Defining Characteristics: Opiate agonists directly depress respiratory center in brain stem, causing decreased sensitivity and responsiveness to increased pCO_2. Also may depress deep breathing and reflex to sigh. Tolerance to respiratory depressant effects occurs with chronic use.

Nursing Implications: Assess baseline pulmonary status, and monitor periodically during drug use. Use cautiously in patients with bronchial asthma, COPD, respiratory depression, and monitor closely.

III.   ALTERATION IN ELIMINATION related to CONSTIPATION, ILEUS

Defining Characteristics: Opium agonists bind to opiate receptors in bowel, slowing peristalsis, leading to constipation. Untreated constipation may result in bowel perforation.

Nursing Implications: Assess baseline elimination, fluid intake, diet, and exercise patterns. Instruct patient about prevention of constipation: goal is to move bowels at least every 2 days by increasing fluids to 3 L/day, following a diet high in fiber (beans, vegetables, fruit), and taking moderate exercise. Assess need for bowel softeners, bulk-forming laxatives, and osmotic cathartics, and discuss prescription with physician. Teach patient self-administration of medications.

IV.   ALTERATION IN NUTRITION related to GI TOXICITY

Defining Characteristics: Nausea, vomiting, and dry mouth may occur. Gastric, biliary, and pancreatic secretions are decreased by opiate agonists; digestion is delayed. Biliary tract muscle tone is increased, and spasm of Oddi's sphincter may occur (morphine > meperidine > codeine).

Nursing Implications: Assess patient tolerance of GI side effects. Teach patient to report side effects. If nausea/vomiting occur, change to another opioid, or premedicate with antiemetic to prevent nausea/vomiting. Assess GI pain, biliary spasm, and consider alternative opioid.

V.   ALTERATION IN CARDIAC OUTPUT related to HYPOTENSION, BRADYCARDIA

Defining Characteristics: Orthostatic hypotension, bradycardia due to cholinergic effect, and peripheral vasodilation may occur with rapid IV dosing. There may be histamine-related flushing, pruritus, diaphoresis with chronic drug usage; tolerance develops to this effect.

Nursing Implications: Assess baseline cardiovascular status. Teach patient to change position slowly and to hold onto stable, nearby structure for support as needed. Be careful when giving IV push opioids, and caution patient to remain in supine position for 15–20 minutes after injection. Monitor cardiovascular status after injection.

VI.   ALTERATION IN URINE ELIMINATION related to URINARY RETENTION

Defining Characteristics: Increased smooth muscle tone in urinary tract and spasm may occur. Bladder tone is increased, which may cause urgency. Vesical sphincter tone may be

MANAGEMENT

increased, leading to difficulty urinating. Increased risk of urinary retention in patients with prostatic hypertrophy or urethral stricture.

Nursing Implications: Assess baseline urinary elimination pattern. Teach patient to increase fluids to 3 L/day, and encourage voiding every 2–3 hours. Instruct patient to report problems with urination.

VII.   KNOWLEDGE DEFICIT related to DRUG ADMINISTRATION, POTENTIAL FOR TOLERANCE, AND DEPENDENCY

Defining Characteristics: Psychological dependence (addiction) occurs rarely in patients taking opioid agonists for cancer pain (> 1%). Physical dependence (precipitation of withdrawal symptoms) occurs with chronic use of the drug for the relief of chronic cancer pain. In addition, tolerance, or less analgesic effect over time with the same drug dose, occurs and requires increased dosage of drug.

Nursing Implications: Assess baseline knowledge of opioid analgesics and attitude about their use for cancer pain management. Teach patient about proper self-administration, possible side effects, and self-care measures. Suggest patient maintain diary of pain intensity, precipitating and alleviating factors, drug dose and time taken, and relief. Teach patient to self-administer opioid agonists for relief of chronic cancer pain around-the-clock, not PRN, to prevent pain. Explain use of prescribed short-acting opioid for rescue or to manage BTP. Discuss with physician dose increase or change in frequency of administration if tolerance develops. Teach patient that withdrawal symptoms may occur if chronic, around-the-clock dosing is interrupted. Withdrawal (abstinence) symptoms that may be seen are restlessness, lacrimation, rhinorrhea, yawning, perspiration, gooseflesh, restless sleep, mydriasis in first 24 hours. These are followed by twitching and leg spasm; severe aching of the back, abdomen, and legs; cramping in abdomen and legs; hot/cold flashes; insomnia; nausea/vomiting, diarrhea; severe sneezing; and increased heart rate, BP, T, which peak at 36–72 hours. Withdrawal syndrome can be prevented by administration of at least one-quarter of previous opioid dose.

VIII.   SEXUAL DYSFUNCTION related to IMPOTENCE, ↓ LIBIDO

Defining Characteristics: Opiate agonists may suppress gonadotropin, causing impotence and decreased libido.

Nursing Implications: Assess baseline sexual pattern. Discuss potential toxicity and impact on sexuality. Provide information, emotional support, and referral as needed.

Drug: hydromorphone HCl extended-release tablets (Exalgo)

Class: Opioid analgesic (opioid agonist).

Mechanism of Action: Agonist of mu-opioid receptors, having a weak affinity for K-receptors. Drug binds to the mu-receptor in the CNS (limbic system, thalamus, striatum, hypothalamus, midbrain, spinal cord), altering pain perception at level of spinal cord and higher centers as well as the emotional response to pain. Also suppresses cough reflex by direct effect on the cough center in the medulla. It is five times more potent (by weight) than morphine. Respiratory depression occurs via direct action on cerebral respiratory control center (brainstem) and may cause nausea/vomiting by direct stimulation of the chemoreceptor trigger zone (posterior medulla).

Metabolism: Uses OROS push-pull osmotic delivery system so that drug is released at a controlled rate, with gradual increase in drug serum concentrations. After a single dose, plasma concentrations increase gradually over 6–8 hours and are sustained for approximately 18–24 hours after drug is given. Median T_{max} is 12–16 hours, and mean half-life is about 11 hours (range 8–5 hr). Steady state plasma concentrations approximately twice those observed following the first dose, with steady state reached after 3–4 days of once-daily dosing. Once reached, steady state serum levels maintained with once-daily dosing, within the same concentration range as immediate-release tablets given 4 times daily, but without the peaks and troughs seen with immediate-release drug dosing. Drug absorption is unaffected by food or fluid. Drug has extensive tissue distribution. 27% of drug binds to plasma proteins. Immediate-release formulation undergoes extensive first-pass metabolism, primarily by the liver (glucuronidation), forming hydromorphone in plasma. 75% of the administered dose is excreted in the urine, mostly as metabolites; 7% of unchanged drug is excreted in the urine, and 1% in the feces. Females have approximately 10% higher mean systemic exposure (C_{max}, AUC).

Indication: In opioid-tolerant patients for the management of pain severe enough to require daily, around-the-clock, long-term opioid treatment and for which alternative treatment options are inadequate. A patient who is considered tolerant is taking at least 60 mg oral morphine/day; or 30 mg oral oxycodone/day; 8 mg oral hydromorphone/day; or an equianalgesic dose of another opioid for a week or longer.

Limitations of use: Because of potential risks of addiction, abuse, and misuse with opioids, the drug should be reserved for use in patients for whom alternative treatment options are ineffective/intolerable. Drug is not indicated as an as-needed (PRN) analgesic.

Contraindications: (1) Opioid nontolerant patients; (2) significant respiratory depression; (3) acute or severe bronchial asthma; (4) known or suspected paralytic ileus; (5) narrowed or obstructed GI tract; (6) known hypersensitivity to any components, including hydromorphone HCl and sulfites.

Dosage/Range:
- Once-daily administration; patient must swallow tablets intact.
- Dose must be individualized for each patient and should NEVER be administered as a first opioid (opioid-naïve patient).
  - To convert to Exalgo from another opioid, use available conversion factors to obtain estimated dose.
  - Dose may be increased using increments of 4–8 mg every 3–4 days, as needed, to achieve adequate analgesia.

Dose Reductions:
- Moderate and severe hepatic dysfunction (fourfold increase in patients with moderate liver impairment) and patients with moderate renal impairment: consider alternate analgesic if

severe renal impairment (twofold to fourfold increase in plasma concentrations, as well as delayed excretion increasing the terminal half-life to 40 hours). Start patients with moderate hepatic impairment on 25% of the normal dose. Closely monitor patient for respiratory and CNS depression.

- Moderate renal impairment: start patient on 50% of the normal dose; if severe renal impairment, start patient at 25% of the normal dose daily and closely monitor for effect and toxicity.
- Concurrent administration of CNS depressants: assess duration of use of the CNS depressant, patient's response including tolerance to CNS depression, use of alcohol or illicit drugs that can cause CNS depression; if the decision to use Exalgo is made, start with one-third to one-half the calculated starting dose, monitor for signs of sedation and respiratory depression, and consider using a lower dose of the concomitant CNS depressant.
- See conversion chart below when converting from another opioid to extended-release hydromorphone HCl. Patients vary in their tolerance and drug effect; it is safer to underdose and provide rescue medication (e.g., immediate-release hydromorphone) than to overestimate and manage an adverse reaction.

Conversion Chart to Exalgo

Previous Oral Opioid	Oral Conversion Ratio
Hydromorphone	1
Codeine	0.06
Hydrocodone	0.4
Methadone*	0.6
Morphine	0.2
Oxycodone	0.4
Oxymorphone	0.6

*Monitor the patient closely when converting from methadone to other opioid agonists, as the ratio varies widely as a function of the previous dose exposure, and methadone has a long half-life, tending to accumulate in the plasma. Use only for conversion of current opioid therapy to extended-release hydromorphone.
Transdermal fentanyl conversion: 18 hours after removal of the fentanyl patch, begin extended-release hydromorphone HCl. For each 25 micrograms/hr fentanyl transdermal dose, the equianalgesic dose of extended-release hydromorphone is 12 mg every 24 hrs.
Select opioid, sum the total daily dose, and then multiply the dose by the conversion ratio to calculate the approximate oral hydromorphone equivalent.
Source: From Exalgo Package Insert, April 2014. Dublin, MI: Covidien Pharmaceuticals.

- When converting from another opioid, calculate a starting dose equivalent to the patient's total daily oral hydromorphone dose, taken once daily. Carefully titrate the dose of extended-release hydromorphone, in increments of 4–8 mg every 3–4 days until adequate pain relief with tolerable side effects is achieved (plasma levels of EXALGO are sustained for 18–24 hours).
- Consider dosage increases of 25–50% of the current daily dose for each titration step. If more than two rescue doses of immediate-release analgesic are needed within a 24-hour

period for 2 consecutive days, the dose of extended-release hydromorphone may need to be titrated upward. Do not administer extended-release hydromorphone more than once a day.

- For patients taking more than one opioid, calculate the approximate oral hydromorphone dose for each opioid and sum the totals to obtain the approximate total hydromorphone daily dose.
- Breakthrough pain (BTP): ensure patient has a prescription for short-acting hydromorphone for rescue, and have patient keep a pain diary. If possible, it is important to try to identify the source of increased pain before increasing the Exalgo dose.
- Maintain frequent contact with the patient/family when titrating dose to assess tolerance and efficacy.
- When the drug is no longer needed, taper doses gradually, by 25–50% every 2–3 days down to a dose of 8 mg/day, before discontinuing therapy to prevent symptoms of withdrawal in the physically dependent patient. Signs and symptoms of withdrawal are restlessness, lacrimation, rhinorrhea, yawning, perspiration, chills, piloerection, myalgia, mydriasis, irritability, anxiety, backache, joint pain, weakness, abdominal cramps, insomnia, nausea, anorexia, vomiting, diarrhea, BP, respiratory rate, heart rate. Infants born to mothers who are physically dependent on opioids will also exhibit respiratory difficulties and withdrawal symptoms.
- Do not give mixed agonist/antagonist with this drug (e.g., pentazocine, nalbuphine, and butorphanol), as it may precipitate withdrawal as well as decrease the analgesic effect.
- Drug is not to be used for (1) PRN analgesic, (2) pain that is mild or not expected to persist for an extended time, (3) acute pain, (4) postoperative pain, unless already receiving chronic opioid therapy prior to surgery, or if postoperative pain is expected to be moderate to severe and persisting for an extended period of time.

Drug Preparation:
- Oral. Available as 8-mg, 12-mg, 16-mg, or 32-mg strengths. Store at 59–86°F (25–30°C).
- Ensure that pharmacist knows that this drug (extended-release form) is different from immediate-release hydromorphone 8-mg tablets.

Drug Administration:
- Oral, swallowed whole, with adequate water or liquid, once every 24 hours, with or without food.
- Teach patient that drug must not be broken, crushed, dissolved, or chewed before swallowing.
- Discontinue or taper all other extended-release opioids when beginning this drug.
- USE CAUTION WHEN ADMINISTERING, AND ENSURE THAT CORRECT drug and dose are prescribed, as hydromorphone *immediate release* is also available as an 8-mg tablet. When extended-release hydromorphone HCl is no longer needed, unused tablets should be destroyed by flushing them down the toilet (per FDA).
- Teach patient that opioid analgesics may impair the mental and/or physical ability to drive and use machines, and to avoid these activities until the effect of the drug is known.
- Disposal: flush all remaining tablets down the toilet or remit to authorities at a certified drug take-back program.

MANAGEMENT

Drug Interactions:
- CNS depressants (e.g., hypnotics, sedatives, general anesthetics, antipsychotics, alcohol): may cause additive depressant effects and respiratory depression, hypotension, profound sedation, coma; if must use concurrently, reduce dose of one or both agents. Do not take drug when drinking alcohol.
- MAO inhibitors: MAO inhibitors may cause CNS excitation or depression, hypotension, or hypertension if used concurrently. Do not use concurrently, and separate by at least 14 days after stopping the MAO inhibitor.
- Mixed agonist/antagonist opioid analgesics (e.g., buprenorphine, nalbuphine, pentazocine) may reduce analgesic effect by competitive blockade of receptors ± precipitate withdrawal symptoms. Do not use concurrently.
- Anticholinergic drugs may ↑ risk of urinary retention and/or severe constipation leading to paralytic ileus.
- Cytochrome P450 enzymes: minimal potential to inhibit CYP3A4, -2C9, -2C19, -2D6, and -4A11.

Lab Effects/Interference:
- None known.

Special Considerations:
- Individualize dose for each patient when starting dosing regimen. Overestimating the initial dose when converting from another opioid can result in overdosage and death.
  - Balance between pain control and adverse effects.
  - Risk factors for abuse, addiction, or diversion, including a prior history of abuse, addiction, or diversion.
  - Monitor closely for respiratory depression, especially within the first 24–72 hours of starting therapy.
- Drug can be associated with clinically significant respiratory depression, which can result in death when not used as recommended or abused; monitor patients closely.
- Drug is contraindicated in patients with known or suspected paralytic ileus, or preexisting or actual narrowed or obstructed GI tract (e.g., esophageal motility disorders, small bowel inflammatory disease, "short gut" syndrome due to adhesions or decreased transit time, past history of peritonitis, strictures, cystic fibrosis, chronic intestinal pseudo-obstruction, Meckel's diverticulum), as tablet does not change in shape and may cause obstruction. Drug may obscure the diagnosis or clinical course of patients with an acute abdomen.
- Drug is not recommended during labor and delivery, pregnancy, or nursing. Prolonged use of the drug during pregnancy can result in neonatal opioid withdrawal syndrome, which may be life-threatening if not recognized and treated by established neonatal protocols.
- Administer drug with caution, and in reduced dosages, to elderly patients, especially those with cardiovascular, pulmonary, renal, or hepatic disease.
- Monitor patients with head injury or increased intracranial pressure closely for signs of sedation and respiratory depression, as they may be susceptible to intracranial effects of CO_2 retention.

- Use with caution in patients with adrenocortical insufficiency (e.g., Addison's disease), delirium tremens, myxedema or hypothyroidism, prostatic hypertrophy, urethral stricture, psychosis. Drug worsens seizures in patients with convulsive disorders.
- **Teach patient/caregiver to keep out of reach of children and pets, as accidental ingestion can result in a fatal overdose.**
- Drug can be abused; use caution when prescribing and monitor closely if there is an increased risk of misuse, abuse, or diversion. Addiction is defined as psychological dependence. This is different from physical dependence (goes into withdrawal if drug is abruptly discontinued).
- Drug may have additive effects when taken in conjunction with alcohol or other CNS depressants. Use drug with extreme caution in patients susceptible to intracranial effects of CO_2 retention.
- Drug may cause hypotension; use with caution in patients with circulatory shock.
- Most common side effects (> 10%) are constipation, nausea, vomiting, somnolence, headache, dizziness.
- Drug should not be abruptly discontinued, as it may precipitate withdrawal symptoms.
- If acute overdosage occurs, respiratory depression, somnolence progressing to stupor or coma, skeletal muscle flaccidity, cold and clammy skin, constricted pupils, sometimes bradycardia, hypotension, and death may occur. Once emergently reversed, patient will require continued monitoring for 24–48 hours or more due to delayed peak plasma level, which occurs at 16 hours from time of dose, as well as 11-hour mean elimination half-life.

Potential Toxicities/Side Effects and the Nursing Process

I.   SENSORY/PERCEPTUAL ALTERATIONS related to CNS DEPRESSION

Defining Characteristics: Drowsiness, sedation, mood changes, euphoria, dysphoria, dizziness, mental clouding may occur. At high doses, may cause seizures. Miosis (pupillary constriction) may occur.

Nursing Implications: Assess baseline neurologic status. Use cautiously, if at all, in patients with head injury, increased ICP, severe CNS depression, acute alcoholism, the elderly, and the debilitated. Assess other concurrent medications. Use with caution in patients receiving other opioids, tranquilizers, hypnotics, or MAO inhibitors, since increasing CNS depressant effects can be dangerous. Monitor neurologic status closely. Teach patient to avoid driving and operating machinery while taking the medicine and to AVOID concurrent alcohol. Recall that drug can produce changes in pupillary response, which can obscure neurologic signs of increasing intracranial pressure in patients with head injuries.

II.   ALTERATION IN OXYGENATION related to RESPIRATORY DEPRESSION

Defining Characteristics: Opiate agonists directly depress respiratory center in brain stem, causing decreased sensitivity and responsiveness to increased pCO_2. Also may depress deep breathing. Patients have a reduced urge to breathe, a decreased respiratory rate, and often have a "sighing" pattern of breathing (deep breaths separated by abnormal, long pauses). CO_2 retention can also exacerbate opioid sedation. Tolerance to respiratory depressant effects occurs with chronic use. Patients at risk are the elderly, debilitated, suffering from conditions causing hypoxia or hypercapnia. Drug may decrease respiratory drive while simultaneously increasing airway resistance so that apnea occurs in patients at risk. Methadone is challenging, as the drug conversion ratio varies widely based on its long half-life. Consider alternative analgesic in patients with significant COPD, cor pulmonale, or patients with substantially decreased respiratory reserve, hypoxia, hypercapnia, or pre-existing respiratory depression.

Nursing Implications: Assess baseline pulmonary status, and monitor periodically during drug use. Ensure that dose calculations when converting patient to drug are conservative, with underdosing and use of rescue medications for BTP preferable to overdosing with increased toxicity. It is easier to dose-increase than to have to dose-reduce given the long drug half-life. Special consideration and close monitoring is needed for (1) patients being converted from methadone, (2) elderly, cachectic, or debilitated patients with COPD, cor pulmonale, or with substantially reduced respiratory reserve, hypoxia, hypercapnia, or pre-existing respiratory depression. Monitor patients closely at this time, as well as any change in dose. Interventions include close observation, supportive measures, and use of opioid antagonists to reverse the respiratory depression.

III.   ALTERATION IN ELIMINATION related to CONSTIPATION, ILEUS

Defining Characteristics: Opium agonists bind to opiate receptors in bowel, slowing peristalsis, leading to constipation. Untreated constipation may result in bowel perforation.

Nursing Implications: Assess baseline elimination, fluid intake, diet, and exercise patterns. Instruct patient about prevention of constipation: goal is to move bowels at least every 2 days by increasing fluids to 3 L/day, following a diet high in fiber (beans, vegetables, fruit), and doing moderate exercise. Assess need for bowel softeners, bulk-forming laxatives, and osmotic cathartics, and discuss prescription with physician. Teach patient self-administration of medications.

IV.   ALTERATION IN NUTRITION related to GI TOXICITY

Defining Characteristics: Nausea, vomiting, and dry mouth may occur. Gastric, biliary, and pancreatic secretions are decreased by opiate agonists; digestion is delayed. Biliary tract muscle tone is increased and spasm of Oddi's sphincter may occur, increasing biliary tract pressure (morphine > meperidine > codeine).

Nursing Implications: Assess patient tolerance of GI side effects. Teach patient to report side effects. If nausea/vomiting occur, change to another opioid, or premedicate with antiemetic to prevent nausea/vomiting. Assess GI pain, biliary spasm, and consider alternative opioid. The drug must be used cautiously if at all in patients with inflammatory or obstructive bowel disorders, patients with acute pancreatitis secondary to biliary tract disease, and patients about to undergo biliary surgery.

V. ALTERATION IN CARDIAC OUTPUT related to HYPOTENSION, BRADYCARDIA

Defining Characteristics: Orthostatic hypotension, bradycardia due to cholinergic effect, and peripheral vasodilatation may occur. There may be histamine-related flushing, pruritus, and diaphoresis with chronic drug usage; tolerance develops to this effect. Syncope may occur. Risk is increased in patients with reduced blood volume or concomitant administration of some CNS-depressing medications (e.g., phenothiazines, general anesthetics).

Nursing Implications: Assess baseline cardiovascular status. Teach patient to change position slowly and to hold onto stable, nearby structure for support as needed.

Be careful when giving IV push opioids, and caution patient to remain in supine position for 15–20 minutes after injection. Monitor cardiovascular status after injection.

VI. ALTERATION IN URINE ELIMINATION related to URINARY RETENTION

Defining Characteristics: Increased smooth muscle tone in urinary tract and spasm may occur. Bladder tone is increased, which may cause urgency. Vesical sphincter tone may be increased, leading to difficulty urinating. Increased risk of urinary retention in patients with prostatic hypertrophy or urethral stricture.

Nursing Implications: Assess baseline urinary elimination pattern. Teach patient to increase fluids to 3 L/day, and encourage voiding every 2–3 hours. Instruct patient to report problems with urination.

VII. KNOWLEDGE DEFICIT related to DRUG ADMINISTRATION, POTENTIAL FOR TOLERANCE, AND DEPENDENCY

Defining Characteristics: Psychological dependence (addiction) occurs rarely in patients taking opioid agonists for cancer pain (> 1%). Physical dependence (precipitation of withdrawal symptoms) occurs with chronic use of the drug for the relief of chronic cancer pain. In addition, tolerance, or less analgesic effect over time with the same drug dose, occurs and requires increased dosage of drug.

Nursing Implications: Assess baseline knowledge of opioid analgesics and attitude about their use for cancer pain management. Teach patient about proper self-administration, possible side effects, and self-care measures. Suggest patient maintain diary of pain intensity, precipitating and alleviating factors, drug dose and time taken, and relief. Teach patient to self-administer opioid agonists for relief of chronic cancer pain around-the-clock, not PRN, to prevent pain. Explain use of prescribed short-acting opioid for rescue or to manage BTP. Discuss with physician dose increase or change in frequency of administration if tolerance develops. Teach patient that withdrawal symptoms may occur if chronic, around-the-clock dosing is interrupted. Withdrawal (abstinence) symptoms that may be seen are restlessness, lacrimation, rhinorrhea, yawning, perspiration, gooseflesh, restless sleep, mydriasis in first 24 hours. These are followed by twitching and leg spasm; severe aching of the back, abdomen, and legs; cramping in abdomen and legs; hot/cold flashes; insomnia; nausea/vomiting, diarrhea; severe sneezing; and increased heart rate, BP, and T, which peak at 36–72 hours. Withdrawal syndrome can be prevented by administration of at least ¼ of previous opioid dose.

VIII.   SEXUAL DYSFUNCTION related to IMPOTENCE, ↓ LIBIDO

Defining Characteristics: Opiate agonists may suppress gonadotropin, causing impotence and decreased libido.

Nursing Implications: Assess baseline sexual pattern. Discuss potential toxicity and impact on sexuality. Provide information, emotional support, and referral as needed.

Drug: methadone (Dolophine, Methadose)

Class: Opioid analgesic (opioid agonist).

Mechanism of Action: A synthetic opioid agonist, methadone resembles morphine but has milder action; binds to opiate receptors in CNS (limbic system, thalamus, striatum, hypothalamus, midbrain, spinal cord), altering pain perception at level of spinal cord and higher centers, as well as the emotional response to pain. Also suppresses cough reflex.

Metabolism: Well absorbed from GI tract; onset and duration of single dose similar to morphine. Short-term duration of analgesic action is 4–8 hours. With chronic administration, plasma elimination half-life is substantially longer, (e.g., 8–59 hours, median 22–48 hours). Peak respiratory depressant effects occur later and persist longer than its peak analgesic effects. With repeated dosing, methadone may be retained in the liver, then slowly released, prolonging the duration of action despite low plasma concentrations. Highly tissue-bound; metabolized by liver, excreted by renal filtration, then is reabsorbed (pH dependent). Steady-state plasma concentrations and full analgesic effects are usually not apparent until 3–5 days after dosing.

Indication: For the treatment of moderate-to-severe pain not responsive to nonopioid analgesics, and for the detoxification treatment of opioid addiction.

Dosage/Range: *For moderate to severe pain:*
• Because of long half-life with long-term dosing, management is complex and requires meticulous patient assessment to prevent overdosage.
• PO: 5–20 mg q 6–8 h, or more for severe cancer pain.
• Subcutaneous, IM (10 mg/mL): 2.5–10 mg q 3–4 h.

Drug Preparation:
- Store tablets in tight, light-resistant containers at 15–30°C (59–86°F).
- Injection should be protected from light and stored at 15–40°C (59–104°F).
- At home, teach patient to store oral doses in a safe place away from children and pets.

Drug Administration:
- PO, IM, subcutaneous.
- Teach patient that opioid analgesics may impair the mental and/or physical ability to drive and use machines, and to avoid these activities until the effect of the drug is known.

Drug Interactions:
- Injection incompatible with solutions containing aminophylline, ammonium chloride, amobarbital sodium, chlorothiazide sodium, heparin sodium, methicillin sodium, nitrofurantoin, phenobarbital sodium, sodium bicarbonate.
- Alcohol, CNS depressants: additive effects.
- Opioid antagonists, mixed agonist/antagonists, partial agonists: may precipitate withdrawal symptoms and reduce analgesia.
- Anti-retroviral agents (abacavir, amprenavir, efavirenz, nelfinavir, nevirapine, ritonavir, lopinavir + ritonavir combination): increased clearance with decreased methadone plasma levels, and decreased methadone effectiveness. Monitor patient for signs/symptoms of withdrawal and discuss methadone dose adjustment with physician or NP/PA.
- Didanosine and stavudine: methadone decreases the AUC of these drugs.
- Zidovudine: methadone increases the AUC of zidovudine, which can result in increased zidovudine toxicity.
- CYP3A4 inducers (e.g., rifampin, phenytoin, St. John's wort): decrease methadone serum level, increasing the risk for withdrawal and decreased pain relief. Assess patient and discuss methadone dose adjustment with physician or NP/PA. Teach patient NOT to take St. John's wort.
- CYP3A4 inhibitors (e.g., ketoconazole, erythromycin, voriconazole; also sertraline, fluvoxamine): decrease methadone clearance, resulting in increased methadone serum level and risk of toxicity. Monitor patient closely and assess need for dose adjustment if coadministration is medically necessary.
- Monamine oxidase inhibitors (MAOIs): MAO inhibitors may cause CNS excitation or depression, hypotension, or hypertension if used concurrently. Do not use concurrently, and separate by at least 14 days after stopping the MAO inhibitor.

Lab Effects/Interference:
- Prolonged QTc interval.

Special Considerations:
- Oral dose is twice parenteral dose (equianalgesic effect).
- May produce similar or slightly greater respiratory depression than equivalent doses of morphine.
- Additive benefit when combined with acetaminophen or aspirin.
- Give smallest effective dose to prevent development of tolerance, physical dependency.
- Reduce dose in debilitated patients or patients receiving other CNS depressants.

MANAGEMENT

- Use with caution in patients with hepatic or renal dysfunction, hypothyroidism, Addison's disease, severe CNS depression, respiratory depression, head injury, elevated ICP.
- Drug is Pregnancy Category C and not recommended during pregnancy unless the potential benefit justifies the potential risk to the fetus.
- Drug should not be used by nursing mothers.
- If required, naloxone HCl will reverse opiate toxicity (e.g., respiratory depression). However, it is important that acute withdrawal symptoms be prevented by giving only enough naloxone to reverse respiratory depression and that this be continued for opioid drug half-life.

Potential Toxicities/Side Effects and the Nursing Process

I.   SENSORY/PERCEPTUAL ALTERATIONS related to CNS DEPRESSION

Defining Characteristics: Drowsiness, sedation, mood changes, euphoria, dysphoria, dizziness, mental clouding may occur. At high doses, may cause seizures. Miosis (papillary constriction) may occur.

Nursing Implications: Assess baseline neurologic status. Use cautiously, if at all, in the elderly, the debilitated, and patients with head injury, increased ICP, severe CNS depression, acute alcoholism. Assess other concurrent medications. Use with caution in patients receiving other opioids, tranquilizers, hypnotics, MAO inhibitors, since increasing CNS depressant effects can occur. Monitor neurologic status closely. Instruct patient to avoid driving and operating machinery while taking the medicine, and to AVOID concurrent alcohol.

II.   ALTERATION IN OXYGENATION related to RESPIRATORY DEPRESSION

Defining Characteristics: Opiate agonists directly depress respiratory center in brain stem, causing decreased sensitivity and responsiveness to increased pCO_2. Also may depress deep breathing and reflex to sigh. Tolerance to respiratory depressant effects occurs with chronic use.

Nursing Implications: Assess baseline pulmonary status, and periodically during drug use. Use cautiously in patients with bronchial asthma, COPD, respiratory depression, and monitor closely.

III.   ALTERATION IN ELIMINATION related to CONSTIPATION, ILEUS

Defining Characteristics: Opium agonists bind to opiate receptors in bowel, slowing peristalsis, leading to constipation. Untreated constipation may result in bowel perforation.

Nursing Implications: Assess baseline elimination, fluid intake, diet, and exercise patterns. Instruct patient regarding prevention of constipation: goal is to move bowels at least every 2 days by increasing fluids to 3 L/day, following a diet high in fiber (beans, vegetables, fruit), and taking moderate exercise. Assess need for bowel softeners, bulk-forming laxatives, and osmotic cathartics, and discuss prescription with physician. Teach patient self-administration of medications.

IV. ALTERATION IN NUTRITION, LESS THAN BODY REQUIREMENTS, related to GI TOXICITY

Defining Characteristics: Nausea, vomiting, and dry mouth may occur. Gastric, biliary, and pancreatic secretions are decreased by opiate agonists; digestion is delayed. Biliary tract muscle tone is increased, and spasm of Oddi's sphincter may occur (morphine > meperidine > codeine).

Nursing Implications: Assess patient tolerance of GI side effects. Instruct patient to report side effects. If nausea/vomiting occur, change to another opioid, or premedicate with antiemetic to prevent nausea/vomiting. Assess GI pain, biliary spasm, and consider alternative opioid.

V. ALTERATION IN CARDIAC OUTPUT related to HYPOTENSION, BRADYCARDIA

Defining Characteristics: Orthostatic hypotension, bradycardia due to cholinergic effect, and peripheral vasodilation may occur with rapid IV dosing. There may be histamine-related flushing, pruritus, diaphoresis with chronic drug usage; tolerance develops to this effect.

Nursing Implications: Assess baseline cardiovascular status. Teach patient to change position slowly and to hold onto stable, nearby structure for support as needed. Be careful when giving IV push opioids, and caution patient to remain in supine position for 15–20 minutes after injection. Monitor cardiovascular status after injection.

VI. ALTERATION IN URINE ELIMINATION related to URINARY RETENTION

Defining Characteristics: Increased smooth muscle tone in urinary tract and spasm may occur. Bladder tone is increased, which may cause urgency. Vesical sphincter tone may be increased leading to difficulty urinating. Increased risk of urinary retention in patients with prostatic hypertrophy or urethral stricture.

Nursing Implications: Assess baseline urinary elimination pattern. Teach patient to increase fluids to 3 L/day, and encourage voiding every 2–3 hours. Instruct patient to report problems with urination.

VII. KNOWLEDGE DEFICIT related to DRUG ADMINISTRATION, POTENTIAL FOR TOLERANCE, AND DEPENDENCY

Defining Characteristics: Psychological dependence (addiction) occurs rarely in patients taking opioid agonists for cancer pain (> 1%). Physical dependence (precipitation of withdrawal symptoms) occurs with chronic use of the drug for the relief of chronic cancer pain. In addition, tolerance, or less analgesic effect over time with the same drug dose, occurs and requires increased dosage of drug.

Nursing Implications: Assess baseline knowledge of opioid analgesics, and attitude about their use for cancer pain management. Teach patient about proper self-administration, possible side effects, and self-care measures. Suggest patient maintain diary of pain intensity, precipitating and alleviating factors, drug dose and time taken, and relief. Teach patient to self-administer opioid agonists for relief of chronic cancer pain around-the-clock, not PRN, to prevent pain. Explain use of prescribed short-acting opioid for rescue or to manage BTP. Discuss with physician dose increase or change in frequency of administration if tolerance develops. Teach patient that withdrawal symptoms may occur if chronic, around the-clock dosing is interrupted. Withdrawal (abstinence) symptoms that may be seen are restlessness, lacrimation, rhinorrhea, yawning, perspiration, gooseflesh, restless sleep, mydriasis in first 24 hours. These are followed by twitching and leg spasm; severe aching of the back, abdomen, and legs; cramping in abdomen and legs; hot/cold flashes; insomnia; nausea/vomiting, diarrhea; severe sneezing; and increased heart rate, BP, T, which peak at 36–72 hours. Withdrawal syndrome can be prevented by administration of at least ¼ of previous opioid dose.

VIII. SEXUAL DYSFUNCTION related to IMPOTENCE, ↓ LIBIDO

Defining Characteristics: Opiate agonists may suppress gonadotropin, causing impotence and decreased libido.

Nursing Implications: Assess baseline sexual pattern. Discuss potential toxicity and impact on sexuality. Provide information, emotional support, and referral as needed.

Drug: morphine (Astramorph, Avinza, Duramorph, Infumorph, Kadian Morphine Sulfate Sustained Release, MS Contin, MSIR, Morphelan, Oramorph, Roxanol)

Class: Opioid analgesic (opioid agonist).

Mechanism of Action: Binds to opiate receptors in CNS (limbic system, thalamus, striatum, hypothalamus, midbrain, spinal cord). This opioid agonist alters pain perception at level of spinal cord and higher centers, as well as the emotional response to pain. Also suppresses cough reflex.

Metabolism: Variable absorption from GI tract; increased absorption when taken with food. Peak analgesia 60 minutes (oral), 20–60 minutes (rectal), 50–90 minutes (subcutaneous), 30–60 minutes (IM), 20 minutes (IV). Duration is 4–7 hours. Maximum respiratory depression is 30 minutes (IM), 7 minutes (IV), 90 minutes (subcutaneous). Drug is slowly absorbed into systemic circulation after intrathecal (IT) administration. Peak CSF concentrations occur 60–90 minutes after epidural dose. Metabolized by liver and excreted in urine and, to a small degree, feces.

Indication: For the relief of severe, acute pain or severe, chronic pain (e.g., in terminally ill patients). Used also parenterally for preoperative sedation, as a supplement to anesthesia, and for analgesia during labor. Also used in patients with acute pulmonary edema for its cardiovascular effects and to allay anxiety. Morphine should not be used in the treatment of pulmonary edema resulting from a chemical respiratory irritant. Morphine is the drug of choice in relieving pain of MI.

Contraindications: (1) Known hypersensitivity to the drug; (2) in convulsive states (e.g., status epilepticus, tetanus, and strychnine poisoning), as it has a stimulating effect on the spinal cord; (3) heart failure secondary to chronic lung disease; (4) cardiac arrhythmias; (5) brain tumor; (6) acute alcoholism; (7) delirium tremens; (8) if prior idiosyncratic reaction to the drug; (9) premature infants, or during delivery when premature infant is anticipated.

Dosage/Range: *For moderate to severe pain:*
- Oral: 10–60 mg PO q 3–4 h titrated to pain; 10–240 mg sustained release q 8–12 h, titrated to pain.
- Rectal: 10–60 mg q 4 h.
- Subcutaneous, IM: 4–15 mg q 3–4 h.
- IV: 1–100 mg/h, and higher, titrated to need in physically dependent patients.
- Intrathecal: dose is 1/10 the epidural dose.
- Epidural: 5 mg q 24 h.
- At home, teach patient to store oral doses in a safe place away from children and pets.

Drug Preparation:
- Store tablets in tight, light-resistant containers at 15–30°C (59–86°F).
- Injection should be protected from light, and stored at 15–40°C (59–104°F).

Drug Administration:
- Begin morphine therapy using immediate-release oral preparations and increase dose to control pain; once optimal dose identified, convert to sustained-release formulation by dividing 24-hour total morphine dose by 2, giving two (q 12 h) doses.
- Intrathecal or epidural: use preservative-free morphine only, e.g., Astramorph PF, Duramorph PF, Infumorph; consult individual policies/procedures for administration.
- Teach patient that opioid analgesics may impair the mental and/or physical ability to drive and use machines, and to avoid these activities until the effect of the drug is known.

Drug Interactions:
- Injection incompatible with solutions containing aminophylline, ammonium chloride, amobarbital sodium, chlorothiazide sodium, heparin sodium, methicillin sodium, nitrofurantoin, phenobarbital sodium, sodium bicarbonate.
- Alcohol, CNS depressants: additive effects.

Lab Effects/Interference:
- None known.

Special Considerations:
- Oral to parenteral dose is 3–6 to 1 (equianalgesic dose).
- Highly concentrated formulations are available and are for use in continuous infusion pumps.

MANAGEMENT

- Do not crush sustained-release formulations (e.g., MS Contin, Oramorph).
- When epidural or intrathecal route is used, refer to institutional policy/procedure for administration and patient monitoring.
- Additive benefit when combined with acetaminophen or aspirin.
- Give smallest effective dose to prevent development of tolerance, physical dependency.
- Reduce dose in debilitated patients, or patients receiving other CNS depressants.
- Ensure that patients and caregivers are taught the dose and amount of opioid analgesic to self-administer. It is reported that a patient misunderstood and thought he was taking a 5-mg dose of morphine = 5 mL, when in fact the formulation the patient had was a solution of 100 mg/5 mL. This resulted in a 20-fold overdose. To prevent further errors, the drug has since been repackaged, and requires a Medication Guide be dispensed to each patient with the drug (Roxane Laboratories, December 2010).
- Use with caution in patients with hepatic or renal dysfunction, hypothyroidism, Addison's disease, severe CNS depression, respiratory depression, head injury, elevated intracranial pressure.
- If required, naloxone HCl will reverse opiate toxicity (e.g., respiratory depression). However, it is important that acute withdrawal symptoms be prevented by giving only enough naloxone to reverse respiratory depression and that this be continued for opioid drug half-life.
- Kadian as well as Avinza are sustained-release morphine formulated for once-a-day dosing; available in 20-, 50-, and 100-mg tablets (Kadian) and 30-, 60-, 90-, and 120-mg capsules (Avinza).

Potential Toxicities/Side Effects and the Nursing Process

I.   SENSORY/PERCEPTUAL ALTERATIONS related to CNS DEPRESSION

Defining Characteristics: Drowsiness, sedation, mood changes, euphoria, dysphoria, dizziness, mental clouding may occur. At high doses, may cause seizures. Miosis (papillary constriction) may occur.

Nursing Implications: Assess baseline neurologic status. Use cautiously, if at all, in the elderly, the debilitated, and patients with head injury, increased intracranial pressure, severe CNS depression, acute alcoholism. Assess other concurrent medications. Use with caution in patients receiving other opioids, tranquilizers, hypnotics, MAO inhibitors, since increasing CNS depressant effects can occur. Monitor neurologic status closely. Instruct patient to avoid driving and operating machinery while taking the medicine, and to AVOID concurrent alcohol.

II.   ALTERATION IN OXYGENATION related to RESPIRATORY DEPRESSION

Defining Characteristics: Opiate agonists directly depress respiratory center in brain stem, causing decreased sensitivity and responsiveness to increased pCO_2. Also may depress deep breathing and reflex to sigh. Tolerance to respiratory depressant effects occurs with chronic use.

Nursing Implications: Assess baseline pulmonary status, and periodically during drug use. Use cautiously in patients with bronchial asthma, COPD, respiratory depression, and monitor closely.

III. ALTERATION IN ELIMINATION related to CONSTIPATION, ILEUS

Defining Characteristics: Opium agonists bind to opiate receptors in bowel, slowing peristalsis, leading to constipation. Untreated constipation may result in bowel perforation.

Nursing Implications: Assess baseline elimination, fluid intake, diet, and exercise patterns. Instruct patient regarding prevention of constipation: goal is to move bowels at least every 2 days by increasing fluids to 3 L/day, following a diet high in fiber (beans, vegetables, fruit), and taking moderate exercise. Assess need for bowel softeners, bulk-forming laxatives, and osmotic cathartics, and discuss prescription with physician. Teach patient self-administration of medications.

IV. ALTERATION IN NUTRITION, LESS THAN BODY REQUIREMENTS, related to GI TOXICITY

Defining Characteristics: Nausea, vomiting, and dry mouth may occur. Gastric, biliary, and pancreatic secretions are decreased by opiate agonists; digestion is delayed. Biliary tract muscle tone is increased, and spasm of Oddi's sphincter may occur (morphine > meperidine > codeine).

Nursing Implications: Assess patient tolerance of GI side effects. Teach patient to report side effects. If nausea/vomiting occur, change to another opioid, or premedicate with antiemetic to prevent nausea/vomiting. Assess GI pain, biliary spasm, and consider alternative opioid.

V. ALTERATION IN CARDIAC OUTPUT related to HYPOTENSION, BRADYCARDIA

Defining Characteristics: Orthostatic hypotension, bradycardia due to cholinergic effect, and peripheral vasodilation may occur with rapid IV dosing. There may be histamine-related flushing, pruritus, diaphoresis with chronic drug usage; tolerance develops to this effect.

Nursing Implications: Assess baseline cardiovascular status. Teach patient to change position slowly and to hold onto stable, nearby structure for support as needed. Be careful when giving IV push opioids, and caution patient to remain in supine position for 15–20 minutes after injection. Monitor cardiovascular status after injection.

MANAGEMENT

VI.   ALTERATION IN URINE ELIMINATION related to URINARY RETENTION

Defining Characteristics: Increased smooth muscle tone in urinary tract and spasm may occur. Bladder tone is increased, which may cause urgency. Vesical sphincter tone may be increased, leading to difficulty urinating. Increased risk of urinary retention in patients with prostatic hypertrophy or urethral stricture.

Nursing Implications: Assess baseline urinary elimination pattern. Teach patient to increase fluids to 3 L/day, and encourage voiding every 2–3 hours. Instruct patient to report problems with urination.

VII.   KNOWLEDGE DEFICIT related to DRUG ADMINISTRATION, POTENTIAL FOR TOLERANCE, AND DEPENDENCY

Defining Characteristics: Psychological dependence (addiction) occurs rarely in patients taking opioid agonists for cancer pain (< 1%). Physical dependence (precipitation of withdrawal symptoms) occurs with chronic use of the drug for the relief of chronic cancer pain. In addition, tolerance, or less analgesic effect over time with the same drug dose, occurs and requires increased dosage of drug.

Nursing Implications: Assess baseline knowledge of opioid analgesics, and attitude about their use for cancer pain management. Teach patient about proper self-administration, possible side effects, and self-care measures. Suggest patient maintain diary of pain intensity, precipitating and alleviating factors, drug dose and time taken, and relief. Teach patient to self-administer opioid agonists for relief of chronic cancer pain around-the-clock, not PRN, to prevent pain. Explain use of pre-scribed short-acting opioid for rescue or to manage breakthrough pain. Discuss with physician dose increase or change in frequency of administration if tolerance develops. Teach patient that withdrawal symptoms may occur if chronic, around-the-clock dosing is interrupted. Withdrawal (abstinence) symptoms that may be seen are restlessness, lacrimation, rhinorrhea, yawning, perspiration, gooseflesh, restless sleep, mydriasis in first 24 hours. These are followed by twitching and leg spasm; severe aching of the back, abdomen, and legs; cramping in abdomen and legs; hot/cold flashes; insomnia; nausea/vomiting, diarrhea; severe sneezing; and increased heart rate, BP, T, which peak at 36–72 hours. Withdrawal syndrome can be prevented by administration of at least one-quarter of previous opioid dose.

VIII.   SEXUAL DYSFUNCTION related to IMPOTENCE, ↓ LIBIDO

Defining Characteristics: Opiate agonists may suppress gonadotropin, causing impotence and decreased libido.

Nursing Implications: Assess baseline sexual pattern. Discuss potential toxicity and impact on sexuality. Provide information, emotional support, and referral as needed.

Drug: oxycodone (Percodan, Endodan, Roxiprin, Oxecta)

Class: Opioid analgesic (opioid agonist).

Mechanism of Action: A synthetic opioid agonist, oxycodone resembles morphine but has milder action; binds to opiate receptors in CNS (limbic system, thalamus, striatum, hypothalamus, midbrain, spinal cord), altering pain perception at level of spinal cord and higher centers, as well as the emotional response to pain. Drug is relatively selective for the mu receptor, and can interact with other opioid receptors at high doses. Also suppresses cough reflex. Oxecta formulation uses Aversion Technology, which discourages abuse of the drug (e.g., the active ingredient gels when improperly used thus discourage injection, and they irritate the nasal passages to discourage inhalation). However, it still can be abused by crushing, chewing, snorting, or injecting the product.

Metabolism: Onset of analgesia in 10–15 minutes, peaks 30–60 minutes, duration 3–6 hours. Metabolized by liver and kidney; excreted in urine.

Indications: Management of moderate-to-severe pain where the use of an opioid anaglesic is appropriate.

Contraindications: (1) Known hypersensitivity to oxycodone, (2) situations where opioids are contraindicated (e.g., significant respiratory depression in unmonitored settings/ absence of resuscitative equipment), (3) patients with acute or severe bronchial asthma or hypercarbia, (4) patient suspected of having paralytic ileus.

Dosage/Range: *For moderate to moderately severe pain:*
- 5 mg q 6 h (Roxicodone).
- 5 mg q 6 h, combined with acetaminophen: 300 mg (e.g., Oxycet, Percocet, Roxicet caplets), OR 500 mg (e.g., Roxicet caplets, Tylox); OR combined with aspirin: 325 mg (e.g., Percodan, Codoxy, Roxiprin); OR combined with ibuprofen 5 mg/400 mg (e.g., Combunox).
- Oral solution: 5 mg/5 mL (Roxicodone); 20 mg/mL (Roxicodone, Intensol).
- 5 mg to 15 mg every 4–6 hr as needed for pain (Oxecta).

Drug Preparation:
- Store tablets in tight, light-resistant containers at 15–30°C (59–86°F) and protect from light.
- At home, teach patient to store oral doses in a safe place away from children and pets.

Drug Administration:
- Oral.
- Percocet: 2.5/325 (2.5 mg oxycodone plus 325 mg acetaminophen); 5/325, 7.5/325, 7.5/500, 10/325, 10/650. Acetaminophen cumulative dose should not exceed 4,000 mg a day.
- Oxecta available in 5-mg and 7.5-mg tablets. Must be swallowed whole and cannot be crushed or dissolved. Thus it cannot be administered via nasogastric, gastric, or other feeding tubes as it may occlude the tube.
- Teach patient that opioid analgesics may impair the mental and/or physical ability to drive and use machines, and to avoid these activities until the effect of the drug is known.

Drug Interactions:
- Alcohol, CNS depressants: additive CNS depressant effects.
- Anticoagulants, chemotherapy: aspirin-oxycodone combination may increase bleeding risk; AVOID concurrent use.

Lab Effects/Interference:
- None known.

Special Considerations:
- Adverse effects are milder than morphine.
- Preparations may contain sodium metabisulfite and may cause allergic reactions, including anaphylaxis and severe asthma-like reactions.
- Additive benefit when combined with acetaminophen or aspirin.
- Give smallest effective dose to prevent development of tolerance, physical dependency.
- Reduce dose in debilitated patients or patients receiving other CNS depressants.
- Use with caution in patients with hepatic or renal dysfunction, hypothyroidism, Addison's disease, severe CNS depression, respiratory depression, head injury, elevated ICP.
- If required, naloxone HCl will reverse opiate toxicity (e.g., respiratory depression). However, it is important that acute withdrawal symptoms be prevented by giving only enough naloxone to reverse respiratory depression and that this be continued for opioid drug half-life.

Potential Toxicities/Side Effects and the Nursing Process

I.   SENSORY/PERCEPTUAL ALTERATIONS related to CNS DEPRESSION

Defining Characteristics: Drowsiness, sedation, mood changes, euphoria, dysphoria, dizziness, mental clouding may occur. At high doses, may cause seizures. Miosis (papillary constriction) may occur.

Nursing Implications: Assess baseline neurologic status. Use cautiously, if at all, in the elderly, the debilitated, and patients with head injury, increased ICP, severe CNS depression, acute alcoholism. Assess other concurrent medications. Use with caution in patients receiving other opioids, tranquilizers, hypnotics, MAO inhibitors, since increasing CNS depressant effects can occur. Monitor neurologic status closely. Instruct patient to avoid driving and operating machinery while taking the medicine, and to AVOID concurrent alcohol.

II.   ALTERATION IN OXYGENATION related to RESPIRATORY DEPRESSION

Defining Characteristics: Opiate agonists directly depress respiratory center in brain stem, causing decreased sensitivity and responsiveness to increased pCO_2. Also may depress deep breathing and reflex to sigh. Tolerance to respiratory depressant effects occurs with chronic use.

Nursing Implications: Assess baseline pulmonary status, and periodically during drug use. Use cautiously in patients with bronchial asthma, COPD, respiratory depression, and monitor closely.

III. ALTERATION IN ELIMINATION related to CONSTIPATION, ILEUS

Defining Characteristics: Opium agonists bind to opiate receptors in bowel, slowing peristalsis, leading to constipation. Untreated constipation may result in bowel perforation.

Nursing Implications: Assess baseline elimination, fluid intake, diet, and exercise patterns. Instruct patient regarding prevention of constipation: goal is to move bowels at least every 2 days by increasing fluids to 3 L/day, following a diet high in fiber (beans, vegetables, fruit), and taking moderate exercise. Assess need for bowel softeners, bulk-forming laxatives, and osmotic cathartics, and discuss preparation with physician. Teach patient self-administration of medications. Monitor for decreased bowel motility in postoperative patients.

IV. ALTERATION IN NUTRITION, LESS THAN BODY REQUIREMENTS, related to GI TOXICITY

Defining Characteristics: Nausea, vomiting, dry mouth may occur. Gastric, biliary, and pancreatic secretions are decreased by opiate agonists; digestion is delayed. Biliary tract muscle tone is increased, and spasm of Oddi's sphincter may occur (morphine > meperidine > codeine).

Nursing Implications: Assess patient tolerance of GI side effects. Teach patient to report side effects. If nausea/vomiting occur, change to another opioid, or premedicate with antiemetic to prevent nausea/vomiting. Assess GI pain, biliary spasm, and consider alternative opioid.

V. ALTERATION IN CARDIAC OUTPUT related to HYPOTENSION, BRADYCARDIA

Defining Characteristics: Orthostatic hypotension, bradycardia due to cholinergic effect, and peripheral vasodilation may occur with rapid IV dosing. There may be histamine-related flushing, pruritus, diaphoresis with chronic drug usage; tolerance develops to this effect.

Nursing Implications: Assess baseline cardiovascular status. Teach patient to change position slowly and to hold onto stable, nearby structure for support as needed. Teach patient to report dizziness, any falls, or other problems.

VI. ALTERATION IN URINE ELIMINATION related to URINARY RETENTION

Defining Characteristics: Increased smooth muscle tone in urinary tract and spasm may occur. Bladder tone is increased, which may cause urgency. Vesical sphincter tone may be increased, leading to difficulty urinating. Increased risk of urinary retention in patients with prostatic hypertrophy or urethral stricture.

Nursing Implications: Assess baseline urinary elimination pattern. Teach patient to increase fluids to 3 L/day, and encourage voiding every 2–3 hours. Instruct patient to report problems with urination.

VII.   KNOWLEDGE DEFICIT related to DRUG ADMINISTRATION, POTENTIAL FOR TOLERANCE, AND DEPENDENCY

Defining Characteristics: Psychological dependence (addiction) occurs rarely in patients taking opioid agonists for cancer pain (> 1%). Physical dependence (precipitation of withdrawal symptoms) occurs with chronic use of the drug for the relief of chronic cancer pain. In addition, tolerance, or less analgesic effect over time with the same drug dose, occurs and requires increased dosage of drug.

Nursing Implications: Assess baseline knowledge of opioid analgesics, and attitude about their use for cancer pain management. Teach patient about proper self-administration, possible side effects, and self-care measures. Suggest patient maintain diary of pain intensity, precipitating and alleviating factors, drug dose and time taken, and relief. Teach patient to self-administer for relief of chronic cancer pain around-the-clock, not PRN, to prevent pain. Explain use of prescribed short-acting opioid for rescue or to manage breakthrough pain. Discuss with physician dose increase or change in frequency of administration if tolerance develops. Teach patient that withdrawal symptoms may occur if chronic, around-the-clock dosing is interrupted. Withdrawal (abstinence) symptoms that may be seen are restlessness, lacrimation, rhinorrhea, yawning, perspiration, gooseflesh, restless sleep, mydriasis in first 24 hours. These are followed by twitching and leg spasm; severe aching of the back, abdomen, and legs; cramping in abdomen and legs; hot/cold flashes; insomnia; nausea/vomiting, diarrhea; severe sneezing; and increased heart rate, BP, T, which peak at 36–72 hours. Withdrawal syndrome can be prevented by administration of at least ¼ of previous opioid dose.

VIII.   POTENTIAL FOR INJURY related to DRUG ABUSE

Defining Characteristics: Oxycodone has been significantly abused in the past. Opiate antagonists are sought after by people with addiction disorders and drug abusers. Addiction is a psychological dependence characterized by compulsive use of an opiate for nonmedical purposes, and despite potential harm. "Drug seeking" behavior is common in addicts and drug abusers, and often involves "doctor shopping," or loss of prescriptions. Newer formulations incorporate tamper-proof technology, such as Aversion Technology used in Oxecta. Additives discourage abuse by forming a gel if a user tries to prepare it for injection, and it irritates the nasal passages if a user tries to snort it (Oxecta). In addition, opioids now require Risk Evaluation and Mitigation Strategy (REMS) education of prescribers and patients.

Nursing Implications: REMS requires healthcare professionals to complete education about the risks and benefits of prescribing controlled-release opiates, and strategies to prevent abuse or illicit use, in addition to a very detailed patient education guide. Some also require patient agreements. Strategies to prevent abuse include careful record-keeping of prescribing information (e.g., quantity, frequency, renewal requests). Patients should be assessed regularly, and repeated requests to obtain a prescription early before it is due should be explored further, along with "lost prescriptions." In the event the patient is abusing the drug, it is important to develop a contract with the patient stating the expected behaviors and sequelae if they are not adhered to.

IX. SEXUAL DYSFUNCTION related to IMPOTENCE, ↓ LIBIDO

Defining Characteristics: Opiate agonists may suppress gonadotropin, causing impotence and decreased libido.

Nursing Implications: Assess baseline sexual pattern. Discuss potential toxicity and impact on sexuality. Provide information, emotional support, and referral as needed.

Drug: oxycodone controlled-release formulation (OxyContin)

Class: Opioid analgesic (opioid agonist).

Mechanism of Action: A synthetic mu-receptor opioid agonist, oxycodone resembles morphine but has milder action; binds to opiate receptors in CNS (limbic system, thalamus, striatum, hypothalamus, midbrain, spinal cord), altering pain perception at level of spinal cord and higher centers, as well as the emotional response to pain. Also suppresses cough reflex.

Metabolism: About 60–87% of oral dose of oxycodone reaches the central compartment compared to a parenteral dose. High bioavailability due to low presystemic and/or first pass metabolism. Drug has biphasic absorption pattern with half-lives of 0.6 and 6.9 hours, corresponding to an initial release of oxycodone from the tablet, followed by a prolonged release. Steady state plasma concentrations are reached within 24–36 hours of initiation of dosing. Food has no significant effect on extent of absorption of oxycodone from OxyContin. Once absorbed, oxycodone is distributed to skeletal muscle, liver, intestinal tract, lungs, spleen, and brain. Drug has been found in breast milk. Oxycodone HCl is extensively metabolized to noroxycodone, primarily via CYP3A4-mediated N-demethylation, and to a lesser degree (to oxymorphone) via CYP2D6-mediated, O-demethylation Oxycodone and its metabolites are excreted primarily via the kidney. The elimination half-life of oxycodone following the administration of OxyContin was 4.5 hours compared to 3.2 hours for immediate-release oxycodone. The elderly have plasma concentrations of oxycodone 15% higher as compared to younger subjects, and females have a plasma concentration 25% higher than males.

Indications: For the management of moderate-to-severe pain when a continuous, around-the-clock analgesic is needed for an extended period of time. Drug is NOT intended for use as a PRN analgesic.

Dosage/Range:
- Treatment must be individualized in every case.
- Start on lowest appropriate dose. Initiate dosing regimen individually for each patient. OxyContin 60-mg and 80-mg tablets and single doses > 40 mg, or total daily doses > 80 mg should ONLY be used in opioid-tolerant patients. Teach patient to ensure the drug is used only by the patient for whom it is prescribed. Prescribers must complete OxyContin Risk Evaluation and Mitigation Strategy training (www.oxycontinrems.com): Healthcare Professional Letter, Healthcare Provider Training Guide, Education Confirmation Form. Patients and caregivers can go on this site to obtain the OxyContin Medication Guide.
- Nonopioid-tolerant patient:
  - Use low initial doses. For example, dosage for a nonopioid-tolerant patient who requires around-the-clock analgesia is 10 mg every 12 hours. In patients who are not already opioid-tolerant, especially if also receiving concurrent treatment with muscle relaxants, sedatives, and other CNS-active drugs, start low and proceed very cautiously.
  - Do not begin treatment with OxyContin 60-mg or 80-mg tablets, a single dose > 40 mg, or a total daily dose > 80 mg, as these may cause fatal respiratory depression.
- For patients who are opioid-tolerant (e.g., taking at least 60 mg oral morphine/day, 25 mcg transdermal fentanyl/hour, 30 mg oral oxycodone/day, 8 mg oral hydromorphone/day, 25 mg oral oxymorphone/day, or an equianalgesic dose of another opioid for > one week), use standard conversion ratio estimates. Titrate dose to adequate analgesia with minimal/acceptable side effects.
  - Calculate 24-hour requirement of opioid, then convert to oxycodone. Standard conversion estimates may be used but are approximate. It is safer to underestimate the equianalgesic dose, and supplement oxycodone for breakthrough pain; then calculate the equivalent total daily dose of combined drug, and divide by two, to obtain the 12-hour dose of oxycontin.
  - When converting from oxycodone, divide the 24-hour oxycodone dose in half to obtain the twice-a-day (q 12 h) of OxyContin. Round down to a dose that is appropriate for the tablet strengths available.
  - Discontinue all other around-the-clock opioid drugs when OxyContin is initiated.
- Close observation and frequent titration are indicated until the patient is stable on the new therapy.
- In all cases, patients should also receive a short-acting analgesic for breakthrough pain.
- To convert transdermal fentanyl to OxyContin, use 10 mg OxyContin every 12 hours for each 25-µg fentanyl transdermal patch. Initiate OxyContin 18 hours after removal of the patch(s). Follow the patient closely for early titration to find the optimal dose, as there are limited clinical data about dose conversion.
- If patient no longer requires therapy with OxyContin, taper the dose gradually to prevent withdrawal in the physically dependent patient.
- Frequently assess pain relief and opioid side effects. Titrate to adequate effect (usually mild or no pain), with use of no more than 2 doses of rescue or breakthrough pain medication per 24 hours. Titrate dosage every 1–2 days, as steady state concentrations are approximated within 24–36 hours. Increase the dose, NOT the dosing frequency, as there are no data about administering the drug any sooner than every 12 hours. Increase the

total daily dose of oxycodone by 25–50% of the current dose at each increase. If signs of excessive opioid-related side effects occur, reduce the next dose; however, if the pain increases, patient should take a supplemental dose of immediate-release oxycodone, or a non-opioid analgesic adjuvant drug.

- Maintain close contact with the patient/family during dose titration to assess tolerance and effect.
- Oxycontin 60-mg, 80-mg, 160-mg tablets, or a single dose > 40 mg or a total daily dose > 80 mg, are to be used ONLY in opiate-tolerant patients (see Special Considerations), as they will be tolerant to the respiratory depressant effects of the drug.
- Oxycontin is contraindicated in patients with significant respiratory depression, acute or severe bronchial asthma in an uncontrolled setting, known or suspected paralytic ileus and GI obstruction, or hypersensitivity to oxycodone.

Dose Modification:
- Elderly: initial dose may need to be reduced to one-third to one-half of the usual dose.
- Hepatic impairment: start therapy at one-third to one-half of the usual dose with careful dose titration.
- Renal impairment (creatinine clearance < 60 mL/min): start therapy conservatively, as plasma concentrations may be 50% higher than in patients with normal renal function.
- Debilitated, nontolerant patients: start at one-third to one-half of the usual dose with careful dose titration.

Drug Preparation: Available as 10-mg, 15-mg, 20-mg, 30-mg, 40-mg, 60-mg, 80-mg, controlled-release tablets.

Drug Administration:
- Oral.
- Patient should be instructed to swallow the tablet whole, and to NOT chew, break, crush, dissolve, or cut the tablet, as this can cause overdosage. Tablets should be taken one tablet at a time with enough water to ensure complete swallowing after placing in mouth. Doses of 160 mg should be taken on an empty stomach.
- When OxyContin is no longer needed, unused tablets should be destroyed by flushing them down the toilet (per FDA).
- Teach patient that opioid analgesics may impair the mental and/or physical ability to drive and use machines, and to avoid these activities until the effect of the drug is known.

Drug Interactions: All cytochrome P450 3A4 inhibitors (macrolide antibiotics like erythromycin, azole antifungal agents like ketoconazole, protease inhibitors like ritonavir) may decrease oxycodone metabolism and result in an increase in oxycodone plasma concentrations; do not give concurrently if possible; otherwise monitor the patient closely for an extended period of time and with each dosage adjustment.
- CNS depressants (e.g., hypnotics, sedatives, general anesthetics, antipsychotics, alcohol) may cause additive depressant effects and respiratory depression, hypotension, profound sedation, coma; if must use concurrently, reduce dose of one or both agents. Otherwise respiratory depression, hypotension, and profound sedation or coma may occur. Do not take drug when drinking alcohol.

MANAGEMENT

- MAO inhibitors: MAO inhibitors may cause CNS excitation or depression, hypotension, or hypertension if used concurrently. Do not use concurrently, and separate by at least 14 days after stopping the MAO inhibitor.
- OxyContin may enhance the neuromuscular blocking action of skeletal muscle relaxants and produce an increased degree of respiratory depression.
- Mixed agonist/antagonist opioid analgesics (e.g., buprenorphine, nalbuphine, pentazocine) may reduce analgesic effect by competitive blockade of receptors ± precipitate withdrawal symptoms. Do not use concurrently.
- Anticholinergic drugs may increase risk of urinary retention and/or severe constipation leading to paralytic ileus.

Lab Effects/Interference:
- Increased serum amylase level caused by spasm of sphincter of Oddi.

Special Considerations:
- Individualize dose for each patient when starting dosing regimen. Overestimating the initial dose when converting from another opioid can result in overdosage and death. Also remember that the drug has a high risk of abuse. In calculating the initial dose, consider:
  - Risk factors for abuse, addiction, or diversion, including a prior history or family history of abuse, addiction, or diversion.
  - Age, general condition, medical status of the patient.
  - Daily dose, potency, and specific characteristics of the patient's current opioid.
  - Reliability of the relative potency estimate used to calculate the equivalent dose of oxycodone needed.
  - Patient's degree of opioid exposure and opioid tolerance.
  - Concurrent nonopioid analgesics and other medications, such as those with CNS activity.
  - Type and severity of the patient's pain.
  - The balance between pain control and adverse effects.
- Drug is not recommended during labor and delivery, pregnancy, or nursing.
- Administer drug with caution, and in reduced dosages, to elderly patients, especially those with cardiovascular, pulmonary, renal, or hepatic disease. May cause hypotension; use cautiously in patients at increased risk of hypotension or in circulatory shock.
- Special instructions for OxyContin 60-mg, 80-mg tablets or a single dose > 40 mg, or total dose > 80 mg/24 hours: should be prescribed ONLY for opioid-tolerant patients.
- Opioid-tolerant is defined as taking at least 60 mg oral morphine daily, 25 µg transdermal fentanyl/hr, 30 mg oral oxycodone/day, 8 mg hydromorphone/day, 25 mg oral oxymorphone/day, or an equianalgesic dose of another opioid for a week or longer.
- OxyContin tablets are indicated for the management of moderate to severe pain when a continuous, around-the-clock opioid analgesic is needed for an extended period of time. It is NOT intended for use on an as-needed basis. Drug is NOT indicated for pain relief in the immediate postoperative period (first 12–24 hours after surgery), or if the pain is mild or not expected to persist for an extended period of time. If the surgical patient has been receiving OxyContin prior to surgery, or if the postsurgery pain is moderate to severe and expected to last for an extended period of time, then the drug can be used.

- As OxyContin was used illicitly in the last decade (see the introduction to this chapter), a new formulation was released in April 2010 that is very difficult to chew, break, crush, or dissolve, thereby decreasing its abuse potential.
- Drug must be swallowed whole, as taking broken, chewed, dissolved, or crushed drug or its contents leads to rapid release and absorption of a potentially fatal dose of oxycodone. **Keep out of reach of children and pets.**
- Use with caution in patients with adrenocortical insufficiency (e.g., Addison's disease), delirium tremens, myxedema or hypothyroidism, prostatic hypertrophy, urethral stricture, toxic psychosis, severe impairment of hepatic, pulmonary, or renal function, patients at risk for ileus. Drug worsens seizures in patients with convulsive disorders.
- Drug may cause spasm of the sphincter of Oddi, and should be used with caution, if at all, in patients with biliary tract disease, including acute pancreatitis.
- Drug not approved in the treatment of addiction. In addition, not every urine drug test for "opioids" or "opiates" detects oxycodone reliably.
- Most common adverse effects (> 5%) are constipation, nausea, somnolence, dizziness, vomiting, pruritus, headache, dry mouth, asthenia, and sweating.

Potential Toxicities/Side Effects and the Nursing Process

I. SENSORY/PERCEPTUAL ALTERATIONS related to CNS DEPRESSION

Defining Characteristics: Drowsiness, sedation, mood changes, euphoria, dysphoria, dizziness, alterations in judgment and levels of consciousness, and mental clouding may occur. The respiratory depressant effects of opioids includes CO_2 retention and secondary increase of CSF; it may be magnified in the presence of head injury, intracranial lesions, or other pre-existing causes of increased intracranial pressure. At high doses, may cause seizures. Miosis (pupillary constriction) may occur. OxyContin can worsen and obscure neurologic signs (e.g., LOC, pupillary) of increasing intracranial pressure in patients who are head injured.

Nursing Implications: Assess baseline neurologic status. Use cautiously, if at all, in the elderly, the debilitated, and patients with head injury, increased ICP, severe CNS depression, acute alcoholism. Assess other concurrent medications. Use with caution in patients receiving other opioids, tranquilizers, hypnotics, and MAO inhibitors, because increasing CNS depressant effects can occur. Discuss using a lower initial dose of a CNS depressant when given to a patient receiving OxyContin. Teach patient NOT to use alcohol or illicit drugs while taking OxyContin. Monitor neurologic status closely. Instruct patient to avoid driving and operating machinery while taking the medicine, and to AVOID concurrent alcohol.

II. ALTERATION IN OXYGENATION related to RESPIRATORY DEPRESSION

Defining Characteristics: Opiate agonists directly depress respiratory center in brain stem, causing decreased sensitivity and responsiveness to increased pCO_2. Also may depress deep breathing and reflex to sigh. Tolerance to respiratory depressant effects occurs with chronic use.

MANAGEMENT

Nursing Implications: Assess baseline pulmonary status, and periodically during drug use. Use with extreme caution in patients with significant COPD or cor pulmonale; patients with decreased respiratory reserve, hypoxia, or hypercapnia; or patients with preexisting respiratory depression or bronchial asthma. Teach patient and family members to report any "breathlessness" or dyspnea. Monitor patients closely as to analgesic benefit and adverse effects.

III.   ALTERATION IN ELIMINATION related to CONSTIPATION, ILEUS

Defining Characteristics: Opium agonists bind to opiate receptors in bowel, slowing peristalsis, leading to constipation. Untreated constipation may result in bowel perforation.

Nursing Implications: Assess baseline elimination, fluid intake, diet, and exercise patterns. Instruct patient regarding prevention of constipation: goal is to move bowels at least every 2 days by increasing fluids to 3 L/day, following a diet high in fiber (beans, vegetables, fruit), and taking moderate exercise. All patients should be on a bowel regimen. Assess need for bowel softeners, bulk-forming laxatives, and osmotic cathartics, and discuss preparation with physician. Teach patient self-administration of medications.

IV.   ALTERATION IN NUTRITION, LESS THAN BODY REQUIREMENTS, related to GI TOXICITY

Defining Characteristics: Nausea, vomiting, dry mouth may occur. Gastric, biliary, and pancreatic secretions are decreased by opiate agonists; digestion is delayed. Biliary tract muscle tone is increased, and spasm of Oddi's sphincter may occur (morphine > meperidine > codeine).

Nursing Implications: Assess patient tolerance of GI side effects. Teach patient to report side effects. If nausea/vomiting occur, change to another opioid, or premedicate with antiemetic to prevent nausea/vomiting. Assess GI pain, biliary spasm, and consider alternative opioid.

V.   ALTERATION IN URINE ELIMINATION related to URINARY RETENTION

Defining Characteristics: Increased smooth muscle tone in urinary tract and spasm may occur. Bladder tone is increased, which may cause urgency. Vesical sphincter tone may be increased, leading to difficulty urinating. Increased risk of urinary retention in patients with prostatic hypertrophy or urethral stricture.

Nursing Implications: Assess baseline urinary elimination pattern. Teach patient to increase fluids to 3 L/day, and encourage voiding every 2–3 hours. Instruct patient to report problems with urination.

VI.   ALTERATION IN CARDIAC OUTPUT related to HYPOTENSION, BRADYCARDIA

Defining Characteristics: Orthostatic hypotension, bradycardia due to cholinergic effect, and peripheral vasodilitation may occur. Oxycodone may cause orthostatic hypotension in ambulatory patients. There may be histamine-related flushing, pruritus, diaphoresis with chronic drug usage; tolerance develops to this effect.

Nursing Implications: Assess baseline cardiovascular status. Teach patient to change position slowly and to hold onto stable, nearby structure for support as needed. Teach patient to report dizziness, any falls, or other problems. Drug should be administered with caution if at all, in patients in shock as the vasodilitation caused by the drug may further reduce cardiac output and BP.

VII. KNOWLEDGE DEFICIT related to DRUG ADMINISTRATION, POTENTIAL FOR TOLERANCE, AND PHYSICAL DEPENDENCY

Defining Characteristics: Psychological dependence (addiction) occurs rarely in patients taking opioid agonists for cancer pain (< 1%). Physical dependence (precipitation of withdrawal symptoms) occurs with chronic use of the drug for the relief of chronic cancer pain. In addition, tolerance, or less analgesic effect over time with the same drug dose, occurs and requires increased dosage of drug.

Nursing Implications: Assess baseline knowledge of opioid analgesics and attitude about their use for cancer pain management. Teach patient about proper self-administration, possible side effects, and self-care measures. Suggest patient maintain diary of pain intensity, precipitating and alleviating factors, drug dose and time taken, and relief. Teach patient to self-administer opioid agonists for relief of chronic cancer pain around-the-clock, not PRN, to prevent pain. Explain use of prescribed short-acting opioid for rescue or to manage breakthrough pain. Discuss with physician dose increase or change in frequency of administration if tolerance develops. Teach patient that withdrawal symptoms may occur if chronic, around-the-clock dosing is interrupted. Withdrawal (abstinence) symptoms that may be seen are restlessness, lacrimation, rhinorrhea, yawning, perspiration, gooseflesh, restless sleep, mydriasis in first 24 hours. These are followed by twitching and leg spasm; severe aching of the back, abdomen, and legs; cramping in abdomen and legs; hot/cold flashes; insomnia; nausea/vomiting, diarrhea; severe sneezing; and increased heart rate, BP, T, which peak at 36–72 hours. Withdrawal syndrome can be prevented by administration of at least ¼ of previous opioid dose.

VIII. POTENTIAL FOR INJURY related to DRUG ABUSE

Defining Characteristics: OxyContin has been significantly abused in the past. Opiate antagonists are sought after by people with addiction disorders and drug abusers. Addiction is a psychological dependence characterized by compulsive use of an opiate for nonmedical purposes, and despite potential harm. "Drug seeking" behavior is common in addicts and drug abusers, and often involves "doctor shopping," or loss of prescriptions. The FDA requires that Purdue Pharma use the same REMS as hydromorphone extended-release tablets (see Exalgo).

Nursing Implications: Healthcare professionals must complete education about the risks and benefits of prescribing controlled-release opiates, and strategies to prevent abuse or illicit use, in addition to a very detailed patient education guide. The Purdue Pharma guide is called Medical Education Resource Catalogue Online (MERCO), a Web-based resource, and has, among the many programs, ASAP (Addressing Substance Abuse Prevention). It is found at http://www.purduepharmamededresources.com. Strategies to prevent abuse include careful record-keeping of prescribing information (e.g., quantity, frequency, renewal requests). Patients should be assessed regularly, and repeated requests to obtain a prescription early before it is due should be explored further, along with "lost prescriptions." In the event the patient is abusing the drug, it is important to develop a contract with the patient stating the expected behaviors and sequelae if they are not adhered to.

IX.   SEXUAL DYSFUNCTION related to IMPOTENCE, ↓ LIBIDO

Defining Characteristics: Opiate agonists may suppress gonadotropin, causing impotence and decreased libido.

Nursing Implications: Assess baseline sexual pattern. Discuss potential toxicity and impact on sexuality. Provide information, emotional support, and referral as needed.

Drug: oxymorphone hydrochloride (Opana)

Class: Opioid analgesic (opioid agonist).

Mechanism of Action: A semisynthetic opioid agonist, oxymorphone HCl resembles morphine but has milder action; binds to opiate receptors in CNS (limbic system, thalamus, striatum, hypothalamus, midbrain, spinal cord), altering pain perception at level of spinal cord and higher centers, as well as the emotional response to pain. Also suppresses cough reflex.

Metabolism: Absolute oral bioavailability is about 10%, and steady-state serum levels occurred after 3 days of multiple doses. Food increases absorption by 38%, so it should not be taken with food. Drug is not bound to plasma proteins to any degree (10–12%), and is highly metabolized by the liver by reduction or conjugation with glucuronide into active and inactive metabolites. In studies of drug in extended formulation, bioavailability is higher in patients with hepatic or renal impairment, and plasma levels in the elderly were 40% higher than younger controls. Drug and metabolites are excreted in the urine and feces.

Indication: For the relief of moderate-to-severe acute pain where the use of an opioid is appropriate.

Dosage/Range: *For moderate to severe acute pain:*
- Usual initial dose in opioid-naïve patients is 10–20 mg PO q 4–6 hr PRN depending on initial pain intensity; alternatively, a dose of 5 mg may be used initially.
- If patient is receiving parenteral oxymorphone, given the 10% bioavailability, multiply the total parenteral dose of morphone by 10, and administer in 4 or 6 equally divided doses.
- Beginning dose for elderly patient should be 5 mg PO q 4–6 hr PRN.

- Administer cautiously and in reduced doses in patients with creatinine clearance rates < 50 mL/min.
- Drug is contraindicated in patients with moderate and severe hepatic dysfunction; use cautiously and start at the lowest dose in patients with mild hepatic dysfunction, and titrate dose up.
- If patient is receiving CNS depressants (sedatives, hypnotics, general anesthetics, phenothiazines, tranquilizers, or alcohol) concurrently, start at one-third to one-half of the usual dose.
- If opioids are discontinued, drug should be gradually tapered to prevent withdrawal.

Drug Preparation:
- Drug available in 5- and 10-mg tablets.
- At home, teach patient to store oral doses in a safe place away from children and pets.

Drug Administration:
- Oral, on an empty stomach (at least 1 hour before or 2 hours after food ingestion).
- Teach patient that opioid analgesics may impair the mental and/or physical ability to drive and use machines, and to avoid these activities until the effect of the drug is known.

Drug Interactions:
- Alcohol, CNS depressants: Additive CNS depressant effects (hypotension, respiratory depression, profound sedation).
- Mixed agonist/antagonist analgesics (pentazocine, nalbuphine, butorphanol, buprenorphine) should not be given concurrently, as they may reduce the analgesic effect of oxymorphone and/or precipitate withdrawal.

Lab Effects/Interference:
- None known.

Special Considerations:
- Indicated for the relief of moderate-to-severe acute pain.
- Additive benefit when combined with acetaminophen or aspirin.
- Give smallest effective dose to prevent development of tolerance, physical dependency.
- Reduce dose in debilitated patients or patients receiving other CNS depressants.
- If required, naloxone HCl will reverse opiate toxicity (e.g., respiratory depression). However, it is important that acute withdrawal symptoms are prevented by giving only enough naloxone to reverse respiratory depression, and that this be continued for opioid drug half-life.
- Opioids cause peripheral vasodilation, which may cause hypotension; in addition, many cause the release of histamine, which can further intensify the hypotension. Oxymorphone has a lower likelihood of causing histamine release than other opioids.

Potential Toxicities/Side Effects and the Nursing Process

I.   SENSORY/PERCEPTUAL ALTERATIONS related to CNS DEPRESSION

Defining Characteristics: Adverse effects were < 10%: drowsiness, sedation, mood changes, euphoria, dysphoria, dizziness, confusion.

MANAGEMENT

Nursing Implications: Assess baseline neurologic status. Use cautiously in the elderly, and start with lowest dose and titrate up. Use cautiously, if at all, in patients who are debilitated, and patients with head injury, increased ICP, severe CNS depression, or acute alcoholism. Assess other concurrent medications. Use with caution in patients receiving other opioids, tranquilizers, hypnotics, MAO inhibitors, since increasing CNS depressant effects can occur. Monitor neurologic status closely. Instruct patient to avoid driving and operating machinery while taking the medicine, and to AVOID concurrent alcohol.

II.   ALTERATION IN OXYGENATION related to RESPIRATORY DEPRESSION

Defining Characteristics: Opiate agonists directly depress respiratory center in brain stem, causing decreased sensitivity and responsiveness to increased pCO_2. May also depress deep breathing and reflex to sigh. Tolerance to respiratory depressant effects occurs with chronic use.

Nursing Implications: Assess baseline pulmonary status, and periodically during drug use. Use cautiously in patients with bronchial asthma, COPD, respiratory depression, and monitor closely.

III.   ALTERATION IN ELIMINATION related to CONSTIPATION, ILEUS

Defining Characteristics: Opium agonists bind to opiate receptors in bowel, slowing peristalsis, leading to constipation. Untreated constipation may result in bowel perforation. Incidence of constipation in clinical trials was 4%.

Nursing Implications: Assess baseline elimination, fluid intake, diet, and exercise patterns. Instruct patient regarding prevention of constipation: goal is to move bowels at least every 2 days by increasing fluids to 3 L/day, following a diet high in fiber (beans, vegetables, fruit), and taking moderate exercise. Assess need for bowel softeners, bulk-forming laxatives, and osmotic cathartics, and discuss preparation with physician. Teach patient self-administration of medications.

IV.   ALTERATION IN NUTRITION, LESS THAN BODY REQUIREMENTS, related to GI TOXICITY

Defining Characteristics: Nausea, vomiting, dry mouth may occur. Gastric, biliary, and pancreatic secretions are decreased by opiate agonists; digestion is delayed. Biliary tract muscle tone is increased, and spasm of Oddi's sphincter may occur (morphine > meperidine > codeine).

Nursing Implications: Assess patient tolerance of GI side effects. Teach patient to report side effects. If nausea/vomiting occur, change to another opioid, or premedicate with antiemetic to prevent nausea/vomiting. Assess GI pain, biliary spasm, and consider alternative opioid.

V.   ALTERATION IN URINE ELIMINATION related to URINARY RETENTION

Defining Characteristics: Rarely, increased smooth muscle tone in urinary tract and spasm may occur. Bladder tone is increased, which may cause urgency. Vesical sphincter tone may be increased, leading to difficulty urinating. Increased risk of urinary retention in patients with prostatic hypertrophy or urethral stricture.

Nursing Implications: Assess baseline urinary elimination pattern. Teach patient to increase fluids to 3 L/day, and encourage voiding every 2–3 hours. Instruct patient to report problems with urination.

VI.   KNOWLEDGE DEFICIT related to DRUG ADMINISTRATION, POTENTIAL FOR TOLERANCE, AND DEPENDENCY

Defining Characteristics: Psychological dependence (addiction) occurs rarely in patients taking opioid agonists for cancer pain (< 1%). Physical dependence (precipitation of withdrawal symptoms) occurs with chronic use of the drug for the relief of chronic cancer pain. In addition, tolerance, or less analgesic effect over time with the same drug dose, occurs and requires increased dosage of drug.

Nursing Implications: Assess baseline knowledge of opioid analgesics, and attitude about their use for cancer pain management. Teach patient about proper self-administration, possible side effects, and self-care measures. Suggest patient maintain diary of pain intensity, precipitating and alleviating factors, drug dose and time taken, and relief. Teach patient to self-administer opioid agonists for relief of chronic cancer pain around-the-clock, not PRN, to prevent pain. Explain use of prescribed short-acting opioid for rescue or to manage breakthrough pain. Discuss with physician dose increase or change in frequency of administration if tolerance develops. Teach patient that withdrawal symptoms may occur if chronic, around-the-clock dosing is interrupted. Withdrawal (abstinence) symptoms that may be seen in the first 24 hours are restlessness, lacrimation, rhinorrhea, yawning, perspiration, gooseflesh, restless sleep, mydriasis. These are followed by twitching and leg spasms; severe aching of the back, abdomen, and legs; cramping in abdomen and legs; hot/cold flashes; insomnia; nausea/vomiting, diarrhea; severe sneezing; and increased heart rate, BP, T, which peak at 36–72 hours. Withdrawal syndrome can be prevented by administration of at least ¼ of previous opioid dose.

Drug: oxymorphone hydrochloride extended release (Opana ER)

Class: Opioid analgesic (opioid agonist).

Mechanism of Action: A semisynthetic opioid agonist, oxymorphone HCl resembles morphine but has milder action; binds to opiate receptors in CNS (limbic system, thalamus, striatum, hypothalamus, midbrain, spinal cord), altering pain perception at level of spinal cord and higher centers, as well as the emotional response to pain. Also suppresses cough reflex.

Metabolism: Absolute oral bioavailability is about 10%, and steady-state serum levels occurred after 3 days of multiple doses. Food increases absorption by 38% so it should not be taken with food. Drug is not bound to plasma proteins to any degree (10–12%), and is highly metabolized by the liver by reduction or conjugation with glucuronide into active and inactive metabolites. In studies of drug in extended formulation, bioavailability is higher in patients with hepatic or renal impairment, and plasma levels in the elderly were 40% higher than younger controls. Drug and metabolites are excreted in the urine and feces.

Indication: For the relief of moderate-to-severe pain in patients requiring continuous, around-the-clock opioid treatment for an extended period of time. Drug is not intended for PRN use, for pain in the immediate postoperative period if the pain is mild, or not expected to persist for an extended period of time. Drug is only indicated for the postoperative use if the patient is already receiving the drug prior to surgery or if the postoperative pain is expected to be moderate or severe and persist for an extended period of time. Physicians should individualize treatment, moving from parenteral to oral analgesics as appropriate.

Dosage/Range: *For moderate to severe pain:*
- Usual initial dose in opioid-naïve patients is 5 mg every 12 hours; thereafter, the dose should be individually titrated in increments of 5–10 mg q 12 hours every 3–7 days to an effective dose that provides adequate analgesia and minimal side effect.
- To convert a patient from oxymorphone immediate release (Opana), give half the total daily dose of Opana as Opana ER every 12 hours.
- If patient is receiving parenteral oxymorphone, given the 10% bioavailability, multiply the total parenteral dose of oxymorphone by 10 and administer in two equally divided doses.
- Beginning dose for elderly patient should be 5 mg PO q 4–6 hr PRN.
- Administer cautiously and in reduced doses in patients with creatinine clearance rates < 50 mL/min.
- Drug is contraindicated in patients with moderate and severe hepatic dysfunction; use cautiously and start at the lowest dose in patients with mild hepatic dysfunction, and titrate dose up.
- If patient is receiving CNS depressants (sedatives, hypnotics, general anesthetics, phenothiazines, tranquilizers, or alcohol) concurrently, start at one-third to one-half of the usual dose.
- If opioids are discontinued, drug should be gradually tapered to prevent withdrawal.
- If converting from other opioids to oxymorphone, use the following equianalgesic table (Opana ER package insert, June 2006); generally, start oxymorphone ER by giving half of the calculated total daily dose in two divided doses, every 12 hours; gradually titrate dose until pain is adequately controlled.

Opioid	Approximate Equivalent Dose (Oral)	Oral Conversion Ratio
Oxymorphone	10 mg	1
Hydrocodone	20 mg	0.5
Oxycodone	20 mg	0.5
Methadone	20 mg	0.5
Morphine	30 mg	0.333

Drug Preparation:
- Drug available in 5-, 10-, 20-, and 40-mg tablets.
- At home, teach patient to store oral doses in a safe place away from children and pets.

Drug Administration:
- Oral on an empty stomach (at least 1 hour before or 2 hours after food ingestion); drug must be swallowed whole and is not to be broken, chewed, dissolved, or crushed, as this would lead to a rapid release and absorption of a potentially fatal dose of oxymorphone.
- Teach patient that opioid analgesics may impair the mental and/or physical ability to drive and use machines, and to avoid these activities until the effect of the drug is known.

Drug Interactions:
- Alcohol, CNS depressants: Additive CNS depressant effects (hypotension, respiratory depression, profound sedation); alcohol must NOT be used concurrently as it may result in a potentially fatal overdose of oxymorphone.
- Mixed agonist/antagonist analgesics (pentazocine, nalbuphine, butorphanol, buprenorphine) should not be given concurrently, as they may reduce the analgesic effect of oxymorphone and/or precipitate withdrawal.
- Anticholinergic medications: If used concurrently, may increase risk of urinary retention, and/or severe constipation, which may lead to paralytic ileus.
- Cimetidine: Reported increase in CNS side effects (confusion, disorientation, respiratory depression, apnea, seizures).

Lab Effects/Interference:
- None known.

Special Considerations:
- Indicated for the relief of moderate to severe pain when a continuous, around-the-clock opioid analgesic is needed for an extended period of time.
- Drug is contraindicated in patients who (1) have acute pain and need a PRN analgesic, as this drug is intended only for extended analgesia; (2) are in immediate postoperative period (12–24 hours after surgery); (3) have hypersensitivity to morphine analogues, such as codeine; (4) have postop pain that is mild and not expected to persist; (5) have other contraindications to opioids (e.g., acute/severe bronchial asthmas, hypercarbia, paralytic ileus); (6) have moderate or severe hepatic impairment.
- Additive benefit when combined with acetaminophen or aspirin.
- Opioids cause peripheral vasodilation, which may cause hypotension; in addition, may cause the release of histamine, which can further intensify the hypotension. Oxymorphone has a lower likelihood of causing histamine release than other opioids.
- Give smallest effective dose to prevent development of tolerance, physical dependency.
- Reduce dose in debilitated patients or patients receiving other CNS depressants.
- If required, naloxone HCl will reverse opiate toxicity (e.g., respiratory depression). However, it is important that acute withdrawal symptoms are prevented by giving only enough naloxone to reverse respiratory depression, and that this be continued for opioid drug half-life.

MANAGEMENT

Potential Toxicities/Side Effects and the Nursing Process

I.   SENSORY/PERCEPTUAL ALTERATIONS related to CNS DEPRESSION

Defining Characteristics: Adverse effects were < 10% drowsiness, sedation, mood changes, euphoria, dysphoria, dizziness, confusion.

Nursing Implications: Assess baseline neurologic status. Use cautiously in the elderly, and start with lowest dose and titrate up. Use cautiously, if at all, in patients who are debilitated, and patients with head injury, increased ICP, severe CNS depression, or acute alcoholism. Assess other concurrent medications. Use with caution in patients receiving other opioids, tranquilizers, hypnotics, MAO inhibitors, since increasing CNS depressant effects can occur. Monitor neurologic status closely. Instruct patient to avoid driving and operating machinery while taking the medicine, and to AVOID concurrent alcohol.

II.   ALTERATION IN OXYGENATION related to RESPIRATORY DEPRESSION

Defining Characteristics: Opiate agonists directly depress respiratory center in brain stem, causing decreased sensitivity and responsiveness to increased pCO_2. May also depress deep breathing and reflex to sigh. Tolerance to respiratory depressant effects occurs with chronic use.

Nursing Implications: Assess baseline pulmonary status, and periodically during drug use. Use cautiously in patients with bronchial asthma, COPD, respiratory depression, and monitor closely.

III.   ALTERATION IN ELIMINATION related to CONSTIPATION, ILEUS

Defining Characteristics: Opium agonists bind to opiate receptors in bowel, slowing peristalsis, leading to constipation. Untreated constipation may result in bowel perforation. Incidence of constipation in clinical trials was 4%.

Nursing Implications: Assess baseline elimination, fluid intake, diet, and exercise patterns. Instruct patient regarding prevention of constipation: goal is to move bowels at least every 2 days by increasing fluids to 3 L/day, following a diet high in fiber (beans, vegetables, fruit), and taking moderate exercise. Assess need for bowel softeners, bulk-forming laxatives, and osmotic cathartics, and discuss preparation with physician. Teach patient self-administration of medications.

IV.   ALTERATION IN NUTRITION, LESS THAN BODY REQUIREMENTS, related to GI TOXICITY

Defining Characteristics: Nausea, vomiting, and dry mouth may occur. Gastric, biliary, and pancreatic secretions are decreased by opiate agonists; digestion is delayed. Biliary tract muscle tone is increased, and spasm of Oddi's sphincter may occur (morphine > meperidine > codeine).

Nursing Implications: Assess patient tolerance of GI side effects. Teach patient to report side effects. If nausea/vomiting occur, change to another opioid, or premedicate with antiemetic to prevent nausea/vomiting. Assess GI pain, biliary spasm, and consider alternative opioid.

V. ALTERATION IN URINE ELIMINATION related to URINARY RETENTION

Defining Characteristics: Rarely, increased smooth muscle tone in urinary tract and spasm may occur. Bladder tone is increased, which may cause urgency. Vesical sphincter tone may be increased, leading to difficulty urinating. Increased risk of urinary retention in patients with prostatic hypertrophy or urethral stricture.

Nursing Implications: Assess baseline urinary elimination pattern. Teach patient to increase fluids to 3 L/day, and encourage voiding every 2–3 hours. Instruct patient to report problems with urination.

VI. KNOWLEDGE DEFICIT related to DRUG ADMINISTRATION, POTENTIAL FOR TOLERANCE, AND DEPENDENCY

Defining Characteristics: Psychological dependence (addiction) occurs rarely in patients taking opioid agonists for cancer pain (< 1%). Physical dependence (precipitation of withdrawal symptoms) occurs with chronic use of the drug for the relief of chronic cancer pain. In addition, tolerance, or less analgesic effect over time with the same drug dose, occurs and requires increased dosage of the drug.

Nursing Implications: Assess baseline knowledge of opioid analgesics, and attitude about their use for cancer pain management. Teach patient about proper self-administration, possible side effects, and self-care measures. Suggest patient maintain diary of pain intensity, precipitating and alleviating factors, drug dose and time taken, and relief. Teach patient to self-administer opioid agonists for relief of chronic cancer pain around-the-clock, not PRN, to prevent pain. Explain use of prescribed short-acting opioid for rescue or to manage breakthrough pain. Discuss with physician dose increase or change in frequency of administration if tolerance develops. Teach patient that withdrawal symptoms may occur if chronic, around-the-clock dosing is interrupted. Withdrawal (abstinence) symptoms that may be seen in the first 24 hours are restlessness, lacrimation, rhinorrhea, yawning, perspiration, gooseflesh, restless sleep, mydriasis. These are followed by twitching and leg spasms; severe aching of the back, abdomen, and legs; cramping in abdomen and legs; hot/cold flashes; insomnia; nausea/vomiting, diarrhea; severe sneezing; and increased heart rate, BP, T, which peak at 36–72 hours. Withdrawal syndrome can be prevented by administration of at least ¼ of previous opioid dose.

MANAGEMENT

ADJUVANT AGENTS

Drug: modafinil (Provigil)

Class: Wakeful promoting agent, symptom management.

Mechanism of Action: Promotes wakefulness without generalized CNS stimulation by an unknown mechanism. Drug acts in selected brain areas thought to regulate normal wakefulness in the hypothalamus: increased neuronal activity in tuberomammillary nucleus (wake-promoting center), which then projects into cerebral cortex; decreases activity in the ventrolateral preoptic area (sleep promoting); does not affect suprachiasmatic nucleus (regulated circadian rhythm). Action is different from amphetamines.

Metabolism: Rapidly absorbed from the GI system with peak plasma concentrations in 2–4 hours. Taking with food delays absorption by 1 hour, but does not affect bioavailability. About 60% protein-bound (albumin), but at steady state does not displace protein binding of warfarin. Metabolized in the liver, with renal excretion of metabolites. Drug clearance may be reduced in the elderly. Drug is a reversible inhibitor of drug-metabolizing enzyme CYP2C19. Elimination half-life 15 hours.

Indication: To improve wakefulness in adult patients with excessive sleepiness associated with narcolepsy, obstructive sleep apnea, and shift work disorder.

Contraindication: Individuals with known hypersensitivity to modafinil.

Dosage/Range:
- 200 mg as a single dose in the morning for OSA and narcolepsy. For shift-work disorder, it should be taken approximately 1 hour prior to the start of the patient's work shift.
- 50% dose reduction in patients with severe liver impairment.
- Consider dose reduction in elderly patients with renal impairment and/or hepatic impairment.

Drug Preparation:
- Oral, available in 100-mg and 200-mg tablets.

Drug Administration:
- Oral, in the morning, with a glass of water.

Drug Interactions:
- Potentially, due to reversible inhibition of CYP2C19 enzyme system:
  - Diazepam, phenytoin, propranolol: drug may increase serum levels of these drugs; monitor closely for toxicity and dose reduce if needed.
  - Patients with CYP2C19 deficiency: increased serum levels of tricyclic antidepressants, SSRIs; monitor closely for toxicity and dose-reduce if needed.
  - Patients taking drug chronically may have increased induction of metabolism enzyme CYP3A4, resulting in theoretic decreased serum levels of steroidal contraceptives, cyclosporine, theophylline: monitor closely and dose-increase as necessary.
  - Methylphenidate: delays absorption of modafinil by 1 hour when given together.
  - Use in pregnancy or breastfeeding women only if benefit outweighs risk, as drug is potentially teratogenic.

Lab Effects/Interference:
* Unknown.

Special Considerations:
* Use with caution in patients who have had a recent MI or unstable angina.
* Use cautiously in patients with a history of psychosis.
* Women using steroidal contraceptives should use alternative or concomitant methods of contraception while taking the drug and for 1 month following discontinuation of the drug.
* Drug may produce psychoactive and euphoric effects, alterations in mood, perception, thinking, and feelings typical of other CNS stimulants. Drug binds to dopamine reuptake site and causes an increase in extracellular dopamine but no increase in dopamine release. Drug is reinforcing.
* Incidence of insomnia was 3% (placebo 1%).
* Drug is indicated to improve wakefulness in adult patients with excessive sleepiness associated with narcolepsy, obstructive sleep apnea, and shift work disorder. Drug does not cause withdrawal when discontinued.

Potential Toxicities/Side Effects (dose- and schedule-dependent) and the Nursing Process

I.   ALTERATION IN COMFORT related to HEADACHE, NAUSEA, DEPRESSION, NERVOUSNESS, RHINITIS

Defining Characteristics: In controlled clinical trials, headache occurred 10% more frequently than placebo, nausea occurred 9% more than placebo, depression 1% more than placebo, rhinitis 11% (placebo 8%), and nervousness 2% more than placebo. The few patients who discontinued the drug did so due to headache (1%), nausea (1%), depression (1%), and nervousness (1%).

Nursing Implications: Teach patient that these effects are rare but may occur. Teach symptom management strategies and if these do not work, to notify provider. If this occurs, discuss drug discontinuance versus more aggressive symptom management if drug is effective in reducing fatigue.

II.   ALTERATION IN NUTRITION, POTENTIAL, related to NAUSEA, DRY MOUTH, DIARRHEA, ANOREXIA, THIRST

Defining Characteristics: Although rare, these symptoms may occur: nausea occurs in 13% (placebo 4%), diarrhea 8% (placebo 4%), dry mouth 5% (placebo 1%), anorexia 5% (placebo 1%), and thirst 1%.

Nursing Implications: Perform baseline patient nutritional assessment, history of nausea and vomiting, bowel elimination pattern, oral assessment, and usual appetite. Teach patient these are rare, but to report these side effects so that they can be evaluated. Teach patient self-care measures, including dietary modification, local comfort measures as well as pharmacologic management as determined by the nurse/physician team. Teach patient to report symptoms that persist and do not respond to the planned therapy.

MANAGEMENT

Chapter 7
Nausea and Vomiting

Nausea and/or vomiting can occur commonly during the course of the cancer experience, related to disease, such as liver metastases, or to treatment, such as with chemotherapy or radiation to the abdomen. In addition, if acute nausea and vomiting are not prevented following cancer chemotherapy, delayed nausea and vomiting often follow. This problem continues. Nausea is often underreported and underassessed (Wickham, 2003). A replication of the Coates et al. (1983) study by de Boer-Dennert et al. (1997) showed that patients rated nausea as more distressing than vomiting since much has been done to prevent and control chemotherapy-induced vomiting. In 2003, Hofman et al. showed that fatigue was the top patient concern, followed by nausea, and then sleep disturbance. Complete control of chemotherapy-induced nausea and vomiting (CINV) has improved greatly with the advent of serotonin 5-hydroxytryptamine type 3 (5-HT$_3$) receptor antagonists used in combination with dexamethasone, bringing complete control to about 70% for patients receiving high-dose cisplatin. This new century of genomics has led to the understanding that the effectiveness of many drugs, and 5-HT$_3$ receptor antagonists in particular, is influenced by the recipient's genotype. This is because the liver's microenzyme system, cytochrome P450, and subtypes are determined by an individual's genotype. If the genotype is an ultrarapid metabolizer, the drug is rapidly cleared and eliminated from the body with decreased effect and undertreatment, while slow or poor metabolizers slowly clear the drug from the body with the risk of overtreatment. A study by Kaiser et al. (2002) evaluated whether patients who vomited after receiving their first cycle of emetogenic chemotherapy with 5-HT$_3$ receptor antagonist protection by either ondansetron or tropisetron were either ultrarapid or slow metabolizers of the P450 subsystem CYP2D6. They found that 30% had nausea and vomiting. The ultrarapid metabolizers had a higher incidence of nausea and vomiting, which was more marked for tropisetron- than ondansetron-receiving patients, and the poor metabolizers had higher serum concentrations and were protected. As we look to the future, not only do we see patients having genotypic evaluation of their tumors for an individualized prescription of anticancer treatment, but it will also include individual prescription of antiemetic dose based on genotype.

CHEMOTHERAPY-INDUCED NAUSEA AND VOMITING

CINV is primarily determined by the type of chemotherapy being administered, including the dose, schedule, and route of administration. For example, patients receiving cisplatin 100 mg/m^2 have been used as clinical subjects in antiemetic studies, as 100% of patients will vomit without antiemetic premedication. The risk of CINV can be predicted by the drug; in general, highly emetogenic drugs have a risk of 90% or higher of causing emesis, moderately emetogenic drugs have a risk of 30–90%, low-risk drugs have a risk of 10–30%, and minimal-risk drugs have < 10% risk. In combination therapy, however, the addition of one with another agent can increase the risk. For example, doxorubicin and cyclophosphamide are both moderately emetogenic, but when combined, the risk increases to highly emetogenic. It is much easier to prevent a patient's nausea and vomiting than it is to try to control it afterwards.

CINV appears mediated by multiple pathways. Nausea usually precedes vomiting, and it is controlled by cerebral and autonomic input, with common accompanying signs and symptoms of tachycardia, pallor, and diaphoresis. Vomiting involves the ejection of stomach contents and is a critical protection mechanism that helps the body excrete poisons. Most commonly, receptors in the gut enterochromaffin cells are stimulated and release serotonin. Serotonin binds to 5-HT$_3$ receptors, which stimulate the vagus nerve. This leads to stimulation of the chemotherapy trigger zone (CTZ) in the area postrema on the floor of the fourth ventricle, leading to activation of the vomiting center (VC) in the medulla, or to stimulation of the vomiting center directly. The 5-HT$_3$ receptor antagonists, such as granisetron and ondansetron, block the emetic impulses from reaching the CTZ and VC. In addition, other neuroreceptors in the CTZ can transmit impulses to the VC, such as dopamine, endorphin, and substance P. Other neuroreceptors that are found in the VC and vestibular center and that appear to have a role in emesis are acetylcholine, corticosteroid, histamine, cannabinoid, opiate, and neurokinin-1 (NK$_1$). Dopamine antagonists include phenothiazines and butyrophenones, and substance P/NK$_1$ receptor antagonist antiemetics include aprepitant and its IV formulation fosaprepitant, which has been FDA-approved, as well as the investigational agent casopitant. Emotional and cognitive factors can influence the occurrence and severity of CINV through a descending pathway from the cerebral cortex to the vomiting center, such as with anticipatory nausea and vomiting. Here a conditioned response is set up based on three to four past episodes of severe nausea and/or vomiting. The benzodiazepine lorazepam has been effective in preventing or lessening this effect through the drug's amnesiac qualities.

Dexamethasone has long been known to reduce the incidence of CINV, through a probable anti-inflammatory effect, leading to a closing of spaces in the gut wall that would permit leakage of emetogens into the bloodstream (Wickham, 2003). However, the exact mechanism is unknown.

Delayed nausea and vomiting are difficult to control but appear to be influenced by slowed gastric emptying. Thus, delayed antiemetic regimens usually include metoclopramide to speed gastric emptying, along with dexamethasone, and a phenothiazine or serotonin antagonist. It has become clear that substance P and its receptor NK$_1$, in the gut and brainstem, are important mediators in delayed CINV. The NK$_1$ receptors are located near the vomiting center, the "final common pathway" for emesis, so it is expected the NK$_1$ receptor antagonists will have broader application (Wickham, 2003). Although great strides have been made in the prevention and control of CINV, even with maximal pharmacologic blockade of known pathways, 100% protection is not obtained, so it is clear that other pathways await discovery. See Figure 7.1 for a review of pathophysiology of CINV. See Table 7.1 for the emetogenicity of cancer chemotherapy agents, and Table 7.2 for a schematic for antiemetic drugs and doses for CINV.

MANAGEMENT

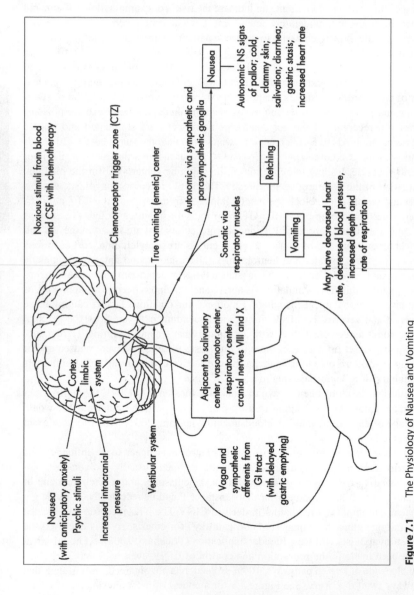

Figure 7.1 The Physiology of Nausea and Vomiting

Source: Reproduced from Burke MM, Wilkes GM, Ingwersen K, et al. *Chemotherapy and the Nursing Process.* Sudbury, MA: Jones and Bartlett Publishers; 1996. *Drawing adapted from original by Gail Wilkes.*

Table 7.1   Emetogenic Risk by Antineoplastic Agent

A. Intravenous Agents

High Risk > 90%	Moderate Risk 30–90%	Low Risk 10–30%	Minimal Risk < 10%
AC combination [doxorubicin or epirubicin plus cyclophosphamide] Carmustine > 250 mg/m²	Aldesleukin > 12–15 million IU/m² Amifostine > 300 mg/m² Arsenic trioxide Azacitidine Bendamustine Busulfan Carboplatin Carmustine ≤ 250 mg/m²	Ado-trastuzumab emtansine Aldesleukin ≤ 12 million IU/m² Amifostine ≤ 300 mg/m² Belinostat Blinatumomab Brentuximab vedotin	Alemtuzumab Asparaginase Bevacizumab Bleomycin Bortezomib Cetuximab Cladribine Cytarabine <100 mg/m²
Cisplatin	Clofarabine	Cabazitaxel Carfilzomib Cytarabine 100–200 mg/m²	Decitabine Denileukin diftitox Dexrazoxane
Cyclophosphamide > 1,500 mg/m²	Cyclophosphamide </ = 1,500 mg/m²	Docetaxel	Fludarabine
Dacarbazine		Doxorubicin (liposomal) Eribulin	Fludarabine Interferon alpha ≤ 5 million IU/m² Ipilimumab
	Cytarabine > 200 mg/m² Dactinomycin Daunorubicin	Etoposide	Methotrexate ≤ 50 mg/m² Nelarabine Nivolumab Obinutuzumab Ofatumumab Panitumumab
Doxorubicin >/ = 60 mg/m² Epirubicin > 90 mg/m²			Pegaspargase Peginterferon Pembrolizumab Pertuzumab
Ifosfamide ≥ 2 g/m² per dose	Doxorubicin </ = 60 mg/m²	5-Fluorouracil Floxuridine	Ramucirumab Rituximab Siltuximab Temsirolimus Trastuzumab
Mechlorethamine	Epirubicin ≤ 90 mg/m²	Gemcitabine Interferon alfa > 5 < 10 million IU/m² Ixabepilone	
		Methotrexate > 50 mg/m² < 250 mg/m²	Valrubicin

(continued)

MANAGEMENT

Table 7.1   *(Continued)*

A. Intravenous Agents

High Risk > 90%	Moderate Risk 30–90%	Low Risk 10–30%	Minimal Risk < 10%
Streptozocin	Idarubicin	Mitomycin C	Vinblastine Vincristine Vincristine liposomal

	Ifosfamide < 2 g/m²
	  per dose
	Interferon alfa
	  ≥ 10 million IU/m²
		Mitoxantrone
		Omacetaxine
			Vinorelbine

	Irinotecan	Paclitaxel Paclitaxel-albumin bound	
	Melphalan Methotrexate ≥ 250 mg/m²	Pemetrexed Pentostatin Pralatrexate	
	Oxaliplatin Temozolomide	Romidepsin Thiotepa Topotecan Ziv-aflibercept	

B. Oral Agents

Moderate to High	Minimal to Low
Altretamine Busulfan (≥ 4 mg/day) Ceritinib Crizotnib Cyclophosphamide (≥ 100 mg/m²/day)	Afatinib Axitinib Bexarotene Bosutinib Busulfan (< 4 mg/day) Cabozantinib Capecitabine
Estramustine Etoposide Lenvatinib Lomustine (single day)	Chlorambucil Cyclophosphamide (< 100 mg/m²/day) Dasatinib
Mitotane Olaparib	Dabrafenib Erlotinib Everolimus Fludarabine
Panobinostat Procarbazine	Gefitinib Hydroxyurea Ibrutinib Idelalisib Imatinib Lenalidomide

Table 7.1 *(Continued)*

B. Oral Agents

Moderate to High	Minimal to Low
Temozolomide (> 75 mg/m²/day)	Melphalan
	Mercaptopurine
	Methotrexate
	Nilotinib
	Palbociclib
	Pazopanib
	Pomalidomide
	Ponatinib
	Regorafenib
	Ruxolitinib
	Sonidegib
Vismodegib	Sorafenib
	Sunitinib
	Temozolomide (≤ 75 mg/m²/day)
	Thalidomide
	Thioguanine
	Topotecan
	Trametinib
	Tretinoin
	Vandetanib
	Vemurafenib
	Vorinostat

Key: High: > 90% risk of emesis; Moderate: 30–90% risk of emesis; low risk: 10–30% risk of emesis; minimal risk: < 10% risk of emesis.

Data from: National Comprehensive Cancer Network, Inc. NCCN Guidelines Version 1.2015 Antiemesis, available at http://www.nccn.org/professionals/physician_gls/pdf/antiemesis.pdf, accessed 9.18.14; Multinational Association of Supportive Care in Cancer (MASCC). MASCC/ESMO Antiemetic Guidelines 2011, available at http://www.mascc.org/assets/documents/mascc_guidelines_english_2013.pdf, accessed 8.22.13; Grunberg SM, Warr D, Gralla RJ et al. (2011). Evaluation of new antiemetic agents and definition of antineoplastic agent emetogenicity—state of the art. *Support Care Cancer* 19 Suppl 1: S43–47.

Table 7.2   Antiemetic Agents Used in CINV

Antiemetic Agent	IV Doses (Acute)	Oral Doses (Acute)	Oral (Delayed)
Serotonin Receptor Antagonists			
• Dolasetron		100 mg (acute)	100 mg qd delayed
• Granisetron	0.01 mg/kg or 1 mg IV	1–2 mg oral (acute)	1 mg bid delayed
• Ondansetron	0.15 mg/kg q 4 h × 4 h mg/kg q IV per dose	24 mg oral (acute)	8 mg bid delayed
• Palonosetron	0.25 mg IV day 1		

(continued)

Table 7.2   *(Continued)*

Antiemetic Agent	IV Doses (Acute)	Oral Doses (Acute)	Oral (Delayed)
Corticosteroids			
• Dexamethasone	20 mg	20 mg	8 mg bid days 2–4 highly emeto-genic, 4–8 mg bid days 2–3 moderately emetogenic
Substance P/NK1 Receptor Antagonist			
• Aprepitant		125 mg PO day 1 with dexamethasone 12 mg PO with serotonin receptor antagonist	80 mg day 2, 3 with dexamethasone 8 mg PO
• Fosaprepitant		150 mg IV day 1 with dexamethasone 12 mg PO with serotonin receptor antagonist	Dexamethasone 8 mg PO/IV day 2, then 8 mg PO/IV bid days 3,4
Substance P/NK1 Receptor Antagonist/Serotonin-3 Receptor Antagonist			
• Netupitant/ palonosetron		(A) Highly emetogenic: 300 mg/0.5 mg PO 1 h before chemo-therapy with dexa-methasone 12 mg PO given 30 min before chemotherapy on day 1	Dexamethasone 8 mg PO days 2–4
		(B) Anthracyclines/ cyclophosphamide not considered emetogenic: 300 mg/ 0.5 mg PO 1 h before chemotherapy with dexamethasone 12 mg PO given 30 min before chemo-therapy on day 1 only	
Dopamine Receptor Antagonists			
• Metoclopramide			20–40 mg bid–qid
• Prochlorperazine			15–30 mg LA spansules bid PRN
Benzodiazepines			
• Lorazepam	0.5–1 mg	1–2 mg	

Data from Wickham R. Nausea and Vomiting, chapter 11. In Yarbro CH, Goodman M, Frogge MH. Cancer Symptom Management, 3rd ed. Sudbury MA: Jones & Bartlett Publishers, 2003; NCCN (2015).

CINV can occur *acutely*, during the first 24 hours following chemotherapy administration; *delayed*, occurring after the first 24 hours; or *anticipatory*, occurring before chemotherapy, in anticipation of nausea and vomiting.

Factors that influence the occurrence and severity of CINV include gender (females have higher risk than males), age (younger people have a higher risk than older people), drug dose and emetogenic potential, combination of drugs versus single agent, history of alcohol intake (increased alcohol intake confers protection), and past experience with nausea and vomiting, such as air sickness, which increases risk.

Delayed nausea and vomiting are influenced by the effectiveness of control/prevention of the acute phase of CINV (Roila, 2000; Koeller et al., 2002), as well as the half-life of the antineoplastic agent. For example, the metabolites of cisplatin continue to be excreted for 3–5 days after drug administration, so protection must be provided for that period of time; for cyclophosphamide, the half-life is at least 12 hours, so only half the drug is excreted by that time, and full antiemetic protection must continue for at least 24 hours to prevent delayed nausea and vomiting. Common delayed regimens begin on days 2–4 for highly emetogenic regimens (aprepitant 80 mg PO daily × 2 plus dexamethasone 8 mg PO daily × 3; or a serotonin antagonist such as granisetron 1 mg PO bid or ondansetron 8 mg PO twice daily, plus dexamethasone 8 mg PO daily × 3; or metoclopramide 30–40 mg PO twice daily plus dexamethasone 8 mg PO twice daily × 3 days). For moderately emetogenic regimens, delayed emesis regimens are given on days 2–3 and include a serotonin antagonist, or dexamethasone, or metoclopramide alone or in combination (Grunberg and Siebel, 2007).

Insofar as CINV involves multiple pathways, multiple antiemetics to block these pathways are needed, especially for aggressive antiemesis. Antiemetics must be administered to prevent nausea and vomiting, so the drug(s) should be administered prior to chemotherapy administration in order to block stimulation of the pathways. Oral antiemetics should be administered 30–40 minutes before treatment; rectal (PR) preparations 60 minutes before; intramuscular (IM) injections 20–30 minutes before; and intravenous bolus (IVB) 10–30 minutes prior to chemotherapy (Barton-Burke et al., 2001).

In order to better identify treatment approaches for CINV, American Society for Clinical Oncology (ASCO) published "Recommendations for the Use of Antiemetics: Evidence-Based Clinical Practice Guidelines" and stated that "at equivalent doses, serotonin-receptor antagonists have equivalent safety and efficacy and can be used interchangeably based on convenience, availability, and cost" (Gralla et al., 1999). They listed four agents in this class; three of these agents are commercially available in the United States: dolasetron, granisetron, and ondansetron. This does not include palonosetron, which has a long half-life, and which is effective in preventing delayed as well as acute nausea/vomiting. Finally, key members of the Supportive Care in Cancer organization have developed consensus guidelines for the study and prescription of antiemetic care (Koeller et al., 2002).

In addition, the National Community Network (NCCN, 2015) has developed supportive care guidelines for antiemesis, which identify the following principles of emesis control in patients with cancer:

- The goal is the prevention of nausea/vomiting.
- Patients have risk of nausea and vomiting for at least 3 days when receiving highly emetogenic chemotherapy and 2 days for moderately emetogenic chemotherapy after the last dose. They should receive antiemetic protection for the full period of risk.

- Oral and IV antiemetics have equivalent efficacy.
- Use the lowest fully efficacious dose before chemotherapy or radiation therapy.
- Choose antiemetic(s) based on emetogenicity of the therapy, prior experience with antiemetics, patient factors, and antiemetic(s) potential side effect(s).
- Consider an H_2 blocker or proton pump inhibitor to prevent dyspepsia, which can be mistaken for nausea.
- Ensure that other potential causes of emesis in patients with cancer are not overlooked:
  - Partial or complete bowel obstruction.
  - Vestibular dysfunction.
  - Brain metastases.
  - Electrolyte imbalance (hypercalcemia, hyperglycemia, hyponatremia).
  - Uremia.
  - Concomitant drug treatment, including opiates.
  - Gastroparesis (tumor, chemotherapy such as vincristine) or other causes, such as diabetes.
  - Psychophysiologic causes (anxiety, anticipatory nausea/vomiting).
- For multi-drug regimens, select antiemetic therapy based on drug with highest emetic risk.
- Lifestyle measures may help to alleviate nausea/vomiting such as eating small, frequent meals, controlling amount of food consumed, and eating foods at room temperature.

Aprepitant (Emend) is the first substance P/NK_1 receptor antagonist indicated for the prevention of acute and delayed nausea and vomiting related to highly emetogenic chemotherapy, in combination with other antiemetic agents. First identified in 1931 and reaching notoriety in 1950 when linked with pain transmission, substance P has continued to be prominent in the symptom management field. Substance P is a member of the tachykinin family of peptides and, together with NK_1 receptors, is found in high concentrations in the chemotherapy trigger zone (CTZ, in the medulla oblongata) and the dorsal horn of the spinal cord (posterior column of gray matter), as well as the gut. Substance P is released from peripheral sensory as well as central sensory nerve endings and plays a key role in transmitting noxious sensory information to the brain. Substance P initiates its activity by binding to the NK_1 receptor, a site distinctly different from the serotonin-mediated $5\text{-}HT_3$ site (Hesketh, 2001).

In an effort to design a serotonin antagonist with a long half-life and activity against delayed chemotherapy-induced nausea and vomiting, palonosetron (Aloxi) was created and approved for the prevention of chemotherapy-induced nausea and vomiting. More recently, a hybrid composed of both a serotonin-receptor antagonist (palonosetron) and a substance P/NK_1 receptor antagonist (netupitant) was FDA approved for the prevention of acute and delayed nausea and vomiting associated with initial and repeat courses of cancer chemotherapy.

Given these advances, complete protection from chemotherapy-induced nausea and vomiting should be the standard (Hesketh, 2008); however, there continues to be a minority of patients who have significant nausea and vomiting. The NCCN (v1.2015) recommends the following plan for the prevention of IV chemotherapy-induced emesis:

Highly emetogenic chemotherapy:
- Start prior to chemotherapy, using a serotonin ($5\text{-}HT_3$) antagonist, steroid, $\pm$ NK_1 antagonist.

- **DAY 1:**
  - *Serotonin-receptor antagonist:* ondansetron 16–24 mg PO or 8–16* mg IV, day 1; OR granisetron 2 mg PO daily or 1 mg PO bid or 0.01 mg/kg (max 1 mg) IV day 1, or transdermal patch as 3.1 mg/24 h patch (containing 34.3 mg granisetron total dose) applied 24–48 hours prior to first dose of chemotherapy (maximum duration of patch is 7 days); OR dolasetron 100 mg PO; OR palonosetron 0.25 mg IV day 1 (preferred); WITH
  - *Steroid:* dexamethasone 12 mg PO or IV day 1; 8 mg PO or IV daily on days 2–4 with aprepitant 125 mg PO; OR dexamethasone 12 mg PO or IV day 1, 8 mg PO day 2, then 8 mg PO bid days 3 and 4 with fosprepitant 150 mg day 1, AND
  - *Neurokinin-1 antagonist:* aprepitant 125 mg PO day 1, 80 mg PO days 2–3; OR fosprepitant 150 mg IV day 1 only, with or without lorazepam 0.5–2mg PO or IV or sublingual either every 4 hours or every 6 hours days 1–4, ± H$_2$ blocker or proton pump inhibitor (PPI); OR
  - *Netupitant-containing regimen:* Netupitant 300 mg/palonosetron 0.5 mg PO once, with dexamethasone 12 mg PO once; OR
  - *Olanzapine-containing regimen:* olanzapine 10 mg PO days 1–4, palonosetron 0.25 mg IV day 1, dexamethasone 20 mg IV day 1, with or without lorazepam and with or without H$_2$ blocker or proton pump inhibitor (PPI).

Moderately emetogenic chemotherapy:
- Start before chemotherapy: serotonin 5-HT$_3$ antagonist, steroid, with/without NK$_1$ antagonist day 1; days 2 and 3: serotonin (5-HT$_3$) antagonist OR steroid monotherapy or NK$_1$ antagonist ± steroid.
  - **DAY 1:**
    - *Serotonin-receptor antagonist:* ondansetron 16–24 mg PO or 8–16* mg IV day 1; OR granisetron 2 mg PO or 1 mg PO bid or 0.01 mg/kg (max 1 mg) IV day 1, or transdermal patch as 3.1 mg/24 patch (containing 34.3 mg granisetron/day) applied approximately 24–48 hours prior to first dose of chemotherapy (maximum duration of patch is 7 days); OR dolasetron 100 mg PO; OR palonosetron 0.25 mg IV day 1 (preferred); PLUS
    - *Steroid:* dexamethasone 12 mg PO or IV day 1; WITH OR WITHOUT
    - *NK1 antagonist:* aprepitant 125 mg PO or fosaprepitant 150 mg IV day 1; WITH OR WITHOUT
    - Lorazepam 0.5–2 mg PO or IV or SL every 6 hours on days 1–4, as needed WITH OR WITHOUT
    - H$_2$ blocker or proton pump inhibitor; OR
    - *Netupitant-containing regimen*: Netupitant 300 mg/palonosetron 0.5 mg PO once, with dexamethasone 12 mg PO once; OR
    - *Olanzapine-containing regimen:* Day 1: olanzapine 10 mg PO, palonosetron 0.25 mg IV, dexamethasone 20 mg IV, with or without lorazepam and with or without H$_2$ blocker or proton pump inhibitor (PPI).
  - **DAYS 2–3:**
    - *Serotonin-receptor antagonist:* monotherapy unless palonsetron used on day 1: dolasetron 100 mg PO daily; OR granisetron 1–2 mg PO daily or 1 mg PO bid, or

0.01 mg/kg IV (maximum 1 mg); OR ondansetron 8 mg PO bid or 16 mg PO daily or 8–16 mg IV, with or without Lorazepam 0.5–2 mg PO or IV or SL either every 4 or 6 hours on days 1–4, as needed ±.
- H$_2$ blocker or proton pump inhibitor, OR
- *Steroid monotherapy:* dexamethasone 8 mg, OR
- *NK1 antagonist:* ± steroid if NK$_1$ antagonist used on day 1: aprepitant used day 1: aprepitant 80 mg PO ± dexamethasone 8 mg PO or IV daily; OR fosaprepitant used day 1: ± dexamethasone 8 mg PO or IV daily; OR olanzapine 10 mg PO days 2–4 (if given day 1), with or without lorazepam and with or without H$_2$ blocker or proton pump inhibitor (PPI).
- *Olanzapine:* olanzapine 10 mg PO days 2–3

Low emetogenic chemotherapy:
- Start antiemesis before chemotherapy; repeat daily for multiday doses of chemotherapy.
  - Dexamethasone 12 mg PO or IV daily; OR metoclopramide 10–40 mg PO or IV, then either every 4 or 6 hours PRN or prochlorperazine 10 mg PO or IV, then every 4 or 6 hours (maximum 40 mg a day); OR serotonin-receptor antagonist dolasetron 100 mg PO PRN daily; OR granisetron 2 mg PO daily or 1 mg PO PRN bid; OR ondansetron 16–24 mg PO PRN daily; with or without lorazepam 0.5–2 mg every 6 hours PRN with or without H2 blocker or proton pump inhibitor.

Minimal emetogenic chemotherapy:
- No routine prophylaxis.
- If nausea or emesis within 24 hours, consider using drugs in low emetogenicity category.

Oral chemotherapy:
High to moderate emetic risk:
- Start before chemotherapy and continue daily.
- Serotonin receptor antagonist: dolasetron 100 mg PO daily or granisetron 2 mg PO daily or 1 mg PO bid or ondansetron 16–24 mg PO (total dose) daily with or without lorazepam 0.5–2 mg PO or sublingual every 6 hours PRN with or without H2 blocker or proton pump inhibitor.

Low to minimal emetic risk: PRN recommended; if nausea/vomiting.
- Start before chemotherapy and continue daily.
  - Metoclopramide 10-40 mg PO and then every 4 or every 6 hours PRN or Prochlorperazine 10 mg PO or IV and then every 6 hours PRN (maximum 40 mg/ day) or haloperidol 1–2 mg PO every 4 hours or every 6 hours PRN or a serotonin receptor antagonist [dolasetron 100 mg PO daily or granisetron 2 mg PO daily or 1 mg PO bid or ondansetron 16–24 mg PO daily] with or without lorazepam 0.5–2 mg PO or sublingual every 6 hours PRN with or without H2 blocker or proton pump inhibitor.

Rescue or breakthrough emesis management (some patients may require one or several agents utilizing differing mechanisms of action):
- Add an additional agent from a different drug class to the current regimen.
- Atypical antipsychotic: olanzapine 10 mg PO daily × 3 days.
- Benzodiazepine: lorazepam 0.5–2.0 mg PO every 4 or 6 hours PO or IV.

- Phenothiazine: prochlorperazine (25 mg supp PR every 12 hours or 10 mg PO or IV every 4 or 6 hours); OR promethazine 12.5–25 mg PO or IV via central line only every 4 hours.
- Other: metoclopramide 10–40 mg PO or IV, either every 4 or 6 hours using diphenhydramine 25–50 mg PO, or IV every 4 or 6 hours to manage dystonic reactions; OR haloperidol 0.5–2mg PO or IV every 4–6 hours; OR scopalamine transdermal patch every 72 hours. Serotonin-receptor antagonist (different from drug previously used), such as ondansetron 16 mg PO or IV daily; OR granisetron 1–2 mg PO daily or 1 mg PO bid or 0.01 mg/kg (maximum 1 mg IV); OR dolasetron 100 mg PO daily.
- Cannabinoid: dronabinol 5–10 mg PO every 3 or 6 hours; OR Nabilone 1–2 mg PO bid.
- Steroid: dexamethasone 12 mg PO or IV daily.
- If the patient has dyspepsia, consider antacid therapy (H_2 blocker or proton pump inhibitor).
- Ensure adequate hydration or fluid repletion, along with correction of any electrolyte imbalance.
- FOR THE NEXT CYCLE, consider changing the regimen (both day 1 and postchemotherapy regimen) to higher level of primary antiemetic treatment.
- Monitor for dystonic reactions when phenothiazines are used, and administer diphenhydramine as needed to resolve reaction.
- Olanzapine has been shown to be superior to metoclopramide for the treatment of breakthrough emesis in patients receiving highly emetogenic chemotherapy who had also received the highest level of primary antiemesis; dose was olanzapine 10 mg PO × 3 days (Navari et al., 2012).
- Consider anxiolytic therapy to prevent anticipatory emesis (e.g., alprazolam 0.5–1 mg or lorazepam 0.5–2 mg PO) beginning on the night before treatment and then repeated the next day 1–2 hours before chemotherapy begins.
- Consider the transdermal antiemetic route for managing multiday emetogenic chemotherapy regimens.

RADIATION-INDUCED NAUSEA AND VOMITING

Radiation therapy to the gastrointestinal tract usually causes nausea and vomiting. Highest risk (90%) is when total body irradiation (TBI) or external beam radiation is administered to the upper or total abdomen or upper hemithorax, with emesis occurring within 10–15 minutes with TBI or hemithorax treatment, and within 1–2 hours when external beam therapy is administered to the upper abdomen (Wickham, 2003). Antiemesis is effective using serotonin antagonists with or without dexamethasone, which should be administered at a time before RT when the drug can be absorbed (NCCN Antiemesis Guidelines, 2013). NCCN (2013) recommends to protect against upper abdomen RT: granisetron 2 mg PO daily, or ondansetron 8 mg PO bid with or without dexamethasone 4 mg PO daily prior to RT. Recommended prophylaxis for TBI is ondansetron 8 mg PO bid–tid or granisetron 2 mg PO daily with or without dexamethasone 4 mg PO daily. For breakthrough nausea and vomiting from RT to other sites, use agents described above for breakthrough antiemesis. Antiemesis for patients receiving combined chemotherapy and RT, refer to recommended antiemetics for the chemotherapy agent.

MANAGEMENT

DISEASE-INDUCED NAUSEA AND VOMITING

Site of advanced disease is a strong predictor of the risk for nausea and vomiting. Metastases to the liver are often associated with difficult-to-control nausea and vomiting. Pressure from ascites or obstruction of a hollow viscus, as with advanced ovarian cancer, can also lead to intractable nausea and vomiting. A factor here, along with advanced pancreatic cancer, may be delayed gastric emptying, or gastric outlet syndrome. Increased intracranial pressure (ICP) from a malignant brain tumor often causes nausea and vomiting. Other conditions related to disease that cause nausea and vomiting include hypercalcemia, hyperglycemia, electrolyte imbalance, and severe constipation. Strategies to relieve nausea and vomiting in these circumstances vary with the cause; they range from aggressive antiemesis to correction of delayed gastric emptying (metoclopramide) or the obstruction (stent if possible, or if not, release of gastric contents via a gastrostomy tube), to correction of electrolyte abnormalities.

Currently, antiemetics are available as oral, intravenous, rectal suppositories, transdermal, and transmucosal.

In summary then, nausea and/or vomiting can arise from treatment or complications of disease. There are a variety of agents useful for blocking a number of neurotransmitter pathways to prevent or control nausea and vomiting in cancer. Specifically, it is known that chemotherapy stimulates nausea and vomiting via multiple pathways and often, therefore, multiple drugs are necessary for the prevention of nausea and vomiting associated with aggressive chemotherapy.

References

Barton-Burke M, Wilkes G, Berg D., et al. *Cancer Chemotherapy: A Nursing Process Approach,* 3rd ed., Sudbury, MA, Jones and Bartlett Publishers 2001.

Coates A, Abraham S, Kaye SB., et al. On the Receiving End—Patient Perception of the Side-effects of Cancer Chemotherapy. *Eur J Cancer Clin Oncol* 1983; 19 203–208.

Cotanch PM, Stum S. Progressive Muscle Relaxation as Antiemetic Therapy for Cancer Patients. *Oncol Nurs Forum* 1987; 14(1) 33–37.

de Boer-Dennert M, de Wit R, Schmitz PIM., et al. Patient Perceptions of the Side-effects of Chemotherapy: The Influence of 5HT₃ Antagonists. *Br J Cancer* 1997; 76 1055–1061.

Eisai Inc. Akynzeo (netupitant/palonosetron) [package insert]. Woodcliff Lake, NJ, December 2014.

Eisai Inc. Aloxi (palonostron) [package insert]. Woodcliff Lake, NJ. May 2014.

Food and Drug Administration, et al. 2012; FDA Drug Safety Communication: New information regarding QT prolongation with ondansetron Zofran_http://www.fda.gov/Drugs/DrugSafety/ucm310190.htm, accessed July 3, 2012.

Grunberg SM, Aziz Z, Shaharyar A., et al. Phase III Results of a Novel Neurokinin-1 (NK₁) Receptor Antagonist, Casopitant: Single Oral and 3-Day Oral Dosing Regimens for Chemotherapy-induced Nausea and Vomiting (CINV) in Patients (Pts) Receiving Moderately Emetogenic Chemotherapy (MEC). *J Clin Oncol* 26: 2008 (May 20 suppl: abstract #9540).

Grunberg SM, Gabrial NY, Clark G. Phase III Trial of Transdermal Granisetron Patch (Sancuso) Compared With Oral Granisetron in the Management of Chemotherapy-Induced Nausea and Vomiting (CINV). Multinational Association of Supportive Care (MASCC) 20th Annual Symposium, abstract #18, 2007.

Grunberg SM, Siebel M. Management of Nausea and Vomiting. Pazdur R, Coia LR, Hoskins WJ, Wagman LD (eds). *Cancer Management: A Multidisciplinary Approach,* 10th ed. Lawrence, KS, CMP Healthcare Media LLC; 2007.

Herrstedt J, Grunberg SM, Rolski J, et al. Phase III Results for the Novel Neurokinin-1 (NK$_1$) Receptor Antagonist, Casopitant: Single Oral Dosing Regimen for Chemotherapy-induced Nausea and Vomiting (CINV) in Patients (Pts) Receiving Highly Emetogenic Chemotherapy (HEC). *J Clin Oncol* 26 2008 (May 20 suppl: Abstract #9549).

Hesketh PJ. Chemotherapy-induced Nausea and Vomiting. *N Engl J Med* 2008; 358 2482–2494.

Hesketh PJ. Potential Role of the NK1 Receptor Antagonists in Chemotherapy-induced Nausea and Vomiting. *Supportive Care Cancer* 2001; 9 350–354.

Hesketh PJ, Beck TM, Uhlenhopp M, et al. Adjusting the Dose of Intravenous Ondansetron plus Dexamethasone to the Emetogenic Potential of the Chemotherapy Regimen. *J Clin Oncol* 1995; 13(8) 2117–2122.

Hesketh P, Rossi G, Rizzi G, et al. Efficacy and safety of NEPA, an oral combination of netupitant and palonosetron, for prevention of chemotherapy-induced nausea and vomiting following highly emetogenic chemotherapy: a randomized dose ranging pivotal study. *Ann Oncol* 2014; 35(7) 1340–1346.

Hofman M, Morrow GR, Roscoe JA, et al. 2004; Cancer patients' expectations of experiencing treatment-related side effects. *Cancer* 101 (4) 851–857.

Kaiser R, Sezer O, Papies A, et al. Patient-tailored Antiemetic Treatment with 5-hydroxytryptamine Type 3 Receptor Antagonists According to Cytochrome P-450 Genotypes. *J Clin Oncol* 2002; 20(12) 2805–2811.

Meda Pharmaceuticals Inc. Cesamet package insert (nabilone) [package insert]. Somerset, NJ, February 2010.

National Comprehensive Cancer Network. *Clinical Practice Guideline Antiemesis*, version 2.2015; http://www.nccn.org. Accessed June 14, 2015.

Navari RM, Nagy CK, Gray SE, et al. 2012; The use of olanzapine versus metoclopramide for the treatment of breakthrough chemotherapy-induced nausea and vomiting (CINV) in patients receiving highly emetogenic chemotherapy. *J Clin Oncol 30, 2012* (suppl; abstr 9064).

Sylvester RK, Etzell R, Levitt R, et al. Comparison of 16-mg vs 32-mg Ondansetron and Dexamethasone in Patients Receiving Cisplatin. *Proc Am Soc Clin Oncol* 1996; 15 547 (abstract 1781).

VanBelles, Cocquyt V, DeSmet M, et al. Comparison of a Neurokinin-1 Antagonist L-758, 298 to Ondansetron in the Prevention of Cisplatin-induced Emesis. *Proc Am Soc Clin Oncol* 1998; 17 51a (abstract 198).

Wickham R. Nausea and Vomiting, *Chapter 11*. Yarbro CH, Frogge MH, Goodman M. *Cancer Symptom Management,* 3rd ed. Sudbury, MA: Jones and Bartlett Publishers 2003.

Drug: aprepitant (Emend oral formulation)

Class: Substance P/neurokinin-1 (NK$_1$) receptor antagonist. For IV preparation, see fosaprepitant dimeglumine.

Mechanism of Action: Selective substance P/neurokinin-1 (NK$_1$) receptor antagonist (high affinity). Drug has no affinity for 5-HT$_3$, dopamine, or corticosteroid receptors. Drug crosses the blood–brain barrier to saturate brain NK$_1$ receptors. Drug increases the activity of serotonin-receptor antagonists and corticosteroids in preventing acute nausea and vomiting, and inhibits both acute and delayed nausea and vomiting related to cisplatin chemotherapy.

Metabolism: Drug is well absorbed after oral administration with 60–65% bioavailability. Drug is 95% bound to plasma proteins and crosses the placenta and blood–brain barrier. Aprepitant undergoes extensive metabolism in the liver by the P450 hepatic microenzyme system, specifically CYP3A4, and minor metabolism by CYP1A2 and CYP2C19. Seven inactive metabolites have been found in the plasma. The drug is excreted in the urine (57%) and the feces (45%). The terminal half-life of the drug is 9–13 hours.

Indication: (1) In combination with other antiemetic agents, for the prevention of (a) acute and delayed nausea and vomiting associated with initial and repeat courses of highly emetogenic cancer chemotherapy, including high-dose cisplatin; (b) nausea and vomiting associated with initial and repeat courses of moderately emetogenic cancer chemotherapy; and (2) for the prevention of postoperative nausea and vomiting (POVN). CIVN is chemotherapy-induced nausea and vomiting.

Dosage/Range:
- 3-day regimen for CINV: Day 1, 125 mg PO 1 hour before chemotherapy, together with a serotonin (HT_3) receptor antagonist and dexamethasone (dose reduced to 12 mg day 1, 8 mg days 2 and 3); days 2 and 3, 80 mg PO each morning. Fosaprepitant dimeglumine for injection may be substituted for oral aprepitant on day 1 only as part of the regimen.
- PONV: 40 mg within 3 hours prior to induction of anesthesia.

Drug Preparation:
- Oral drug supplied as (1) 80-mg capsules in bottle of 30 capsules or in unit-dose packs of 5 capsules; (2) 125-mg tablets in bottle of 30 capsules or in unit-dose packs of 5 capsules; and (3) trifold pack containing one 125-mg capsule and two 80-mg capsules. Capsules should be stored at room temperature.
- Day 1: give 125-mg capsule PO 1 hour before chemotherapy, and then the 80-mg capsule in the morning on days 2 and 3. Give with or without food.

Drug Interactions:
- Drugs that inhibit the CYP3A4 isoenzyme system can increase the serum level of aprepitant: ketoconazole, itraconazole, nefazodone, clarithromycin, ritonavir, nelfinavir; diltiazem (twofold increase in aprepitant plasma concentration), so coadminister cautiously and monitor for aprepitant toxicity or dose-reduce aprepitant.
- Drugs that strongly induce CYP3A4 isoenzyme system can lower aprepitant serum levels: rifampin, carbamazepine, phenytoin; assess for efficacy of aprepitant and need for drug dose increase.
- Drug is a moderate inhibitor of P450 hepatic isoenzyme system CYP3A4, so the plasma concentrations of the following drugs can theoretically be increased if coadministered:
  - Chemotherapy agents are docetaxel, paclitaxel, etoposide, irinotecan, ifosfamide, imatinib, vinorelbine, vinblastine, and vincristine.
  - Dexamethasone (dose-reduce dexamethasone by 50%).
  - Methylprednisolone (dose-reduce 25% if IV, 50% if PO).
  - Benzodiazepines: midazolam, lorazepam, alprazolam, triazolam.
- Drug is an inducer of CYP2C9, and the plasma concentrations of the following drugs can theoretically be decreased if coadministered:

- Warfarin (34% decrease with 14% decrease in INR; closely monitor INR 7–10 days after 3-day antiemetic regimen, and modify warfarin dose as needed).
- Phenytoin, tolbutamide, oral contraceptives.

Lab Effects/Interference:
- Decreased INR if patient taking warfarin.

Special Considerations:
- Contraindications: do not give concomitantly with pimozide, terfenadine, astemizole, or cisapride; do not give if hypersensitive to aprepitant or any of its components; use cautiously if at all during pregnancy or breastfeeding; no studies have been done in patients with severe liver failure.
- Significant drug interactions (see above).
- Drug is well-tolerated with few side effects.

Potential Toxicities/Side Effects and the Nursing Process

I. ALTERATION IN NUTRITION, LESS THAN BODY REQUIREMENTS, related to CONSTIPATION, DIARRHEA, NAUSEA, ANOREXIA, HICCUPS

Defining Characteristics: Gastrointestinal side effects may occur but are infrequent with the following incidences: constipation (10.3%), diarrhea (10.3%), nausea (12.7%), vomiting (7.5%), hiccups (10.8%), and anorexia (10.1%).

Nursing Implications: Teach patient that these side effects may occur, and to report them if unrelieved by symptom-management measures. Teach patient self-care measures to manage and prevent symptoms.

II. ALTERATION IN COMFORT related to ASTHENIA/FATIGUE, ABDOMINAL PAIN, HEADACHE

Defining Characteristics: Asthenia/fatigue occurred in 17.8% of patients; abdominal pain 4.6%; headache 8.5%.

Nursing Implications: Teach patient that these side effects may occur and measures to minimize their occurrence. Teach energy-conserving measures, management of abdominal pain and headache. Teach patient to report signs and symptoms that worsen or are unrelieved.

Drug: dexamethasone (Decadron)

Class: Glucocorticoid steroid.

Mechanism of Action: May inhibit prostaglandin release by stabilizing lysosomal membranes, thereby interrupting hypothalamic prostaglandin release and subsequent stimulation of nausea and vomiting. Causes demargination of marginated WBCs, with leukocytosis. Decreases inflammation by suppression of migration of polymorphonuclear leukocytes.

Metabolism: Half-life is 3–4 hours; oral dose peaks in 1–2 hours, with duration of 2 days; IM peaks in 8 hours, with duration of 6 days.

Indication: For management of (1) endocrine disorders (e.g., primary or secondary adrenocortical insufficiency); (2) rheumatic disorders (short-term); (3) collagen diseases; (4) dermatologic diseases; (5) allergic states; (6) ophthalmic diseases; (7) GI diseases (e.g., ulcerative colitis); (8) respiratory diseases; (9) hematologic disorders; (10) neoplastic diseases; (11) edematous states; (12) other diseases or treatments.

Dosage/Range:
Adult (as antiemetic):
- *Oral:* 4 mg q 4 h × four doses beginning 1–8 hours before chemotherapy.
- *IV:* 10–20 mg prior to chemotherapy, then q 4–6 h.

Drug Preparation:
- *Oral:* administer with food or milk.
- *IV:* may be given with H_2-antagonist (e.g., ranitidine) to prevent gastric irritation.

Drug Interactions:
- Indomethacin, aspirin: increased GI irritation and bleeding; avoid concurrent administration.
- Barbiturates, phenytoin, rifampin: decreased dexamethasone effect; increase dose as needed.

Lab Effects/Interference:
- Increased WBC may occur due to demargination.
- Increased serum glucose level.
- May cause decreased K.

Special Considerations:
- Contraindicated in patients with psychosis, hypersensitivity, idiopathic thrombocytopenia, acute glomerulonephritis, amebiasis, fungal infections, and nonasthmatic bronchial disease.
- Indicated in the management of inflammation, allergies, neoplasms, cerebral edema, and in combination antiemetic therapy.
- If patient received dexamethasone chronically, drug must be tapered to prevent withdrawal (i.e., signs/symptoms of adrenal insufficiency, rebound weakness, arthralgia, fever, dizziness, orthostatic hypotension, dyspnea, hypoglycemia).

Potential Toxicities/Side Effects and the Nursing Process

I.   ALTERATION IN NUTRITION, LESS THAN BODY REQUIREMENTS, related to GI TOXICITY

Defining Characteristics: Increased appetite, abdominal distension, pancreatitis, GI hemorrhage; diarrhea may occur.

Nursing Implications: Assess baseline nutritional status and monitor throughout therapy. Discuss symptomatic management of diarrhea, abdominal distension, and increased appetite with patient. Assess stool for occult blood and notify physician if positive. Monitor Hgb and HCT values.

II. ALTERATIONS IN SENSORY/PERCEPTUAL PATTERNS related to CHANGES IN MOOD, VASODILATION, CATARACTS

Defining Characteristics: Euphoria, insomnia, depression, flushing, sweating, headache, mood changes, and cataracts may occur.

Nursing Implications: Assess baseline mental status and monitor during therapy. Discuss symptomatic management or drug discontinuance, based on severity, with physician.

III. ALTERATION IN CARDIAC OUTPUT related to CHF

Defining Characteristics: Congestive heart failure (CHF), hypertension, fluid retention, and edema may occur.

Nursing Implications: Assess baseline vital signs (VS), and monitor during therapy. Discuss hypertension with physician, monitor daily weights, and assess for edema.

IV. ALTERATION IN CARBOHYDRATE METABOLISM related to CARBOHYDRATE INTOLERANCE

Defining Characteristics: May cause hyperglycemia, hypokalemia, and carbohydrate intolerance.

Nursing Implications: Assess baseline blood glucose, K, and monitor during therapy. Teach patient signs/symptoms of hyperglycemia (polyuria, polydipsia), especially if receiving drug for extended period.

Drug: diphenhydramine hydrochloride (Benadryl)

Class: Antihistamine.

Mechanism of Action: Inhibits histamine, and has slight, if any, antiemetic activity by blocking the CTZ and decreasing vestibular stimulation. Acts on blood vessels, GI, respiratory systems by competing with histamine for H_1-receptor site; decreases allergic response by blocking histamine.

Metabolism: Biologically transformed in the liver; half-life is 2.4–9.3 hours; 80–85% protein-bound; excreted by the kidney. Metabolized in the liver, crosses placenta, and is excreted in breastmilk.

MANAGEMENT

Indications: Useful in the management of allergic reactions, prevention of allergic reactions, motion sickness, and parkinsonism.

Contraindications: In neonates, nursing mothers, as a local anesthetic and if hypersensitive to the drug or its components.

Dosage/Range:
Adult:
- *Oral:* 25–50 mg q 4 h.
- *IM:* 25–50 mg q 4 h.
- *IV:* 50 mg prior to chemotherapy or 25 mg q 4 h × 4 doses, beginning prior to antiemetic.

Drug Preparation:
- Available forms include 25-, 50-mg capsules; elixir 12.5 mg/mL; syrup 12.5 mg/mL; injection available as 10 mg/mL and 50 mg/mL.
- Administer IM deep in large muscle mass.

Drug Interactions:
- CNS depressants: increased sedation; monitor patient closely.

Lab Effects/Interference:
- None known.

Special Considerations:
- Useful in treatment or prevention of extrapyramidal side effects (EPS) related to antiemetics (dopamine antagonists).
- Contraindicated in patients with prior hypersensitivity to H_1-receptor antagonist, acute asthma attack, or lower respiratory tract disease.

Potential Toxicities/Side Effects and the Nursing Process

I.   ALTERATIONS IN SENSORY/PERCEPTUAL PATTERNS related to CNS CHANGES

Defining Characteristics: Sedation/drowsiness, dizziness, confusion (especially in the elderly), hyperexcitability, blurred vision/diplopia, tinnitus, dry mouth/nose/throat all may occur.

Nursing Implications: Assess patient's level of consciousness and risk for increased sedation (i.e., elderly, concomitant CNS depressant drugs). Monitor neurologic VS closely if sedated. Instruct patient to avoid alcohol ingestion, operation of equipment, or driving a car while drowsy. Teach strategies to protect safety.

II.   ALTERED URINARY ELIMINATION related to URINARY RETENTION, DYSURIA

Defining Characteristics: Urinary retention, dysuria, frequency may occur.

Nursing Implications: Assess baseline urinary elimination pattern. Teach patient potential side effects and instruct to report them. Use drug cautiously in men with prostatic hypertrophy; if side effects occur, instruct patient not to take drug and discuss with physician.

III. ALTERATION IN COMFORT related to RASH

Defining Characteristics: Rash, urticaria, photosensitivity, hypotension, palpitations may occur.

Nursing Implications: Assess baseline drug allergy history. Instruct patient to report rash, itching, and to avoid sunlight while taking the drug. Assess VS and monitor patient closely for hypotension, especially if patient is elderly, sedated, or taking other sedating drugs.

IV. POTENTIAL FOR INJURY related to BONE MARROW DEPRESSION

Defining Characteristics: Thrombocytopenia, agranulocytosis, hemolytic anemia may occur rarely.

Nursing Implications: Assess baseline CBC, platelet count. Discuss abnormalities with physician.

Drug: dolasetron mesylate (Anzemet)

Class: Serotonin-receptor antagonist.

Mechanism of Action: Together with the active metabolite hydrodolasetron, drug is a selective serotonin 5-HT$_3$ receptor antagonist, blocking transmission of impulses via the vagus nerve peripherally and centrally in the chemotherapy receptor trigger zone (CTZ). Blocks chemotherapy-induced nausea and vomiting produced by the release of serotonin from the enterochromaffin cells of the small intestines, which otherwise would stimulate the 5-HT$_3$ receptors on the vagus efferents that begin the vomiting reflex.

Metabolism: IV: Parent drug is rapidly eliminated from the plasma and completely metabolized into the major metabolite hydrodolasetron, as is the oral drug. Hydrodolasetron is metabolized by the cytochrome P450 enzyme system in the liver, with an approximate half-life of 7.3 hours. Oral and orally administered IV solution are bioequivalent, and apparent absolute bioavailability of oral dolasetron is 75%, determined by the active metabolite; 66% of drug is excreted in the urine unchanged, and 33% in the feces. Metabolite is 77% protein-bound.

Indication: For the prevention of nausea and vomiting associated with moderately emetogenic cancer chemotherapy, including initial and repeat courses in adults and children 2 years and older.

Dosage/Range:
- For the prevention of cancer chemotherapy-induced nausea and vomiting:
  - *Adult:* 100 mg PO given within 1 hour prior to chemotherapy.
  - *Pediatric* (2–16 years of age): 1.8 mg/kg given within 1 hour before chemotherapy up to a maximum of 100 mg.

Drug Preparation:
- Tablets available in 50-mg and 100-mg doses, each in a 5-count bottle or blister pack, or in a 10-count unit dose.
- Anzemet (dolonestron) IV is contraindicated in adult and pediatric patients for the prevention of CINV prevention due to its dose-dependent QT prolongation.

Drug Administration:
- Oral: administer within 1 hour before chemotherapy.

Drug Interactions:
- Anzemet injection has been recalled due to prolongation of QTc interval on the ECG.
- Increased hydrodolasetron serum levels (24%) when given with cimetidine (nonselective inhibitor of cytochrome P450 enzyme system).
- Decreased hydrodolasetron serum levels (28%) when combined with rifampin (potent inducer of P450 enzyme system).

Lab Effects/Interference:
- Transient increased liver transaminases (AST, ALT) in < 1% of patients; rare increase in bili, GGT, all phos.
- Prolonged QTc interval.

Special Considerations:
- Administer with caution in patients who have or may develop cardiac conduction defects, especially prolongation of QT interval (e.g., patients with hypokalemia, hypomagnesemia, receiving diuretics, congenital QT syndrome, receiving antiarrhythmic drugs or other drugs causing QT segment prolongation, and with high cumulative doses of anthracycline chemotherapy).
  - Prolongation of PR, QRS, and QTc intervals was observed in some patients.
  - These changes are mild, transient, asymptomatic, and do not require medical treatment.
  - Of note, this is a class effect of serotonin-receptor antagonists, and other drugs were also associated with less severe/similar electrocardiographic changes.
- Rare anaphylaxis, facial edema, urticaria.
- No dosage modifications necessary in elderly or patients with hepatic or renal impairment.

Potential Toxicities/Side Effects and Nursing Process

I.   ALTERATION IN COMFORT related to HEADACHE

Defining Characteristics: Headache (24%), fever (4%), fatigue (4%), and, rarely, arthralgia/myalgia occur.

Nursing Implications: Assess baseline comfort. Teach patient to report any unusual occurrence. Provide symptomatic management.

II. ALTERATION IN NUTRITION, LESS THAN BODY REQUIREMENTS, related to CONSTIPATION, DYSPEPSIA

Defining Characteristics: Constipation, dyspepsia, anorexia, and, rarely, pancreatitis may occur. In less than 1% of patients, there is an increase in LFTs.

Nursing Implications: Assess baseline weight, nutritional pattern. Instruct patient to report alterations, and manage symptomatically. Discuss alterations in LFTs and/or abdominal pain suggestive of pancreatitis with physician.

III. POTENTIAL ALTERATIONS IN SENSORY/PERCEPTUAL PATTERNS related to VERTIGO, PARESTHESIA

Defining Characteristics: Rarely, flushing, vertigo, paresthesia, agitation, sleep disorder, depersonalization may occur, as may ataxia, twitching, confusion, anxiety, abnormal dreams.

Nursing Implications: Teach patient to report any changes, and assess patient safety. Discuss any significant alterations with physician and consider alternative antiemetics.

Drug: dronabinol (Marinol)

Class: Cannabinoid.

Mechanism of Action: Active ingredient is d-9-tetrahydrocannabinol (THC). Probably depresses CNS and may disrupt higher cortical input, inhibit prostaglandin synthesis, or bind to opiate receptors in the brain to indirectly block the VC.

Metabolism: Metabolized by the liver.

Indication: For the treatment of (1) anorexia associated with weight loss in patients with AIDS, and (2) nausea and vomiting associated with cancer chemotherapy in patients who have failed to respond adequately to conventional antiemetic treatments.

Dosage/Range:
Adult:
- *Oral:* 5 mg/m^2 given 1–3 hours prior to chemotherapy, then every 2–4 hours post-chemotherapy for a total of 4–6 doses per day.
- If ineffective at above dose and no significant toxicity, dose may be increased by 2.5 mg/m^2 increments to a maximum of 15 mg/m^2 per dose.

Drug Preparation:
- Available in 2.5-, 5-, or 10-mg gel capsules that harden under refrigeration.

Drug Administration:
- Oral.

Drug Interactions:
- CNS depressants: increased sedation; avoid concurrent use.

Lab Effects/Interference:
- None known.

Special Considerations:
- More effective than placebo and, in some instances, may be better than prochlorperazine. Can produce physical and psychological dependency.
- May increase appetite; may produce dry mouth.
- Contains sesame oil, so should not be used by patients allergic to sesame oil.
- **Warnings and Precautions:**
  - Teach patient not to drive, operate machinery, or engage in hazardous activity until it is clear they can tolerate the drug and perform these tasks.
  - Use cautiously and only if benefit outweighs risk in patients with:
    - Seizure disorder, as drug may lower seizure threshold.
    - Cardiac disorders, as occasional hypotension, HTN, syncope, and/or tachycardia may occur.
    - History of substance abuse, as drug has abuse potential.
    - History of mania, depression, schizophrenia, as drug may exacerbate these conditions; monitor patients closely.
    - Patients receiving concomitant CNS depressants (e.g., sedatives, hypnotics, other psychoactive drugs), as CNS effects may be additive or synergistic.
    - Elderly, as they may be more sensitive to the neurological, psychoactive, and postural hypotensive effects of the drug.
    - Pregnant women, nursing mothers, pediatric patients, as drug has not been studied in these patient populations.

Potential Toxicities/Side Effects and the Nursing Process

I.   ALTERATIONS IN SENSORY/PERCEPTUAL PATTERNS related to CNS CHANGES

Defining Characteristics: Mood changes, disorientation, drowsiness, muddled thinking, dizziness, and brief impairment of perception, coordination, and sensory functions may occur. Increased toxicity in elderly (up to 35%).

Nursing Implications: Explain to patient these changes may occur to decrease anxiety, fear. Assess baseline mental status, and monitor during therapy. Assess patient safety and implement measures to ensure this. Avoid use in the elderly.

II.   ALTERATION IN CARDIAC OUTPUT related to TACHYCARDIA

Defining Characteristics: Tachycardia, orthostatic hypotension may occur.

Nursing Implications: Assess baseline VS, and monitor during therapy. If hypotension occurs, notify physician and anticipate increasing rate of IV fluids to increase BP.

Drug: fosaprepitant dimeglumine (Emend for injection)

Class: Substance P/neurokinin-1 receptor antagonist. For oral formulation, see aprepitant.

Mechanism of Action: Drug is a prodrug of aprepitant. Selective substance P/neurokinin-1 (NK_1) receptor antagonist (high affinity). Drug has no affinity for 5-HT_3, dopamine, or corticosteroid receptors. Drug crosses the blood–brain barrier to saturate brain NK_1 receptors. Drug increases the activity of serotonin-receptor antagonists and corticosteroids in preventing acute nausea and vomiting and inhibits both acute and delayed nausea and vomiting related to cisplatin chemotherapy.

Metabolism: Drug is rapidly converted to aprepitant after IV administration, and the pro-drug is negligible 30 minutes following administration. The mean aprepitant serum concentrations at 24 hours postdose were similar between a 125-mg oral dose and a 115-mg IV fosaprepitant dose. Aprepitant is 95% bound to plasma proteins and crosses the placenta and blood–brain barrier. Aprepitant undergoes extensive metabolism in the liver by the P450 hepatic microenzyme system, specifically CYP3A4, and minor metabolism by CYP1A2 and CYP2C19. Seven inactive metabolites have been found in the plasma The drug is excreted in the urine (57%) and the feces (45%). The terminal half-life of the drug is 9–13 hours. The C_{max} is 16% higher for females than males, and the half-life of aprepitant is lower in females than males; however, this is not believed to be clinically important. No dosage adjustment necessary for patients with renal insufficiency or requiring dialysis or patients with mild to moderate hepatic insufficiency.

Indication: In combination with other antiemetic agents, for the (a) prevention of acute and delayed nausea and vomiting associated with initial and repeat courses of highly emetogenic cancer chemotherapy, including high-dose cisplatin, (b) prevention of nausea and vomiting associated with initial and repeat courses of moderately emetogenic cancer chemotherapy.

Dosage/Range:
- *Highly emetogenic chemotherapy:* Day 1: 150 mg IV over 20–30 minutes, started 30 minutes before chemotherapy, together with a serotonin- (HT_3-) receptor antagonist and dexamethasone 12 mg PO on day 1, 8 mg PO day 2, and 8 mg bid on days 3 and 4.
- *Highly emetogenic chemotherapy (3-day dosing regimen):* Day 1: fosaprepitant 115 mg IV as a 15- minute infusion 30 minutes before chemotherapy. Days 2 and 3: aprepitant 80-mg capsules are given orally; serotonin-receptor antagonist day 1; dexamethasone 12 mg PO day 1, 8 mg PO days 2–4.
- *Moderately emetogenic chemotherapy (3-day dosing regimen):* Day 1: fosaprepitant 115 mg IV as a 15-minute infusion 30 minutes before chemotherapy. Days 2 and 3: aprepitant 80-mg capsules are given orally; serotonin-receptor antagonist day 1; dexamethasone 12 mg PO day 1 only.
- Do not use fosaprepitant concurrently with pimozide or cisapride.

Drug Preparation:
- IV formulation supplied as single dose of 115-mg lyophilized white to off-white solid and single dose of 150-mg lyophilized white to off-white solid formulations. Vial should be stored at 2–8°C (36–46°F). Aseptically add 5-mL 0.9% sodium chloride for injection into the vial; gently swirl the contents until dissolved (do not shake or jet the diluent into the vial). Aseptically withdraw entire contents, and add 115-mg dose to previously prepared 110-mL bag of 0.9% sodium chloride infusion bag, or 150-mg dose to a 145-mL infusion bag of 0.9% sodium chloride infusion bag. This results in a final concentration of 1 mg/mL.

Drug Interactions:
- Drugs that inhibit the CYP3A4 isoenzyme system can increase the serum level of aprepitant: ketoconazole, itraconazole, nefazodone, clarithromycin, ritonavir, nelfinavir; diltiazem (twofold increase in aprepitant plasma concentration); thus, coadminister cautiously and monitor for aprepitant toxicity or dose-reduce aprepitant.
- Drugs that strongly induce CYP3A4 isoenzyme system can lower aprepitant serum levels: rifampin, carbamazepine, phenytoin; assess for efficacy of aprepitant and need for drug dose increase.
- Drug is a moderate inhibitor of P450 hepatic isoenzyme system CYP3A4; thus, the plasma concentrations of the following drugs can theoretically be increased if coadministered:
  - Chemotherapy agents are docetaxel, paclitaxel, etoposide, irinotecan, ifosfamide, imatinib, vinorelbine, vinblastine, and vincristine.
  - Dexamethasone (dose-reduce dexamethasone by 50%).
  - Methylprednisolone (dose-reduce 25% if IV, 50% if PO).
  - Pimozide, terfenadine, astemizole: do not use together.
  - Benzodiazepines: midazolam, lorazepam, alprazolam, triazolam.
- Drug is an inducer of CYP2C9, and the plasma concentrations of the following drugs can theoretically be decreased if coadministered:
  - Warfarin (34% decrease with 14% decrease in INR; closely monitor during 2 weeks following antiemetic treatment, especially as the INR and PT 7–10 days after 3-day antiemetic regimen may be significantly lowered; assess INR, PT frequently and manage warfarin dose closely.
  - Phenytoin, tolbutamide serum levels can be decreased.
- Hormonal contraceptives can become ineffective during and for 28 days following last dose of fosaprepitant or aprepitant; alternative or backup methods of contraception should be used.

Lab Effects/Interference:
- Decreased INR, PT if patient taking warfarin.

Special Considerations:
- Contraindications: do not give concomitantly with pimozide, terfenadine, astemizole, or cisapride. Do not give if hypersensitive to aprepitant or any of its components. Use cautiously if at all during pregnancy or breastfeeding. No studies have been done in patients with severe liver failure.
- Significant drug interactions (discussed previously here).
- Most common side effects: hiccups, asthenia/fatigue, increased AST/ALT, headache, constipation, anorexia, dyspepsia, diarrhea, eructation, infusion-site reactions.

Potential Toxicities/Side Effects and the Nursing Process

I. ALTERATION IN NUTRITION, LESS THAN BODY REQUIREMENTS, related to CONSTIPATION, DIARRHEA, NAUSEA, ANOREXIA, HICCUPS

Defining Characteristics: Gastrointestinal side effects may occur but are infrequent with the following incidences: constipation (10.3%), diarrhea (10.3%), nausea (12.7%), vomiting (7.5%), hiccups (10.8%), and anorexia (10.1%).

Nursing Implications: Teach patient that these side effects may occur and to report them if unrelieved by symptom management measures. Teach patient self-care measures to manage and prevent symptoms.

II. ALTERATION IN COMFORT related to ASTHENIA/FATIGUE, ABDOMINAL PAIN, HEADACHE

Defining Characteristics: Asthenia/fatigue occurred in 17.8% of patients; abdominal pain 4.6%; headache 8.5%.

Nursing Implications: Teach patient that these side effects may occur and measures to minimize their occurrence. Teach energy-conserving measures and management of abdominal pain and headache. Teach patient to report signs and symptoms that worsen or are unrelieved.

Drug: granisetron hydrochloride (Kytril)

Class: Serotonin-receptor antagonist.

Mechanism of Action: Binds to vagal afferents (serotonin receptors) adjacent to the enterochromaffin cells in the GI mucosa, thus preventing the stimulation of afferent fibers that would otherwise stimulate the VC and CTZ. In addition, granisetron inhibits a positive feedback loop located on the enterochromaffin cells that normally responds to high levels of serotonin released from chemotherapy injury to the gut mucosa by releasing a surge of additional serotonin. Thus, granisetron blocks two pathways of serotonin release to prevent chemotherapy-induced nausea and vomiting.

Metabolism: Rapidly and extensively metabolized by the liver using the P450 cytochrome enzymes; 12% of unchanged drug is eliminated in the urine at 48 hours. The half-life of IV granisetron in cancer patients is 9 hours.

Indication: *Oral formulation* indicated for (1) prevention of nausea and/or vomiting associated with initial and repeat courses of emetogenic cancer chemotherapy, including high-dose cisplatin; and (2) prevention of nausea and vomiting associated with radiation, including total body irradiation and fractionated abdominal radiation. *IV formulation* indicated for (1) prevention of nausea and/or vomiting associated with initial and repeat courses of emetogenic cancer chemotherapy, including high-dose cisplatin; and (2) prevention and treatment of postoperative nausea and vomiting in adults.

MANAGEMENT

Dosage/Range:
- *IV:* 10 mcg/kg IV over 5 minutes, beginning within 30 minutes prior to chemotherapy.
- *Oral:* 2 mg PO or 1 mg bid (q 12 h) beginning up to 1 hour before chemotherapy.
- *Oral:* 2 mg PO once daily taken within1 hour of radiation.

Drug Preparation:
- Dilute in 20–50 mL 0.9% sodium chloride or 5% dextrose.

Drug Administration:
- IV infusion over 5 minutes.
- Drug can also be given IV push over 5 minutes.

Drug Interactions:
- None known; however, because the drug is metabolized by the P450 cytochrome enzymes, drugs that induce or inhibit this may theoretically change the drug serum levels and half-life.

Lab Effects/Interference:
- Rarely, increased AST, ALT.

Special Considerations:
- Useful in the management of high-dose cisplatin, in combination with dexamethasone, either with oral tablets or IV preparation.
- Preliminary study data showed little difference in efficacy between oral dosing of 1 mg bid versus a single dose of 2 mg.
- Both IV and tablet formulation are indicated for the prevention of nausea and vomiting associated with initial and repeat courses of emetogenic chemotherapy, including cisplatin.

Potential Toxicities/Side Effects and the Nursing Process

I.   ALTERATION IN COMFORT related to HEADACHE, ASTHENIA, SOMNOLENCE

Defining Characteristics: Side effects are uncommon but may include headache, asthenia, and somnolence.

Nursing Implications: Teach patient that side effects may occur. Headache is usually relieved by OTC analgesics such as acetaminophen.

II.   ALTERATION IN ELIMINATION related to CONSTIPATION OR DIARRHEA

Defining Characteristics: A small percentage of patients may experience constipation or diarrhea.

Nursing Implications: Assess baseline elimination pattern. Instruct patient to report alterations. Identify patients at risk, such as those receiving narcotic analgesics for cancer pain, who may develop constipation. Assist patient in modifying bowel regimen.

Drug: granisetron hydrochloride transdermal (Sancuso)

Class: Serotonin-receptor antagonist.

Mechanism of Action: Drug, in a transdermal patch, is delivered via the transdermal route. Granisetron binds to vagal afferents (serotonin receptors) adjacent to the enterochromaffin cells in the GI mucosa, thus preventing the stimulation of afferent fibers that would otherwise stimulate the VC and CTZ. In addition, granisetron inhibits a positive feedback loop located on the enterochromaffin cells that normally responds to high levels of serotonin released from chemotherapy injury to the gut mucosa by releasing a surge of additional serotonin. Thus, granisetron blocks two pathways of serotonin release to prevent chemotherapy-induced nausea and vomiting.

Metabolism: Drug contains 34 mg of drug and delivers drug over 5 days. Once absorbed, drug is rapidly and extensively metabolized by the liver using the P450 cytochrome enzymes; 12% of unchanged drug is eliminated in the urine at 48 hours. The half-life of IV granisetron in cancer patients is 9 hours.

Indication: For the prevention of nausea and vomiting in patients receiving moderately and/or highly emetogenic chemotherapy for up to 5 consecutive days.

Dosage/Range:
- 34.3-mg transdermal patch providing antiemesis for 7 days, delivering 3.1 mg per 24 hours.

Drug Preparation:
- None.

Drug Administration:
- Remove plastic backing and apply to clean, dry skin.
- Apply to the upper outer arm a minimum of 24 hours and a maximum of 48 hours before chemotherapy. Remove the patch a minimum of 24 hours after completion of chemotherapy. The patch can be worn up to 7 days depending upon the duration of the chemotherapy regimen.

Drug Interactions:
- None known, but because the drug is metabolized by the P450 cytochrome enzymes, drugs that induce or inhibit this may theoretically change the drug serum levels and half-life.

Lab Effects/Interference:
- Rarely, increased AST, ALT.

Special Considerations:
- Patch can mask a progressive ileus and/or gastric distention caused by the underlying condition.
- In a noninferiority trial, transdermal formulation was as good as oral granisetron in the management of patients with cancer receiving first cycle of multiday (3–5 day), moderate or

highly emetogenic chemotherapy (Grundberg et al., 2007). This phase III trial was a random-ized, double-blind, multinational (nine countries) trial that enrolled 641 patients. Complete protection was achieved in 60.2% of patients receiving the transdermal granisetron and 64.9% of those receiving oral granisetron. Ninety percent of the patients in the transdermal granisetron arm had ≥ 75% patch adherence. Side effects were identical (constipation and headache were most common), and there was no significant irritation at the patch site.

Potential Toxicities/Side Effects and the Nursing Process

I.   ALTERATION IN COMFORT related to HEADACHE, ASTHENIA, SOMNOLENCE

Defining Characteristics: Side effects are uncommon but may include headache, asthenia, and somnolence.

Nursing Implications: Teach patient that side effects may occur. Headache is usually relieved by OTC analgesics such as acetaminophen.

II.   ALTERATION IN ELIMINATION related to CONSTIPATION OR DIARRHEA

Defining Characteristics: A small percentage of patients may experience constipation or diarrhea.

Nursing Implications: Assess baseline elimination pattern. Instruct patient to report alterations. Identify patients at risk, such as those receiving narcotic analgesics for cancer pain, who may develop constipation. Assist patient in modifying bowel regimen.

Drug: haloperidol (Haldol)

Class: Butyrophenone.

Mechanism of Action: Tranquilizer that depresses cerebral cortex, hypothalamus, limbic system (controls activity and aggression); appears to block dopamine receptors in CTZ, giving antiemetic activity.

Metabolism: Metabolized by the liver, excreted in the urine, bile, and crosses placenta. Enters breastmilk. Half-life is 21 hours.

Indication: For the management of manifestations of psychotic disorders; control of tics and vocal utterances of Tourette's disorder in children and adults. May be useful in the management of chemotherapy-induced nausea and vomiting refractory to other agents.

Dosage/Range:
Adult:

- *Oral:* 3–5 mg q 2 h × 3–4 doses, beginning 30 minutes before chemotherapy.
- *IM:* 0.5–2 mg (dose-reduce in older patients).

Drug Preparation:
- Available as 0.5-, 1-, 2-, 5-, 10-, 20-mg tablets; injection: 5 mg/mL.

Drug Interactions:
- *Epinephrine:* reversal of vasopressor effects; avoid concurrent use.
- *CNS depressants:* increased sedation; monitor patient closely.

Lab Effects/Interference:
- Rarely, increased alk phos, bili, serum transaminases (AST, ALT).
- Rarely, decreased PT (if patient on warfarin).
- Rarely, decreased serum cholesterol.
- Prolongs QTc interval on ECG.

Special Considerations:
- Indicated for the management of psychotic disorders, short-term treatment of hyperactive children showing excessive motor activity, schizophrenia; may be used in the management of nausea and vomiting.
- Contraindicated in severe toxic CNS depression or comatose states; individuals with hypersensitivity; patients with Parkinson's disease, blood dyscrasias, brain damage, bone marrow depression, and alcohol or barbiturate withdrawal states.
- Shown to be equivalent to THC and superior to phenothiazines when tested as an antiemetic.

Potential Toxicities/Side Effects and the Nursing Process

I. ALTERATIONS IN SENSORY/PERCEPTUAL PATTERNS related to TARDIVE DYSKINESIA

Defining Characteristics: With chronic use, tardive dyskinesia syndrome occurs, characterized by involuntary, dyskinetic movements; sedation, EPS may occur when used as an antiemetic.

Nursing Implications: Assess baseline level of consciousness and monitor during therapy. Assess for signs/symptoms of EPS (dystonia, tongue protrusion, trismus, opisthotonus), and administer diphenhydramine as ordered.

II. ALTERATION IN OXYGENATION related to LARYNGOSPASM

Defining Characteristics: Laryngospasm and respiratory depression occur rarely.

Nursing Implications: Assess baseline pulmonary status, and monitor during therapy. Identify risk factors (concomitant narcotics, CNS depressants). Notify physician, and hold drug if respiratory depression occurs or is suspected. Be prepared to institute respiratory support if necessary and to reverse opiate.

III.   ALTERATION IN CARDIAC OUTPUT/PERFUSION related to ORTHOSTATIC HYPOTENSION

Defining Characteristics: Orthostatic hypotension may occur and may precipitate angina; also, tachycardia, EKG changes, and rare cardiac arrest may occur.

Nursing Implications: Assess VS baseline, and monitor during therapy. If hypotension occurs, notify physician and anticipate increasing rate of IV fluids to increase BP. Epinephrine should NOT be used because the drug reverses vasopressor effect; rather, metaraminol or norepinephrine should be used.

Drug: metoclopramide hydrochloride (Reglan)

Class: Substituted benzamide.

Mechanism of Action: Procainamide derivative without cardiac effects. Acts both centrally and peripherally. Acts peripherally to enhance the action of acetylcholine at muscarinic synapses and in the CNS to antagonize dopamine. Is primarily a dopamine antagonist blocking the CTZ; also stimulates upper GI tract motility, thus increasing gastric emptying, and opposes retrograde peristalsis of retching.

Metabolism: Metabolized by the liver, excreted in the urine, with a half-life of 4 hours.

Indication: *Oral:* for the (1) prevention and management of acute and recurrent diabetic gastroparesis; (2) short-term therapy of symptomatic, documented gastroesophageal reflux disease in adults who fail to respond to conventional therapy. *IV:* (1) prevention of nausea and vomiting associated with emetogenic cancer chemotherapy; (2) prevention of post-operative nausea and vomiting when nasogastric suction is undesirable; (3) facilitation of small bowel intubation when tube does not pass pylorus with conventional maneuvers; (4) acute and recurrent diabetic gastric stasis; (5) stimulation of gastric emptying and intestinal transit or barium where delayed emptying interferes with radiological examination of the stomach and/or small intestines.

Dosage/Range:
Adult:
- *Oral:* 10 mg qid (gastroparesis) administered 30 minutes before each meal and at bedtime for 2–8 weeks.
- *IV:* Highly emetogenic chemotherapy: 2 mg/kg q 2 h × 3–5 doses OR 3 mg/kg q 2 h × 2 doses, beginning 30 minutes prior to chemotherapy. Dose-reduce 50% renal insufficiency (CrCl < 40 mL/min). Moderately emetogenic chemotherapy: 1 mg/kg given 30 minutes before beginning cancer chemotherapy, and repeat every 2 hours × 2 doses, then every 3 hours × 3 doses.
- *IM:* Postoperative nausea and vomiting: 10–20 mg IM near end of surgery.

Drug Preparation:
- *IV:* available as 5 mg/mL; further dilute in 50 mL 0.9% sodium chloride or 5% dextrose and administer over 15 minutes.

Drug Interactions:
- Digoxin: may decrease absorption; monitor digoxin effectiveness and modify dose as needed.
- Aspirin, acetaminophen, tetracycline, ethanol, levodopa, diazepam: may increase absorption; monitor for drug toxicity.
- CNS depressants: increased depressant effects; monitor patient closely.

Lab Effects/Interference:
- None known.

Special Considerations:
- Indicated as an antiemetic to prevent nausea and vomiting from chemotherapy, delayed gastric emptying, gastroesophageal reflux.
- Increased incidence of dystonic reactions in men under 35 years old. Consider diphenhydramine q 4 h or lorazepam and decadron to minimize dystonic reactions.
- Efficacy as an antiemetic: 60% complete protection against high-dose cisplatin, and increased to 66% with the addition of steroids and lorazepam.
- Contraindicated in patients with prior hypersensitivity to this drug, procaine, or procainamide; patients with seizure disorder, pheochromocytoma, GI obstruction.
- Use cautiously in patients with breast cancer, as may increase prolactin levels, and in patients with renal insufficiency.

Potential Toxicities/Side Effects and the Nursing Process

I. ALTERATIONS IN SENSORY/PERCEPTUAL PATTERNS related to SEDATION, EPS

Defining Characteristics: Sedation, akathisia (restlessness), adverse dystonic, or extrapyramidal effects may occur; increased risk in patients < 30 years old.

Nursing Implications: Assess baseline neurologic status, and monitor during therapy. Protect patient safety, and keep all necessary patient equipment at the bedside (e.g., commode). Assess for extrapyramidal side effects, and administer diphenhydramine as ordered. In addition, lorazepam administered as part of combination antiemetics helps to decrease akathisia.

II. POTENTIAL FOR ALTERED BOWEL ELIMINATION related to DIARRHEA

Defining Characteristics: Increase in both esophageal sphincter pressure and gastric emptying, leading to diarrhea with high doses. Action antagonized by narcotics.

Nursing Implications: Assess baseline bowel elimination status. Teach patient to report diarrhea, and administer kaolin/pectin as ordered, or other antidiarrheals. Arrange for commode at the bedside if bathroom far from bed. Also, diarrhea may be prevented by administration of dexamethasone as part of antiemetic regimen.

III.   ALTERATION IN COMFORT related to DRY/MOUTH, RASH

Defining Characteristics: Dry mouth, rash, urticaria, hypotension may occur.

Nursing Implications: Assess baseline comfort. Teach patient to report rash, urticaria, and treat symptomatically. Monitor VS, and slow infusion rate if hypotensive, as well as replace IV fluids per physician's order.

Drug: nabilone (Cesamet)

Class: Cannabinoid antiemetic.

Mechanism of Action: Drug acts as an omnineuromodulator, interacting with the cannabinoid receptors CB1 and CB2, which are involved in regulating nausea and vomiting. CB1 and CB2 receptors are found throughout the human body.

Metabolism: After oral administration, drug and its carbinol metabolite achieve peak plasma levels in 2 hours, but this amount represents only 10–20% of total drug. Plasma half-life of nabilone is about 2 hours, while that of the total radiocarbon dose was 35 hours. Drug is highly protein-bound. Drug is primarily metabolized by direct enzymatic oxidation in the liver (first pass), and excreted via the biliary system. Drug and its metabolites are excreted primarily in the feces (65%), with 20% excreted in the urine.

A substantial number of patients experience disturbing psychotomimetic reactions not experienced with other antiemetic agents (Cesamet package insert, 2010). Use of nabilone requires close supervision of the patient during initiation and dose adjustments. It is not intended to be used PRN or as the first antiemetic agent the patient has been prescribed.

Dosage/Range:
- 1 or 2 mg PO bid, beginning 1–3 hours before planned chemotherapy; beginning with the lower dose is recommended, with dose increase as needed. Some patients have benefited from a beginning dose the night before chemotherapy.
- Give drug during the entire course of each cycle of chemotherapy, and if needed, for 48 hours after the last dose of each cycle of chemotherapy.
- The maximum daily dose is 6 mg, given orally in divided doses 3 times a day.

Drug Preparation:
- None, oral capsule.

Drug Administration:
- Teach patients that they:
  - May experience mood changes and other adverse behavioral effects, so they should not become alarmed when it occurs; patients should be with a responsible (supervisory) person while using the drug, especially initially and during dose adjustments.

- Should not drive, operate machinery, or engage in any hazardous activity while receiving nabilone.
- Should not take other substances or drugs that depress the CNS (e.g., alcohol, benzodiazepines, barbiturates).

Drug Interactions:
- Additive CNS depressant effects with alcohol, sedatives, hypnotics, or other psychotomimetic substances. DO NOT give concomitantly.
- Diazepam: significantly impairs psychomotor function; DO NOT give concurrently.
- Amphetamines, cocaine, other sympathomimetic agents: additive HTN, tachycardia, possible cardiotoxicity.
- Atropine, scopolamine, antihistamines, other anticholinergic agents: additive or super-additive tachycardia, drowsiness.
- Amitriptyline, amoxapine, desipramine, and other tricyclic antidepressants: additive tachycardia, HTN, drowsiness.
- Disulfiram: reversible hypomanic reaction possible.
- Opioids: cross-tolerance and mutual potentiation.
- Naltrexone: oral THC effects were enhanced by opioid receptor blockade (THC is active ingredient in marijuana).
- Alcohol: increase in the positive subjective mood effects of smoked marijuana.

Lab Effects/Interference:
- Leukopenia.

Special Considerations:
- Nabilone drug effects may persist for an unpredictable length of time after oral administration. Adverse psychiatric reactions can last 48–72 hours after last dose of treatment.
- Drug may affect the CNS, causing dizziness, drowsiness, euphoria "high," ataxia, anxiety, disorientation, depression, hallucinations, and psychosis.
- Use cautiously, if at all, in patients with severe liver or renal dysfunction.
- Use cautiously in patients with a history of current or previous psychiatric disorders, including bipolar disorder, depression, and schizophrenia, as the symptoms of these disease states may be unmasked by the use of cannabinoids.
- Use cautiously in patients with a substance abuse history. Drug is a controlled substance; monitor patients for signs of excessive use, abuse, and misuse.
- Use with caution in patients with a history of substance abuse, including alcohol abuse or dependence and marijuana, as nabilone contains a similar active compound to marijuana.
- Drug should not be taken with alcohol, sedatives, hypnotics, or other psychotomimetic substances.
- Adverse psychiatric reactions can persist for 48–72 hours after drug is taken.
- Use cautiously in elderly patients with hypertension or heart disease, as drug elevates supine and standing heart rates; it also causes postural hypotension, as well as tachycardia.
- Drug should not be used during pregnancy, in nursing mothers, or in pediatric patients, as safety has not been established.
- Common side effects are unsteadiness, dizziness, difficulty concentrating, drowsiness, mouth dryness, and/or headache.

Potential Toxicities/Side Effects and the Nursing Process

I.   ALTERATIONS IN SENSORY/PERCEPTUAL PATTERNS related to SEDATION, EPS

Defining Characteristics: Frequency of symptoms was drowsiness (66%), psychological high (39%), depression (14%), ataxia (13%), blurred vision (13%), sensation disturbance (12%), euphoria (4%), and hallucinations (2%). Rarely, syncope, nightmares, distortion in the perception of time, confusion, disassociation, dysphoria, psychotic reactions, and seizures occurred in < 1% of patients. Anxiety, insomnia, and emotional lability may all occur. Increased toxicity in the elderly.

Nursing Implications: Explain to patient these changes may occur and give strategies to decrease anxiety, fear. Assess baseline mental status, and monitor during therapy. Assess patient's comfort and ability to cope with side effects that occur. Assess patient safety and implement measures to ensure this. Teach patient to avoid driving a car and operating machinery until effect of drug is known and safety assured. Develop safety plan for home care, and involve family or significant caregiver in plan. Avoid use of drug in the elderly. Teach patient to notify physician or NP immediately if patient experiences changes in mood (depression, anxiety), confusion, difficulty breathing, fainting, irregular heartbeats, tremors, hallucinations, and increased blood pressure, as they may indicate an overdose.

If psychotic episodes occur, manage patient conservatively if possible. If moderate episode or anxiety reaction, provide verbal support and comforting. If severe, discuss need for antipsychotic drugs, although this has not been studied. Monitor patient closely for additive CNS depressant effects if antipsychotic therapy is used. Protect patient's airway, and support ventilation and perfusion. Consider administration of activated charcoal to decrease GI absorption of drug and to hasten drug elimination.

II.   ALTERATION IN CARDIAC OUTPUT related to TACHYCARDIA, ORTHOSTATIC HYPOTENSION

Defining Characteristics: Tachycardia, syncope, orthostatic hypotension may rarely occur.

Nursing Implications: Assess baseline VS, and monitor during therapy. Teach patient to change position from lying to sitting gradually and from sitting to standing so that dizziness is minimized. If hypotension occurs, notify physician and anticipate increasing IV fluids to increase BP during chemotherapy administration.

Drug: netupitant/palonosetron (Akynzeo)

Class: Antiemetic. Netupitant is a substance P/neurokinin 1 (NK$_1$) receptor antagonist, and palonosetron is a serotonin-3 (5-HT$_3$) receptor antagonist.

Mechanism of Action: Drug is a fixed combination of netupitant, a substance P/neurokinin 1 (NK$_1$) receptor antagonist, and palonosetron, a serotonin-3 (5-HT$_3$) receptor antagonist.

It blocks the mechanism by which chemotherapy causes nausea and vomiting: (1) blocks the release of serotonin from enterochromaffin cells in the small intestines, which is stimulated by chemotherapy, thereby preventing stimulation of serotonin-3 (5-HT$_3$) receptors on vagal efferents, and preventing stimulation of the vomiting center; (2) prevents delayed antiemesis by blocking substance P activation of tachykinin family neurokinin 1 (NK$_1$) receptors in the central and peripheral nervous systems.

Metabolism: After oral administration, the peak plasma concentration for each drug is achieved in approximately 5 hours. Netupitant and its metabolites are highly plasma protein bound. Once absorbed, netupitant is extensively metabolized to three active, major metabolites primarily by CYP3A4, and to a lesser degree by CYP2C9 and CYP2D6. Netupitant is eliminated primarily in the feces (70.7%) and urine (3.95%), with an elimination half-life of 80 ± 29 hours. Palonosetron is metabolized by CYP2D6 and others, with 50% metabolized to two primary, non-active metabolites (< 1%). Palonosetron is eliminated via the urine (85–93%), with an elimination half-life of 48 ± 19 hours.

Indication: Indicated for the prevention of acute and delayed nausea and vomiting associated with initial and repeat courses of cancer chemotherapy, including, but not limited to, highly emetogenic chemotherapy. Oral palonosetron prevents nausea and vomiting during the acute phase, and netupitant prevents nausea and vomiting during both the acute and delayed phases.

Dosage/Range:
- 300 mg netupitant/0.5 mg palonosetron 1 hour prior to the start of chemotherapy.
  - **Highly emetogenic chemotherapy,** including cisplatin-based chemotherapy: One capsule administered 1 hour prior to the start of chemotherapy, with dexamethasone 12 mg administered PO 30 minutes prior to chemotherapy on day 1, and 8 mg PO administered on days 2–4.
  - **Anthracycline- and cyclophosphamide-based chemotherapy and chemotherapy not considered highly emetogenic:** One capsule administered 1 hour prior to the start of chemotherapy, with dexamethasone 12 mg PO administered 30 minutes prior to chemotherapy on day 1 only. Dexamethasone on days 2–4 is not necessary.
- The drug can be taken with or without food.
- The drug should *not* be used in patients with severe hepatic or renal impairment.

Drug Preparation: None. Store at room temperature.

Drug Administration:
- Teach the patient to take the capsule 1 hour before the start of chemotherapy, and to take it either with or without food.
- Review the patient's medication profile for potential serotonergic drugs (e.g., SSRIs, SNRIs, dextromethorphan, fentanyl, linezolid, tramadol); discuss changing serotonergic drugs to alternative agents, to prevent possible serotonin syndrome. Teach the patient to *not* take any cold medication (over the counter) that contains dextromethorphan.
- Teach the patient that two rare, potentially life-threatening reactions may occur, and the patient should get emergency help **right away if either occurs**:

- An allergic, or hypersensitivity reaction, including anaphylaxis: If hives, swollen face, trouble breathing, or chest pain occurs.
- Serotonin syndrome: Happens when drugs that block serotonin are given with drugs that increase serotonin levels, such as certain antidepressants and cough medicine ingredients. Signs and symptoms include the following:
  - Altered mental status (e.g., agitation, hallucinations, delirium, coma)
  - Autonomic instability (e.g., tachycardia, labile BP, dizziness, diaphoresis, flushing hyperthermia)
  - Neuromuscular symptoms (e.g., tremor, rigidity, myoclonus, hyperreflexia, incoordination)
  - Seizures, with or without GI symptoms (e.g., nausea, vomiting, diarrhea)
- Serotonin syndrome has been described in patients taking a 5-HT$_3$ receptor antagonist and a serotonergic drug (e.g., selective serotonin reuptake inhibitors [SSRIs] and serotonin and noradrenaline reuptake inhibitors [SNRIs]).
- If either hypersensitivity or serotonin syndrome occurs, discontinue netupitant/palonosetron and provide immediate supportive/emergency care.
- Teach the patient not to start any new medication, such as SSRIs or SNRIs, if prescribed by another physician, until after discussing it with the provider.
- Assess geriatric patients closely, as they may have more hepatic or renal impairment, cardiac issues, concomitant disease, or other drug therapy.
- Pregnancy Category C: Not recommended unless the potential benefit exceeds the potential risk to the fetus.
- It is unknown if the drug is excreted in human milk; a decision should be made whether to discontinue nursing or to discontinue the drug, taking into account the importance to the mother.

Drug Interactions:
- Netupitant is a moderate inhibitor of CYP3A4.
- **CYP3A4 substrates** (e.g., dexamethasone; midazolam; chemotherapy agents—docetaxel, paclitaxel, etoposide, irinotecan, cyclophosphamide, ifosfamide, imatinib, vinorelbine, vinblastine, vincristine): Inhibition of CYP3A4 by netupitant can result in increased plasma concentrations of the concomitant drug lasting at least 4 days; use with caution.
- **CYP3A4 inducers** (e.g., rifampin): Decreased plasma concentrations of netupitant; avoid concomitant use.
- **CYP3A4 inhibitors** (e.g., ketoconazole): Can result in significantly increased plasma concentrations of netupitant; no dosage adjustment necessary for a single dose.
- **Serotonergic drugs** (e.g., SSRIs, SNRIs, dextromethorphan, fentanyl, linezolid, tramadol): Serotonin syndrome may occur; do not use together concomitantly.

Lab Effects/Interference: Increased transaminases (ALT, AST), total bilirubin.

Special Considerations:
- Most common adverse reactions (incidence ≥ 3% and greater than that with palonosetron alone): headache, asthenia, dyspepsia, fatigue, constipation, erythema.

- Hypersensitivity reactions, including anaphylaxis, have been reported in patients taking palonosetron. Monitor the patient closely.
- Serotonin syndrome may occur in patients who take 5-HT$_3$ receptor antagonists and serotonergic drugs. Review the patient's medication profile for concomitant administration of an SSRI or SNRI, and discuss changing the antidepressant.
- Avoid use of the drug in patients with severe hepatic or renal impairment including ESRD.

Potential Toxicities/Side Effects and the Nursing Process

I.   ALTERATION IN COMFORT related to HEADACHE, ASTHENIA, FATIGUE, OR DYSPEPSIA

Defining Characteristics: Headache occurs in 9% of patients. Dyspepsia occurs in 4%, fatigue in 4–7%, and asthenia in 8%.

Nursing Implications: Teach the patient that these symptoms may occur, offer self-care strategies to use, and tell them to report symptoms that do not resolve.

II.   ALTERATION IN BOWEL ELIMINATION related to CONSTIPATION

Defining Characteristics: Constipation occurs in approximately 3% of patients.

Nursing Implications: Assess baseline bowel elimination status. Teach patients that constipation may occur, and suggest the use usual strategies to prevent constipation. If constipation occurs, teach the patient to use bowel softeners and laxatives, and to report if these measures are ineffective.

Drug: ondansetron hydrochloride (zofran)

Class: Serotonin-receptor antagonist.

Mechanism of Action: Selective 5-HT$_3$ (serotonin) receptor antagonist and may block 5-HT$_3$ receptors found peripherally on the vagus nerve terminals and centrally in the CTZ, thus preventing chemotherapy-induced vomiting.

Metabolism: Extensively metabolized, with only 5% of parent compound found in urine. Metabolized by hepatic cytochrome P-450 enzymes CYP3A4, CYP2D6, and CYP1A2.

Indication: *IV:* (1) Prevention of nausea and vomiting associated with initial and repeat courses of emetogenic cancer chemotherapy, including high-dose cisplatin; and (2) Prevention of postoperative nausea and/or vomiting. *Oral:* (1, 2) Prevention of nausea and vomiting associated with highly and moderately emetogenic cancer chemotherapy;

(3) Prevention of nausea and vomiting associated with radiotherapy in patients receiving either total body irradiation, single high-dose fraction to the abdomen, or daily fractions to the abdomen; (4) Prevention of postoperative nausea and vomiting.

Contraindications: (1) Concomitant use of apomorphine (causes profound hypotension and loss of consciousness), and in patients with a known hypersensitivity to ondansetron.

Dosage/Range:

CINV *Adult and pediatric patients (6 months to 18 years):*
- *IV:* 0.15 mg/kg (max 16 mg/dose) in 50 mL 5% dextrose or 0.9% sodium chloride injection USP given over 15 min q 4 h × 3 doses, beginning 30 minutes prior to chemotherapy.
- *Oral:*
  - Adult, highly emetogenic chemo: 24 mg PO 30 minutes before chemotherapy. This dose has not been studied in children.
  - Adult, children age 12 and older: Moderately emetogenic chemotherapy: 8 mg PO twice daily, starting 30 min before chemotherapy, the second dose given 8 hours later; one 8-mg tablet PO bid (every 12 hr) for 1–2 days after chemotherapy.
  - Children age 4–11 years: Moderately emetogenic chemotherapy: 4-mg tablet PO three times a day, the first 30 minutes before chemotherapy, then doses at 4 and 8 hours after the first dose. One 4-mg tablet PO every 8 hours for 1–2 days after chemotherapy.
- *Radiation therapy (RT):* Ondansetron 8 mg PO tid.
  - TBI: Give 8 mg tablet 1–2 hours prior to each fraction of radiation each day.
  - Single high-dose fraction: 8 mg 1–2 hours prior to RT, then every 8 hours after the first dose for 1–2 days after completion of RT.
  - Daily fractionated RT to abdomen: 8 mg PO 1–2 hours prior to RT, with subsequent doses every 8 hours after first dose for each day RT is given.

PONV *Adult and pediatric patients (age 1 month and older for IV):*
- *IV Adults:* 4 mg IVP (undiluted) over > 30 seconds before induction of anesthesia, or postoperatively if patient did not receive prophylactic antiemetics and experiences nausea and/or vomiting occurring within 2 hours of surgery; may also be given IM.
- *IV Pediatric* (age 1 month–12 years): weight ≤ 40 kg is 0.1-mg/kg single dose or if > 40 kg, a single 4-mg IV dose, IV over 2–5 minutes (at least 30 sec) immediately prior to or following anesthesia induction, or postoperatively if no previous prophylactic antiemetics and patient experiences nausea.
- *Oral Adults:* 16 mg (two 8-mg tablets or ODT) 1 hour before induction of anesthesia.

Patients with severe hepatic dysfunction (Child-Pugh score ≥ 10): maximum total daily dose of 8 mg.

Drug Preparation:

- The 4-mg and 8-mg doses of Zofran oral solution or Zofran oral disintegrating tablet (ODT) are bioequivalent to corresponding doses of Zofran tablets and may be used interchangeably. One Zofran 24-mg tablet is bioequivalent to and interchangeable with three 8-mg Zofran tablets.

* IV available as 2 mg/mL as single- or multi-dose vial; mix prescribed dose in 50 mL 5% dextrose or 0.9% sodium chloride and infuse over 15 minutes.
* Tablets available as either regular tablet or ODT (oral disintegrating tablet), which is freeze-dried and dissolves instantly on the tongue, available in 4-mg and 8-mg strengths.
* Zofran ODT available as 4-mg and 8-mg disintegrating tablets in unit packs of 30 tabs.
* Zofran Oral Solution available as 5 mg of ondansetron HCL dihydrate, equivalent to 4 mg of ondansetron per 5 mL, in glass bottles of 50 mL with child-resistant closures. Protect from light and store bottles upright.

Drug Administration:
* *IV:* Infuse over 15–30 minutes as above, or IVP in prevention of postoperative nausea/vomiting.
* *PO:* Administer per dosing above.
* Orally disintegrating tablet (Zofran ODT): with dry hands, peel back the foil backing of 1 blister and gently remove the tablet; immediately place the tablet on top of the tongue where it will dissolve in seconds; then swallow with saliva. Administer per dosing above.
* Oral Solution: Available as an oral solution, 4 mg/5 mL; 10 mL (2 tsp) is equivalent to one 8-mg Zofran tablet. Administer per dosing section above.
* Rarely, hypersensitivity reactions, including anaphylaxis and bronchospasm, have been reported in patients taking serotonin-receptor antagonists. Teach patient to stop taking drug and notify healthcare provider right away, or seek immediate medical help if reaction serious.

Drug Interactions:
* Apomorphine: concurrent use may result in profound hypotension and loss of consciousness; DO NOT give concurrently (contraindicated).
* Potent inducers of CYP3A4 (e.g., phenytoin, carbamazepine, rifampin): decrease serum levels of ondansetron but no dosage changes recommended for ondansetron.
* Tramadol: potential decreased analgesic effect when drugs are coadministered.
* Alkaline IV solutions: precipitate may form.

Lab Effects/Interference:
* Rarely, increased LFTs.

Special Considerations:
* Maximum IV dose is 16 mg. No larger dose should be given, as there is a dose-related increased risk of prolongation of QTc with potential for torsades de pointes.
* Avoid drug in patients with congenital long QT syndrome. Use ECG to monitor patients with electrolyte abnormalities (e.g., hypomagnesemia, hypokalemia), CHF, bradyarrhythmias, or patients taking other medication that prolongs the QT interval.
* Does not affect the dopamine system, so does not cause EPS.

MANAGEMENT

- Drug is excreted in breastmilk; use caution if administering to a woman who is nursing. Drug should be used during pregnancy only if clearly needed.
- Drug can mask a progressive ileus and gastric distention; drug does not stimulate gastric or intestinal peristalsis.

Potential Toxicities/Side Effects and the Nursing Process

I.   ALTERATION IN ELIMINATION related to DIARRHEA OR CONSTIPATION

Defining Characteristics: Patients may experience diarrhea (22%) or constipation (11%).

Nursing Implications: Assess baseline elimination status. Teach patient to report alterations, and treat symptomatically.

II.   ALTERATION IN COMFORT related to HEADACHE

Defining Characteristics: Headache may occur (16%).

Nursing Implications: Assess comfort level. Teach patient to report headache. Administer acetaminophen as ordered.

III.   ALTERATION IN NUTRITION, LESS THAN BODY REQUIREMENTS, related to LFTs

Defining Characteristics: Transient increases in LFTs may occur (5%).

Nursing Implications: Assess LFTs baseline, and monitor during therapy.

Drug: ondansetron oral soluble film (Zuplenz)

Class: Serotonin-receptor antagonist.

Mechanism of Action: Selective 5-HT$_3$ (serotonin) receptor antagonist and may block 5-HT$_3$ receptors found peripherally on the vagus nerve terminals and centrally in the CTZ, thus preventing chemotherapy-induced vomiting. Novel formulation.

Metabolism: Extensively metabolized, with only 5% of parent compound found in urine.

Indication: FDA-indicated for (1) prevention of nausea and vomiting associated with highly emetogenic cancer chemotherapy; (2) prevention of nausea and vomiting associated with initial and repeat courses of moderately emetogenic cancer chemotherapy; (3) prevention of nausea and vomiting associated with radiotherapy in patients receiving TBI, single high-dose fraction to abdomen, or daily fractions to the abdomen; (4) prevention of postoperative nausea and/or vomiting.

Contraindications: Patients hypersensitive to ondansetron, or concomitant use of apomorphine.

Dosage/Range:

Adult:

- *Prevention of nausea and vomiting associated with **highly emetogenic** cancer chemotherapy:* 24 mg given as successive 8-mg films, administered 30 minutes before the start of single-day highly emetogenic chemotherapy. Allow each oral soluble film to dissolve completely before administering the next film.
- *Prevention of nausea and vomiting associated with **moderately emetogenic** cancer chemotherapy:* One 8-mg film administered 30 minutes before start of emetogenic chemotherapy, with a subsequent dose 8 hours after the first dose. One 8-mg oral soluble film should be administered twice daily (every 12 hours) for 1–2 days after completion of chemotherapy.
- *Prevention of nausea and vomiting associated with radiotherapy:* One 8-mg film given three times a day.
- *Total body irradiation (TBI):* One 8-mg oral soluble film given 1–2 hours before each fraction of radiotherapy.
- *Single high-dose fraction radiotherapy to the abdomen:* One 8-mg oral soluble film given 1–2 hours before radiotherapy, with subsequent doses every 8 hours after the first dose for 1–2 days after completion of radiotherapy.
- *Daily fractionated radiotherapy to the abdomen:* One 8-mg oral soluble film given 1–2 hours before radiotherapy, with subsequent doses every 8 hours after the first dose for each day radiotherapy is given.
- *Prevention of postoperative nausea and/or vomiting:* 16 mg given successively as two 8-mg films 1 hour before induction of anesthesia. Allow the first oral soluble film to dissolve completely before administering the second film.
- *Dosage adjustment for patients with impaired hepatic function (Child-Pugh score > 10):* Do not exceed a total daily dose of 8 mg.

Pediatric (4–11 years of age):

- *Prevention of nausea and vomiting associated with moderately emetogenic cancer chemotherapy:* One 8-mg oral soluble film should be administered three times daily, starting 30 minutes before the start of emetogenic chemotherapy, with subsequent doses 4 and 8 hours after the first dose. One 4-mg oral soluble film should be administered three times a day (every 8 hours) for 1–2 days after the completion of chemotherapy.

Drug Preparation:

- Available in 4-mg and 8-mg oral soluble films, labeled with the dose, in a pouch package.

Drug Administration:

- With dry hands, fold the pouch along the dotted line to expose the tear notch. While still folded, tear the pouch carefully along the edge and remove the oral soluble film for the pouch. Immediately place the film on the top of the tongue, where it will dissolve in 4–20 seconds. Once dissolved, have the patient swallow with or without liquid. Wash hands after administering or taking the oral soluble film.

* Teach patient self-administration: see package insert and patient teaching tool.
* Rarely, hypersensitivity reactions, including anaphylaxis and bronchospasm, have been reported in patients taking serotonin-receptor antagonists. Teach patient to stop taking drug, and notify healthcare provider right away or seek immediate medical help if serious reaction occurs.

Drug Interactions:
* Apomorphine: profound hypotension and loss of consciousness.
* Phenytoin, carbamazepine, rifampicin: these are potent inducers of CYP3A4, and ondansetron clearance is significantly increased, with lower ondansetron serum levels. However, there are no data to show the soluble film dose should be increased.
* Tramadol: concomitant use may reduce analgesic activity of tramadol.

Lab Effects/Interference:
* Rarely, increased LFTs.

Special Considerations:
* Does not affect the dopamine system, so does not cause EPS.
* Hypersensitivity reactions, including anaphylaxis and bronchospasm, have been reported in patients with hypersensitivity to other selective 5-HT$_3$ receptor antagonists.
* Transient ECG changes, including QT interval prolongation, have been reported rarely, predominantly with IV ondansetron.
* The use of ondansetron in patients following abdominal surgery or in patients with chemotherapy-induced nausea and vomiting may mask a progressive ileus and/or gastric distention.
* The most common adverse drug reactions (> 5%) in chemotherapy- or radiotherapy-induced nausea and vomiting in trials were headache, mailaise/fatigue, constipation and diarrhea.
* The most common adverse drug reaction (> 5%) in postoperative nausea and vomiting trials was headache.

Potential Toxicities/Side Effects and the Nursing Process

I.   ALTERATION IN ELIMINATION related to DIARRHEA OR CONSTIPATION

Defining Characteristics: Patients may experience diarrhea (3–6%) or constipation (6–9%).

Nursing Implications: Assess baseline elimination status. Teach patient to report alterations, and treat symptomatically.

II.   ALTERATION IN COMFORT related to HEADACHE

Defining Characteristics: Headache may occur (11–27%).

Nursing Implications: Assess comfort level. Teach patient to report headache, and administer acetaminophen as ordered.

III. ALTERATION IN NUTRITION, LESS THAN BODY REQUIREMENTS, related to LFTs

Defining Characteristics: Rare, transient increases in LFTs may occur, especially in patients receiving cyclophosphamide-based chemotherapy (1–2%).

Nursing Implications: Assess LFTs baseline, and monitor during therapy.

Drug: palonosetron (Aloxi)

Class: Serotonin subtype 3 (5-HT$_3$) receptor antagonist antiemetic.

Mechanism of Action: Selective serotonin antagonist with strong binding affinity to receptor.

Metabolism: Drug is excreted via renal and metabolic pathways.

Indication: *Adults:* for (1) moderately emetogenic cancer chemotherapy-prevention of acute and delayed nausea and vomiting associated with initial and repeat courses; (2) highly emetogenic cancer chemotherapy-prevention of acute and delayed nausea and vomiting associated with initial and repeat courses; (3) prevention of postoperative nausea and vomiting (PONV) for up to 24 hours after surgery. Efficacy beyond 24 hours has not been demonstrated. *Pediatrics:* ages 1 month to < 17 years for (1) prevention of nausea and vomiting associated with initial and repeat courses of emetogenic cancer chemotherapy, including highly emetogenic cancer chemotherapy.

Dosage/Range:
- *Chemotherapy induced nausea and vomiting (CINV):*
  - *Adults*: single 0.25-mg IV over 30 **seconds**, given 30 minutes before the start of chemotherapy. Give once every 7 days.
  - *Pediatrics:* 20 mcg/kg (max 1.5 mg) × 1; infuse over 15 **minutes** beginning approximately 30 minutes before the start of chemotherapy.
- *Postoperative nausea and vomiting, Adult (PONV, Adult):*
  - A single 0.075-mg dose given IV over 10 **seconds** immediately before the induction of anesthesia.

Drug Preparation:
- Available at a concentration of 0.05 mg/mL (50 mcg/mL) and supplied as a single-use sterile glass vial that provides 0.25 mg/5mL (free base) and 0.075 mg/1.5 mL (free base).
- Draw up in a syringe to administer IVP, or draw up prescribed dose and place in appropriate pediatric pump for slow infusion over 15 minutes.

MANAGEMENT

Drug Administration:
- Inspect drug for particulate matter and discoloration, and do not use if found. Drug should be colorless without particulate matter.
- *Adult:* IV over 30 seconds (CINV) or 10 seconds (PONV) as above dosage section; flush line with normal saline prior to and after drug administration.
- *Pediatric:* IV Infuse over 15 minutes as above dosage section; flush line with normal saline prior to and after drug administration.
- Asssess for hypersensitivity reaction, including anaphylaxis, which has been reported in patients with or without known hypersensitivity to other selective 5-HT$_3$ receptor antagonists.

Drug Interactions:
- None known.

Lab Effects/Interference:
- Rare prolongation of QTc interval on ECG (> 500 msec, changes > 60 msec from baseline).

Special Considerations:
- Palonosetron has greater potency, higher binding affinity to the 5-HT$_3$ receptor, and has a longer half-life (40 hours) than any of the first-generation serotonin-receptor antagonists.
- Rarely, patients hypersensitive to other HT$_3$ receptor antagonists may be hypersensitive to palonosetron.
- Most common side effects are:
  - CINV (occurring in > 5%): headache, constipation.
  - PONV (occurring in > 2%): QT prolongation, bradycardia, headache, constipation.

Potential Toxicities/Side Effects and the Nursing Process

I.   ALTERATION IN COMFORT related to HEADACHE

Defining Characteristics: Headache occurs in 3.7% (capsule) 0–9% (IV) of patients.

Nursing Implications: Teach patients that this may occur, and to take acetaminophen to relieve headache if it occurs.

II.   ALTERATION IN BOWEL ELIMINATION related to CONSTIPATION

Defining Characteristics: Constipation occurs in about 0.6% (capsule) to 5% (injection) of patients.

Nursing Implications: Assess baseline bowel elimination status. Teach patients that constipation may occur, and to use usual strategies to prevent constipation. If constipation occurs, teach patient to use bowel softeners, laxatives as needed, and to increase oral fluids, fiber, and exercise to promote peristalsis.

III.   ALTERATION IN OXYGENATION related to RARE CARDIAC EVENTS

Defining Characteristics: Cardiovascular events are rare and occur in 1% of patients. These include nonsustained tachycardia, bradycardia, hypotension or hypertension, sinus arrhythmia, supraventricular extrasystoles, sinus tachycardia, and QT prolongation. The relationship to palonosetron was not clear in all instances. In nonclinical studies, palonosetron has the ability to block ion channels involved in ventricular depolarization and repolarization and to prolong action potential duration.

Nursing Implications: Assess baseline cardiac status, and monitor closely during therapy. Teach patient to notify the provider if any abnormalities occur, such as rapid or slow heartbeat.

Drug: prochlorperazine (Compazine)

Class: Phenothiazine.

Mechanism of Action: Blocks dopamine receptors in CTZ; also decreases vagal stimulation of VC by peripheral afferents.

Metabolism: Metabolized by liver, excreted in kidney, crosses placenta, excreted in breastmilk. Onset of action for oral is 30–40 minutes, duration 3–4 hours; extended release 30–40 minutes with duration 10–13 hours; PR onset 60 minutes, duration 3–4 hours; and IM onset 10–20 minutes, duration 12 hours.

Indication: (1) For the control of severe nausea and vomiting; and (2) treatment of schizophrenia.

Contraindication: Do not use (1) in patients with known hypersensitivity to phenothiazines; (2) in patients with comatose states or in the presence of large amounts of CNS depressants (e.g., alcohol, barbiturates, opioids); (3) in pediatric surgery; (4) in pediatric patients < 2 years of age or weighing < 20 lbs, or in children with conditions for which dosage has not been established. Drug is NOT indicated for the treatment of elderly patients with dementia-related psychosis treated with antipsychotic drugs, as there is an increased mortality in these patients.

Dosage/Range:
Adult:
- *Oral:* 5–25 mg q 4–6 h; slow-release: 10–75 mg q 12 h.
- *IM/IV:* 5–40 mg q 3–4 h; dilute in 50 mL 5% dextrose or 0.9% sodium chloride and administer IV over 20–30 minutes.
- *PR:* 25 mg q 4–6 h.

Drug Preparation:
- Store in tight, light-resistant containers. Administer IM injection deep into large muscle mass.

MANAGEMENT

Drug Interactions:
- Antacids: decreased prochlorperazine absorption; take 2 hours before or after antacid.
- Antidepressants: increased parkinsonian symptoms; avoid concomitant use or use cautiously.
- Barbiturates: decreased prochlorperazine effect; may need to increase dose of prochlorperazine.

Lab Effects/Interference:
- Rarely, may cause increased LFTs.

Special Considerations:
- Increased risk of dystonic reactions in men under 35 years old. Consider diphenhydramine or lorazepam and decadron q 4 h to minimize risk of dystonia.
- Dose-reduce in the elderly.
- Use cautiously in combination with CNS depressants.

Potential Toxicities/Side Effects and the Nursing Process

I.   ALTERATIONS IN SENSORY PERCEPTUAL PATTERN related to SEDATION, EPS

Defining Characteristics: Sedation, blurred vision, EPS reactions may occur, especially dystonia; also, seizure threshold may be lowered.

Nursing Implications: Assess baseline mental status. Teach patient to report signs/symptoms of EPS and assess for them during treatment (tongue protrusion, trismus, akathisia or restlessness, tremor, insomnia, dizziness). Administer diphenhydramine as ordered to reverse reaction. Diphenhydramine may be ordered prior to drug to prevent EPS.

II.   ALTERATION IN NUTRITION related to CONSTIPATION, APPETITE, CHOLESTATIC JAUNDICE

Defining Characteristics: Dry mouth, constipation, increased appetite and weight gain, cholestatic jaundice may occur.

Nursing Implications: Assess baseline nutritional patterns, moistness of mucous membranes, and elimination pattern. Assess baseline liver function, and monitor during therapy.

III.   ALTERATION IN SKIN INTEGRITY related to RASH

Defining Characteristics: Mild photosensitivity, rash, urticaria, and, rarely, exfoliative dermatitis may occur.

Nursing Implications: Assess baseline skin integrity. Teach patient to report any changes.

IV. ALTERATION IN CARDIAC OUTPUT related to ORTHOSTATIC HYPOTENSION

Defining Characteristics: Orthostatic hypotension, tachycardia, and EKG changes may occur.

Nursing Implications: Assess baseline VS prior to and during IV infusions, especially with high doses. Discuss with physician and anticipate increasing IV fluid rate if hypotensive.

Drug: scopolamine transdermal patch (Transderm Scop, The Travel Patch)

Class: Anti-muscarinic; used as an antiemetic.

Mechanism of Action: Appears to prevent nausea/vomiting associated with motion sickness by blocking cholinergic impulses, thus preventing stimulation of the VC.

Metabolism: Drug is well-absorbed percutaneously behind the ear, and circulating plasma levels detectable at 4 hours, and peak levels within 24 hours. Drug crosses placenta and blood–brain barrier, and may be reversibly bound to plasma proteins. Drug is extensively metabolized and conjugated, with < 10% of total dose excreted in the urine over 108 hours. Half-life of drug after patch removal is 9.5 hours.

Indication: In adults (1) for the prevention of nausea and vomiting associated with motion sickness; and (2) recovery from anesthesia and surgery. The patch should be applied only to the skin in the postauricular area.

Contraindication: For patients (1) who are hypersensitive to the drug scopolamine, to other belladonna alkaloids, or to other component ingredients in the drug or delivery system; and (2) with angle-closure (narrow-angle) glaucoma.

Dosage/Range:
Adult:
- Patch: transdermal patch 1.5 mg every 72 h.
- Drug releases 1 mg scopolamine over 3 days.

Drug Preparation:
- Available as a tan-colored circular patch, 2.5 cm^2 on a clear, oversized hexagonal peel strip, which is removed prior to use.
- Each patch contains 1.5 mg scopolamine and is programmed to deliver 1.0 mg scopolamine over 3 days.
- Available in packages of 4 patches, each individually wrapped.

MANAGEMENT

Drug Administration:
- Apply 4 hours prior to time protection is needed.
- To prevent postoperative nausea/vomiting, the patch should be applied the night before scheduled surgery.
- Apply to clean and dry hairless area behind ear; remove clear plastic cover, exposing adhesive layer; apply directly to skin behind ear and press firmly; wash hands.
- If patch falls off, wash area; then reapply new patch in another location behind the ear.
- If therapy is required for > 3 days, the first patch should be removed and a fresh one placed on the hairless area behind the other ear.
- For perioperative use, the patch should be kept in place for 24 hours after surgery, then removed and discarded.
- If patient needs an MRI, patch should be removed to avoid skin burns (patch contains aluminum).

Drug Interactions:
- None significant.

Lab Effects/Interference:
- None known.

Special Considerations:
- Wash hands after handling patch to prevent exposure to scopolamine.
- Use cautiously in:
  - Elderly patients with urinary bladder-neck obstruction.
  - Patients with history of seizures or psychosis, as drug can potentially aggravate both disorders.
  - Patients with impaired liver or renal function; there is increased likelihood of CNS effects.
  - Patients with chronic, open-angle glaucoma; monitor closely, as mydriatic effect of drug may increase intraocular pressure.
- Drug should not be used in children and should be used with caution in the elderly.
- Teach patients that drowsiness, disorientation, and confusion may occur with this drug, and to avoid activities that require mental alertness, such as driving a motor vehichle or operating dangerous machinery.
- Rarely, idiosyncratic reactions have occurred, including acute toxic psychosis, confusion, agitation, rambling speech, hallucinations, paranoid behaviors, and delusions.

Potential Toxicities/Side Effects and the Nursing Process

I.   ALTERATION IN MUCOUS MEMBRANE INTEGRITY related to DRY MOUTH

Defining Characteristics: Dry mouth occurs in 67% of patients.

Nursing Implications: Teach patient this may occur. Suggest patient suck ice chips, sugar-free candy, or practice usual oral hygiene regimen more frequently.

II. ALTERATIONS IN SENSORY/PERCEPTUAL PATTERNS related to DROWSINESS, BLURRED VISION

Defining Characteristics: Drowsiness, blurred vision, mydriasis may occur; rarely, disorientation, restlessness, confusion may occur.

Nursing Implications: Assess baseline mental status. Instruct patient to report changes in vision or feeling state. Assess patient safety needs, and provide safe environment.

Chapter 8
Anorexia and Cachexia

Anorexia and weight loss may be presenting symptoms of cancer, or symptoms of advanced disease. No other symptoms may cause more powerful distress to a patient than being confronted with weight loss and inability to eat due to anorexia. Consequences of severe anorexia include nutritional depletion and further weight loss, which result in decreased functional status, diminished treatment responses to chemotherapy, and apparent decreased quality of life. Primary cachexia, or wasting syndrome, occurs in at least two-thirds of patients with advanced cancer or human immunodeficiency virus (HIV) disease. The associated extreme weakness and fatigue lead to incapacity, dependency, social isolation, and again, apparent diminished quality of life.

Anorexia and cachexia can be terrifying and frustrating to family members. The patient's spouse may be used to nurturing the patient and preparing meals, and feel rejected and frightened by a loved one's inability to eat. This may symbolize personal failure on the part of the spouse, as well as failure of current treatment to reverse the disease process and a poor prognosis.

Fearon et al. (2011) report on international consensus development of definition and classification: a multifactorial syndrome defined an ongoing loss of skeletal muscle mass (with or without loss of fat mass) that cannot be fully reversed by traditional nutritional support interventions, and it leads to progressive functional impairment. Pathophysiology was attributed to negative protein and energy balance related to abnormal metabolism and decreased food intake. Diagnostic criterion for cachexia was a weight loss > 5% or weight loss > 2% in patients already depleted (BMI < 20 kg/m^2 or decreased skeletal muscle mass [sarcopenia]). The group also identified that the cachexia syndrome can progress through stages: from precachexia to cachexia to refractory cachexia.

In the literature, metabolically, cachexia appears to result from chronic, systemic inflammation with the release of acute-phase proteins and orchestration by cytokines such as tumor necrosis factor, IL-1 and IL-6 (Laviano et al., 2002). Morley et al. (2006) suggest that other potential mediators of cachexia are testosterone, insulin-like growth factor I deficiency, excess myostatin, and excess glucocorticoids. This leads to the preferential breakdown of skeletal muscle protein and body fat, resulting in the profound wasting syndrome characterized by anorexia, early satiety, weight loss, decreased function, and death (Inui, 2002). Secondary cachexia is simple starvation from decreased food intake or defective nutrient absorption, and results from situations such as nausea, vomiting, and anorexia due to chemotherapy. As expected, patients responding to chemotherapy will show a weight gain.

Pharmacologic agents used to stimulate appetite are varied in mechanism of action, efficacy, and strength of evidence. Corticosteroids have been tried for many years, with usual effect within 1–3 weeks (Ottery et al., 1998; Loprinzi et al., 1999). However, side effects, such as insomnia, muscle catabolism, and hyperglycemia, have limited their usefulness. When compared with megestrol acetate 800 mg/day, dexamethasone (0.75 mg four times daily) patients had similar responses but different toxicities: megestrol acetate caused thromboembolism, whereas dexamethasone caused myopathy, peptic ulcers, and problems related to Cushingoid side effects (Loprinzi et al., 1999). Of the studies of pharmacologic agents in the treatment of anorexia and cachexia in cancer, megestrol acetate has shown statistical improvement in nonfluid weight gain (Ottery, 1998). Mantovani et al. (1998) suggest that megestrol acetate, in fact, downregulates cytokine production, resulting in increased appetite and anabolism. There appears to be a dose-response effect, and Loprinzi et al. (1992) showed optimal weight gain at a dose of 800 mg/day. Patients showed increased appetite, increased food intake, weight gain, and less nausea and vomiting. The incidence of thrombophlebitis was 6%. Loprinzi et al. also demonstrated that the weight gain resulting from megestrol acetate is increased fat and lean body mass, not water gain (i.e., edema, ascites).

Metoclopramide, at low doses for stimulation of GI motility, has been shown to decrease early satiety and postprandial fullness, and may be helpful for some patients (Kris et al., 1985). Cannabinoid derivatives, such as δ-9-tetrahydrocannabinol (THC) and dronabinol, appear to stimulate appetite and possible weight gain in some patients (Beal et al., 1997; Kaplan et al., 1998; Klausner et al., 1996; Jatoi, 2006). Eicosapentaenoic acid (EPA) (fish oil, thought to stabilize acute phase proteins) in a nutritional supplement was compared with megestrol acetate or a combination of both; megestrol acetate was found more effective in stimulating appetite (Jatoi et al., 2004). Studies continue to explore whether other agents, such as melatonin (regulation of circadian rhythm), can be of benefit (Cunningham, 2003).

The ONS Putting Evidence into Practice (PEP) cards for anorexia recommend for practice, based on strong evidence from rigorously conducted studies, corticosteroids (reserved for those with anorexia with advanced disease or who may have disease regression, where a short-term benefit is needed), and progestins. In addition, they point out that dietary counseling is likely to be effective, as individual dietary counseling has been shown to improve nutritional intake and body weight. They point out that effectiveness is not established for cyproheptadine, EPA, erythropoietin, ghrelin, metoclopramide, oral branched chain amino acids, pentoxifylline, and thalidomide. Effectiveness is unlikely with cannabinoids, hydrazine sulfate, and melatonin (Adams et al., 2008).

It is exciting to think that perhaps nutritional stimulation might improve the patient's ability to tolerate aggressive therapy or in some way improve efficacy of the treatment; however, a randomized, double-blind, controlled trial compared megestrol acetate or placebo together with chemotherapy and radiation therapy for newly diagnosed patients with extensive small cell lung cancer (SCLC), and there was no difference in patient response (efficacy), quality of life, or overall survival between the two groups (Loprinzi & Jatoi, 2007). In an earlier study (1999) with chemotherapy only, patients receiving megestrol acetate had more thromboembolic events and edema, and inferior response to chemotherapy and survival (Rowland et al., 1996).

MANAGEMENT

References

Adams L, Cunningham R, Caruso RA, Norling M, Shepard N. *Anorexia: What Interventions Are Effective in Managing Anorexia in People with Cancer.* Pittsburgh, PA, Oncology Nursing Society, 2008.

Beal JE. Long-term Efficacy and Safety of Dronabinol for Acquired Immunodeficiency Syndrome-associated Anorexia. *J Pain Symptom Manage* 1997; 14(1) 7–14.

Cunningham RS. (2014). The Cancer Cachexia Syndrome, Chapter 17 in Yarbro CH, Wujuk D, Gobel BH (eds). *Cancer Symptom Management*, 4th ed. Burlington, MA: Jones & Bartlett Learning, 351–384.

Fearon K, Strasser F, Anker SD et al. (2011). Definition and classification of cancer cachexia: An international consensus. *Lancet Oncol* 12(5): 489–95.

Inui A. Cancer Anorexia-Cachexia Syndrome: Current Issues in Research and Management. *CA Cancer J Clin* 2002; 52 72–91.

Jatoi A, Rowland K, Loprinzi CL, et al. An Eicosapentaenoic Acid Supplement Versus Megestrol Acetate Versus Both for Patients with Cancer-Associated Wasting: A North Central Cancer Treatment Group and National Cancer Institute of Canada Collaborative Effort. *J Clin Oncol* 2004; 22 2469–2476.

Jatoi A. Pharmacologic Therapy for the Cancer Anorexia/Weight Loss Syndrome: A Data Driven, Practical Approach. *J Support Oncol* 2006; 4(10) 499–502.

Klausner JD, Makonkawkeyoon S, Akarasewi P, et al. The Effect of Thalidomide on the Pathogenesis of Human Immunodeficiency Virus Type 1 and *M. tuberculosis* Infection. *J Acquir Immune Defic Syndr Hum Retrovirology* 1996; 11 247–257.

Kornblith AB, Hollis D, Phillips CA, et al. Effect of Megestrol Acetate upon Quality of Life in Advanced Breast Cancer Patients in a Dose Response Trial. *Proc Am Soc Clin Oncol* 1992; 11 377.

Kris MG, Yeh SDJ, Gralla RJ, et al. Symptomatic Gastroparesis in Cancer Patients: Possible Cause of Anorexia That Can Be Improved with Oral Metoclopramide. *Proc Am Soc Clin Oncol* 1985; 4 267.

Laviano A, Russo M, Freda F, et al. Neurochemical Mechanisms for Cancer Cachexia. *Nutrition* 2002; 18 100–105.

Loprinzi C, Jatoi A. Anorexia and Cachexia. In Pazdur R, Coia LR, Hoskins WJ, Wagman LD (eds). *Cancer Management: A Multidisciplinary Approach*, 10th ed. Lawrence, KS: CMP Healthcare Media LLC; 2007.

Loprinzi CL, Ellison NM, Schard OJ, et al. Controlled Trial of Megestrol Acetate for the Treatment of Cancer Anorexia and Cachexia. *J Natl Cancer Inst* 1990; 82 1127–1132.

Loprinzi CL, Jensen M, Burnham N, et al. Body Composition Changes in Cancer Patients Who Gain Weight from Megestrol Acetate. *Proc Am Soc Clin Oncol* 1992; 11 378.

Loprinzi CL, Kugler JW, Sloan JA, et al. Randomized Comparison of Megestrol Acetate Versus Dexamethasone Versus Fluoxymesterone for the Treatment of Cancer Anorexia/Cachexia. *J Clin Oncol* 1999; 17 3299–3306.

Loprinzi CL, Mailliard J, Schaid D, et al. Dose/Response Evaluation of Megestrol Acetate for the Treatment of Cancer Anorexia/Cachexia: A Mayo Clinic and North Central Cancer Treatment Group Trial. *Proc Am Soc Clin Oncol* 1992; 11 378.

Mantovani G, Maccio A, Paola L, et al. Cytokine Activity in Cancer-related Anorexia/Cachexia: Role of Megestrol Acetate and Medroxyprogesterone Acetate. *Semin Oncol* 1998; 25 (suppl) 45–52.

Morley JE, Thomas DR, Wilson MMG. Cachexia: Pathophysiology and Relevance. *Am J Clin Nutr* 2006; 83 735–743.

Ottery FD, Walsh D, Strawford A. Pharmacologic Management of Anorexia/Cachexia. *Semin Oncol* 1998; 25 (suppl) 35–44.

Rowland KM, Loprinzi CL, Shaw EG, et al. Randomized Double Blind Placebo Controlled Trial of Cisplatin and Etoposide Plus Megestrol Acetate/Placebo in Extensive-Stage Small Cell Lung Cancer: A North Central Cancer Treatment Group Study. *J Clin Oncol* 1996; 14 135–141.

Drug: dronabinol (Marinol)

Class: Cannabinoid.

Mechanism of Action: Stimulates appetite in acquired immunodeficiency syndrome (AIDS) patients, leading to trends toward improved body weight and mood.

Metabolism: 90–95% absorption after oral dose, but because of first-pass effect of the liver and high lipid solubility, only about 20% of the dose reaches the systemic circulation. Large area of distribution so that drug continues to be excreted for a long period of time. The appetite stimulation effect may persist for 24 hours from a single dose.

Indication: For the treatment of (1) anorexia associated with weight loss in patients with AIDS; and (2) nausea and vomiting associated with cancer chemotherapy in patients who have failed to respond adequately to conventional antiemetic treatments.

Dosage/Range:
- 2.5 mg bid before lunch and supper, or if patient is intolerant, a single 2.5-mg dose may be taken in the evening or at bedtime.
- If clinically indicated and if no significant adverse effects, dose may be gradually increased to a maximum of 20 mg/day.

Drug Preparation:
- Available in 2.5-, 5-, or 10-mg gel capsules that harden under refrigeration.

Drug Administration:
- Oral.

Drug Interactions:
- Amphetamines, cocaine: additive hypertension, tachycardia.
- Atropine, scopolamine: tachycardia, drowsiness.
- Amitriptyline, tricyclic antidepressants: additive tachycardia, hypertension.
- Barbiturates, CNS depressants, buspirone: drowsiness and additive CNS depression.
- Theophylline: increased metabolism.

Lab Effects/Interference:
- None known.

Special Considerations:
- Contains sesame oil, so should not be used by patients allergic to sesame oil.
- Can produce physical and psychological dependency.
- Can cause dry mouth.
- Warnings and Precautions:
  - Teach patient not to drive, operate machinery, or engage in hazardous activity until it is clear they can tolerate the drug and perform these tasks.
  - Use cautiously and only if benefit outweighs risk in patients with:
    - Seizure disorder, as drug may lower seizure threshold.

MANAGEMENT

- Cardiac disorders, as occasional hypotension, HTN, syncope, and/or tachycardia may occur.
- History of substance abuse, as drug has abuse potential.
- History of mania, depression, schizophrenia, as drug may exacerbate these conditions; monitor patients closely.
- Patients receiving concomitant CNS depressants (e.g., sedatives, hypnotics, other psychoactive drugs), as CNS effects may be additive or synergistic.
- Elderly, as they may be more sensitive to the neurological, psychoactive, and postural hypotensive effects of the drug.
- Pregnant women, nursing mothers, and pediatric patients, as drug has not been studied in these patient populations.
- Drug has antiemetic qualities.

Potential Toxicities/Side Effects and the Nursing Process

I.   ALTERATIONS IN SENSORY/PERCEPTUAL PATTERNS related to CNS CHANGES

Defining Characteristics: Drug can cause changes in mood, cognition, memory, and perception. In addition, nervousness, anxiety, confusion, dizziness, depersonalization, euphoria, paranoid reaction, somnolence, and thinking abnormalities can occur. Drug has abuse potential.

Nursing Implications: Assess appropriateness of drug for patient, as this would not be the drug of choice for a substance abuser, either one who is actively using or who has withdrawn and is abstaining because of abuse potential. Teach patient of possible side effects, as well as self-care strategies to avoid heightened fear or anxiety.

II.   POTENTIAL FOR ALTERATION IN OXYGENATION related to SYMPATHOMIMETIC EFFECTS

Defining Characteristics: Tachycardia and conjunctival infection may occur. Drug interactions may cause hypertension.

Nursing Implications: Review patient medication profile to identify any possible drug interactions. Monitor appetite stimulation effects, and weigh these against any sympathomimetic changes.

Drug: megestrol acetate oral suspension (Megace OS)

Class: Synthetic progestin.

Mechanism of Action: Alters malignant cell environment in hormonally sensitive tumors, discouraging tumor cell proliferation; appears to stimulate appetite and weight gain in cancer cachexia directly or indirectly through antagonism of TNF. Designated as orphan drug by FDA for management of anorexia, cachexia, or weight loss > 10% of baseline. Approved for AIDS-related cachexia.

Metabolism: Well-absorbed from GI tract. Metabolized in liver and excreted by kidneys.

Indication: Treatment of anorexia, cachexia, or an unexplained, significant weight loss in patients with a diagnosis of acquired immunodeficiency syndrome (AIDS).

Contraindication: Megace ES: known hypersensitivity, known or suspected pregnancy.

Dosage/Range:
- Optimal dose for management of cachexia is 800 mg/day in a single dose.
- Studies showed that daily doses of 400 mg and 800 mg a day were found to be clinically effective.
- Available in:
  - Megace OS 40 mg/mL.
  - Megace ES formulation (concentrated suspension) delivering 625 mg (125 mg/mL), which has been shown equivalent to the 800 mg of Megace oral suspension (40 mg/mL) (in volunteers under federally approved conditions).

Drug Preparation:
- Store in tight container at temperature 15°–25°C (59°–77°F).
- Available in bottles of 240 mL (8 fl oz).
- Oral administration: shake container well before using.

Drug Administration:
- 20 mL Megase OS (800 mg) PO once a day; OR
- 5 mL of Megace ES (625 mg) once a day.

Drug Interactions:
- None.

Lab Effects/Interference:
- May increase glucose, lactic dehydrogenase (LDH).
- Rare leukopenia.

Special Considerations:
- One-third of patients with metastatic cancer gain weight.
- Weight gain appears to be from increased fat stores rather than from water gain (Loprinzi et al., 1992).
- Warnings and Precautions:
  - Drug can cause fetal harm. Teach women to avoid pregnancy; if used during pregnancy, the patient should be apprised of the potential hazard to the fetus.
  - Drug is not intended for prophylactic use to avoid weight loss.
  - Drug has glucocorticoid activity and may exacerbate or lead to new onset diabetes mellitus; care should be taken if the drug is stopped to prevent adrenal insufficiency (slowly withdraw drug).
  - Use cautiously in diabetics and patients with a history of thromboembolic disease.
- Breakthrough vaginal bleeding may occur in women.

- Women of reproductive age who are sexually active should use effective contraception to avoid pregnancy.
- Nursing mothers should make a decision to stop nursing or stop the drug, taking into consideration the importance of the drug to the mother's health.
- Most common adverse events in > 5% of patients receiving 800 mg/20 mL Megace OS in 2 clinical efficacy trials were nausea, diarrhea, impotence, rash, flatulence, HTN, and asthenia.

Potential Toxicities/Side Effects and the Nursing Process

I.   ALTERATIONS IN PERFUSION related to DEEP VEIN THROMBOSIS

Defining Characteristics: Rarely, 6% of patients may experience deep vein thrombosis (DVT) or pulmonary emboli.

Nursing Implications: Assess baseline peripheral vascular status and monitor during therapy. Teach patient to report immediately pain in calf, erythema, shortness of breath, chest pain.

II.   ALTERATION IN NUTRITION related to HYPERGLYCEMIA

Defining Characteristics: Hyperglycemia is uncommon but may be significant if it occurs.

Nursing Implications: Assess baseline FBS, and monitor during therapy. Teach patient signs and symptoms of hyperglycemia and to report them (polydipsia, polyuria, polyphagia).

III.   ALTERATION IN COMFORT related to CARPAL TUNNEL SYNDROME, NAUSEA AND VOMITING, TUMOR FLARE

Defining Characteristics: Carpal tunnel syndrome, nausea, vomiting, tumor flare may occur rarely.

Nursing Implications: Instruct patient to report any signs/symptoms. Discuss with patient, physician symptomatic measures.

IV.   ANXIETY related to ABNORMAL UTERINE BLEEDING

Defining Characteristics: Breakthrough vaginal bleeding, discharge often occur in females, and can cause anxiety.

Nursing Implications: Teach female patient that this is an expected side effect. Encourage patient to verbalize feelings, provide patient with emotional support and information about cause and management.

Chapter *9*
Anxiety *and* Depression

Anxiety and depression in response to uncertainty and hopelessness are frequently associated with the cancer experience. Studies have shown that anxiety increases with the cancer diagnosis and remains elevated to some degree throughout treatment, regardless of modality or setting (Clark, 1990). Drugs such as CNS stimulants, psychotropics, steroids, and caffeine may cause anxiety (Rucker and Gobel, 2014). The American Society of Clinical Oncology (ASCO) (Andersen et al., 2014) promulgates screening, assessment, and care of anxiety and depressive symptoms in adult patients with cancer, using available evidence-based tools, which can be found on their website. These include management algorithms for both anxiety and depression. The ASCO/Oncology Nursing Society (ONS) Chemotherapy Administration Safety Standards (2013) include assessment of psychosocial concerns, including anxiety and depression, and need for support, with action taken as needed.

Nursing efforts are aimed at anxiety-reducing strategies, such as helping the patient explore the anxiety and find anxiety-reducing activities (e.g., relaxation exercises, verbalization of feelings). Nurses can also refer patients for specialized support if necessary, and, as appropriate, teach patients and their families about prescribed anxiolytic medications. Depression is an often expected response to the cancer experience, to an actual or perceived loss of health, role, and life. The reported incidence of depression in hospitalized cancer patients is 25–42% (Trask, 2004). It also may be associated with chronic cancer pain and can clearly adversely affect quality of life. Prominent features may be perceived loss of self-esteem, worthlessness, hopelessness, guilt, and sadness. There is a continuum of depression, ranging from everyday sadness to severe, debilitating depression with physical and/or psychological symptoms that constitute a major depressive disorder (Valentine, 2007). Pyter et al. (2009) postulated that malignant tumors released substances that contribute to depression. Although the study was conducted with rats, it showed that these animals were less eager to eat and had increased levels of cytokines in both blood and the hippocampus, compared to healthy rats. Certain antineoplastic medications can be associated with depression, such as docetaxel, interferon- alpha, interleukin-2, leuprolide, paclitaxel, and tamoxifen (Fulcher, 2014). Most commonly in practice, nurses assess patient symptoms of changes in appetite, sleeplessness, lethargy, and social withdrawal. Nurses use caring and compassion to help patients who are depressed acknowledge and explore their feelings. Through patient teaching and supportive counseling, short-term realistic and achievable goals can often be negotiated by patient and nurse. Now, nurses are helping patients to make the "mountain" more manageable.

Patients cope individually with the multiple threats that cancer brings. Patients with depression may have a variety of symptoms that fall within one or more categories of functioning, with symptoms that may include (ASCO, 2007):

- Mood symptoms: feelings of sadness, helplessness, hopelessness; irritability; feelings of guilt or worthlessness.
- Cognitive symptoms: decreased ability to concentrate, decreased memory, suicidal thoughts.
- Physical symptoms: fatigue or low energy, poor appetite, inability to experience pleasure.
- Behavioral symptoms: social withdrawal, crying spells, loss of interest in activities or hobbies, decreased sex drive.

In 2007, the Institute of Medicine published a report called *Cancer Care for the Whole Patient,* and proposed a model based on the NCCN model of psychosocial care that should be incorporated into routine cancer care: screening for distress and psychosocial needs, making a treatment plan to address the needs and implementing it, referring to specialists/services as needed, and reevaluating and revising the plan as needed (IOM, 2007). Nurses have been using the nursing process to do this routinely, but now it has become a team responsibility. Long thought to be an integral component in the clinical management of cancer patients, today, national organizations committed to outstanding oncology care have developed standards to ensure that the consistent assessment of patient's psychosocial issues is routinely performed during the cancer experience, such as NCCN, The Joint Commission, and Quality Oncology Performance Initiative (QOPI, ASCO's quality arm) (NCCN, 2012). In Canada, emotional distress is called the 6th vital sign that is routinely assessed (Bultz & Carlson, 2005).

Of course, pharmacotherapy is also very important. It is generally accepted that depression results from a deficiency in key neurotransmitters, resulting in either an overexpression or underexpression of neurotransmitters that control the release or breakdown of the neurotransmitters (Barsevick & Much, 2003).

The tricyclic antidepressant (TCA) medications once were the cornerstone of managing cancer-related depression, partially because of their ability to improve sleeplessness and to enhance analgesia. These drugs include amitriptyline (Elavil). However, these drugs also have undesirable side effects, such as dry mouth, constipation, and blurred vision related to their anticholinergic, α-adrenergic–blocking, and antihistamine properties (Valentine, 2007). Serotonin antagonist reuptake inhibitors (SARIs) raise serotonin levels and include trazodone (Desyrel). Common side effects include dry mouth, dizziness, sedation, orthostasis, and rarely priapism in men. Monoamine oxidase inhibitors (MAOIs) are not used often because of the many drug interactions that can occur. These drugs are phenelzine (Nardil) and tranylcypromine (Parnate) and prevent the breakdown of neurotransmitters, thus increasing their levels. Side effects include insomnia and orthostasis.

Newer antidepressant medications are more commonly used and have found a firm niche in oncology care. The selective serotonin reuptake inhibitors (SSRIs) are quite effective for many patients and have few side effects, together with a short half-life. In addition, they differ from the TCAs in that they are generally less lethal if a patient accidentally overdoses (except citalopram hydrobromide). They also do not possess anticholinergic or α-adrenergic–blocking properties and thus are safer in medically complex patients (Valentine, 2007). These agents block serotonin reuptake, and thus, more serotonin is available as a neurotransmitter; they include fluoxetine (Prozac), sertraline (Zoloft), citalopram

(Celexa), escitalopram (Lexapro), and paroxetine (Paxil). Common side effects are nausea, insomnia, headache, and sexual problems. The serotonin-norepinephrine reuptake inhibitors (SNRIs) increase the levels of norepinephrine as well as serotonin to act as neurotransmitters. Drugs in this category are venlafaxine (Effexor), duloxetine (Cymbalta), and mirtazapine (Remeron), and common side effects are nausea, dry mouth, headache, and sedation. Another SNRI, desvenlafaxine (Pristiq) is a synthetic form of the active metabolite of venlafaxine that is being studied as a nonhormonal treatment for menopausal symptoms.

Because of an increased risk of suicidality (suicidal thinking and behavior) in young adults 18–24 years old during the initial treatment (first 1–2 months), the FDA has required that all antidepressant drugs indicate this risk as a black box warning (FDA, 2007).

Massie and Popkin (1998) suggest principles to guide antidepressant therapy in patients with cancer: start with a lower dose, slowly increase the dose, as the therapeutic dose may be lower than that in noncancer patients, and monitor very carefully for side effects, as there may be overlapping toxicity in organ systems (with chemotherapy, the malignancy).

In addition, it is important to do a thorough assessment of herbs used in the management of anxiety and depression, as these may be interacting with anticancer drug therapy. For example, St. John's wort is both an inducer and/or inhibitor of the key metabolic CYP3A4, CYP2C9, and CYP2D6 pathways. It induces the metabolism of irinotecan primary active metabolite SN-38 via the cytochrome P450 CYP3A4 subsystem, lowering serum levels by up to 42% with an effect lasting up to 3 weeks (Mathijssen et al., 2002). Table 9.1 depicts antianxiety and antidepressant agents commonly prescribed.

Table 9.1   Agents Commonly Used in the Management of Anxiety and Depression in Patients with Cancer

Drug	Dose Range (Oral)	Half-Life or Onset of Therapeutic Effect	Common Side Effects	Comments
Antianxiety				
Alprazolam (Xanax)	0.25–1.0 mg PO every 6–24 hours	10–15 hours half-life	Sedation, confusion, motor incoordination, somnolence	Short half-life; rapid onset; tolerance may develop rapidly
Clonazepam (Klonopin)	0.5–2.0 PO every 6–24 hours	Peak serum level 1–2 hours; half-life 18–60 hours, median 30–40 hours	Drowsiness, dizziness, motor incoordination, orthostasis, ↓ mental alertness	Increased CNS depressant effects when combined with CNS depressants
Chlorazepate (Tranxene)	15–30 mg a day, maximum 60 mg/day	48 hours	Dizziness, blurred vision, insomnia, nausea, muscle weakness, amnesia	Long half-life leads to accumulation of active metabolites

(continued)

Table 9.1   *(Continued)*

Drug	Dose Range (Oral)	Half-Life or Onset of Therapeutic Effect	Common Side Effects	Comments
Diazepam (Valium, Valrelease)	2–10 mg every 6–24 hours PO, IM, IV	20–70 hours half-life	Drowsiness, fatigue, lethargy, weakness, rash, vivid dreams, feeling "hung over"	Long half-life, so accumulation of active metabolites; fast absorption; difficult to use in older patients
Lorazepam (Ativan)	0.5–2.0 mg PO, IM, IV every 4–12 hours	10–20 hours half-life	Drowsiness, fatigue, lethargy, weakness, rash, vivid dreams	Short half-life with intermediate absorption; continuous IV infusion in severe cases
Oxazepam (Serax)	30–120 mg/day (usual max dose 60 mg/day)	5–15 hours	Drowsiness, fatigue, lethargy, weakness, rash, vivid dreams	Short half-life

Antidepressants SSRIs

Drug	Dose Range (Oral)	Half-Life or Onset of Therapeutic Effect	Common Side Effects	Comments
Paroxetine (Paxil)	20 mg to start PO (morning) to 50 mg every day 62.5 mg if paroxetine CR	Onset 3–10 days	Nausea, dry mouth, rash, headache, drowsiness, loss of libido, postural hypotension, mild nausea, anxiety; sedation	Caution in elderly, patients with renal or hepatic dysfunction, suicidal ideation; dose ↑ if needed after 2–3 weeks; if renal or hepatic dysfunction, begin with one-half to one-fourth of the normal starting dose to start
Sertraline (Zoloft)	50 PO to start (morning), up to 200 mg every day	Onset 7 days	Same as paroxetine, except, no sedation, sexual dysfunction	Same
Fluoxetine (Prozac)		Onset 2–4 weeks	Same as paroxetine; sexual dysfunction	Same
Escitalopram (Lexapro)	10 mg PO daily; if ↑ to 20 mg daily, do so after at least 1 week	Half-life of 27–32 hours; steady-state plasma levels in 1 week	Same as paroxetine, no sedation	Same
Citalopram hydrobromide (Celexa)	20 mg PO to start (morning); 40 mg PO daily after at least 1 week	Terminal half-life of 25 hours; steady state in 1 week	Same as paroxetine, except may be fatal if overdosed	Same

Table 9.1   *(Continued)*

Drug	Dose Range (Oral)	Half-Life or Onset of Therapeutic Effect	Common Side Effects	Comments
TCAs				
Amitriptyline (Elavil)	25–250 mg	Onset 4–6 weeks	Anticholinergic (urinary retention, dry mouth, thirst, blurred vision, sedation) and antihistaminic (sedation); tachycardia, orthostatic hypotension, arrhythmia; withdrawal reaction	Caution in patients with suicidal ideation, cardiac/renal or hepatic dysfunction; don't stop drug abruptly; do baseline EKG and assess toxicity
Desipramine (Norpramin)	25–150 mg	4–6 weeks	Same as amitriptyline	Same as amitriptyline; serum level correlates with therapeutic effect
Doxepin (Sinequan)	50–150 mg	4–6 weeks	Same as amitriptyline	Same as amitriptyline
Imipramine (Tofranil)	25–150 mg	4–6 weeks	Same as amitriptyline	Same as amitriptyline; serum level correlates with therapeutic effect
Nortriptyline (Pamelor)	50–150 mg	4–6 weeks	Same as amitriptyline	Same as amitriptyline; serum level correlates with therapeutic effect
Trazodone (Dyseril)	50–250 mg	1–4 weeks	Same as amitriptyline	Same as amitriptyline
SNRI				
Venlafaxine HCl (Effexor)	75–225 mg/day	1–4 weeks	Emotional lability, vertigo, trismus, nausea	Use cautiously in elderly, patients with cardiac/renal or hepatic dysfunction; also helpful with hot flashes
Nefazodone HCl (Serzone)	200–600 mg/day	1–4 weeks	Dizziness, drowsiness, dry mouth, headache	Use cautiously in elderly, patients with cardiac/renal or hepatic dysfunction
Duloxetine (Cymbalta)	40 mg daily to start, ↑ to 60 mg PO daily	Half-life of 12 hours, steady-state achieved in 3 days	Nausea, dry mouth, constipation, diarrhea, insomnia, decreased appetite, somnolence	Contraindicated if narrow angle glaucoma; indicated in patients with peripheral neuropathic pain

MANAGEMENT

(continued)

Table 9.1 *(Continued)*

Drug	Dose Range (Oral)	Half-Life or Onset of Therapeutic Effect	Common Side Effects	Comments
Mirtazapine (Remeron)	15 mg PO daily to start; ↑ to 45 mg PO daily after 2–4 weeks if needed	Elimination half-life of 20–40 hours; steady state in 3–4 days	↑ appetite, weight gain, peripheral edema; CNS effects, drowsiness, orthostasis	Use cautiously and monitor closely hepatic or renal insufficiency, epilepsy, organic brain syndrome, heart disease, BPH, acute narrow angle glaucoma, DM; rare BMD
Desvenlafaxine (Pristiq)	50 mg recommended dose; may slowly ↑ dose to 400 mg in clinical trials	Elimination half-life 11 hrs; time to steady state 4–5 days	Nausea, headache, dry mouth, sweating, dizziness, insomnia	Dose reduction for severe renal impairment; use cautiously in older persons or in patients with cardiac/renal or hepatic dysfunction
Atypical (unknown MOA)				
Bupropion hydrochloride (Wellbutrin)	100 mg PO twice daily for at least 3 days, may ↑ to 100 mg three times daily; after 4 weeks may ↑ to 150 mg three times daily if needed	Half-life of 14 hours	Weight loss, restlessness, agitation, insomnia, dizziness, tachycardia, changes in BP, dry mouth, anorexia, nausea, vomiting, urinary retention	Drug increases activity, so useful if psychomotor slowing; rare sexual dysfunction; may cause seizures; contraindicated if history of seizures, bulimia, anorexia nervosa

BPH: benign prostatic hypertrophy, DM: diabetes mellitus, BMD: bone marrow depression.
Data from Rucker Y, Gobel BH (2014). Anxiety. Yarbro CH, Wujuk D, Gobel BH (Eds). *Cancer Symptom Management* (4th ed.). Jones & Bartlett Learning, Burlington, MA, pp. 619–637; Fulcher CD (2014). Depression. Yarbro CH, Wujuk D, Gobel BH (Eds). *Cancer Symptom Management* (4th ed.). Jones & Bartlett Learning, Burlington, MA, pp. 655–673.

References

Adler NE, Page NEK, Institute of Medicine (IOM): http://www.iom.edu/Reports/2007/Cancer-Care-for-the-Whole-Patient-Meeting-Psychosocial-Health-Needs.aspx; assessed 7/7/12 2008 Cancer Care for the Whole Patient: Meeting Psychosocial Health Needs.

Andersen BL, DeRubeis RJ, Berman BS et al. Screening, assessment, and care of anxiety and depressive symptoms in adults with cancer: an American Society of Clinical Oncology guideline adaptation. *J Clin Oncol* 2014;32(15):1605–1619. Tools available at http://www.asco.org/screening-assessment-and-care-anxiety-and-depressive-symptoms-adults-cancer-american-society, accessed September 21, 2014.

Bultz BD, Carlson LE, 2005. *J Clin Oncol 23* 6440-6441 Emotional distress: The sixth vital sign in cancer care.

Clark J. Psychosocial Dimensions: The Patient. Groenwald S, Frogge MH, Goodman M, Yarbro CH. *Cancer Nursing Principles and Practice,* 2nd ed. Sudbury, MA: Jones and Bartlett Publishers 1990.

Federal Drug Administration. FDA Proposes New Warnings About Suicidal Thinking, Behavior in Young Adults Who Take Antidepressant Medications. http://www.fda.gov/bbs/topics/NEWS/2007/NEW01624.html. Accessed 2 July 2007.

Fulcher CD, (2014). Depression, chapter 31 In Yarbro CH, Wujuk D, Gobel BH (Eds.), *Cancer Symptom Management,* 4th ed., Burlington, MA: Jones & Bartlett Learning, pp 655–673.

Lacouture ME, Anadkat MJ, Bensadoun RJ, et al. (2011). Clinical practice guidelines for the prevention and treatment of EGFR inhibitor-associated dermatologic toxicities. *Support Care Cancer* 19:1079–1095.

Loprinzi CL, Sloan J, Stearns V et al. (2009). New antidepressants and gabapentin for hot flashes: An individual patient pooled analysis. *J Clin Oncol* 27(17): 2831–2837.

Massie MJ, Popkin MK. Depressive Disorders, *Chapter 10.* Holland JC. *Psycho-Oncology,* New York, NY: Oxford University Press 1998; 518–540.

Mathijssen RH, Verweij J, de Bruijn P, et al. Effects of St. John's Wort on Irinotecan Metabolism. *J Natl Cancer Inst* 2002; 94(16) 1247–1249.

Neuss MN, Polovich M, McNiff K et al. 2013 Updated American Society of Clinical Oncology/Oncology Nursing Society chemotherapy administration safety standards including standards for the safe administration and management of oral chemotherapy. *J Oncology Practice* 2013;9(2s) 5s–13s.

Pyter LM, Pineros V, Galang JA. Peripheral Tumors Induce Depressive-like Behaviors and Cytokine Production and Alter Hypothalamic-Pituitary-Adrenal Axis Regulation. *Proceedings of the National Academy of Sciences (PNAS)* 2009; 106: 9069–9074.

Rucker Y, Gobel BH (2014). Anxiety, chapter 29 In Yarbro CH, Wujuk D, Gobel BH (Eds.), *Cancer Symptom Management,* 4th ed., Burlington, MA: Jones & Bartlett Learning, pp. 619–637.

Smith EM, Pang H, Cirrincione C et al. (2013) Effect of duloxetine on pain, function, and quality of life among patients with chemotherapy-induced painful peripheral neuropathy JAMA 309(13) 1359–1367.

Trask PC. Assessment of Depression in Cancer Patients. *J Natl Cancer Inst* 2004; 32 80–92.

Valentine A. Depression, Anxiety, and Delirium. In Pazdur R, Coia LR, Hoskins WJ, Wagman LD (eds). *Cancer Management: A Multidisciplinary Approach.* Lawrence, KS: CMP Media LLC; 2007.

Drug: alprazolam (Xanax)

Class: Benzodiazepine (anxiolytic).

Mechanism of Action: Binds to benzodiazepine receptors in the CNS (limbic and cortical areas, cerebellum, brain stem, and spinal cord), resulting in the following effects: anxiolytic, ataxia, anticonvulsant, muscle relaxation. Appears to potentiate the effects of γ-aminobutyric acid (GABA).

MANAGEMENT

Metabolism: Well absorbed from GI tract. Widely distributed in body tissues and fluids, including CSF. Crosses placenta and is excreted in breastmilk. Highly bound to plasma proteins. Metabolized in liver and excreted in urine. Short elimination time; half-life of 12–15 hours. May produce psychological and physical dependence. Indicated for management of anxiety, the short-term relief of anxiety associated with depression, and panic disorder.

Indication: For the management of patients with (1) anxiety disorder; (2) panic disorder, with or without agoraphobia.

Contraindications: In (1) patients with known sensitivity to the drug or other benzodiazepines; (2) in combination with ketoconazole or itraconaxole, as these drugs impair metabolism of alprazolam.

Dosage/Range:
Adult:
- Anxiety: 0.25–0.5 mg PO tid (may gradually increase dose q 3–4 days over time to maximum 4 mg/day in divided doses).
- Elderly/debilitated: 0.25 mg PO bid.
- Discontinue drug by decreasing dose by 0.25–0.5 mg q 3–7 days.
- Drug should be used for short-term use only (< 4 months).
- Panic: optimal dosage not determined; titrate dose and increase slowly.

Drug Preparation:
- Available in 0.25-mg, 0.50-mg and 1 mg tablets.
- Store in tight, light-resistant containers at 15–30°C (59–86°F).

Drug Administration:
- Orally, in divided doses.
- May take with food if stomach upset occurs.

Drug Interactions:
- CNS depressants (alcohol, anticonvulsants, phenothiazines, opiates): additive CNS depression; avoid concurrent use or use cautiously and monitor carefully.
- Smoking: may decrease alprazolam serum level by up to 50%.
- CYP3A potent inhibitors (e.g., ketoconazole, itraconazole, nefazodone, fluvoxamine, erythromycin): increase alprazolam serum levels by decreasing drug metabolism; avoid coadministration or monitor closely for toxicity.
- CYP3A inducers (e.g., cabamazepine, HIV protease inhibitors such as ritonivir): may decrease alprazolam serum levels by inducing metabolism of the drug.
- Tricyclic antidepressants: increased serum levels of antidepressant possible; use together cautiously.
- Digoxin: may decrease renal excretion of digoxin; monitor for overdosage; may need to decrease digoxin.

Lab Effects/Interference:
- No consistent pattern of interaction between benzodiazepines and laboratory tests.

Special Considerations:
- Wide margin of safety between therapeutic and toxic doses.
- May impair ability to perform activities requiring mental alertness (e.g., driving a car, operating machinery).
- May produce psychological and physical dependence.
- Administer cautiously in patients with liver or renal impairment.
- Use cautiously in patients with chronic pulmonary disease or sleep apnea.
- Contraindicated in patients with depressive neuroses, psychotic reactions (without prominent anxiety), acute alcoholic intoxication (with depressed VS), known hypersensitivity to the drug, or acute angle-closure glaucoma.
- May cause fetal damage so should not be used during pregnancy or if the mother is breastfeeding.
- Withdrawal symptoms (including seizure, delirium) can occur with rapid drug discontinuance in patients taking high or chronic doses.
- If manic episodes or hyperactivity occur soon after drug started, drug should be discontinued.
- Drug should not be used to manage "everyday stress."

Potential Toxicities/Side Effects and the Nursing Process

I.   ALTERATIONS IN SENSORY/PERCEPTUAL PATTERNS related to CNS DEPRESSION

Defining Characteristics: CNS depressant effects include drowsiness, fatigue, lethargy, confusion, weakness, headache, which may occur initially and resolve with continued therapy or dose reduction. Vivid dreams, suicidal ideation, and bizarre behavior also may occur. Patient risk factors: elderly, debilitated, liver dysfunction, low serum albumin.

Nursing Implications: Assess baseline neurologic status and risk factors, and monitor during treatment. Instruct patient to report signs/symptoms and discuss drug modification with physician. Evaluate patient satisfaction with drug efficacy. If patient expresses suicidal ideation (more common in panic disorders), refer patient for psychiatric evaluation and drug modification. Instruct patient to avoid alcohol while taking drug. Teach patient prescribed schedule for discontinuing drug when used chronically: assess for signs/symptoms of withdrawal (increased anxiety, rebound insomnia; may also include agitation, dysphoria, nausea/vomiting, irritability, muscle cramps, hallucinations, seizures).

II.   ALTERATION IN NUTRITION, LESS THAN BODY REQUIREMENTS, related to GI SIDE EFFECTS

Defining Characteristics: Nausea, vomiting, weight increase or decrease, dry mouth, constipation may occur; also, elevated serum LFTs.

Nursing Implications: Assess baseline nutrition and elimination patterns and LFTs, and monitor during therapy. Discuss abnormalities and drug modification with physician. Teach patient to self-administer prescribed antiemetics as appropriate.

III.   POTENTIAL FOR INJURY related to DECREASE IN MENTAL ALERTNESS, PHYSICAL COORDINATION

Defining Characteristics: Drug may cause drowsiness, dizziness, and impair physical coordination, mental alertness.

Nursing Implications: Assess other medications that may increase risk (e.g., opiates, phenothiazines) and response to drug. Instruct patient to avoid potentially hazardous activities, including driving a car, operating machinery.

IV.   ALTERATIONS IN CARDIAC OUTPUT related to RHYTHM DISTURBANCES, VASODILATION

Defining Characteristics: Drug may cause bradycardia, tachycardia, hyper- or hypotension, palpitations, edema.

Nursing Implications: Assess baseline VS, and monitor during therapy. Discuss abnormalities with physician. Instruct patient to report dizziness on standing or other changes.

V.   ALTERATIONS IN SKIN INTEGRITY related to RASH

Defining Characteristics: Urticaria, pruritus, rash (morbilliform, urticarial, or maculopapular) may occur.

Nursing Implications: Assess baseline skin integrity, and instruct patient to report changes. Teach symptomatic skin management, and discuss drug discontinuance with physician if severe.

Drug: amitriptyline hydrochloride (Elavil)

Class: Tricyclic antidepressant.

Mechanism of Action: Blocks reuptake of neurotransmitters at neuronal membrane, thus increasing available serotonin and norepinephrine in CNS, and potentiating their effects. Appears to have analgesic effect separate from antidepressant action. May increase bioavailability of morphine. Indicated in the treatment of depressive (affective) mood disorders. Also used as an adjuvant analgesic in cancer pain management.

Metabolism: Well absorbed from GI tract. Distributed to lungs, heart, brain, liver; highly bound to plasma, proteins. Plasma half-life of 10–50 hours. Metabolized in liver, excreted in urine and, to a lesser degree, in bile and feces.

Indication: For the relief of symptoms of depression.

Dosage/Range:
Adult:
- Oral: 25–100 mg PO hs divided or single dose; may increase to 200–300 mg/day (300 mg maximum).
- Cancer pain: 25 mg/day hs; may increase by 25 mg of 1–2 days to 75–150 mg, when desired relief level is reached; may start at 10 mg in elderly.
- Elderly: 30 mg/day in divided doses.
- Intramuscular (IM): 20–30 mg qid or as single dose at bedtime.

Drug Preparation:
- Oral: store in well-closed containers at 15–30°C (59–86°F); store Elavil 10-mg capsules away from light. Administer as a single bedtime dose.
- IM: administer IM in large muscle mass; change to oral as soon as possible.

Drug Interactions:
- Monoamine oxidase inhibitors (MAOIs): increased excitation, hyperpyrexia, seizures; use together cautiously (especially if high dose is used).
- CNS depressants (alcohol, sedatives, hypnotics): increase CNS depression; use together cautiously.
- Sympathomimetic (epinephrine, amphetamines): increased hypertension; AVOID concurrent use.
- Cimetidine methylphenidate: increased amitriptyline levels, increased toxicity; use cautiously and monitor for increased toxicity.
- Warfarin: may increase PT; monitor closely and decrease dose of warfarin as needed.

Lab Effects/Interference:
- None known; bone marrow depression uncommon.

Special Considerations:
- Antidepressant effect may take 2 weeks or longer.
- Adjuvant analgesic useful in cancer pain management.
- May also decrease depression associated with chronic cancer pain and promote improved sleep.
- Contraindicated in patients with myocardial infarction, seizure disorder, or benign prostatic hypertrophy.
- Use cautiously in patients with urine retention, narrow-angle glaucoma, hyperthyroidism, hepatic dysfunction, or suicidal ideation.
- Drug should be gradually discontinued rather than abruptly withdrawn to prevent anxiety, malaise, dizziness, nausea/vomiting.
- May be helpful in treating hiccups.
- Increased anticholinergic side effects in older persons.

MANAGEMENT

- Teach all patients/families to call provider right away if thoughts of suicide or dying; attempts to commit suicide; new or worse depression; new or worse anxiety; feeling very agitated or restless; panic attacks; trouble sleeping (insomnia); new or worse irritability; aggressive, angry, or violent behavior; acting on dangerous impulses; extreme increase in activity or talking (mania); any unusual changes in behavior or mood.

Potential Toxicities/Side Effects and the Nursing Process

I.   ALTERATIONS IN SENSORY/PERCEPTUAL PATTERNS related to DROWSINESS, FATIGUE, EPS

Defining Characteristics: Drowsiness, dizziness, weakness, lethargy, and fatigue are common; confusion, disorientation, hallucinations may occur in the elderly. Extrapyramidal symptoms may occur (fine tremor, rigidity, dystonia, dysarthria, dysphagia), as may peripheral neuropathy and blurred vision.

Nursing Implications: Assess baseline gait, neurologic and mental status, and monitor during therapy. Instruct patient to report signs/symptoms; discuss benefit/risk ratio with physician. Assess for signs/symptoms of suicidal ideation; if they occur, refer for psychiatric evaluation. Inform patient that drowsiness, dizziness will resolve after 1–2 weeks; instruct to avoid hazardous activities while drowsy (e.g., driving a car, operating machinery).

II.   ALTERATION IN CARDIAC OUTPUT related to POSTURAL HYPOTENSION, TACHYCARDIA

Defining Characteristics: Postural hypotension, EKG changes, tachycardia, hypertension may occur.

Nursing Implications: Assess baseline orthostatic BP, heart rate, and monitor during therapy. Instruct patient to report abnormalities, including postural dizziness, palpitations. Drug should be stopped several days before surgery to prevent hypertensive crisis, especially if high dose.

III.   ALTERATION IN NUTRITION, LESS THAN BODY REQUIREMENTS, related to GI SIDE EFFECTS

Defining Characteristics: Dry mouth, anorexia, nausea, vomiting, diarrhea, abdominal cramping may occur; also, elevated LFTs.

Nursing Implications: Assess baseline nutrition and elimination patterns and LFTs, and monitor during therapy. Discuss abnormalities with physician, and discuss drug modification. Teach patient to self-administer prescribed antiemetics as appropriate. LFTs should be repeated, and if still elevated, the drug should be discontinued. Teach patient to take full dose at bedtime. Suggest patient use sugar-free hard candy, frequent ice chips, or artificial saliva for dry mouth.

IV. ALTERATION IN URINARY ELIMINATION related to URINARY RETENTION

Defining Characteristics: Urinary retention may occur. Increased risk if patient has history of urinary retention.

Nursing Implications: Assess baseline urinary elimination pattern and risk. Assess for urinary retention, and instruct patient to report signs/symptoms. Discuss alternative drug with physician if this occurs.

V. ALTERATIONS IN SKIN INTEGRITY related to ALLERGY

Defining Characteristics: Urticaria, erythema, rash, and photosensitivity may occur.

Nursing Implications: Assess baseline drug allergy history and skin integrity. Instruct patient to report skin changes. If angioedema of face or tongue develops, discuss drug discontinuance with physician. Instruct patient to avoid sunlight or to use sunblock protection.

Drug: bupropion hydrochloride (Wellbutrin)

Class: Aminoketone antidepressant.

Mechanism of Action: Unknown. Does block reuptake of serotonin, norepinephrine, and dopamine weakly; does not inhibit MAO; has CNS stimulant effects.

Metabolism: Peak plasma level 2 hours after oral administration, and it appears that only a small percentage of the dose reaches the systemic circulation. Half-life about 14 hours (8–24 hours average). Four major metabolites, with significantly longer elimination half-lives. Primarily excreted in the urine (87%) and to a lesser extent in the feces (10%).

Indication: For the treatment of major depressive disorder.

Contraindications: (1) Seizure disorder; (2) current or prior diagnosis of bulimia or anorexia nervosa; (3) abrupt discontinuation of alcohol, benzodiazepines, barbiturates, antiepileptic drugs; (4) monoamine oxidase inhibitors (MAOIs) during or within 14 days of stopping treatment with buproprion HCL, or within 14 days of stopping an MAOI intended to treat psychiatric disorders; (5) patients being treated with linezolid or IV methylene blue; (6) known hypersensitivity to drug or other ingredients.

Dosage/Range:
Adult:
- Initial dose: 100 mg bid (200 mg/day) for at least 3 days.
- After 3 days, may increase dose to 100 mg PO 3 times daily (300 mg/day) with at least 6 hours between doses. Usual target dose is 300 mg/day in 3 divided doses.

- Maximum dose is 450 mg/day given as 150 mg 3 times a day.
- Gradually titrate dose to reduce seizure risk.
- Periodically reassess the dose and need for maintenance treatment.
- Mild to moderate hepatic impairment: reduce dose and/or frequency of dosing.
- Renal impairment: reduce dose and/or frequency.
- If after 4 weeks of treatment there is no clinical response, may increase to a maximum of 450 mg/day (150 mg tid).

Drug Preparation:
- Available in 75-mg and 100-mg tablets.
- Protect tablets from light and moisture.
- Ensure at least 6 hours between doses (optimally, give in morning and evening).

Drug Interactions:
- Because of extensive drug metabolism by liver, when given with other drugs that have hepatic metabolism may have decreased effect of that drug (e.g., carbamazepine, cimetidine, phenobarbital, phenytoin).
- MAOIs may increase drug toxicity.
- Use cautiously in patients receiving L-dopa, starting with small initial dose, and slowly increasing dose.
- Use cautiously in patients receiving other seizure-threshold-lowering drugs, starting with small initial dose, and slowly and gradually increasing dose.
- Bupropion (Zyban; smoking cessation aid): DO NOT USE TOGETHER, as will increase risk of seizures.

Lab Effects/Interference:
- Rarely, anemia and pancytopenia.

Special Considerations:
- Warnings and Precautions:
  - Seizure risk is dose-related; minimize risk by gradually increasing dose and limiting dose to 450 mg/day. Discontinue if seizures occur.
  - Hypertension: can occur; monitor BP before starting treatment and periodically during treatment.
  - Activation of mania/hypomania: screen patients for bipolar disorder and monitor for these symptoms.
  - Psychosis and other neuropsychiatric reactions: Teach patient to contact a healthcare professional right away if this occurs.
- Teach patient to avoid alcohol when taking drug.
- Use cautiously, if at all, in individuals:
  - Who are underweight, as drug may cause weight loss of at least 2.25 kg (5 lb) (28% of patients), and most patients do not gain weight (only 9% of patients gain weight).
  - With a recent history of myocardial infarction or unstable heart disease.
- Drug contains same ingredient found in bupropion, which is used in smoking cessation. DO NOT USE TOGETHER.

• Teach all patients/families to call provider right away if thoughts of suicide or dying; attempts to commit suicide; new or worse depression; new or worse anxiety; feeling very agitated or restless; panic attacks; trouble sleeping (insomnia); new or worse irritability; aggressive, angry, or violent behavior; acting on dangerous impulses; extreme increase in activity or talking (mania); any unusual changes in behavior or mood.

Potential Toxicities/Side Effects and the Nursing Process

I. ALTERATIONS IN SENSORY/PERCEPTUAL PATTERNS related to RESTLESSNESS, AGITATION, INSOMNIA

Defining Characteristics: Many patients experience increased restlessness, agitation, anxiety, and insomnia, especially after initiation of therapy. This may be severe enough to require treatment with sedative/hypnotic or drug discontinuation. Restlessness, agitation, hostility, decreased concentration, ataxia, incoordination, confusion, paranoia, anxiety, manic episodes in bipolar manic depressives, migraine, insomnia, euphoria, and psychoses may occur. Akathisia, dyskinesia, dystonia, muscle spasms, bradykinesia, and sensory disturbances may occur.

Nursing Implications: Assess baseline gait, neurologic and mental status, and monitor during therapy. Teach patient to report signs/symptoms; discuss benefit/risk ratio with physician. Assess for signs/symptoms of suicidal ideation; if they occur, refer for psychiatric evaluation. Inform patient that drowsiness, dizziness will resolve after 1–2 weeks; instruct to avoid hazardous activities while drowsy (e.g., driving a car, operating machinery). Instruct patient to avoid alcohol ingestion, as this may precipitate seizures.

II. ALTERATION IN CARDIAC OUTPUT related to CHANGES IN BP, HR

Defining Characteristics: Dizziness, tachycardia, hypertension or hypotension, palpitations, edema, syncope, and cardiac arrhythmias may occur.

Nursing Implications: Assess baseline orthostatic BP, heart rate, presence of peripheral edema, and monitor during therapy. Patient should have a baseline EKG. Instruct patient to report abnormalities including postural dizziness, palpitations. Discuss any significant changes with physician, and discuss interventions. If the patient has had a recent myocardial infarction, expect that dose of drug may be reduced.

III. ALTERATION IN NUTRITION, LESS THAN BODY REQUIREMENTS, related to GI SIDE EFFECTS

Defining Characteristics: Dry mouth, anorexia, nausea, vomiting, diarrhea, constipation, weight loss of up to 2.25 kg (5 lb), dyspepsia, weight gain and increased appetite, increased salivation, taste changes, stomatitis may occur rarely.

MANAGEMENT

Nursing Implications: Assess baseline nutrition and elimination patterns, weight, and monitor during therapy. Discuss abnormalities with physician, and discuss drug modification. Teach patient to self-administer prescribed antiemetics as appropriate. Suggest patient use sugar-free hard candy, frequent ice chips, or artificial saliva for dry mouth.

IV.   ALTERATION IN URINARY ELIMINATION related to URINARY RETENTION

Defining Characteristics: Urinary retention, frequency, and nocturia may occur. Increased risk in patients with history of urinary retention.

Nursing Implications: Assess baseline urinary elimination pattern and risk. Assess for urinary retention, and instruct patient to report signs/symptoms. Discuss alternative drug with physician if this occurs.

V.   ALTERATIONS IN SKIN INTEGRITY related to ALLERGY

Defining Characteristics: Urticaria, erythema, rash, pruritus may occur.

Nursing Implications: Assess baseline drug allergy history and skin integrity. Instruct patient to report skin changes. If angioedema of face or tongue develops, tell patient to stop drug and discuss drug discontinuance with physician.

VI.   POTENTIAL SEXUAL DYSFUNCTION related to IMPOTENCE, IRREGULAR MENSES

Defining Characteristics: Impotence in men and irregular menses in women may occur.

Nursing Considerations: Assess baseline sexual functioning. Inform patient that alterations may occur, and instruct to report them. If severe, discuss dysfunction with physician, and whether another antidepressant would provide equal benefit with less dysfunction.

Drug: buspirone hydrochloride (BuSpar)

Class: Antianxiety agent.

Mechanism of Action: Unclear; drug is considered a midbrain modulator and affects many neurotransmitters (serotonin, dopamine, and cholinergic and noradrenergic systems).

Metabolism: Rapid and complete GI absorption. Food may delay absorption but does not affect total serum drug level. Distributed to body tissues and fluids, especially brain. Metabolized in liver and excreted in urine.

Indication: For the management of anxiety disorders or the short-term relief of symptoms of anxiety.

Dosage/Range:
Adult:
- Oral: 10–15 mg in 2–3 divided doses.
- May be increased in 5-mg increments every 2–4 days to achieve goal (maximum 60 mg/day).
- Maintenance: usual is 5–10 mg tid.

Drug Preparation:
- Store tablets in tight, light-resistant containers at < 30°C (86°F).
- Administer with food.

Drug Interactions:
- MAOIs: increased BP; AVOID CONCURRENT USE.
- Haloperidol: increased haloperidol serum levels; AVOID CONCURRENT USE or reduce haloperidol dose.
- Alcohol: may increase fatigue, drowsiness, dizziness; AVOID CONCURRENT USE.
- Other CNS depressants (analgesics, sedatives): may increase fatigue, drowsiness, dizziness; AVOID CONCURRENT USE.

Lab Effects/Interference:
- None known.

Special Considerations:
- Selective anxiolytic; causes little sedation or psychomotor dysfunction.
- Anxiolytic effect comparable to oral diazepam.
- Onset slower, so patients should be told to expect full anxiolytic effect in 3–4 weeks.
- Use with caution if renal insufficiency; dose-reduce in anuric patients.

Potential Toxicities/Side Effects and the Nursing Process

I. ALTERATIONS IN SENSORY/PERCEPTUAL PATTERNS related to DIZZINESS, DROWSINESS

Defining Characteristics: Far less sedation than with other anxiolytics. May cause dizziness, drowsiness, headache in 10% of patients; fatigue, nightmares, weakness, paresthesia occur less frequently.

Nursing Implications: Assess baseline neurologic status, and monitor during therapy. Instruct patient to report signs/symptoms, and discuss drug modification with physician. Instruct patient to avoid alcohol while taking drug.

II. ALTERATION IN NUTRITION, LESS THAN BODY REQUIREMENTS, related to GI SIDE EFFECTS

Defining Characteristics: Nausea occurs in 8% of patients; less common is dry mouth, vomiting, diarrhea, or constipation.

Nursing Implications: Assess baseline nutrition and elimination patterns, and monitor during therapy. Instruct patient to report signs/symptoms.

Drug: citalopram hydrobromide (Celexa)

Class: Antidepressant.

Mechanism of Action: Selective serotonin reuptake inhibitor (SSRI) with unique structure unlike other antidepressants (racemic bicyclic phthalane derivative). Drug inhibits the reuptake of neurotransmitter serotonin in the CNS, thus potentiating serotonin activity in the CNS and relieving depressive symptoms.

Metabolism: Steady-state plasma level reached in 1 week. Bioavailability is 80% following single daily dose, unaffected by food intake, and peak plasma level is reached in 4 hours. Metabolism is primarily hepatic, with a terminal half-life of 25 hours. Renal excretion accounts for 20% of drug excretion. In the elderly, drug is more slowly cleared, with increases in area under the curve (AUC) by 23% and half-life by 30%. Patients with hepatic dysfunction have reduced drug clearance (37%), with half-life of drug extended to 8 hours.

Indication: For the treatment of depression.

Dosage/Range:
Adult:
- 20 mg daily, increased 40 mg daily after at least 1 week.
- Patients with hepatic dysfunction or elderly: 20 mg daily.
- If changing to or from monoamine oxidase inhibitor therapy, wait at least 14 days between drugs.

Drug Preparation:
- Oral: available in 20-mg (pink) and 40-mg (white) oval, scored tablets.

Drug Administration:
- Administer orally in morning or evening, without regard to food.

Drug Interactions:
- Monoamine oxidase inhibitors: potential for serious, sometimes fatal interactions (hyper-thermia, rigidity, myoclonus, autonomic instability, mental status changes, including coma). DO NOT USE TOGETHER, and if changing to/from citalopram HBr, drugs MUST be separated by at least 14 days.
- Alcohol: possible potentiation of depression of cognitive and motor function; DO NOT USE TOGETHER.
- Cimetidine: increases AUC of citalopram HBr by 43%. Use together with caution, if at all; assess for toxicity and reduce dose as needed if must use together.
- Lithium: use together cautiously, and monitor serum lithium levels if used together.
- Warfarin: monitor INR, PT closely.
- Carbamazepine, ketoconazole, itraconazole, fluconazole, erythromycin: possible increase in clearance of citalopram HBr, monitor drug effectiveness and increase dose as needed.

- Metoprolol: may increase metoprolol levels; monitor BP and HR.
- Tricyclic antidepressants (e.g., imipramine): possible increases in plasma tricyclic antidepressant level; use together cautiously, if at all.

Lab Effects/Interference:
- Infrequently, increased liver function tests, alk phos, and abnormal glucose tolerance test.
- Rarely, bilirubinemia, hypokalemia, and hypoglycemia.

Special Considerations:
- At high doses in animals, drug is teratogenic, and, in some tests, mutagenic and carcinogenic (> 20 times the human maximum dose). DO NOT give to pregnant women or nursing mothers.
- Most responses occur within 1–4 weeks of therapy, but if no benefit has yet occurred, patients should be taught to continue taking medicine as prescribed.
- Use cautiously in patients with a seizure disorder, and monitor closely during therapy.
- Teach all patients/families to call provider right away if thoughts of suicide or dying; attempts to commit suicide; new or worse depression; new or worse anxiety; feeling very agitated or restless; panic attacks; trouble sleeping (insomnia); new or worse irritability, aggressive, angry, or violent behavior; acting on dangerous impulses; extreme increase in activity or talking (mania); any unusual changes in behavior or mood.

Potential Toxicities/Side Effects and the Nursing Process

I.   ALTERATION IN NUTRITION related to GI SIDE EFFECTS

Defining Characteristics: Nausea (21%) and dry mouth (20%) are common. Less common are diarrhea (8%), dyspepsia (5%), vomiting (4%), and abdominal pain (3%). Infrequent are gastritis, stomatitis, erructation, dysphagia, teeth grinding, change in weight, and gingivitis. The following were rare: colitis, cholecystitis, gastroesophageal reflux, diverticulitis, and hiccups.

Nursing Implications: Assess baseline nutrition and elimination patterns, and monitor during therapy. Discuss abnormalities with physician, and discuss drug modification. Teach patient to self-administer prescribed antiemetics as appropriate. Suggest patient use sugar-free hard candy, frequent ice chips, or artificial saliva for dry mouth.

II.   ALTERATION IN CARDIAC OUTPUT, POTENTIAL, related to CHANGES IN BLOOD PRESSURE

Defining Characteristics: Tachycardia, postural hypotension, and hypotension are common. The following are infrequent: hypertension, bradycardia, peripheral edema, angina, arrhythmias, flushing, and cardiac failure. Rarely, transient ischemic attacks, phlebitis, changes in cardiac conduction (atrial fibrillation, bundle branch block), and cardiac arrest.

Nursing Implications: Assess baseline orthostatic BP, heart rate, and monitor during therapy. Teach patient to report abnormalities, including postural dizziness, palpitations.

Discuss significant changes with physician. If patient has orthostatic hypotension, teach patient to change position slowly and to hold on to support.

III.   SENSORY/PERCEPTUAL ALTERATIONS related to CHANGES IN MENTAL STATUS

Defining Characteristics: The following may occur: somnolence (18%), insomnia (15%), agitation (3%), impaired concentration, amnesia, apathy, confusion, taste perversion, abnormal ocular accommodation, and possibly worsening depression and suicide attempt. Infrequently, increased libido, aggressive reaction, depersonalization, hallucination, euphoria, paranoia, emotional lability, and panic reaction may occur.

Nursing Implications: Assess baseline gait, neurologic, affective, and mental status, and monitor during therapy. Teach patient to report signs and symptoms; discuss benefit/risk ratio with physician. Assess for signs and symptoms of suicidal ideation; if they occur, refer for psychiatric evaluation. Teach patient that drowsiness may occur, and teach to avoid hazardous activities while drowsy (e.g., driving a car, operating machinery).

IV.   POTENTIAL FOR INJURY related to DRUG OVERDOSE

Defining Characteristics: Although rare, drug overdoses have resulted in fatalities (total drug 3,920 mg and 2,800 mg in two cases resulting from this drug only) while other total doses of 6,000 mg have not resulted in death. Symptoms resulting from overdose include dizziness, sweating, nausea, vomiting, tremor, somnolence, sinus tachycardia, amnesia, confusion, coma, convulsions, hyperventilation, cyanosis, rhabdomyolysis, and EKG changes (QT interval prolongation, nodal rhythm, and ventricular arrhythmias).

Nursing Implications: Teach patient self-administration schedule and to keep drug in tightly closed container out of reach of children and pets. Teach patient not to double doses if a dose is missed. Give prescriptions in smallest number of pills possible (e.g., 1 month's worth at a time). In the event of an overdosage, teach patient to come to nearest emergency department where focus is on maintaining a patent airway and oxygenation, gastric evacuation by lavage and use of activated charcoal, and close monitoring of cardiac and overall status. Because of large area of drug distribution, dialysis is unlikely to be beneficial.

V.   ALTERATIONS IN SKIN INTEGRITY related to RASH, SKIN CHANGES

Defining Characteristics: Rash and pruritus may occur. Less commonly, photosensitivity, urticaria, eczema, acne, dermatitis, alopecia, and dry skin may occur. Rarely, angioedema, epidermal necrolysis, erythema multiforme have been reported.

Nursing Implications: Assess baseline skin integrity. Teach patient to report skin changes. If angioedema of face or tongue develops, discuss drug discontinuance with physician. Assess impact of changes on patient and discuss strategies to minimize distress and preserve skin integrity and comfort.

VI. SEXUAL DYSFUNCTION, POTENTIAL, related to ↓ LIBIDO, IMPOTENCE, ANORGASMIA

Defining Characteristics: While difficult to separate from sexual dysfunction related to depression, the following have been reported in men: decreased ejaculation disorder (6.1%), decreased libido (3.8%), and impotence (2.8%); and in women: decreased libido (1.3%) and anorgasmia (1.1%). Dysmenorrhea and amenorrhea may occur in female patients.

Nursing Implications: Assess baseline sexual functioning. Teach patient that alterations may occur and to report them. If severe, discuss dysfunction with physician and whether an antidepressant other than an SSRI would provide equal benefit with less dysfunction.

VII. ALTERATION IN URINE ELIMINATION related to CHANGES IN PATTERNS

Defining Characteristics: Polyuria is common. Less commonly, the following may occur: urinary frequency, incontinence, retention, and dysuria. Rarely, hematuria, liguria, pyelonephritis, renal calculus, and renal pain have been reported.

Nursing Implications: Assess baseline urinary elimination pattern and risk for alterations. Assess for changes in urinary elimination and teach patient to report signs and symptoms. Discuss alternative drug with physician if severe or bothersome symptoms occur.

Drug: clonazepam (Klonopin)

Class: Benzodiazepine.

Mechanism of Action: Appears to enhance the activity of γ-aminobutyric acid (GABA), which inhibits neurotransmitter activity in the CNS. Drug is able to suppress absence seizures (petit mal) and decrease the frequency, amplitude, and duration of minor motor seizures. Unclear mechanism in relieving panic episodes.

Metabolism: Completely absorbed after oral administration, with peak plasma levels of 1–2 hours. Drug half-life is 18–60 hours (typically 30–40 hours), and therapeutic serum level is 20–80 ng/mL; 80% protein-bound, metabolized by the liver via the P450 cytochrome enzyme system, and inactive metabolites are excreted in the urine.

Indication: (1) Alone or as an adjunct in the treatment of Lennox-Gastaut syndrome (petit mal), akinetic and myoclonic seizures; (2) panic disorder.

Dosage/Range:
Adult (panic attacks):
- Initial: 0.25 mg bid.
- May increase as needed to target dose of 1 mg/day after at least 3 days on the previous dose. Some individuals may require doses of up to 4 mg/day in divided doses, and dose

is titrated up to that dose in increments of 0.125–0.25 mg bid every 3 days until panic disorder is controlled or as limited by side effects.
* Withdrawal of treatment must be gradual, with a decrease of 0.125 mg bid every 3 days until drug is completely withdrawn.

Adult (seizure disorders):
* Initial dose: 1.5 mg/day in three divided doses.
* Dosage may be increased in increments of 0.5–1 mg every 3 days until seizures are controlled or as limited by side effects.
* Maximum recommended daily dose is 20 mg/day.

Drug Preparation:
* Oral.
* Available in 0.5-, 1-, and 2-mg tablets.
* Discontinuance of drug when used for panic attacks: gradually discontinue, by 0.125 mg bid every 3 days, until drug is completely withdrawn.

Drug Interactions:
* CNS depressants (narcotics, barbiturates, hypnotics, anxiolytics, phenothiazines): potentiation of CNS depressive effects; use together cautiously, if at all, and monitor patient closely.
* Alcohol: potentiates CNS depressant effects; DO NOT use together.
* Phenobarbital: increases hepatic metabolism of clonazepam so that decreased serum levels lead to decreased clonazepam effect; assess patient for drug efficacy and need for increased drug dose.
* Phenytoin: increased hepatic metabolism of clonazepam so that decreased serum levels lead to decreased clonazepam effect; assess patient for drug efficacy and need for increased drug dose.
* Valproic acid: increased risk of absence seizure activity.

Lab Effects/Interference:
* Rarely, anemia, leukopenia, thrombocytopenia, eosinophilia.
* Transient elevation of liver function studies (serum transaminases and alk phos).

Special Considerations:
* Contraindicated during pregnancy, for breastfeeding mothers, and patients with severe liver dysfunction or acute narrow-angle glaucoma.
* May cause psychological and physical dependency.

Potential Toxicities/Side Effects and the Nursing Process

I.   ALTERATIONS IN SENSORY/PERCEPTUAL PATTERNS related to CNS DEPRESSION

Defining Characteristics: CNS depressant effects include drowsiness (37%), and, less commonly, dizziness (8%); abnormal coordination (6%); ataxia (5%); dysarthria (2%); depression (7%); memory disturbance (4%); nervousness (3%); decreased intellectual ability (2%); emotional lability; confusion; paresthesia; feeling of drunkenness; paresis; tremor; head fullness; hyperactivity, or hypoactivity. Rarely, suicidal ideation.

Nursing Implications: Assess baseline gait, neurologic status, affects, and monitor during treatment. Instruct patient to report signs/symptoms, and discuss drug modification with physician. Evaluate patient satisfaction with drug efficacy. Instruct patient to avoid alcohol while taking drug. Instruct patient prescribed schedule for discontinuing drug when used chronically: assess for signs/symptoms of withdrawal. Assess patient risk for suicide, and if at risk, refer to psychiatry for supportive counseling.

II. ALTERATION IN NUTRITION, LESS THAN BODY REQUIREMENTS, related to GI SIDE EFFECTS

Defining Characteristics: Constipation (1%), decreased appetite (1%), and less commonly, abdominal pain, flatulence, increased salivation, dyspepsia, decreased appetite; also elevated serum transaminases and alk phos.

Nursing Implications: Assess baseline nutrition and elimination patterns and serum transaminases, alk phos, and monitor during therapy. Assess degree of discomfort and interference with nutrition. Discuss significant abnormalities with physician and discuss drug modification.

III. INJURY related to DECREASE IN MENTAL ALERTNESS, PHYSICAL COORDINATION

Defining Characteristics: Drug may cause drowsiness, dizziness, and impair physical coordination, mental alertness.

Nursing Implications: Assess other medications that may increase risk (e.g., opiates, phenothiazines) and response to drug. Instruct patient to avoid potentially hazardous activities, including driving a car, operating machinery. Instruct patient to avoid alcohol.

IV. ALTERATIONS IN CARDIAC OUTPUT related to POSTURAL HYPOTENSION

Defining Characteristics: Drug may cause postural hypotension, palpitations, chest pain, edema.

Nursing Implications: Assess baseline VS, and monitor during therapy. Discuss abnormalities with physician. Instruct patient to report dizziness on standing or other changes, and to change position slowly and hold on to support if this occurs.

V. ALTERATIONS IN SKIN INTEGRITY related to SKIN DISORDERS

Defining Characteristics: Acne flare, xeroderma, contact dermatitis, pruritus, skin disorders may occur.

MANAGEMENT

Nursing Implications: Assess baseline skin integrity, and instruct patient to report changes. Teach symptomatic skin management, and discuss drug discontinuance with physician if severe.

VI.   SEXUAL DYSFUNCTION related to CHANGES IN LIBIDO, MENSTRUAL IRREGULARITIES

Defining Characteristics: Loss or increase in libido, menstrual irregularities in women; decreased ejaculation in men.

Nursing Implications: Assess baseline sexual functioning. Inform patient that alterations may occur, and instruct to report them. If severe, discuss dysfunction with physician, and whether another antidepressant would provide equal benefit with less dysfunction.

VII.   ALTERATION IN ELIMINATION, URINARY, related to DYSURIA, BLADDER DYSFUNCTION

Defining Characteristics: Dysuria, polyuria, cystitis, urinary incontinence, bladder dysfunction, urinary retention, urine discoloration, and urinary bleeding may occur uncommonly.

Nursing Implications: Assess baseline urinary elimination pattern. Instruct patient to report any changes. Discuss impact on patient, and severity, and discuss significant problems with physician.

Drug: desipramine hydrochloride (Norpramin, Pertofrane)

Class: Tricyclic antidepressant.

Mechanism of Action: Blocks reuptake of neurotransmitters at neuronal membrane, thus increasing available serotonin and norepinephrine in CNS, and potentiating their effects. Appears to have analgesic effect separate from antidepressant action. May increase bioavailability of morphine. Indicated in the treatment of depressive (affective) mood disorders. Also used as an adjuvant analgesic in cancer pain management.

Metabolism: Well absorbed from GI tract. Highly protein-bound. Plasma half-life of 7–60 hours. Metabolized in liver, and primarily excreted in urine.

Indication: For the treatment of depression.

Dosage/Range:
Adult:
• Oral: 75–150 mg hs, or in divided doses.
• May be gradually increased to 300 mg/day if needed.
• Elderly: 25–50 mg/day, maximum 150 mg/day.

Drug Preparation:
- Store in tight containers at < 40°C (104°F).
- Administer as a single bedtime dose.

Drug Interactions:
- MAOIs: increased excitation, hyperpyrexia, seizures; use together cautiously (especially if high dose used).
- Sympathomimetic (epinephrine, amphetamines): increased hypertension; AVOID concurrent use.
- Cimetidine methylphenidate: increased amitriptyline levels, increased toxicity; use cautiously and monitor for increased toxicity.
- Warfarin: may increase PT; monitor closely and decrease dose of warfarin as needed.
- Barbiturates: may decrease desipramine serum level; monitor for decreased antidepressant effect; may need increased dose.
- Alcohol: may antagonize antidepressant effects; AVOID CONCURRENT USE.

Lab Effects/Interference:
- Rarely, altered liver function studies.
- Rarely, increased or decreased serum glucose levels.
- Rarely, increased pancreatic enzymes.
- Rarely, bone marrow depression with agranulocytosis, eosinophilia, purpura, thrombocytopenia.

Special Considerations:
- Antidepressant effect may take 2 weeks or longer.
- Adjuvant analgesic useful in cancer pain management.
- May also decrease depression associated with chronic cancer pain and promote improved sleep.
- Contraindicated in patients with myocardial infarction, seizure disorder, or benign prostatic hypertrophy.
- Use cautiously in patients with urine retention, narrow-angle glaucoma, hyperthyroidism, hepatic dysfunction, or suicidal ideation.
- Drug should be gradually discontinued rather than abruptly withdrawn to prevent anxiety, malaise, dizziness, nausea/vomiting.
- May be helpful in treating hiccups.
- Increased anticholinergic side effects in elderly.
- Teach all patients/families to call provider right away if thoughts of suicide or dying; attempts to commit suicide; new or worse depression; new or worse anxiety; feeling very agitated or restless; panic attacks; trouble sleeping (insomnia); new or worse irritability; aggressive, angry, or violent behavior; acting on dangerous impulses; extreme increase in activity or talking (mania); any unusual changes in behavior or mood.

Potential Toxicities/Side Effects and the Nursing Process

I. ALTERATIONS IN SENSORY/PERCEPTUAL PATTERNS related to DROWSINESS, EPS

Defining Characteristics: Drowsiness, dizziness, weakness, lethargy, fatigue are common; confusion, disorientation, hallucinations may occur in the elderly. Extrapyramidal symptoms may occur (fine tremor, rigidity, dystonia, dysarthria, dysphagia), as may peripheral neuropathy and blurred vision. Less sedation than amitriptyline.

Nursing Implications: Assess baseline gait, neurologic and mental status, and monitor during therapy. Instruct patient to report signs/symptoms; discuss benefit/risk ratio with physician. Assess for signs/symptoms of suicidal ideation; if they occur, refer for psychiatric evaluation. Inform patient that drowsiness, dizziness will resolve after 1–2 weeks; instruct to avoid hazardous activities while drowsy (e.g., driving a car, operating machinery).

II.   ALTERATION IN CARDIAC OUTPUT related to POSTURAL HYPOTENSION, TACHYCARDIA

Defining Characteristics: Postural hypotension, EKG changes, tachycardia, hypertension may occur. Less severe than with other tricyclics.

Nursing Implications: Assess baseline orthostatic BP, heart rate, and monitor during therapy. Instruct patient to report abnormalities, including postural dizziness, palpitations. Drug should be stopped several days before surgery to prevent hypertensive crisis, especially if high dose is used.

III.   ALTERATION IN NUTRITION, LESS THAN BODY REQUIREMENTS, related to GI SIDE EFFECTS

Defining Characteristics: Dry mouth, anorexia, nausea, vomiting, diarrhea, abdominal cramping may occur; also, elevated LFTs.

Nursing Implications: Assess baseline nutrition and elimination patterns and LFTs, and monitor during therapy. Discuss abnormalities with physician, and discuss drug modification. Teach patient to self-administer prescribed antiemetics as appropriate. LFTs should be repeated, and if still elevated, the drug should be discontinued. Instruct patient to take full dose at bedtime. Suggest patient use sugar-free hard candy, frequent ice chips, or artificial saliva for dry mouth.

IV.   ALTERATION IN URINARY ELIMINATION related to URINARY RETENTION

Defining Characteristics: Urinary retention may occur. Increased risk in patients with history of urinary retention.

Nursing Implications: Assess baseline urinary elimination pattern and risk. Assess for urinary retention, and instruct patient to report signs/symptoms. Discuss alternative drug with physician if this occurs.

V.   ALTERATIONS IN SKIN INTEGRITY related to ALLERGY

Defining Characteristics: Urticaria, erythema, rash, and photosensitivity may occur.

Nursing Implications: Assess baseline drug allergy history and skin integrity. Instruct patient to report skin changes. If angioedema of face or tongue develops, discuss drug discontinuance with physician. Instruct patient to avoid sunlight or to use sunblock protection.

Drug: desvenlafaxine succinate (Pristiq)

Class: Serotonin-norepinephrine reuptake inhibitor (SNRI) antidepressant.

Mechanism of Action: Drug is synthetic active metabolite of venlafaxine. It appears to potentiate neurotransmitter activity by inhibiting neuronal serotonin and norepinephrine reuptake.

Metabolism: Drug is well absorbed after oral administration (80% bioavailability, with mean time to peak plasma level of 7.5 hours after the dose). With once-daily dosing, steady state is reached in 4–5 days. The terminal half-life is 11 hours. Drug is 30% protein-bound. Metabolized primarily by conjugation (UGT isoforms) and to a minor extent through oxidation (CYP3A4); 45% of the drug is excreted unchanged in the urine 72 hours after oral administration. Elimination half-lives significantly prolonged in severe renal dysfunction or end-stage renal disease (ESRD), and thus, dose should be adjusted in this population.

Indication: For the treatment of major depressive disorder.

Dosage/Range:
- Adult (indicated for the treatment of depression): extended-release tablet 50 mg daily, with or without meals.
- In clinical studies, doses 50–400 mg daily were used. There is no evidence a dose higher than 50 mg daily offers increased benefit.
- Patients with hepatic dysfunction: do not escalate dose above 100 mg/day.
- Patients with renal impairment:
  - Mild (CrCl 50–80 mL/min): no dose adjustment.
  - Moderate (CrCl 30–50 mL/min) dysfunction: 50 mg PO daily but do not escalate dose.
  - Severe renal dysfunction (CrCl M 30 mL/min) or ESRD, 50 mg PO every other day; do not escalate dose. Do not give supplemental doses after hemodialysis.
- In older patients, ensure renal function when considering dose.

Drug Preparation:
- XL capsule available in 50- and 100-mg strengths.
- Administer PO daily with or without food at about the same time each day; tablets must be swallowed whole (DO NOT dissolve, crush, divide, or chew).
- Drug can cause HTN: monitor BP and correct HTN before initiating treatment, and monitor BP during therapy.
- When changing from an MAOI to venlafaxine HCl, wait at least 14 days after MAOI is stopped; when stopping desvenlafaxine and beginning an MAOI, wait at least 7 days.
- If drug is discontinued, taper with gradual dose reduction if possible (e.g., decrease frequency).

Drug Interactions:
- MAOIs: tremor, myoclonus, diaphoresis, nausea, vomiting, flushing, dizziness, hyperthermia resembling neuroleptic malignant syndrome, and may be fatal. DO NOT USE TOGETHER. See Administration section.
- CNS-active agents: concomitant use has not been studied; use cautiously and monitor closely if required.
- Serotonergic drugs: use cautiously together if at all, and monitor closely.
- Drugs interfering with hemostasis (aspirin, NSAIDs, warfarin): serotonin important in hemostasis, and when reuptake blocked, risk of upper GI bleeding increased.
  - Aspirin, NSAIDs: increased risk of bleeding; do not use together concomitantly if possible.
  - Warfarin: altered anticoagulant effects, including increased bleeding; monitor INR and signs/symptoms bleeding closely, especially when drug started or stopped.
- Ethanol: no increased impairment, but because of CNS-active drug interaction, patients should be instructed not to drink alcohol.
- Venlafaxine: desvenlafaxine is the active metabolite in venlafaxine, and thus, the patient will overdose; do not coadminister.
- Inhibitors of CYP3A4 (e.g., ketoconazole increases area under the curve of desvenlafaxine by 43%): may increase serum level of desvenlafaxine, and thus, do not coadminister if possible.
- Drugs metabolized by CYP2D6: concomitant administration with desvenlafaxine may increase concentration of that drug.

Lab Effects/Interference:
- Elevated cholesterol, low-density lipids (LDL), and triglycerides: monitor baseline and throughout therapy.
- Hyponatremia.
- Rare abnormal LFTs, increased prolactin serum level.

Special Considerations:
- Drug is indicated for the treatment of patients with major depressive disorder.
- Avoid drug use during pregnancy and in nursing mothers. Drug exposure to fetus in third trimester resulted in neonates developing complications requiring prolonged hospitalization with respiratory support and tube feedings.
- Contraindicated in patients hypersensitive to desvenlafaxine succinate, venlafaxine HCl, or any excipients of drug; patients receiving MAO inhibitors (see Administration).
- Warnings:
  - Mydriasis may occur, and thus, patients with angle-closure and narrow angle glaucoma are at risk: monitor patients with raised intraocular pressure (or at risk of developing it) closely.
  - Drug can activate mania/hypomania states. Use cautiously in patients with bipolar disorder; screen patients initially for bipolar disorder, as drug is not approved for treatment of related depression. The risk of mania is 0.1%. Use cautiously in patients with a history of or family history of mania or hypomania and inform about the risk of activation of mania/hypomania.

- Use cautiously in patients with cardiovascular, cerebrovascular, or lipid metabolism diseases.
- Rarely seizures can occur: use cautiously in patients with a history of seizures.
- Rarely interstitial lung disease and eosinophilic pneumonia can occur; if patients develop progressive dyspnea, cough, or chest discomfort, stop drug and fully evaluate patient's pulmonary status.
- Monitor for clinical worsening and suicide risk.
- Drug was studied for short-term (8-week) treatment; monitor continued need of drug past that time.
- Rarely, serotonin syndrome may occur with desvenlafaxine (Pristiq), especially when used together with SSRIs, SNRIs, 5-hydroxytryptamine receptor agonists (triptans), and with drugs that reduce serotonin metabolism (including MAOIs), characterized by mental status changes (agitation, hallucinations, coma), autonomic instability (labile BP, hyperthermia), neuromuscular abnormalities (hyperreflexia, incoordination), with or without gastrointestinal symptoms (nausea, vomiting, diarrhea). Caution patient not to take other antidepressants or tryptophan supplements (serotonin precursors) while taking this drug.
- Teach all patients/families to call provider right away if thoughts of suicide or dying; attempts to commit suicide; new or worse depression; new or worse anxiety; feeling very agitated or restless; panic attacks; trouble sleeping (insomnia); new or worse irritability; aggressive, angry, or violent behavior; acting on dangerous impulses; extreme increase in activity or talking (mania); any unusual changes in behavior or mood.

MANAGEMENT

Potential Toxicities/Side Effects and the Nursing Process

I. ALTERATION IN OXYGENATION, POTENTIAL, related to CHANGES IN BP, TACHYCARDIA, HYPERLIPIDEMIA

Defining Characteristics: At all doses, some patients experienced sustained hypertension defined as a treatment-emergent diastolic BP of ≥ 90 mm Hg and ≥ 10 mm Hg above baseline for three consecutive visits. This occurred at all doses with the following incidence: placebo 0.5%, 50 mg/day: 1.3%, 100 mg/day: 0.7%, 200 mg/day, 1.1%, and 400 mg/day 2.3%. Orthostatic hypotension also occurred. Rarely, small increases in heart rate occurred in patients during clinical studies (incidence 1–2%). Patients with a history of MI, unstable heart disease, uncontrolled HTN were excluded from studies. Dose-related increases in LDL, total serum cholesterol, and triglycerides were seen during clinical studies, affecting 3–10% of patients depending on dose.

Nursing Implications: Assess baseline weight, cardiac status and BP at each visit. If BP elevated, reassess × 3, and if patient has three successive episodes as defined previously here, discuss dose reduction or change to another antidepressant with physician. Teach patient to change position slowly as risk of orthostatic hypotension. Instruct patient to report any headache, edema, palpitations, chest pain, or any changes in condition. Discuss any symptoms with the physician depending on severity. Monitor baseline cholesterol, LDL, and triglycerides, and monitor during therapy.

II.   ALTERATIONS IN SENSORY/PERCEPTUAL PATTERNS related to DIZZINESS, INSOMNIA, SOMNOLENCE, ANXIETY

Defining Characteristics: Infrequently, dizziness, fatigue, or somnolence can occur. Insomnia occurs in 9–15% of patients depending on dose. Anxiety occurs in 3–5% of patients. Rarely, blurred vision, mydriasis (2% incidence at 50-mg dose and 6% at 400-mg dose), tinnitus, taste perversion, irritability, manic or hypomanic reaction, seizure, depersonalization, syncope, extrapyramidal disorder, and abnormal dreams may occur.

Nursing Implications: Assess baseline neurologic status, affective state, and risk factors, and monitor during treatment. Instruct patient to avoid alcohol while taking drug. Assess effect on older persons and/or patients with hepatic or renal dysfunction. Assess for symptoms at each visit, and instruct patient to report changes. If symptoms occur, discuss strategies to ensure patient safety and comfort.

III.   ALTERATION IN NUTRITION, LESS THAN BODY REQUIREMENTS, related to GI SIDE EFFECTS, HYPONATREMIA

Defining Characteristics: Nausea (22–41% of patients), vomiting (3–9% compared with 3% placebo), dry mouth (11–25%), diarrhea (11%), constipation (9–14%), and decreased appetite (5–10%). Hyponatremia is rare and appears related to syndrome of inappropriate antidiuretic hormone (SIADH). Rarely, cases of serum sodium < 110 mmol/L have occurred. Patients at risk are older persons who are volume-depleted or on diuretic therapy.

Nursing Implications: Assess baseline nutrition and gastrointestinal functional status, and instruct the patient to report any GI disturbances or changes. Discuss measures to reduce nausea and/or stimulate appetite. Assess baseline serum sodium and risk factors for developing hyponatremia (SIADH), and monitor closely during therapy. Teach patients at risk signs and symptoms (headache, difficulty concentrating, memory impairment, confusion, weakness and unsteadiness; severe signs and symptoms are hallucination, syncope, seizure, coma) and to call their provider (mild) or to come to the emergency room or clinic right away (severe) if they occur.

IV.   SEXUAL DYSFUNCTION, POTENTIAL, related to EJACULATORY DISTURBANCES

Defining Characteristics: Anorgasmia occurred in 0% at the 50-mg dose, 3% at the 100-mg dose, 5% at 200-mg dose, and 8% at 400-mg dose; decreased libido in 3–6% of patients, abnormal orgasm in 1–3%, and delayed ejaculation in 1–7% of patients; and ejaculation dysfunction in 3–11% of patients depending on the dose. Women rarely experienced anorgasmia (1–3%).

Nursing Implications: Assess baseline sexual functioning. Inform patient that alterations may occur, and instruct to report them. If severe, discuss dysfunction with physician and whether another antidepressant would provide equal benefit with less dysfunction.

V.   ALTERATION IN COMFORT related to HYPERHIDROSIS, HEADACHE

Defining Characteristics: Hyperhidrosis (excessive sweating) occurs in 10% at a 50-mg dose, 18% at 200-mg dose, and 21% at a 400-mg dose. Headache may occur uncommonly.

Nursing Implications: Assess baseline comfort level. Instruct patient to report any changes in comfort, and discuss strategies to reduce discomfort. If hyperhidrosis is severe, teach patient to change clothes frequently to see if this increases comfort.

Drug: diazepam (Valium)

Class: Benzodiazepine (anxiolytic).

Mechanism of Action: Binds to benzodiazepine receptors in the CNS (limbic and cortical areas, cerebellum, brain stem, and spinal cord), resulting in the following effects: anxiolytic, ataxia, anticonvulsant, muscle relaxation. Appears to potentiate the effects of GABA.

Metabolism: Well absorbed from GI tract. Widely distributed in body tissues and fluids, including CSF. Crosses placenta and is excreted in breastmilk. Highly bound to plasma proteins. Metabolized in liver and excreted in urine. Half-life of 20–80 hours. May produce psychological and physical dependence. Indicated for management of anxiety, the relief of reflex spasm or spasticity, and as an anticonvulsant for termination of status epilepticus.

Indication: (1) Management of anxiety disorders or for the short-term relief of anxiety symptoms; (2) acute alcohol withdrawal; (3) relief of skeletal muscle spasm due to reflex spasm; (4) adjunctive in the management of convulsive disorders.

Dosage/Range:
Adult:
- Oral: 2–10 mg tid–qid or 15–30 mg/day extended-release preparation.
- Intravenous (IV) (tension): 5–10 mg IV, maximum 30 mg/8 h.
- IV (seizures): 5–10 mg IV, maximum 30 mg; may repeat in 2–4 hours if needed.
- IV (status epilepticus): 5–20 mg slow IV push (IVP) (2–5 mg/min), q 5–10 min, maximum 60 mg.
- IV (elderly, debilitated): 2–5 mg slow IVP.

Drug Preparation:
- Oral: protect tablets from light and store at 15–30°C (59–86°F).
- IV: Do not administer with other drugs; drug may absorb to sides of plastic syringe or to plastic IV bag and tubing if added to IV infusion bag; consult hospital pharmacist for IV infusion protocol; administer IVP slowly 2–5 mg/min; have emergency equipment available.

Drug Interactions:
- CNS depressants (alcohol, anticonvulsants, phenothiazines, opiates): additive CNS depression; avoid concurrent use or use cautiously and monitor carefully.
- Oral contraceptives, isoniazid, ketoconazole, or cimetidine: decrease plasma clearance of diazepam so may increase effect (e.g., sedation); monitor patient closely.

- Tricyclic antidepressants: increased serum levels of antidepressant possible; use together cautiously.
- Digoxin: may decrease renal excretion of digoxin; monitor for overdosage; may need to decrease digoxin.
- Levodopa: may decrease levodopa effect; monitor patient response; may have to increase levodopa dose.

Lab Effects/Interference:
- Rarely, altered liver function studies.
- Rarely, neutropenia.

Special Considerations:
- Wide margin of safety between therapeutic and toxic doses.
- May impair ability to perform activities requiring mental alertness (e.g., driving a car, operating machinery).
- May produce psychological and physical dependence.
- Administer cautiously in patients with liver or renal impairment.
- Use cautiously in patients with chronic pulmonary disease or sleep apnea.
- Contraindicated in patients with depressive neuroses, psychotic reactions (without prominent anxiety), acute alcoholic intoxication (with depressed VS), known hypersensitivity to the drug, or acute angle-closure glaucoma.
- May cause fetal damage, so should not be used during pregnancy or if the mother is breastfeeding.
- Withdrawal symptoms (including seizure, delirium) can occur with rapid drug discontinuance in patients taking high or chronic doses.

Potential Toxicities/Side Effects and the Nursing Process

I.   ALTERATIONS IN SENSORY/PERCEPTUAL PATTERNS relating to CNS DEPRESSION

Defining Characteristics: CNS depressant effects include drowsiness, fatigue, lethargy, confusion, weakness, headache, which may occur initially and resolve with continued therapy or dose reduction. Vivid dreams, visual disturbances, slurred speech, "hangover," and bizarre behavior may also occur. Patient risk factors: elderly, debilitated, liver dysfunction, low serum albumin.

Nursing Implications: Assess baseline neurologic status and risk factors, and monitor during treatment. Instruct patient to report signs/symptoms and discuss drug modification with physician. Evaluate patient satisfaction with drug efficacy. Instruct patient to avoid alcohol while taking drug. Teach patient prescribed schedule for discontinuing drug when used chronically: assess for signs/symptoms of withdrawal (increased anxiety, rebound insomnia; may also include agitation, dysphoria, nausea/vomiting, irritability, muscle cramps, hallucinations, seizures).

II. ALTERATION IN NUTRITION, LESS THAN BODY REQUIREMENTS, related to GI SIDE EFFECTS

Defining Characteristics: Nausea, vomiting, abdominal discomfort may occur; also, elevated LFTs.

Nursing Implications: Assess baseline nutrition and elimination patterns and LFTs, and monitor during therapy. Discuss abnormalities with physician and discuss drug modification. Teach patient to self-administer prescribed antiemetics as appropriate.

III. INJURY related to DECREASE IN MENTAL ALERTNESS, PHYSICAL COORDINATION

Defining Characteristics: Drug may cause drowsiness, dizziness, and impair physical coordination, mental alertness.

Nursing Implications: Assess other medications that may increase risk (e.g., opiates, phenothiazines) and response to drug. Instruct patient to avoid potentially hazardous activities, including driving a car, operating machinery.

IV. ALTERATIONS IN PERFUSION related to CARDIOPULMONARY COMPROMISE

Defining Characteristics: Drug may cause transient hypotension, bradycardia, cardiovascular collapse, respiratory depression.

Nursing Implications: Assess baseline VS; have resuscitation equipment nearby. Monitor q 5–15 min and before IV dose of drug. Discuss abnormalities with physician.

V. ALTERATIONS IN SKIN INTEGRITY related to RASH

Defining Characteristics: Urticaria, rash may occur; also phlebitis, pain at injection site.

Nursing Implications: Assess baseline skin integrity, and instruct patient to report changes. Teach symptomatic skin management, and discuss drug discontinuance with physician if severe. Assess IV site for evidence of pain, phlebitis, and change site; apply heat as needed.

Drug: doxepin hydrochloride (Sinequan)

Class: Antidepressant of the dibenzoxepine tricyclic class.

Mechanism of Action: Appears to exert adrenergic effect at the synapses, preventing deactivation of norepinephrine by reuptake into the nerve terminals.

MANAGEMENT

Metabolism: Metabolized in the liver by the P450 enzyme system, into active metabolite. Effective serum level of doxepin and metabolite is 100–200 mg/mL. Takes 2–8 days to reach steady state.

Indication: For the relief of depression; relief of insomnia.

Dosage/Range:
Adult:
- Initial dose of 75 mg/day is recommended; in elderly, dose should start at 25–50 mg/day.
- Dose may be titrated up or down based on response. Usual dose is 75–150 mg/day. Patients with mild symptoms may require only 25–50 mg/day.
- Patients with severe symptoms may require gradual titration up to 300 mg/day.

Drug Preparation:
- Oral, taken in a single dose (maximum 150-mg dose) or in divided doses. Single dose given at bedtime enhances sleep.
- Available in 10-, 25-, 50-, 75-, 100-, and 150-mg capsules.
- If changing a patient from MAOI to doxepin HCl, wait at least 14 days before the careful initiation of doxepin.

Drug Interactions:
- Alcohol: do not use concomitantly, as increases drug toxicity.
- MAOI: severe reaction, including death may occur; DO NOT USE TOGETHER.
- Cimetidine: increased serum levels of drug and anticholinergic side effects (severe dry mouth, urinary retention, blurred vision); avoid concurrent use.
- Tolazamide: may cause severe hypoglycemia; monitor patient's serum glucose carefully.

Lab Effects/Interference:
- Rarely, eosinophilia, bone marrow depression (e.g., agranulocytosis, leukopenia, thrombocytopenia, purpura).
- Increased or decreased blood glucose levels.

Special Considerations:
- Contraindicated in patients with glaucoma or urinary retention.
- Antianxiety effect appears before the antidepressant effect, which takes 2–3 weeks.
- Most sedating of antidepressants, so useful in enhancing sleep, and single dose (up to 150 mg) should be taken at bedtime.
- Recommended for the treatment of depression accompanied by anxiety and insomnia, depression associated with organic illness or alcohol, psychotic depressive disorders with associated anxiety.
- Teach all patients/families to call provider right away if thoughts of suicide or dying; attempts to commit suicide; new or worse depression; new or worse anxiety; feeling very agitated or restless; panic attacks; trouble sleeping (insomnia); new or worse irritability; aggressive, angry, or violent behavior; acting on dangerous impulses; extreme increase in activity or talking (mania); any unusual changes in behavior or mood.
- Doxepin has been studied, and it has been found to reduce pruritis from EGFRI rash (Lacouture et al., 2011).

Potential Toxicities/Side Effects and the Nursing Process

I.   ALTERATIONS IN SENSORY/PERCEPTUAL related to DROWSINESS, EPS

Defining Characteristics: Drowsiness, which may disappear as therapy continues. Rarely, dizziness, confusion, disorientation, hallucinations, numbness, paresthesia, ataxia, extrapyramidal symptoms, seizures, blurred vision, tardive dyskinesia, tremor may occur.

Nursing Implications: Assess baseline gait, neurologic, affective and mental status, and monitor during therapy. Instruct patient to report signs/symptoms; discuss benefit/risk ratio with physician and measures to reduce extrapyramidal side effects if they occur. Assess for signs/symptoms of suicidal ideation; if they occur, refer for psychiatric evaluation. Inform patient that drowsiness will decrease after 1–2 weeks, and instruct to avoid hazardous activities while drowsy (e.g., driving a car, operating machinery). Instruct patient to avoid alcohol while taking drug.

II.   ALTERATION IN CARDIAC OUTPUT related to BLOOD PRESSURE CHANGES

Defining Characteristics: Hypotension or hypertension, tachycardia may occur.

Nursing Implications: Assess baseline orthostatic BP, heart rate, and monitor during therapy. Instruct patient to report abnormalities, including postural dizziness, palpitations.

III.   ALTERATION IN NUTRITION, LESS THAN BODY REQUIREMENTS, related to GI SIDE EFFECTS

Defining Characteristics: Dry mouth, anorexia, nausea, vomiting, diarrhea, indigestion, taste changes, aphthous stomatitis may occur rarely.

Nursing Implications: Assess baseline nutrition and elimination patterns. Discuss abnormalities with physician, and discuss drug modification. Teach patient to self-administer prescribed antiemetics as appropriate. Instruct patient to take full dose at bedtime (if 150 mg or less). Suggest patient use sugar-free hard candy, frequent ice chips, or artificial saliva for dry mouth.

IV.   ALTERATION IN URINARY ELIMINATION related to URINARY RETENTION

Defining Characteristics: Urinary retention may occur. Increased risk in patients with history of urinary retention.

Nursing Implications: Assess baseline urinary elimination pattern and risk. Assess for urinary retention, and instruct patient to report signs/symptoms. Discuss alternative drug with physician if this occurs.

V.   ALTERATIONS IN SKIN INTEGRITY related to ALLERGY

Defining Characteristics: Urticaria, erythema, rash, and photosensitivity may occur.

Nursing Implications: Assess baseline drug allergy history and skin integrity. Instruct patient to report skin changes. If severe changes occur, discuss drug discontinuance with physician. Instruct patient to avoid sunlight or to use sunblock protection.

VI.   SEXUAL DYSFUNCTION related to CHANGES IN LIBIDO

Defining Characteristics: Increased or decreased libido, testicular swelling, gynecomastia in males; enlargement of breasts and galactorrhea in women.

Nursing Implications: Assess baseline sexual functioning. Inform patient that alterations may occur, and instruct to report them. If severe, discuss dysfunction with physician and whether another antidepressant would provide equal benefit with less dysfunction.

Drug: duloxetine hydrochloride (Cymbalta)

Class: Antidepressant.

Mechanism of Action: Selective serotonin and norepinephrine uptake inhibitor (SSNRI), resulting in potentiation of serotonergic and noradrenergic activity in the CNS, and antidepressant, central pain inhibition, and anxiolytic qualities.

Metabolism: After oral ingestion, drug undergoes extensive metabolism, but metabolites do not appear to contribute to the drug effect. The drug is highly protein-bound. Elimination half-life is about 12 hours, achieving steady-state plasma levels in 3 days of dosing. When taken with food, the time to reach peak concentration increases from 6 to 10 hours and reduces absorption by about 10%. When the drug is taken in the evening, there is a 3-hour delay in absorption and a 33% increase in drug clearance compared with taking the drug in the morning. The drug is metabolized by the CYP1A2 and CYP2D6P450 hepatic enzymes. Metabolites are excreted in the urine primarily (70%) with 20% excreted in the feces. Drug area under the curve is about 25% higher, and the half-life of the drug about 4 hours longer in older women. Smoking reduces the bioavailability by 33%, but the manufacturer does not recommend dose modification in smokers. Drug is not recommended for patients with severe renal impairment (urinary creatinine clearance < 30 mL/min), including patients on dialysis or patients with hepatic insufficiency.

Indication: (1) Major depressive disorder; (2) generalized anxiety disorder; (3) diabetic peripheral neuropathic pain; (4) fibromyalgia; (5) chronic musculoskeletal pain.

Dosage/Range:
Adult (depression):
- 20 mg orally twice daily to 60 mg/day (given either once a day or as 30 mg twice daily) without regard to meals.

Adult (diabetic peripheral neuropathy):
- 60 mg orally once daily without regard to meals (start with a lower dose if renal impairment and gradually increase dose).

Adult (generalized anxiety disorder):
- 60 mg orally once daily without regard to meals.

Drug Preparation:
- Oral, available as delayed release capsules in 20-, 30-, and 60-mg strengths.
- When discontinuing fluoxetine, the drug should be gradually reduced in dose (tapered), as otherwise, discontinuation symptoms such as dizziness, nausea, headache, paresthesia, vomiting, irritability, nightmares, insomnia, diarrhea, anxiety, hyperhidrosis, and vertigo may occur.
- Allow at least 14 days between stopping an MAOI and beginning fluoxetine; when stopping fluoxetine to begin an MAOI, wait at least 5 days after stopping fluoxetine before beginning the MAOI.

Drug Interactions:
- CYP1A2 inhibitors (cimetidine, ciprofloxacin, levofloxacin, enoxacin): increased serum levels and terminal half-life of duloxetine; avoid concurrent administration.
- CYP2D6 inhibitors (paroxetine, quinidine): increased duloxetine serum levels by 60%; avoid concurrent use.
- Drugs metabolized by CYP1A2: no effect on the other drugs.
- Drugs metabolized by CYP2D6 (tricyclic antidepressants [TCA], phenothiazines, type 1C antiarrhythmics such as propafenone and flecainide): increased serum levels of these drugs; use together cautiously if at all and monitor TCA serum levels; do not give concurrently with thioridazine as increased risk of ventricular arrhythmias and sudden death.
- Alcohol: DO NOT USE CONCOMITANTLY, as this may increase the risk of hepatic injury in heavy alcohol imbibers.
- CNS-acting drugs: use together cautiously, if at all.
- Serotonergic drugs (triptans, linezolid, lithium, tramadol, St. John's wort): increased risk for serotonin syndrome (mental status changes such as agitation, hallucinations, coma); autonomic instability such as tachycardia, labile BP, hyperthermia; neuromuscular aberrations such as hyperreflexia, incoordination; and/or GI symptoms such as nausea, vomiting, diarrhea. DO NOT use concurrently.
- Drugs that affect gastric acidity: drug requires a pH of 5.5 to dissolve the enteric coating. No effect with magnesium or aluminum containing antacids, but caution advised in patients with slow gastric emptying (diabetics). It is not known whether concurrent administration with proton-pump inhibitors affects drug absorption.
- MAOIs: when drug is given concomitantly or within a short time period, severe, potentially life-threatening interactions may occur, including symptoms resembling neuroleptic malignant syndrome. DO NOT GIVE TOGETHER, AND END SEPARATELY, as stated in the Administration section.

Lab Effects/Interference:
- Increased liver transaminases.
- Rare anemia, leucopenia, thrombocytopenia.

- Rare hypercholesteremia, hyperlipidemia, hypoglycemia, dyslipidemia, hypertriglyceridemia.
- Rare increased serum creatinine.

Special Considerations:
- Duloxetine significantly reduced painful chemotherapy-induced peripheral neuropathy compared to placebo (Smith et al., 2013).
- FDA-approved for the treatment of major depressive disorder, the management of neuropathic pain associated with diabetic peripheral neuropathy, and the treatment of generalized anxiety disorder (associated with at least three symptoms such as restlessness, easy fatigability, difficulty concentrating, irritability, muscle tension, and/or sleep disturbance).
- Contraindicated in patients who are (1) taking MAOIs, (2) have uncontrolled narrow-angle glaucoma, (3) have end-stage renal disease or severe renal impairment (urinary creatinine clearance < 30 mL/min), (4) have hepatic insufficiency, and (5) nursing mothers.
- Women who are pregnant in the third trimester: neonates exposed to SSRIs, SNRIs developed complications requiring prolonged hospitalization; must consider risk versus benefit, and consider tapering drug during third trimester.
- Increased risk of suicidality (thinking and behavior) in young adults aged 18–24 years, as well as children and adolescents, especially during the first 2 months of treatment; monitor closely for signs/symptoms of suicidality (emergency of agitation, irritability, unusual changes in behavior, emergence of suicidality).
- Teach all patients/families to call provider right away if thoughts of suicide or dying; attempts to commit suicide; new or worse depression; new or worse anxiety; feeling very agitated or restless; panic attacks; trouble sleeping (insomnia); new or worse irritability; aggressive, angry, or violent behavior; acting on dangerous impulses; extreme increase in activity or talking (mania); any unusual changes in behavior or mood.

Potential Toxicities/Side Effects and the Nursing Process

I.   ALTERATIONS IN SENSORY/PERCEPTUAL PATTERNS related to CNS EFFECTS

Defining Characteristics: Blurred vision, vertigo, lethargy, dizziness, somnolence, tremor, paresthesia/hypoesthesia, hot flushes, agitation, anxiety, nervousness, nightmare/abnormal dreams, sleep disorder may occur in at least 1 of 100 patients. Patients aged 18–24 years are at risk for suicide, or others at risk for suicide may commit suicide during initial period of treatment.

Nursing Implications: Assess baseline neurologic status and risk factors, and monitor during treatment. Instruct patient to report signs/symptoms, and discuss drug modification with physician. Evaluate patient satisfaction with drug efficacy. Instruct patient to avoid alcohol while taking drug. Assess suicide risk, and if at high risk, monitor closely and provide supportive counseling and referral to a psychiatrist. The patient should receive only a small number of pills to prevent overdose.

II. ALTERATION IN NUTRITION, LESS THAN BODY REQUIREMENTS, related to GI SIDE EFFECTS

Defining Characteristics: Nausea and less commonly vomiting, diarrhea, constipation, dry mouth, dyspepsia, anorexia, abdominal discomfort, flatulence, taste changes, and gastroenteritis may occur.

Nursing Implications: Assess baseline nutrition and elimination patterns. Discuss abnormalities with physician and discuss drug modification. Teach patient to self-administer prescribed antiemetics as appropriate. If patient is losing weight, instruct patient to report this and involve nutritionist in care.

III. SEXUAL DYSFUNCTION, POTENTIAL, related to IMPOTENCE

Defining Characteristics: Sexual dysfunction and anorgasmia and erectile dysfunction in men can occur uncommonly.

Nursing Implications: Assess baseline sexual functioning. Inform patient that alterations may rarely occur and that they should be reported. If severe, discuss dysfunction with a physician and whether another antidepressant would provide equal benefit with less dysfunction.

Drug: escitalopram oxalate (Lexapro)

Class: Antidepressant.

Mechanism of Action: Selective inhibitor of neuronal reuptake of serotonin (SSRI) in the CNS, resulting in potentiation of serotonin activity in the CNS; has minimal effect on reuptake of norepinephrine or dopamine.

Metabolism: After oral administration, 80% of the drug is absorbed, with peak plasma levels in 5 hours and steady-state plasma concentrations in about 1 week. Drug is 56% bound to plasma proteins. The terminal half-life of the drug is 27–32 hours. Drug undergoes hepatic biotransformation, with CYP3A4 and CYP2C19 liver microsomes primarily involved in drug metabolism. Bioavailability of tablet is the same as the oral solution.

Indication: For the acute and maintenance treatment of major depressive disorder; acute treatment of generalized anxiety disorder.

Dosage/Range:
- Recommended dose is 10 mg/day orally (20 mg daily has not shown improved benefit); however, if dose is increased to 20 mg daily, wait at least 1 week before increasing the dose.

Drug Preparation:
- Available in 5-, 10-, and 20-mg tablets, as well as 5-mg/5-mL oral solution.
- May be given in morning or evening and with or without food.
- When discontinuing drug, the dose should be gradually tapered rather than abruptly stopped.

MANAGEMENT

Drug Interactions:
- CYP1A2 inhibitors (cimetidine): increased serum levels of escitalalopram oxalate by 43%; avoid concurrent administration.
- Drugs metabolized by CYP2D6 (tricyclic antidepressants [TCA], phenothiazines, metoprolol): possible, increased serum levels of these drugs; use together cautiously and monitor TCA serum levels.
- Alcohol: DO NOT USE CONCOMITANTLY, as this may increase the risk of hepatic injury in heavy alcohol imbibers.
- CNS-acting drugs: use together cautiously if at all.
- Serotonergic drugs (triptans, linezolid, lithium, tramadol, St. John's wort): increased risk for serotonin syndrome (mental status changes such as agitation, hallucinations, coma); autonomic instability such as tachycardia, labile BP, hyperthermia; neuromuscular aberrations such as hyperreflexia, incoordination; and/or GI symptoms such as nausea, vomiting, diarrhea. DO NOT use concurrently.
- Drugs that interfere with hemostasis (NSAIDs, aspirin, warfarin): increased risk of upper-GI bleeding; use cautiously if at all, and monitor closely.
- MAOIs: when drug is given concomitantly or within a short time period, severe, potentially life-threatening interactions may occur, including symptoms resembling neuroleptic malignant syndrome. DO NOT GIVE TOGETHER AND END SEPARATELY, as stated in the Administration section.
- Lithium: enhanced serotonergic effects, monitor patient closely; monitor lithium levels.
- Pimozide: increased QTc by 10 msec; avoid concurrent use.
- Sumatriptan: weakness, hyperreflexia, and incoordination; avoid concurrent use.

Lab Effects/Interference:
- None known.

Special Considerations:
- FDA-approved for the treatment of major depressive disorder, the management of neuropathic pain associated with diabetic peripheral neuropathy, and the treatment of generalized anxiety disorder (associated with at least three symptoms, such as restlessness, easy fatigability, difficulty concentrating, irritability, muscle tension, and/or sleep disturbance).
- Contraindicated in patients who are (1) taking MAOIs, (2) have uncontrolled narrow-angle glaucoma, (3) have end-stage renal disease or severe renal impairment (urinary creatinine clearance < 30 mL/min), (4) have hepatic insufficiency, and (5) nursing mothers.
- Women who are pregnant in the third trimester: neonates exposed to SSRIs, SNRIs developed complications requiring prolonged hospitalization; must consider risk versus benefit and consider tapering drug during third trimester.
- Increased risk of suicidality (thinking and behavior) in young adults aged 18–24, as well as children and adolescents, especially during the first 2 months of treatment; monitor closely for signs/symptoms of suicidality (emergency of agitation, irritability, unusual changes in behavior, emergence of suicidality).

- Teach all patients/families to call provider right away if thoughts of suicide or dying; attempts to commit suicide; new or worse depression; new or worse anxiety; feeling very agitated or restless; panic attacks; trouble sleeping (insomnia); new or worse irritability; aggressive, angry, or violent behavior; acting on dangerous impulses; extreme increase in activity or talking (mania); any unusual changes in behavior or mood.

Potential Toxicities/Side Effects and the Nursing Process

I. ALTERATIONS IN SENSORY/PERCEPTUAL PATTERNS related to CNS EFFECTS

Defining Characteristics: Somnolence (13%), insomnia (12%), abnormal dreaming (3%), lethargy (3%), and dizziness (2%) may occur. Patients age 18–24 years are at risk for suicide, or others at risk for suicide may commit suicide during initial period of treatment.

Nursing Implications: Assess baseline neurologic status, sleep patterns, and risk factors, and monitor during treatment. Instruct patient to report signs/symptoms, and discuss drug modification with physician. Evaluate patient satisfaction with drug efficacy. Instruct patient to avoid alcohol while taking drug. Assess suicide risk, and if at high risk, monitor closely and provide supportive counseling and referral to a psychiatrist. The patient should receive only a small number of pills to prevent overdose.

II. ALTERATION IN NUTRITION, LESS THAN BODY REQUIREMENTS, related to GI SIDE EFFECTS

Defining Characteristics: Nausea (18%), dry mouth (9%), diarrhea (8%), constipation (5%), indigestion (3%), vomiting (3%), and rarely abdominal discomfort and flatulence may occur. Weight changes were no different from placebo group.

Nursing Implications: Assess baseline nutrition and elimination patterns. Discuss abnormalities with physician, and discuss drug modification. Teach patient to self-administer prescribed antiemetics as appropriate. If patient is losing weight, instruct patient to report this and involve nutritionist in care.

III. SEXUAL DYSFUNCTION, POTENTIAL, related to IMPOTENCE

Defining Characteristics: Sexual dysfunction, including ejaculation disorder (primarily ejaculatory delay), decreased libido, and impotence in men and decreased libido and anorgasmia in women can occur uncommonly. SSRIs have a rare incidence of priapism.

Nursing Implications: Assess baseline sexual functioning. Inform patient that alterations may rarely occur and should be reported. If severe, discuss dysfunction with physician and whether another antidepressant would provide equal benefit with less dysfunction.

MANAGEMENT

Drug: fluoxetine hydrochloride (Prozac)

Class: Antidepressant.

Mechanism of Action: Inhibits CNS neuronal uptake of serotonin.

Metabolism: Well absorbed after oral administration, and peak serum levels occur in 6–8 hours. Peak plasma concentrations are 15–55 mg/mL. Time to steady state in serum level is 2–4 weeks; 94.5% protein-bound. Drug is extensively metabolized in the liver to norfluoxetine and other metabolites using P450 enzyme pathway; inactive metabolites are excreted in the urine. Elimination half-life is 1–3 days when administered acutely, and 4–6 days with chronic administration.

Indication: For the treatment of (1) major depressive disorder; (2) panic disorder.

Dosage/Range:
Adult (for depression):
• 20 mg/day initially.
• After several weeks of therapy, if no response, may increase dose gradually to a maximum dose of 80 mg/day.
• Patients with hepatic dysfunction, elderly, or patients with concurrent diseases: start at lower dose or give less frequently.
• Weekly 90-mg tablets: begin 7 days after last 20-mg daily dose.

Drug Preparation:
• Give orally with or without food in the morning; with higher doses, e.g., 80 mg/day, may give two doses, one in the morning and one at noon.
• Available in pulvules of 10 mg and 20 mg; liquid/oral solution available as 20 mg/5 mL; weekly 90-mg tablets.
• Allow at least 14 days between stopping an MAOI and beginning fluoxetine; when stopping fluoxetine to begin an MAOI, wait at least 5 weeks before beginning the MAOI.

Drug Interactions:
• Alcohol: DO NOT USE CONCOMITANTLY, as increases impaired judgment, thinking, and motor skills.
• Tricyclic antidepressants (TCAs): decreased metabolism and increased serum levels of TCA; monitor for increased toxicity and dose-reduce TCA as necessary when drug is given concomitantly with fluoxetine.
• MAOIs: when drug is given concomitantly or within a short time period, severe, potentially life-threatening interactions may occur, including symptoms resembling neuroleptic malignant syndrome. DO NOT GIVE TOGETHER, AND END SEPARATELY, as stated in Administration section.
• Buspirone: reduced effects of buspirone; assess need to increase dose.
• Carbamazepine: increased serum levels of carbamazepine, with potential increased toxicity; monitor closely and dose-reduce as necessary.
• Cyproheptadine: decreased fluoxetine serum levels, so that effect was reduced or reversed; avoid concomitant administration if possible.

- Dextromethorphan: increased risk of hallucinations.
- Diazepam: increased diazepam half-life with increased circulating serum levels, leading to increased toxicity (e.g., excessive sedation or impaired psychomotor skills); dose-reduce diazepam or avoid concurrent administration.
- Digoxin: displaces fluoxetine from plasma protein binding, leading to increased fluoxetine serum levels and effect; monitor for toxicity and dose reduce as necessary.
- Lithium: increased lithium serum levels leading to possible increased neurotoxicity; monitor patient closely, and reduce lithium dose as needed.
- Phenytoin: increased phenytoin serum levels; monitor effect and serum levels, and modify dose accordingly.
- Tamoxifen: study indicates that taking this drug with tamoxifen may negate the benefit of tamoxifen; do not use together. Tamoxifen is a prodrug that requires metabolism by the CYP2D6 enzymes, which are inhibited by SSRIs including fluoxetine hydrochloride.
- Thioridazine: DO NOT administer together. Discontinue fluoxetine at least 5 weeks before starting thioridazine.
- Tryptophan: increased risk of CNS toxicity (e.g., headache, sweating, dizziness, agitation, aggressiveness) and peripheral toxicity (e.g., nausea, vomiting); use together cautiously if at all; avoid if possible.
- Warfarin: displaces fluoxetine from plasma protein binding sites, leading to increased fluoxetine serum levels, and effect; monitor for toxicity and dose-reduce as necessary.
- Teach all patients/families to call provider right away if thoughts of suicide or dying; attempts to commit suicide; new or worse depression; new or worse anxiety; feeling very agitated or restless; panic attacks; trouble sleeping (insomnia); new or worse irritability; aggressive, angry, or violent behavior; acting on dangerous impulses; extreme increase in activity or talking (mania); any unusual changes in behavior or mood.

Lab Effects/Interference:
- None known.

Special Considerations:
- Weekly dosing is for patients whose depression is stable on daily dosing. Diarrhea and cognitive changes are more common with weekly dosing.
- May take up to 4 weeks of therapy before benefit is seen.
- Possibility of suicide attempt may exist in depression and persist until depression managed by drug; monitor high-risk patients closely and give smallest prescription of tablets possible to ensure frequent follow-up and reduce the risk of overdosage.
- Has slight-to-no anticholinergic, sedative, or orthostatic hypotensive side effects.
- Avoid use in women who are pregnant or breastfeeding.
- Drug is also indicated for treatment of obsessive-compulsive disorder and bulimia disorder.

Potential Toxicities/Side Effects and the Nursing Process

I. ALTERATIONS IN SKIN INTEGRITY related to RASH

Defining Characteristics: Urticaria, rash may occur (7%). In initial trials, in one-third of patients developing rash, rash was associated with fever, leukocytosis, arthralgias,

MANAGEMENT

edema, carpal tunnel syndrome, respiratory distress, lymphadenopathy, proteinuria, and/or mildly elevated liver transaminase levels that required drug discontinuation, which largely resolved symptoms.

Nursing Implications: Assess baseline skin integrity, and instruct patient to report rash immediately. Discuss drug discontinuance with physician if severe or associated with other symptoms as above. Teach symptomatic skin management.

II.   ALTERATIONS IN SENSORY/PERCEPTUAL PATTERNS related to CNS EFFECTS

Defining Characteristics: CNS effects include headache and, less commonly, activation of mania or hypomania, insomnia, anxiety, decreased ability to concentrate, tremor, sensory disturbances, abnormal dreams, nervousness, dizziness, fatigue, sedation, lightheadedness, blurred vision. Rarely, seizures may occur. Patients at risk for suicide may commit suicide during initial period of treatment.

Nursing Implications: Assess baseline neurologic status and risk factors, and monitor during treatment. Instruct patient to report signs/symptoms, and discuss drug modification with physician. Evaluate patient satisfaction with drug efficacy. Instruct patient to avoid alcohol while taking drug. Assess suicide risk, and if at high risk, monitor closely, provide supportive counseling, and prescribe only small numbers of pills to prevent overdosage. May take up to 4 weeks for therapeutic effect to be seen.

III.   ALTERATION IN NUTRITION, LESS THAN BODY REQUIREMENTS, related to GI SIDE EFFECTS

Defining Characteristics: Nausea and, less commonly, vomiting, diarrhea, constipation, dry mouth, dyspepsia, anorexia, abdominal discomfort, flatulence, taste changes, gastroenteritis, and increased hunger may occur. Significant weight loss can occur in underweight, depressed patients.

Nursing Implications: Assess baseline nutrition and elimination patterns. Discuss abnormalities with physician and discuss drug modification. Teach patient to self-administer prescribed antiemetics as appropriate. If patient is losing weight, instruct patient to report this immediately, and discuss benefit of continuation of drug with physician.

IV.   INJURY related to DECREASE IN MENTAL ALERTNESS, PHYSICAL COORDINATION

Defining Characteristics: Drug may cause drowsiness, dizziness, and impair physical coordination, mental alertness.

Nursing Implications: Assess other medications that may increase risk (e.g., opiates, phenothiazines) and response to drug. Instruct patient to avoid potentially hazardous activities, including driving a car, operating machinery.

V.   SEXUAL DYSFUNCTION, POTENTIAL, related to IMPOTENCE

Defining Characteristics: Sexual dysfunction, impotence, anorgasmia may occur.

Nursing Implications: Assess baseline sexual functioning. Inform patient that alterations may occur, and instruct to report them. If severe, discuss dysfunction with physician, and whether another antidepressant would provide equal benefit with less dysfunction.

VI.   ALTERATION IN OXYGENATION, POTENTIAL, related to ALTERED BREATHING PATTERNS

Defining Characteristics: Bronchitis, upper respiratory infections, pharyngitis, cough, dyspnea, rhinitis, nasal congestion, and sinusitis may occur infrequently.

Nursing Implications: Assess baseline respiratory status, and instruct patient to report any changes. Discuss serious changes with physician, and interventions necessary.

VII.   ALTERATION IN COMFORT, POTENTIAL, related to PAIN

Defining Characteristics: Pain in muscles, joints, or back may occur; flulike symptoms are infrequent, as are asthenia, chest pain, and limb pain.

Nursing Implications: Assess baseline comfort level; instruct patient to report any changes. Discuss symptom management strategies, unless severe, and then discuss benefit of changing to another antidepressant medicine.

Drug: imipramine pamoate (Tofranil-PM)

Class: Tricyclic antidepressant.

Mechanism of Action: Blocks reuptake of neurotransmitters at neuronal membrane, thus increasing available serotonin and norepinephrine in CNS, and potentiating their effects. Appears to have analgesic effect separate from antidepressant action. May increase bioavailability of morphine. Indicated in the treatment of depressive (affective) mood disorders. Also used as an adjuvant analgesic in cancer pain management.

Metabolism: Completely absorbed from GI tract; highly protein-bound. Plasma half-life is 8–16 hours. Metabolized in liver; excreted in urine and, to lesser degree, in bile and feces.

Indication: For the relief of symptoms of depression.

MANAGEMENT

Dosage/Range:
Adult:
- Oral: 75–100 mg/day (may increase on patient response, to maximum 300 mg; reduce dose in elderly, 30–40 mg/day, to maximum 100 mg).
- IM: used only when oral route cannot be used.

Drug Preparation:
- Oral: store in well-closed containers at 15–30°C (59–86°F). Administer as a single bedtime dose.
- IM: administer IM in large muscle mass; change to oral as soon as possible.

Drug Interactions:
- MAOIs: increased excitation, hyperpyrexia, seizures; use together cautiously (especially if high dose is used).
- CNS depressants (alcohol, sedatives, hypnotics): increase CNS depression; use together cautiously.
- Sympathomimetic (epinephrine, amphetamines): increased hypertension; AVOID concurrent use.
- Cimetidine methylphenidate: increased imipramine levels, increased toxicity; use cautiously and monitor for increased toxicity.
- Warfarin: may increase PT; monitor closely and decrease dose of warfarin as needed.
- Barbiturates: may decrease imipramine level; monitor patient response; may need to increase dose.

Lab Effects/Interference:
- Increased metanephrine (Pisano test).
- Decreased urinary 5-HIAA.

Special Considerations:
- Antidepressant effect may take 2 weeks or longer.
- Adjuvant analgesic useful in cancer pain management.
- May also decrease depression associated with chronic cancer pain and promote improved sleep.
- Contraindicated in patients with myocardial infarction, seizure disorder, or benign prostatic hypertrophy.
- Use cautiously in patients with urine retention, narrow-angle glaucoma, hyperthyroidism, hepatic dysfunction, or suicidal ideation.
- Drug should be gradually discontinued rather than abruptly withdrawn to prevent anxiety, malaise, dizziness, nausea/vomiting.
- May be helpful in treating hiccups.
- Increased anticholinergic side effects in elderly.
- Some preparations may contain sodium bisulfite, which can cause allergic reactions, including anaphylaxis, in hypersensitive individuals. Check ingredients. Assess allergy history.
- Teach all patients/families to call provider right away if thoughts of suicide or dying; attempts to commit suicide; new or worse depression; new or worse anxiety; feeling

very agitated or restless; panic attacks; trouble sleeping (insomnia); new or worse irritability; aggressive, angry, or violent behavior; acting on dangerous impulses; extreme increase in activity or talking (mania); any unusual changes in behavior or mood.

Potential Toxicities/Side Effects and the Nursing Process

I.　ALTERATIONS IN SENSORY/PERCEPTUAL PATTERNS related to DROWSINESS, CNS EFFECT

Defining Characteristics: Drowsiness, dizziness, weakness, lethargy, fatigue are common; confusion, disorientation, hallucinations may occur in the elderly. Extrapyramidal symptoms may occur (fine tremor, rigidity, dystonia, dysarthria, dysphagia), as may peripheral neuropathy and blurred vision.

Nursing Implications: Assess baseline gait, neurologic and mental status, and monitor during therapy. Instruct patient to report signs/symptoms; discuss benefit/risk ratio with physician. Assess for signs/symptoms of suicidal ideation; if they occur, refer for psychiatric evaluation. Inform patient that drowsiness, dizziness will resolve after 1–2 weeks; instruct to avoid hazardous activities while drowsy (e.g., driving a car, operating machinery).

II.　ALTERATION IN CARDIAC OUTPUT related to POSTURAL HYPOTENSION, TACHYCARDIA

Defining Characteristics: Postural hypotension, EKG changes, tachycardia, hypertension may occur.

Nursing Implications: Assess baseline orthostatic BP, heart rate, and monitor during therapy. Instruct patient to report abnormalities, including postural dizziness, palpitations. Drug should be stopped several days before surgery to prevent hypertensive crisis (especially if high dose is used).

III.　ALTERATION IN NUTRITION related to GI SIDE EFFECTS

Defining Characteristics: Dry mouth, anorexia, nausea, vomiting, diarrhea, and abdominal cramping may occur; also, elevated LFTs.

Nursing Implications: Assess baseline nutrition and elimination patterns and LFTs, and monitor during therapy. Discuss abnormalities with physician, and discuss drug modification. Teach patient to self-administer prescribed antiemetics as appropriate. LFTs should be repeated, and if still elevated, the drug should be discontinued. Instruct patient to take full dose at bedtime. Suggest patient use sugar-free hard candy, frequent ice chips, or artificial saliva for dry mouth.

MANAGEMENT

IV.   ALTERATION IN URINARY ELIMINATION related to URINARY RETENTION

Defining Characteristics: Urinary retention may occur. Increased risk in patients with history of urinary retention.

Nursing Implications: Assess baseline urinary elimination pattern and risk. Assess for urinary retention, and instruct patient to report signs/symptoms. Discuss alternative drug with physician if this occurs.

V.   ALTERATIONS IN SKIN INTEGRITY related to ALLERGY

Defining Characteristics: Urticaria, erythema, rash, photosensitivity may occur.

Nursing Implications: Assess baseline drug allergy history and skin integrity. Instruct patient to report skin changes. If angioedema of face or tongue develops, discuss drug discontinuance with physician. Instruct patient to avoid sunlight or to use sunblock protection.

Drug: lorazepam (Ativan)

Class: Benzodiazepine (anxiolytic).

Mechanism of Action: Binds to benzodiazepine receptors in the CNS (limbic and cortical areas, cerebellum, brain stem, and spinal cord), resulting in the following effects: anxiolytic, ataxia, anticonvulsant, muscle relaxation. Appears to potentiate the effects of GABA.

Metabolism: Well absorbed from GI tract. Widely distributed in body tissues and fluids, including CSF. Crosses placenta and is excreted in breastmilk. Highly bound to plasma proteins. Metabolized in liver and excreted in urine. Short half-life of 10–20 hours. May produce psychological and physical dependence. Indicated for management of anxiety and short-term relief of anxiety associated with depression.

Indication: (1) Treatment of status epilepticus; (2) preanesthetic in adult patients.

Dosage/Range:
Adult:
- Oral: 1–6 mg/day in divided doses (maximum 10 mg/day).
- IM: 0.044 mg/kg or 2 mg, whichever is smaller (initial dose).
- IV: 0.044 mg/kg (up to 2 mg) given 15–20 minutes prior to surgery; 1.4 mg/m² given 30 minutes prior to chemotherapy; or 0.05 mg/kg (maximum 4 mg) if perioperative amnesia is desired.
- Use maximum dose (2 mg) in patients > 50 years old.

Drug Preparation:
- Oral: may administer with food to decrease stomach upset; has been given sublingually for more rapid onset (investigational).
- IM and IV: store drug in refrigerator until use.

- IM: administer undiluted, deep IM in large muscle mass (e.g., gluteus maximus).
- IV: dilute in equal volume of 0.9% sodium chloride or 5% dextrose for IVP administration (administer slowly; not > than 2 mg/min) OR dilute in 50 mL 0.9% sodium chloride or 5% dextrose immediately prior to administering IVB over 15 minutes.

Drug Interactions:
- CNS depressants (alcohol, anticonvulsants, phenothiazines, opiates): additive CNS depression; avoid concurrent use or use cautiously and monitor carefully.
- Oral contraceptives, isoniazid, ketoconazole: decrease plasma clearance of lorazepam so may increase effect (e.g., sedation); monitor patient closely.
- Tricyclic antidepressants: increased serum levels of antidepressant possible; use together cautiously.
- Digoxin: may decrease renal excretion of digoxin; monitor for overdosage; may need to decrease digoxin.

Lab Effects/Interference:
- Rarely, leukopenia, elevated LDH.
- Less frequently, elevated liver function studies.

Special Considerations:
- Wide margin of safety between therapeutic and toxic doses.
- May impair ability to perform activities requiring mental alertness (e.g., driving a car, operating machinery).
- May produce psychological and physical dependence.
- Administer cautiously in patients with liver or renal impairment.
- Use cautiously in patients with chronic pulmonary disease or sleep apnea.
- Contraindicated in patients with depressive neuroses, psychotic reactions (without prominent anxiety), acute alcoholic intoxication (with depressed VS), known hypersensitivity to the drug, or acute angle-closure glaucoma.
- May cause fetal damage, so should not be used during pregnancy or if the mother is breastfeeding.
- Withdrawal symptoms (including seizure, delirium) can occur with rapid drug discontinuance in patients taking high or chronic doses.
- If manic episodes or hyperactivity occur soon after drug started, drug should be discontinued.
- Drug should not be used to manage "everyday stress."
- Causes anterograde amnesia.

Potential Toxicities/Side Effects and the Nursing Process

I. ALTERATIONS IN SENSORY/PERCEPTUAL PATTERNS related to CNS DEPRESSION

Defining Characteristics: CNS depressant effects include drowsiness, fatigue, lethargy, confusion, weakness, headache, which may occur initially and resolve with continued therapy or dose reduction. Vivid dreams, suicidal ideation, and bizarre behavior may also occur. Patient risk factors: elderly, debilitated, liver dysfunction, low serum albumin.

Nursing Implications: Assess baseline neurologic status and risk factors, and monitor during treatment. Instruct patient to report signs/symptoms and discuss drug modification with physician. Evaluate patient satisfaction with drug efficacy. If patient expresses suicidal ideation (more common in panic disorders), refer patient for psychiatric evaluation and drug modification. Instruct patient to avoid alcohol while taking drug. Teach patient prescribed schedule for discontinuing drug when used chronically; assess for signs/symptoms of withdrawal (increased anxiety, rebound insomnia; may also include agitation, dysphoria, nausea/vomiting, irritability, muscle cramps, hallucinations, seizures).

II.   ALTERATION IN NUTRITION, LESS THAN BODY REQUIREMENTS, related to GI SIDE EFFECTS

Defining Characteristics: Nausea, vomiting, weight increase or decrease, dry mouth, constipation may occur; also elevated serum LFTs.

Nursing Implications: Assess baseline nutrition and elimination patterns and LFTs, and monitor during therapy. Discuss abnormalities with physician and discuss drug modification. Teach patient to self-administer prescribed antiemetics as appropriate.

III.   INJURY related to DECREASE IN MENTAL ALERTNESS, PHYSICAL COORDINATION

Defining Characteristics: Drug may cause drowsiness, dizziness, and impair physical coordination, mental alertness. Sedation, amnesia may last hours, impaired thinking and coordination 24–48 hours, and longer in the elderly.

Nursing Implications: Assess other medications that may increase risk (e.g., opiates, phenothiazines) and response to drug. Instruct patient to avoid potentially hazardous activities, including driving a car, operating machinery. For 8 hours following IV injection, assess level of consciousness and instruct patient to call nurse for assistance in ambulating if needed. Instruct patient to avoid alcohol for 24–48 hours after drug injection.

IV.   ALTERATIONS IN CARDIAC OUTPUT related to CHANGES IN BP, HR

Defining Characteristics: Drug may cause bradycardia, tachycardia, hypertension or hypotension, palpitations, edema.

Nursing Implications: Assess baseline VS, and monitor during therapy. Discuss abnormalities with physician. Instruct patient to report dizziness upon standing or other changes.

V. ALTERATIONS IN SKIN INTEGRITY related to RASH

Defining Characteristics: Urticaria, pruritus, rash (morbilliform, urticarial, or maculo-papular) may occur.

Nursing Implications: Assess baseline skin integrity, and instruct patient to report changes. Teach symptomatic skin management, and discuss drug discontinuance with physician if severe.

Drug: mirtazapine (Remeron)

Class: Antidepressant.

Mechanism of Action: Centrally active presynaptic α_2-antagonist, which increases central noradrenergic and serotonergic neurotransmission (via 5-HTs$_1$ receptors). Drug also blocks 5-HT$_2$ and 5-HT$_3$ receptors that contribute to antidepressant action. Thus, drug increases brain levels of both serotonin and norepinephrine. Antagonizes histamine H$_1$ causing some sedation but has limited anticholinergic or cardiovascular effects.

Metabolism: Active ingredient mirtazapine is rapidly absorbed from the GI tract with > 50% bioavailability. Peak plasma level is reached in about 2 hours, with approximately 85% of drug protein-bound. Mean elimination half-life is 20–40 hours with rare variation (up to 65 hours vs shorter in young men). Steady state reached in 3–4 days. Drug extensively metabolized (demethylation, oxidation, conjugation) and eliminated via urine and feces in a few days. Renal or hepatic insufficiency can delay drug clearance.

Indication: For the treatment of major depressive disorder.

Dosage/Range:
Adults:
- 15 mg PO daily to start, increasing in 2–4 weeks to a maximum of 45 mg daily if no response.
- If no response at maximal dose in 2–4 weeks, stop drug.
- Monitor elderly patients during dose titration. Use lowest dose, and monitor patients with renal or hepatic insufficiency closely due to reduced drug clearance.
- Response should be seen in 2–4 weeks of treatment at optimal dose.
- Once a response is obtained, drug is usually continued until the patient is symptom free for 4–6 months, and then the drug is gradually discontinued.

Drug Preparation:
- Tablets available in 15-, 30-, and 45-mg strengths, as well as in SolTab Orally Disintegrating Tablets (ODT), which dissolve on the tongue within 30 seconds.
- Administer tablets in a single daily dose at bedtime or in two divided doses (morning and evening).
- Administer SolTab ODT with or without water, to be chewed or allowed to disintegrate on the tongue.
- Store drug in the dark at 2–30°C.

Drug Interactions:
- Alcohol: AVOID concurrent use as potentiation of CNS depressant effects.
- Monoamine oxidase inhibitors (MAOI): AVOID concurrent use; DO NOT start mirtazapine until at least 2 weeks after the cessation of MAOI, and do not start an MAOI until at least 2 weeks after cessation of mirtazapine.
- Benzodiazepines: Potentiate CNS depressant effects of drug. Use together cautiously, if at all.

Lab Effects/Interference:
- Transient increase in hepatic transaminases (SGOT/AST and SGPT/ALT).

Special Considerations:
- Rarely, granulocytopenia or agranulocytosis may occur, usually after 4–6 weeks of treatment.
- Possibility of suicide attempt may exist in depression and persist until depression is managed by drug. Monitor high-risk patients closely and give smallest prescription of tablets to ensure frequent follow-up and reduce the risk of overdosage.
- Avoid use in women who are pregnant or breastfeeding.
- Discontinue the drug if jaundice develops.
- Abrupt termination of drug after long-term therapy can result in nausea, headache, and malaise.
- Drug at low doses enhances sleep.
- Patients requiring close monitoring for toxicity include those with epilepsy or organic brain syndrome; hepatic or renal insufficiency; heart disease, including conduction disturbances, and angina pectoris, or history of myocardial infarction; hypotension; prostatic hypertrophy or other voiding (micturition) disturbances; acute narrow-angle glaucoma; and diabetes mellitus.
- Teach all patients/families to call provider right away if thoughts of suicide or dying; attempts to commit suicide; new or worse depression; new or worse anxiety; feeling very agitated or restless; panic attacks; trouble sleeping (insomnia); new or worse irritability; aggressive, angry, or violent behavior; acting on dangerous impulses; extreme increase in activity or talking (mania); any unusual changes in behavior or mood.

Potential Toxicities/Side Effects and the Nursing Process

I.   ALTERATION IN NUTRITION, MORE THAN BODY REQUIREMENTS, related to INCREASED APPETITE, WEIGHT GAIN, EDEMA

Defining Characteristics: Increased appetite and weight gain are common. Peripheral edema may occur, resulting in increased weight. Drug may be chosen for its appetite stimulation in patients with advanced cancer who are depressed and losing weight.

Nursing Implications: Assess baseline nutrition pattern and weight, and monitor during therapy. Assess baseline fluid status and presence of edema, and monitor during therapy. Teach patient that these side effects may occur and to report them, especially edema. If patient develops significant edema, assess cardiopulmonary status (heart rate, orthostatic blood pressure, respiratory rate at rest and with activity, oxygen saturation). Discuss significant edema with physician.

II. ALTERATIONS IN SENSORY/PERCEPTUAL PATTERNS related to CNS EFFECTS

Defining Characteristics: CNS effects include drowsiness and sedation, especially during the first few weeks of treatment. Rarely, seizure, tremor, or myoclonus may occur. Worsening of psychotic symptoms may occur in patients with schizophrenia or other psychotic disturbances, and paranoid thoughts may become intensified. Mania may become activated in patients with manic depressive psychosis. Patients at risk for suicide may attempt/commit suicide during initial period of treatment.

Nursing Implications: Assess baseline neurologic status and risk factors, and monitor during treatment. Instruct patient to report signs/symptoms, and discuss drug modification with physician. Evaluate patient satisfaction with drug efficacy. Teach patient to avoid alcohol while taking drug, and to avoid benzodiazepines unless physician feels benefits outweigh risks. Assess suicide risk, and if at high risk, monitor closely, provide supportive counseling, and prescribe only a small number of pills to prevent overdosage. May take up to 4 weeks for therapeutic effect to be seen.

III. POTENTIAL FOR INJURY related to DECREASE IN MENTAL ALERTNESS, PHYSICAL COORDINATION, ORTHOSTATIC HYPOTENSION

Defining Characteristics: Drug may cause drowsiness, decreased mental alertness, and orthostatic hypotension.

Nursing Implications: Assess other medications patient is taking that may increase the risk (e.g., opiates, phenothiazines) and response to drug. Instruct patient to avoid potentially hazardous activities, such as driving a car or other vehicle, and operating machinery. Assess baseline orthostatic blood pressure and heart rate, and monitor during therapy. Teach patient that orthostatic hypotension may occur, and to report symptoms such as dizziness when changing position. Teach patient self-care measures to minimize risk of injury, such as changing position slowly over the course of 5 minutes, going from lying to sitting, and then from sitting to standing positions, holding on to walls or fixed railings when walking, and removing scatter rugs from walkways.

IV. POTENTIAL FOR INFECTION, BLEEDING, AND FATIGUE related to RARE BONE MARROW DEPRESSION

Defining Characteristics: Rare granulocytopenia or agranulocytosis may occur, usually after 4–6 weeks of treatment. If it occurs, it is usually reversible following drug discontinuance.

Nursing Implications: Teach patient that this rare side effect may occur. Instruct patient to stop the drug and to report signs and symptoms of infection, such as fever, sore throat, productive cough, or dysuria right away. If the patient develops any signs and symptoms of infection, the drug should be stopped and a complete blood count with differential checked.

Assess baseline CBC/differential, and periodically during therapy, especially at 4–6 weeks after drug initiated.

V.   POTENTIAL ALTERATION IN SKIN INTEGRITY related to EXANTHEMA

Defining Characteristics: Rarely, skin rash resembling chickenpox, measles, or rubella may develop.

Nursing Implications: Assess baseline skin integrity, and instruct patient to report rash immediately. Discuss drug cessation or discontinuance with physician. Teach patient symptomatic skin management.

Drug: nefazodone HCl (Serzone)

Class: Antidepressant, synthetically derived phenylpiperazine.

Mechanism of Action: Appears to inhibit neuronal uptake of serotonin and norepinephrine. Drug occupies central serotonin ($5\text{-}HT_2$) receptors and acts as an antagonist. In addition, it antagonizes α-adrenergic receptors that may explain the associated postural hypotension.

Metabolism: Rapidly and completely absorbed after oral administration, but extensively metabolized by the liver using the P450 cytochrome enzyme system. Food delays absorption and decreases bioavailability by 20%. Peak plasma concentrations occur at 1 hour, and half-life of the drug is 2–4 hours. Drug is extensively protein-bound (> 99%). Time to steady state is 4–5 days. Only 1% of drug is excreted unchanged in the urine.

Indication: For the treatment of depression.

Dosage/Range:
Adult:
- Initial: 200 mg/day, administered in two divided doses.
- If no or slight response, increase dose by 100–200 mg/day in two divided doses after at least 1 week at the previous dose; usual dose requirements are 300–600 mg/day in two divided doses.
- Elderly (especially women) or debilitated patients: begin at 50% of dose or 100 mg/day in two divided doses, and titrate up to therapeutic dose very slowly and gradually.

Drug Preparation:
- Oral, total dose given in two divided, bid doses on an empty stomach.
- Available in 100-, 150-, 200-, and 250-mg tablets.
- If changing from an MAOI to nefazodone HCl, allow at least 14 days after discontinuance of the MAOI before starting nefazodone; if changing from nefazodone to an MAOI, allow at least 7 days after stopping nefazodone before starting the MAOI.

Drug Interactions:
- Terfenadine, astemizole, cisapride: are metabolized by the P450 hepatic enzyme system; nefazodone can inhibit their metabolism, resulting in QT elongation and potential cardiac arrest; DO NOT GIVE CONCOMITANTLY WITH NEFAZODONE.
- MAOIs: may cause symptoms resembling neuroleptic malignant syndrome, including death. DO NOT USE CONCURRENTLY. See Administration guidelines when changing from/to MAOIs.
- Alprazolam: increased serum levels of alprazolam; monitor effect and toxicity, and determine need for dose reduction.
- Digoxin: increased plasma levels of digoxin; assess effect and toxicity, and need for dose reduction of digoxin.
- Propranolol: decreased plasma levels of propranolol; assess effect and need for increased dosage.
- Triazolam: increased plasma levels of triazolam; assess effect, toxicity, and need for dosage reduction.

Lab Effects/Interference:
- Rarely, increased AST, ALT, LDH.
- Rarely, decreased HCT, anemia, leukopenia.
- Rarely, hypercholesterolemia, hypoglycemia.

Special Considerations:
- Contraindications: coadministration with terfenadine, astemizole, cisapride, or MAOIs.
- Drug produces slight anticholinergic effects, moderate sedation, and slight orthostatic hypotension.
- May take several weeks until therapeutic effect is known.
- Use with caution in patients recovering from myocardial infarction, who have unstable heart disease and are taking digoxin, and patients with a history of mania.
- Monitor patients at risk for suicide carefully, as attempts may be made during initial period before significant antidepressant effects of the drug are seen.
- Avoid use during pregnancy or in nursing mothers.
- Teach all patients/families to call provider right away if thoughts of suicide or dying; attempts to commit suicide; new or worse depression; new or worse anxiety; feeling very agitated or restless; panic attacks; trouble sleeping (insomnia); new or worse irritability; aggressive, angry, or violent behavior; acting on dangerous impulses; extreme increase in activity or talking (mania); any unusual changes in behavior or mood.

Potential Toxicities/Side Effects and the Nursing Process

I. **ALTERATIONS IN SENSORY/PERCEPTUAL PATTERNS related to DROWSINESS, DIZZINESS**

Defining Characteristics: Dizziness (17% incidence), drowsiness (25%), insomnia (17%), lightheadedness (10%), activation of mania or hypomania, agitation, blurred vision (9%), confusion (7%), decreased concentration (3%), memory impairment (4%), paresthesia (4%), ataxia (2%), incoordination (2%), psychomotor retardation (2%), tremor (1%), hypertonia (1%), vertigo, twitching, hallucinations, abnormal dreams (3%), and paranoia may occur. Neuroleptic malignant syndrome is rare (e.g., hyperthermia, seizures).

Nursing Implications: Assess baseline gait, neurologic and mental status, and monitor during therapy. Instruct patient to report signs/symptoms; depending upon severity and dysfunction, discuss benefit/risk ratio with physician. Assess for signs/symptoms of suicidal ideation; if they occur, refer for psychiatric evaluation. Inform patient that drowsiness, dizziness will resolve after 1–2 weeks; instruct to avoid hazardous activities while drowsy (e.g., driving a car, operating machinery).

II.   ALTERATION IN CARDIAC OUTPUT related to POSTURAL HYPOTENSION, TACHYCARDIA

Defining Characteristics: Infrequent postural hypotension (4% incidence), hypotension (2%), tachycardia, hypertension, syncope, ventricular ectopic beats, angina pectoris, and CVA may occur rarely.

Nursing Implications: Assess baseline orthostatic BP, heart rate, and monitor during therapy. Instruct patient to report abnormalities, including postural dizziness, palpitations. If patient has orthostatic hypotension, teach patient to change position slowly and to hold on to supportive structure. If symptoms are significant, discuss changing to another antidepressant with physician.

III.   ALTERATION IN NUTRITION, LESS THAN BODY REQUIREMENTS, related to GI SIDE EFFECTS

Defining Characteristics: Dry mouth (25% incidence), nausea (22%), vomiting (rare), diarrhea (5%), constipation (14%), dyspepsia (9%), and rarely eructation, gastritis, stomatitis, peptic ulceration, rectal hemorrhage have been reported.

Nursing Implications: Assess baseline nutrition and elimination patterns and LFTs, and monitor during therapy. Discuss abnormalities with physician, and discuss drug modification. Teach patient to self-administer prescribed antiemetics, and other symptom management interventions, as ordered. Suggest patient use sugar-free hard candy, frequent ice chips, or artificial saliva for dry mouth.

IV.   ALTERATION IN URINARY ELIMINATION related to URINARY FREQUENCY

Defining Characteristics: Infrequently (2% incidence), urinary frequency, urinary retention, and urinary tract infections may occur.

Nursing Implications: Assess baseline urinary elimination pattern and risk. Assess for urinary frequency, retention, and infection, and instruct patient to report signs/symptoms. Discuss alternative drug with physician if this occurs.

V. ALTERATION IN COMFORT related to HEADACHE

Defining Characteristics: Headache (36% incidence), asthenia (11%), arthralgia (1%) may occur.

Nursing Implications: Assess baseline comfort. Instruct patient to report unrelieved symptoms, and consider symptom-management strategies. Discuss severe discomfort that is unrelieved with physician and consider alternative antidepressant therapy.

Drug: nortriptyline hydrochloride (Aventyl, Pamelor)

Class: Tricyclic antidepressant.

Mechanism of Action: Blocks reuptake of neurotransmitters at neuronal membrane, thus increasing available serotonin and norepinephrine in CNS, and potentiating their effects. May increase bioavailability of morphine. Indicated in the treatment of depressive (affective) mood disorders. Also used as an adjuvant analgesic in cancer pain management.

Metabolism: Distributed to lungs, heart, brain, liver; highly bound to plasma, proteins. Plasma half-life is 16–90 hours. Metabolized in liver, excreted in urine, and, to a lesser degree, in bile and feces.

Indication: For the relief of depressive symptoms.

Dosage/Range:
Adult:
- Oral: 75–100 mg/day (maximum 100 mg or serum levels should be monitored; therapeutic dose: 50–150 mg/mL).
- Elderly: 30–50 mg/day.

Drug Preparation:
- Store oral solution in tight, light-resistant containers; store tablets in tight containers; keep at temperature of 15–30°C (59–86°F).
- Administer in single bedtime dose.

Drug Interactions:
- MAOIs: increased excitation, hyperpyrexia, seizures; use together cautiously (especially if high dose is used).
- CNS depressants (alcohol, sedatives, hypnotics): increase CNS depression; use together cautiously.
- Sympathomimetic (epinephrine, amphetamines): increased hypertension; AVOID concurrent use.
- Cimetidine methylphenidate: increased nortriptyline levels, increased toxicity; use cautiously and monitor for increased toxicity.

- Warfarin: may increase PT; monitor closely and decrease dose of warfarin as needed.
- Barbiturates: may decrease nortriptyline levels; monitor patient response; may need to increase dose.

Lab Effects/Interference:
- Rarely, bone marrow depression (agranulocytosis, eosinophilia, purpura, thrombocy-topenia).
- Rarely, increased or decreased serum glucose levels.

Special Considerations:
- Antidepressant effect may take 2 weeks or longer.
- Adjuvant analgesic useful in cancer pain management.
- May also decrease depression associated with chronic cancer pain and promote improved sleep.
- Contraindicated in patients with myocardial infarction, seizure disorder, or benign prostatic hypertrophy.
- Use cautiously in patients with urine retention, narrow-angle glaucoma, hyperthyroidism, hepatic dysfunction, or suicidal ideation.
- Drug should be gradually discontinued rather than abruptly withdrawn to prevent anxiety, malaise, dizziness, nausea/vomiting.
- May be helpful in treating hiccups.
- Increased anticholinergic side effects in elderly.
- Some preparations may contain sodium bisulfite, which can cause allergic reactions, including anaphylaxis, in hypersensitive individuals. Check ingredients and assess allergy history.
- Teach all patients/families to call provider right away if thoughts of suicide or dying; attempts to commit suicide; new or worse depression; new or worse anxiety; feeling very agitated or restless; panic attacks; trouble sleeping (insomnia); new or worse irritability; aggressive, angry, or violent behavior; acting on dangerous impulses; extreme increase in activity or talking (mania); any unusual changes in behavior or mood.

Potential Toxicities/Side Effects and the Nursing Process

I.   ALTERATIONS IN SENSORY/PERCEPTUAL PATTERNS related to DROWSINESS, DIZZINESS

Defining Characteristics: Drowsiness, dizziness, weakness, lethargy, fatigue are common; confusion, disorientation, hallucinations may occur in the elderly. Extrapyramidal symptoms may occur (fine tremor, rigidity, dystonia, dysarthria, dysphagia), as may peripheral neuropathy and blurred vision.

Nursing Implications: Assess baseline gait, neurologic and mental status, and monitor during therapy. Instruct patient to report signs/symptoms; discuss benefit/risk ratio with physician. Assess for signs/symptoms of suicidal ideation; if they occur, refer for psychiatric evaluation. Inform patient that drowsiness, dizziness will resolve after

1–2 weeks; instruct to avoid hazardous activities while drowsy (e.g., driving a car, operating machinery).

II. ALTERATION IN CARDIAC OUTPUT related to POSTURAL HYPOTENSION, TACHYCARDIA

Defining Characteristics: Low incidence of postural hypotension; EKG changes, tachycardia, and hypertension may occur.

Nursing Implications: Assess baseline orthostatic BP, heart rate, and monitor during therapy. Instruct patient to report abnormalities, including postural dizziness, palpitations. Drug should be stopped several days before surgery to prevent hypertensive crisis (especially if high dose is used).

III. ALTERATION IN NUTRITION, LESS THAN BODY REQUIREMENTS, related to GI SIDE EFFECTS

Defining Characteristics: Dry mouth, anorexia, nausea, vomiting, diarrhea, abdominal cramping may occur; also, elevated LFTs.

Nursing Implications: Assess baseline nutrition and elimination patterns and LFTs, and monitor during therapy. Discuss abnormalities with physician, and discuss drug modification. Teach patient to self-administer prescribed antiemetics as appropriate. LFTs should be repeated, and if still elevated, the drug should be discontinued. Instruct patient to take full dose at bedtime. Suggest patient use sugar-free hard candy, frequent ice chips, or artificial saliva for dry mouth.

IV. ALTERATION IN URINARY ELIMINATION related to URINARY FREQUENCY

Defining Characteristics: Urinary retention may occur. Increased risk if history of urinary retention.

Nursing Implications: Assess baseline urinary elimination pattern and risk. Assess for urinary retention, and instruct patient to report signs/symptoms. Discuss alternative drug with physician if this occurs.

V. ALTERATIONS IN SKIN INTEGRITY related to ALLERGY

Defining Characteristics: Urticaria, erythema, rash, photosensitivity may occur.

Nursing Implications: Assess baseline drug allergy history and skin integrity. Instruct patient to report skin changes. If angioedema of face or tongue develops, discuss drug discontinuance with physician. Instruct patient to avoid sunlight or to use sunblock protection.

MANAGEMENT

Drug: oxazepam (Serax)

Class: Benzodiazepine (anxiolytic).

Mechanism of Action: Binds to benzodiazepine receptors in the CNS (limbic and cortical areas, cerebellum, brain stem, and spinal cord), resulting in the following effects: anxiolytic, ataxia, anticonvulsant, muscle relaxation. Appears to potentiate the effects of GABA.

Metabolism: Well absorbed from GI tract. Widely distributed in body tissues and fluids, including CSF. Crosses placenta and is excreted in breastmilk. Highly bound to plasma proteins. Metabolized in liver and excreted in urine. Short half-life of 5–20 hours. May produce psychological and physical dependence. Indicated for management of anxiety, the short-term relief of anxiety associated with depression, and alcohol withdrawal.

Indication: Management of (1) anxiety disorders or for the short-term relief of symptoms of anxiety; (2) alcoholics with acute tremulousness, confusional state, or anxiety associated with alcohol withdrawal.

Dosage/Range:
Adult:
- Oral: 10–30 mg tid–qid.
- Elderly: 10 mg tid OR 15 mg tid–qid.

Drug Preparation:
- Store tablets in tight container at < 40°C (104°F).

Drug Interactions:
- CNS depressants (alcohol, anticonvulsants, phenothiazines, opiates): additive CNS depression; avoid concurrent use or use cautiously and monitor carefully.
- Oral contraceptives, isoniazid, ketoconazole, or cimetidine: decrease plasma clearance of oxazepam, so may increase effect (e.g., sedation); monitor patient closely.
- Tricyclic antidepressants: increased serum levels of antidepressant possible; use together cautiously.
- Digoxin: may decrease renal excretion of digoxin; monitor for overdosage; may need to decrease digoxin.

Lab Effects/Interference:
- Rarely, leukopenia.
- Rarely, altered liver function studies.

Special Considerations:
- Wide margin of safety between therapeutic and toxic doses.
- May impair ability to perform activities requiring mental alertness (e.g., driving a car, operating machinery).
- May produce psychological and physical dependence.
- Administer cautiously in patients with liver or renal impairment.
- Use cautiously in patients with chronic pulmonary disease or sleep apnea.

- Contraindicated in patients with depressive neuroses, psychotic reactions (without prominent anxiety), acute alcoholic intoxication (with depressed VS), known hypersensitivity to the drug, or acute angle-closure glaucoma.
- May cause fetal damage, so should not be used during pregnancy or if the mother is breastfeeding.
- Withdrawal symptoms (including seizure, delirium) can occur with rapid drug discontinuance in patients taking high or chronic doses.
- If manic episodes or hyperactivity occur soon after drug started, drug should be discontinued.
- Drug should not be used to manage "everyday stress."
- Serax 15-mg tablet contains dye tartrazine, which may cause allergic reactions in sensitive individuals, especially if sensitive to aspirin.

Potential Toxicities/Side Effects and the Nursing Process

I.   ALTERATIONS IN SENSORY/PERCEPTUAL PATTERNS related to CNS DEPRESSION

Defining Characteristics: CNS depressant effects include drowsiness, fatigue, lethargy, weakness. Cumulative effects are less, as there is a short plasma half-life. Risk factors: elderly, debilitated, liver dysfunction, low serum albumin.

Nursing Implications: Assess baseline neurologic status and risk factors, and monitor during treatment. Instruct patient to report signs/symptoms. Instruct patient to avoid alcohol while taking drug. Teach patient prescribed schedule for discontinuing drug when drug is used chronically.

II.   ALTERATION IN NUTRITION, LESS THAN BODY REQUIREMENTS, related to GI SIDE EFFECTS

Defining Characteristics: Nausea, vomiting, weight increase or decrease, dry mouth, constipation may occur; also, elevated LFTs.

Nursing Implications: Assess baseline nutrition and elimination patterns and LFTs, and monitor during therapy. Discuss abnormalities with physician and discuss drug modification. Teach patient to self-administer prescribed antiemetics as appropriate.

III. INJURY related to DECREASE IN MENTAL ALERTNESS, PHYSICAL COORDINATION

Defining Characteristics: Drug may cause drowsiness, dizziness, and impair physical coordination, mental alertness.

Nursing Implications: Assess other medications that may increase risk (e.g., opiates, phenothiazines) and response to drug. Instruct patient to avoid potentially hazardous activities, including driving a car, operating machinery.

IV.   ALTERATIONS IN CARDIAC OUTPUT related to TRANSIENT
      HYPOTENSION

Defining Characteristics: Transient hypotension may occur.

Nursing Implications: Assess baseline VS, and monitor during therapy. Discuss abnormalities with physician. Instruct patient to report dizziness on standing or other changes.

V.   ALTERATIONS IN SKIN INTEGRITY related to RASH

Defining Characteristics: Urticaria, pruritus, rash (morbilliform, urticarial, or maculo-papular) may occur.

Nursing Implications: Assess baseline skin integrity, and instruct patient to report changes. Teach symptomatic skin management, and discuss drug discontinuance with physician if severe.

Drug: paroxetine hydrochloride (Paxil)

Class: Antidepressant with mechanism of action different from selective serotonin reuptake inhibitors, tricyclic, or tetracyclic antidepressants.

Mechanism of Action: Appears to potentiate serotonergic activity of the CNS by potent and selective inhibition of serotonin reuptake by the neurons.

Metabolism: Completely absorbed after oral administration and metabolized to some degree by the P450 hepatic enzyme system. Distributed throughout the body, including the CNS, and is extensively protein-bound (95%). Increased serum levels occur in patients with hepatic or renal dysfunction (twofold), and in elderly patients. Time to peak plasma levels 5.2 hours, and time to reach steady state is 10–24 days. Largely excreted in the urine (64%) over a 10-day period, and approximately 36% is excreted in the feces.

Indication: For the treatment of (1) major depressive disorder; (2) obsessive and compulsive disorder; (3) panic disorder; (4) generalized anxiety disorder.

Dosage/Range:
Adult (depression):
- Initial: 20 mg/day PO in the morning. Initial response may be delayed; if no response, may increase dose in 10-mg/day increments after an interval of at least 1 week, to a maximum of 50 mg/day.
- Patients who are elderly, or who have severe hepatic or renal dysfunction: initial dose of 10 mg/day, with increased dose adjustments made after at least 1 week, in 10-mg/day increments up to a maximum of 40 mg/day.

Drug Preparation:
- Oral, available in 10-, 20-, 30-, and 40-mg tablets.
- Administer as a single daily dose, usually in the morning.
- Allow at least 14 days when changing from an MAOI to paroxetine, or when changing from paroxetine to an MAOI.

Drug Interactions:
- Tryptophan: when administered concomitantly, headache, nausea, sweating, and dizziness may occur; avoid concomitant administration.
- MAOIs: reactions including death have occurred (hyperthermia, rigidity, myoclonus, autonomic instability, mental status changes including delirium/coma); allow at least 14 days between changing to or from paroxetine to an MAOI.
- Warfarin: increased bleeding despite a normal PT; give together cautiously, if at all.
- Sumatriptan: may cause hyperreflexia, weakness; incoordination may occur; monitor patient closely.
- Drugs inhibiting the P450 cytochrome hepatic metabolic pathway (e.g., cimetidine): paroxetine serum levels may be increased by up to 50%; assess response and toxicity carefully and need to decrease paroxetine dosage.
- Drugs inducing the P450 cytochrome hepatic metabolic pathway (e.g., phenobarbital, phenytoin): paroxetine serum levels may be reduced by up to 25–50%; assess response and need to increase paroxetine dosage.
- Drugs metabolized by the P450 cytochrome hepatic metabolic pathway (other antidepressant medications, phenothiazines, type IC antiarrhythmics): paroxetine may inhibit the metabolism of these drugs, resulting in increased toxicity.
- Tricyclic antidepressants should be given together with caution, and the dose of the tricyclic antidepressant may need to be reduced.
- Drugs that are highly bound to plasma proteins: paroxetine may displace the other drug from serum proteins, thus increasing the serum level of the other drug, resulting in toxicity. Give together cautiously and monitor/reduce drug as needed.
- Alcohol: avoid concurrent administration.
- Lithium, digoxin: use together cautiously; digoxin levels may be reduced.
- Procyclidine: increased anticholinergic effects possible; decrease dose of procyclidine if necessary to coadminister.
- Tamoxifen: study indicates that taking this drug with tamoxifen may negate the benefit of tamoxifen; do not use together. Tamoxifen is a prodrug that requires metabolism by the CYP2D6 enzymes, which are inhibited by SSRIs including fluoxetine hydrochloride. See *tamoxifen* in *Chapter 1*.
- Theophylline: may elevate serum theophylline levels; monitor and adjust dose accordingly.

Lab Effects/Interference:
- None known.

Special Considerations:
- Drug excreted in breastmilk; drug should be administered cautiously, if at all, in breastfeeding mothers.
- Drug is teratogenic, so women of childbearing age should use contraception if sexually active.

- Drug indicated for the treatment of depression, panic disorder, obsessive-compulsive disorder.
- Teach all patients/families to call provider right away if thoughts of suicide or dying; attempts to commit suicide; new or worse depression; new or worse anxiety; feeling very agitated or restless; panic attacks; trouble sleeping (insomnia); new or worse irritability; aggressive, angry, or violent behavior; acting on dangerous impulses; extreme increase in activity or talking (mania); any unusual changes in behavior or mood.

Potential Toxicities/Side Effects and the Nursing Process

I.   ALTERATIONS IN SENSORY/PERCEPTUAL PATTERNS related to DIZZINESS, SOMNOLENCE

Defining Characteristics: Somnolence, dizziness, insomnia, tremor, nervousness, and asthenia occur in more than 5% of patients. Less common are headache, agitation, seizures, anxiety, activation of mania or hypomania, paresthesia, confusion, impaired concentration, emotional lability, depression.

Nursing Implications: Assess baseline neurologic status, affective state, and risk factors, and monitor during treatment. Instruct patient to avoid alcohol while taking drug. Assess effect on elderly and/or patients with hepatic or renal dysfunction. Inform patient that daytime drowsiness may occur, and instruct to use caution if driving or operating heavy machinery. Assess for symptoms at each visit, and instruct patient to report changes. If symptoms occur, discuss strategies to ensure patient safety and comfort.

II.   ALTERATION IN NUTRITION, LESS THAN BODY REQUIREMENTS, related to GI SIDE EFFECTS

Defining Characteristics: Nausea and decreased appetite may occur.

Nursing Implications: Assess baseline nutrition status, and instruct patient to report any nausea or loss of appetite. Discuss measures to reduce nausea and/or stimulate appetite.

III. ALTERATION IN COMFORT related to SWEATING

Defining Characteristics: Sweating may occur.

Nursing Implications: Inform patient that this may occur, and assess impact on patient and need for intervention.

IV.   SEXUAL DYSFUNCTION, POTENTIAL, related to EJACULATORY DISTURBANCES

Defining Characteristics: Incidence of ejaculatory disturbances is 13%; other disorders may occur (10%), including erectile difficulties, delayed ejaculation/orgasm, impotence, and other sexual dysfunction.

Nursing Implications: Assess baseline sexual functioning. Inform patient that alterations may occur, and instruct to report them. If severe, discuss dysfunction with physician, and whether another antidepressant would provide equal benefit with less dysfunction.

Drug: sertraline hydrochloride (Zoloft)

Class: Antidepressant.

Mechanism of Action: Inhibits CNS neuronal uptake of serotonin.

Metabolism: Undergoes extensive first-pass metabolism by the liver and is excreted in the urine (45% by 9 days) and the feces (40–45%). Time to peak plasma levels is 4.5–8.4 hours, and peak plasma levels are 20–55 mg/mL. Food reduces time to reach peak serum levels. Highly protein-bound (98%). Time to steady-state plasma levels is 7 days but is increased to 2–3 weeks in the elderly.

Indication: For the treatment of (1) major depressive disorder in adults; (2) obsessive-compulsive disorder; (3) panic disorder; (4) post-traumatic stress disorder; (5) premenstrual dysphoria disorder; (6) social anxiety disorder.

Dosage/Range:
Adult:
- Initial: 50 mg/day. If no response after a period of 1–2 weeks, may titrate gradually up to a maximum dose of 200 mg/day.

Drug Preparation:
- Oral, once daily in morning or evening.
- Available in 25-, 50-, and 100-mg tablets.
- When changing from an MAOI to sertraline HCl, wait at least 14 days after stopping the MAOI before initiating sertraline; when changing from sertraline HCl to an MAOI, wait at least 14 days after stopping sertraline before beginning the MAOI.

Drug Interactions:
- MAOIs: Severe reactions, similar to neuroleptic malignant syndrome, including death may occur; DO NOT ADMINISTER CONCURRENTLY; see Administration section.
- Alcohol: DO NOT give concurrently.
- Benzodiazepines: Decreased metabolism of benzodiazepine drugs, which are metabolized by the P450 enzyme system in the liver, resulting in increased serum levels and toxicity; monitor for toxicity and adjust dose accordingly.
- Tamoxifen: Study indicates that taking this drug with tamoxifen may negate the benefit of tamoxifen; do not use together. Tamoxifen is a prodrug that requires metabolism by the CYP2D6 enzymes, which are inhibited by SSRIs including fluoxetine hydrochloride.
- Tolbutamide: Decreased clearance with increased serum levels; monitor blood-sugar levels closely.

MANAGEMENT

- Warfarin: Increased PT and delayed normalization of same; monitor PT values closely.
- CNS-active drugs: Monitor effects closely and modify drug doses accordingly (e.g., lithium).

Lab Effects/Interference:
- Increased AST or ALT, total cholesterol, triglycerides.
- Decreased serum uric acid.

Special Considerations:
- Teach all patients/families to call provider right away if thoughts of suicide or dying; attempts to commit suicide; new or worse depression; new or worse anxiety; feeling very agitated or restless; panic attacks; trouble sleeping (insomnia); new or worse irritability; aggressive, angry, or violent behavior; acting on dangerous impulses; extreme increase in activity or talking (mania); any unusual changes in behavior or mood.

Potential Toxicities/Side Effects and the Nursing Process

I.   ALTERATIONS IN SENSORY/PERCEPTUAL PATTERNS related to HEADACHE, INSOMNIA

Defining Characteristics: Commonly, headache, insomnia. Less commonly, drowsiness, dizziness, agitation, nervousness, anxiety, tremor, fatigue, impaired concentration, paresthesia, yawning, hypoesthesia, twitching, confusion, abnormal coordination (ataxia), abnormal gait, hyperesthesia, hyperkinesia, abnormal dreams, amnesia, apathy, hallucinations. Suicidal ideation or attempt is uncommon, but patients at risk may attempt suicide during initial treatment before therapeutic effects of drug are felt.

Nursing Implications: Assess baseline gait, neurologic, affective, and mental status, and monitor during therapy. Instruct patient to report signs/symptoms; discuss benefit/risk ratio with physician. Assess for signs/symptoms of suicidal ideation; if they occur, refer for psychiatric evaluation. Inform patient that drowsiness may occur, and instruct to avoid hazardous activities while drowsy (e.g., driving a car, operating machinery).

II.   ALTERATION IN CARDIAC OUTPUT, POTENTIAL, related to CHANGES IN BP

Defining Characteristics: Rarely, palpitations, edema, hypertension or hypotension, peripheral ischemia, postural hypotension, tachycardia, and syncope may occur.

Nursing Implications: Assess baseline orthostatic BP, heart rate, and monitor during therapy. Instruct patient to report abnormalities, including postural dizziness, palpitations. Discuss significant changes with physician. If patient has orthostatic hypotension, teach patient to change position slowly and to hold on to support.

III. ALTERATION IN NUTRITION, LESS THAN BODY REQUIREMENTS, related to GI SIDE EFFECTS

Defining Characteristics: Nausea and diarrhea are common. Less common are dry mouth, constipation, dyspepsia, increased or decreased appetite, vomiting, increased salivation, abdominal pain, gastroenteritis, dysphagia, eructation, taste changes; also, elevated LFTs.

Nursing Implications: Assess baseline nutrition and elimination patterns and LFTs, and monitor during therapy. Discuss abnormalities with physician, and discuss drug modification. Teach patient to self-administer prescribed antiemetics as appropriate. Suggest patient use sugar-free hard candy, frequent ice chips, or artificial saliva for dry mouth.

IV. ALTERATION IN URINARY ELIMINATION related to URINARY FREQUENCY

Defining Characteristics: Urinary frequency, dysuria, urinary incontinence, nocturia, polyuria may occur.

Nursing Implications: Assess baseline urinary elimination pattern and risk. Assess for changes in urinary elimination, and instruct patient to report signs/symptoms. Discuss alternative drug with physician if this occurs.

V. ALTERATIONS IN SKIN INTEGRITY related to RASH

Defining Characteristics: Maculopapular rash, acne, facial edema, pruritus, excessive sweating, alopecia, and dry skin may occur rarely.

Nursing Implications: Assess baseline skin integrity. Instruct patient to report skin changes. If angioedema of face or tongue develops, discuss drug discontinuance with physician. Assess impact of changes on patient and discuss strategies to minimize distress.

VI. SEXUAL DYSFUNCTION, POTENTIAL, related to MENSTRUAL IRREGULARITY, ↓ LIBIDO

Defining Characteristics: Menstrual disorders, dysmenorrhea, intermenstrual bleeding, sexual dysfunction, decreased libido may occur.

Nursing Implications: Assess baseline sexual functioning. Inform patient that alterations may occur, and instruct to report them. If severe, discuss dysfunction with physician, and whether another antidepressant would provide equal benefit with less dysfunction.

MANAGEMENT

Drug: trazodone hydrochloride (Desyrel, Trialodine)

Class: Antidepressant.

Mechanism of Action: Appears to selectively inhibit the uptake of serotonin by brain synaptosomes and potentiates the behavioral changes induced by the serotonin precursor, 5-hydroxytryptophan.

Metabolism: Well absorbed after oral administration, with peak plasma levels occurring at 1 hour when taken on an empty stomach and at 2 hours when taken with food. Metabolized by the liver and excreted in the urine and feces. Time to steady state is 3–7 days. Elimination half-life initially is 3–6 hours, followed by slower phase with a half-life of 5–9 hours.

Indication: For the treatment of major depressive disorder in adults.

Dosage/Range:
Adult:
- Initial dose of 150 mg in divided doses.
- Increase dose by 50 mg/day q 3–4 days (maximum outpatient dosage is 300 mg/day, and inpatient is 600 mg/day in divided doses).

Maintenance:
- Lowest possible dose; once therapeutic effect reached, may be able to gradually reduce dose.

Elderly:
- 75 mg/day in divided doses; increase dose as needed and tolerated, every 3–4 days.

Drug Preparation:
- Oral administration, shortly after a meal or light snack, in divided doses.
- If drowsiness, may take majority of dose at bedtime.

Drug Interactions:
- Alcohol, CNS depressants: increased CNS depression; DO NOT GIVE TOGETHER.
- Antihypertensives: additive hypotension; evaluate and modify dose of antihypertensive as needed.
- Barbiturates: increased CNS depression; avoid concomitant use.
- Clonidine: reduced effect of clonidine; assess need for increased clonidine dosage.
- Digoxin: trazodone may increase serum digoxin levels; assess effects, and need to decrease digoxin dosage.
- MAOIs: initiate combined therapy cautiously and monitor patient for toxicity.
- Phenytoin: serum phenytoin levels may be increased; monitor levels and therapeutic effect and need for reduced phenytoin dosage.

Lab Effects/Interference:
- Occasional decreased WBC and neutrophil count.

Special Considerations:
- 75% of patients will respond within 2 weeks of therapy, and the remainder within 2–4 weeks.
- Drug causes moderate sedative effects and orthostatic hypotension, with slight anticholinergic effects.

- Contraindicated in patients during recovery from myocardial infarction, or patients receiving electroshock therapy.
- Elderly may be more vulnerable to sedative and hypotensive effects of drug.
- Teach all patients/families to call provider right away if thoughts of suicide or dying; attempts to commit suicide; new or worse depression; new or worse anxiety; feeling very agitated or restless; panic attacks; trouble sleeping (insomnia); new or worse irritability; aggressive, angry, or violent behavior; acting on dangerous impulses; extreme increase in activity or talking (mania); any unusual changes in behavior or mood.

Potential Toxicities/Side Effects and the Nursing Process

I.   SEXUAL DYSFUNCTION related to PRIAPISM

Defining Characteristics: Priapism (prolonged or inappropriate penile erection) may occur, and has required surgical intervention in some cases, and in others there was permanent dysfunction.

Nursing Implications: Teach male patients that this may occur. If it does, patient should immediately discontinue the drug and call physician. Make certain the patient understands the instructions and knows how to contact the physician. If priapism has persisted for 24 hours or more, a urologist should be consulted.

II.   ALTERATIONS IN SENSORY/PERCEPTUAL PATTERNS related to CNS DEPRESSION

Defining Characteristics: CNS depressant effects include drowsiness, fatigue, nightmares, confusion, anger, excitement, decreased ability to concentrate, disorientation, insomnia, nervousness, impaired memory, dizziness, lightheadedness; rarely, hallucinations, impaired speech, hypomania, incoordination, tremors, paresthesias may occur.

Nursing Implications: Assess baseline gait, neurologic status, affective state, and risk factors, and monitor during treatment. Instruct patient to report worsening depression, and assess for any suicidal ideation. Instruct patient to avoid alcohol while taking drug. Assess effect on elderly and/or debilitated patients (cognition, motor function, other sensitivities). Assess effect of drug side effects on patient, and weigh against benefit. Inform patient that daytime drowsiness may occur, and instruct to use caution if driving or operating heavy machinery. If sleep problems, have patient take majority of dose at bedtime to enhance sleep.

III.   ALTERATION IN NUTRITION, LESS THAN BODY REQUIREMENTS, related to GI SIDE EFFECTS

Defining Characteristics: Diarrhea, nausea, vomiting, flatulence may occur rarely.

Nursing Implications: Assess baseline nutrition status, and instruct the patient to report any nausea or vomiting. If required, discuss with physician antiemetic to manage symptoms. If severe, discuss alternative antidepressant medications.

MANAGEMENT

IV.   INJURY related to DECREASE IN MENTAL ALERTNESS, PHYSICAL COORDINATION

Defining Characteristics: Drug may cause drowsiness, dizziness, blurred vision, and impair physical coordination, mental alertness.

Nursing Implications: Assess baseline mental alertness, and teach patient to assess tolerance of medication before driving a car or operating heavy machinery. Assess medication profile to identify other medications that may increase risk (e.g., opiates, phenothiazines) and response to drug.

V.   ALTERATION IN OXYGENATION, POTENTIAL, related to CHANGES IN BP, SYNCOPE

Defining Characteristics: Rarely, hypotension or hypertension, syncope, palpitations, tachycardia, shortness of breath, and chest pain may occur.

Nursing Implications: Assess baseline cardiovascular status, and vital signs, and monitor during therapy at each visit. Instruct patient to report any palpitations, chest pain, or any changes in condition. Discuss significant symptoms with the physician. If patient is hypotensive and receiving antihypertensive medication, discuss with physician discontinuing or dose-reducing the antihypertensive medication. Prior to elective surgery, because interaction with anesthesia is unknown, temporarily discontinue drug.

Drug: venlafaxine hydrochloride (Effexor, Effexor XR)

Class: Serotonin-norepinephrine reuptake inhibitor (SNRI) antidepressant.

Mechanism of Action: Appears to potentiate neurotransmitter activity by inhibiting neuronal serotonin and norepinephrine reuptake.

Metabolism: Well absorbed after oral administration, and eliminated via the kidneys; time to reach steady state is 3–4 days. Drug and metabolite half-lives are 5 ± 2 and 11 ± 2 hours. Increased drug serum levels in patients with renal or hepatic dysfunction.

Indications: XR: treatment of (1) major depressive disorder; (2) generalized anxiety disorder; (3) social anxiety disorder; (4) panic disorder. Immediate release: treatment of (1) major depressive disorder; (2) hot flashes.

Dosage/Range:
Adult (indicated for the treatment of depression and generalized anxiety disorder):
• Initial (extended-release capsule): 75 mg once a day, at the same time each day; if indicated, can start dose at 37.5 mg once daily for 4–7 days, increasing to 75-mg capsule strength; if no response after adequate trial at 75 mg per day, may increase dose in 75-mg

increments after at least a 4-day trial at the previous dose, up to a maximum of 225 mg per day in a single dose.
- Initial (immediate-release tablets): 75 mg/day in two or three divided doses.
- If little or no response, dose may be increased in dose increments of up to 75 mg/day after at least 4 days at the previous dose, to 150 mg/day, and up to a maximum of 225 mg/day for moderately depressed patients. Severely depressed patients may need up to 350–375 mg/day in three divided doses.
- Patients with hepatic dysfunction: daily dose should be reduced at least 50%.
- Patients with renal impairment: Mild to moderate dysfunction: reduce daily dose by 25%; patients receiving hemodialysis: 50% dose reduction; dose is given after dialysis.

Drug Preparation:
- Effexor XR tablets available in a 225-mg dose (uses Osmodex controlled-release technology).
- XL capsule available in 37.5-mg, 75-mg, and 150-mg strengths.
- Immediate-release tablets available as 25-, 37.5-, 50-, 75-, and 100-mg tablets.
- Drug should be administered orally with food in a single dose in morning or at night (same time every day) for extended-release capsule, or in two to three divided doses for tablets.
- When changing from an MAOI to venlafaxine HCl, wait at least 14 days after MAOI is stopped; when stopping venlafaxine HCl and beginning an MAOI, wait at least 7 days.
- When discontinuing drug after > 1 week of therapy, taper dose. If more than 6 weeks of therapy, taper over 2 weeks.

Drug Interactions:
- MAOIs: tremor, myoclonus, diaphoresis, nausea, vomiting, flushing, dizziness, hyperthermia resembling neuroleptic malignant syndrome, and may be fatal. DO NOT USE TOGETHER. See Administration section.
- Cimetidine: may increase venlafaxine HCl serum levels that are significant in patients with existing hypertension, hepatic dysfunction, or who are elderly; use with caution in these patients and monitor closely.
- Haloperidol: may increase haloperidol serum levels; monitor patient when drugs are administered concomitantly.

Lab Effects/Interference:
- Infrequent increased alk phos, creatinine, transaminases AST, ALT.
- Infrequent hyperglycemia with glycosuria, hyperlipemia, bilirubinemia, hyperuricemia, hypercholesterolemia, hypoglycemia, hypokalemia, hyperkalemia, hyperphosphatemia, hyponatremia, hypophosphatemia, hypoproteinemia, uremia, albuminuria.

Special Considerations:
- Avoid drug use during pregnancy and in nursing mothers.
- Dose-reduce in patients with hepatic or renal dysfunction.

MANAGEMENT

* Use caution in patients with mania.
* Use for more than 4–6 weeks has not been evaluated.
* Contraindicated in patients receiving MAOIs.
* Studies have shown equal efficacy to fluoxetine (Costa, 1998; Silverstone & Ravindran, 1999).
* Drug has been shown to reduce hot flashes (vasomotor symptoms) (Loprinzi et al., 2009).
* Serious adverse reactions have occurred in patients changing from MAOIs to venlafaxine HCl or from venlafaxine to an MAOI. It is imperative to wait 14 days changing from MAOIs to venlafaxine HCl or 7 days after stopping venlafaxine before starting an MAOI.
* Teach all patients/families to call provider right away if thoughts of suicide or dying; attempts to commit suicide; new or worse depression; new or worse anxiety; feeling very agitated or restless; panic attacks; trouble sleeping (insomnia); new or worse irritability; aggressive, angry, or violent behavior; acting on dangerous impulses; extreme increase in activity or talking (mania); any unusual changes in behavior or mood.

Potential Toxicities/Side Effects and the Nursing Process

I.   ALTERATION IN OXYGENATION, POTENTIAL, related to CHANGES IN BP

Defining Characteristics: Rarely, hypertension, vasodilation, tachycardia, postural hypotension, angina, extrasystoles, syncope, thrombophlebitis, peripheral edema occur. Migraine headaches are frequent.

Nursing Implications: Assess baseline weight, presence of peripheral edema, cardiac status and vital signs, and monitor during therapy at each visit. Instruct patient to report any edema, palpitations, chest pain, or any changes in condition. Discuss any symptoms with the physician depending on severity.

II.   ALTERATIONS IN SENSORY/PERCEPTUAL PATTERNS related to EMOTIONAL LABILITY, VERTIGO

Defining Characteristics: Emotional lability, trismus, vertigo occur frequently; infrequently, apathy, ataxia, circumoral paresthesia, CNS stimulation, euphoria, hallucinations, hostility, blurred vision, abnormal accommodation, photophobia, tinnitus, taste perversion, manic reaction, psychosis, sleep disturbance, abnormal dreams, and stupor may occur.

Nursing Implications: Assess baseline neurologic status, affective state, and risk factors, and monitor during treatment. Instruct patient to avoid alcohol while taking drug. Assess effect on elderly and/or patients with hepatic or renal dysfunction. Assess for symptoms at each visit, and instruct patient to report changes. If symptoms occur, discuss strategies to ensure patient safety and comfort.

III. ALTERATION IN NUTRITION, LESS THAN BODY REQUIREMENTS, related to GI SIDE EFFECTS

Defining Characteristics: Nausea (37% of patients), anorexia (11%), constipation (15%) may occur. Less commonly, dry mouth, diarrhea, dyspepsia, flatulence, dysphagia, melena, gastroenteritis, and eructation may occur.

Nursing Implications: Assess baseline nutrition and gastrointestinal functional status, and instruct the patient to report any GI disturbances or changes. Discuss measures to reduce nausea and/or stimulate appetite.

IV. SEXUAL DYSFUNCTION, POTENTIAL, related to EJACULATORY DISTURBANCES

Defining Characteristics: Incidence of ejaculatory disturbances is 12%, and other disorders may occur (1–6%), including erectile difficulties, delayed ejaculation/orgasm, impotence, and other sexual dysfunction. Rarely, women with uterine fibroids may develop enlargement, uterine hemorrhage, or vaginal hemorrhage; in addition, women may develop vaginitis and metrorrhagia and, rarely, amenorrhea.

Nursing Implications: Assess baseline sexual functioning. Inform patient that alterations may occur, and instruct to report them. If severe, discuss dysfunction with physician, and whether another antidepressant would provide equal benefit with less dysfunction.

V. ALTERATION IN COMFORT related to PAIN

Defining Characteristics: Malaise, neck pain, hangover-like effect, arthritis, bone pain may occur infrequently.

Nursing Implications: Assess baseline comfort level. Instruct patient to report any changes in comfort, and discuss strategies to reduce discomfort.

VI. ALTERATION IN OXYGENATION, POTENTIAL, related to ALTERED BREATHING PATTERNS

Defining Characteristics: Bronchitis, dyspnea may occur frequently; infrequently, asthma, chest congestion, hyperventilation, laryngitis may occur.

Nursing Implications: Assess baseline respiratory status, and instruct patient to report any changes. Discuss serious changes with physician, and interventions necessary.

MANAGEMENT

VII. ALTERATION IN SKIN INTEGRITY, POTENTIAL, related to RASH

Defining Characteristics: Infrequently, acne, alopecia, brittle nails, contact dermatitis, dry skin, maculopapular rash, urticaria, and herpes simplex and zoster may occur.

Nursing Implications: Assess baseline skin integrity, and instruct patient to report any changes. Discuss serious changes with the physician, and need for changing to another antidepressant depending on severity.

VIII. POTENTIAL FOR INJURY related to EFFECTS ON BLOOD CELL ELEMENTS

Defining Characteristics: Frequently, ecchymosis may occur; less commonly, anemia, leucocytosis, leukopenia, lymphadenopathy, lymphocytosis, thrombocytopenia, thrombocythemia may occur.

Nursing Implications: Assess baseline CBC and presence of bruising on skin. Instruct patient to report any bleeding, bruising, infection, or any changes in condition. Check CBC as indicated and discuss any changes with physician.

IX. ALTERATION IN URINARY ELIMINATION related to DYSURIA

Defining Characteristics: Frequently, dysuria, hematuria, metrorrhagia, impaired urination, or vaginitis may occur. Infrequently, albuminuria, kidney calculus, cystitis, nocturia, bladder pain, kidney pain, polyuria, prostatitis, pyelonephritis, pyuria, incontinence, urinary urgency may occur.

Nursing Implications: Assess baseline urinary status. Instruct patient to report any changes, and discuss interventions with physician.

Drug: zolpidem tartrate (Ambien)

Class: Benzodiazepine-like hypnotic.

Mechanism of Action: Despite a chemical structure unlike the benzodiazepines, it selectively binds to one of the GABA complexes that the benzodiazepines non-selectively bind to, producing deep sleep (stages 3 and 4) without muscle relaxant or anticonvulsant properties.

Metabolism: Well absorbed from GI tract, with 70% of drug reaching the systemic circulation. Absorption and distribution affected by food intake. Widely distributed in body tissues and fluids, including CSF. Crosses placenta and is excreted in breastmilk. Highly bound to plasma proteins. Metabolized in liver and excreted in urine, bile, and feces. Onset of action in 7–27 minutes, with a peak of 0.5–2.3 hours, and duration of 6–8 hours. Elimination half-life is 1.7–2.5 hours.

Indication: For the short-term treatment of insomnia characterized by difficulties with sleep initiation. Ambien has been shown to decrease sleep latency for up to 35 days.

Dosage/Range:
Adult (for insomnia):
• Oral: 10–20 mg PO at hs.
• Elderly or debilitated individuals: 5 mg PO.

Drug Preparation:
• Store tablets in tight container at < 40°C (104°F).
• Administer on an empty stomach immediately before bedtime.

Drug Interactions:
• CNS depressants (e.g., alcohol, phenothiazines): additive CNS depression; avoid concurrent use or use cautiously and monitor carefully.

Lab Effects/Interference:
• None.

Special Considerations:
• Indicated for the short-term treatment of insomnia, generally 7–10 days of use.
• Contraindications: nursing mothers.
• Administer cautiously in patients with liver or renal dysfunction, pregnancy, pulmonary compromise, or who are depressed.
• May cause increased depression in patients who are already depressed.

Potential Toxicities/Side Effects and the Nursing Process

I. ALTERATIONS IN SENSORY/PERCEPTUAL PATTERNS related to CNS DEPRESSION

Defining Characteristics: CNS depressant effects include drowsiness, fatigue, lethargy, drugged feeling, depression, anxiety, irritability.

Nursing Implications: Assess baseline neurologic status, affective state, and risk factors, and monitor during treatment. Instruct patient to report worsening depression, and assess for any suicidal ideation. Instruct patient to avoid alcohol while taking drug. Assess effect on elderly and/or debilitated patients (cognition, motor function, other sensitivities). Assess effect of drug side effects on patient, and weigh against benefit. Inform patient that daytime drowsiness may occur, and instruct to use caution if driving or operating heavy machinery.

MANAGEMENT

II.   ALTERATION IN NUTRITION, LESS THAN BODY REQUIREMENTS, related to GI SIDE EFFECTS

Defining Characteristics: Nausea, vomiting, dyspepsia may occur.

Nursing Implications: Assess baseline nutrition status, and instruct the patient to report any nausea or vomiting.

III.   INJURY related to DECREASE IN MENTAL ALERTNESS, PHYSICAL COORDINATION

Defining Characteristics: Drug may cause drowsiness, dizziness, diplopia, and impair physical coordination, mental alertness. At doses > 10 mg, patients may experience antero-grade amnesia or memory impairment.

Nursing Implications: Assess other medications that may increase risk (e.g., opiates, phe-nothiazines) and response to drug. Instruct patient to avoid potentially hazardous activities, including driving a car, operating machinery.

Section 3
Complications

Chapter *10*
Managing Tumor-Related Skeletal Events and Hypercalcemia

Metastases to bone can significantly alter a patient's quality of life related to pain, disability, hypercalcemia, and complications such as fracture (Roodman, 2004). Fortunately, there has been significant progress in the management of tumor-related skeletal events as the biology underlying metastases to bone is better understood. To review, bones normally undergo constant remodeling where osteoclasts break down bone cells (a process called resorption), followed by the building of new bone by osteoblasts. The process is tightly regulated by the body, and osteoclastic activity—as well as osteoblastic activity—is controlled by both systemic and local factors. For example, osteoclasts (breakdown) are stimulated by the parathyroid hormone-related peptide (PTHrP) hormone, 1,25-dihydroxyvitamin D_3, and thyroxine (T_4). This happens by inducing the bone marrow stromal cells and the osteoblasts to express the receptor activator of nuclear factor-kB ligand (RANKL, or osteoclast differentiation factor). RANKL is also important in immune function, as it is a survival factor for dendritic cells, and RANKL has an important role in cell migration to bone and in specific metastatic behaviors of cancer cells (Jones et al., 2008). Locally, osteoblasts secrete interleukin-6 (IL-6), IL-1, prostaglandin Es, and colony-stimulating factors (CSFs), which lead to the formation of osteoclasts. Epidermal growth factor (EGF) and tumor necrosis factor (TNF) stimulate osteoclastic activity, as do thymocyte-dependent lymphocytes (T-cells), which produce IL-17. The microenvironment of the bone includes the stromal cells, which produce macrophage CSF and RANKL, as do osteoblasts. This stimulates monocyte-macrophage precursors to produce osteoclasts. The systemic factors upregulate or increase the expression of RANKL on the marrow stromal cells and the osteoblasts. RANKL binds to the RANK receptor on the osteoclast precursors made by the monocyte-macrophage precursors.

Osteoclastic activity can be halted by local and systemic factors, such as corticosteroids (which kill osteoblasts) and osteoprotegerin (called osteoclastogenesis inhibitory factor, a member of the TNF superfamily). These inhibit the differentiation of macrophages into osteoclasts, and osteoprotegerin binds to RANKL on osteoblast/stromal cells and osteoclast precursor cells. Thus, it is the balance between RANKL and osteoprotegerin that moves osteoclast activity. The osteoclasts act on the trabecular bone surface and break down the minerals and matrix by releasing proteases that dissolve the matrix, leaving small holes in the bone trabecula or framework of bone on the surface. Then the osteoclasts undergo apoptosis. Now the scales favor osteoblastic activity, and the osteoblasts fill the bone holes with new bone that still needs to be mineralized or calcified. Mesenchymal stem cells produce the osteoblasts and a transcription factor called Runx-2, which turns on the genes responsible for the differentiation or maturation of the osteoblasts. Systemic factors (e.g., parathyroid hormone, prostaglandins, cytokines, platelet-derived growth factor (PDGF)) and local factors that are released from the bone matrix (e.g., bone morphogenetic proteins [BMPs]), insulin-like-growth factor (IGF), fibrocyte growth factor, vascular endothelial growth factor (VEGF), and prostate-specific antigen (PSA) all increase osteoblastic proliferation and differentiation. Old bone is replaced systematically, so building and tearing down of bone are always balanced without damaging the integrity of the skeleton. As women get older and reach menopause, the osteoblastic process (buildup) lags behind osteoclastic (breakdown) activity, so these women are at risk for osteoporosis. In addition, women being treated with hormones for breast cancer with selective estrogen receptor modulators (SERMs) are at risk for bone density loss and are thus advised to take calcium and vitamins, and to exercise regularly. Patients with cancers that metastasize to bone are at risk for skeletal lesions: patients with breast cancer have primarily osteoblastic with about 15–20% having osteolytic, and patients with prostate cancer have largely osteoblastic lesions. Patients with multiple myeloma have only osteoblastic bone lesions. Only osteoblastic processes (active bone formation) show on bone scans (Roodman, 2004).

As more is understood about the process of bone resorption and metastases, agents are targeted against the malignant pathways, such as denosumab (Xgeva), a human monoclonal antibody that blocks RANKL. Denosumab has been FDA-approved for the prevention of skeletal-related events in patients with bone metastases from solid tumors. It is not indicated for prevention of skeletal events in patients with multiple myeloma. Osteoclast differentiation, activation, and survival are regulated by three molecules: receptor activator of nuclear factor kB (RANK), the cytokine RANKL, and osteoprotegerin, a soluble decoy receptor of RANKL, which can turn off RANKL to stop bone loss (Body et al., 2006). RANKL binds to RANK on premature and mature osteoclasts and regulates their differentiation, function, and survival (Body et al., 2006). The seed and soil hypothesis suggests that breast or prostate cancer cells are the "seeds," which secrete substances that create a microenvironment in the skeleton (bone), where various cytokines and growth factors make a very rich "soil" that attracts circulating tumor cells and fosters tumor growth in the bone. RANKL appears to regulate cancer cell migration and bone metastases in cells that express the receptor RANK, such as breast cancer cells (Jones et al., 2006). RANK is also expressed by prostate cancer cells where again RANKL has been found to act directly on RANK-expressing prostate tumor cells, guiding tumor cell migration to bone, and expressing tumor metastases genes that further stimulate tumor growth (Armstrong et al., 2008). Bisphosphonates have been shown to directly inhibit tumor growth in laboratory studies of human breast cancer cell lines. In addition, disseminated tumor cells in the bone marrow in early stage breast cancer are reduced with treatment by zoledronic acid (Zometa) (Rack et al., 2007).

In 2013, Xgeva was FDA-indicated for the treatment of adults and skeletally mature adolescents with giant cell tumor of bone that is unresectable or where surgical resection will likely be disfiguring. Although now being used as an anti-tumor treatment, it has been left in this chapter as the mechanism of action, and the drug's other uses are best described here.

Hypercalcemia is a metabolic complication of malignant disease and is evidenced by a serum calcium of > 10.5 mg/dL. Potentially fatal, hypercalcemia occurs in 10–20% of

COMPLICATIONS

patients with cancer, principally in patients with breast cancer; multiple myeloma; squamous cell cancers of head, neck, and esophagus; prostate cancer; and adult T-cell lymphoma. Hypercalcemia is compounded by problems of advanced disease, such as immobility and dehydration. Hypercalcemia of malignancy is either humoral or related to tumor invasion of bone. In humoral hypercalcemia, osteoclasts are activated and break down bone (resorption) as a result of tumor-released factors, such as parathyroid hormone-related protein, as shown in Figure 10.1. This type may occur in patients with squamous-cell malignancies of the lung, head and neck, or with genitourinary cancers, such as renal cell or ovarian cancer. This group of patients in most cases does not have bony involvement by tumor. In contrast, patients with bony metastases in which a tumor has invaded the bone have tumors that release local substances that cause the bone to undergo resorption by osteoclasts (bone is broken down) with the release of calcium. Malignancies commonly associated with this type of hypercalcemia are breast cancer and multiple myeloma.

In reviewing normal calcium homeostasis, calcium is found primarily in bone. As such, 99% of the body's calcium is in the form of insoluble crystals, giving the human skeleton strength and durability. The remaining 1% is distributed between the body's intracellular and extracellular fluids: 45% is ionized in the serum, 45% is bound by protein, and 10% is found in insoluble complexes.

The ionized fraction of calcium is necessary for excitation of nerves, voluntary skeletal muscle, cardiac muscle, and involuntary muscles in the gut. If the body has too much

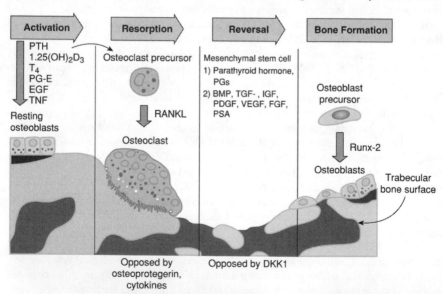

Figure 10.1   Process of Bone Building and Breakdown

Source: Data from Loberg RD, Logothetis CJ, Keller ET, Pienta KJ. Pathogenesis and treatment of prostate cancer bone metastases: Targeting the lethal phenotype. *J Clin Oncol* 2005; 23(32) 8232–8241; Logothetis CJ, Lin SH. Osteoblasts in prostate cancer metastasis to bone. *Nat Rev Cancer* 2005; 5(1) 21–28; Roodman GD. Mechanisms of bone metastasis. *N Engl J Med* 2004; 350(16) 1655–1664.

ionized calcium, there is decreased excitability of these tissues. For instance, symptoms of early hypercalcemia (calcium of 10–12 mg/dL) are fatigue, lethargy, constipation, anorexia, nausea and vomiting, and polyuria. Later symptoms, when the calcium is > 12 mg/dL, are altered mental status, coma, decreased deep tendon reflexes, increased cardiac contractility, and oliguric renal failure. In contrast, if there is too little ionized calcium in the body, there is increased excitability of nerves and muscle. The body attempts to regain more calcium to raise the level of ionized calcium by "raiding" the bone matrix.

Because 45% of the calcium outside of bone is bound to albumin, it is important to correct the value of ionized calcium in the serum if the albumin is low (normally bound calcium is now free in the serum, and the serum level may actually be higher than the laboratory value). The formula to determine ionized serum calcium, corrected for low serum albumin is:

$$\text{Corrected serum calcium} = \text{measured total serum calcium (mg/dL)} + [4.0 - \text{serum albumin (g/dL)}] \times 0.8$$

For example, a patient has a serum calcium of 10.0 mg/dL but has a serum albumin of 2.2 (normal is 3.5–5.5 g/dL). The corrected serum calcium is 10.0 mg/dL + (4.0 – 2.2 = 1.8 g/dL) × 0.8 + 10.0 + 1.44 = 11.44 mg/dL. Thus, a serum calcium level that appears normal may be abnormal (high) in the presence of a low serum albumin level.

The human skeleton undergoes constant remodeling, where there is an exquisite balance between bone formation and bone resorption (breakdown). Bone formation is mediated by osteoblasts and bone resorption by osteoclasts. Calcium balance is maintained by a number of factors. First, parathyroid hormone (PTH) released by the parathyroid gland increases serum calcium levels by stimulating bone resorption, increasing renal absorption of calcium, and stimulating the production of $1,25(OH)_2D_3$, which increases the intestinal absorption of calcium. In contrast, calcitonin balances these effects by reducing serum calcium: it inhibits bone resorption (breakdown) and decreases renal absorption of calcium. Normally, intestinal absorption of calcium is balanced by an approximately equal loss of calcium through urinary excretion. In most individuals before midlife, bone formation balances bone resorption.

There are many potential causes of hypercalcemia of malignancy. These include:

- Secretion of parathyroid-related protein by tumor.
- Secretion of other bone-resorbing substances by tumor (i.e., cytokines, transforming growth factor [TGF-α], IL-1, TNF).
- Conversion of 25-hydroxyvitamin D_3 to 1,25-dihydroxyvitamin D_3 by tumor.
- Local effects of osteolytic bony metastasis.

Therapeutic efforts to lower serum calcium in hypercalcemia of malignancy are based on rehydration to restore glomerular filtration and excretion of calcium (normally up to 600 mg/day), and drugs that promote calcium excretion or inhibit osteoclastic bone resorption. Today, bisphosphonate agents have been shown to decrease the development of osteoclastic bone lesions from breast and prostate cancer metastases and multiple myeloma. For patients with advanced disease, general management principles are based on palliation of symptoms. Diet restriction of calcium is not necessary, as calcium absorbed from the

COMPLICATIONS

gut is often less than normal and patients are malnourished. Patients with T-cell lymphoma, who have increased 1,25-dihydroxyvitamin D_3, are an exception to this rule. These patients have high levels of 1,25-dihydroxyvitamin D_3 and should avoid intake of dairy products. It is important for patients to bear weight if possible, since immobility increases osteoclastic activity and decreases osteoblastic activity. Since calcium is a potent diuretic, patients are often dehydrated with the loss of sodium and water. Further, as the serum calcium increases, the distal renal tubules become less able to retain sodium, and there is further sodium loss from the kidneys. Patients are usually rehydrated with 3–4 liters per day of 0.9% sodium chloride over 48 hours to restore fluid volume. Loop diuretics are administered, such as furosemide (Lasix), which increase calcium excretion. Thiazide diuretics are avoided, since they increase tubular reabsorption of calcium. This usually provides symptomatic improvement, but it is important to monitor the patient closely for possible fluid overload on the one hand, or intravascular dehydration with electrolyte imbalance on the other.

A number of drugs inhibit osteoclastic bone activity. The bisphosphonates have potent hypocalcemic activity, binding tightly to the calcified bone matrix. Some of the drugs inhibit lymphokine- and prostaglandin-mediated bone resorption, and the drugs vary in their inhibition of bone mineralization. Pamidronate (Aredia) and zoledronic acid (Zometa) inhibit bone resorption at low doses without decreasing mineralization and normalizing serum calcium in 80–90% of patients within 48–96 hours (Fitton and McTavish, 1991). Pamidronate and zolendronic acid are effective in reducing pain from bony metastases and decrease the incidence of bone metastasis in patients with multiple myeloma or breast cancer. Zolendronic acid was shown to reduce skeletal events in patients with prostate cancer (Berenson et al., 2001). More recently, studies have determined that bone resorption markers such as N-telopeptide of type I collagen (NTX) correlate with the extent of bone metastases and reflect the extent of bony metastases in patients (Lipton et al., 2007). Furthermore, studies have suggested that the normalization of NTX as a result of bisphosphonate therapy results in decreased progression of bony metastases and lower incidence of fractures (Brown et al., 2005). Lipton et al. (2007) demonstrated in a retrospective subset analysis of a phase III randomized controlled trial patients with breast cancer that early normalization of elevated baseline NTX through zolendronic acid therapy was associated with higher event-free survival (e.g., fewer fractures) and higher overall survival. Similarly, Hirsch et al. (2008) found statistically significant correlations between zolendronic acid and increased survival compared to placebo in patients with high baseline NTX levels. Well, what about prevention of bony metastases and improved survival in the adjuvant breast cancer setting? In a very exciting presentation, Ghant (2009) reported that in a randomized, open-label phase III trial of patients with early premenopausal breast cancer, there was improved outcome when zoledronic acid was added to endocrine therapy (either tamoxifen or anastrozole) (Austrian Breast and Colorectal Cancer Study Group, ABCSG-12). Adjuvant zolendronic acid was included in the study, both to counter the significant bone loss associated with ovarian suppression (goserelin) and to see whether the antitumor effects seen in the metastatic setting would be seen in the adjuvant setting as well as measured by time to disease recurrence and overall survival. At a median follow-up of 60 months, patients receiving zolendronic acid had improved disease-free survival ($p = .011$), as evidenced by less contralateral breast cancer, distant metastases, and local regional recurrence, as well as longer relapse-free survival ($p = .014$) and a trend toward improved overall survival ($p = .101$). However, in the final analysis, there was no significant difference in overall survival. There were no reported renal toxicity or confirmed osteonecrosis of the jaw during the study. Although the initial study report from the ABCSG-12 trial (Ghant et al., 2009) showed that zolendronic acid reduced breast cancer recurrence and breast cancer death by 33%, the *Adjuvant Zoledronic Acid to Reduce Recurrence* (AZURE) study reported in 2010 showed no effect on breast cancer recurrence or suvival overall (Coleman et al., 2010). However, a subset analysis did show that in postmenopausal women (> 5 years menopausal), zolendronic acid did show a significant benefit on overall survival, reducing the risk for death by 29% ($p = 0.017$). There was no benefit in younger (< 5 years postmenopausal) or premenopausal women. Studies are ongoing to further define the role of bisphosphonates on cancer recurrence (NSABP B-34, SWOG SO307), and adjuvant treatment of breast cancer with zolendronic acid is not recommended at this time.

Etidronate (Didronel) inhibits osteoclastic resorption, but with long-term use, the drug inhibits bone mineralization, causing osteomalacia and pathologic fractures. A class effect of the drugs is potential renal insufficiency (zolendronic acid > pamidronate) and also rarely osteonecrosis of the jaw. Patients should have a serum creatinine assessed before each treatment, as well as serial urinalyses for protein. In addition, patients should have a baseline oral exam by a dentist or oral surgeon, and patients at highest risk for osteonecrosis of the jaw (e.g., poor dental health) should be seen regularly. As more patients are treated with bisphosphonates, and for longer periods of time, osteonecrosis of the jaw is emerging as a more significant problem. Dental surgery appears to be a risk factor so that a dental screening with necessary extractions and implants should be done prior to begin ning bisphosphonate therapy. The risk of developing osteonecrosis of the jaw increases the longer a patient is on therapy. Oncology nurses should continue to assess patients for any signs or symptoms of dental problems during bisphosphonate therapy.

Table 10.1 shows staging and recommendations from the American Association of Oral and Maxillofacial Surgeons.

Other hypocalcemic agents include the following, but are less often used. Oral phosphates inhibit bone resorption and stimulate bone formation, as well as precipitate calcium.

Table 10.1   Staging and Recommendations for Treatment of Bisphosphonate-Related Osteonecrosis of the Jaw

Stage	Recommended Treatment
At risk: No apparent necrotic bone in patients who have been treated with either oral or IV bisphosphonates	Teach patient about risk and close need for monitoring; no treatment indicated
Stage 0: No clinical evidence of necrotic bone, but nonspecific clinical findings and symptoms	Systemic management, including the use of analgesics and antibiotics
Stage 1: Exposed and necrotic bone in patients who are asymptomatic and have no evidence of infection	Antibacterial mouth rinse, clinical follow-up on a quarterly basis, patient education, and review of indications for continued bisphosphate therapy

(continued)

Table 10.1   *(Continued)*

Stage	Recommended Treatment
Stage 2: Exposed and necrotic bone associated with infection, as evidenced by pain and erythema in the region of exposed bone with or without purulent discharge	Symptomatic treatment with oral antibiotics, oral antibacterial mouth rinses, pain control, and superficial debridement to relieve soft-tissue irritation
Stage 3: Exposed and necrotic bone in patients with pain, infection, and one or more of the following: exposed and necrotic bone extending beyond the region of the alveolar bone; pathologic fracture; extra-oral fistulae; oral-antral or oral-nasal communication; or osteolysis extending to the inferior border of the mandible of the sinus floor	Antibacterial mouth rinse, antibiotic therapy and pain control, and surgical debridement/resection for longer-term palliation of infection and pain

Data from: American Association of Oral and Maxillofacial Surgeons, Position Paper, January 2009.

However, the side effect of diarrhea limits their usefulness. Glucocorticoids have an unpredictable effect, and their value is limited by side effects of high drug doses. However, they are often used in steroid-responsive malignancies such as multiple myeloma and lymphoma. Calcitonin inhibits bone resorption and promotes urinary calcium excretion with a rapid, but brief, response (2–3 days). Plicamycin (mithramycin) inhibits osteoclastic bone resorption by killing the osteoclasts. It is potent, lowering calcium in 24–72 hours, but rebound hypercalcemia often occurs within 1 week. The high toxicity of the drug prevents wide usage.

After symptomatic hypercalcemia is resolved, the malignant disease is treated if appropriate to prevent recurrence (e.g., with chemotherapy or radiotherapy to lytic bone lesions). Nursing implications revolve around management of the patient receiving aggressive hydration and hypocalcemic medications. Patient education is prominent, as patients and their families are taught about the disease, as well as self-assessment of signs and symptoms of hypercalcemia, fluid balance, activity, and oral care. For patients receiving bisphosphonates for the prevention of bony metastases, nursing priorities include assessment of renal function before each treatment, oral assessment and patient education about potential, albeit rare, osteonecrosis of the jaw, and teaching patients about self-administration of calcium and vitamin D supplements to prevent osteoporosis.

References

American Association of Oral and Maxillofacial Surgeons. Position Paper on Bisphosphonate-Related Osteonecrosis of the Jaw, 2009 Update. Available at http://www.aaoms.org/docs/position_papers/bronj_update.pdfg. Accessed August 14, 2009.

Amgen. Xgeva (denosumab) [package insert]. Thousand Oaks, CA, June 2014.

Armstrong AP, Miller RE, Jones JC, Zhang J, Keller ET, Dougall WC. RANKL Acts Directly on RANK-Expressing Prostate Tumor Cells and Mediates Migration and Expression of Tumor Metastasis Genes. *Prostate* 2008; 68(1) 92–104.

Berenson JR, Rosen LS, Howell A. Zoledronic Acid Reduces Skeletal-related Events in Patients with Osteolytic Metastases. A Double-blind, Randomized Dose-response Study. *Cancer* 2001; 91 144–154.

Blum RH, Novetsky D, Shasha D, Fleishman S. The Multidisciplinary Approach to Bone Metastases. *Oncology* 2003; 17 845–857.

Body JJ, Facon T, Coleman RE, et al. A Study of the Biological Receptor Activator of Nuclear Factor kB-Ligand Inhibitor, Denosumab, in Patients with Multiple Myeloma or Bone Metastases from Breast Cancer. *Clin Cancer Res* 2006; 12 1221–1228.

Bone HG, Bolognese MA, Yuen CK, Kendler DL, Wang H, Liu Y, San Martin J. Effects of Denosumab on Bone Mineral Density and Bone Turnover in Postmenopausal Women. *J Clin Endocrinol Metabolism* 2008; 93(6) 2149–2157.

Coleman R, Coleman R, Thorpe H, et al. Adjuvant Treatment with Zoledronic Acid in Stage II/III Breast Cancer. The AZURE Trial (BIG 01/04). *Cancer Res* 2010; 70(24 suppl): Abstract S4–5.

Ghant M, Mlineritsch B, Schippinger W, et al. Adjuvant Ovarian Suppression Combined with Tamoxifen or Anastrozole, Alone or in Combination with Zoledronic Acid, in Premenopausal Women with Hormone-Responsive, Stage I and II Breast Cancer: First Efficacy Results From ABCSG-12. *J Clin Oncol* 26; 2008 (May 20 suppl: abstract LBA4).

Ghant M, Mlineritsch B, Schippinger W, et al. Endocrine Therapy Plus Zoledronic Acid in Premenopausal Breast Cancer. *N Engl J Med* 2009; 360 679–691.

Hirsch V, Major PP, Lipton A, et al. Zoledronic Acid and Survival in Patients with Metastatic Bone Disease from Lung Cancer and Elevated Markers of Osteoclast Activity. *Thorac Oncol* 2008; 3(3) 228–236.

Jones DH, Nakashima T, Sanchez OH, et al. Regulation of Cancer Cell Migration and Bone Metastasis by RANKL. *Nature* 2006; 440(7084) 692–696.

Lipton A, Cook RJ, Major P, Smith MR, Coleman RE. Zoledronic Acid and Survival in Breast Cancer Patients with Bone Metastases and Elevated Markers of Osteoclast Activity. *Oncologist* 2007; 12 1035–1043.

Lipton A, Steger GG, Figueroa J, et al. Randomized Active Controlled Phase II Study of Denosumab Efficacy and Safety in Patients with Breast Cancer Related Bone Metastases. *J Clin Oncol* 2007; 25(28) 4431–4437.

Rack BK, Jueckstock J, Genss E-M, et al. *Effect of Zoledronate on Persisting Isolated Tumor Cells in the Bone Marrow of Patients Without Recurrence of Early Breast Cancer.* Presented at the 30th San Antonio Breast Cancer Symposium, San Antonio, TX; December 13–16, 2007, Abstract 511.

Reich CD. Advances in the Treatment of Bone Metastases. *Clin J Oncol Nurs* 2003; 7 641–646.

Roodman GD. Mechanisms of Bone Metastases. *N Engl J Med* 2004; 350(16) 1655–1664.

Sanofi-aventis. Calcimar (calcitonin-salmon) [Product monograph]. Laval, Quebec. April 15, 2014. Available at http://products.sanofi.ca/en/calcimar.pdf, accessed 6.15.14.

Drug: calcitonin-salmon (Calcimar, Miacalcin)

Class: Thyroid hormone.

Mechanism of Action: Inhibits bone absorption (breakdown) by inhibiting bone osteoclasts and blocking osteolysis. Decreases high serum calcium concentrations in hypercalcemia of malignancy, beginning 2 hours after dose and lasting 6–8 hours. Promotes renal excretion of calcium, phosphate; also acts on GI tract to decrease volume, acidity of gastric fluid, and enzyme content in pancreatic fluid.

Metabolism: Rapidly converted to smaller fragments by kidneys; excreted in urine.

Indication: For the treatment of (1) symptomatic Paget's disease in patients who do not respond to alternative treatments; (2) hypercalcemia.

Dosage/Range:
Adult (hypercalcemia):
- Subcutaneous (SQ) or intramuscular (IM): 4 international units/kg every 12 h × 1–2 days; if no effect, increase dose to 8 international units/kg q 12 h × 1–2 days, then if still unsatisfactory response, can be increased to a maximum of 8 international units/kg every 6 h (maximum).

Drug Preparation:
- Refrigerate for 2–6 hours (36–43°F, 2–6°C).
- Reconstitute according to manufacturer's recommendations.
- If allergy suspected, perform skin test first: withdraw 0.05 mL of the 200 international units/mL solution in tuberculin syringe, then fill syringe with 1 mL 0.9% sodium chloride. After mixing, discard 0.9 mL; inject 0.1 mL intradermally on forearm and inspect for urticaria or wheal at 15 minutes.

Drug Interactions:
- None.

Lab Effects/Interference:
- Decreased alk phos.
- Decreased 24-hour urinary excretion of hydroxyproline.
- Casts in urine (indicate kidney damage).
- Decreased Ca++.

Special Considerations:
- Calcitonin-salmon consists of a foreign protein, so allergic reactions may occur. Perform skin test first if sensitivity is suspected. Do not use drug if wheal forms.
- It is unknown whether drug crosses placenta or is excreted in breastmilk; use cautiously in pregnancy or breastfeeding.
- Patient should receive adequate saline hydration to keep urinary output at ~2 L/day throughout treatment.
- 80% of patients have reduction in calcium in 24 hours.
- Antibodies to drug may develop with long-term use.
- Rapid onset of action and mild side effects.
- Short duration of response.
- Evidence of increased risk of malignancies with long term use of calcitonin so treatment duration should be limited to shortest period of time possible (Sanofi-Aventis, 2014).

Potential Toxicities/Side Effects and the Nursing Process

I.   INJURY related to HYPERSENSITIVITY

Defining Characteristics: Rare hypersensitivity may occur.

Nursing Implications: Perform skin testing as ordered when sensitivity suspected; if positive, suggest use of human calcitonin or other hypocalcemic agent. Assess for signs/ symptoms of hypersensitivity (generalized itching, agitation, dizziness, nausea, sense of impending doom, urticaria, angioedema, respiratory distress, hypotension). If this develops, stop drug immediately, notify physician, maintain IV access, and be prepared to administer epinephrine, hydrocortisone, diphenhydramine.

II.   ALTERATION IN NUTRITION, LESS THAN BODY REQUIREMENTS, related to GI SIDE EFFECTS

Defining Characteristics: Transient nausea/vomiting is mild and tolerance develops; anorexia, diarrhea, epigastric discomfort, and abdominal pain may occur as well.

Nursing Implications: Assess baseline nutrition and elimination patterns. Since nausea/vomiting may occur within 30 minutes after injection, administer at bedtime to decrease distress.

III.   ALTERATION IN COMFORT related to DRUG EFFECTS

Defining Characteristics: Flushing of face, hands, and feet may occur soon after injection, as well as tingling of palms and soles. Rarely, rash (maculopapular), erythema, urticaria, headache, chills have developed. Inflammation may occur at IM or subcutaneous injection site.

Nursing Implications: Assess comfort level. Administer drug at bedtime if possible. If symptoms are uncomfortable, consider symptomatic relief measures (e.g., heat, cold). Reassure patient that flushing lasts ~1 hour and is transient. Assess rash if severe; discuss drug discontinuance with physician.

IV.   ALTERATIONS IN ELECTROLYTES related to HYPOCALCEMIA, HYPERCALCEMIA

Defining Characteristics: Rarely, if drug is very effective, hypocalcemia may occur; conversely, if drug is ineffective, hypercalcemia may occur.

Nursing Implications: Monitor serum Ca^+ closely. Assess for signs/symptoms of hypocalcemia (muscle twitching, spasm tetany, seizures) and hypercalcemia (bone pain, nausea, vomiting, polyuria, polydipsia, constipation, bradycardia, lethargy, muscle weakness, psychosis). Notify physician, recheck serum calcium immediately, and institute corrective measures as ordered.

Drug: cinacalcet HCl (Sensipar)

Class: Hypocalcemic agent.

Mechanism of Action: The calcium-sensing receptor on the surface of the chief cell of the parathyroid gland regulates PTH secretion. PTH is responsible for telling the bones to break down bone (osteoclastic) and release calcium into the blood when it is needed. Cinacalcet HCl directly decreases PTH levels by increasing the sensitivity of calcium-sensing receptors to activation by extracellular calcium. As PTH levels decrease, the level of calcium in the blood decreases.

Metabolism: Oral drug is well absorbed, and maximum plasma levels are achieved in 2–6 hours. Drug AUC levels are increased 82% when ingested with a high-fat meal. Drug is metabolized by CYP3A4, CYP2D6, and CYP1A2 enzymes of the P450 microenzyme system. Drug is excreted in the urine (80%) primarily, and to a lesser degree in the feces (15%). Drug is poorly excreted in patients with moderate-to-severe hepatic impairment, with a half-life prolonged 33% and 70%, respectively. Drug is highly protein-bound so hemodialysis does not treat overdosage.

Indication: Calcium-sensing receptor agonist indicated for (1) secondary hyperparathyroidism (HPT) in patients with chronic kidney disease on dialysis; (2) hypercalcemia in patients with parathyroid carcinoma; (3) severe hypercalcemia in patients with primary HPT who are unable to undergo parathyroidectomy.

Dosage/Range:
- 30 mg PO bid, titrated every 2–4 weeks through sequential doses of 30 mg PO bid, then 60 mg PO bid, then 90 mg PO bid, and 90 mg tid or qid as necessary to normalize serum calcium levels.
- Monitor patients with moderate or severe hepatic impairment closely.
- Do not administer if serum calcium is < 8.4 mg/dL.
- Monitor calcium levels frequently during dose titration.

Drug Preparation:
- Drug available in 30-, 60-, and 90-mg tablets.
- Administer with food or shortly after a meal.

Drug Interactions:
- Drug is a potent inhibitor of CYP2D6: dosage adjustment may be needed for flecainide, vinblastine, thioridazine, tricyclic antidepressants.
- Ketoconazole: increased AUC by 2.3 times of cinacalcet HCl.
- Amitriptyline: increased amitriptyline and nortriptyline by 20% in CYP2D6 extensive metabolizers.
- Warfarin: no effect.

Lab Effects/Interference:
- Hypocalcemia.
- Hyperphosphatemia.

Special Considerations:
- Drug is indicated for treatment of hypercalcemia in patients with parathyroid carcinoma.
- Patients should be monitored for signs and symptoms of hypocalcemia.
- Drug should not be used by pregnant or breastfeeding mothers, unless benefit outweighs risk.

Potential Toxicities/Side Effects and the Nursing Process

I. POTENTIAL FOR INJURY related to HYPOCALCEMIA

Defining Characteristics: Drug lowers serum calcium. Signs and symptoms of hypocalcemia are paresthesia, myalgias, cramping, tetany, and seizures.

Nursing Implications: Assess baseline serum calcium, phosphate, magnesium levels, as well as PTH level. Develop a plan for titration with the patient, and frequency of laboratory monitoring. Teach patient symptoms of hypocalcemia, and to report them right away if they occur. Serum calcium should be assessed within 1 week after initiation or dose adjustment. Once dose has been established, serum calcium should be assessed q month. If serum calcium > 7.5 mg/dL but < 8.4 mg/dL, or if symptoms of hypocalcemia occur, discuss with physician the addition of calcium-containing phosphate binders and/or vitamin D sterols to raise the serum calcium. If the serum calcium falls to < 7.5 mg/dL or if symptoms of hypocalcemia persist, stop drug until serum calcium level reaches 8.0 mg/dL and/or symptoms resolve. Resume dose per physician, at next lowest dose of drug.

II. ALTERATION IN NUTRITION, LESS THAN BODY REQUIREMENTS, related to GI SIDE EFFECTS

Defining Characteristics: Nausea (31%) and vomiting (27%) are most common adverse effects, but diarrhea may also occur (21%).

Nursing Implications: Assess baseline nutritional and elimination status, and monitor during treatment. Ensure adequate hydration and urinary output of 2 L/day. Teach patient to administer oral antiemetics prior to taking drug, and as needed between drug doses. Assess food preferences, and suggest small, frequent feedings. Teach patient to report symptoms that worsen or do not resolve with supportive care.

III. ALTERATION IN COMFORT related to MYALGIA AND DIZZINESS

Defining Characteristics: Myalgia affects about 15% of patients and dizziness 10% of patients.

Nursing Implications: Assess baseline hydration, comfort status, and teach patient that these side effects may occur. Teach patient to change position slowly if dizziness occurs, and to notify nurse or physician if dizziness worsens or does not resolve. Teach patient symptom-management strategies, such as local application of heat for myalgias, and to notify provider if myalgias worsen.

Drug: denosumab (Xgeva)

Class: Inhibitor of osteoclastic bone resorption via inhibition of RANKL (receptor activator of nuclear factor-kB ligand); RANK ligand (RANKL) inhibitor.

COMPLICATIONS

Mechanism of Action: Human monoclonal antibody (IgG_2) with specificity and affinity for RANKL, so it binds to RANKL, thus preventing RANKL from activating its receptor RANK on the surface of osteoclasts and their precursors. This inhibits or turns off osteoclast formation, function, and survival, and decreases bone resorption. Increased osteoclast activity (bone resorption), stimulated by RANKL, is a mediator of bony metastases in solid tumors. It mimics the effect of the RANK modulator osteoprotegerin. The end result is increased bone mass and strength in both cortical and trabecular bone. Giant cell bone tumors consist of stromal cells expressing RANKL, and osteoclast-like giant cells express the RANK receptors. Cell signaling through the RANK receptor enhances osteolysis and tumor growth. Denosumab (Xgeva) prevents RANKL from activating the RANK receptor on osteoclasts, their precursors, and osteoclast-like giant cells so they cannot break down bone.

Metabolism: After subcutaneous dosing, bioavailability of denosumab is 62%, and multiple dosing of 120 mg every 4 weeks resulted in up to a 2.8-fold accumulation of denosumab concentration, with steady state reached by 6 months. The mean elimination half-life is 28 days. Drug clearance and volume of distribution is proportional to body weight: 48% higher in a 100-lb. (45-kg) person, and 46% lower in a 265-lb. (120-kg) person, compared to the 145-lb. (66-kg) person. Renal impairment did not affect drug pharmacokinetics, and no studies were done to evaluate the effect of hepatic impairment.

Indication: For (1) prevention of skeletal-related events in patients with bone metastases from solid tumors; (2) treatment of adults and skeletally mature adolescents with giant cell tumor of bone that is unresectable or where surgical resection is likely to result in severe morbidity. Drug is NOT indicated for the prevention of skeletal-related events in patients with multiple myeloma.

Dosage/Range:
- Prevention of skeletal-related events in patients with bone metastases: 120 mg SQ every 4 weeks.
- Treatment of adults and skeletally mature adolescents with giant cell tumor of bone: 120 mg SQ every 4 weeks, with additional 120 mg doses on days 8 and 15 of the first month of treatment.

Drug Preparation:
- Drug is available as 120 mg per 1.7 mL (70 mg/mL) single-use vial. Drug should be refrigerated at 36–46°F (2–8°C) in its original carton. Do not freeze. Once removed from the refrigerator, drug must not be exposed to temperatures above 25°C(77°F) or direct light, and it must be used within 14 days. Protect from direct light and heat.
  - Prior to administration, remove drug from refrigerator and bring to room temperature, 25°C (77°F), by letting it stand in the original container for 15–30 minutes. Do not warm any other way.
  - Inspect drug for particulate matter or discoloration, and discard if found. Solution should be clear, colorless to pale yellow, and it may contain trace amounts of protein-aceous particles ranging from translucent to white.
  - Using a 27-gauge needle, aseptically draw up entire contents of vial; do not reenter vial. Discard the empty vial.

Drug Administration:
* Administer subcutaneously in the upper arm, upper thigh, or abdomen. Rotate sites. Administer calcium and vitamin D as necessary to treat or prevent hypocalcemia.
* Drug is contraindicated in patients with clinically significant hypersensitivity to drug or its components.
* Same active ingredient in Prolia, so patient should not take Prolia when taking Xgeva.

Drug Interactions:
* No studies have been carried out. There are no identified drug interactions with standard chemotherapy or hormonal therapy.
* Drugs causing hypocalcemia: increased risk for hypocalcemia.

Lab Effects/Interference:
* Hypocalcemia, hypercholesterolemia, hypophosphatemia.

Special Considerations:
* Severe hypocalcemia may occur; hypocalcemia should be corrected prior to starting denosumab. Monitor calcium levels prior to each treatment. Patients with renal impairment (creatinine clearance < 30 mL/min or receiving dialysis) are at increased risk. Patients MUST take adequate calcium and vitamin D supplements, as well as magnesium, as prescribed by their physician or nurse practitioner. Teach patient to report signs/symptoms of hypocalcemia (abdominal cramping, irregular heartbeat, depression, irritability, lethargy or sluggishness, muscle spasms, seizures).
* Osteonecrosis of the jaw (ONJ) may develop. ONJ is characterized by jaw pain, osteomyelitis, osteitis, bone erosion, tooth or periodontal infection, toothache, gingival ulceration or gingival erosion, delayed healing of mouth or jaw after dental surgery. Patient should have an oral exam prior to starting denosumab, have any dental work completed prior to starting the drug, and be monitored closely for symptoms. Patient should avoid invasive dental procedures during treatment with denosumab. If ONJ develops, patient should be referred to a dentist or oral surgeon; however, extensive oral surgery may exacerbate the condition. Risk factors of ONJ are associated with tooth extraction and/or local infection with delayed healing. Teach patients to report any dental or jaw issues, such as pain, right away during therapy. Teach patient to practice good oral hygiene regularly during drug therapy. Consider discontinuance of drug therapy if ONJ develops based on individual patient assessment, and patients should be evaluated and treated by a dentist or oral surgeon.
* Drug may cause atypical femoral fracture, occurring anywhere in the femoral shaft from just below the lesser trochanter to above the supracondylar flare, which may be transverse or short oblique, without communication. Fracture is not usually associated with trauma, or it may occur with minimal trauma to the area. Fractures may be bilateral and patients may report prodromal pain (e.g., dull, aching thigh pain) prior to the diagnosis, weeks to months before complete fracture occurs. Concomitant administration of corticosteroids may increase risk. Teach patients to report any new or unusual thigh, hip, or groin pain immediately. Evaluate patients for incomplete fracture. Also assess patient for signs and symptoms of fracture in the contralateral limb. Consider interrupting denosumab therapy pending a risk/benefit assessment.

COMPLICATIONS

- Hypersensitivity, including anaphylaxis, has been rarely reported. Reactions may include hypotension, dyspnea, upper airway edema, lip swelling, rash, pruritus, and urticaria. If anaphylactic or other significant allergic reaction occurs, provide emergency intervention as ordered; drug should be permanently discontinued.
- The most common adverse reactions (> 25%) were fatigue/asthenia, hypophosphatemia, nausea (in patients with bone metastases), and arthralgia, headache, nausea, back pain, fatigue, and extremity pain (in patients with giant cell tumor).
- Drug may cause fetal harm. Drug should not be used in pregnant women, as it may cause fetal impairment of dentition and bone growth, as well as alteration in maturation of the maternal mammary gland and impaired lactation. It is not known if the drug is excreted in human milk, so patients who are nursing should discontinue nursing or discontinue the drug. Teach female patients of childbearing potential to use highly effective birth control during therapy and for at least 5 months after last dose of Xgeva.
- If the patient becomes pregnant while receiving the drug, Amgen has a Pregnancy Surveillance Program. RANKL and RANK function in other body processes, and thus, the long-term effects of antagonism of this cytokine are unclear.
- Drug is not recommended in pediatric patients, as it may impair bone growth in children with open growth plates, as well as inhibit teeth eruption.

Potential Toxicities/Side Effects and the Nursing Process

I.   ALTERATIONS IN ELECTROLYTES related to HYPOCALCEMIA

Defining Characteristics: Denosumab may cause severe hypocalcemia. In clinical trials, hypocalcemia was reported in 18% (3.1% severe), with hypophosphatemia in 32% (severe in 15.4%). Drug is contraindicated in patients who are hypocalcemic. Drug may worsen hypocalcemia, especially if the patient has severe renal impairment (creatinine clearance < 30 mL/min or receiving dialysis). Patients must take calcium and vitamin D supplements, as well as magnesium, as needed and prescribed. Patients at risk for hypocalcemia are those taking other concomitant drugs that reduce serum calcium, or with a history of hypoparathyroidism, thyroid surgery, parathyroid surgery, malabsorption syndromes, excision of small intestine, or severe renal impairment as above. Post-marketing reports have documented severe symptomatic hypocalcemia, including fatal cases.

Nursing Implications: Assess serum calcium, phosphorus, and magnesium baseline and prior to each treatment. Consider monitoring patients with renal impairment, those who are receiving concomitant drugs that may cause hypocalcemia, or those with other risk for hypocalcemia more closely during therapy. Prior to drug administration, hypocalcemia must be corrected. Teach patient importance of daily calcium and vitamin D supplements and assess adherence (recommended daily calcium 1,000-mg and at least 400-mg vitamin D supplements). Assess for signs/symptoms of hypocalcemia (muscle twitching, spasm tetany, seizures), and teach patient to report any symptoms right away (spasms, twitches, muscle stiffness, or cramps in muscles, numbness or tingling in fingers, toes, or around the mouth).

II.   POTENTIAL FOR INJURY related to ONJ

Defining Characteristics: Patients receiving denosumab are at risk for ONJ, which is associated with RANKL inhibitor and bisphosphonate therapy. The incidence in denosumab clinical trials was 2.2%; of those who developd ONJ, 79% had a history of tooth extraction, poor oral hygiene, or use of a dental appliance, tooth extraction, and/or local infection with delayed healing. Patients at risk for ONJ are those who have had invasive dental procedures, a cancer diagnosis, concomitant therapies with corticosteroids, poor oral hygiene, and preexisting periodontal or dental disease. Patients on clinical trials also had pain in the back, musculoskeleton, and abdomen that was not significantly higher than placebo. Patient symptoms were jaw pain, osteomyelitis, osteitis, bone erosion, tooth or periodontal infection, toothache, gingival ulceration, and gingival erosion.

Nursing Implications: Ensure that patient has a thorough oral exam and dental history prior to starting drug, and periodically during therapy. If the patient has risk factors such as invasive dental procedures (e.g., tooth extraction, dental implants, oral surgery, cancer diagnosis, concomitant therapies such as chemotherapy and corticosteroids, poor oral hygiene, periodontal and/or other preexisting dental disease, anemia, coagulopathy, infection, ill-fitting dentures), patient should have a dental exam with necessary preventive dentistry prior to starting the drug. Any outstanding oral or dental issues must be referred to a dentist or oral surgeon for preventive work prior to starting the drug. Assess patient's baseline oral hygiene practices and ensure that they are effective. Teach patient to practice good oral hygiene consistently, and to report to the nurse or physician any problems that arise in the oral cavity or teeth. Monitor patients at risk closely. If ONJ does develop, consult a dentist or oral surgeon. Unfortunately, extensive dental surgery to treat ONJ may exacerbate the condition. If a patient is suspected to have, or has ONJ, patient should receive care by a dentist or oral surgeon (e.g., extensive dental surgery to treat ONJ may exacerbate it).

III.   ALTERATIONS IN NUTRITION, LESS THAN BODY REQUIREMENTS, related to NAUSEA, DIARRHEA

Defining Characteristics: Nausea occurred in > 25% of patients, while diarrhea occurred less.

Nursing Implications: Assess baseline nutritional and elimination status, and monitor during treatment. Instruct patient to report nausea and diarrhea, and discuss appropriate antiemetic with physician or nurse practitioner. Discuss bowel elimination plan. Teach patient to report any abdominal discomfort.

Drug: etidronate disodium (Didronel)

Class: Bisphosphonate; hypocalcemic agent.

Mechanism of Action: Inhibits osteoclastic bone resorption (bone breakdown), thereby decreasing calcium release, and serum calcium levels. Indicated in the management of hypercalcemia of malignancy.

Metabolism: Oral absorption is variable and decreased by food. Following IV injection, drug is distributed into bone, then excreted unchanged in the urine.

Indication: For the treament of symptomatic Paget's disease of bone and in the prevention and treatment of heterotopic ossification following total hip replacement or due to spinal cord injury. Drug is NOT approved for the treatment of osteoporosis.

Dosage/Range:
Adult (hypercalcemia of malignancy):
- IV (induction): 7.5 mg/kg/day × 3 days (may increase to 7 days; if hypercalcemia recurs, wait at least 7 days before treatment using same induction regimen).
- Oral (maintenance): 20 mg/kg/day beginning on day after last IV dose, for up to 90 days if effective.

Drug Preparation:
- Oral: give as single oral dose (may be advised if GI distress); give at least 2 hours before or after a meal.
- IV: dilute drug in at least 250 mL 0.9% sodium chloride and infuse over at least 2 hours.

Drug Interactions:
- Nephrotoxic drugs: additive nephrotoxicity; AVOID concurrent use.

Lab Effects/Interference:
- Decreased P, decreased Mg.
- Abnormal renal function tests.
- Decreased Ca.

Special Considerations:
- Saline hydration should be maintained during treatment to keep urinary output at 2 L/day.
- Use with caution.
- It is unknown whether drug crosses placenta or is excreted in breastmilk; use with caution, if at all, in pregnant or breastfeeding women.
- 60–70% response rate when given with hydration and diuresis, and one-half of this when based on corrected calcium value.

Potential Toxicities/Side Effects and the Nursing Process

I.   ALTERATIONS IN NUTRITION, LESS THAN BODY REQUIREMENTS, related to GI SIDE EFFECTS

Defining Characteristics: Diarrhea, nausea, vomiting, abdominal discomfort, and guaiac-positive stools may occur rarely.

Nursing Implications: Assess baseline nutritional and elimination status and monitor during treatment. Instruct patient to report nausea and vomiting, and consider dividing dose (if oral) or slowing infusion rate > 2 hours. Guaiac stools and notify physician if positive.

II.   ALTERATION IN URINE ELIMINATION related to NEPHROTOXICITY

Defining Characteristics: Drug is nephrotoxic and may cause rises in serum BUN and creatinine. Increased risk when concurrent nephrotoxic drugs administered.

Nursing Implications: Assess baseline hydration status and total body fluid balance to ensure adequate urinary output (> 2 L/day). Assess baseline serum BUN and creatinine, and monitor throughout treatment. Dose reduction necessitated by renal insufficiency.

III.   ALTERATIONS IN ELECTROLYTES related to HYPOCALCEMIA, HYPERCALCEMIA

Defining Characteristics: Rarely, if drug is very effective, hypocalcemia may occur; conversely, if drug is ineffective, hypercalcemia may occur. Increased sodium phosphate levels may occur during oral therapy but are less frequent with IV dosing (serum phosphate levels are inversely proportional to serum calcium).

Nursing Implications: Monitor serum calcium closely. Assess for signs/symptoms of hypocalcemia (muscle twitching, spasm tetany, seizures) and hypercalcemia (bone pain, nausea, vomiting, polyuria, polydipsia, constipation, bradycardia, lethargy, muscle weakness, psychosis). Notify physician, recheck serum calcium immediately, and institute corrective measures as ordered.

Drug: gallium nitrate (Ganite)

Class: Hypocalcemic agent.

Mechanism of Action: Inhibits calcium release from bone by inhibiting bone resorption and turnover. Indicated for the treatment of hypercalcemia of malignancy refractory to hydration.

Metabolism: Excreted by kidneys.

Indications: For the treatment of clearly symptomatic cancer-related hypercalcemia that has not responded to adequate hydration (corrected serum calcium > 12 mg/dL).

Dosage/Range:
Adult:
- IV: Severe hypercalcemia: 200 mg/m^2 as continuous 24-hour infusion × 5 days (or when serum calcium normalizes if before 5 days). Moderate hypercalcemia: 100 mg/m^2 as continuous 24-hour infusion × 5 days (or less if patient achieves normal serum calcium).

Drug Preparation:
- Dilute daily dose in 1 L 0.9% sodium chloride or 5% dextrose injection, and infuse over 24 hours (42 mL/hour) via infusion pump.

COMPLICATIONS

Drug Interactions:
- Nephrotoxic drugs (amphotericin B, aminoglycosides, and cisplatin): additive nephrotoxicity; avoid concurrent use.

Lab Effects/Interference:
- Increased BUN, creatinine.
- Decreased calcium; transient decrease in phosphorus, decrease in bicarbonate.
- Rarely, anemia, leukopenia.

Special Considerations:
- Contraindicated in patients with severe renal dysfunction (serum creatinine > 2.5 mg/dL).
- Unknown if drug crosses placenta or is excreted in breastmilk; use cautiously in pregnancy, and suggest mother interrupt breastfeeding while taking drug.
- 92% patient response (reduction in serum calcium corrected for albumin), lasting for 7.5 days.
- Saline hydration to maintain urinary output of 2 L/day should be maintained during treatment.

Potential Toxicities/Side Effects and the Nursing Process

I.   ALTERATION IN URINE ELIMINATION related to NEPHROTOXICITY

Defining Characteristics: Increased serum BUN, creatinine in 13% of patients. Decreased risk if concurrent administration of other nephrotoxic drugs.

Nursing Implications: Assess baseline hydration status and total body fluid balance to ensure adequate urinary output (> 2 L/day). Assess baseline serum BUN and creatinine, and monitor throughout treatment. Dose reduction necessitated by renal insufficiency. Drug should NOT be given if serum creatinine > 2.5 mg/dL.

II.   ALTERATIONS IN ELECTROLYTES related to HYPOCALCEMIA, HYPERCALCEMIA

Defining Characteristics: Rarely, if drug is very effective, hypocalcemia may occur; conversely, if drug is ineffective, hypercalcemia may occur. Transient hypophosphatemia occurs in up to 79% of hypercalcemic patients after treatment with drug. Also, decreased serum bicarbonate occurs in 40–50% of patients.

Nursing Implications: Monitor serum calcium closely. Assess for signs/symptoms of hypocalcemia (muscle twitching, spasm tetany, seizures) and hypercalcemia (bone pain, nausea, vomiting, polyuria, polydipsia, constipation, bradycardia, lethargy, muscle weakness, psychosis). Notify physician, recheck serum calcium immediately, and institute corrective measures as ordered. Monitor serum phosphate levels, and administer replacement oral phosphates as ordered.

III. ALTERATIONS IN NUTRITION, LESS THAN BODY REQUIREMENTS, related to GI SIDE EFFECTS

Defining Characteristics: Diarrhea, nausea, vomiting, constipation may occur.

Nursing Implications: Assess baseline nutritional and elimination status, and monitor during treatment. Instruct patient to report nausea and vomiting. Administer ordered anti-emetics. Ensure adequate hydration with urinary output > 2 L/day.

Drug: pamidronate disodium (Aredia)

Class: Bisphosphonate; hypocalcemic agent.

Mechanism of Action: Probably inhibits osteoclast activity in bone (bone breakdown) and may also block dissolution of minerals (hydroxyapatite) in bone, thus preventing calcium release from bone. Does not inhibit bone formation or bone mineralization. Indicated for the treatment of hypercalcemia of malignancy, in conjunction with adequate hydration, as well as prevention of osteolytic lesions in breast cancer and multiple myeloma.

Metabolism: Excreted by kidneys.
Adult (hypercalcemia of malignancy):
- IV (moderate hypercalcemia, 12–13.5 mg/dL corrected): 60–90 mg as continuous infu-sion over 2 24 hours.
- IV (severe hypercalcemia > 13.5 mg/dL): 90 mg as continuous infusion over 2–24 hours.
- If retreatment required, wait a minimum of 7 days between treatments.
Osteolytic bone metastases of breast cancer:
- 90 mg in 250 mL of IV fluid via 2-hour infusion every 3–4 weeks.
Osteolytic lesions of multiple myeloma:
- 90 mg in 500 mL IV fluid via a 2- to 4-hour infusion every month.

Indication: (1) Treatment of moderate or severe hypercalcemia associated with malig-nancy, with or without bone metastases; (2) treatment of moderate to severe Paget's disease of bone; (3) in conjunction with standard antineoplastic therapy, for the treatment of osteo-lytic bone metastases of breast cancer and osteolytic lesions of multiple myeloma.

Drug Preparation/Administration:
- Reconstitute by adding 10 mL sterile water for injection to 30-mg vial. Further dilute in 1 L 0.9% sodium chloride or 5% dextrose injection as per manufacturer's directions.
- Infuse over 2–24 hours via infusion pump or rate controller.
- When drug is given to prevent lytic lesions in the bone, patients should take an oral calcium supplement of 500 mg and a multiple vitamin containing 400 IU of vitamin D daily.

COMPLICATIONS

Drug Interactions:
- Use caution with other potentially nephrotoxic drugs.
- Increased risk of renal function deterioration in multiple myeloma patients also receiving thalidomide.

Lab Effects/Interference:
- Decreased calcium.
- Decreased K+, decreased Mg, decreased P (phosphate).
- Increased serum creatinine, urinary excretion of protein (proteinuria).

Special Considerations:
- Use cautiously when combined with renally toxic drugs, such as aminoglycoside antibiotics or loop diuretics. Use cautiously in patients who have aspirin-sensitive asthma.
- The drug may rarely cause osteonecrosis of the jaw, often in conjunction with a dental procedure, such as tooth extraction. Patients should have an oral examination and preventive dentistry completed before starting bisphosphonate therapy and periodically during treatment if high risk or symptoms arise. Patients should avoid dental work being done while receiving bisphosphonate therapy.
- Drug may rarely cause renal insufficiency: assess serum creatinine at baseline and before each treatment, and perform periodic urinalyses for protein. Hold the drug for increased serum creatinine or proteinuria.
- Saline hydration to maintain urinary output of 2 L/day should be maintained during treatment for hypercalcemia.
- Clinical studies show 64% of patients have corrected serum calcium levels by 24 hours after beginning therapy, and after 7 days 100% of the 90-mg group had normal corrected levels. For some (33–53%), normal or partially corrected calcium levels in 60-mg and 90-mg groups persisted × 14 days.
- Drug may cause atypical femoral fracture, occurring anywhere in the femoral shaft from just below the lesser trochanter to above the supracondylar flare, which may be transverse or short oblique, without communication. Fracture is not usually associated with trauma, or may occur with minimal trauma to the area. Fractures may be bilateral, and patients may report prodromal pain (e.g., dull, aching thigh pain) prior to the diagnosis, weeks to months before complete fracture occurs. Concomitant administration of corticosteroids may increase risk. Teach patients to report any new or unusual thigh, hip, or groin pain immediately. Evaluate patients for incomplete fracture, and suspect atypical fracture in any patient who has/is receiving bisphosphonate therapy and presents with thigh or groin pain without trauma. Also assess patient for signs and symptoms of fracture in the contralatateral limb. Consider discontinuing pamidronate therapy pending a risk/benefit assessment. It is unknown if the atypical femur fracture continues after therapy is stopped. Poor healing of the atypical fracture has been reported.
- Has been shown to reduce bony metastasis in patients with multiple myeloma and to reduce pain.
- Patients with preexisting anemia, leukopenia, or thrombocytopenia should be monitored closely for 2 weeks after pamidronate disodium treatment.

Potential Toxicities/Side Effects and the Nursing Process

I. ALTERATIONS IN NUTRITION, LESS THAN BODY REQUIREMENTS, related to GI SIDE EFFECTS

Defining Characteristics: Nausea, vomiting, abdominal discomfort, constipation, and anorexia may occur rarely.

Nursing Implications: Assess baseline nutritional and elimination status and monitor during treatment. Ensure adequate hydration and urinary output of 2 L/day. Administer ordered antiemetics. Administer oral phosphates as cathartics if ordered. Assess food differences and offer small, frequent feedings.

II. ALTERATION IN ELECTROLYTES related to HYPOCALCEMIA, HYPERCALCEMIA

Defining Characteristics: Rarely, if drug is very effective, hypocalcemia may occur; conversely, if drug is ineffective, hypercalcemia may occur. Hypokalemia, hypomagnesemia, hypophosphatemia may occur. Women with breast cancer taking the drug to prevent lytic lesions are at risk for developing osteoporosis.

Nursing Implications: Monitor serum calcium closely. Assess for signs/symptoms of hypocalcemia (muscle twitching, spasm tetany, seizures) and hypercalcemia (bone pain, nausea, vomiting, polyuria, polydipsia, constipation, bradycardia, lethargy, muscle weakness, psychosis). Notify physician, recheck serum calcium immediately, and institute corrective measures as ordered. Monitor serum potassium, magnesium, phosphate levels and notify physician of abnormalities. Women receiving drug to prevent lytic lesions should receive calcium and vitamin D supplements and should be encouraged to exercise. If a smoker, she should be encouraged to stop smoking to reduce the risk of osteoporosis.

III. ALTERATIONS IN COMFORT related to LOCAL VEIN IRRITATION

Defining Characteristics: Transient fever (1°C or 3°F elevation) may occur 24–48 hours after drug administration (27% of patients), local reactions (pain, irritation, phlebitis) are common with 90-mg dose.

Nursing Implications: Assess baseline temperature, and monitor during and after infusion. Administer antipyretics as ordered. Assess IV site and restart new IV as needed for 90-mg dose in large vein where drug can be rapidly diluted. Apply warm packs as needed to site.

IV. ALTERATIONS IN FLUID BALANCE related to AGGRESSIVE HYDRATION

Defining Characteristics: Patients receive aggressive saline hydration to ensure urinary output of 2 L/day. Hypertension may occur. Patients with history of heart disease or renal insufficiency are at risk for fluid overload.

COMPLICATIONS

Nursing Implications: Assess baseline hydration status, total body fluid balance; monitor q 4 h. Discuss with physician need for diuretics once hydrated to keep body fluid balance equal (I = O). Monitor vital signs q 4 h during hydration, and notify physician of changes.

Drug: zoledronic acid (Zometa)

Class: Bisphosphonate.

Mechanism of Action: Inhibits bone resorption. Inhibits tumor-related osteoclast activity in bone (bone breakdown), promotes apoptosis of osteoclasts, and blocks dissolution of minerals (hydroxyapatite) in bone, thus preventing calcium release from bone, as well as osteoclastic resorption of cartilage. It also inhibits osteoclast activity and the release of calcium from the bones that is caused by tumor-related stimulatory factors. It does not inhibit bone formation or bone mineralization. Drug is very rapidly taken up in the bone, but very slowly released. Drug appears to inhibit endothelial cell proliferation and to inhibit the beta fibroblast growth factor (bFGF)-mediated angiogenesis. The drug is 100–850 times more potent than pamidronate.

Metabolism: Drug is primarily eliminated intact via the kidney. Long terminal half-life in plasma of 167 hours. Rapid injection results in 30% increase in serum drug concentration and renal damage.

Indication:
- Indicated for the treatment of (1) hypercalcemia of malignancy; (2) patients with multiple myeloma and patients with documented bone metastases from solid tumors, in conjunction with standard antineoplastic therapy; (3) patients with prostate cancer with bone metastases who have progressed after treatment with at least one hormonal therapy.

Dosage/Range:
- Hypercalcemia of malignancy (corrected calcium ≥ 12 mg/dL): 4 mg (maximum) IV over at least 15 minutes; if retreatment required, wait at least 7 days before administering again and monitor renal function closely.
- Multiple myeloma and metastatic bone lesions from solid tumors with urinary creatinine clearance of at least 60 mL/min is 4 mg IV over at least 15 minutes every 3–4 weeks.
- Single doses should NOT exceed 4 mg, and duration of infusion should be at least 15 minutes, as otherwise increases risk of renal dysfunction.
- Assess serum creatinine prior to EACH DOSE:
  - If patient has a normal serum creatinine prior to treatment, but has an increase of 0.5 mg/dL within 2 weeks of next dose, hold Zometa until the serum creatinine is at least within 10% of baseline value.
  - If patient has an abnormal serum creatinine prior to treatment, but has an increase of 1.0 mg/dL within 2 weeks of next dose, Zometa should be withheld until the serum creatinine is at least within 10% of baseline value.
- *Dose reductions for renal insufficiency if urinary creatinine clearance (Cr Cl) is:*
  - 50–60 mL/min: dose is 3.5 mg.
  - 40–49 mL/min: dose is 3.3 mg.
  - 30–39 mL/min: dose is 3.0 mg.

- Coadminister oral calcium supplements of 500 mg and a multiple vitamin containing 400 IU of vitamin D daily.

Drug Preparation:
- Drug is available in 4-mg/100 mL single-use ready-to-use bottle, or 4 mg/5 mL single-use vial of concentrate.
- 4 mg/100 mL single-use ready-to-use bottle (contains overfill so can you can withdraw entire 4- mg dose as 100 mLs): Administer 4 mg (100 mL) without further dilution for full dose. To prepare reduced doses for patients with decreased Cr Cl, aseptically remove the specified volume from the vial and discard: 12 mL to make a 3.5-mg dose, 18 mL to make a 3.3-mg dose, and 25 mL to make a 3.0-mg dose. Replace the 0.9% sodium chloride or 5% dextrose injection in the same volume that was withdrawn into the vial, bringing the volume back to 100 mL.
- 4 mg/5 mL single-use vial of concentrate: Withdraw 4-mg dose (5 mL) and immediately dilute in 100 mL 5% dextrose injection, USP or 0.9% sodium chloride injection, USP. DO NOT use any other IV solution, such as lactated Ringer's solution. Administer full dose as ordered over at least 15 minutes. To prepare reduced doses for patients with decreased baseline Cr Cl, withdraw the specified volume from the vial and then immediately dilute in 100 mL 5% dextrose injection, USP or 0.9% sodium chloride injection, USP: 3.5 mg dose = 4.4 mL, 3.3 mg dose = 4.1 mL, and 3.0 mg dose = 3.8 mL.
- If not used immediately, drug may be refrigerated at 2–8°C (36–46°F) for up to 24 hours (make sure the drug mixing time/date are clear on the label, as the nurse must complete administration within 24 hours of the initial dilution).

Drug Administration:
- Administer as a single IV dose over *at least* 15 minutes. Use a separate, vented infusion line from all other drugs; do not allow drug to come into contact with any calcium or divalent cation-containing solutions.
- Do not exceed 4-mg dose.
- *Hypercalcemia of malignancy:*
  - Assure that patient has been adequately rehydrated prior to drug administration and that the BUN and creatinine are WNL. Monitor electrolytes during treatment.
  - Dose adjustments are not necessary in patients presenting with mild-to-moderate renal impairment prior to starting zolendronic acid (serum creatinine < 400 μM/L or 4.5 mg/dL).
- Multiple myeloma and metastatic bone lesions of solid tumors:
  - For patients who require retreatment and who have had altered renal status after receiving the drug, here are manufacturer's recommendations for patients with:
    - Normal serum creatinine before receiving drug, but have an increase of 0.5 mg/dL within 2 weeks of next dose: hold drug until serum creatinine is at least within 10% of baseline value.
    - Abnormal serum creatinine before receiving drug, but have an increase of 1.0 mg/dL within 2 weeks of next dose: drug should be held until serum creatinine is at least within 10% of baseline value.

- Patients should take an oral calcium supplement of 500 mg and a multiple vitamin containing 400 IU of vitamin D daily.

Drug Interactions:
- Incompatible with calcium-containing fluids, such as lactated Ringer's, or divalent-cation-containing solutions.
- Use cautiously together with aminoglycoside antibiotics, as there may be an additive effect resulting in hypocalcemia for prolonged periods, as well as renal toxicity.
- Use cautiously together with loop diuretics, as the risk of hypocalcemia and nephrotoxicity may be increased.
- Reclast: patients should NOT take both zoledronic acid and Reclast.
- Nephrotoxic drugs: use with caution.
- Thalidomide: combination in patients with multiple myeloma may increase risk of renal dysfunction.

Lab Effects/Interference:
- Hypocalcemia.
- Hypophosphatemia.
- Hypomagnesemia.
- Increased BUN and serum creatinine.

Special Considerations:
- Not recommended in patients with bone metastases and severe renal impairment, pregnant women, or nursing mothers. Monitor serum creatinine prior to each dose. Teach women of childbearing age to avoid pregnancy while receiving the drug.
- Severe, incapacitating bone, joint, or muscle pain may occur; discontinue drug if severe symptoms occur.
- Drug is NOT indicated for hyperparathyroidism or non-tumor-associated hypercalcemia.
- Drug is not indicated for pediatric use.
- Use caution and close monitoring of renal function in geriatric patients.
- Use cautiously when combined with renally toxic drugs, such as aminoglycoside antibiotics or loop diuretics. Use drug cautiously in patients who have aspirin-sensitive asthma, as well as in older patients.
- Monitor serum creatinine before each dose; monitor serum electrolytes, magnesium, phosphate, and hematocrit/hemoglobin baseline and regularly during treatment. Discuss abnormal values with physician, as risk must be weighed against benefit. Risk factors for deteriorating renal function, possibly renal failure are (1) impaired renal function and (2) multiple cycles of bisphosphonate therapy.
- Drug may rarely cause osteonecrosis of the jaw, often in conjunction with a dental procedure, such as tooth extraction. Patients should have an oral examination and preventive dentistry completed before starting bisphosphonate therapy, and it should be assessed periodically during treatment if high risk or symptoms arise. Patients should avoid invasive dental work while receiving bisphosphonate therapy.
- Drug may cause atypical femoral fracture, occurring anywhere in the femoral shaft from just below the lesser trochanter to above the supracondylar flare, which may be transverse or short oblique, without communication. Fracture is not usually associated with

trauma, or may occur with minimal trauma to the area. Fractures may be bilateral, and patients may report prodromal pain (e.g., dull, aching thigh pain) prior to the diagnosis, weeks to months before complete fracture occurs. Concomitant administration of corticosteroids may increase risk. Teach patients to report any new or unusual thigh, hip, or groin pain immediately. Evaluate patients for incomplete fracture; assess patient also for signs and symptoms of fracture in the contralateral limb. Consider discontinuing Zometa therapy pending a risk/benefit assessment. It is unknown whether the atypical femur fracture will continue after therapy is stopped. Poor healing of the atypical fracture has been reported.

* Teach patients to use effective birth control measures, as drug can cause fetal harm. Nursing mothers should not receive this drug.
* As compared with pamidronate in the management of hypercalcemia of malignancy, Zometa had a 45.3% response rate by day 4 and an 82.6% response rate by day 7, as compared with a 33.3% response rate and a 63.6% response rate, respectively, when pamidronate was given. Time to relapse was 30 days with Zometa and 17 days with pamidronate.

Potential Toxicities/Skin Effects and the Nursing Process

I. ALTERATION IN COMFORT, related to FEVER, NAUSEA AND VOMITING, INSOMNIA, AND FLU-LIKE SYMPTOMS

Defining Characteristics: Fever occurred in 44% of patients during clinical trials. Flu-like symptoms of chills, bone pain, and/or arthralgias and myalgias may occur less commonly. Nausea occurred in 29% of patients, and vomiting 14%. Insomnia affects 15%. The symptom frequency was similar to the pamidronate and placebo groups.

Nursing Implications: Assess baseline comfort and temperature. Teach patient that these side effects may occur and to report them. Administer or teach patient self-administration of acetaminophen or over-the-counter NSAIDs as appropriate to manage fever, arthralgias, or myalgias if they occur. Teach patient to report if symptoms do not resolve. Administer antiemetics as ordered to minimize nausea and vomiting.

II. ALTERATION IN BOWEL ELIMINATION PATTERN related to CONSTIPATION, DIARRHEA, ABDOMINAL PAIN, AND ANOREXIA

Defining Characteristics: Diarrhea affected 24% (versus 18% placebo) of patients in clinical trials, while 31% developed constipation (compared to 38% in placebo). Fouteen percent of patients developed abdominal pain (versus 11% in placebo), and 22% anorexia (compared to 23% in placebo).

Nursing Implications: Assess baseline bowel elimination status, and teach patient to report alterations. Teach patient to use diet modifications depending upon changes, and over-the-counter antidiarrheals or laxatives as necessary. Teach patient to report persistent diarrhea or constipation (lasting more than 24 hours), presence of blood, abdominal cramping, or pain.

III.   ALTERATION IN ACTIVITY TOLERANCE related to ANEMIA, FATIGUE

Defining Characteristics: Anemia occurred in 33% of patients (compared to 23% in placebo arm) during clinical trials.

Nursing Implications: Assess baseline hemoglobin and hematocrit. Teach patient to report fatigue, and discuss strategies to conserve energy, such as alternating rest and activity. Discuss with physician transfusion if symptoms are severe.

IV.   ALTERATION IN FLUID AND ELECTROLYTE BALANCE
related to CHANGES IN RENAL EXCRETION

Defining Characteristics: Drug will cause renal dysfunction with rise in serum creatinine if drug is given rapidly or in less than 15 minutes. Hypophosphatemia occurred in 13% of patients during clinical trials, hypokalemia in 12%, and hypomagnesemia in 10%.

Nursing Implications: Assess baseline renal function and electrolytes prior to initial therapy, post-therapy, and prior to any additional therapy as needed. Dose reduction necessary in patients with renal insufficiency. Hold drug if renal abnormalities do not correct, as indicated in Administration section.

V.   POTENTIAL FOR INJURY related to OSTEOPOROSIS,
OSTEONECROSIS OF THE JAW (ONJ)

Defining Characteristics: Women with breast cancer and men with prostate cancer are at risk for osteoporosis from various cancer treatments, including hormonal manipulation. ONJ may occur rarely, and it is associated with recent dental procedures, such as tooth extraction.

Nursing Implications: Teach patient to take calcium and vitamin D supplements (or multivitamin) while receiving bisphosphonates, and encourage patient to exercise regularly. If a smoker, encourage the patient to stop smoking to reduce the risk of osteoporosis. Teach patient to have a dental exam and preventive dental work before starting therapy, and to practice excellent oral hygiene.

Chapter *11*
Infection

According to the Centers for Disease Control (CDC), there are over 650,000 cancer patients receiving outpatient chemotherapy yearly. These patients are susceptible to infections related to their treatments. Many cancer chemotherapy regimens cause neutropenia that result in delays or reductions in dosages of chemotherapy for cancer patients. Chemotherapy, radiation therapy, and even the malignancy itself can result in immunosuppression and infection risk. The risk for infection results from damage to bone marrow and stem cells. Additionally, cancer patients receiving newer treatments, such as hematopoietic stem cell transplant, and those receiving high-dose corticosteroids, purine analogues, and alemtuzumab are at risk for life-threatening infection.

Febrile neutropenia is a serious and life-threatening condition resulting from decreased white blood cell count and cancer patients' inabilty to fight infection. Leukocytes, or white blood cells (WBCs), are divided into cells that contain granules in the cytoplasm (granulocytes) and cells that do not (agranulocytes). White blood cells containing granules include neutrophils, basophils, and eosinophils, while the non-granulocyte WBCs (mononuclear leukocytes) include lymphocytes, monocytes, and macrophages. Neutrophils fight against invading microorganisms by migrating to the site of infection. The type and amount of neutrophils are key indicators of both infection and risk associated with infection, especially for the patient with cancer. See Figure 11.1 for maturation of the formed blood cell elements.

The risk of infection is related to the degree and duration of neutropenia, as shown in Table 11.1. The absolute neutrophil count (ANC), the number of neutrophils in the body, determines the risk for infection. This calculation is shown in Table 11.2.

Assessing the risk of infection includes: treatment intent (curative therapy, adjuvant therapy, prolonged survival, better health-related quality of life, symptom management), chemotherapy regimen risk (high, moderate, low) and treatment-related factors (type and kind of mylosuppressive agents, history of surgery, chemotherapy and/or radiation therapy, relative dose intensity), and patient-related factors (age, nutritional status, performance status, immune function, active infection, history of infection or febrile neutropenia, stage and type of cancer, hemoglobin and albumin levels, comorbidities). In non-neutropenic, immunocompromised patients, the level of risk may be more difficult to quantify. Yet, we know that the frequency and severity of infection are inversely proportional to the neutrophil count. Therefore, the rate of decline, and the length of time the patient is neutropenic, results in greater risk of infection. Infection and fever in a neutropenic patient represent a medical emergency, and, if untreated, can result in sepsis and death. Neutropenia-related infections can be life threatening and require aggressive treatment with antibiotic, antifungal, and/or antiviral agents. Additionally, an estimated 8.5% of all cancer deaths in the United States were associated with severe sepsis at a cost of $3.4 billion per year.

1228

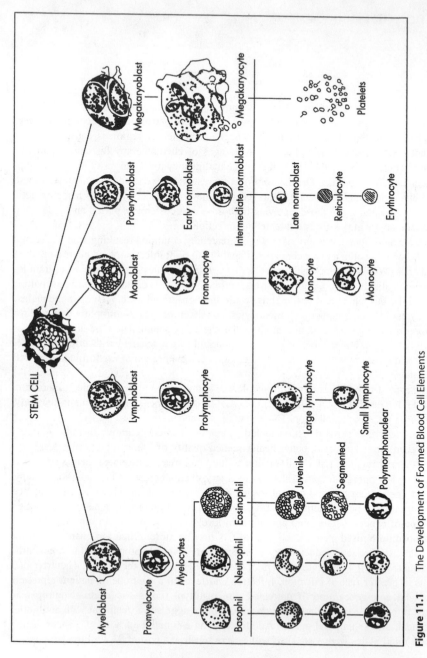

Figure 11.1 The Development of Formed Blood Cell Elements

Table 11.1   Relative Risk of Infection

Risk	Number/Neutrophils
No significant risk	1,500–2,000/mm^3
Minimal risk	1,000–1,500/mm^3
Moderate risk	500–1,000/mm^3
Severe risk	< 500/mm^3

Table 11.2   Calculation of Absolute Neutrophil Count

Patient Example	Normal Values
1. Lab results: total white blood count (WBC) = 4,000/mm^3	5,000–10,000/mm^3
neutrophils = 40	50–70%
lymphocytes = 50	20–40%
monocytes = 6	2–6%
eosinophils = 1	0.5–1%
bands = 2	
2. Total WBC × % (neutrophils + bands)	2,500–7,000/mm^3
4,000 × % (40 + 2) –	
4,000 × 42/100 =	
4,000 × 0.42 = 1,680/mm^3	

Gram-negative bacilli are responsible for the high incidence of life-threatening infections (*Escherichia coli, Klebsiella* spp., *Proteus* spp., and *Pseudomonas aeruginosa*). However, gram-positive organisms such as *Staphylococcus epidermis* and streptococci have increased as a result of decreasing gram-negative sepsis that is treated promptly with empiric antimicrobial therapy. Healthcare-associated infections (HAI) stem from central line–associated bloodstream infections (CLABSI), catheter-associated urinary tract infections (CAUTI), selected surgical-site infections (SSI), hospital-onset *Clostridium difficile* infections, and hospital-onset methicillin-resistant *Staphylococcus aureus* (MRSA) bacteremia.

CENTRAL LINE INFECTIONS

Central venous catheters are common in the oncology patient population. A central line is a catheter whose tip terminates in a great vessel, such as aorta, pulmonary artery, superior vena cava, inferior vena cava, brachiocephalic veins, internal jugular veins, subclavian veins, external iliac veins, and common femoral veins. The Centers for

Disease Control (CDC) *Guidelines for the Prevention of Intravascular Catheter-related Infections* (2011   http://www.cdc.gov/hicpac/pdf/guidelines/bsi-guidelines-2011.pdf) estimated 250,000 cases of central line-associated bloodstream infections (BSIs) occur in hospitals in the United States. Catheter-related bloodstream infections (CRBSI) independently increase hospital costs and length of stay, but have not been shown to independently increase mortality. While 80,000 CRBSIs occur in ICUs each year, a total of 250,000 cases of BSIs are estimated to occur annually. By several analyses, costs of these infections are substantial, both in terms of morbidity and expenditure of financial resources. To improve patient outcomes and reduce healthcare costs, there is considerable interest by healthcare providers, insurers, regulators, and patient advocates in reducing the incidence of these infections (CDC, 2011).

Yet, vascular access is necessary for patients undergoing intensive or cyclic chemotherapy. The risk of infection varies by device used, duration of placement, and extent of the patient's immunosuppression (CDC, 2011; NCCN, v.2.2015). According to NCCN, infections are categorized as entry- or exit-site infections, tunnel or port-pocket infections, septic phlebitis, or catheter-associated bloodstream infections. These infections tend to be caused by gram-positive organisms with coagulase-negative staphylococci being cultured most frequently. Catheter-associated bloodstream infections usually respond without the need for catheter removal except if the causal microorganism is yeast or nontuberculosis mycobacterium. Bloodstream infections caused by Bacillus organisms, *Candida, S. aureus, Acinetobacter, C. jeikeium, P. aeruginosa, S. maltophilia,* and vancomycin-resistant enterococci may be difficult to eradicate with antimicrobial therapy alone, making removal of the catheter imperative (NCCN, v.2.2015).

In addition to a course of antibacterial therapy, research suggests that administering antibiotics into lumens of central venous catheters, using catheters impregnated with minocycline and rifampin or silver-chlorhexadine, using vancomycin-lock solution may reduce vascular access infections. However, studies are not definitive and data are inconclusive to recommend any of these interventions. Instead, hand hygiene, maximal barrier precautions during insertion, using transparent dressings and chlorhexidine, and changing the needleless system device and end cap on a routine basis according to manufacturer guidelines can help minimize the risk of venous access device infections.

INFECTIOUS ORGANISMS

Disease-related immunosuppression is associated with defects in cell-mediated immunity (thymus-dependent lymphocytes), such as with certain lymphomas. This leads to an increased risk for bacterial infections (*Mycobacterium, Nocardia asteroides, Legionella, Salmonella*), as well as infections caused by fungi (*Cryptococcus, Histoplasma, Candida, Aspergillus*), parasites (*Pneumocystis carinii* pneumonia, *Toxoplasma gondii*), and viruses (varicella zoster, cytomegalovirus). Other malignancies may have defects in the humoral immune system (B lymphocytes), as in multiple myeloma and chronic lymphocytic leukemia (CLL). Patients with these malignancies are at risk for infection from bacteria (*Streptococcus pneumoniae, Haemophilus influenzae, Neisseria meningitidis, Klebsiella pneumoniae,* and *Staphylococcus aureus*) and certain enteroviruses. Antibiotic resistance, such as vancomycin-resistant enterococci (VRE) and methicillin-resistant *Staphylococcus aureus* (MRSA), is a concern for cancer patients.

Since 1989, U.S. hospitals report a rapid increase in the incidence of infection and colonization from vancomycin-resistant enterococci (VRE). This increase poses important problems, including (a) the lack of available antimicrobial therapy for VRE infections, since most VRE infections are resistant to drugs previously used to treat these infections (e.g., aminoglycosides and ampicillin); and (b) the possibility that vancomycin-resistant genes present in VRE can be transferred to other gram-positive microorganisms (e.g., *Staphylococcus aureus*). Recommendations regarding management of multidrug-resistant organisms are found in *Guideline for the Management of Multidrug-resistant Organisms in Healthcare Settings* (CDC, 2006), http://www.cdc.gov/hicpac/pdf/guidelines/MDROGuideline2006.pdf.

Increased risk for VRE infection and colonization is associated with previous vancomycin and/or multi-antimicrobial therapy, severe underlying disease or immunosuppression, and intra-abdominal surgery. Enterococci are found in normal gastrointestinal and female genital tracts, thus most enterococcal infections are attributed to endogenous sources. Whenever possible, empiric antimicrobial therapy should be modified based on culture and sensitivity results.

Methicillin-resistant *Staphylococcus aureus* (MRSA), a bacterial infection, is highly resistant to antibiotics. MRSA infections are grouped into types: community-acquired MRSA (CA-MRSA) and hospital- or healthcare-acquired MRSA (HA-MRSA). HA-MRSA infections occur in people who are or have recently been in a hospital or other healthcare facility. Those who have been hospitalized or had surgery within the past year are at increased risk. MRSA bacteria are responsible for a large percentage of hospital-acquired staph infections. Community-acquired MRSA (CA-MRSA) infections occur in otherwise healthy people who have not recently been in the hospital. Infections occur among athletes sharing equipment or personal items (such as towels or razors) and children in daycare facilities. Members of the military and those who get tattoos are at risk, and the number of CA-MRSA cases is on the rise.

ANTIMICROBIAL AGENTS

Antimicrobial medications kill or inhibit the growth of organisms without harming the patient. Antimicrobial agents may be bacteriostatic (inhibit growth of organisms) or bactericidal (kill microorganisms). Drug activity varies, so that at low concentrations a drug may be bacteriostatic but bactericidal in higher concentrations. Usually antimicrobial drugs target some difference between microorganism and host. Overall, antibiotics are prescribed based on patient factors—the condition of both renal and hepatic systems, drug allergies, spectrum of antibiotic activity, and site of infection.

Antimicrobial medications used to treat infections in patients with cancer are considered antibacterial, antiviral, and antifungal. These drugs target specific cellular mechanisms of the infectious agent. For example, sulfonamide antibiotics inhibit para-aminobenzoic acid, an essential requirement for nucleic acid synthesis in many bacteria but not in humans.

COMPLICATIONS

Penicillins and cephalosporins contain a β-lactam ring that disrupts the synthesis of peptidoglycan. Peptidoglycan gives shape and strength to the bacterial cell wall. Table 11.3 provides an overview of older antibacterial agents (penicillins/cephalosporins) to newer categories of antibacterials (streptogramins/oxazolidinones).

Making minor modifications to an existing class of drugs has largely developed newer antibiotics. Daptomycin is the first drug in a new structural class, cyclic lipopeptides. Its mode of action kills gram-positive bacteria rapidly by disrupting multiple

Table 11.3   Comparison of Antibiotic Categories

Antibacterial Category	Examples	Mechanism of Action, Including Differences Among or Between Categories or Unique Characteristics
Penicillins		Penicillins are derived from the fungus *Penicillium* and contain a β-lactam ring.
Natural penicillins	• penicillin V • penicillin G	The first group comprises natural penicillins, which are active against many aerobic gram-positive cocci (*S. aureus, Streptococcus*), gram-negative aerobic cocci (*N. meningitidis,* some *H. influenzae*), and some spirochetes. However, they are resistant to *Pseudomonas,* most *Enterobacter,* and to bacteria that produce the enzyme penicillinase, which inactivates the penicillin molecule.
Penicillinase-resistant penicillins	• cloxacillin • dicloxacillin • nafcillin • oxacillin	The second group contains the penicillinase-resistant penicillins. These are semisynthetic drugs that can withstand the action of the enzyme penicillinase and continue to exert their antibiotic action. They are primarily used to treat *S. aureus* and *S. epidermidis* strains that secrete penicillinase; they also have some activity against gram-negative bacteria and spirochetes.
Aminopenicillins	• amoxicillin • ampicillin • bacampicillin	The third group includes the aminopenicillins; this group has heightened activity against gram-negative bacteria as compared to the first two groups. These drugs are resistant to penicillinase-producing bacteria.
Extended-spectrum penicillins	• carbenicillin • mezlocillin • piperacillin • ticarcillin	The fourth group is composed of the extended-spectrum penicillins; drugs in this group have enhanced activity against gram-negative bacilli, both aerobic and nonaerobic.
Cephalosporins		The cephalosporins are derived from cephalosporin C (produced by a fungus) and have broad bactericidal activity. They contain a β-lactam ring and may also be referred to as β-lactam antibiotics. Bacterial resistance can develop, and a major mechanism is the development by the bacteria of an enzyme, β-lactamase, which inactivates the cephalosporin antibiotic by destroying the β-lactam ring.

Antibacterial Category	Examples	Mechanism of Action, Including Differences Among or Between Categories or Unique Characteristics
First generation	• cefadroxil • cephalothin • cefazolin • cephalexin • cephapirin • cephradine	First-generation cephalosporins are active against gram-positive cocci (*Staphylococcus* and *Streptococcus*) and have only limited activity against gram-negative bacteria (e.g., *E. coli*); they have no activity against enterococci.
Second generation	• cefaclor • cefamandole • cefmetazole • cefonicid • ceforanide • cefotetan • cefoxitin • cefprozil • cefuroxime • cefuroxime axetil	Second-generation cephalosporins are active against the same organisms as the first-generation drugs but are slightly more active against gram-negative bacteria. In addition, they are active against *H. influenzae*.
Third generation	• cefdinir • cefixime • cefoperazone • cefotaxime • cefpodoxime • ceftazidime • ceftibuten • ceftizoxime • ceftriaxone • loracarbef	Third-generation cephalosporins are less active against gram-positive organisms but have broader activity against gram-negative organisms than either first- or second-generation drugs.
Fourth generation	• cefepime • ceftaroline • fosamil	Fourth-generation cephalosporins are projected to have many attributes, including: • Extended spectrum of activity for gram-negative and gram-positive organisms (different from third-generation cephalosporins) • Minimal β-lactamase activity due to rapid periplasmic penetration and high penicillin-binding protein (PBP) access • Spectrum of activity to include gram-negative organisms with multiple drug resistance patterns (*Enterobacter* and *Klebsiella*)
Streptogramins	• quinupristin/ dalfopristin	This new class of antibiotics, the streptogramin group, is a separate family of antimicrobials. Synercid is an intravenous combination of two semisynthetic,

(continued)

COMPLICATIONS

Table 11.3　*(Continued)*

Antibacterial Category	Examples	Mechanism of Action, Including Differences Among or Between Categories or Unique Characteristics
		water-soluble derivatives of naturally occurring pristinamycin. The two distinct compounds are quinupristin and dalfopristin, derived from pristinamycin I and pristinamycin II. These two compounds work synergistically to kill susceptible bacteria through a two-pronged attack on protein synthesis in bacterial cells. Each component of the drug binds irreversibly to different sites on the bacterial cell's ribosomal subunit to form a stable quinupristin-ribosome—dalfopristin complex, which disables the cell's ability to make cellular protein. Without the ability to manufacture new proteins, the bacterial cell dies.
Oxazolidinones	• linezolid	Inhibits initiation of protein synthesis by binding to a site on bacterial 23S ribosomal RNA of the 50S subunit. This mechanism of inhibiting protein synthesis is not shared by other antibacterials. Cross-resistance is unlikely.
Macrolides	• azithromycin • clarithromycin • erythromycin • fidaxomicin	Binds to 50S ribosomal subunit, resulting in inhibition of protein synthesis. In some cases, the drug metabolite is twice as active as the parent compound.
Lipopeptides	• daptomycin	Derived from the fermentation of *Streptomyces roseosporus*. The mechanism of action is not fully understood. Binds to bacterial membranes and causes a rapid depolarization of membrane potential. This loss of membrane potential leads to inhibition of protein, DNA, and RNA synthesis resulting in bacterial cell death.
Ketolide	• telithromycin	Similar to that of macrolides and is related to the 50S-ribosomal subunit binding with inhibition of bacterial protein synthesis. Telithromycin appears to have greater affinity for the ribosomal binding site than macrolides. It concentrates in phagocytes, where it exhibits activity against intracellular respiratory pathogens.

aspects of bacterial membrane function. Telithromycin, a first-in-class antibiotic group called ketolides, is structurally related to macrolide antibiotics; the newest drug of the macrolide antibiotic class is fidaxomicin, which is specifically designed to offer optimal spectrum activity for first-line treatment of upper- and lower-respiratory tract infections. Glycylcyclines are structurally similar to tetracyclines and tigecycline is the first agent in this class to be FDA-approved for treatment of MRSA. There are a growing number of MRSA-resistant agents, including colistimethate.

Another class of antimicrobial agents, echinocandins or glucan synthesis inhibitors, is an option available for treating opportunistic fungal infections. Caspofungin inhibits the synthesis of a key component of the fungal cell wall. Caspofungin demonstrates fungicidal activity against *Candida* species; it is indicated for treatment of invasive *Aspergillus* in patients who are refractory to, or intolerant of, other therapies. Ideal candidates for this drug are patients with amphotericin B–induced nephrotoxicity. Caspofungin appears to be well-tolerated. Another drug, Micafungin, inhibits synthesis of 1,3-b-D-glucan, an essential component of fungal cell walls. Micafungin is indicated for treatment of patients with esophageal candidiasis and as prophylaxis for *Candida* infections in patients undergoing hematopoietic stem cell transplantation.

The latest echinocandin, anidulafungin, was FDA-approved for treatment of candidemia and esophageal candidiasis. All three echinocandins are well-tolerated and have some use in febrile neutropenia. There are anecdotal reports regarding use of these agents to treat less common fungal infections and limited use as a component of antifungal therapy. Anti-infective agents have limited benefits if there are any drug interactions or impaired renal and hepatic function. The echinocandins are an important addition to the antifungal armentarium for treating fungal infections in immunocompromised patients.

Posaconazole, a broad-spectrum triazole, is used for treatment and prevention of invasive fungal infections. It is a lipophilic antifungal triazole similar to other members in this class and effective against *Candida* species, *Cryptococcus neoformans, Aspergillus* species, *Fusarium* species, zygomycetes, and endemic fungi. The compound is available as an oral suspension and appears to be well-tolerated, even in long-term courses of treatment. The latest options in the anti-infective area are combinations of drugs, such as ceftazidime/avibactam (Avycaz) and ceftolozane/tazobactam (Zerbaxa). These drugs use a two-pronged approach for treating infection. Ceftazidime/avibactam combines a next-generation, non-beta-lactam beta-lactamase inhibitor and third-generation, antipseudomonal cephalosporin antibiotic. Ceftolozane/tazobactam is a combination of a cephalosporin-class antibacterial and a beta-lactamase inhibitor.

On the horizon are some agents that are newly discovered and now in development as anti-infective agents, such as platensimycin, a previously unknown class of antibiotics produced by *Streptomyces platensis*. It remains to be seen whether this new class of antibiotics will be effective against microorganisms in humans. New research suggests that anti-microbial peptides isolated from diverse organisms such as amphibians, humans, plants, arthropods (insects and arachnids), and even from other bacteria may be useful for patients with cancer. Several antimicrobial peptides have been isolated from scorpion venoms and/or hemolymphs. One such scorpion venom is Vejovine, a unique and sufficiently different antimicrobial peptide that is showing promise as a new category of antimicrobial agent. Vejovine shows a broad spectrum of activity against representative clones of bacterial clinical isolates in patients from different hospitals in Mexico. Additional experiments are aimed at detecting whether a higher therapeutic index can be obtained; eventually Vejovine could be used for local or topical treatment of infections caused by multidrug-resistant bacteria. Finally, polyketides are a large family of structurally diverse, natural products with a broad range of biologic activities, including antibiotic and pharmacologic properties. Many important antibiotics are polyketides, such as tetracyclines, erythromycin, adriamycin, monensin, rifamycin, and avermectins.

Work is beginning on a general strategy for biosynthesis of polyketides through cloning gene clusters. This fundamentally new strategy for treating infectious disease is being

COMPLICATIONS

bioengineered in the laboratory. One such proposed treatment would modulate the host's immune responses to enhance clearance of infectious agents. Antimicrobial host defense peptides are being investigated for their potential as a new class of antimicrobial drug (Easton et al., 2009). This work has shown promise in the laboratory and, if actualized, modulation of innate immunity by synthetic variants of host defense peptides might be protective without direct antimicrobial action.

Bacteriophage therapy to treat bacterial infections offers a new approach built on top of an old idea. There is growing interest in bacteriophages as treatment for infection, especially in light of growing antibiotic resistance (Kutateladze & Adamia, 2010; Lu & Koeris, 2011). This treatment is underutilized in the United States, but is growing in popularity in other parts of the world. However, advances in biotechnology, bacterial diagnostics, macromolecular delivery, and synthetic biology are providing opportunities to overcome clinical development issues. Some of these issues include regulation, limited host range, bacterial resistance to phages, manufacturing challenges, side effects of bacterial lysis, and delivery mechanisms.

EVIDENCE-BASED GUIDELINES

Infections in patients with cancer are a topic of interest beyond the treatment of infections. Preventing infection or treating early is a key factor in minimizing sequelae for neutropenic cancer patients. There are an ever-expanding number of prevention and treatment evidence-based guidelines. The National Comprehensive Cancer Network (NCCN), the Oncology Nursing Society (ONS) Putting Evidence into Practice (PEP), the American Society of Clinical Oncologists (ASCO), the Multinational Association for Supportive Care in Cancer (MASCC), and the Centers for Disease Control (CDC) report and/or update evidence-based guidelines regularly.

The NCCN Prevention and Treatment of Cancer-related Infections, Version 2.2015, offers comprehensive evidence-based guidelines to prevent and treat cancer-related infections found in the cancer population. The guidelines delineate prevention, diagnosis, and treatment of major common and opportunistic infections, highlighting the risk of infection for cancer patients, presenting fever and neutropenia risk, and recommending antimicrobial prophylaxis. The NCCN Guidelines can be found at http://www.nccn.org.

The ONS PEP Guidelines focus on nursing-sensitive patient outcomes (NSPOs), which are outcomes that are attained through or are significantly impacted by nursing interventions. The interventions must be within the scope of nursing practice and integral to the processes of nursing care. The specific ONS PEP Guidelines are available at http://www.ons.pep.org. These NSPOs validate the value and effectiveness of nursing practice and help nurses demonstrate their contribution to quality patient care. ASCO guidelines focus on how and when to prevent and treat infection in patients receiving outpatient chemotherapy. The guidelines focus on febrile neutropenia and provide advice on identifying patients who have both neutropenia and fever but are at low risk for complications and can be treated at home. ASCO Guidelines can be found at http://www.asco.org/sites/www.asco.org/files/fn_adult_guideline.pdf.

Interestingly, the problem of infections in cancer patients is an international issue as well. MASCC guidelines focus on use of granulocyte-colony stimulating factors and white blood cell growth factors in reducing febrile neutropenia. MASCC validated a risk assessment tool for febrile neutropenia. The Immunocompromised Host Society and MASCC produced a set of guidelines on methodology for clinical trials involving patients with febrile neutropenia. MASCC Guidelines can be found in detail at http://www.mascc.org.

Finally, the CDC has an ongoing initiative related to healthcare-associated infections (HAIs). Several guidelines were developed concerning various aspects of HAIs, including evidence-based guidelines, infection rates, and economic impact of HAIs to the healthcare system. The CDC guidelines can be found at http://www.cdc.gov/HAI. As more and more antibiotic, antibacterial, antiviral, and antifungal agents are discovered, the cost for these drugs continues to rise. It is through the use of the guidelines mentioned above that we can provide evidence-based care to cancer patients while attempting to maintain the costs of health care in today's environment.

References

Agency for Healthcare Research and Quality, Research Activities, 2008; 339 (November) 1. Available at http://www.ahrq.gov/. Accessed June 2012.

American Thoracic Society. Guidelines for the Management of Adults with Hospital acquired, Ventilatory associated and Health Care-associated Pneumonia. *Am J Respiratory Crit Care* 2005; 171 388–416.

Ampicillin Sodium/Sulbactam Sodium. Available at http://hcunviweb05/mdxcgi/quiklocn.cxe? CTL–E:/Mdx/mdxcgi/MEGAT.SYS&SET=1C573 Accessed June 2005.

Avycaz [package insert]. Available at http://pi.actavis.com/data_stream.asp?product_group=1957&p= pi&language=E. Accessed May 2015.

Avycaz. Available at http://www.avycaz.com. Accessed May 2015.

Avycaz. Available at http://www.drugs.com/cdi/avycaz.html. Accessed May 2015.

Avycaz. Available at http://www.drugs.com/history/avycaz.html. Accessed May 2015.

Baden LR, Bensinger W, Angarone M, Casper C et al. (2013). NCCN Prevention and Treatment of Cancer-related Infections v.1.2013. http://www.nccn.org/professionals/physician_gls/pdf/infections.pdf. Accessed June 2013.

Brungs SM, Render ML. Using Evidence-based Practice to Reduce Central Line Infections. *Clin J Oncol Nurs* 2006; 10(6) 723–725.

Centers for Disease Control and Prevention. Basic Infection Control and Prevention Plan Outpatient Oncology Settings. (November 2011). Available at http://www.cdc.gov/HAI/settings/outpatient/basic-infection-control-prevention-plan-2011/.

Centers for Disease Control and Prevention. Guidelines for Preventing Opportunistic Infections Among Hematopoietic Stem Cell Transplant Recipients: Recommendations of CDC, the Infection Disease Society of America, and the American Society of Blood and Marrow Transplant. *Morbidity Mortality Weekly Rep* 2000; 49 (RR-10) 1–126.

Centers for Disease Control and Prevention. Guidelines for the Prevention of Intravascular Catheter-related Infections. Available at http://www.cdc.gov/hicpac/pdf/guidelines/bsi-guidelines-2011.pdf.

COMPLICATIONS

Centers for Disease Control and Prevention. Guide to Infection Prevention in Outpatient Settings: Minimum Expectations for Safe Care (May 2011). Available at http://www.cdc.gov/HAI/settings/outpatient/outpatient-care-guidelines.html.

Centers for Disease Control and Prevention. Management of Multi-drug Resistant Organisms in Healthcare Settings. Available at http://www.cdc.gov/hicpac/pdf/guidelines/MDROGuideline 2006.pdf.

Center Watch. Drug Information: Telavancin. Available at http://www.centerwatch.com/drug-information/fda-approvals/drug-details.aspx?DrugID=1055. Accessed November 1, 2010.

Cresemba [package insert]. Available at http://www.astellas.us/docs/cresemba.pdf. Accessed May 2015.

Cresemba New FDA Drug Approval. Center Watch. Available at http://www.centerwatch.com/drug-information/fda-approved-drugs. Accessed May 2015.

Cresemba. Available at http://www.drugs.com/cresemba.html. Accessed May 2015.

Cooper MA, Shales D. Fix the antibiotics pipeline. *Nature* 2011; 472 7.

Courtney R, Pai S, Laughlin M, Lim J, Batra V. Pharmacokinetics, Safety, and Tolerability of Oral Posaconazole Administered in Single and Multiple Doses in Healthy Adults. *Antimicrobial Agents Chemotherapy* 2003; 47(9) 2788–2795.

Crawford, J, Dale, DC, Kuderer, NM, et al. Risk and Timing of Neutropenic Events in Adult Cancer Patients Receiving Chemotherapy: The Results of a Prospective Nationwide Study of Oncology Practice. *J Natl Compr Canc Netw* 2008; 6: 109–118.

Cubicin [product information]. *Cubist Pharmaceutical Inc* September 2003.

Dalvance [package insert]. Available at http://content.stockpr.com/duratatherapeutics/files/docs/Dalvance+APPROVED+USPI.PDF. Accessed May 2015.

Dalvance new FDA drug approval. Center Watch. Available at http://www.centerwatch.com/drug-information/fda-approved-drugs. Accessed May 2015.

Dalvance. Available at http://www.drugs.com/sfx/dalvance-side-effects.html. Accessed May 2015.

Declomycin. Available at http://www.rxmed.com/b.main/b2.pharmaceutical/b2.1monographs/CPS-Monographs. Accessed June 2004.

Declomycin [product information]. *Lederle Pharmaceutical Division, American Cynamid Co* Pearl River, NY: 2003.

Dificid [product information]. Optimer Pharmaceuticals, Inc., San Diego, CA: 2011.

Doripenem Monograph. *National PBM Drug Monograph, January 2008. VHA Pharmacy Benefits Management Services and the Medical Advisory Panel.* Available at http://www.pbm.va.gov. Accessed June 2010.

Drugs.com. Drug Information Online. *Colistimethate Injection.* Available at http://www.drugs.com/MTM/colistimethate.html. Accessed June 2010.

Drugs.com. Drug Information Online. *Daptomycin* Available at http://www.drugs.com/MTM/daptomycin.html. Accessed June 2004.

Drugs.com. Drug Information Online. *Doripenem* Available at http://www.drugs.com/MTM/doripenem.html. Accessed June 2010.

Drugs.com. Drug Information Online. *Doripenem* Available at http://www.drugs.com/MTM/doripenem.html. Accessed June 2011.

Drugs.com. Drug Information Online. *Norfloxacin* Available at http://www.drugs.com/MTM/norfloxacin.html. Accessed June 2010.

Drugs.com. Drug Information Online. *Telavancin* Available at http://www.drugs.com/MTM/telavancin.html. Accessed June 2010.

Easton DM, Nijnik A, Mayer ML, Hancock REW. Potential of immunomodulatory host defense peptides as novel anti-infectives. *Trends Biotechnol.* 2009; 27(10) 582–590.

Flowers CR, Seidenfeld J, Bow EJ, Karten C, Gleason C, Hawley DK, Kuderer NM, Langston AA, Marr KA, Rolston KVI, & Ramsey SD. (2013). Antimicrobial prophylaxis and outpatient management of fever and neutropenia in adults treated for malignancy: American Society of Clinical Oncology Clinical Practice Guidelines. *J Clin Oncol*, 31 (6 February 20), 794–810.

Freifeld AG, Bow EJ, Sepkowitz KA, Boeckh MJ, Ito JI, Mullen CA, Raad II, Rolston KV, Young JH, & Wingard JR. Clinical practice guideline for the use of antimicrobial agents in neutropenic patients with cancer: 2010 update by the Infectious Diseases Society of America. *Cln Infect Dis* 2011; 52: e56-e93 or 427–431.

Gemifloxacin Mesylate [package insert]. http://hcunviweb05/mdxcgi/quiklocn.exe?CTL=E:/Mdx/mdxcgi/ MEGAT.SYS&SET=1C573. June 2005.

Goh KP. Management of Hyponatremia. *AM Fam Physician* 2004; 69(10) 2387–2394.

Hernandez-Aponte C, Silva-Sanchez J, Quintero-Hernandcz V, Rodriguez-Romera A, Balderas C, Possani LD & Gurrola GB. (2011). Vejovine, a new antibiotic from the scorpion venom of Vaejovis mexicanus. *Toxicon* 57 (2011) 84–92.

Irwin M, Erb C, Williams C, Wilson BJ, & Zitella LJ. (2013). Putting Evidence into Practice (PEP): Improving Oncology Patient Outcomes. Prevention of Infection. Pittsburgh, PA: Oncology Nursing Society.

Ketek [product information]. *Aventis Pharmaceutical Inc* March 2004.

Kutateladze M, Adamia R. Bacteriophages as potential new therapeutics to replace or supplement antibiotics. *Trends Biotechnol.* 2010; 28(12) 591–595.

Lu TK, Koeris MS. The next generation of bacteriophage therapy. *Curr Opin Microbiol.* 2011; 14 524–531.

Malpiedi PJ, Peterson KD, Soe M, Edwards JE, Scott RD, Wise ME, Baggs J, Yi SH, Dudeck MA, Arnold KE, Weiner LM, Rebmann CA, Srinivasan A, Fridkin SK & McDonald LC. (2013). 2011 National and State Healthcare-Associated Infection Standardized Infection Ratio Report. Published February 22, 2013. Available at http://www.cdc.gov/hai/national-annual-sir/index.html.

Medline. *Drug Information: Daptomycin* Available at http://www.nlm.nih.gov/medline. Accessed June 2004.

Medline Plus. *Drug Information: Colistimethate Injection* Available at http://www.nlm.nih.gov/medlineplus/print/druginfo/meds/a682860.html. Accessed June 2010.

Medline Plus. *Drug Information: Doripenem* Available at http://www.nlm.nih.gov/medlineplus/print/druginfo/meds/a608015.html. Accessed June 2010.

Medline Plus. *Drug Information: Norfloxacin* Available at http://www.nlm.nih.gov/medlineplus/print/druginfo/meds/a687006.html. Accessed June 2010.

Meropenem [package insert]. http://hcunviweb05/mdxcgi/quiklocn.exe?CTL=E:/Mdx/mdxcgi/MEGAT.SYS&SET=1C573. Accessed June 2005.

Mycamine [package insert]. Osaka Japan: Fujisawa Pharmaceutical Company LTD 2005.

National Comprehenisve Cancer Network. Prevention and Treatment of Cancer-related Infections. http://www.nccn.org/professionals/physician_gls/pdf/infections.pdf. Accessed May 2015.

Norfloxacin [product information]. Merck & Co. Inc. September 2008.

Orbactiv [package insert]. Available at http://www.themedicinescompany.com/app/webroot/img/orbactiv-prescribing-information.pdf. Accessed May 2015.

Orbactiv. Available at http://www.drugs.com/mtm/orbactiv.html. Accessed May 2015.

Orbactiv. Available at http://www.drugs.com/pro/orbactiv.html. Accessed May 2015.

Orbactiv. Available at http://www.drugs.com/sfx/orbactiv-side-effects.html. Accessed May 2015.

Orbactiv. Available at http://www.drugs.com/cdi/orbactiv.html. Accessed May 2015.

Raad II, Graybill JR, Bustamante AB., et al. Safety of Long-Term Oral Posaconazole Use in the Treatment of Refractory Invasive Fungal Infections. *Clin Infect Dis* 2006; 42(15 June) 1726–1734.

Rifaximin [package insert]. http://hcunviweb05/mdxcgi/quiklocn.exe?CTL=E:/Mdx/mdxcgi/MEGAT.SYS&SET=1C573. June 2005.

COMPLICATIONS

Scott RD. (2009). The Direct Medical Cost of Healthcare-Associated Infections in U.S. Hospitals and the Benefits of Prevention. Atlanta, GA: Center for Disease Control.

Sivextro [package insert]. Available at http://sivextro.com/pdf/sivextro-prescribing-info.pdf. Accessed May 2015.

Spellberg, B. (2012). New antibiotic development: Barriers and opportunities in 2012 in confronting today's crisis in antibiotic development. *The Alliance for the Prudent Use of Antibiotics (APUA) Newsletter,* 30(1) May 2012, pp. 8–10.

TEFLARO® (ceftaroline fosamil) [package insert]. Facta Farmaceutici S.p.A. Nucleo Industriale S. 64020 Teramo, Italy; 2011. Teflaro is a trademark of Forest Laboratories, Inc. Forest Pharmaceuticals, Inc.; Subsidiary of Forest Laboratories, Inc.; St. Louis, MO 63045, USA.

Telithromycin. Available at http://www.centerwatch.com/patient/drugs/dru853.html. Accessed June 2004.

Telithromycin. Thompson Center Watch. *Clinical Trials Listing Service. Drugs approved by the FDA* Available at http://www.mcromedex.com/products/updates/drugdex_updates/de/tilithromycinfull.html. Accessed June 2004.

The United States Pharmacopeial Convention, Inc.; 1998.

Torres HA, Hachem RY, Chemaly RF. et al. Posaconazole: A broad spectrum triazole antifungal. *Lancet Infect Di* 2005; 5(12) 775–785.

Tygacil [package insert]. Philadelphia, PA: Wyeth Pharmaceuticals, Inc.; 2005.

United States Pharmacopeia Drug Information for Health Care Professionals. Rockville, MD: 18th ed.

Valganciclovir [package insert]. San Francisco, CA: Genetech USA, Inc. Available at http://www.gene.com/gene/products/information/valcyte/pdf/pi.pdf. Accessed August 2010.

Vasquez JA, Sobel JD. Anidulafungin: A Novel Echinocandin. *Clin Infect Dis* 2006; 43 215–222.

VHA Pharmacy Benefits Management Strategic Healthcare Group and Medical Advisor Panel. *Daptomycin.*

Warner-Lambert Co. Omnicef [package insert]. Morris Plains, NJ: Parke-Davis 1998.

Williams, MD, Braun, LA, Cooper, LM, et al. Hospitalized Cancer Patients with Severe Sepsis: Analysis of Incidence, Mortality, and Associated Costs of Care. Critical Care 2004; 8: R291-R298 (DOI 10.1186/cc2893). http://ccforum.com/content/8/5/R291. Accessed June 2014.

Zerbaxa [package insert]. Available at http://www.zerbaxa.com/pdf/PrescribingInformation.pdf. Accessed May 2015.

Zerbaxa. Available at http://www.drugs.com/mtm/zerbaxa.html. Accessed May 2015.

Zerbaxa. Available at http://www.drugs.com/pro/zerbaxa.html. Accessed May 2015.

Zerbaxa. Available at http://www.drugs.com/sfx/zerbaxa-side-effects.html. Accessed May 2015.

ANTIBIOTICS

Drug: amikacin sulfate (Amikin)

Class: Aminoglycoside antibacterial antibiotic.

Mechanism of Action: Synthetic antibiotic derived from kanamycin; bactericidal, most probably by inhibition of protein synthesis. Active against aerobic microorganisms: many sensitive gram-negative organisms (including *Acinetobacter, Citrobacter, Enterobacter,*

E. coli, Klebsiella, Proteus, Pseudomonas, Salmonella, Serratia, and *Shigella*), and some sensitive gram-positive organisms (*S. aureus* and *S. epidermidis*). Over time bacterial resistance may develop, either naturally or acquired.

Metabolism: Well-absorbed following parenteral administration, but variability in absorption after IM injection (peak serum level 0.5–2 hours, duration 8–12 hours). Widely distributed into body fluids. Minimally protein-bound. Readily crosses placenta and into breastmilk. Drug excreted unchanged in the urine.

Indication: For the treatment of infections caused by susceptible strains of microorganisms, especially gram-negative bacteria.

Dosage/Range:
- 15 mg/kg/day given in 8-hour or 12-hour doses IV or IM.
- Desired peak serum concentration is 15–30 mg/mL, and trough serum concentration is 5–10 mg/mL.

Drug Preparation:
- Store injectable at < 40°C (104°F).
- Potency not affected by pale yellow color that may develop.
- Stable for 24 hours at concentrations of 0.25 and 5 mg/mL in 0.9% sodium chloride, 5% dextrose.

Drug Administration:
- IV: in 100–200 mL IV fluid (e.g., 0.9% sodium chloride or 5% dextrose injection), infused over 30–60 minutes.

Drug Interactions:
- Increased risk of toxicity with other ototoxic drugs: acyclovir, other aminoglycosides, amphotericin B, bacitracin, cephalosporins, colistin, cisplatin, ethacrynic acid, furosemide, vancomycin.
- Potentiation of neuromuscular blockade when given concurrently with general anesthetics (succinylcholine, tubocurarine)—use cautiously; observe for signs/symptoms of respiratory depression.
- Synergism with extended-spectrum penicillins but must be administered separately.

Lab Effects/Interference:
- Serum ALT, serum alk phos, serum AST, serum bili, and serum LDH values all may be increased.
- BUN and serum creatinine values may be increased.
- Serum Ca+, serum Mg+, serum K+, and serum Na+ concentrations may be decreased.

Special Considerations:
- Used as first-line treatment in short-term treatment of serious gram-negative infections (e.g., septicemia, respiratory tract infections).
- Use against gram-positive organisms only as second-line treatment.
- Use in pregnancy only if infection is life-threatening and no safer drug exists; drug crosses placenta and may cause fetal toxicity.

Potential Toxicities/Side Effects and the Nursing Process

I.   ALTERATIONS IN SENSORY/PERCEPTUAL PATTERNS
   related to OTOTOXICITY

Defining Characteristics: Damage to eighth cranial nerve (auditory) may result in dizziness, nystagmus, vertigo, ataxia (vestibular damage), and less commonly, tinnitus, roaring sound in ears, and impaired hearing (auditory damage). Hearing loss usually begins with high-frequency loss, followed by clinical hearing loss, then permanent hearing loss if damage continues. Increased risk in elderly or renally impaired patients.

Nursing Implications: Assess baseline hearing (ability to hear spoken voice) and continue during therapy. Teach patient potential side effects, and instruct patient to report any hearing/perceptual problems (e.g., tinnitus, vertigo, decreased hearing). Discuss drug discontinuance and audiogram with physician to confirm hearing dysfunction if symptoms arise. Assess for increased risk if given concurrently with other ototoxic medications (e.g., cisplatin, furosemide).

II.   ALTERATION IN URINARY ELIMINATION related to NEPHROTOXICITY

Defining Characteristics: Renal damage characterized by tubular necrosis with increased serum BUN, creatinine; decreased urine creatinine clearance and specific gravity; proteinuria and casts in urine. Azotemia usually not associated with oliguria. Rarely, electrolyte wasting with hypomagnesemia, hypocalcemia, and hypokalemia may occur. Renal dysfunction usually reversible after drug discontinuance. Increased risk in elderly and in patients with preexisting renal dysfunction. Risk is low in well-hydrated patients with normal renal function when normal doses given.

Nursing Implications: Assess baseline renal function and electrolytes, and monitor periodically during therapy. Discuss any abnormalities with physician, as drug should be dose-reduced or discontinued if renal dysfunction develops. Assess baseline total body fluid balance, weight, and monitor periodically during antibiotic therapy. Monitor hydration status to keep patient well hydrated. Assess drug peak and trough levels as ordered so that drug dosage is correctly titrated. Increased risk of toxicity if peak serum concentration > 30–35 mg/mL. Draw blood for peak drug concentration 30 minutes after completion of 30-minute infusion or at the end of a 60-minute infusion; draw trough immediately before next dose.

III.   ALTERATIONS IN SENSORY/PERCEPTUAL PATTERNS related to
   CNS EFFECTS, NEUROMUSCULAR BLOCKADE

Defining Characteristics: Headache, tremor, lethargy may occur. Peripheral neuropathy or encephalopathy (numbness, skin-tingling, muscle-twitching) may occur rarely. Neuromuscular blockade is dose related, self-limiting, and uncommon: risk is greater with topical application or when drug is administered to patient with neuromuscular disease (myasthenia gravis) or hypocalcemia.

Nursing Implications: Assess baseline neurologic status. Assess coexisting risk factors, neuroblockade medications. Teach patient about side effects, and instruct to report headache, tremor, and lethargy. Observe for respiratory depression. If signs/symptoms arise, discuss drug discontinuance with physician.

IV. POTENTIAL FOR INJURY related to HYPERSENSITIVITY

Defining Characteristics: Rash, urticaria, pruritus, fever, and eosinophilia have occurred rarely. CROSS-SENSITIVITY between AMINOGLYCOSIDES exists.

Nursing Implications: Assess for drug allergies to any aminoglycoside—amikacin, gentamicin, kanamycin, neomycin, netilmicin, streptomycin, tobramycin—prior to drug administration. Instruct patient to report any allergic reactions. Assess for signs/symptoms of allergic reaction after drug dose.

V. ALTERATION IN NUTRITION, LESS THAN BODY REQUIREMENTS, related to GI SIDE EFFECTS

Defining Characteristics: Nausea, vomiting, anorexia have occurred rarely. Also, transient hepatomegaly with elevated LFTs—AST, ALT, LDH, alk phos—has occurred.

Nursing Implications: Assess baseline nutritional status, preexisting nausea/vomiting, anorexia. Assess baseline LFTs and monitor periodically during treatment. Instruct patient to report side effects. Provide symptomatic interventions if side effects occur; discuss with physician use of alternative drug(s).

VI. POTENTIAL FOR FATIGUE, INFECTION, AND BLEEDING related to BONE MARROW INJURY

Defining Characteristics: Anemia, leukopenia, granulocytopenia, and thrombocytopenia may occur. Also, patients receiving antibiotics are at risk for overgrowth of nonsusceptible microorganisms, such as fungi (superinfection). Rare.

Nursing Implications: Assess baseline CBC, differential, and monitor periodically during treatment. Instruct patient to report signs/symptoms of fatigue, infection, or bleeding immediately. Assess for signs/symptoms of superinfection. Discuss any adverse effects with physician.

COMPLICATIONS

Drug: amoxicillin (Amoxil, Polymox, Trimox, Wymox; amoxicillin plus potassium clavulanate is Augmentin)

Class: Penicillin (aminopenicillin antibiotic); β-lactam.

Mechanism of Action: Semisynthetic antibiotic prepared from fungus *Penicillium*. Contains β-lactam ring and is bactericidal by inhibiting cell wall synthesis. Aminopenicillins have increased activity against gram-negative bacilli (*H. influenzae, E. coli*), as well as some activity against gram-positive bacilli (*Streptococci* and *Staphylococci*).

Metabolism: Well-absorbed from GI tract; rate of absorption slowed by food, but total amount of drug absorbed remains unchanged. Widely distributed in body tissues and fluids. Crosses placenta and is found in breastmilk. Excreted in urine and bile.

Indication: For the treatment of infections of upper and lower respiratory tract, genito-urinary (GU) tract, and skin caused by sensitive organisms. Infections caused by bacteria, such as tonsillitis, bronchitis, pneumonia, and gonorrhea, in ear, nose, throat, skin, or urinary tract. Sometimes used in combination with clarithromycin (Biaxin) to treat stomach ulcers caused by *Helicobacter pylori*.

Dosage/Range:
Adult:
- 125–500 mg PO q 8 h 48–72 hours after infection eradicated; for uncomplicated urinary tract infection, may use single dose of 3 g PO.
- Drug dose should be reduced if severe renal failure occurs.
- Augmentin dose: mild to moderate infection: 500 mg PO bid; severe infection: 875 mg PO bid.

Drug Preparation:
- Store capsules in tight container at 15–30°C (59–86°F).
- Administer on empty stomach.

Drug Interactions:
- Aminoglycosides: synergism.
- Aminoglycosides (e.g., gentamicin): incompatible when mixed together; administer at separate sites at different times. Penicillinase-resistant penicillins can inactivate aminoglycoside serum samples from patients receiving both drugs.
- Rifampin: possible antagonism, only at high doses of penicillin.
- Probenecid: increased serum level of penicillin; may be coadministered to exert this effect.
- Allopurinol: increased incidence of rash; avoid concurrent administration if possible.
- Clavulanic acid (β-lactamase inhibitor): synergistic bactericidal effect. Amoxicillin plus potassium clavulanate = Augmentin.

Lab Effects/Interference:
Major clinical significance:
- Urine glucose: high urinary concentrations of a penicillin may produce false-positive or falsely elevated test results with copper-reduction tests (Benedict's, Clinitest, or Fehling's); glucose enzymatic tests (Clinistix or Testape) are not affected.

Clinical significance:
- Coombs' tests: false-positive result may occur during therapy with any penicillin.
- ALT, alk phos, AST, serum bili, and serum LDH values may be increased.
- Estradiol, total-conjugated estriol, estriol-glucuronide, or conjugated estrone concentrations may be transiently decreased in pregnant women following administration of amoxicillin.
- WBC: leukopenia or neutropenia is associated with the use of all penicillins; the effect is more likely to occur with prolonged and severe hepatic function impairment.

Special Considerations:
* Contraindicated in patients with prior hypersensitivity to penicillins. Use with caution in patients sensitive to other β-lactams (e.g., cephalosporins) since partial cross-allergenicity exists.
* Obtain ordered specimen and send for culture and sensitivity prior to first antibiotic dose.
* Consider alternative antibiotic therapy if eosinophilia, drug fever or rash, arthralgia, hematuria, or unexplained rise in BUN and serum creatinine occur.
* Monitor electrolytes and renal, hepatic, and hematologic laboratory parameters during extended treatment periods.
* Use with caution in pregnancy or with nursing women.
* Amoxicillin rash may occur that is distinct from drug-allergic rash; increased risk if concurrent use of allopurinol.
* Lower incidence of diarrhea as a GI side effect than ampicillin.
* May cause false-positive with Clinitest glucose testing.

Potential Toxicities/Side Effects and the Nursing Process

I. POTENTIAL FOR INJURY related to HYPERSENSITIVITY REACTION

Defining Characteristics: Urticaria, pruritus, rash (maculopapular or erythematous), fever and chills, eosinophilia, myalgia, edema, erythema, angioedema, Stevens-Johnson syndrome, and exfoliative skin reactions occur in 5% of patients. Increased risk in individuals allergic to cephalosporin antibiotics A nonimmunologic rash may occur 3–14 days after drug started, characterized as a generalized erythematous/maculopapular rash, and worse over pressure areas of elbows and knees. Rash usually subsides in 6–14 days, even if drug is continued. If drug is stopped, resolves in 1–7 days.

Nursing Implications: Assess allergy to cephalosporin antibiotics and penicillin: if patient states "yes," determine actual response (e.g., "swollen lips = angioedema"). If angioedema, patient SHOULD NOT receive drug. Discuss other patient responses with physician to determine whether drug should be given. Assess baseline skin condition, including integrity and allergy history to drugs. Instruct patient to report rash, itching, other skin changes. Teach patient skin care and symptomatic measures as appropriate. If skin rash develops, discuss drug discontinuance with physician. If rash progresses, drug should be discontinued, as fatal Stevens-Johnson syndrome may develop. Be prepared to treat severe acute hypersensitivity reactions with airway management, oxygen, epinephrine, corticosteroids, and antihistamines as ordered.

II. ALTERATION IN NUTRITION, LESS THAN BODY REQUIREMENTS, related to GI SIDE EFFECTS

Defining Characteristics: Nausea, vomiting, diarrhea, and anorexia may occur; rarely, pseudomembranous colitis caused by *Clostridium difficile* resistant to the antibiotic occurs. Rarely, transient increases in LFTs—AST, ALT, alk phos, bili—may occur.

Nursing Implications: Assess baseline nutritional status. Instruct patient to report GI disturbances. Administer and instruct patient to self-administer antiemetics as needed and as ordered. Teach patient importance of nutritious diet and suggest small, frequent, high-calorie, high-protein meals as appropriate. Assess baseline LFTs and monitor periodically during treatment. Discuss abnormalities and drug interruption with physician.

III.   FUNGAL SUPERINFECTION related to OVERGROWTH OF ENDOGENOUS MICROORGANISMS

Defining Characteristics: Vaginal candidiasis, vaginitis may occur as endogenous bacteria are eliminated and normal fungal population expands.

Nursing Implications: Teach female patient to report vaginal itching or discharge. Discuss appropriate antifungal treatment with physician. Teach perineal hygiene and symptomatic management.

IV.   ALTERATIONS IN PROTECTIVE MECHANISMS (RARE) related to TRANSIENT LEUKOPENIA

Defining Characteristics: Rarely, transient leukopenia, lymphocytosis, anemia, eosinophilia may occur. Prolonged PT, prolonged activated partial thromboplastin time (aPTT), and hypoprothrombinemia have occurred rarely, especially in elderly or debilitated patients, or in individuals with vitamin K deficiency.

Nursing Implications: Assess baseline laboratory parameters and monitor periodically during treatment. Assess patient for response to antibiotics. Discuss abnormalities with physician.

V.   KNOWLEDGE DEFICIT related to SELF-ADMINISTRATION OF MEDICATION

Defining Characteristics: Increased compliance when patient is instructed in self-care activities.

Nursing Implications: Assess knowledge regarding infection and planned treatment. Teach drug action, potential side effects, and when and how to take drug (take medication as directed, 1 hour before or 2 hours after food). Instruct patient to report any possible drug side effects that occur.

Drug: ampicillin sodium/sulbactam sodium (UNASYN)

Class: Penicillin (aminopenicillin antibiotic).

Mechanism of Action: Semisynthetic antibiotic prepared from fungus *Penicillium*. Contains β-lactam ring and is bactericidal by inhibiting cell wall synthesis. Aminopenicillins have increased activity against gram-negative bacilli (*H. influenzae, E. coli*), as well as some activity against gram-positive bacilli (*Streptococci* and *Staphylococci*). Although sulbactam alone possesses little useful antibacterial activity, whole organism studies have shown that sulbactam restores ampicillin activity against beta lactamase-producing strains of bacteria.

Metabolism: Well-absorbed from GI tract, but rate and amount of drug absorbed is decreased with food. Widely distributed in body tissues and fluids. Crosses placenta and is found in breastmilk. Excreted in urine and bile.

Indication: For treatment of infections of the skin, intra-abdominal infections, and gynecologic infections caused by sensitive organisms. In combination with sulbactam, there is irreversible inhibition of beta lactamases, thus making ampicillin effective against beta lactamase bacteria that would otherwise be resistant to it.

Dosage/Range:
Adult:
* Dose modification necessary if renal impairment occurs. See manufacturer's package insert.
* UNASYN: 1.5–3 g ampicillin and 0.5–1 g sulbactam IV/IM every 6 hours (dose not to exceed 4 g sulbactam a day).

Drug Preparation:
* IV dilute with normal saline only; give over 10–30 minutes.
* IM: reconstitute per manufacturer's directions and use within 1 hour after reconstitution.

Drug Interactions:
* Aminoglycosides: synergism.
* Aminoglycosides (e.g., gentamicin): incompatible when mixed together; administer at separate sites at different times. Also, penicillinase-resistant penicillins can inactivate aminoglycoside serum samples from patients receiving both drugs.
* Rifampin: possible antagonism, only at high doses of ampicillin.
* Probenecid: decreases renal tubular secretion of ampicillin and sulbactam.
* Oral contraceptives: may decrease efficacy of contraceptive and increase incidence of breakthrough bleeding. Suggest additional use of barrier contraception.
* Sulbactam: broadens antibacterial coverage of ampicillin against resistant beta lactamase-producing microorganisms.
* Concurrent administration of allopurinol and ampicillin increases the incidence of rashes.

Lab Effects/Interference:
* Urine glucose: high urinary concentrations of penicillin may produce false-positive or falsely elevated test results with copper-reduction tests (Benedict's Clinitest, or Fehling's); glucose enzymatic tests (Clinistix or Testape) are not affected.
* Estradiol, total conjugated estriol, estriol-glucuronide or conjugated estrone concentrations may be transiently decreased in pregnant women following administration of ampicillin.
* Increased AST (SGOT), ALT (SGPT), alkaline phosphatase, and LDH.
* Decreased serum albumin and total protein.

COMPLICATIONS

- WBC: leukopenia or neutropenia is associated with the use of all penicillins; the effect is more likely to occur with prolonged and severe hepatic function impairment.
- BUN and serum creatinine: increased concentrations have been associated with ampicillin.

Special Considerations:
- Contraindicated in patients with prior hypersensitivity to penicillins. Use with caution in patients sensitive to other β-lactams (e.g., cephalosporins) since partial cross-allergenicity exists.
- Obtain ordered specimen and send for culture and sensitivity prior to first antibiotic dose.
- Consider alternative antibiotic therapy if eosinophilia, drug fever or rash, arthralgia, hematuria, or unexplained rise in BUN and serum creatinine occur.
- Monitor electrolytes and renal, hepatic, and hematologic laboratory parameters during extended treatment periods.
- Use with caution in pregnancy or with nursing women.
- Renal dysfunction: Unasyn dose must be reduced.

Potential Toxicities/Side Effects and the Nursing Process

I.   POTENTIAL FOR INJURY related to HYPERSENSITIVITY REACTION AND LOCAL REACTIONS (pain at injection site and thrombophlebitis)

Defining Characteristics: Urticaria, pruritus, rash (maculopapular or erythematous), fever and chills, eosinophilia, myalgia, edema, erythema, angioedema, Stevens-Johnson syndrome, and exfoliative skin reactions occur in 5% of patients. Increased risk in individuals allergic to cephalosporin antibiotics.

Nursing Implications: Assess allergy to cephalosporin antibiotics and penicillin: if patient states "yes," determine actual response (e.g., "swollen lips = angioedema"). If angioedema, patient SHOULD NOT receive drug. Discuss other patient responses with physician to determine whether drug should be given. Assess baseline skin condition including integrity and allergy history to drugs. Instruct patient to report rash, itching, other skin changes. Teach patient skin care and symptomatic measures as appropriate. If skin rash develops, discuss drug discontinuance with physician. If rash progresses, drug should be discontinued, as fatal Stevens-Johnson syndrome may develop. Be prepared to treat severe acute hypersensitivity reactions with airway management, oxygen, epinephrine, corticosteroids, and antihistamines as ordered.

II.   ALTERATION IN NUTRITION, LESS THAN BODY REQUIREMENTS, related to GI SIDE EFFECTS

Defining Characteristics: Nausea, vomiting, diarrhea may occur; rarely, pseudomembranous colitis caused by *C. difficile* resistant to the antibiotic occurs. Rarely, transient increases in LFTs—AST, ALT, alk phos, bili—may occur.

Nursing Implications: Assess baseline nutritional status. Instruct patient to report GI disturbances. Administer and teach patient to self-administer antiemetics as needed and as ordered. Teach patient importance of nutritious diet and suggest small, frequent, high-calorie, high-protein meals as appropriate. Assess baseline LFTs, and monitor periodically during treatment. Discuss abnormalities and drug interruption with physician.

III. FUNGAL SUPERINFECTION related to REDISTRIBUTION OF ENDOGENOUS MICROORGANISMS

Defining Characteristics: Vaginal candidiasis, vaginitis may occur as endogenous bacteria are eliminated and normal fungal population expands.

Nursing Implications: Instruct female patient to report vaginal itching or discharge. Discuss appropriate antifungal treatment with physician. Teach perineal hygiene and symptomatic management.

IV. KNOWLEDGE DEFICIT related to SELF-ADMINISTRATION OF MEDICATION

Defining Characteristics: Increased compliance when patient is instructed in self-care activities.

Nursing Implications: Assess knowledge regarding infection and planned treatment. Teach about drug action, potential side effects, and when and how to take drug. (Take medication as directed, 1 hour before or 2 hours after food.) Instruct patient to report any possible drug side effects.

Drug: azithromycin (Zithromax)

Class: Antibacterial (macrolide).

Mechanism of Action: Azithromycin binds to the 50S ribosomal subunit of the 70S ribosome of susceptible organisms, thereby inhibiting RNA-dependent protein synthesis. Bactericidal for *S. pyogenes, S. pneumoniae,* and *H. influenzae*. It is bacteriostatic for staphylococci and most aerobic gram-negative species.

Metabolism: Rapidly and widely distributed throughout the body; concentrates intracellularly, resulting in tissue concentrations 10 to 100 times those in plasma and serum. Rapidly absorbed with decreased absorption when given with food. Azithromycin is highly concentrated in phagocytes and fibroblasts. Over 50% of the dose is eliminated through biliary excretion as unchanged drug; approximately 4.5% of the dose is excreted unchanged in the urine within 72 hours.

Indication: For treatment of many different types of infections caused by bacteria, such as respiratory infections, skin infections, ear infections, and sexually transmitted diseases.

Dosage/Range:
- Oral: loading dose of 500 mg as a single dose on day 1, then 250 mg once a day on days 2–5.

COMPLICATIONS

- No adjustment in dose is required in patients with mild renal function impairment. No data available for patients with more severe renal function impairment.
- IV: if indicated, 500 mg may be given daily × 1–2 days, then followed by oral therapy 250 mg to complete course.

Drug Preparation:
- Reconstitute 500-mg vial with 4.8 mL sterile water for concentration of 100 mg/mL.
- Further dilute with 250 or 500 mL of compatible IV solution.

Drug Administration:
- Oral: give at least 1 hour before and 2 hours after meals. Give at least 1 hour before and 2 hours after aluminum- and magnesium-containing antacids.
- IV: infuse 500 mg/500 mL over 3 hours and 500 mg/250 mL over 1 hour.

Drug Interactions:
- Concurrent use with antacids has decreased peak serum concentration by approximately 24%.

Lab Effects/Interference:
- Serum SGPT, serum SGOT values may be increased.
- Creatinine clearance ≥ 40 mL per minute is desired.

Special Considerations:
- Do not use when there is a known hypersensitivity to erythromycins or other macrolides.
- Use with caution in patients with severe, impaired hepatic function.

Potential Toxicities/Side Effects and the Nursing Process

I.   POTENTIAL FOR INJURY related to HYPERSENSITIVITY

Defining Characteristics: Rarely, serious allergic reactions such as anaphylaxis and angioedema have been known to occur. Fever, joint pain, skin rash, urticaria, pruritus, difficulty breathing, swelling of face, mouth, neck, hands, and feet have occurred rarely.

Nursing Implications: Assess for drug allergies to erythromycin or macrolide antibiotic prior to drug administration. Teach patient to report any allergic reactions. Assess for signs/symptoms of allergic reaction after drug dose.

II.   ALTERATION IN NUTRITION related to GI SIDE EFFECTS

Defining Characteristics: Abdominal pain, diarrhea, nausea, and vomiting have occurred rarely.

Nursing Implications: Assess baseline nutritional status, preexisting nausea/vomiting, anorexia. Assess baseline LFTs and monitor periodically during treatment. Teach patient to report side effects. Provide symptomatic interventions if side effects occur; discuss with physician use of alternative drug(s).

III.   ALTERATION IN URINARY ELIMINATION related to
ACUTE INTERSTITIAL NEPHRITIS

Defining Characteristics: Risk is low, but patient may manifest symptoms of acute interstitial nephritis—fever, joint pain, skin rash.

Nursing Implications: Assess baseline renal function and electrolytes, and monitor periodically during therapy. Monitor hydration status to keep patient well hydrated.

IV.   SENSORY/PERCEPTUAL ALTERATIONS related to CNS EFFECTS OF
DIZZINESS AND HEADACHE

Defining Characteristics: Dizziness and headache may occur.

Nursing Implications: Assess baseline neurologic status. Teach patient about side effects and to report dizziness or headache. If signs/symptoms arise, discuss drug discontinuance with physician.

Drug: aztreonam (Azactam)

Class: Antibacterial (systemic).

Mechanism of Action: Bactericidal by inhibition of cell wall synthesis, which results in cell wall disintegration, lysis, and cell death. Narrow spectrum of activity against aerobic, gram-negative microorganisms (*Enterobacteriaceae* and *Pseudomonas aeruginosa*).

Metabolism: Poorly absorbed from GI tract. Widely distributed in body tissue and fluids, including CSF and peritoneal fluid. Crosses placenta and is excreted in breastmilk. Partially metabolized and excreted primarily in urine.

Indication: For treatment of gram-negative infections of urinary and lower respiratory tract, septicemia, and gynecologic and intra-abdominal infections. Drug improves breathing symptoms in cystic fibrosis (CF) patients with lung infections caused by *P. aeruginosa*.

Dosage/Range:
- Given IV or IM (IV preferred for doses > 1 g, and for serious infections).
- Adults: 500 mg–2 g IV/IM q 6–12 h (maximum 8 g/day).
- Dose modification needed for renal dysfunction (creatinine clearance < 30 mL/min); may need to modify dosage in hepatic impairment.

Drug Preparation:
- IV: reconstitute by adding 10 mL sterile water for injection or compatible IV fluid. Further dilute by adding to a volume of IV fluid (50 mL for each gram of drug) so final concentration is < 20 mg/mL. Administer over 20–60 minutes. Flush line with plain IV fluid before and after drug infusion to prevent incompatibilities.

COMPLICATIONS

• IM: reconstitute drug with 3 mL for each gram of drug using sterile or bacteriostatic water for injection, or 0.9% sodium chloride. Do not mix with local anesthetics. Administer deep IM in large muscle mass (e.g., gluteus maximus).

Drug Interactions:
• Probenecid: increased serum concentrations of antibiotic; monitor and decrease dose if needed.
• Aminoglycosides, penicillins: may have synergistic antibacterial effect against some organisms.
• Nephrotoxic drugs (aminoglycosides, colistin, vancomycin): may increase risk of renal dysfunction; avoid if possible.
• Magnesium, calcium: incompatible in IV fluid.
• Oral anticoagulants, ASPIRIN: may increase risk of bleeding.
• Alcohol: disulfiram-like reaction (flushing, throbbing headache, dyspnea, nausea, vomiting, diaphoresis, chest pain, palpitation, hyperventilation, tachycardia, hypertension, syncope, weakness, blurred vision) when alcohol is ingested within 48–72 hours of aztreonam; does not occur if alcohol is ingested prior to first antibiotic dose. If no alcohol prior to first dose, avoid alcohol for 72 hours after last dose.

Lab Effects/Interference:
• Coombs' (antiglobulin) tests may become positive during therapy.
• Serum ALT, serum alk phos, serum AST, and serum LDH values may be transiently increased during therapy.
• Serum creatinine concentrations may be transiently increased during therapy.
• PTT and PT may be prolonged during therapy.

Special Considerations:
• Obtain and send specimen for culture and sensitivity prior to first drug dose.
• May cause false-positive Clinitest glucose result.
• Use with caution in patients with renal or hepatic dysfunction.
• Drug crosses placenta and is excreted in breastmilk. Use with caution if patient is pregnant; weigh potential risks and benefits carefully if lactating; suggest interruption of breastfeeding during antibiotic therapy.
• Use cautiously if prior immediate hypersensitivity reaction to penicillins or cephalosporins; little risk of cross-allergenicity, but monitor patient closely.
• Comparable anti-infective effectiveness to aminoglycosides against gram-negative organisms without ototoxicity or nephrotoxicity.

Potential Toxicities/Side Effects and the Nursing Process

I.   ALTERATIONS IN SKIN INTEGRITY related to ALLERGY HYPERSENSITIVITY REACTION

Defining Characteristics: 1–2% incidence of rash that is mild, transient, pruritic, and/or erythematous. Less than 1% of patients develop purpura, erythema multiforme, urticaria, or exfoliative dermatitis. Less than 1% incidence occurs of immediate hypersensitivity reaction characterized by angioedema, bronchospasm, severe shock. Little cross-allergenicity with penicillins, cephalosporins (less than 1%).

Nursing Implications: Assess baseline skin integrity and presence of drug allergies; if anaphylactic reaction to penicillins or cephalosporins, monitor patient closely during drug infusions. Instruct patient to report immediately signs/symptoms of rash, pruritus, shortness of breath, and adverse sensation. Teach patient skin care and symptomatic measures as appropriate. If skin rash develops, discuss drug discontinuance with physician. If rash progresses, especially in HIV-infected patients, drug should be discontinued, as fatal Stevens-Johnson syndrome may develop. Be prepared to treat severe acute hypersensitivity reactions with airway management, oxygen, epinephrine, corticosteroids, antihistamines as ordered.

II.   ALTERATION IN NUTRITION, LESS THAN BODY REQUIREMENTS, related to GI SIDE EFFECTS

Defining Characteristics: Nausea, vomiting, diarrhea, anorexia may occur; rarely, pseudomembranous colitis caused by *C. difficile* resistant to the antibiotic occurs. Rarely, transient increases in LFTs—AST, ALT, alk phos—may occur. May develop taste alteration and halitosis.

Nursing Implications: Assess baseline nutritional status. Instruct patient to report GI disturbances. Administer and teach patient to self-administer antiemetics as needed and as ordered. Teach patient importance of nutritious diet and suggest small, frequent, high-calorie, high-protein meals as appropriate. Assess baseline LFTs and monitor periodically during treatment. Discuss abnormalities and drug interruption with physician. Encourage oral hygiene after meals and at bedtime.

III.   FUNGAL SUPERINFECTION related to REDISTRIBUTION OF ENDOGENOUS MICROORGANISMS

Defining Characteristics: Vaginal candidiasis, vaginitis may occur as endogenous bacteria are eliminated and normal fungal population expands.

Nursing Implications: Instruct female patient to report vaginal itching or discharge. Discuss appropriate antifungal treatment with physician. Teach perineal hygiene and symptomatic management.

IV.   ALTERATIONS IN PROTECTIVE MECHANISMS (RARE) related to PANCYTOPENIA

Defining Characteristics: Pancytopenia, neutropenia, thrombocytopenia, anemia, leukocytosis, thrombocytosis may occur rarely. Eosinophilia occurs in 11% of patients. May have slight prolongation of bleeding time with high doses (e.g., 2-g IV q 6 h).

COMPLICATIONS

Nursing Implications: Assess baseline laboratory parameters, and monitor periodically during treatment. Assess patient for response to antibiotics. Discuss abnormalities with physician. Assess for signs/symptoms of bleeding. If taking anticoagulants, assess for increased PT, signs/symptoms of bleeding.

V.   ALTERATIONS IN SENSORY/PERCEPTUAL PATTERNS related to DIZZINESS, SOMNOLENCE

Defining Characteristics: Dizziness, headache, somnolence, seizures occur rarely.

Nursing Implications: Assess baseline neurologic function and comfort, and monitor during treatment. Instruct patient to report any changes. Discuss any abnormalities with physician.

VI.   ALTERATIONS IN COMFORT related to LOCAL INJECTION IRRITATION

Defining Characteristics: 2–3% incidence of phlebitis and thrombophlebitis when administering IV; 3% incidence of pain and swelling at injection site when given IM.

Nursing Implications: Rotate IM injection sites and administer drug deep IM in large muscle mass (e.g., gluteus maximus). Use IM injection when IV administration is not possible. Change IV sites q 48 h and assess for signs/symptoms of phlebitis prior to each administration. Administer drug slowly. Apply warm packs to increase comfort.

VII.   ALTERATIONS IN CARDIAC OUTPUT related to CARDIOVASCULAR CHANGES

Defining Characteristics: Rare, ~1% incidence of hypotension, transient EKG changes (e.g., premature ventricular contractions), bradycardia, flushing, and chest pain.

Nursing Implications: Assess baseline heart rate and BP; monitor during therapy, at least with initial dose.

Drug: carbenicillin indanyl sodium (Geocillin, Geopen)

Class: Extended-spectrum penicillin antibacterial.

Mechanism of Action: Semisynthetic penicillin prepared from fungus *Penicillium*. Contains β-lactam ring and is bactericidal by inhibiting cell wall synthesis.

Metabolism: After oral administration, rapidly converted to carbenicillin by hydrolysis. Widely distributed in body tissues and fluids. Crosses placenta and is excreted in breast-milk. Excreted via urine and bile.

Indication: For treatment of acute and chronic infections of the upper and lower urinary tract or for asymptomatic bacteriuria caused by susceptible *Enterobacter, E. coli, Morganella morganii, Proteus mirabilis, Proteus vulgaris, Providencia rettgeri, Pseudomonas,* or *enterococci.* Active against gram-positive and gram-negative organisms, but most active against *Pseudomonas* and *Proteus,* except those organisms that have developed resistance to carbenicillin.

Dosage/Range:
Adult:
- 1 tablet (382 mg).
- Urinary tract infections:
  - *E. coli, Proteus* species, *Enterobacter:* 1–2 tabs qid.
  - *Pseudomonas, Enterococcus:* 2 tabs qid.
- Prostatitis due to *E. coli, Proteus mirabilis, Enterobacter, Enterococcus:* 2 tabs qid.

Drug Preparation:
- Oral, none.

Drug Interactions:
- Probenecid: increased serum level of penicillin; may be coadministered to exert this effect.

Lab Effects/Interference:
Major clinical significance:
- Urine glucose: high urinary concentrations of a penicillin may produce false positive or falsely elevated test results with copper sulfate tests (Benedict's, Clinitest, or Fehling's); glucose enzymatic tests (Clinistix or Testape) are not affected.
- PTT and PT: an increase has been associated with IV carbenicillin.

Clinical significance:
- Coombs' (direct antiglobulin) tests: false-positive result may occur during therapy with any penicillin.
- ALT, alk phos, AST, and serum LDH values may be decreased.
- WBC: leukopenia or neutropenia is associated with use of all penicillins; effect is more likely to occur with prolonged therapy and severe hepatic function impairment.

Special Considerations:
- Contraindicated in patients with prior hypersensitivity to penicillins. Use with caution in patients sensitive to other β-lactams (e.g., cephalosporins) since partial cross-allergenicity exists.
- Obtain ordered specimen and send for culture and sensitivity prior to first antibiotic dose.
- Consider alternative antibiotic therapy if eosinophilia, drug fever or rash, arthralgia, hematuria, or unexplained rise in BUN and serum creatinine occur.
- Use with caution in pregnancy or with nursing women.

COMPLICATIONS

Potential Toxicities/Side Effects and the Nursing Process

I.   POTENTIAL FOR INJURY related to HYPERSENSITIVITY REACTION

Defining Characteristics: Urticaria, pruritus, rash (maculopapular or erythematous), fever and chills, eosinophilia, myalgia, edema, erythema, angioedema, Stevens-Johnson syndrome, and exfoliative skin reactions occur in 5% of patients. Increased risk in individuals allergic to cephalosporin antibiotics.

Nursing Implications: Assess allergy to cephalosporin antibiotics and penicillin: if patient states "yes," determine actual response (e.g., "swollen lips = angioedema"). If angioedema, patient SHOULD NOT receive drug. Discuss other patient responses with physician to determine whether drug should be given. Assess baseline skin condition, including integrity and allergy history to drugs. Instruct patient to report rash, itching, other skin changes. Teach patient skin care and symptomatic measures as appropriate. If skin rash develops, discuss drug discontinuance with physician. If rash progresses, drug should be discontinued, as fatal Stevens-Johnson syndrome may develop.

II.   ALTERATION IN NUTRITION, LESS THAN BODY REQUIREMENTS, related to GI SIDE EFFECTS

Defining Characteristics: Nausea, vomiting, diarrhea may occur; rarely, "furry" tongue, abdominal cramps, transient increases in LFTs—AST, ALT, alk phos, bili—may occur.

Nursing Implications: Assess baseline nutritional status. Instruct patient to report GI disturbances. Administer and teach patient to self-administer antiemetics as needed and as ordered. Teach patient importance of nutritious diet and suggest small, frequent, high-calorie, high-protein meals as appropriate. Assess baseline LFTs and monitor periodically during treatment. Discuss abnormalities and drug interruption with physician.

III.   FUNGAL SUPERINFECTION related to REDISTRIBUTION OF ENDOGENOUS MICROORGANISMS

Defining Characteristics: Vaginal candidiasis, vaginitis may occur as endogenous bacteria are eliminated and normal fungal population expands.

Nursing Implications: Instruct female patient to report vaginal itching or discharge. Discuss appropriate antifungal treatment with physician. Teach perineal hygiene and symptomatic management.

IV.   ALTERATIONS IN PROTECTIVE MECHANISMS (RARE) related to LEUKOPENIA

Defining Characteristics: Rarely, transient leukopenia, lymphocytosis, anemia, eosinophilia may occur. Prolonged PT, prolonged aPTT, and hypoprothrombinemia have occurred rarely, especially in elderly or debilitated patients, or in individuals with vitamin K deficiency.

Nursing Implications: Assess baseline laboratory parameters and monitor periodically during treatment. Assess patient for response to antibiotics. Discuss abnormalities with physician. Assess for signs/symptoms of bleeding.

Drug: cefaclor (Ceclor)

Class: Second-generation cephalosporin antibiotic.

Mechanism of Action: Semisynthetic derivative of cephalosporin C (produced by fungus); contains β-lactam ring and is related to penicillins and cephamycins (e.g., cefoxitin). Bactericidal through inhibition of cell wall synthesis with resulting cell wall instability and cell lysis.

Metabolism: Well-absorbed from GI tract; delayed GI absorption if taken with food but total amount of drug absorption is the same. Widely distributed in body tissues, fluids except CSF; readily crosses placenta and is excreted in breastmilk. Unchanged drug rapidly excreted by the kidneys.

Indication: For treatment of certain infections caused by bacteria, such as pneumonia and infections of the ears, lungs, throat, urinary tract, and skin. Active against organisms causing lower respiratory tract infections (*Haemophilus influenzae, Klebsiella, Proteus, Staphylococcus aureus, Streptococcus pneumoniae*); urinary tract infections (*Enterobacter, E. coli*); skin and soft-tissue infections (*S. aureus, E. coli*); septicemia; and biliary infections.

Dosage/Range:
- Oral: 250–500 mg q 8 h (maximum total 4 g/day).

Drug Preparation:
- Store in tight container at 15–30°C (59–86°F).

Drug Interactions:
- Probenecid: increased serum concentrations of cefaclor, but does not usually require dose reduction of antibiotic.

Lab Effects/Interference:
Major clinical significance:
- Coombs' (antiglobulin) tests: a positive reaction frequently appears in patients who receive large doses of cephalosporins; hemolysis rarely occurs, but it has been reported; test may be positive in neonates whose mothers received cephalosporins before delivery.
- Urine glucose: cefaclor may produce false-positive or falsely elevated test results with copper sulfate tests (Benedicts, Clinitest, or Fehling's); glucose enzymatic tests (Clinistix or Testape) are not affected.
- PT: may be prolonged; cephalosporins may inhibit vitamin K synthesis by suppressing gut flora.

Clinical significance:
- Serum ALT, serum alk phos, serum AST, serum bili, or serum LDH values may be increased.
- BUN and serum creatinine concentrations may be increased.
- CBC or platelet count: transient leukopenia, neutropenia, agranulocytosis, thrombocytopenia, eosinophilia, lymphocytosis, and thrombocytosis have been seen on rare occasions.

Special Considerations:
- Use cautiously if renal impairment is present.
- Contraindicated if hypersensitive to other cephalosporins, or if has had angioedema response to penicillin.
- Urine glucose testing with Clinitest may result in false-positive.

Potential Toxicities/Side Effects and the Nursing Process

I.   POTENTIAL FOR INJURY related to HYPERSENSITIVITY REACTION

Defining Characteristics: Urticaria, pruritus, rash (maculopapular or erythematous), fever and chills, eosinophilia, myalgia, edema, erythema, angioedema, Stevens-Johnson syndrome, and exfoliative skin reactions occur in 5% of patients. Increased risk in individuals allergic to penicillin.

Nursing Implications: Assess allergy to cephalosporin antibiotics and penicillin: if patient states "yes," determine actual response (e.g., "swollen lips = angioedema"). If angioedema, patient SHOULD NOT receive drug. Discuss other patient responses with physician to determine whether drug should be given. Assess baseline skin condition including integrity and allergy history to drugs. Instruct patient to report rash, itching, and other skin changes. Teach patient skin care and symptomatic measures as appropriate. If skin rash develops, discuss drug discontinuance with physician. If rash progresses, drug should be discontinued, as fatal Stevens-Johnson syndrome may develop. Be prepared to treat severe acute hypersensitivity reactions with airway management, oxygen, epinephrine, corticosteroids, antihistamines as ordered.

II.   ALTERATION IN NUTRITION, LESS THAN BODY REQUIREMENTS, related to GI SIDE EFFECTS

Defining Characteristics: Nausea, vomiting, diarrhea, and anorexia may occur; rarely, pseudomembranous colitis caused by *C. difficile* resistant to the antibiotic occurs. May cause transient increases in LFTs.

Nursing Implications: Assess baseline nutritional status. Instruct patient to report GI disturbances. Administer and teach patient to self-administer antiemetics as needed and as ordered. Teach patient importance of nutritious diet and suggest small, frequent, high-calorie, high-protein meals as appropriate. Assess baseline LFTs and monitor periodically during treatment. Discuss abnormalities and drug interruption with physician.

III.   FUNGAL SUPERINFECTION related to REDISTRIBUTION OF ENDOGENOUS MICROORGANISMS

Defining Characteristics: Vaginal candidiasis, vaginitis may occur as endogenous bacteria are eliminated and normal fungal population expands.

Nursing Implications: Instruct female patient to report vaginal itching or discharge. Discuss appropriate antifungal treatment with physician. Teach perineal hygiene and symptomatic management.

IV. ALTERATIONS IN PROTECTIVE MECHANISMS (RARE) related to CHANGES IN BLOOD CELL ELEMENTS, CLOTTING FACTOR

Defining Characteristics: Rarely, transient leukopenia, lymphocytosis, anemia, eosinophilia may occur. Prolonged PT, prolonged aPTT, and hypoprothrombinemia have occurred rarely, especially in elderly or debilitated patients, or in individuals with vitamin K deficiency.

Nursing Implications: Assess baseline laboratory parameters and monitor periodically during treatment. Assess patient for response to antibiotics. Discuss abnormalities with physician.

V. ALTERATIONS IN SENSORY/PERCEPTUAL PATTERNS related to DIZZINESS, SOMNOLENCE

Defining Characteristics: Dizziness, headache, somnolence occur rarely.

Nursing Implications: Assess baseline neurologic function and comfort and monitor during treatment. Instruct patient to report any changes. Discuss any abnormalities with physician.

VI. KNOWLEDGE DEFICIT related to SELF-ADMINISTRATION OF MEDICATION

Defining Characteristics: Increased compliance when patient is instructed in self-care activities.

Nursing Implications: Assess knowledge regarding infection and planned treatment. Teach about drug action, potential side effects, and when and how to take drug. Instruct patient to report any possible side effects that occur.

Drug: cefadroxil (Duracef)

Class: First-generation cephalosporin antibacterial.

Mechanism of Action: Semisynthetic derivative of cephalosporin C, contains β-lactam ring, and is related to penicillins and cephamycins. Bactericidal through inhibition of cell wall synthesis by binding to one or more of the penicillin-binding proteins (PBPs) that in turn inhibit final transpeptidation step of peptidoglycan synthesis in bacterial cell walls, thus inhibiting cell wall biosynthesis. Bacteria eventually lyse due to ongoing activity of cell wall autolytic enzymes (autolysins and murein hydrolases) while cell wall assembly is arrested.

Metabolism: Well-absorbed from GI tract; delayed GI absorption if taken with food but total amount of drug absorption is the same. Widely distributed in body tissues, fluids except cerebrospinal fluid; readily crosses placenta and is excreted in breastmilk. Unchanged drug rapidly excreted by the kidneys.

Indication: For treatment of certain infections caused by bacteria, such as skin, throat, and urinary tract infections.

COMPLICATIONS

Dosage/Range:
- Adults: 1–2 g/day every 12 hours.
- Dose: reduce if creatinine clearance is reduced per manufacturer's recommendations.

Drug Preparation:
- Store suspension in refrigerator, discard after 14 days.
- Oral administration.

Drug Interactions:
- Furosemide and aminoglycosides increase nephrotic potential and increase toxicity.
- Probenecid may decrease cephalosporin elimination and increase effect.

Lab Effects/Interference:
- Serum SGPT, serum alk phos, serum SGOT, serum bilirubin, or serum LDH—values may be increased.
- BUN and serum creatinine—concentrations may be increased.

Special Considerations:
- Use with caution in patients with renal dysfunction—dose reduction required if severe impairment exists.
- Contraindicated in patients hypersensitive to other cephalosporin antibiotics.
- Use cautiously if sensitive to penicillin; contraindicated if angioedema reaction to penicillin.
- Obtain ordered specimen and send for culture and sensitivity prior to first drug dose.

Potential Toxicities/Side Effects and the Nursing Process

I.   POTENTIAL FOR INJURY related to HYPERSENSITIVITY REACTION

Defining Characteristics: Urticaria, pruritus, rash (maculopapular or erythematous), fever and chills, eosinophilia, myalgia, edema, erythema, angioedema. Increased risk in individuals allergic to penicillin.

Nursing Implications: Assess allergy to cephalosporin antibiotics and penicillin: if patient states "yes," determine actual response (e.g., "swollen lips = angioedema"). If angioedema, patient SHOULD NOT receive drug. Discuss other patient responses with physician to determine whether drug should be given. Assess baseline skin condition including integrity and allergy history to drugs. Teach patient to report rash, itching, other skin changes. Teach patient skin care and symptomatic measures as appropriate. If skin rash develops, discuss drug discontinuance with physician.

II.   ALTERATION IN NUTRITION, LESS THAN BODY REQUIREMENTS, related to GI SIDE EFFECTS

Defining Characteristics: Nausea and vomiting, diarrhea, and anorexia may occur. Rarely, transient increases in LFTs—AST (SGOT), ALT (SGPT), ALK PHOS, bilirubin—may occur.

Nursing Implications: Assess baseline nutritional status. Teach patient to report GI disturbances. Administer and teach patient to self-administer medication as needed and as ordered. Teach patient importance of nutritious diet and suggest small, frequent, high-calorie, high-protein meals as appropriate. Assess baseline LFTs and monitor periodically during treatment. Discuss abnormalities and drug interruption with physician.

III. FUNGAL SUPERINFECTION related to REDISTRIBUTION OF ENDOGENOUS MICROORGANISMS

Defining Characteristics: Vaginal moniliasis, vaginitis may occur as endogenous bacteria are eliminated and normal fungal population expands.

Nursing Implications: Teach female patient to report vaginal itching or discharge. Discuss appropriate antifungal treatment with physician. Teach perineal hygiene and symptomatic management.

Drug: cefamandole nafate (Mandol)

Class: Second-generation cephalosporin antibacterial.

Mechanism of Action: Semisynthetic derivative of cephalosporin C (produced by fungus); contains β-lactam ring and is related to penicillins and cephamycins (e.g., cefoxitin). Bactericidal through inhibition of cell wall synthesis with resulting cell wall instability and cell lysis.

Metabolism: Not absorbed from GI tract, so must be given IV or IM. Rapidly hydrolyzed to active metabolite. Widely distributed to body tissues and fluids except CSF; 65–75% bound to serum proteins. Readily crosses placenta and is excreted in breastmilk. Rapidly excreted by kidneys in urine.

Indication: For treatment of serious infections caused by susceptible strains of micoorganisms. Active against organisms causing lower respiratory tract infections (*H. influenzae, Klebsiella, Proteus, S. aureus, S. pneumoniae*); urinary tract infections (*Enterobacter, E. coli*); skin and soft-tissue infections (*S. aureus, E. coli*); septicemia; and biliary infections.

Dosage/Range:
Adult:
- 500 mg–1 g q 4–8 h; severe infections: 1–2 g q 4–6 h.
- Dose modification if renal impairment, based on creatinine clearance: refer to manufacturer's package insert.

Drug Preparation:
- Store powder for injection at T < 40°C (104°F). Reconstituted solution stable for 24 hours at room temperature, or 96 hours refrigerated.
- IV or deep IM injection. IV: reconstitute with 10 mL sterile water for injection, 5% dextrose or 0.9% sodium chloride injection, then further dilute in 100-mL piggyback set

COMPLICATIONS

and infuse over 30 minutes. IM: reconstitute 1-g vial with 3 mL sterile or bacteriostatic water for injection, 0.9% sodium chloride. Administer deep IM into large muscle mass (e.g., gluteus maximus).

Drug Interactions:
- Probenecid: increased serum concentrations of antibiotic; monitor and decrease dose if needed.
- Aminoglycosides, penicillins: may have synergistic antibacterial effect against some organisms.
- Nephrotoxic drugs (aminoglycosides, colistin, vancomycin): may increase risk of renal dysfunction; avoid if possible.
- Magnesium, calcium: incompatible in IV fluid.
- Oral anticoagulants, ASPIRIN: may increase risk of bleeding.
- Alcohol: disulfiram-like reaction (flushing, throbbing headache, dyspnea, nausea, vomiting, diaphoresis, chest pain, palpitations, hyperventilation, tachycardia, hypertension, syncope, weakness, blurred vision) when alcohol ingested within 48–72 hours of cefamandole; does not occur if alcohol ingested prior to first antibiotic dose. If no alcohol prior to first dose, avoid alcohol for 72 hours after last dose.

Lab Effects/Interference:
Major clinical significance:
- Coombs' (antiglobulin) tests: a positive reaction frequently appears in patients who receive large doses of cephalosporins; hemolysis rarely occurs, but it has been reported; test may be positive in neonates whose mothers received cephalosporins before delivery.
- Urine glucose: cefamandole may produce false-positive or falsely elevated test results with copper sulfate tests (Benedicts, Clinitest, or Fehling's); glucose enzymatic tests (Clinistix or Testape) are not affected.
- PT: may be prolonged; cephalosporins may inhibit vitamin K synthesis by suppressing gut flora; also, cephalosporins with NMTT side chain (cefamandole) have been associated with an increased incidence of hypoprothrombinemia; patients who are critically ill, malnourished, or have liver function impairment may be at highest risk of bleeding.

Clinical significance:
- Urine protein may produce false-positive tests for proteinuria with acid and denaturization-precipitation tests.
- Serum ALT, serum alk phos, serum AST, serum bili, or serum LDH values may be increased.
- BUN and serum creatinine concentrations may be increased.
- CBC or platelet count: transient leukopenia, neutropenia, agranulocytosis, thrombocytopenia, eosinophilia, lymphocytosis, and thrombocytosis have been seen on rare occasions.

Special Considerations:
- Use with caution in patients with renal dysfunction—dose reduction required if severe impairment exists.
- Use cautiously if history of colitis exists.
- Contraindicated in patients hypersensitive to other cephalosporin antibiotics.

- Use cautiously if sensitive to penicillin; contraindicated if angioedema reaction to penicillin.
- Obtain ordered specimen and send for culture and sensitivity prior to first drug dose.
- May cause false-positive direct Coombs' test.
- May cause false-positive Clinitest glucose result.

Potential Toxicities/Side Effects and the Nursing Process

I.   POTENTIAL FOR INJURY related to HYPERSENSITIVITY REACTION

Defining Characteristics: Urticaria, pruritus, rash (maculopapular or erythematous), fever and chills, eosinophilia, myalgia, edema, erythema, angioedema, Stevens-Johnson syndrome, and exfoliative skin reactions occur in 5% of patients. Increased risk in individuals allergic to penicillin.

Nursing Implications: Assess allergy to cephalosporin antibiotics and penicillin: if patient states "yes," determine actual response (e.g., "swollen lips = angioedema"). If angioedema, patient SHOULD NOT receive drug. Discuss other patient responses with physician to determine whether drug should be given. Assess baseline skin condition including integrity and allergy history to drugs. Instruct patient to report rash, itching, other skin changes. Teach patient skin care and symptomatic measures as appropriate. If skin rash develops, discuss drug discontinuance with physician. If rash progresses, drug should be discontinued, as fatal Stevens-Johnson syndrome may develop. Be prepared to treat severe acute hypersensitivity reactions with airway management, oxygen, epinephrine, corticosteroids, antihistamines as ordered.

II.   ALTERATION IN NUTRITION, LESS THAN BODY REQUIREMENTS, related to GI SIDE EFFECTS

Defining Characteristics: Nausea, vomiting, diarrhea, anorexia may occur; rarely, pseudomembranous colitis caused by *C. difficile* resistant to the antibiotic occurs. Rarely, transient increases in LFTs—AST, ALT, alk phos, bilirubin—may occur.

Nursing Implications: Assess baseline nutritional status. Instruct patient to report GI disturbances. Administer and teach patient to self-administer antiemetics as needed and as ordered. Teach patient importance of nutritious diet and suggest small, frequent, high-calorie, high-protein meals as appropriate. Assess baseline LFTs and monitor periodically during treatment. Discuss abnormalities and drug interruption with physician.

III.   FUNGAL SUPERINFECTION related to REDISTRIBUTION OF ENDOGENOUS MICROORGANISMS

Defining Characteristics: Vaginal candidiasis, vaginitis may occur as endogenous bacteria are eliminated and normal fungal population expands.

COMPLICATIONS

Nursing Implications: Teach female patient to report vaginal itching or discharge. Discuss appropriate antifungal treatment with physician. Teach perineal hygiene and symptomatic management.

IV.   ALTERATIONS IN PROTECTIVE MECHANISMS (RARE) related to TRANSIENT LEUKOPENIA

Defining Characteristics: Rarely, transient leukopenia, lymphocytosis, anemia, eosinophilia may occur. Prolonged PT, prolonged aPTT, and hypoprothrombinemia have occurred rarely, especially in elderly or debilitated patients, or in individuals with vitamin K deficiency.

Nursing Implications: Assess baseline laboratory parameters and monitor periodically during treatment. Assess patient for response to antibiotics. Discuss abnormalities with physician. Assess for signs/symptoms of bleeding. If they occur, especially in elderly or debilitated patients, discuss vitamin K administration with physician. Instruct patient to avoid aspirin. If taking oral anticoagulants, assess for increased PT, signs/symptoms of bleeding.

V.   ALTERATIONS IN SENSORY/PERCEPTUAL PATTERNS related to DIZZINESS, HEADACHE, SOMNOLENCE

Defining Characteristics: Dizziness, headache, somnolence occur rarely.

Nursing Implications: Assess baseline neurologic function and comfort and monitor during treatment. Instruct patient to report any changes. Discuss any abnormalities with physician.

VI.   ALTERATIONS IN COMFORT related to LOCAL INJECTION IRRITATION

Defining Characteristics: Pain, induration, sterile abscesses may form in IM injection sites; phlebitis may develop in IV sites.

Nursing Implications: Rotate IM injection sites and administer drug deep IM in large muscle mass (e.g., gluteus maximus). Use IM injection when IV administration is not possible. Change IV sites q 48 h and assess for signs/symptoms of phlebitis prior to each administration. Administer drug slowly. Apply warm packs to increase comfort.

Drug: cefazolin sodium (Ancef)

Class: First-generation cephalosporin antibacterial.

Mechanism of Action: Semisynthetic derivative of cephalosporin C (produced by fungus); contains β-lactam ring and is related to penicillins and cephamycins (e.g., cefoxitin).

Bactericidal through inhibition of cell wall synthesis, with resulting cell wall instability and cell lysis.

Metabolism: Not absorbed from GI tract, so must be given IV or IM. Widely distributed to body tissues and fluids, including bile; 74–86% bound to serum proteins. Excreted unchanged in urine. Crosses placenta and is excreted in breastmilk.

Indication: For the treatment of biliary tract infections caused by susceptible *E. coli, Klebsiella, P. mirabillis, S. aureus,* or various streptococci. Active against many gram-positive aerobic cocci (*S. aureus,* groups A and B streptococci); some susceptible gram-negative organisms (*E. coli, H. influenzae, Klebsiella, Proteus*); and gram-negative organisms causing intra-abdominal and biliary infections.

Dosage/Range:
- IV is same as IM.
- Adults: 250 mg–1.5 g q 6–8 h (maximum 12 g/day in life-threatening infections).
- May give loading dose of 500 mg.
- Dose-reduce if serum creatinine = 1.5 mg/dL according to manufacturer's package insert.

Drug Preparation:
- Store powder at < 40°C (104°F) and protect from light. Is available as frozen solution that should be stored at T < −20°C (−4°F).
- Reconstitute powder with sterile water for injection, bacteriostatic water for injection, or 0.9% sodium chloride, solution stable for 24 hours at room temperature or 96 hours at 5°C (41°F).
- Further dilute in 50–100 mL 0.9% sodium chloride or 5% dextrose for IV administration.
- For IM administration, reconstitute with 2–2.5 mL sterile or bacteriostatic water for injection or 0.9% sodium chloride injection. Administer deep IM in large muscle mass (e.g., gluteus maximus).

Drug Interactions:
- Probenecid: increased serum concentrations of antibiotic; monitor and decrease dose if needed.
- Aminoglycosides, penicillins: may have synergistic antibacterial effect against some organisms.
- Nephrotoxic drugs (aminoglycosides, colistin, vancomycin): may increase risk of renal dysfunction; avoid if possible.

Lab Effects/Interference:
Major clinical significance:
- Coombs' (antiglobulin) tests: a positive reaction frequently appears in patients who receive large doses of cephalosporins; hemolysis rarely occurs but it has been reported; test may be positive in neonates whose mothers received cephalosporins before delivery.
- Urine glucose: cefazolin may produce false-positive or falsely elevated test results with copper sulfate tests (Benedicts, Clinitest, or Fehling's); glucose enzymatic tests (Clonistix or Testape) are not affected.

- PT may be prolonged; cephalosporins may inhibit vitamin K synthesis by suppressing gut flora.

Clinical significance:
- Serum ALT, serum alk phos, serum AST, serum bili, or serum LDH values may be increased.
- BUN and serum creatinine concentrations may be increased.
- CBC or platelet count: transient leukopenia, neutropenia, agranulocytosis, thrombocytopenia, eosinophilia, lymphocytosis, and thrombocytosis have been seen on rare occasions.

Special Considerations:
- Used in treatment of serious infections of respiratory tract, urinary tract, skin and soft tissues, and biliary tree.
- Use with caution in patients with renal dysfunction—dose reduction required if severe impairment exists.
- Use cautiously if history of colitis exists.
- Contraindicated in patients hypersensitive to other cephalosporin antibiotics.
- Use cautiously if sensitive to penicillin; contraindicated if angioedema reaction to penicillin.
- Obtain ordered specimen and send for culture and sensitivity prior to first drug dose.
- May cause false-positive direct Coombs' test.
- May cause false-positive Clinitest glucose result.

Potential Toxicities/Side Effects and the Nursing Process

I.   POTENTIAL FOR INJURY related to HYPERSENSITIVITY REACTION

Defining Characteristics: Urticaria, pruritus, rash (maculopapular or erythematous), fever and chills, eosinophilia, myalgia, edema, erythema, angioedema, Stevens-Johnson syndrome, and exfoliative skin reactions occur in 5% of patients. Increased risk in individuals allergic to penicillin.

Nursing Implications: Assess allergy to cephalosporin antibiotics and penicillin: if patient states "yes," determine actual response (e.g., "swollen lips = angioedema"). If angioedema, patient SHOULD NOT receive drug. Discuss other patient responses with physician to determine whether drug should be given. Assess baseline skin condition including integrity and allergy history to drugs. Instruct patient to report rash, itching, other skin changes. Teach patient skin care and symptomatic measures as appropriate. If skin rash develops, discuss drug discontinuance with physician. If rash progresses, drug should be discontinued, as fatal Stevens-Johnson syndrome may develop. Be prepared to treat severe acute hypersensitivity reactions with airway management, oxygen, epinephrine, corticosteroids, antihistamines as ordered.

II. ALTERATION IN NUTRITION, LESS THAN BODY REQUIREMENTS, related to GI SIDE EFFECTS

Defining Characteristics: Nausea, vomiting, diarrhea, anorexia may occur; rarely, pseudomembranous colitis caused by *C. difficile* resistant to the antibiotic occurs. Rarely, transient increases in LFTs—AST, ALT, alk phos, bili—may occur.

Nursing Implications: Assess baseline nutritional status. Instruct patient to report GI disturbances. Administer and teach patient to self-administer antiemetics as needed and as ordered. Teach patient importance of nutritious diet and suggest small, frequent, high-calorie, high-protein meals as appropriate. Assess baseline LFTs and monitor periodically during treatment. Discuss abnormalities and drug interruption with physician.

III. FUNGAL SUPERINFECTION related to REDISTRIBUTION OF ENDOGENOUS MICROORGANISMS

Defining Characteristics: Vaginal candidiasis, vaginitis may occur as endogenous bacteria are eliminated and normal fungal population expands.

Nursing Implications: Teach female patient to report vaginal itching or discharge. Discuss appropriate antifungal treatment with physician. Teach perineal hygiene and symptomatic management.

IV. ALTERATIONS IN PROTECTIVE MECHANISMS (RARE) related to CHANGES IN FORMED BLOOD CELL ELEMENTS

Defining Characteristics: Rarely, transient leukopenia, lymphocytosis, anemia, eosinophilia may occur. Prolonged PT, prolonged aPTT, and hypoprothrombinemia have occurred rarely, especially in elderly or debilitated patients, or in individuals with vitamin K deficiency.

Nursing Implications: Assess baseline laboratory parameters and monitor periodically during treatment. Assess patient for response to antibiotics. Discuss abnormalities with physician. Assess for signs/symptoms of bleeding. If they occur, especially in elderly or debilitated patients, discuss vitamin K administration with physician. Instruct patient to avoid aspirin. If taking oral anticoagulants, assess for increased PT, signs/symptoms of bleeding.

V. ALTERATIONS IN SENSORY/PERCEPTUAL PATTERNS related to DIZZINESS, SOMNOLENCE

Defining Characteristics: Dizziness, headache, somnolence occur rarely.

Nursing Implications: Assess baseline neurologic function and comfort and monitor during treatment. Teach patient to report any changes. Discuss any abnormalities with physician.

VI.   ALTERATIONS IN COMFORT related to LOCAL INJECTION IRRITATION

Defining Characteristics: Pain, induration, sterile abscesses may form in IM injection sites; phlebitis may develop in IV sites.

Nursing Implications: Rotate IM injection sites, and administer drug deep IM in large muscle mass (e.g., gluteus maximus). Use IM injection when IV administration is not possible. Change IV sites q 48 h, and assess for signs/symptoms of phlebitis prior to each administration. Administer drug slowly. Apply warm packs to increase comfort.

Drug: cefdinir (Omnicef)

Class: Cephalosporin broad-spectrum antibiotic.

Mechanism of Action: Inhibits cell wall synthesis, thus destroying microorganisms. Stable in presence of some β-lactamase enzymes, so active against many microorganisms that are resistant to the penicillins and other cephalosporin antibiotics.

Metabolism: Well-absorbed from the GI tract following oral dosing, with maximal plasma concentration in 2–4 hours. Drug largely unmetabolized and eliminated by the kidneys. Mean plasma half-life is 1.7 hours. Dose must be adjusted in patients with severe renal dysfunction or who receive hemodialysis.

Indication: For treatment of moderate infections caused by certain bacteria.

Dosage/Range:
Adults with:
- Community-acquired pneumonia: 300 mg PO q 12 h × 10 days.
- Acute exacerbation of chronic bronchitis: 300 mg PO q 12 h or 600 mg PO q 24 h × 10 days.
- Acute maxillary sinusitis: 300 mg PO q 12 h or 600 mg PO q 24 h × 10 days.
- Pharyngitis/tonsillitis: 300 mg PO q 12 h × 5–10 days or 600 mg PO q 24 h × 10 days.
- Uncomplicated skin/skin structures: 300 mg PO q 12 h × 10 days.
- Patients with renal insufficiency (creatinine clearance < 30 mL/min) is 300 mg PO q 24 h.
- Patients on hemodialysis: 300 mg PO every other day with 300 mg given at the end of each dialysis.

Drug Preparation:
- Oral, available as 300-mg tablets or oral suspension that, when reconstituted as directed, results in 125 mg/5 mL in 60- or 100-mL bottles.

Drug Administration:
- Take orally without regard to meals or food intake.

Drug Interactions:
- Antacids containing magnesium or aluminum decrease absorption of cefdinir; take cefdinir at least 2 hours before or after the antacid.
- Iron or iron supplements decrease absorption by up to 80%; separate drugs by at least 2 hours.

- Probenecid inhibits the renal excretion of cefdinir, increasing peak plasma levels by 54% and prolonging half-life by 50%; decrease cefdinir dose if must use together.

Lab Effects/Interference:
- False-positive reaction for ketones in testing using nitroprusside.
- False-positive test for glucose in the urine using Clinitest, Benedict's solution, or Fehling's solution (suggest using Clinistix or Testape).
- False-positive Coombs' test (rare).
- Increased gamma glutamyltransferase (1%); rarely other liver function tests.

Special Considerations:
- Indicated for the treatment of adults with mild-to-moderate infections:
- Community-acquired pneumonia caused by *H. influenzae* (including β-lactamase–producing strains), penicillin-susceptible strains of *Streptococcus pneumoniae*, *Moraxella catarrhalis* (including β-lactamase–producing strains).
- Acute exacerbation of chronic bronchitis caused by *H. influenzae* (including β-lactamase–producing strains), penicillin-susceptible strains of *Streptococcus pneumoniae*, *Moraxella catarrhalis* (including β-lactamase–producing strains).
- Acute maxillary sinusitis caused by *H. influenzae* (including β-lactamase–producing strains), penicillin-susceptible strains of *Streptococcus*, *pneumoniae*, *Moraxella catarrhalis* (including β-lactamase–producing strains).
- Pharyngitis/tonsillitis caused by *S. pyogenes*.
- Uncomplicated skin and skin structure infections caused by *Staphylococcus aureus* (including β-lactamase–producing strains) and *S. pyogenes*.
- Contraindicated in patients with an allergy to the cephalosporin class of antibiotics as well as penicillin (cross-sensitivity in 10% of patients).
- Use cautiously, if at all, in patients with a history of colitis.
- Use in pregnancy only when benefits outweigh risks.
- If patient has severe renal dysfunction as evidenced by creatinine clearance < 30 mL/min, the dose should be reduced to 300 mg q day.
- Diabetic patients should know that the oral suspension has 2.86 g of sucrose per teaspoon.

COMPLICATIONS

Potential Toxicities/Side Effects and the Nursing Process

I.   ALTERATION IN NUTRITION related to GI SIDE EFFECTS

Defining Characteristics: Diarrhea occurs in approximately 16% of patients, and nausea in 3%. Less common are abdominal discomfort (1%), vomiting < 1%, anorexia (< 1%). The following rarely occur: dyspepsia, flatulence, constipation, abnormal stools (red-colored in patients taking iron). As with all antibiotics, pseudomembranous colitis may occur, ranging in severity from mild to life-threatening. Treatment with antibiotics changes the intestinal microflora, so *C. difficile* bacteria may overgrow. Once diagnosis is made, mild diarrhea may stop with cessation of drug; if moderate to severe, it will require, in addition, hydration, electrolyte replacement, nutritional support, and antibacterial coverage against *C. difficile*.

Nursing Implications: Assess baseline nutritional and elimination status. Teach patient to report GI disturbances. Teach patient to report diarrhea immediately, consider whether this is pseudomembranous colitis, and send stool specimen for *C. difficile;* if positive, discuss drug discontinuance with physician. Administer and teach patient to self-administer anti-emetics, antidiarrheals as needed and as ordered. Teach patient importance of nutritious diet and suggest small, frequent, high-calorie, high-protein meals as appropriate. Assess baseline LFTs and monitor periodically during treatment. Discuss abnormalities and drug interruption with physician.

II.   SENSORY/PERCEPTUAL ALTERATIONS related to CNS EFFECTS

Defining Characteristics: Headaches occur in 2% of patients, and less common (< 1%) are dizziness, asthenia, insomnia, somnolence.

Nursing Implications: Assess baseline neurologic function and comfort and monitor during treatment. Teach patient to report any changes. Teach patient how to manage symptoms. If unrelieved or persistent, discuss any abnormalities with physician.

III.   ALTERATION IN SKIN INTEGRITY related to ALLERGY/HYPERSENSITIVITY

Defining Characteristics: Uncommonly (< 1%) rash and pruritus may occur; other manifestations include eosinophilia, urticaria, flushing, fever, chills, photosensitivity, angioedema. Rarely, Stevens-Johnson syndrome reaction, toxic epidermal necrolysis, and exfoliative dermatitis have occurred. Anaphylactic reactions have occurred rarely.

Nursing Implications: Assess baseline skin condition including integrity and drug allergy history. Teach patient to report rash, itching, other skin changes. Teach patient skin care and symptomatic measures as appropriate. If skin rash develops, discuss drug discontinuance with physician. If rash progresses, drug should be discontinued, as fatal Stevens-Johnson syndrome may develop. Be prepared to treat severe acute hypersensitivity reactions with airway management, oxygen, epinephrine, corticosteroids, antihistamines as ordered.

IV.   FUNGAL SUPERINFECTION related to REDISTRIBUTION OF ENDOGENOUS MICROORGANISMS

Defining Characteristics: Vaginal moniliasis, vaginitis may occur as endogenous bacteria are eliminated and normal fungal population expands.

Nursing Implications: Teach female patient to report vaginal itching or discharge. Discuss appropriate antifungal treatment with physician. Teach perineal hygiene and symptomatic management.

Drug: cefditoren pivoxil (Spectracef)

Class: Cephalosporin antibacterial.

Mechanism of Action: Semisynthetic derivative of cephalosporin C, contains β-lactam ring, and is related to penicillins and cephamycins. Bactericidal through inhibition of cell wall synthesis, with resulting cell wall instability and cell lysis.

Metabolism: Well-absorbed from GI tract.

Indication: For treatment of infections caused by bacteria.

Dosage/Range:
- Oral (adult 12 years and older): 200–400 mg q 12 hours.
- Dose modification if renal impairment, based on creatinine clearance—refer to manufacturer's recommendations.
- Dose modification if hepatic impairment, based on LFTs—refer to manufacturer's recommendations.

Drug Preparation:
- Take with food.

Drug Interactions:
- Probenecid: increased serum concentrations of antibiotic; monitor and decrease dose if needed.
- Histamine H_2 antagonists: Famotidine decreases oral absorption; concomitant use should be avoided.
- Nephrotoxic drugs: may increase risk of renal dysfunction; avoid if possible.
- Magnesium- and aluminum-containing antacids decrease oral absorption; concomitant use should be avoided.

Lab Effects/Interference:
- Serum ALT (SGPT), serum alk phos, serum AST (SGOT), and serum bilirubin—values may be increased.
- BUN and serum creatinine—concentrations may be increased.

Special Considerations:
- Use cautiously if renal impairment is present.
- Contraindicated if hypersensitive to other cephalosporins, or if has had angioedema response to penicillin.

Potential Toxicities/Side Effects and the Nursing Process

I. POTENTIAL FOR INJURY related to HYPERSENSITIVITY REACTION

Defining Characteristics: Urticaria, pruritus, rash (maculopapular or erythematous), fever and chills, eosinophilia, myalgia, edema, erythema, angioedema. Increased risk in individuals allergic to penicillin.

Nursing Implications: Assess allergy to cephalosporin antibiotics and penicillin: if patient states "yes," determine actual response (e.g., "swollen lips = angioedema"). If angioedema, patient SHOULD NOT receive drug. Discuss other patient responses with physician to determine whether drug should be given. Assess baseline skin condition including integrity and allergy history to drugs. Teach patient to report rash, itching, other skin changes. Teach patient skin care and symptomatic measures as appropriate. If skin rash develops, discuss drug discontinuance with physician.

II.   ALTERATION IN NUTRITION, LESS THAN BODY REQUIREMENTS, related to GI SIDE EFFECTS

Defining Characteristics: Nausea, vomiting, diarrhea, and anorexia may occur.

Nursing Implications: Assess baseline nutritional status. Teach patient to report GI disturbances. Administer and teach patient to self-administer antiemetics as needed and as ordered. Teach patient importance of nutritious diet and suggest small, frequent, high-calorie, high-protein meals as appropriate. Discuss abnormalities and drug interruption with physician.

III.   FUNGAL SUPERINFECTION related to REDISTRIBUTION OF ENDOGENOUS MICROORGANISMS

Defining Characteristics: Vaginal moniliasis, vaginitis may occur as endogenous bacteria are eliminated and normal fungal population expands.

Nursing Implications: Teach female patient to report vaginal itching or discharge. Discuss appropriate antifungal treatment with physician. Teach perineal hygiene and symptomatic management.

Drug: cefepime (Maxipime)

Class: Fourth-generation cephalosporin antibiotic.

Mechanism of Action: Exerts bactericidal action by inhibiting cell wall synthesis. Highly resistant to hydrolysis by β-lactamases, and exhibits rapid penetration into gram-negative bacterial cells.

Metabolism: Given intramuscularly and parenterally. Widely distributed into body tissues and fluids. Serum protein binding is less than 19% and is independent of its concentration in the serum. Excreted in urine. The average elimination half-life is approximately 2 hours.

Indication: For treatment of moderate to severe nosocomial pneumonia, infections caused by multiple drug-resistant microorganisms (e.g., *P. aeruginosa*) and empirical treatment of febrile neutropenia. Drug is used for treatment of infections in lower respiratory tract, skin, abdomen, and urinary tract. Active against gram-negative and gram-positive organisms. Spectrum of activity includes gram-negative organisms with multiple drug resistance patterns (*Enterobacter* and *Klebsiella*).

Dosage/Range:
Adult:
- IV and IM are similar.
- Mild–mod UTI: 0.5–1 g IV or IM q 12 h × 7–10 days.
- Severe UTI, *Klebsiella pneumoniae:* 2 g IV q 12 h × 10 days.
- Moderate-to-severe pneumonia: 1–2 g IV q 12 h × 10 days.
- Febrile neutropenia: 2 g IV q 8 h × 7 days or neutrophil recovery.

Drug Preparation:
- IV or IM: add diluent recommended by manufacturer into vial.

Drug Interactions:
- Solutions of cefepime should not be added to solutions of metronidazole, vancomycin hydrochloride, gentamicin sulfate, tobramycin sulfate, or netilmicin sulfate and aminophylline because of potential side effects. If necessary, administer each drug separately.

Lab Effects/Interference:
Major clinical significance:
- Coombs' (antiglobulin) tests: a positive reaction has appeared in clinical trials without evidence of hemolysis.
- PT or PTT. may be prolonged; cephalosporins may inhibit vitamin K synthesis by suppressing gut flora.

Clinical significance:
- Serum SGPT, serum alk phos, serum SGOT, serum bilirubin, or serum LDH: values may be increased.
- BUN and serum creatinine: concentrations may be increased.
- CBC or platelet count: transient leukopenia, neutropenia, agranulocytosis, thrombocytopenia, eosinophilia, lymphocytosis, and thrombocytosis have been seen on rare occasions.

Special Considerations:
- Contraindicated in patients hypersensitive to other cephalosporin antibiotics.
- Use cautiously if sensitive to penicillin; contraindicated if angioedema reaction to penicillin.
- Obtain specimen and send for culture and sensitivity prior to first drug dose.
- May cause false-positive Clinitest glucose result.

Potential Toxicities/Side Effects and the Nursing Process

I.   POTENTIAL FOR INJURY related to HYPERSENSITIVITY REACTION

Defining Characteristics: Urticaria, pruritus, rash (maculopapular or erythematous), fever and chills, eosinophilia, myalgia, edema, erythema, angioedema, Stevens-Johnson syndrome, and exfoliative skin reactions occur in 5% of patients. Increased risk in individuals allergic to penicillin.

Nursing Implications: Assess allergy to cephalosporin antibiotics and penicillin: if patient states "yes," determine actual response (e.g., "swollen lips = angioedema"). If angioedema, patient SHOULD NOT receive drug. Discuss other patient responses with physician to determine whether drug should be given. Assess baseline skin condition including integrity and allergy history to drugs. Teach patient to report rash, itching, other skin changes. Teach patient skin care and symptomatic measures as appropriate. If skin rash develops, discuss drug discontinuance with physician. If rash progresses, drug should be discontinued, as fatal Stevens-Johnson syndrome may develop. Be prepared to treat severe acute hypersensitivity reactions with airway management, oxygen, epinephrine, corticosteroids, antihistamines as ordered.

II.   ALTERATION IN NUTRITION, LESS THAN BODY REQUIREMENTS, related to GI SIDE EFFECTS

Defining Characteristics: Nausea, vomiting, diarrhea, constipation, abdominal pain, and dyspepsia may occur; rarely, pseudomembranous colitis caused by *C. difficile* resistant to the antibiotic occurs. Rarely, transient increases in LFTs—AST (SGOT), ALT (SGPT), alk phos, bilirubin—may occur.

Nursing Implications: Assess baseline nutritional status. Teach patient to report GI disturbances. Administer and teach patient to self-administer antiemetics, antidiarrheals as needed and as ordered. Teach patient importance of nutritious diet and suggest small, frequent, high-calorie, high-protein meals as appropriate. Assess baseline LFTs and monitor periodically during treatment. Discuss abnormalities and drug interruption with physician.

III.   FUNGAL SUPERINFECTION related to REDISTRIBUTION OF ENDOGENOUS MICROORGANISMS

Defining Characteristics: Vaginal moniliasis, vaginitis may occur as endogenous bacteria are eliminated and normal fungal population expands.

Nursing Implications: Teach female patient to report vaginal itching or discharge. Discuss appropriate antifungal treatment with physician. Teach perineal hygiene and symptomatic management.

IV.   ALTERATIONS IN PROTECTIVE MECHANISMS (RARE) related to CHANGES IN FORMED BLOOD CELL ELEMENTS

Defining Characteristics: Rarely, transient leukopenia, lymphocytosis, anemia, eosinophilia may occur. Prolonged PT, prolonged aPTT, and hypoprothrombinemia have occurred rarely, especially in elderly or debilitated patients, or in individuals with vitamin K deficiency.

Nursing Implications: Assess baseline laboratory parameters and monitor periodically during treatment. Assess patient for response to antibiotics. Discuss abnormalities with physician. Assess for signs and symptoms of bleeding. If they occur, especially in elderly or debilitated patients, discuss vitamin K administration with physician. Teach patient to avoid aspirin. If taking oral anticoagulants, assess for increased PT, signs and symptoms of bleeding.

V.   SENSORY/PERCEPTUAL ALTERATIONS related to DIZZINESS, SOMNOLENCE

Defining Characteristics: Dizziness, headache, somnolence occur rarely.

Nursing Implications: Assess baseline neurologic function and comfort and monitor during treatment. Teach patient to report any changes. Discuss any abnormalities with physician.

Drug: cefixime (Suprax)

Class: Third-generation cephalosporin antibacterial.

Mechanism of Action: Semisynthetic derivative of cephalosporin C (produced by fungus); contains β-lactam ring and is related to penicillins and cephamycins (e.g., cefoxitin). Bactericidal through inhibition of cell wall synthesis, with resulting cell wall instability and cell lysis.

Metabolism: 30–50% absorbed from GI tract; rate of absorption slowed by food but does not affect total dose absorbed; 65–70% protein-bound. Eliminated unchanged in urine, and to a lesser degree in bile and feces.

Indication: For treatment of infections caused by bacteria, such as pneumonia, bronchitis, gonorrhea; and ear, lung, throat, and urinary infections. Active against a wide spectrum of bacteria such as *S. aureus, S. pyogenes, Morxella catarrhalis, E. coli, P. mirabilis, Salmonella, Shigella, Neisseria gonorrhoeae*, and sensitive gram-negative bacteria (e.g., urinary tract infections caused by *E. coli, Proteus, H. influenzae*), as well as *S. pneumoniae* and *H. influenzae* related to acute bronchitis and acute exacerbations of chronic bronchitis.

Dosage/Range:
Adult:
- 400 mg/day PO (single, or two divided doses q 12 h).
- Duration: 5–10 days for uncomplicated urinary tract infection or upper respiratory infection; 10–14 days for lower respiratory tract infections.
- Dose-reduce if creatinine clearance < 60 mL/min per manufacturer's package insert.

Drug Preparation:
- Store tablets in tight container at 15–30°C (59–86°F).
- Oral administration.

COMPLICATIONS

Drug Interactions:
- Probenecid: increased serum concentrations of antibiotic; monitor and decrease dose if needed.

Lab Effects/Interference:
Major clinical significance:
- Coombs' (antiglobulin) tests: a positive reaction frequently appears in patients who receive large doses of cephalosporins; hemolysis rarely occurs, but it has been reported; test may be positive in neonates whose mothers received cephalosporins before delivery.
- PT: may be prolonged; cephalosporins may inhibit vitamin K synthesis by suppressing gut flora.

Clinical significance:
- Serum ALT, serum alk phos, serum AST, serum bili, or serum LDH values may be increased.
- BUN and serum creatinine concentrations may be increased.
- CBC or platelet count: transient leukopenia, neutropenia, agranulocytosis, thrombocytopenia, eosinophilia, lymphocytosis, and thrombocytosis have been seen on rare occasions.

Special Considerations:
- Use with caution in patients with renal dysfunction; dose reduction required if severe impairment exists.
- Use cautiously if history of colitis exists.
- Contraindicated in patients hypersensitive to other cephalosporin antibiotics.
- Use cautiously if sensitive to penicillin; contraindicated if angioedema reaction to penicillin.
- Obtain ordered specimen and send for culture and sensitivity prior to first drug dose.
- May cause false-positive direct Coombs' test.
- May cause false-positive Clinitest glucose result.

Potential Toxicities/Side Effects and the Nursing Process

I.   POTENTIAL FOR INJURY related to HYPERSENSITIVITY REACTION

Defining Characteristics: Urticaria, pruritus, rash (maculopapular or erythematous), fever and chills, eosinophilia, myalgia, edema, erythema, angioedema, Stevens-Johnson syndrome, and exfoliative skin reactions occur in 5% of patients. Increased risk in individuals allergic to penicillin.

Nursing Implications: Assess allergy to cephalosporin antibiotics and penicillin: if patient states "yes," determine actual response (e.g., "swollen lips = angioedema"). If angioedema, patient SHOULD NOT receive drug. Discuss other patient responses with physician to determine whether drug should be given. Assess baseline skin condition including integrity and allergy history to drugs. Instruct patient to report rash, itching, other skin changes. Teach patient skin care and symptomatic measures as appropriate. If skin rash develops, discuss drug discontinuance with physician. If rash progresses, drug should be discontinued, as fatal Stevens-Johnson syndrome may develop. Be prepared to treat severe acute hypersensitivity reactions with airway management, oxygen, epinephrine, corticosteroids, antihistamines as ordered.

II. ALTERATION IN NUTRITION, LESS THAN BODY REQUIREMENTS, related to GI SIDE EFFECTS

Defining Characteristics: Nausea, vomiting, diarrhea, anorexia may occur; rarely, pseudomembranous colitis caused by *C. difficile* resistant to the antibiotic occurs. Rarely, transient increases in LFTs—AST, ALT, alk phos, bili—may occur.

Nursing Implications: Assess baseline nutritional status. Instruct patient to report GI disturbances. Administer and teach patient to self-administer antiemetics as needed and as ordered. Teach patient importance of nutritious diet and suggest small, frequent, high-calorie, high-protein meals as appropriate. Assess baseline LFTs and monitor periodically during treatment. Discuss abnormalities and drug interruption with physician.

III. FUNGAL SUPERINFECTION related to REDISTRIBUTION OF ENDOGENOUS MICROORGANISMS

Defining Characteristics: Vaginal candidiasis, vaginitis may occur as endogenous bacteria are eliminated and normal fungal population expands.

Nursing Implications: Teach female patient to report vaginal itching or discharge. Discuss appropriate antifungal treatment with physician. Teach perineal hygiene and symptomatic management.

IV. ALTERATIONS IN PROTECTIVE MECHANISMS (RARE) related to TRANSIENT LEUKOPENIA

Defining Characteristics: Rarely, transient leukopenia, lymphocytosis, anemia, eosinophilia may occur. Prolonged PT, prolonged aPTT, and hypoprothrombinemia have occurred rarely, especially in elderly or debilitated patients, or in individuals with vitamin K deficiency.

Nursing Implications: Assess baseline laboratory parameters and monitor periodically during treatment. Assess patient for response to antibiotics. Discuss abnormalities with physician. Assess for signs/symptoms of bleeding. If they occur, especially in elderly or debilitated patients, discuss vitamin K administration with physician. Instruct patient to avoid aspirin. If taking oral anticoagulants, assess for increased PT, signs/symptoms of bleeding.

V. ALTERATIONS IN SENSORY/PERCEPTUAL PATTERNS related to DIZZINESS, SOMNOLENCE

Defining Characteristics: Dizziness, headache, somnolence occur rarely.

Nursing Implications: Assess baseline neurologic function and comfort and monitor during treatment. Instruct patient to report any changes. Discuss any abnormalities with physician.

COMPLICATIONS

Drug: cefoperazone sodium (Cefobid)

Class: Third-generation cephalosporin antibacterial.

Mechanism of Action: Semisynthetic derivative of cephalosporin C, contains β-lactam ring, and is related to penicillins and cephamycins. Bactericidal through inhibition of cell wall synthesis, with resulting cell wall instability and cell lysis.

Metabolism: Not absorbed from GI tract so must be given IV or IM. Widely distributed in body fluids, including bile and cerebrospinal fluid at high doses, and body tissues. Metabolized by liver and excreted by kidneys into urine.

Indication: For treatment of susceptible infections, such as respiratory tract infection, infections of the skin, and skin structures, urinary tract infections, pelvic inflammatory disease, endometritis, and other infections. Commonly used against gram-negative bacteria.

Dosage/Range:
- IV route when possible, but IV and IM doses are the same.
- Adults: 2–12 g q 6–12 hours IM/IV; MAX 16 g/day.
- Pediatrics: 100–150 mg/kg/day q 8–12 hours IV; MAX 6 g/day.

Drug Preparation:
- Store vial containing powder at < 30°C (86°F).
- IV: Reconstitute with sterile water for injection, and further dilute in 50–100 mL of 0.9% sodium chloride or 5% dextrose injection and infuse over 15–30 minutes at maximum concentration of 50 mg/mL.
- IM: Reconstitute by adding sterile or bacteriostatic water for injection. Depending on dose, divide dose and give in separate IM sites; may need to administer large doses to avoid discomfort. Administer IM injections deeply into large muscle (e.g., gluteus maximus).

Drug Interactions:
- Probenecid: increased serum concentrations of antibiotic; monitor and decrease dose if needed.
- Aminoglycosides, penicillins: may have synergistic antibacterial effect against some organisms.
- Nephrotoxic drugs (aminoglycosides, colistin, vancomycin): may increase risk of renal dysfunction; avoid if possible.
- Heparin and warfarin-cephalosporins may inhibit vitamin K synthesis by suppressing gut flora.
- Typhoid vaccine.

Lab Effects/Interference:
- PT: may be prolonged; cephalosporins may inhibit vitamin K synthesis by suppressing gut flora.
- Serum SGPT, serum alk phos, serum SGOT, serum bilirubin, or serum LDH: values may be increased.
- BUN and serum creatinine: concentrations may be increased.

Special Considerations:
- Use with caution in patients with renal dysfunction; dose reduction required if severe impairment exists.
- Contraindicated in patients hypersensitive to other cephalosporin antibiotics.
- Use cautiously if sensitive to penicillin; contraindicated if angioedema reaction to penicillin.
- Obtain ordered specimen and send for culture and sensitivity prior to first drug dose.

Potential Toxicities/Side Effects and the Nursing Process

I.   POTENTIAL FOR INJURY related to HYPERSENSITIVITY REACTION

Defining Characteristics: Urticaria, pruritus, rash (maculopapular or erythematous), fever and chills, eosinophilia, myalgia, edema, erythema, and angioedema. Increased risk in individuals allergic to penicillin.

Nursing Implications: Assess allergy to cephalosporin antibiotics and penicillin: if patient states "yes," determine actual response (e.g., "swollen lips = angioedema"). If angioedema, patient SHOULD NOT receive drug. Discuss other patient responses with physician to determine whether drug should be given. Assess baseline skin condition including integrity and allergy history to drugs. Teach patient to report rash, itching, or other skin changes. Teach patient skin care and symptomatic measures as appropriate. If skin rash develops, discuss drug discontinuance with physician.

II.   ALTERATION IN NUTRITION, LESS THAN BODY REQUIREMENTS, related to GI SIDE EFFECTS

Defining Characteristics: Diarrhea or anorexia may occur.

Nursing Implications: Assess baseline nutritional status. Teach patient to report GI disturbances. Administer and teach patient to self-administer antidiarrheal agent as needed and as ordered.

III.   FUNGAL SUPERINFECTION related to REDISTRIBUTION OF ENDOGENOUS MICROORGANISMS

Defining Characteristics: Vaginal moniliasis, vaginitis may occur as endogenous bacteria are eliminated and normal fungal population expands.

Nursing Implications: Teach female patient to report vaginal itching or discharge. Discuss appropriate antifungal treatment with physician. Teach perineal hygiene and symptomatic management.

COMPLICATIONS

IV.   ALTERATIONS IN PROTECTIVE MECHANISMS (RARE)

Defining Characteristics: Prolonged PT, prolonged aPTT, and hypoprothrombinemia have occurred rarely, especially in elderly or debilitated patients, or in individuals with vitamin K deficiency.

Nursing Implications: Assess baseline laboratory parameters, and monitor periodically during treatment. Assess patient for response to antibiotics. Discuss abnormalities with physician. Assess for signs/symptoms of bleeding. If they occur, especially in elderly or debilitated patients, discuss vitamin K administration with physician. Teach patient to avoid aspirin. If taking oral anticoagulants, assess for increased PT, signs/symptoms of bleeding.

V.   ALTERATIONS IN COMFORT related to LOCAL INJECTION IRRITATION

Defining Characteristics: Pain, induration, and sterile abscesses may form in IM injection sites; phlebitis may develop in IV sites.

Nursing Implications: Rotate IM injection sites, and administer drug deep IM in large muscle mass (e.g., gluteus maximus). Use IM injection when IV administration is not possible. Change IV sites q 48 hours, and assess for signs/symptoms of phlebitis prior to each administration. Administer drug slowly. Apply warm packs to increase comfort.

Drug: cefotaxime sodium (Claforan)

Class: Third-generation cephalosporin antibacterial.

Mechanism of Action: Semisynthetic derivative of cephalosporin C (produced by fungus); contains β-lactam ring and is related to penicillins and cephamycins (e.g., cefoxitin). Bactericidal through inhibition of cell wall synthesis, with resulting cell wall instability and cell lysis.

Metabolism: Not absorbed from GI tract, so must be given IV or IM. Widely distributed in body fluids, including bile and CSF at high doses, and body tissues. Crosses placenta and is excreted in breastmilk. Metabolized by liver and excreted by kidneys into urine.

Indication: For treatment of infections of lower respiratory tract, including pneumonia; urinary tract; skin and skin structures; peritonitis; gynecological infections, including pelvic inflammatory disease, endometritis, and pelvic cellulitis caused by susceptible strains of specific microorganisms; perioperative prophylaxis. Active against gram-negative cocci (*Enterobacter,* some strains of *Pseudomonas, E. coli, Klebsiella, Serratia*), as well as gram-positive *S. aureus* and *Staphylococcus epidermidis,* and *S. pneumoniae.* Used to treat serious lower respiratory tract, urinary tract, gynecologic, CNS, blood, and skin infections caused by sensitive bacteria.

Dosage/Range:
- IV route when possible, but IV and IM doses are the same.
- Adults: 1–2 g q 6–8 h (severe, 2 g q 4 h) × 48–72 hours after infection eradicated.

Drug Preparation:
- Store vial containing powder at < 30°C (86°F).
- Frozen injection should be stored at < −20°C (−4°F).
- IV: reconstitute with 10 mL sterile water for injection, and further dilute in 50–100 mL of 0.9% sodium chloride or 5% dextrose injection and infuse over 20–30 minutes.
- IM: reconstitute by adding 2–5 mL sterile or bacteriostatic water for injection. Depending on dose, divide dose and give in separate IM sites; may need to administer large doses (2 g) IV to avoid discomfort. Administer IM injections deeply into large muscle (e.g., gluteus maximus).

Drug Interactions:
- Probenecid: increased serum concentrations of antibiotic; monitor and decrease dose if needed.
- Aminoglycosides, penicillins: may have synergistic antibacterial effect against some organisms.
- Nephrotoxic drugs (aminoglycosides, colistin, vancomycin): may increase risk of renal dysfunction; avoid if possible.

Lab Effects/Interference:
Major clinical significance:
- Coombs' (antiglobulin) tests: a positive reaction frequently appears in patients who receive large doses of cephalosporins; hemolysis rarely occurs, but it has been reported, test may be positive in neonates whose mothers received cephalosporins before delivery.
- PT· may be prolonged; cephalosporins may inhibit vitamin K synthesis by suppressing gut flora.

Clinical significance:
- Serum ALT, serum alk phos, serum AST, serum bili, or serum LDH values may be increased.
- BUN and serum creatinine concentrations may be increased.
- CBC or platelet count: transient leukopenia, neutropenia, agranulocytosis, thrombocytopenia, eosinophilia, lymphocytosis, and thrombocytosis have been seen on rare occasions.

Special Considerations:
- Use with caution in patients with renal dysfunction; dose reduction required if severe impairment exists.
- Use cautiously if history of colitis exists.
- Contraindicated in patients hypersensitive to other cephalosporin antibiotics.
- Use cautiously if sensitive to penicillin; contraindicated if angioedema reaction to penicillin.
- Obtain ordered specimen and send for culture and sensitivity prior to first drug dose.
- May cause false-positive direct Coombs' test.

Potential Toxicities/Side Effects and the Nursing Process

I. POTENTIAL FOR INJURY related to HYPERSENSITIVITY REACTION

Defining Characteristics: Urticaria, pruritus, rash (maculopapular or erythematous), fever and chills, eosinophilia, myalgia, edema, erythema, angioedema, Stevens-Johnson

COMPLICATIONS

syndrome, and exfoliative skin reactions occur in 5% of patients. Increased risk in individuals allergic to penicillin.

Nursing Implications: Assess allergy to cephalosporin antibiotics and penicillin: if patient states "yes," determine actual response (e.g., "swollen lips = angioedema"). If angioedema, patient SHOULD NOT receive drug. Discuss other patient responses with physician to determine whether drug should be given. Assess baseline skin condition including integrity and allergy history to drugs. Instruct patient to report rash, itching, other skin changes. Teach patient skin care and symptomatic measures as appropriate. If skin rash develops, discuss drug discontinuance with physician. If rash progresses, drug should be discontinued, as fatal Stevens-Johnson syndrome may develop. Be prepared to treat severe acute hypersensitivity reactions with airway management, oxygen, epinephrine, corticosteroids, antihistamines as ordered.

II.   ALTERATION IN NUTRITION, LESS THAN BODY REQUIREMENTS, related to GI SIDE EFFECTS

Defining Characteristics: Nausea, vomiting, diarrhea, anorexia may occur; rarely, pseudomembranous colitis caused by *C. difficile* resistant to the antibiotic occurs. Rarely, transient increases in LFTs—AST, ALT, alk phos, bili—may occur.

Nursing Implications: Assess baseline nutritional status. Instruct patient to report GI disturbances. Administer and teach patient to self-administer antiemetics as needed and as ordered. Teach patient importance of nutritious diet and suggest small, frequent, high-calorie, high-protein meals as appropriate. Assess baseline LFTs, and monitor periodically during treatment. Discuss abnormalities and drug interruption with physician.

III.   FUNGAL SUPERINFECTION related to REDISTRIBUTION OF ENDOGENOUS MICROORGANISMS

Defining Characteristics: Vaginal candidiasis, vaginitis may occur as endogenous bacteria are eliminated and normal fungal population expands.

Nursing Implications: Instruct female patient to report vaginal itching or discharge. Discuss appropriate antifungal treatment with physician. Teach perineal hygiene and symptomatic management.

IV.   ALTERATIONS IN PROTECTIVE MECHANISMS (RARE) related to TRANSIENT LEUKOPENIA

Defining Characteristics: Rarely, transient leukopenia, lymphocytosis, anemia, eosinophilia may occur. Prolonged PT, prolonged aPTT, and hypoprothrombinemia have occurred rarely, especially in elderly or debilitated patients, or in individuals with vitamin K deficiency.

Nursing Implications: Assess baseline laboratory parameters, and monitor periodically during treatment. Assess patient for response to antibiotics. Discuss abnormalities with physician. Assess for signs/symptoms of bleeding. If they occur, especially in elderly or debilitated patients, discuss vitamin K administration with physician. Instruct patient to avoid aspirin. If taking oral anticoagulants, assess for increased PT, signs/symptoms of bleeding.

V.   ALTERATIONS IN SENSORY/PERCEPTUAL PATTERNS related to DIZZINESS, SOMNOLENCE

Defining Characteristics: Dizziness, headache, somnolence occur rarely.

Nursing Implications: Assess baseline neurologic function and comfort and monitor during treatment. Instruct patient to report any changes. Discuss any abnormalities with physician.

VI.   ALTERATIONS IN COMFORT related to LOCAL INJECTION IRRITATION

Defining Characteristics: Pain, induration, and sterile abscesses may form in IM injection sites; phlebitis may develop in IV sites.

Nursing Implications: Rotate IM injection sites, and administer drug deep IM in large muscle mass (e.g., gluteus maximus). Use IM injection when IV administration is not possible. Change IV sites q 48 h, and assess for signs/symptoms of phlebitis prior to each administration. Administer drug slowly. Apply warm packs to increase comfort.

Drug: cefotetan (Cefotan)

Class: Second-generation cephalosporin antibiotic.

Mechanism of Action: Semisynthetic derivative of cephalosporin C; contains β-lactam ring, and is related to penicillins and cephamycins. Bactericidal through inhibition of cell wall synthesis by binding to one or more of the penicillin-binding proteins (PBPs) that in turn inhibit the final transpeptidation step of peptidoglycan synthesis in bacterial cell walls, thus inhibiting cell wall biosynthesis. Bacteria eventually lyse due to ongoing activity of cell wall autolytic enzymes (autolysins and murein hydrolases) while cell wall assembly is arrested.

Metabolism: Widely distributed in body tissues, fluids except cerebrospinal fluid; readily crosses placenta and is excreted in breastmilk. Unchanged drug rapidly excreted by the kidneys.

Indication: For treatment of infections of the lungs, skin, bones, joints, stomach area, blood, female reproductive organs, and urinary tract. Used before surgery to prevent infections.

Dosage/Range:
- Oral (adult): 1–6 g/day in divided doses every 12 hours, usual dose: 1–2 g every 12 hours for 5–10 days; 1–2 g may be given every 24 hours for urinary tract infection.
- Oral (child): 20–40 mg/kg/dose q 12 hours.

Drug Preparation:
• Refrigerate suspension.

Drug Interactions:
• Probenecid: increased serum concentrations of cefotetan but does not usually require dose reduction of antibiotic.
• Aminoglycosides and furosemide can increase nephrotoxicity.
• Disulfiram-like reaction has been reported when taken within 72 hours of ethanol consumption.

Lab Effects/Interference:
• Serum ALT (SGPT), serum alk phos, serum AST (SGOT), and serum bilirubin—values may be increased.
• BUN and serum creatinine—concentrations may be increased.

Special Considerations:
• Use cautiously if renal impairment is present.
• Contraindicated if hypersensitive to other cephalosporins, or if has had angioedema response to penicillin.

Potential Toxicities/Side Effects and the Nursing Process

I.   POTENTIAL FOR INJURY related to HYPERSENSITIVITY REACTION

Defining Characteristics: Urticaria, pruritus, rash (maculopapular or erythematous), fever and chills, eosinophilia, myalgia, edema, erythema, angioedema. Increased risk in individuals allergic to penicillin.

Nursing Implications: Assess allergy to cephalosporin antibiotics and penicillin: if patient states "yes," determine actual response (e.g., "swollen lips = angioedema"). If angioedema, patient SHOULD NOT receive drug. Discuss other patient responses with physician to determine whether drug should be given. Assess baseline skin condition including integrity and allergy history to drugs. Teach patient to report rash, itching, and other skin changes. Teach patient skin care and symptomatic measures as appropriate. If skin rash develops, discuss drug discontinuance with physician.

II.   ALTERATION IN NUTRITION, LESS THAN BODY REQUIREMENTS, related to GI SIDE EFFECTS

Defining Characteristics: Nausea, vomiting, diarrhea, and anorexia may occur. May cause transient increases in LFTs.

Nursing Implications: Assess baseline nutritional status. Teach patient to report GI disturbances. Administer and teach patient to self-administer antiemetics as needed and as ordered. Teach patient importance of nutritious diet and suggest small, frequent, high-calorie, high-protein meals as appropriate. Assess baseline LFTs and monitor periodically during treatment. Discuss abnormalities and drug interruption with physician.

III. FUNGAL SUPERINFECTION related to REDISTRIBUTION OF ENDOGENOUS MICROORGANISMS

Defining Characteristics: Vaginal moniliasis, vaginitis may occur as endogenous bacteria are eliminated and normal fungal population expands.

Nursing Implications: Teach female patient to report vaginal itching or discharge. Discuss appropriate antifungal treatment with physician. Teach perineal hygiene and symptomatic management.

IV. KNOWLEDGE DEFICIT related to SELF-ADMINISTRATION OF MEDICATION

Defining Characteristics: Increased compliance when patient is instructed in self-care activities.

Nursing Implications: Assess knowledge regarding infection and planned treatment. Teach about drug action, potential side effects, and when and how to take drug. Teach patient to report any possible side effects that occur.

Drug: cefoxitin sodium (Mefoxin)

Class: Considered second-generation cephalosporin based on activity spectrum; technically, a cephamycin antibacterial.

Mechanism of Action: β-lactam antibiotic that inhibits bacterial cell wall synthesis, leading to cell lysis.

Metabolism: Not absorbed from GI tract, so must be administered IV or IM.

Indication: For treatment of infections of the lower respiratory tract, urinary tract, skin and skin structures, bone and joint, intra-abdominal infections, gynecological infections, septicemia caused by susceptible microorganisms, and perioperative prophylaxis. Active against sensitive gram-negative bacteria causing lower respiratory infections (*H. influenzae, E. coli, Klebsiella*); GU infections (*E. coli, Klebsiella, Proteus*); septicemia; pelvic infections (*E. coli, Neisseria gonorrheae*); or skin infections (*E. coli, Klebsiella*). Also, some gram-positive infections, including lower respiratory tract infections (*S. aureus, S. pneumoniae*, streptococci).

Dosage/Range:
- IV route preferred; IV and IM dosages the same.
- Adult: 1–2 g q 6–8 h (maximum 12 g/day in divided doses).
- Dose-reduce for renal compromise (based on manufacturer's package insert).

Drug Preparation:
- Store sterile powder at < 30°C (86°F); frozen injection should be stored at < −20°C (−4°F).
- IV: reconstitute drug by adding 10 mL sterile water for injection. Further dilute in 50–100 mL 0.9% sodium chloride or 5% dextrose injection and infuse over 30–60 minutes.

COMPLICATIONS

- IM: reconstitute drug by adding 2 mL sterile water for injection or 0.5% or 1% lidocaine HCl injection without epinephrine to 1 g of cefoxitin. Administer IM deeply into large muscle mass (e.g., gluteus maximus). Using proper technique, ensure that injection is not into blood vessel. (Make certain patient is NOT ALLERGIC to lidocaine.)

Drug Interactions:
- Probenecid: increased serum concentrations of antibiotic; monitor and decrease dose if needed.
- Aminoglycosides, penicillins: may have synergistic antibacterial effect against some organisms.
- Nephrotoxic drugs (aminoglycosides, colistin, vancomycin): may increase risk of renal dysfunction; avoid if possible.
- Magnesium, calcium: incompatible in IV fluid.
- Oral anticoagulants, ASPIRIN: may increase risk of bleeding.
- Alcohol: disulfiram-like reaction (flushing, throbbing headache, dyspnea, nausea, vomiting, diaphoresis, chest pain, palpitation, hyperventilation, tachycardia, hypertension, syncope, weakness, blurred vision) when alcohol ingested within 48–72 hours of cefoxitin; does not occur if alcohol ingested prior to first antibiotic dose. If no alcohol prior to first dose, avoid alcohol for 72 hours after last dose.

Lab Effects/Interference:
Major clinical significance:
- Coombs' (antiglobulin) tests: a positive reaction frequently appears in patients who receive large doses of cephalosporins; hemolysis rarely occurs, but it has been reported; test may be positive in neonates whose mothers received cephalosporins before delivery.
- Urine glucose: some cephalosporins (cefoxitin) may produce false-positive or falsely elevated test results with copper sulfate tests (Benedict's, Fehling's, or Clinitest); glucose enzymatic tests (Clinistix and Testape) are not affected.
- PT: may be prolonged; cephalosporins may inhibit vitamin K synthesis by suppressing gut flora.

Clinical significance:
- Serum and urine creatinine may falsely elevate test values when the Jaffe reaction is used; serum samples should not be obtained within 2 hours of administration.
- Serum ALT, serum alk phos, serum AST, serum bili, or serum LDH values may be increased.
- BUN and serum creatinine concentrations may be increased.
- CBC or platelet count: transient leukopenia, neutropenia, agranulocytosis, thrombocytopenia, eosinophilia, lymphocytosis, and thrombocytosis have been seen on rare occasions.

Special Considerations:
- Use with caution in patients with renal dysfunction; dose reduction required if severe impairment exists.
- Use cautiously if history of colitis exists.
- Contraindicated in patients hypersensitive to other cephalosporin antibiotics.
- Use cautiously if sensitive to penicillin; contraindicated if angioedema reaction to penicillin.

- Obtain ordered specimen and send for culture and sensitivity prior to first drug dose.
- May cause false-positive direct Coombs' test.
- May cause false-positive Clinitest glucose result.

Potential Toxicities/Side Effects and the Nursing Process

I. POTENTIAL FOR INJURY related to HYPERSENSITIVITY REACTION

Defining Characteristics: Urticaria, pruritus, rash (maculopapular or erythematous), fever and chills, eosinophilia, myalgia, edema, erythema, angioedema, Stevens-Johnson syndrome, and exfoliative skin reactions occur in 5% of patients. Increased risk in individuals allergic to penicillin.

Nursing Implications: Assess allergy to cephalosporin antibiotics and penicillin: if patient states "yes," determine actual response (e.g., "swollen lips = angioedema"). If angioedema, patient SHOULD NOT receive drug. Discuss other patient responses with physician to determine whether drug should be given. Assess baseline skin condition including integrity and allergy history to drugs. Instruct patient to report rash, itching, and other skin changes. Teach patient skin care and symptomatic measures as appropriate. If skin rash develops, discuss drug discontinuance with physician. If rash progresses, drug should be discontinued, as fatal Stevens-Johnson syndrome may develop. Be prepared to treat severe acute hypersensitivity reactions with airway management, oxygen, epinephrine, corticosteroids, antihistamines as ordered.

II. ALTERATION IN NUTRITION, LESS THAN BODY REQUIREMENTS, related to GI SIDE EFFECTS

Defining Characteristic: Nausea, vomiting, diarrhea, anorexia may occur; rarely, pseudomembranous colitis caused by *C. difficile* resistant to the antibiotic occurs. Rarely, transient increases in LFTs—AST, ALT, alk phos, bili—may occur.

Nursing Implications: Assess baseline nutritional status. Instruct patient to report GI disturbances. Administer and teach patient to self-administer antiemetics as needed and as ordered. Teach patient importance of nutritious diet, and suggest small, frequent, high-calorie, high-protein meals as appropriate. Assess baseline LFTs and monitor periodically during treatment. Discuss abnormalities and drug interruption with physician.

III. FUNGAL SUPERINFECTION related to REDISTRIBUTION OF ENDOGENOUS MICROORGANISMS

Defining Characteristics: Vaginal candidiasis, vaginitis may occur as endogenous bacteria are eliminated and normal fungal population expands.

Nursing Implications: Instruct female patient to report vaginal itching or discharge. Discuss appropriate antifungal treatment with physician. Teach perineal hygiene and symptomatic management.

COMPLICATIONS

IV.   ALTERATIONS IN PROTECTIVE MECHANISMS (RARE) related to TRANSIENT LEUKOPENIA

Defining Characteristics: Rarely, transient leukopenia, lymphocytosis, anemia, eosinophilia may occur. Prolonged PT, prolonged aPTT, and hypoprothrombinemia have occurred rarely, especially in elderly or debilitated patients, or in individuals with vitamin K deficiency.

Nursing Implications: Assess baseline laboratory parameters, and monitor periodically during treatment. Assess patient for response to antibiotics. Discuss abnormalities with physician. Assess for signs/symptoms of bleeding. If they occur, especially in elderly or debilitated patients, discuss vitamin K administration with physician. Instruct patient to avoid aspirin. If taking oral anticoagulants, assess for increased PT, signs/symptoms of bleeding.

V.   ALTERATIONS IN SENSORY/PERCEPTUAL PATTERNS related to DIZZINESS, SOMNOLENCE

Defining Characteristics: Dizziness, headache, somnolence occur rarely.

Nursing Implications: Assess baseline neurologic function and comfort and monitor during treatment. Instruct patient to report any changes. Discuss any abnormalities with physician.

VI.   ALTERATIONS IN COMFORT related to LOCAL INJECTION IRRITATION

Defining Characteristics: Pain, induration, sterile abscesses may form in IM injection sites; phlebitis may develop in IV sites.

Nursing Implications: Rotate IM injection sites and administer drug deep IM in large muscle mass (e.g., gluteus maximus). Use IM injection when IV administration is not possible. Change IV sites q 48 h, and assess for signs/symptoms of phlebitis prior to each administration. Administer drug slowly. Apply warm packs to increase comfort.

Drug: cefpodoxime proxetil (Vantin)

Class: Cephalosporin antibacterial.

Mechanism of Action: Semisynthetic derivative of cephalosporin C; contains β-lactam ring and is related to penicillins and cephamycins. Bactericidal through inhibition of cell wall synthesis, with resulting cell wall instability and cell lysis.

Metabolism: Well-absorbed from GI tract.

Indication: For treatment of infections of the respiratory tract, urinary tract, skin and skin structures, and treatment of sexually transmitted diseases caused by susceptible strains of specific microorganisms.

Dosage/Range:
- Oral (adult 13 years and older): 100–400 mg q 12 hours.
- Oral (gonorrhea indication): 200-mg single dose.

- Oral (child 6 months–12 years): 10 mg/kg/daily (divided daily–bid) (MAX 400 mg/day).
- Dose modification if renal impairment, based on creatinine clearance: refer to manufacturer's recommendations.

Drug Preparation:
- Take with food.

Drug Interactions:
- Probenecid: increased serum concentrations of antibiotic; monitor and decrease dose if needed.
- Aminoglycosides, penicillins: may have synergistic antibacterial effect against some organisms.
- Nephrotoxic drugs: may increase risk of renal dysfunction; avoid if possible.
- Magnesium and aluminum.

Lab Effects/Interference:
- Serum ALT (SGPT), serum alk phos, serum AST (SGOT), and serum bilirubin: values may be increased.
- BUN and serum creatinine: concentrations may be increased.

Special Considerations:
- Use cautiously if renal impairment is present.
- Contraindicated if hypersensitive to other cephalosporins, or if has had angioedema response to penicillin.

Potential Toxicities/Side Effects and the Nursing Process

I. POTENTIAL FOR INJURY related to HYPERSENSITIVITY REACTION

Defining Characteristics: Urticaria, pruritus, rash (maculopapular or erythematous), fever and chills, eosinophilia, myalgia, edema, erythema, angioedema. Increased risk in individuals allergic to penicillin.

Nursing Implications: Assess allergy to cephalosporin antibiotics and penicillin: if patient states "yes," determine actual response (e.g., "swollen lips = angioedema"). If angioedema, patient SHOULD NOT receive drug. Discuss other patient responses with physician to determine whether drug should be given. Assess baseline skin condition including integrity and allergy history to drugs. Teach patient to report rash, itching, other skin changes. Teach patient skin care and symptomatic measures as appropriate. If skin rash develops, discuss drug discontinuance with physician.

II. ALTERATION IN NUTRITION, LESS THAN BODY REQUIREMENTS, related to GI SIDE EFFECTS

Defining Characteristics: Nausea, vomiting, diarrhea, and anorexia may occur.

Nursing Implications: Assess baseline nutritional status. Teach patient to report GI disturbances. Administer and teach patient to self-administer antiemetics as needed and as ordered. Teach patient importance of nutritious diet and suggest small, frequent,

COMPLICATIONS

high-calorie, high-protein meals as appropriate. Discuss abnormalities and drug interruption with physician.

III.   FUNGAL SUPERINFECTION related to REDISTRIBUTION OF ENDOGENOUS MICROORGANISMS

Defining Characteristics: Vaginal moniliasis, vaginitis may occur as endogenous bacteria are eliminated and normal fungal population expands.

Nursing Implications: Teach female patient to report vaginal itching or discharge. Discuss appropriate antifungal treatment with physician. Teach perineal hygiene and symptomatic management.

Drug: cefprozil (Cefzil)

Class: Second-generation cephalosporin antibiotic.

Mechanism of Action: Semisynthetic derivative of cephalosporin C; contains β-lactam ring, and is related to penicillins and cepha-mycins. Bactericidal through inhibition of cell wall synthesis, with resulting cell wall instability and cell lysis.

Metabolism: Well-absorbed from GI tract; delayed GI absorption if taken with food, but total amount of drug absorption is the same. Widely distributed in body tissues and fluids, except cerebrospinal fluid; readily crosses placenta and is excreted in breastmilk. Unchanged drug rapidly excreted by the kidneys.

Indication: For treatment of certain infections caused by bacteria, such as bronchitis and infections of the ears, throat, sinuses, and skin.

Dosage/Range:
- Oral (adult 13 years and older): 250–500 mg q 12–24 hours.
- Oral (child 7 months–12 years): 7.5–15 mg/kg q 12 hours (MAX 1 g/day).

Drug Preparation:
- Refrigerate suspension.
- Discard after 14 days.

Drug Interactions:
- Probenecid: increased serum concentrations of cefprozil but does not usually require dose reduction of antibiotic.
- Aminoglycosides, penicillins: may have synergistic antibacterial effect against some organisms.
- Typhoid vaccine.

Lab Effects/Interference:
- Serum ALT (SGPT), serum alk phos, serum AST (SGOT), and serum bilirubin: values may be increased.
- BUN and serum creatinine: concentrations may be increased.

Special Considerations:
- Use cautiously if renal impairment is present.
- Contraindicated if hypersensitive to other cephalosporins, or if has had angioedema response to penicillin.

Potential Toxicities/Side Effects and the Nursing Process

I. POTENTIAL FOR INJURY related to HYPERSENSITIVITY REACTION

Defining Characteristics: Urticaria, pruritus, rash (maculopapular or erythematous), fever and chills, eosinophilia, myalgia, edema, erythema, angioedema. Increased risk in individuals allergic to penicillin.

Nursing Implications: Assess allergy to cephalosporin antibiotics and penicillin: if patient states "yes," determine actual response (e.g., "swollen lips = angioedema"). If angioedema, patient SHOULD NOT receive drug. Discuss other patient responses with physician to determine whether drug should be given. Assess baseline skin condition, including integrity and allergy history to drugs. Teach patient to report rash, itching, and other skin changes. Teach patient skin care and symptomatic measures as appropriate. If skin rash develops, discuss drug discontinuance with physician.

II. ALTERATION IN NUTRITION, LESS THAN BODY REQUIREMENTS, related to GI SIDE EFFECTS

Defining Characteristics: Nausea, vomiting, diarrhea, and anorexia may occur. May cause transient increases in LFTs.

Nursing Implications: Assess baseline nutritional status. Teach patient to report GI disturbances. Administer and teach patient to self-administer antiemetics as needed and as ordered. Teach patient importance of nutritious diet and suggest small, frequent, high-calorie, high-protein meals as appropriate. Assess baseline LFTs and monitor periodically during treatment. Discuss abnormalities and drug interruption with physician.

III. FUNGAL SUPERINFECTION related to REDISTRIBUTION OF ENDOGENOUS MICROORGANISMS

Defining Characteristics: Vaginal moniliasis, vaginitis may occur as endogenous bacteria are eliminated and normal fungal population expands.

Nursing Implications: Teach female patient to report vaginal itching or discharge. Discuss appropriate antifungal treatment with physician. Teach perineal hygiene and symptomatic management.

COMPLICATIONS

IV.   KNOWLEDGE DEFICIT related to SELF-ADMINISTRATION OF MEDICATION

Defining Characteristics: Increased compliance when patient is instructed in self-care activities.

Nursing Implications: Assess knowledge regarding infection and planned treatment. Teach about drug action, potential side effects, and when and how to take drug. Teach patient to report any possible side effects that occur.

Drug: ceftaroline fosamil (Telfaro)

Class: Third-generation cephalosporin antibacterial.

Mechanism of Action: Semisynthetic, broad-spectrum, prodrug antibacterial of cephalosporin class of β-lactams; contains β-lactam ring and is related to penicillins and cephamycins (e.g., cefoxitin). Bactericidal through inhibition of cell wall synthesis, with resulting cell wall instability and cell lysis.

Metabolism: Widely distributed in body fluids, including bile and CSF at high doses, and body tissues. Not known whether ceftaroline fosamil is excreted in breastmilk. Because many drugs are excreted in breastmilk, caution should be exercised when ceftaroline fosamil is administered to a nursing woman. Metabolized by liver and excreted by kidneys into urine. The risk of adverse reactions may be greater in patients with impaired renal function. Because elderly patients are more likely to have decreased renal function, care should be taken in dose selection in this age group; monitor renal function. Elderly subjects had greater ceftaroline fosamil exposure relative to non-elderly subjects when administered the same single dose. Higher exposure in elderly subjects attributed to age-related changes in renal function. Dosage adjustment for elderly patients should be based on renal function.

Indication: For treatment of patients with acute bacterial skin and skin structure infections (ABSSSI) caused by susceptible isolates of the following gram-positive and gram-negative microorganisms: *S. aureus,* including methicillin-susceptible and -resistant isolates (MRSA; also known as oxacillin-resistant *S. aureus*, ORSA), *S. pyogenes* (group A beta-hemolytic streptococci), *Streptococcus agalactiae* (group B streptococci), *E. coli, Klebsiella pneumoniae,* and *Klebsiella oxytoca.*

It is also indicated for treatment of community-acquired bacterial pneumonia (CABP) caused by susceptible isolates of gram-positive and gram-negative microorganisms: *Streptococcus pneumonia,* including cases with concurrent bacteremia, *S. aureus* (methicillin-susceptible isolates only), *H. influenzae, Klebsiella pneumoniae, Klebsiella oxytoca,* and *E. coli.*

Dosage/Range:

*   The recommended dosage of Teflaro is 600 mg administered every 12 hours by intravenous (IV) infusion over 1 hour in patients > 18 years of age. The duration of therapy

guided by severity and site of infection and patient's clinical and bacteriological progress. Recommended dosage and administration by infection are described in the table below:

Infection	Dosage	Frequency	Infusion Time (hours)	Recommended Duration of Total Antimicrobial Treatment
Acute Bacterial Skin and Skin Structure Every Infection (ABSSSI)	600 mg	Every 12 hours	1	5–14 days
Community-Acquired Bacterial Pneumonia (CABP)	600 mg	Every 12 hours	1	5–7 days

Drug Preparation:
- Supplied in single-use, clear glass vials containing either 600 mg or 400 mg of sterile ceftaroline fosamil powder. Constituted solution further diluted in 250 mL before infusion. Resulting solution administered IV over approximately 1 hour.
- Appropriate infusion solutions include:
  - 0.9% Sodium Chloride Injection, USP (normal saline).
  - 5% Dextrose Injection, USP.
  - 2.5% Dextrose Injection, USP.
  - 0.45% Sodium Chloride Injection.
  - Lactated Ringer's Injection.

Drug Interactions:
- No clinical drug-drug interaction studies conducted with ceftaroline fosamil.
- Minimal potential for drug-drug interactions between ceftaroline fosamil and CYP450 substrates, inhibitors, or inducers; drugs known to undergo active renal secretion; and drugs that may alter renal blood flow.
- Safety and effectiveness in pediatric patients not established.

Lab Effects/Interference:
- Coombs' (antiglobulin) tests: a positive reaction frequently appears in patients who receive large doses of cephalosporins.
- If anemia develops during or after therapy, a diagnostic workup for drug-induced hemolytic anemia should be performed; consideration given to discontinuation of Ceftaroline fosamil.

Special Considerations:
- Known serious hypersensitivity to ceftaroline fosamil or other members of the cephalosporin class. Serious hypersensitivity (anaphylactic) reactions have been reported with β-lactam antibiotics, including ceftaroline fosamil.

COMPLICATIONS

- Caution in patients with known hypersensitivity to β-lactam antibiotics.
- Clostridium difficile-associated diarrhea (CDAD) reported with nearly all systemic antibacterial agents, including ceftaroline fosamil. Evaluate if diarrhea occurs.
- Use with caution in patients with renal dysfunction.
- Contraindicated in patients hypersensitive to other cephalosporin antibiotics.
- Use cautiously if sensitive to penicillin; contraindicated if angioedema reaction to penicillin.
- Obtain ordered specimen and send for culture and sensitivity prior to first drug dose.
- May cause false-positive direct Coombs' test.

Potential Toxicities/Side Effects and the Nursing Process

I.   POTENTIAL FOR INJURY related to HYPERSENSITIVITY REACTION

Defining Characteristics: Urticaria, pruritus, rash (maculopapular or erythematous), fever and chills, eosinophilia, myalgia, edema, erythema, and angioedema have been known to occur. Increased risk in individuals allergic to penicillin.

Nursing Implications: Assess allergy to cephalosporin antibiotics and penicillin: if patient states "yes," determine actual response (e.g., "swollen lips = angioedema"). If angioedema, patient SHOULD NOT receive drug. Discuss other patient responses with physician to determine whether drug should be given. Assess baseline skin condition, including integrity and allergy history to drugs. Instruct patient to report rash, itching, other skin changes. Teach patient skin care and symptomatic measures as appropriate. If skin rash develops, discuss drug discontinuance with physician. If rash progresses, drug should be discontinued, as fatal Stevens-Johnson syndrome may develop. Be prepared to treat severe acute hypersensitivity reactions with airway management, oxygen, epinephrine, corticosteroids, antihistamines as ordered.

II.   ALTERATION IN NUTRITION, LESS THAN BODY REQUIREMENTS, related to GI SIDE EFFECTS

Defining Characteristics: Nausea, vomiting, diarrhea, anorexia may occur; rarely, pseudomembranous colitis caused by *C. difficile* resistant to the antibiotic occurs.

Nursing Implications: Assess baseline nutritional status. Instruct patient to report GI disturbances. Administer and teach patient to self-administer antiemetics as needed and as ordered. Teach patient importance of nutritious diet, and suggest small, frequent, high-calorie, high-protein meals as appropriate. Assess baseline LFTs, and monitor periodically during treatment. Discuss abnormalities and drug interruption with physician.

III.   FUNGAL SUPERINFECTION related to REDISTRIBUTION OF ENDOGENOUS MICROORGANISMS

Defining Characteristics: Vaginal candidiasis, vaginitis may occur as endogenous bacteria are eliminated and normal fungal population expands.

Nursing Implications: Instruct female patient to report vaginal itching or discharge. Discuss appropriate antifungal treatment with physician. Teach perineal hygiene and symptomatic management.

IV.　ALTERATIONS IN PROTECTIVE MECHANISMS (RARE) related to TRANSIENT LEUKOPENIA

Defining Characteristics: Rarely, transient leukopenia, lymphocytosis, anemia, eosinophilia may occur. Prolonged PT, prolonged aPTT, and hypoprothrombinemia have occurred rarely, especially in elderly or debilitated patients, or in individuals with vitamin K deficiency.

Nursing Implications: Assess baseline laboratory parameters, and monitor periodically during treatment. Assess patient for response to antibiotics. Discuss abnormalities with physician. Assess for signs/symptoms of bleeding. If they occur, especially in elderly or debilitated patients, discuss vitamin K administration with physician. Instruct patient to avoid aspirin. If taking oral anticoagulants, assess for increased PT, signs/symptoms of bleeding.

Drug: ceftazidime (Fortaz, Tazicef, Tazidime)

Class: Third-generation cephalosporin antibacterial.

Mechanism of Action: Semisynthetic derivative of cephalosporin C (produced by fungus); contains β-lactam ring and is related to penicillins and cephamycins (e.g., cefoxitin). Bactericidal through inhibition of cell wall synthesis, with resulting cell wall instability and cell lysis.

Metabolism: Not absorbed from GI tract so must be administered parenterally. Small degree of protein binding (5–24%). Widely distributed in body fluids (including CSF and bile) and body tissues. Crosses placenta and is excreted unchanged in urine.

Indication: For treatment of infections caused by susceptible strains of organisms in lower respiratory tract, skin and skin structures, urinary tract, bacterial septicemia, bone and joint infections, gynecologic infections, intra-abdominal infections including peritonitis, and central nervous system infections including meningitis. Active against sensitive microorganisms causing lower respiratory tract, urinary tract, skin, bone and joint, gynecologic, intra-abdominal infections. These include primarily gram-negative bacteria (*Enterobacter, E. coli, Klebsiella, Proteus, Serratia,* and *Pseudomonas*) and, to a lesser degree, some gram-positive bacteria (*S. aureus, S. epidermidis,* streptococci).

Dosage/Range:
- IV and IM doses are the same.
- Adult: maximum 6 g/d.
- Uncomplicated pneumonia, skin/structure infections: 0.5–1 g IV q 8 h.

COMPLICATIONS

• Bone, joint infection: 2 g q 12 h.
• Severe GYN, abdominal infections or febrile neutropenia: 2 g IV q 8 h.
• Lung infection by pseudomonas in patients with cystic fibrosis: 30–50 mg/kg q 8 h.
• Dose should be reduced in renal insufficiency according to manufacturer's package insert.

Drug Preparation:
• Store sterile powder vials at 15–30°C (59–86°F) and protect from light; frozen injection containers should be stored at < −20°C (−4°F).
• IV: reconstitute according to manufacturer's package insert, as some preparations contain sodium carbonate. Further dilute in 100 mL of 0.9% sodium chloride or 5% dextrose and infuse over 30–60 minutes.
• IM: reconstitute according to manufacturer's package insert, which may suggest the addition of 0.5–1% lidocaine HCl to decrease discomfort. Make certain patient is NOT ALLERGIC to lidocaine. Administer deep IM in large muscle mass (e.g., gluteus maximus).

Drug Interactions:
• Probenecid: increased serum concentrations of antibiotic; monitor and decrease dose if needed.
• Aminoglycosides, penicillins: may have synergistic antibacterial effect against some organisms.
• Nephrotoxic drugs (aminoglycosides, colistin, vancomycin): may increase risk of renal dysfunction; avoid if possible.
• Sodium bicarbonate: incompatible; DO NOT administer concurrently through same IV site.

Lab Effects/Interference:
Major clinical significance:
• Coombs' (antiglobulin) tests: a positive reaction frequently appears in patients who receive large doses of cephalosporins; hemolysis rarely occurs, but it has been reported; test may be positive in neonates whose mothers received cephalosporins before delivery.
• PT: may be prolonged; cephalosporins may inhibit vitamin K synthesis by suppressing gut flora.

Clinical significance:
• Serum ALT, serum alk phos, serum AST, serum bili, or serum LDH values may be increased.
• BUN and serum creatinine concentrations may be increased.
• CBC or platelet count: transient leukopenia, neutropenia, agranulocytosis, thrombocytopenia, eosinophilia, lymphocytosis, and thrombocytosis have been seen on rare occasions.

Special Considerations:
• Empiric use in management of febrile neutropenic patient appears to be as effective as combination antibiotic regimens; vancomycin may need to be added to ceftazidime to better cover gram-positive bacteria (e.g., *S. epidermidis*).

- Has excellent coverage against *P. aeruginosa.*
- Use with caution in patients with renal dysfunction; dose reduction required if severe impairment exists.
- Use cautiously if history of colitis exists.
- Contraindicated in patients hypersensitive to other cephalosporin antibiotics.
- Use cautiously if sensitive to penicillin; contraindicated if angioedema reaction to penicillin.
- Obtain specimen and send for culture and sensitivity prior to first drug dose.
- May cause false-positive direct Coombs' test.
- May cause false-positive Clinitest glucose result.

Potential Toxicities/Side Effects and the Nursing Process

I.   POTENTIAL FOR INJURY related to HYPERSENSITIVITY REACTION

Defining Characteristics: Urticaria, pruritus, rash (maculopapular or erythematous), fever and chills, eosinophilia, myalgia, edema, erythema, angioedema, Stevens-Johnson syndrome, and exfoliative skin reactions occur in 5% of patients. Increased risk in individuals allergic to penicillin.

Nursing Implications: Assess allergy to cephalosporin antibiotics and penicillin: if patient states "yes," determine actual response (e.g., "swollen lips – angioedema"). If angioedema, patient SHOULD NOT receive drug. Discuss other patient responses with physician to determine whether drug should be given. Assess baseline skin condition including integrity and allergy history to drugs. Instruct patient to report rash, itching, other skin changes. Teach patient skin care and symptomatic measures as appropriate. If skin rash develops, discuss drug discontinuance with physician. If rash progresses, drug should be discontinued, as fatal Stevens-Johnson syndrome may develop. Be prepared to treat severe acute hypersensitivity reactions with airway management, oxygen, epinephrine, corticosteroids, antihistamines as ordered.

II.   ALTERATION IN NUTRITION, LESS THAN BODY REQUIREMENTS, related to GI SIDE EFFECTS

Defining Characteristics: Nausea, vomiting, diarrhea, anorexia may occur; rarely, pseudomembranous colitis caused by *C. difficile* resistant to the antibiotic occurs. Rarely, transient increases in LFTs—AST, ALT, alk phos, bili—may occur.

Nursing Implications: Assess baseline nutritional status. Instruct patient to report GI disturbances. Administer and teach patient to self-administer antiemetics as needed and as ordered. Teach patient importance of nutritious diet and suggest small, frequent, high-calorie, high-protein meals as appropriate. Assess baseline LFTs, and monitor periodically during treatment. Discuss abnormalities and drug interruption with physician.

COMPLICATIONS

III.   FUNGAL SUPERINFECTION related to REDISTRIBUTION OF
        ENDOGENOUS MICROORGANISMS

Defining Characteristics: Vaginal candidiasis, vaginitis may occur as endogenous bacteria are eliminated and normal fungal population expands.

Nursing Implications: Instruct female patient to report vaginal itching or discharge. Discuss appropriate antifungal treatment with physician. Teach perineal hygiene and symptomatic management.

IV.   ALTERATIONS IN PROTECTIVE MECHANISMS (RARE) related to
       TRANSIENT LEUKOPENIA

Defining Characteristics: Rarely, transient leukopenia, lymphocytosis, anemia, eosinophilia may occur. Prolonged PT, prolonged aPTT, and hypoprothrombinemia have occurred rarely, especially in elderly or debilitated patients, or in individuals with vitamin K deficiency.

Nursing Implications: Assess baseline laboratory parameters, and monitor periodically during treatment. Assess patient for response to antibiotics. Discuss abnormalities with physician.

V.   ALTERATIONS IN SENSORY/PERCEPTUAL PATTERNS related to
       DIZZINESS, SOMNOLENCE

Defining Characteristics: Dizziness, headache, somnolence occur rarely.

Nursing Implications: Assess baseline neurologic function and comfort and monitor during treatment. Instruct patient to report any changes. Discuss any abnormalities with physician.

VI.   ALTERATIONS IN COMFORT related to LOCAL INJECTION IRRITATION

Defining Characteristics: Pain, induration, sterile abscesses may form in IM injection sites; phlebitis may develop in IV sites.

Nursing Implications: Rotate IM injection sites and administer drug deep IM in large muscle mass (e.g., gluteus maximus). Use IM injection when IV administration is not possible. Change IV sites q 48 h, and assess for signs/symptoms of phlebitis prior to each administration. Administer drug slowly. Apply warm packs to increase comfort.

Drug: ceftazidime/avibactam (Avycaz)

Class: Antibacterial.

Mechanism of Action: An antibacterial combination product consisting of the semisynthetic cephalosporin ceftazidime pentahydrate and the beta-lactamase inhibitor avibactam sodium for intravenous administration.

Metabolism: Ceftazidime is mostly (80–90% of the dose) eliminated as unchanged drug. No metabolism of avibactam was observed in liver microsomes and hepatocytes. Avibactam was found in human plasma. Both ceftazidime and avibactam are excreted mainly by the kidneys.

Indications: Complicated intra-abdominal infections (cIAI), used in combination with metronidazole; complicated urinary tract infections (cUTI), including pyelonephritis.

As only limited clinical safety and efficacy data for ceftazidime/avibactam are currently available, reserve use for patients who have limited or no alternative treatment options.

To reduce the development of drug-resistant bacteria and maintain the effectiveness of this and other antibacterial drugs, ceftazidime/avibactam should be used only to treat infections that are proven or strongly suspected to be caused by susceptible bacteria.

Dosage/Range: The recommended dosage is 2.5 g (2 g ceftazidime and 0.5 g avibactam) administered every 8 hours by IV infusion over 2 hours in patients 18 years or older. For treatment of cIAI, metronidazole should be given concurrently. Guidelines for dosage in patients with normal renal function are listed in Table 11.4.

Drug Preparation:
- Ceftazidime/avibactam for injection is available in single-use vials containing 2 g ceftazidime and 0.5 g avibactam.
- Constitute powder in 10 mL of sterile water for injection, USP; 0.9% of sodium chloride injection, USP (normal saline); 5% of dextrose injection, USP; all combinations of dextrose injection and sodium chloride injection, USP, containing up to 2.5% dextrose, USP; and 0.45% sodium chloride, USP, or lactated Ringer's injection, USP.

Table 11.4   Dosage of Ceftazidime-Avibactam by Indication

Infection	Dosage	Frequency	Infusion Time (hours)	Recommended Duration of Total Antimicrobial Treatment
Complicated IAI (used in combination with metronidazole)	2.5 g (2 g/0.5 g)	Every 8 hr	2	5–14 days
Complicated UTI including pyelonephritis	2.5 g (2 g/0.5 g)	Every 8 hr	2	7–14 days

COMPLICATIONS

- Mix gently. With same diluent used for constitution of powder (except sterile water for injection), dilute reconstituted solution further to achieve a total volume of 50–250 mL before infusion.
- Mix gently and ensure that contents are dissolved completely. Visually inspect diluted solution (for administration) for particulates and discoloration prior to administration (color of infusion solution for administration ranges from clear to light yellow).
- Use diluted solution in infusion bags within 12 hours when stored at room temperature. Diluted solution in infusion bags may be stored under refrigeration at 2–8°C (36–46°F) up to 24 hours following dilution; use within 12 hours of subsequent storage at room temperature.

Drug Interactions: As a potent OAT (organic anion transport) inhibitor, probenecid inhibits OAT uptake of avibactam by 56% to 70% in vitro and has potential to decrease elimination of avibactam when coadministered. Because a clinical interaction the study of avibactam alone with probenecid has not been conducted, coadministration of avibactam with probenecid is not recommended.

Lab Effects/Interference: Administration of ceftazidime may result in a false-positive reaction for glucose in urine with certain methods. Recommend glucose tests based on enzymatic glucose oxidase reaction.

Special Considerations:
- Ceftazidime/avibactam is contraindicated in patients with known serious hypersensitivity to avibactam-containing products, ceftazidime, or other members of the cephalosporin class.
- Drug has decreased efficacy in patients with baseline CrCl of 30–50 mL/min. Monitor CrCl at least daily in patients with changing renal function and adjust the dose of ceftazidime/avibactam accordingly.
- Hypersensitivity reactions include: anaphylaxis and serious skin reactions. Cross-hypersensitivity may occur in patients with history of penicillin allergy. If an allergic reaction occurs, discontinue drug.
- *Clostridium difficile*–associated diarrhea (CDAD): CDAD has been reported with nearly all systemic antibacterial agents, including ceftazidime/avibactam. Evaluate if diarrhea occurs.
- Central nervous system reactions: Seizures and other neurologic events may occur, especially in patients with renal impairment. Adjust dose in patients with renal impairment.

Potential Toxicities/Side Effects and the Nursing Process

I.　POTENTIAL FOR INJURY related to HYPERSENSITIVITY REACTION

Defining Characteristics: Urticaria, pruritus, rash (maculopapular or erythematous), fever and chills, eosinophilia, myalgia, edema, erythema, angioedema, Stevens-Johnson syndrome, and exfoliative skin reactions occur in 5% of patients. Increased risk in individuals allergic to penicillin.

Nursing Implications: Assess allergy to cephalosporin antibiotics and penicillin; if patient states "yes," determine actual response (e.g., "swollen lips angioedema"). If angioedema is present, patient *should not* receive drug. Discuss other patient responses with physician to determine whether drug should be given. Assess baseline skin condition, including integrity, and allergy history to drugs. Instruct patient to report rash, itching, or other skin changes. Teach patient skin care and symptomatic measures as appropriate. If skin rash develops, discuss drug discontinuance with physician. If rash progresses, drug should be discontinued, as fatal Stevens-Johnson syndrome may develop. Be prepared to treat severe acute hypersensitivity reactions with airway management, oxygen, epinephrine, corticosteroids, and antihistamines as ordered.

II.   ALTERATION IN NUTRITION, LESS THAN BODY REQUIREMENTS, related to GI SIDE EFFECTS

Defining Characteristics: Nausea, vomiting, diarrhea, and anorexia may occur; rarely, pseudomembranous colitis caused by *C. difficile* resistant to the antibiotic occurs.

Nursing Implications: Assess baseline nutritional status. Instruct patient to report GI disturbances. Administer, and teach patient to self-administer, antiemetics as needed and as ordered. Teach patient importance of a nutritious diet, and suggest small, frequent, high-calorie, high-protein meals as appropriate. Assess baseline LFTs, and monitor periodically during treatment. Discuss abnormalities and drug interruption with physician.

III.   FUNGAL SUPERINFECTION related to REDISTRIBUTION OF ENDOGENOUS MICROORGANISMS

Defining Characteristics: Vaginal candidiasis or vaginitis may occur as endogenous bacteria are eliminated and normal fungal population expands.

Nursing Implications: Instruct female patients to report vaginal itching or discharge. Discuss appropriate antifungal treatment with physician. Teach perineal hygiene and symptomatic management.

Defining Characteristics: Pain or phlebitis may develop in IV sites.

Nursing Implications: Change IV sites every 48 hours, and assess for signs and symptoms of phlebitis prior to each administration. Administer drug slowly. Apply warm packs to increase comfort.

IV.   ALTERATIONS IN COMFORT related to LOCAL INJECTION-SITE IRRITATION

Defining Characteristics: Pain or phlebitis may develop in IV sites.

Nursing Implications: Change IV sites every 48 hours, and assess for signs and symptoms of phlebitis prior to each administration. Administer drug slowly. Apply warm packs to increase comfort.

COMPLICATIONS

Drug: ceftibuten (Cedax)

Class: Third-generation cephalosporin antibacterial.

Mechanism of Action: Semisynthetic derivative of cephalosporin C, contains β-lactam ring, and is related to penicillins and cephamycins. Bactericidal through inhibition of cell wall synthesis, with resulting cell wall instability and cell lysis.

Metabolism: Well-absorbed from GI tract; delayed GI absorption if taken with food, but total amount of drug absorption is the same. Widely distributed in body tissues and fluids, except cerebrospinal fluid; readily crosses placenta and is excreted in breastmilk. Unchanged drug rapidly excreted by the kidneys.

Indication: For treatment of certain mild to moderate infections caused by susceptible bacteria, such as bronchitis and ear and throat infections caused by *S. pyogenes* (Group A beta-hemolytic streptococci).

Dosage/Range:
- Adults: 400 mg orally daily × 10 days.
- Dose-reduce if creatinine clearance is reduced per manufacturer's recommendations.

Drug Preparation:
- Store suspension in refrigerator; discard after 14 days.
- Oral administration.

Drug Interactions:
- Aminoglycosides, penicillins: may have synergistic antibacterial effect against some organisms.
- Typhoid vaccine.

Lab Effects/Interference:
- Serum SGPT, serum alk phos, serum SGOT, serum bilirubin, or serum LDH: values may be increased.
- BUN and serum creatinine: concentrations may be increased.

Special Considerations:
- Use with caution in patients with renal dysfunction; dose reduction required if severe impairment exists.
- Contraindicated in patients hypersensitive to other cephalosporin antibiotics.
- Use cautiously if sensitive to penicillin; contraindicated if angioedema reaction to penicillin.
- Obtain ordered specimen and send for culture and sensitivity prior to first drug dose.

Potential Toxicities/Side Effects and the Nursing Process

I.   POTENTIAL FOR INJURY related to HYPERSENSITIVITY REACTION

Defining Characteristics: Urticaria, pruritus, rash (maculopapular or erythematous), fever and chills, eosinophilia, myalgia, edema, erythema, angioedema. Increased risk in individuals allergic to penicillin.

Nursing Implications: Assess allergy to cephalosporin antibiotics and penicillin: if patient states "yes," determine actual response (e.g., "swollen lips = angioedema"). If angioedema, patient SHOULD NOT receive drug. Discuss other patient responses with physician to determine whether drug should be given. Assess baseline skin condition including integrity and allergy history to drugs. Teach patient to report rash, itching, other skin changes. Teach patient skin care and symptomatic measures as appropriate. If skin rash develops, discuss drug discontinuance with physician.

II. ALTERATION IN NUTRITION, LESS THAN BODY REQUIREMENTS, related to GI SIDE EFFECTS

Defining Characteristics: Nausea, vomiting, diarrhea, and anorexia may occur. Rarely, transient increases in LFTs—AST (SGOT), ALT (SGPT), alk phos, bili—may occur.

Nursing Implications: Assess baseline nutritional status. Teach patient to report GI disturbances. Administer and teach patient to self-administer medication as needed and as ordered. Teach patient importance of nutritious diet and suggest small, frequent, high-calorie, high-protein meals as appropriate. Assess baseline LFTs and monitor periodically during treatment. Discuss abnormalities and drug interruption with physician.

III. FUNGAL SUPERINFECTION related to REDISTRIBUTION OF ENDOGENOUS MICROORGANISMS

Defining Characteristics: Vaginal moniliasis, vaginitis may occur as endogenous bacteria are eliminated and normal fungal population expands.

Nursing Implications: Teach female patient to report vaginal itching or discharge. Discuss appropriate antifungal treatment with physician. Teach perineal hygiene and symptomatic management.

Drug: ceftolozane/tazobactam (Zerbaxa)

Class: Antibacterial.

Mechanism of Action: Combination product consisting of a cephalosporin-class antibacterial drug and a beta-lactamase inhibitor.

Metabolism: Ceftolozane is eliminated in urine unchanged and does not appear to be metabolized to any appreciable extent. The beta-lactam ring of tazobactam is hydrolyzed to form a pharmacologically inactive tazobactam metabolite M1. Ceftolozane and tazobactam metabolite M1 are eliminated by kidneys.

Indications: Treatment of complicated intra-abdominal infections, used in combination with metronidazole caused by gram-negative and gram-positive microorganisms—*Enterobacter cloacae, Escherichia coli, Klebsiella oxytoca, Klebsiella pneumoniae, Proteus mirabilis,*

Pseudomonas aeruginosa, Bacteroides fragilis, Streptococcus anginosus, Streptococcus constellatus, and *Streptococcus salivarius.* Treatment of complicated urinary tract infections, including pyelonephritis, caused by gram-negative microorganisms—*Escherichia coli, Klebsiella pneumoniae, Proteus mirabilis,* and *Pseudomonas aeruginosa.*

Dosage/Range:
- Ceftolozane 1 g and tazobactam 0.5 g (Zerbaxa 1.5 g) for injection, every 8 hours, by IV infusion administered over 1 hour, for patients 18 years or older with creatinine clearance (CrCl) greater than 50 mL/min.
- Dosage in patients with impaired renal function:

Estimated CrCl (mL/min)*	Recommended Dosage Regimen for Ceftolozane and Tazobactam**
30–50	Ceftolozane and tazobactam 750 mg (500 mg and 250 mg) intravenously every 8 hr
15–29	Ceftolozane and tazobactam 375 mg (250 mg and 125 mg) intravenously every 8 hr
End-stage renal disease (ESRD) on hemodialysis (HD)	A single loading dose of ceftolozane and tazobactam 750 mg (500 mg and 250 mg), followed by ceftolozane and tazobactam 150 mg (100 mg and 50 mg) maintenance dose administered IV every 8 hr, for remainder of treatment period (on hemodialysis days, administer dose at earliest possible time following completion of dialysis)

*CrCl estimated using Cockcroft-Gault formula.
**All doses of ceftolozane and tazobactam are administered over 1 hour.

Drug Preparation:
- Does not contain a bacteriostatic preservative. Aseptic technique must be followed in preparing infusion solution.
- Preparation of doses: Constitute the vial with sterile water for injection or 0.9% sodium chloride for injection, USP and gently shake to dissolve. Final volume is approximately 11.4 mL.
- Caution: The **constituted solution is not for direct injection**.
- To prepare required dose, withdraw appropriate volume per manufacturer's prescribing information. Add the withdrawn volume to an infusion bag containing 0.9% sodium chloride for injection, USP or 5% dextrose injection, USP.

Drug Interactions: No significant drug–drug interactions are anticipated between ceftolozane and tazobactam and substrates, inhibitors, and inducers of cytochrome P450 enzymes (CYPs).

Lab Effects/Interference: Serum ALT (SGPT), serum alkaline phosphatase, serum AST (SGOT), and serum bilirubin values may be increased. BUN and serum creatinine: concentrations may be increased.

Special Considerations:
- Contraindicated in patients with known serious hypersensitivity to ceftolozane and tazobactam, piperacillin/tazobactam, or other members of beta-lactam class.

- Decreased efficacy in patients with baseline CrCl of 30–50 mL/min. Monitor CrCl at least daily in patients with changing renal function and adjust dose accordingly.
- Serious hypersensitivity (anaphylactic) reactions have been reported with beta-lactam antibacterial drugs. Exercise caution in patients with known hypersensitivity to beta-lactam antibacterial drugs.
- *Clostridium difficile*–associated diarrhea (CDAD) has been reported with nearly all systemic antibacterial agents. Evaluate if diarrhea occurs.
- Most common adverse reactions (≥ 5% in either indication) are nausea, diarrhea, headache, and pyrexia.
- Drug has not been studied in pediatric patients.
- Dosage adjustment is required in patients with moderately or severely impaired renal function and in patients with end-stage renal disease on hemodialysis.
- Higher incidence of adverse reactions was observed in patients aged 65 years and older. In complicated intra-abdominal infections, cure rates were lower in patients aged 65 years and older.

Potential Toxicities/Side Effects and the Nursing Process

I. POTENTIAL FOR INJURY related to HYPERSENSITIVITY REACTION

Defining Characteristics: Urticaria, pruritus, rash (maculopapular or erythematous), fever and chills, eosinophilia, myalgia, edema, erythema, angioedema. Increased risk exists in individuals allergic to penicillin cephalosporin antibiotics.

Nursing Implications: Assess allergy to cephalosporin antibiotics and penicillin; if patient states "yes," determine actual response (e.g., "swollen lips angioedema"). If angioedema is present, patient *should not* receive drug. Discuss other patient responses with physician to determine whether drug should be given. Assess baseline skin condition, including integrity, and allergy history to drugs. Teach patient to report rash, itching, and other skin changes. Teach patient skin care and symptomatic measures as appropriate. If skin rash develops, discuss drug discontinuance with physician.

II. ALTERATION IN NUTRITION, LESS THAN BODY REQUIREMENTS, related to GI SIDE EFFECTS

Defining Characteristics: Nausea, vomiting, diarrhea, and anorexia may occur. Drug may cause transient increases in LFTs.

Nursing Implications: Assess baseline nutritional status. Teach patient to report GI disturbances. Administer, and teach patient to self-administer, antiemetics as needed and as ordered. Teach patient importance of a nutritious diet; suggest small, frequent, high-calorie, high-protein meals as appropriate. Assess baseline LFTs and monitor periodically during treatment. Discuss abnormalities and drug interruption with physician.

III.   FUNGAL SUPERINFECTION related to REDISTRIBUTION OF ENDOGENOUS
MICROORGANISMS

Defining Characteristics: Vaginal candidiasis and vaginitis may occur as endogenous
bacteria are eliminated and normal fungal population expands.

Nursing Implications: Instruct female patients to report vaginal itching or discharge.
Discuss appropriate antifungal treatment with physician. Teach perineal hygiene and
symptomatic management.

IV.   ALTERATIONS IN PROTECTIVE MECHANISMS (RARE) related to RARE
LEUKOPENIA

Defining Characteristics: Rarely, hemolytic anemia, leukopenia, or thrombocytopenia
may occur.

Nursing Implications: Assess baseline laboratory parameters, and monitor periodically during
treatment. Assess patient for response to antibiotics. Discuss abnormalities with physician.

V.   ALTERATIONS IN COMFORT related to LOCAL INJECTION-SITE IRRITATION

Defining Characteristics: Pain and phlebitis may develop in IV sites.

Nursing Implications: Change IV sites every 48 hours, and assess for signs and symptoms
of phlebitis prior to each administration. Administer drug slowly. Apply warm packs to
increase comfort.

VI.   KNOWLEDGE DEFICIT related to SELF-ADMINISTRATION OF MEDICATION

Defining Characteristics: Increased compliance when patient is instructed in self-care
activities.

Nursing Implications: Assess knowledge regarding infection and planned treatment.
Teach about drug action, potential side effects, and when and how to take drug. Teach
patient to report any possible side effects that occur.

Drug: ceftriaxone sodium (Rocephin)

Class: Third-generation cephalosporin antibacterial.

Mechanism of Action: Semisynthetic derivative of cephalosporin C (produced by fungus);
contains β-lactam ring and is related to penicillins and cephamycins (e.g., cefoxitin).
Bactericidal through inhibition of cell wall synthesis, with resulting cell wall instability
and cell lysis.

Metabolism: Not absorbed from GI tract and must be given parenterally. Widely distributed into body tissues and fluids, including bile and CSF. Crosses placenta and excreted in breastmilk. Protein binding depends on drug concentration, and varies from 58–96%. Excreted in urine and feces to a lesser extent. Has a long half-life.

Indication: For treatment of acute bacterial otitis media, infections in lower respiratory tract, skin, bone and joint, abdomen, urinary tract, and pelvis (gonorrhea), as well as for treatment of meningitis and sepsis and as preoperative prophylaxis. Active primarily against gram-negative cocci (*H. influenzae, Enterobacter, E. coli, Klebsiella, Proteus, Pseudomonas*) and, to a lesser degree, gram-positive cocci (*S. aureus* and streptococci).

Dosage/Range:
• IV and IM doses same.
• 1–2 g/day, or in equally divided doses q 12 h.
• CNS infections may require maximum recommended of 4 g/day in divided doses.

Drug Preparation:
• Store vial of sterile drug powder at ≤ 25°C (77°F) and protect from light. Frozen injection containers should be stored at ≤ −20°C (−4°F).
• IV: Add diluent recommended by manufacturer into vial, then further dilute in 100 mL 0.9% sodium chloride or 5% dextrose. Infuse over 30–60 minutes.
• IM: Add 0.9–7.2 mL of sterile or bacteriostatic water for injection, or 1% lidocaine HCl without epinephrine to appropriate vial, resulting in 250 mg/mL. Administer deep IM into large muscle mass (e.g., gluteus maximus). Make certain patient is NOT ALLERGIC to lidocaine.

Drug Interactions:
• Probenecid: increased serum concentrations of antibiotic; monitor and decrease dose if needed.
• Aminoglycosides, penicillins: may have synergistic antibacterial effect against some organisms.
• Nephrotoxic drugs (aminoglycosides, colistin, vancomycin): may increase risk of renal dysfunction; avoid if possible.

Lab Effects/Interference:
Major clinical significance:
• Coombs' (antiglobulin) tests: a positive reaction frequently appears in patients who receive large doses of cephalosporins; hemolysis rarely occurs, but it has been reported; test may be positive in neonates whose mothers received cephalosporins before delivery.
• PT: may be prolonged; cephalosporins may inhibit vitamin K synthesis by suppressing gut flora.

Clinical significance:
• Serum ALT, serum alk phos, serum AST, serum bili, or serum LDH values may be increased.
• BUN and serum creatinine concentrations may be increased.

COMPLICATIONS

- CBC or platelet count: transient leukopenia, neutropenia, agranulocytosis, thrombocytopenia, eosinophilia, lymphocytosis, and thrombocytosis have been seen on rare occasions.

Special Considerations:
- Use cautiously if history of colitis exists.
- Contraindicated in patients hypersensitive to other cephalosporin antibiotics.
- Use cautiously if sensitive to penicillin; contraindicated if angioedema reaction to penicillin.
- Obtain specimen and send for culture and sensitivity prior to first drug dose.
- May cause false-positive direct Coombs' test.
- May cause false-positive Clinitest glucose result.

Potential Toxicities/Side Effects and the Nursing Process

I.   POTENTIAL FOR INJURY related to HYPERSENSITIVITY REACTION

Defining Characteristics: Urticaria, pruritus, rash (maculopapular or erythematous), fever and chills, eosinophilia, myalgia, edema, erythema, angioedema, Stevens-Johnson syndrome, and exfoliative skin reactions occur in 5% of patients. Increased risk in individuals allergic to penicillin.

Nursing Implications: Assess allergy to cephalosporin antibiotics and penicillin: if patient states "yes," determine actual response (e.g., "swollen lips = angioedema"). If angioedema, patient SHOULD NOT receive drug. Discuss other patient responses with physician to determine whether drug should be given. Assess baseline skin condition including integrity and allergy history to drugs. Instruct patient to report rash, itching, other skin changes. Teach patient skin care and symptomatic measures as appropriate. If skin rash develops, discuss drug discontinuance with physician. If rash progresses, drug should be discontinued, as fatal Stevens-Johnson syndrome may develop. Be prepared to treat severe acute hypersensitivity reactions with airway management, oxygen, epinephrine, corticosteroids, antihistamines as ordered.

II.   ALTERATION IN NUTRITION, LESS THAN BODY REQUIREMENTS, related to GI SIDE EFFECTS

Defining Characteristics: Nausea, vomiting, diarrhea, anorexia may occur; rarely, pseudomembranous colitis caused by *C. difficile* resistant to the antibiotic occurs. Rarely, transient increases in LFTs—AST, ALT, alk phos, bili—may occur.

Nursing Implications: Assess baseline nutritional status. Instruct patient to report GI disturbances. Administer and teach patient to self-administer antiemetics, antidiarrheals as needed and as ordered. Teach patient importance of nutritious diet and suggest small, frequent, high-calorie, high-protein meals as appropriate. Assess baseline LFTs and monitor periodically during treatment. Discuss abnormalities and drug interruption with physician.

III. FUNGAL SUPERINFECTION related to REDISTRIBUTION OF ENDOGENOUS MICROORGANISMS

Defining Characteristics: Vaginal candidiasis, vaginitis may occur as endogenous bacteria are eliminated and normal fungal population expands.

Nursing Implications: Instruct female patient to report vaginal itching or discharge. Discuss appropriate antifungal treatment with physician. Teach perineal hygiene and symptomatic management.

IV. ALTERATIONS IN PROTECTIVE MECHANISMS (RARE) related to TRANSIENT LEUKOPENIA

Defining Characteristics: Rarely, transient leukopenia, lymphocytosis, anemia, eosinophilia may occur. Prolonged PT, prolonged aPTT, and hypoprothrombinemia have occurred rarely, especially in elderly or debilitated patients, or in individuals with vitamin K deficiency.

Nursing Implications: Assess baseline laboratory parameters, and monitor periodically during treatment. Assess patient for response to antibiotics. Discuss abnormalities with physician. Assess for signs/symptoms of bleeding. If they occur, especially in elderly or debilitated patients, discuss vitamin K administration with physician. Instruct patient to avoid aspirin. If taking oral anticoagulants, assess for increased PT, signs/symptoms of bleeding.

V. ALTERATIONS IN SENSORY/PERCEPTUAL PATTERNS related to DIZZINESS, SOMNOLENCE

Defining Characteristics: Dizziness, headache, somnolence occur rarely.

Nursing Implications: Assess baseline neurologic function and comfort and monitor during treatment. Instruct patient to report any changes. Discuss any abnormalities with physician.

VI. ALTERATIONS IN COMFORT related to LOCAL INJECTION IRRITATION

Defining Characteristics: Pain, induration, and sterile abscesses may form in IM injection sites; phlebitis may develop in IV sites.

Nursing Implications: Rotate IM injection sites, and administer drug deep IM in large muscle mass (e.g., gluteus maximus). Use IM injection when IV administration is not possible. Change IV sites q 48 h, and assess for signs/symptoms of phlebitis prior to each administration. Administer drug slowly. Apply warm packs to increase comfort.

COMPLICATIONS

Drug: cefuroxime (Ceftin, Kefurox, Zinacef)

Class: Second-generation cephalosporin antibiotic.

Mechanism of Action: Semisynthetic derivative of cephalosporin C; contains β-lactam ring, and is related to penicillins and cephamycins. Bactericidal through inhibition of cell wall synthesis by binding to one or more of the penicillin-binding proteins PBPs that in turn inhibit the final transpeptidation step of peptidoglycan synthesis in bacterial cell walls, thus inhibiting cell wall biosynthesis. Bacteria eventually lyse due to ongoing activity of cell wall autolytic enzymes (autolysins and murein hydrolases) while cell wall assembly is arrested.

Metabolism: Widely distributed in body tissues, fluids; crosses blood–brain barrier; therapeutic concentrations achieved in cerebro-spinal fluid even when meninges are not inflamed; readily crosses placenta and is excreted in breastmilk. Unchanged drug rapidly excreted by the kidneys.

Indication: For treatment of certain bacterial infections such as gonorrhea, Lyme disease, and infections of the ears, throat, sinuses, urinary tract, and skin. Active against a wide variety of bacteria, such as *S. aureus, S. pneumoniae, H. influenza, E. coli, Neisseria gonorrhea,* and many others.

Dosage/Range:
- Oral (adult): 250–500 mg twice daily for 10 days.
- IM and IV (adult): 750 mg to 1.5 g/dose every 8 hours or 100–150 mg/kg/day in divided doses every 6–8 hours; maximum dose—6 g/24 hours.

Drug Preparation:
- Refrigerate suspension; solution stable for 48 hours.
- IV infusion in NS or D_5W solution stable for 7 days when refrigerated.

Drug Interactions:
- Probenecid: increased serum concentrations of cefotetan, but does not usually require dose reduction of antibiotic.
- Aminoglycosides: can increase nephrotoxicity.

Lab Effects/Interference:
- Serum ALT (SGPT), serum alk phos, serum AST (SGOT), and serum bilirubin—values may be increased.
- BUN and serum creatinine—concentrations may be increased.

Special Considerations:
- Use cautiously if renal impairment is present.
- Contraindicated if hypersensitive to other cephalosporins, or if has had angioedema response to penicillin.

Potential Toxicities/Side Effects and the Nursing Process

I.   POTENTIAL FOR INJURY related to HYPERSENSITIVITY REACTION

Defining Characteristics: Urticaria, pruritus, rash (maculopapular or erythematous), fever and chills, eosinophilia, myalgia, edema, erythema, angioedema. Increased risk in individuals allergic to penicillin.

Nursing Implications: Assess allergy to cephalosporin antibiotics and penicillin: if patient states "yes," determine actual response (e.g., "swollen lips = angioedema"). If angioedema, patient SHOULD NOT receive drug. Discuss other patient responses with physician to determine whether drug should be given. Assess baseline skin condition including integrity and allergy history to drugs. Teach patient to report rash, itching, and other skin changes. Teach patient skin care and symptomatic measures as appropriate. If skin rash develops, discuss drug discontinuance with physician.

II. ALTERATION IN NUTRITION, LESS THAN BODY REQUIREMENTS, related to GI SIDE EFFECTS

Defining Characteristics: Nausea, vomiting, diarrhea, and anorexia may occur. May cause transient increases in LFTs.

Nursing Implications: Assess baseline nutritional status. Teach patient to report GI disturbances. Administer and teach patient to self-administer antiemetics as needed and as ordered. Teach patient importance of nutritious diet and suggest small, frequent, high-calorie, high-protein meals as appropriate. Assess baseline LFTs and monitor periodically during treatment. Discuss abnormalities and drug interruption with physician.

III. FUNGAL SUPERINFECTION related to REDISTRIBUTION OF ENDOGENOUS MICROORGANISMS

Defining Characteristics: Vaginal moniliasis, vaginitis may occur as endogenous bacteria are eliminated and normal fungal population expands.

Nursing Implications: Teach female patient to report vaginal itching or discharge. Discuss appropriate antifungal treatment with physician. Teach perineal hygiene and symptomatic management.

IV. KNOWLEDGE DEFICIT related to SELF-ADMINISTRATION OF MEDICATION

Defining Characteristics: Increased compliance when patient is instructed in self-care activities.

Nursing Implications: Assess knowledge regarding infection and planned treatment. Teach about drug action, potential side effects, and when and how to take drug. Teach patient to report any possible side effects that occur.

Drug: cephalexin (Biocef, Keflex, Keftab)

Class: First-generation cephalosporin antibacterial.

Mechanism of Action: Semisynthetic derivative of cephalosporin C, contains β-lactam ring, and is related to penicillins and cephamycins. Bactericidal through inhibition of cell wall synthesis by binding to one or more of the penicillin-binding proteins (PBPs) that in turn inhibits the final transpeptidation step of peptidoglycan synthesis in bacterial cell walls, thus inhibiting cell wall biosynthesis. Bacteria eventually lyse due to ongoing activity of

COMPLICATIONS

cell wall autolytic enzymes (autolysins and murein hydrolases) while cell wall assembly is arrested.

Metabolism: Well-absorbed from GI tract; delayed GI absorption if taken with food, but total amount of drug absorption is the same. Widely distributed in body tissues, fluids except cerebrospinal fluid; readily crosses placenta and is excreted in breastmilk. Unchanged drug rapidly excreted by the kidneys.

Indication: For treatment of bacterial infections of the upper respiratory tract, otitis media, skin infections, and urinary tract infections. Active against *S. aureus, S. pneumoniae, H. influenza, E. coli*, and several other bacteria.

Dosage/Range:
- Adults: 250–1,000 mg every 6 hours, maximum—4 g/day.
- Dose-reduce if creatinine clearance is reduced per manufacturer's recommendations.

Drug Preparation:
- Store suspension in refrigerator, discard after 14 days.
- Oral administration.

Drug Interactions:
- Aminoglycosides increase nephrotic potential and increase toxicity.
- Probenecid may decrease cephalosporin elimination and increase effect.

Lab Effects/Interference:
- Serum SGPT, serum alk phos, serum SGOT, serum bilirubin, or serum LDH—values may be increased.
- BUN and serum creatinine—concentrations may be increased.

Special Considerations:
- Use with caution in patients with renal dysfunction—dose reduction required if severe impairment exists.
- Contraindicated in patients hypersensitive to other cephalosporin antibiotics.
- Use cautiously if sensitive to penicillin; contraindicated if angioedema reaction to penicillin.
- Obtain ordered specimen and send for culture and sensitivity prior to first drug dose.

Potential Toxicities/Side Effects and the Nursing Process

I.   POTENTIAL FOR INJURY related to HYPERSENSITIVITY REACTION

Defining Characteristics: Urticaria, pruritus, rash (maculopapular or erythematous), fever and chills, eosinophilia, myalgia, edema, erythema, angioedema. Increased risk in individuals allergic to penicillin.

Nursing Implications: Assess allergy to cephalosporin antibiotics and penicillin: if patient states "yes," determine actual response (e.g., "swollen lips = angioedema"). If angioedema, patient SHOULD NOT receive drug. Discuss other patient responses with physician to determine whether drug should be given. Assess baseline skin condition including integrity and allergy history to drugs. Teach patient to report rash, itching, other skin changes. Teach patient skin care and symptomatic measures as appropriate. If skin rash develops, discuss drug discontinuance with physician.

II. ALTERATION IN NUTRITION, LESS THAN BODY REQUIREMENTS, related to GI SIDE EFFECTS

Defining Characteristics: Nausea, vomiting, diarrhea, and anorexia may occur. Rarely, transient increases in LFTs—AST (SGOT), ALT (SGPT), alk phos, bili—may occur.

Nursing Implications: Assess baseline nutritional status. Teach patient to report GI disturbances. Administer and teach patient to self-administer medication as needed and as ordered. Teach patient importance of nutritious diet and suggest small, frequent, high-calorie, high-protein meals as appropriate. Assess baseline LFTs and monitor periodically during treatment. Discuss abnormalities and drug interruption with physician.

III. FUNGAL SUPERINFECTION related to REDISTRIBUTION OF ENDOGENOUS MICROORGANISMS

Defining Characteristics: Vaginal moniliasis, vaginitis may occur as endogenous bacteria are eliminated and normal fungal population expands.

Nursing Implications: Teach female patient to report vaginal itching or discharge. Discuss appropriate antifungal treatment with physician. Teach perineal hygiene and symptomatic management.

Drug: cephapirin (Cefadyl, cephapirin sodium)

Class: First-generation cephalosporin antibacterial.

Mechanism of Action: Semisynthetic derivative of cephalosporin C, contains β-lactam ring, and is related to penicillins and cephamycins. Bactericidal through inhibition of cell wall synthesis by binding to one or more of the penicillin-binding proteins (PBPs) that in turn inhibit the final transpeptidation step of peptidoglycan synthesis in bacterial cell walls, thus inhibiting cell wall biosynthesis. Bacteria eventually lyse due to ongoing activity of cell wall autolytic enzymes (autolysins and murein hydrolases) while cell wall assembly is arrested.

Metabolism: Well-absorbed from GI tract; delayed GI absorption if taken with food, but total amount of drug absorption is the same. Widely distributed in body tissues, fluids except cerebrospinal fluid; readily crosses placenta and is excreted in breastmilk. Unchanged drug rapidly excreted by the kidneys.

Indication: For treatment of infections caused by susceptible bacteria. Active in respiratory tract infections (*S. pneumoniae, Klebsiella species, H. influenza, S. aureus*, group A beta-hemolytic streptococci); skin infections (*S. aureus, S. epidermidis, E. coli, P. mirabilis*,

COMPLICATIONS

Klebsiella species, group A beta-hemolytic streptococci); urinary tract infections (*E. coli, Klebsiella species, P. mirabilis, S. aureus*); septicemia (*S. viridans, S. aureus, Klebsiella species, E. coli*, group A beta-hemolytic streptococci); endocarditis (*S. aureus, S. viridans*); osteomyelitis (*S. aureus, P. mirabilis, Klebsiella species*, group A beta-hemolytic streptococci).

Dosage/Range:
- Adults: 500–1,000 mg every 6 hours, maximum—4 g/day.
- Dose-reduce if creatinine clearance is reduced per manufacturer's recommendations.

Drug Preparation:
- Reconstituted solution is stable for 10 days when refrigerated.
- IV infusion in NS or D_5W solution stable for 10 days when refrigerated.

Drug Interactions:
- Aminoglycosides increase nephrotic potential and increase toxicity.
- Probenecid may decrease cephalosporin elimination and increase effect.

Lab Effects/Interference:
- Serum SGPT, serum alk phos, serum SGOT, serum bilirubin, or serum LDH—values may be increased.
- BUN and serum creatinine—concentrations may be increased.

Special Considerations:
- Use with caution in patients with renal dysfunction—dose reduction required if severe impairment exists.
- Contraindicated in patients hypersensitive to other cephalosporin antibiotics.
- Use cautiously if sensitive to penicillin; contraindicated if angioedema reaction to penicillin.
- Obtain ordered specimen and send for culture and sensitivity prior to first drug dose.

Potential Toxicities/Side Effects and the Nursing Process

I.   POTENTIAL FOR INJURY related to HYPERSENSITIVITY REACTION

Defining Characteristics: Urticaria, pruritus, rash (maculopapular or erythematous), fever and chills, eosinophilia, myalgia, edema, erythema, angioedema. Increased risk in individuals allergic to penicillin.

Nursing Implications: Assess allergy to cephalosporin antibiotics and penicillin: if patient states "yes," determine actual response (e.g., "swollen lips = angioedema"). If angioedema, patient SHOULD NOT receive drug. Discuss other patient responses with physician to determine whether drug should be given. Assess baseline skin condition including integrity and allergy history to drugs. Teach patient to report rash, itching, other skin changes. Teach patient skin care and symptomatic measures as appropriate. If skin rash develops, discuss drug discontinuance with physician.

II. ALTERATION IN NUTRITION, LESS THAN BODY REQUIREMENTS, related to GI SIDE EFFECTS

Defining Characteristics: Nausea, vomiting, diarrhea, and anorexia may occur. Rarely, transient increases in LFTs—AST (SGOT), ALT (SGPT), alk phos, bili—may occur.

Nursing Implications: Assess baseline nutritional status. Teach patient to report GI disturbances. Administer and teach patient to self-administer medication as needed and as ordered. Teach patient importance of nutritious diet and suggest small, frequent, high-calorie, high-protein meals as appropriate. Assess baseline LFTs and monitor periodically during treatment. Discuss abnormalities and drug interruption with physician.

III. FUNGAL SUPERINFECTION related to REDISTRIBUTION OF ENDOGENOUS MICROORGANISMS

Defining Characteristics: Vaginal moniliasis, vaginitis may occur as endogenous bacteria are eliminated and normal fungal population expands.

Nursing Implications: Teach female patient to report vaginal itching or discharge. Discuss appropriate antifungal treatment with physician. Teach perineal hygiene and symptomatic management.

Drug: cephradine (Anspor, Velosef)

Class: First-generation cephalosporin antibacterial.

Mechanism of Action: Semisynthetic derivative of cephalosporin C (produced by fungus); contains β-lactam ring and is related to penicillins and cephamycins (e.g., cefoxitin). Bactericidal through inhibition of cell wall synthesis, with resulting cell wall instability and cell lysis.

Metabolism: Poorly absorbed from GI tract so must be given parenterally. Widely distributed throughout body tissues and fluids, including CSF; 65–79% protein-bound. Crosses placenta and is excreted in breastmilk. Metabolized in liver and kidneys and is excreted in the urine.

Indication: For treatment of bacterial infections, including upper respiratory infections, ear infections, skin infections, and urinary tract infections. Active against many gram-positive aerobic cocci (streptococci, staphylococci) and has limited gram-negative activity (*Klebsiella, H. influenzae, E. coli, Proteus*). Used in treatment of infections of respiratory tract, GU tract, skin, bone and joint, meningitis, and sepsis.

Dosage/Range:
Adult:
- 500 mg–1 g IM or IV q 4–6 h; and in life-threatening infections, 2 g q 4 h.
- Dose reduction in renal insufficiency according to manufacturer's package insert.

COMPLICATIONS

Drug Preparation:
- Store vial of powder for injection at < 40°C (< 104°F), and frozen injection containers at ≤ −20° (−4°F).
- IV: Reconstitute with at least 10 mL sterile water for injection according to manufacturer's package insert. Further dilute in 100 mL 0.9% sodium chloride or 5% dextrose injection and administer over 30–60 minutes.
- IM: Reconstitute each gram of drug with 4 mL sterile water for injection. Administer deep IM in large muscle mass (e.g., gluteus maximus).

Drug Interactions:
- Probenecid: increased serum concentrations of antibiotic; monitor and decrease dose if needed.
- Aminoglycosides, penicillins: may have synergistic antibacterial effect against some organisms.
- Nephrotoxic drugs (aminoglycosides, colistin, vancomycin): may increase risk of renal dysfunction; avoid if possible.

Lab Effects/Interference:
Major clinical significance:
- Coombs' (antiglobulin) tests: a positive reaction frequently appears in patients who receive large doses of cephalosporins; hemolysis rarely occurs, but it has been reported; test may be positive in neonates whose mothers received cephalosporins before delivery.
- Urine glucose: some cephalosporins (cephradine) may produce a false-positive or falsely elevated test results with copper sulfate tests (Benedict's, Fehling's, or Clinitest); glucose enzymatic tests (Clinistix and Testape) are not affected.
- PT: may be prolonged; cephalosporins may inhibit vitamin K synthesis by suppressing gut flora.

Clinical significance:
- Serum ALT, serum alk phos, serum AST, serum bili, or serum LDH values may be increased.
- BUN and serum creatinine concentrations may be increased.
- CBC or platelet count: transient leukopenia, neutropenia, agranulocytosis, thrombocytopenia, eosinophilia, lymphocytosis, and thrombocytosis have been seen on rare occasions.

Special Considerations:
- Use with caution in patients with renal dysfunction; dose reduction required if severe impairment exists.
- Use cautiously if history of colitis exists.
- Contraindicated in patients hypersensitive to other cephalosporin antibiotics.
- Use cautiously if sensitive to penicillin; contraindicated if angioedema reaction to penicillin.
- Obtain specimen and send for culture and sensitivity prior to first drug dose.
- May cause false-positive direct Coombs' test.
- May cause false-positive Clinitest glucose result.

Potential Toxicities/Side Effects and the Nursing Process

I.   POTENTIAL FOR INJURY related to HYPERSENSITIVITY REACTION

Defining Characteristics: Urticaria, pruritus, rash (maculopapular or erythematous), fever and chills, eosinophilia, myalgia, edema, erythema, angioedema, Stevens-Johnson syndrome, and exfoliative skin reactions occur in 5% of patients. Increased risk in individuals allergic to penicillin.

Nursing Implications: Assess allergy to cephalosporin antibiotics and penicillin: if patient states "yes," determine actual response (e.g., "swollen lips = angioedema"). If angioedema, patient SHOULD NOT receive drug. Discuss other patient responses with physician to determine whether drug should be given. Assess baseline skin condition including integrity and allergy history to drugs. Instruct patient to report rash, itching, other skin changes. Teach patient skin care and symptomatic measures as appropriate. If skin rash develops, discuss drug discontinuance with physician. If rash progresses, drug should be discontinued, as fatal Stevens-Johnson syndrome may develop. Be prepared to treat severe acute hypersensitivity reactions with airway management, oxygen, epinephrine, corticosteroids, antihistamines as ordered.

II.   ALTERATION IN NUTRITION, LESS THAN BODY REQUIREMENTS, related to GI SIDE EFFECTS

Defining Characteristics: Nausea, vomiting, diarrhea, anorexia may occur; rarely, pseudomembranous colitis caused by *C. difficile* resistant to the antibiotic occurs. Rarely, transient increases in LFTs—AST, ALT, alk phos, bili—may occur.

Nursing Implications: Assess baseline nutritional status. Instruct patient to report GI disturbances. Administer and teach patient to self-administer antiemetics as needed and as ordered. Teach patient importance of nutritious diet and suggest small, frequent, high-calorie, high-protein meals as appropriate. Assess baseline LFTs and monitor periodically during treatment. Discuss abnormalities and drug interruption with physician.

III.   FUNGAL SUPERINFECTION related to REDISTRIBUTION OF ENDOGENOUS MICROORGANISMS

Defining Characteristics: Vaginal candidiasis, vaginitis may occur as endogenous bacteria are eliminated and normal fungal population expands.

Nursing Implications: Instruct female patient to report vaginal itching or discharge. Discuss appropriate antifungal treatment with physician. Teach perineal hygiene and symptomatic management.

COMPLICATIONS

IV.   ALTERATIONS IN PROTECTIVE MECHANISMS (RARE) related to TRANSIENT LEUKOPENIA

Defining Characteristics: Rarely, transient leukopenia, lymphocytosis, anemia, eosinophilia may occur. Prolonged PT, prolonged aPTT, and hypoprothrombinemia have occurred rarely, especially in elderly or debilitated patients, or in individuals with vitamin K deficiency.

Nursing Implications: Assess baseline laboratory parameters, and monitor periodically during treatment. Assess patient for response to antibiotics. Discuss abnormalities with physician.

V.   ALTERATIONS IN SENSORY/PERCEPTUAL PATTERNS related to DIZZINESS, SOMNOLENCE

Defining Characteristics: Dizziness, headache, somnolence occur rarely.

Nursing Implications: Assess baseline neurologic function and comfort and monitor during treatment. Instruct patient to report any changes. Discuss any abnormalities with physician.

VI.   ALTERATIONS IN COMFORT related to LOCAL INJECTION IRRITATION

Defining Characteristics: Pain, induration, sterile abscesses may form in IM injection sites; phlebitis may develop in IV sites.

Nursing Implications: Rotate IM injection sites and administer drug deep IM in large muscle mass (e.g., gluteus maximus). Use IM injection when IV administration is not possible. Change IV sites q 48 h, and assess for signs/symptoms of phlebitis prior to each administration. Administer drug slowly. Apply warm packs to increase comfort.

VII.   KNOWLEDGE DEFICIT related to SELF-ADMINISTRATION OF MEDICATION

Defining Characteristics: Increased compliance when patient is instructed in self-care activities.

Nursing Implications: Assess knowledge about infection and planned treatment. Teach about drug action, potential side effects, and when and how to take drug. Teach patient to report any side effects that occur.

Drug: ciprofloxacin (Cipro)

Class: Fluoroquinolone.

Mechanism of Action: Anti-infective; appears to inhibit DNA replication in susceptible bacteria.

Metabolism: Well-absorbed from GI tract; rate decreased by food but not extent of absorption. Widely distributed in body tissues and fluids with highest concentrations in organs, such as liver, kidneys, and lungs. Partially metabolized in liver; excreted in urine and feces. Crosses placenta and is excreted in breastmilk.

Indication: For treatment of different types of bacterial infections. Has a broad spectrum and is active against most gram-negative bacteria (e.g., *Enterobacter, Pseudomonas*), some gram-positive organisms (e.g., methicillin-resistant staphylococci), and some mycobacteria. Also used to treat people who have been exposed to anthrax.

Dosage/Range:
- 250–750 mg q 12 h × 1–2 weeks.
- IV: 200–400 mg q 12 h × 1–2 weeks (IV used if patient unable to take oral formulation).
- Dose modification necessary if renal impairment exists.

Drug Preparation:
- Oral: Take drug with a large glass of fluid, preferably 2 hours after meal/food. Encourage oral fluids of 2–3 qt/day.
- IV: Further dilute drug in 0.9% sodium chloride or 5% dextrose in water to final concentration of < 2 mg/mL. Administer over 60 minutes.

Drug Interactions:
- Antacids (containing magnesium, aluminum, or calcium): decrease oral ciprofloxacin serum level, do not administer concurrently. If must administer antacids, administer at least 2 hours apart.
- Other anti-infectives: potential synergism with clindamycin, aminoglycosides, β-lactam antibiotics against certain organisms.
- Probenecid: 50% increase in ciprofloxacin serum levels; decrease ciprofloxacin dose if given concurrently.
- Theophylline: increases theophylline serum level; avoid if possible, since fatal reactions have occurred. Otherwise, monitor theophylline level very closely and decrease theophylline dose as needed.
- Caffeine: delays caffeine clearance from body. Instruct patient to limit coffee, tea, soft drinks, especially if CNS side effects.

Lab Effects/Interference:
- Serum ALT, serum alk phos, serum AST, and serum LDH values may be increased.

Special Considerations:
- Used in the treatment of infections of urinary and lower respiratory tract, skin, bone and joint, and GI tract, as well as gonorrhea.
- Contraindicated in pregnancy and in women who are breastfeeding.
- Obtain ordered specimen for culture and sensitivity prior to first drug dose.
- Use cautiously in patients with seizure disorders.
- Use cautiously in patients receiving concurrent theophylline, as cardiopulmonary arrest has occurred.

COMPLICATIONS

Potential Toxicities/Side Effects and the Nursing Process

I.   ALTERATION IN NUTRITION, LESS THAN BODY REQUIREMENTS, related to GI SIDE EFFECTS

Defining Characteristics: 2–10% incidence of nausea, vomiting, abdominal discomfort, diarrhea, anorexia.

Nursing Implications: Assess baseline nutritional and elimination status. Instruct patient to report GI disturbances. Administer and teach patient to self-administer antiemetics, antidiarrheals as needed and as ordered. Teach patient importance of nutritious diet and suggest small, frequent, high-calorie, high-protein meals as appropriate. Assess baseline LFTs and monitor periodically during treatment. Discuss abnormalities and drug interruption with physician. Assess whether taking other hepatotoxic drugs. (See Special Considerations section.)

II.   ALTERATIONS IN SENSORY/PERCEPTUAL PATTERNS related to CNS EFFECTS

Defining Characteristics: 1–2% incidence of headache, restlessness. Dizziness, hallucinations, and seizures may also occur. Exacerbated by caffeine, as ciprofloxacin delays caffeine excretion.

Nursing Implications: Assess baseline neurologic function and comfort and monitor during treatment. Instruct patient to report any changes. Discuss any abnormalities with physician. Teach patient to limit or restrict all caffeine-containing fluids, medications, e.g., tea, coffee, soft drinks containing caffeine.

III.   ALTERATION IN SKIN INTEGRITY related to ALLERGY/HYPERSENSITIVITY

Defining Characteristics: 1–4% incidence of rash; other manifestations include eosinophilia, urticaria, flushing, fever, chills, photo-sensitivity, angioedema. Fatal hypersensitivity reactions have occurred rarely. Direct exposure to sunlight can cause sunburn (moderate to severe phototoxicity).

Nursing Implications: Assess baseline skin condition, including integrity and drug allergy history. Instruct patient to report rash, itching, other skin changes. Teach patient skin care and symptomatic measures as appropriate. If skin rash develops, discuss drug discontinuance with physician. If rash progresses, especially in HIV-infected patients, drug should be discontinued as fatal Stevens-Johnson syndrome may develop. Be prepared to treat severe acute hypersensitivity reactions with airway management, oxygen, epinephrine, corticosteroids, antihistamines as ordered. Instruct patient to avoid excessive sun exposure and to use skin protection factor (SPF) 15 or higher.

IV.   ALTERATION IN URINARY ELIMINATION related to RENAL TOXICITY

Defining Characteristics: Increased BUN and creatinine, crystal and stone formation in urine, interstitial nephritis, and renal failure may occur.

Nursing Implications: Assess baseline renal function; expect that drug dose will be decreased in presence of renal dysfunction. Instruct patient to take drug with at least 8 oz (240 mL) of water, and to increase oral fluids to 2–3 qt/day.

V. ALTERATION IN COMFORT related to IV ADMINISTRATION

Defining Characteristics: Drug may cause pain, inflammation, and rare thrombophlebitis at IV site.

Nursing Implications: Change IV site q 48 h. Assess for phlebitis, discomfort, and IV patency prior to each administration. Administer drug slowly over 60–90 minutes in large volume of 5% dextrose (see Drug Preparation). Apply heat to promote comfort.

VI. FUNGAL SUPERINFECTION related to REDISTRIBUTION OF ENDOGENOUS MICROORGANISMS

Defining Characteristics: Vaginal candidiasis, vaginitis may occur as endogenous bacteria are eliminated and normal fungal population expands.

Nursing Implications: Instruct female patient to report vaginal itching or discharge. Discuss appropriate antifungal treatment with physician. Teach perineal hygiene and symptomatic management.

Drug: clarithromycin (Biaxin, Biaxin XL)

Class: Antibacterial (macrolide).

Mechanism of Action: Clarithromycin exerts its antibacterial action by binding to 50S ribosomal subunit resulting in inhibition of protein synthesis. The 14-OH metabolite of clarithromycin is twice as active as the parent compound against certain organisms.

Metabolism: Rapidly and widely distributed throughout the body. Highly stable in presence of gastric acid (unlike erythromycin); food delays but does not affect extent of absorption. Widely distributed in body tissues but does not cross blood–brain barrier into CSF. Metabolized by liver and excreted by kidneys into urine.

Indication: For treatment of certain bacterial infections such as pneumonia, bronchitis, infections of the ears, sinuses, skin, and throat. Used to treat and prevent disseminated mycobacterium avium complex (MAC), a lung infection that often affects people with HIV. May be used in combination to eliminate *H. pylori*.

Dosage/Range:
- Adults: Usual dosage 250–500 mg every 12 hours or 1,000 mg (two 500-mg extended-release tablets) once daily for 7–14 days.
- Children ≥ 6 months: 15 mg/kg/day divided every 12 hours for 10 days.

COMPLICATIONS

Drug Preparation:
- Store tablets and granules for oral suspension at controlled room temperature.
- Reconstituted oral suspension should not be refrigerated because it might gel.
- Microencapsulated particles of clarithromycin in suspension are stable for 14 days when stored at room temperature.

Drug Interactions:
- Alfentanil (and possible other narcotic analgesics): Serum levels may be increased by clarithromycin—monitor for increased effect.
- Astemizole: Concomitant use is contraindicated—may lead to QT prolongation or torsades de pointes.
- Benzodiazepines (those metabolized by CYP3A4, including alprazolam and triazolam): Serum levels may be increased by clarithromycin—somnolence and confusion have been reported.
- Bromocriptine: Serum levels may be increased by clarithromycin—monitor for increased effect.
- Buspirone: Serum levels may be increased by clarithromycin—monitor.
- Calcium channel blockers (felodipine, verapamil, and potentially others metabolized by CYP3A4): Serum levels may be increased by clarithromycin—monitor.
- Carbamazepine: Serum levels may be increased by clarithromycin—monitor.
- Cisapride: Serum levels may be increased by clarithromycin—monitor.
- Cilostazol: Serum levels may be increased by clarithromycin—monitor.
- Clozapine: Serum levels may be increased by clarithromycin—monitor.
- Cyclosporine: Serum levels may be increased by clarithromycin—monitor serum levels.
- Delavirdine: Serum levels may be increased by clarithromycin.
- Digoxin: Serum levels may be increased by clarithromycin; digoxin toxicity and potentially fatal arrhythmias have been reported; monitor digoxin levels.
- Disopyramide: Serum levels may be increased by clarithromycin—monitor.
- Ergot alkaloids: Concurrent use may lead to acute ergot toxicity (severe peripheral vasospasm and dysesthesia).
- Fluconazole: Increases clarithromycin levels and AUC by ~25%.
- Indinavir: Serum levels may be increased by clarithromycin—monitor.
- Loratadine: Serum levels may be increased by clarithromycin—monitor.
- Neuromuscular-blocking agents: May be potentiated by clarithromycin (case reports).
- Oral contraceptives: Serum levels may be increased by clarithromycin—monitor.
- Phenytoin: Serum levels may be increased by clarithromycin; other evidence suggests phenytoin levels may be decreased in some patients—monitor.
- Pimozide: Serum levels may be increased, leading to malignant arrhythmias; concomitant use is contraindicated.
- Quinolone antibiotics (sparfloxacin, gatifloxacin, or moxifloxacin): Concomitant use may increase the risk of malignant arrhythmias—avoid concomitant use.
- Rifabutin: Serum levels may be increased by clarithromycin—monitor.
- Ritonavir: Concurrent use results in a 77% increase in clarithromycin levels (100% increase in metabolite levels); may be given together without dosage adjustment in patients with normal renal function; dosage of clarithromycin must be decreased in renal impairment.
- Sildenafil: Serum levels may be increased by clarithromycin—monitor.

- Tacrolimus: Serum levels may be increased by clarithromycin—monitor serum concentrations.
- Terfenadine: Serum levels may be increased by clarithromycin; may lead to QT prolongation, ventricular tachycardia, ventricular fibrillation or torsades de pointes; concomitant use is contraindicated.
- Theophylline: Serum levels may be increased by clarithromycin (by as much as 20%)—monitor.
- Valproic acid (and derivatives): Serum levels may be increased by clarithromycin—monitor.
- Warfarin: Effects may be potentiated—monitor INR closely and adjust warfarin dose as needed or choose another antibiotic.
- Zidovudine: Peak levels (but not AUC) of zidovudine may be increased—other studies suggest levels may be decreased.
- St. John's wort: May decrease clarithromycin levels.
- CYP3A3/4 enzyme substrate—CYP1A2 and CYP3A3/4 enzyme inhibitor.

Lab Effects/Interference:
- PT/INR—may be prolonged.
- Serum SGPT, serum alk phos, serum SGOT, serum bilirubin, or serum LDH—values may be increased.
- BUN and serum creatinine—concentrations may be increased.

Special Considerations:
- Use with caution in patients with renal dysfunction—dose reduction required if severe impairment exists.
- Do not use when there is known hypersensitivity to erythromycins or other macrolides.
- Obtain ordered specimen and send for culture and sensitivity prior to first drug dose.

Potential Toxicities/Side Effects and the Nursing Process

I. POTENTIAL FOR INJURY related to HYPERSENSITIVITY REACTION

Defining Characteristics: Urticaria, pruritus, rash (maculopapular or erythematous), fever and chills, eosinophilia, myalgia, edema, erythema, angioedema.

Nursing Implications: Assess allergy to erythromycin: if patient states "yes," determine actual response (e.g., "swollen lips = angioedema"). If angioedema, patient SHOULD NOT receive drug. Discuss other patient responses with physician to determine whether drug should be given. Assess baseline skin condition including integrity and allergy history to drugs. Teach patient to report rash, itching, other skin changes. Teach patient skin care and symptomatic measures as appropriate. If skin rash develops, discuss drug discontinuance with physician.

II. ALTERATION IN NUTRITION, LESS THAN BODY REQUIREMENTS, related to GI SIDE EFFECTS

Defining Characteristics: Abdominal pain, diarrhea, nausea, and vomiting may occur.

Nursing Implications: Assess baseline nutritional status, preexisting nausea/vomiting, anorexia. Assess baseline LFTs and monitor periodically during treatment. Teach

COMPLICATIONS

patient to report GI disturbances. Administer and teach patient to self-administer symptomatic interventions if side effects occur; discuss with physician use of alternative drug(s).

III.   FUNGAL SUPERINFECTION related to REDISTRIBUTION OF ENDOGENOUS MICROORGANISMS

Defining Characteristics: Vaginal moniliasis, vaginitis may occur as endogenous bacteria are eliminated and normal fungal population expands.

Nursing Implications: Teach female patient to report vaginal itching or discharge. Discuss appropriate antifungal treatment with physician. Teach perineal hygiene and symptomatic management.

IV.   ALTERATIONS IN PROTECTIVE MECHANISMS (RARE)

Defining Characteristics: Prolonged PT, prolonged INR, and hypoprothrombinemia have occurred rarely, especially in elderly or debilitated patients, or in individuals with vitamin K deficiency.

Nursing Implications: Assess baseline laboratory parameters and monitor periodically during treatment. Assess patient for response to antibiotics. Discuss abnormalities with physician. Assess for signs/symptoms of bleeding. If they occur, especially in elderly or debilitated patients, discuss vitamin K administration with physician. Teach patient to avoid aspirin. If taking oral anticoagulants, assess for increased PT, signs/symptoms of bleeding.

Drug: clindamycin phosphate (Cleocin)

Class: Antibacterial (systemic); antiprotozoal.

Mechanism of Action: Bacteriostatic or bactericidal depending on drug concentration or when used against highly susceptible organisms; binds to bacterial ribosomes and prevents peptide bond formation, thus inhibiting protein synthesis.

Metabolism: Well-absorbed (90% of dose) from GI tract. Food may delay absorption but does not affect amount absorbed. Widely distributed in body tissues and fluids, including bile. Crosses placenta and is excreted in breastmilk. Excreted in urine, bile, and feces.

Indication: For treatment of acute otitis media caused by penicillin-resistant *S. pneumoniae* and to be used in individuals with penicillin hypersensitivity; bone and joint infections including acute hematogenous osteomyelitis caused by *S. aureus* and as adjunct in surgical treatment of chronic bone and joint infections; gynecologic infections (endometritis, nongonococcal tubo-ovarian abscess, pelvic cellulitis, postsurgical vaginal cuff infections), including pelvic inflammatory disease; and intra-abdominal infections (peritonitis, intra-abdominal abscess). Clindamycin is an alternative treatment for pharyngitis and tonsillitis caused by susceptible *S. pyogenes* (group A beta-hemolytic streptococci) in patients who cannot receive beta-lactam anti-infectives and have infections caused by macrolide-resistant *S. pyogenes*. Respiratory tract infections, septicemia, skin and skin structures caused by susceptible anaerobes, *S. pneumoniae, S. pyogenes*, other streptococci, or *S. aureus*. Actinomycosis caused by *Actinomyces israelii*; Babesiosis caused by *Babesia microti*; Bacillus cereus diarrheal-type food poisoning caused by *Bacillus cereus*; bacterial vaginosis; Capnocytophaga infections caused by *Capnocytophaga canimorsus*; clostridial myonecrosis (gas gangrene) caused *Clostridium perfringens* or other Clostridium; malaria caused by chloroquine-resistant *Plasmodium falciparum*; pneumocystis jiroveci (*Pneumocystis carinii*) pneumonia; toxoplasmosis in immunocompromised adults, adolescents, or children (including HIV-infected patients); and anthrax. Active against gram-positive cocci (e.g., staphylococci, streptococci) and many anaerobic gram-positive and gram-negative bacilli (e.g., clostridia, mycobacteria). Prevention of bacterial endocarditis, perinatal group B streptococcal disease, and perioperative prophylaxis.

Dosage/Range:
Adult:
- Oral: 150–450 mg PO q 6 h; IM/IV: 300 mg q 6–12 h (maximum 2.7 g/day).

Drug Preparation:
- Oral: Administer with 8 oz (240 mL) of water to prevent esophageal irritation.
- IM: Single dose should not exceed 600 mg.
- Further dilute in 0.9% sodium chloride or 5% dextrose in water to final concentration < 12 mg/mL, and infuse over 20 minutes (600-mg dose) or 30–40 minutes (1.2-g dose). Maximum 1.2 g in single 1-hour period. May be given as continuous infusion.

Drug Interactions:
- Neuromuscular-blocking agents (tubocurarine, ether, pancuronium): may increase neuromuscular blockade; use concurrently with caution.
- Erythromycin: decreases bactericidal activity of clindamycin.
- Kaolin: decreases GI absorption of clindamycin. Avoid concurrent administration, or administer at least 2 hours apart.

Lab Effects/Interference:
- Serum ALT, serum alk phos, and serum AST concentrations may be increased.

Special Considerations:
- Contraindicated in patients with hypersensitivity to clindamycin or lincomycin; contraindicated in patients with history of colitis.
- Can cause severe, sometimes fatal colitis. Stop drug if diarrhea develops, or if necessary, continue only under close monitoring and endoscopy.
- Used in the treatment of serious infections of respiratory tract, skin/soft tissues, female pelvic/genital tract. May be used investigationally with other drugs in treatment of

Mycobacterium avium complex (MAC); also may be used to treat *P. carinii* pneumonia, crypto-sporidiosis, and toxoplasmosis in AIDS patients.

- Also used for prophylaxis of bacterial endocarditis in penicillin-allergic, erythromycin-intolerant patients.
- DO NOT GIVE rapid IVB: cardiopulmonary arrest has occurred.
- Avoid use in pregnant or breastfeeding women.

Potential Toxicities/Side Effects and the Nursing Process

I.   ALTERATION IN NUTRITION, LESS THAN BODY REQUIREMENTS, related to GI SIDE EFFECTS

Defining Characteristics: Nausea, vomiting, diarrhea, abdominal pain, and tenesmus may occur. Flatulence, bloating, anorexia, and esophagitis may occur as well. Fatal pseudomembranous colitis has occurred, characterized by severe diarrhea, abdominal cramping, and melena. Usually begins 2–9 days after drug is initiated.

Nursing Implications: Assess elimination and nutrition pattern, baseline and during therapy. Instruct patient to report diarrhea and/or abdominal pain immediately. Discuss drug discontinuance with physician if diarrhea occurs. Guaiac stool for occult blood, and notify physician if positive. If severe diarrhea develops, discuss management plan including endoscopy, and fluid and electrolyte replacement. Do not administer antiperistaltic agents such as opiates and diphenoxylate with atropine (Lomotil), since it may worsen condition. Assess for nausea/vomiting, and administer prescribed antiemetic medications. Encourage small, frequent feedings as tolerated. Instruct patient to take oral dose with a full glass of water.

II.   ALTERATION IN SKIN INTEGRITY related to HYPERSENSITIVITY

Defining Characteristics: Maculopapular rash, urticaria may occur. Rarely, erythema multiforme may occur. Increased risk of allergic reaction in asthma patients. Anaphylaxis may rarely occur.

Nursing Implications: Assess baseline allergy history. Assess baseline skin integrity. Instruct patient to report rash, pruritus. Teach patient symptomatic management of rash, pruritus. Assess for hypersensitivity reaction; if it occurs, monitor vital signs (VS), discontinue drug, notify physician, and institute supportive measures.

III.   ALTERATIONS IN COMFORT related to LOCAL ADMINISTRATION EFFECTS

Defining Characteristics: IM administration may cause pain, induration, sterile abscesses, and transient increase in creatine phosphokinase (CPK) due to muscle injury. IV administration may cause erythema, pain, swelling, and thrombophlebitis.

Nursing Implications: Administer maximum 600-mg dose IM deeply in large muscle mass (e.g., gluteus maximus). Rotate sites. Assess IV site prior to each dose for phlebitis or swelling, and change site at least q 48 h. Administer dose slowly: 300–600 mg in 50 mL over 20–30 minutes, and 900-mg to 1200-mg dose in 100 mL IV over 40–60 minutes. Apply heat to painful IV sites as ordered.

IV. ALTERATION IN HEPATIC FUNCTION related to TRANSIENT INCREASES IN LFTs

Defining Characteristics: Transient increases in serum bili, AST, alk phos have occurred.

Nursing Implications: Assess baseline LFTs, and monitor during therapy.

V. FUNGAL SUPERINFECTION related to REDISTRIBUTION OF ENDOGENOUS MICROORGANISMS

Defining Characteristics: Vaginal candidiasis, vaginitis may occur as endogenous bacteria are eliminated and normal fungal population expands.

Nursing Implications: Instruct female patient to report vaginal itching or discharge. Discuss appropriate antifungal treatment with physician. Teach perineal hygiene and symptomatic management.

Drug: colistimethate injection (Coly-Mycin M)

Class: Antibacterial (systemic).

Mechanism of Action: Colistimethate sodium is a surface-active agent that penetrates into and disrupts the bacterial cell membrane.

Metabolism: Partially metabolized, and excreted primarily in urine.

Indication: For treatment of bacterial infections in many different parts of the body, including most strains of aerobic gram-negative microorganisms *Enterobacter aerogenes*, *E. coli*, *Klebsiella pneumoniae*, and *P. aeruginosa*.

Dosage/Range:
- Given IV or IM (IV preferred for doses > 1 g, and for serious infections).
- Adults: Maximum daily dose should not exceed 5 mg/kg/day (2.3 mg/lb) with normal renal function. Should be given in 2 to 4 divided doses at dose levels of 2.5 to 5 mg/kg per day for patients with normal renal function, depending on the severity of the infection.
- In obese individuals, dosage should be based on ideal body weight.
- Dose modification needed for renal dysfunction and may need to modify dosage in hepatic impairment.

COMPLICATIONS

Suggested Modification of Dosage Schedules of Colistimethate for Injection, USP for Adults with Impaired Renal Function

Acute Bacterial Exacerbation of:	Chronic Bronchitis, Community-Acquired	Pneumonia, Acute Maxillary Sinusitis, Uncomplicated Skin Infections
Renal status	Initial dose	Subsequent dose
Cr cl 20–49 mL/min	500 mg	250 mg q 24 h
Cr cl 10–19 mL/min	500 mg	250 mg q 48 h
Hemodialysis	500 mg	250 mg q 48 h
CAPD	500 mg q 48 h	250 mg q 48 h
Uncomplicated UTI/Acute Pyelonephritis		
Cr cl 10–19 mL/min	250 mg	250 mg q 48 h

Drug Preparation:

- The 150-mg vial should be reconstituted with 2 mL sterile water for injection, USP. The reconstituted solution provides colistimethate sodium at a concentration equivalent to 75 mg/mL colistin base activity.
- During reconstitution swirl gently to avoid frothing.
- Parenteral drug products should be inspected visually for particulate matter and discoloration prior to administration, whenever solution and container permit. If these conditions are observed, the product should not be used.
- *Direct intermittent administration:* Slowly inject one-half of the total daily dose over a period of 3 to 5 minutes every 12 hours.
- *Continuous infusion:* Slowly inject one-half of the total daily dose over 3 to 5 minutes. Add the remaining half of the total daily dose of colistimethate for injection, USP, to one of the following: 0.9% NaCl; 5% dextrose in 0.9% NaCl; 5% dextrose in water; 5% dextrose in 0.45% NaCl; 5% dextrose in 0.225% NaCl; lactated Ringer's solution; 10% invert sugar solution.
- Insufficient data to recommend usage of colistimethate for injection, USP, with other drugs or other than the previously listed infusion solutions.
- Administer the second half of the total daily dose by slow IV infusion, starting 1 to 2 hours after the initial dose, over the next 22 to 23 hours.
- In the presence of impaired renal function, reduce the infusion rate depending on the degree of renal impairment. The choice of IV solution and the volume to be employed are dictated by the requirements of fluid and electrolyte management.
- Any infusion solution containing colistimethate sodium should be freshly prepared and used for no longer than 24 hours.

Drug Interactions:

- Curariform muscle relaxants (e.g., tubocurarine) and other drugs, including ether, succinylcholine, gallamine, decamethonium, and sodium citrate, potentiate the neuromuscular blocking effect and should be used with extreme caution in patients being treated with colistimethate.

Drug: colistimethate injection **1329**

- Aminoglycosides and penicillins have been reported to interfere with nerve transmission at the neuromuscular junction. They should not be given with colistimethate.
- Nephrotoxic drugs (aminoglycosides, colistin, vancomycin) may increase risk of renal dysfunction; avoid if possible.

Lab Effects/Interference:
- None well-documented.

Special Considerations:
- The use of colistimethate for injection, USP, is contraindicated for patients with a history of sensitivity to the drug or any of its components.
- Transient neurologic disturbances may occur. These include circumoral paresthesia or numbness, tingling or formication of the extremities, generalized pruritus, vertigo, dizziness, and slurring of speech. For these reasons, patients should be warned not to drive vehicles or use hazardous machinery while on therapy. Reduction of dosage may alleviate symptoms. Therapy need not be discontinued, but such patients should be observed with particular care.
- Nephrotoxicity can occur and is probably a dose-dependent effect of colistimethate sodium. These manifestations of nephrotoxicity are reversible following discontinuation of the antibiotic.
- Respiratory arrest has been reported following IM administration of colistimethate sodium. Impaired renal function increases the possibility of apnea and neuromuscular blockade following administration of colistimethate sodium. Follow recommended dosing guidelines.
- Obtain and send specimen for culture and sensitivity prior to first drug dose.
- Use cautiously if prior immediate hypersensitivity reaction to penicillins or cephalosporins; little risk of cross-allergenicity, but monitor patient closely.
- Use with caution in patients with renal or hepatic dysfunction.

Potential Toxicities/Side Effects and the Nursing Process

I. ALTERATIONS IN SKIN INTEGRITY related to ALLERGY HYPERSENSITIVITY REACTION

Defining Characteristics: Incidence of rash that is mild, transient, pruritic, and/or erythematous. Incidence of immediate hypersensitivity reaction characterized by angioedema, bronchospasm, severe shock. Little cross-allergenicity with penicillins, cephalosporins (less than 1%).

Nursing Implications: Assess baseline skin integrity and presence of drug allergies; if anaphylactic reaction to penicillins or cephalosporins, monitor patient closely during drug infusions. Instruct patient to report immediately signs/symptoms of rash, pruritus, shortness of breath, and adverse sensation. Teach patient skin care and symptomatic measures as appropriate. If skin rash develops, discuss drug discontinuance with physician. If rash progresses, especially in HIV-infected patients, drug should be discontinued, as fatal Stevens-Johnson syndrome may develop. Be prepared to treat severe acute hypersensitivity reactions with airway management, oxygen, epinephrine, corticosteroids, antihistamines as ordered.

II.   ALTERATION IN NUTRITION, LESS THAN BODY REQUIREMENTS, related to GI SIDE EFFECTS

Defining Characteristics: Nausea, vomiting, diarrhea, anorexia may occur; rarely, pseudomembranous colitis caused by *C. difficile* resistant to the antibiotic occurs. Rarely, transient increases in LFTs—AST, ALT, alk phos—may occur.

Nursing Implications: Assess baseline nutritional status. Instruct patient to report GI disturbances. Administer and teach patient to self-administer antiemetics as needed and as ordered. Teach patient importance of nutritious diet and suggest small, frequent, high-calorie, high-protein meals as appropriate. Assess baseline LFTs, and monitor periodically during treatment. Discuss abnormalities and drug interruption with physician. Encourage oral hygiene after meals and at bedtime.

III.   FUNGAL SUPERINFECTION related to REDISTRIBUTION OF ENDOGENOUS MICROORGANISMS

Defining Characteristics: Vaginal candidiasis, vaginitis may occur as endogenous bacteria are eliminated and normal fungal population expands.

Nursing Implications: Instruct female patient to report vaginal itching or discharge. Discuss appropriate antifungal treatment with physician. Teach perineal hygiene and symptomatic management.

IV.   ALTERATIONS IN SENSORY/PERCEPTUAL PATTERNS related to DIZZINESS, SOMNOLENCE

Defining Characteristics: Tingling of extremities and tongue, slurred speech, dizziness, vertigo, and paresthesia have occurred.

Nursing Implications: Assess baseline neurologic function and comfort and monitor during treatment. Instruct patient to report any changes. Discuss any abnormalities with physician.

V.   ALTERATIONS IN COMFORT related to LOCAL INJECTION IRRITATION

Defining Characteristics: Potential for incidence of phlebitis and thrombophlebitis when administering IV; potential incidence of pain and swelling at injection site when given IM.

Nursing Implications: Rotate IM injection sites and administer drug deep IM in large muscle mass (e.g., gluteus maximus). Use IM injection when IV administration is not possible. Change IV sites q 48 h and assess for signs/symptoms of phlebitis prior to each administration. Administer drug slowly. Apply warm packs to increase comfort.

Drug: co-trimoxazole; trimethoprim and sulfamethoxazole (Bactrim, Bactrim DS, Cotrim, Septra)

Class: Sulfonamide antibacterial (systemic); antiprotozoal.

Mechanism of Action: Bactericidal by preventing folic acid synthesis so microorganism cannot undergo cell division (sequential inhibition of folic acid synthesis, first by sulfamethoxazole, then by trimethoprim).

Metabolism: Rapidly absorbed from GI tract. Widely distributed into body tissues and fluids; crosses the placenta and is excreted in breastmilk. Highly protein-bound. Metabolized by the liver and excreted in the urine.

Indication: For treatment of many bacterial infections, such as pneumonia, bronchitis (*S. pneumoniae, H. influenzae, Legionella micdadei, L. pittsburgensis,* or *L. pneumoniae*), infections of the urinary tract (*E. coli, Klebsiella, Enterobacter, Morganella morganii, P. mirabilis,* or *P. vulgaris*), ears (*S. pneumoniae* or *H. influenza*), and intestines (susceptible enterotoxigenic *E. coli,* enteroinvasive *E. coli, Shigella flexneri* or *Shigella sonnei, Yersinia enterocolitica, Yersinia pseudotuberculosis*). Active against gram-positive bacteria (streptococci, *S. aureus, Nocardia*), gram-negative bacteria (*Enterobacter, E. coli, Proteus, Klebsiella, Shigella*), and protozoa (*P. carinii*).

Dosage/Range:
Adult:
- Oral: Trimethoprim 160 mg and sulfamethoxazole 800 mg (double-strength tablet DS) q 12 h × 7–14 days (depending on infection).
- Oral: *P. carinii* pneumonia prophylaxis: one DS tablet twice daily 2 days per week (typically consecutive) or one DS tablet every other day.
- IV: 10–20 mg/kg in two to four divided doses q 6–8 h (usually 21 days for *P. carinii* pneumonia in AIDS patients).
- Dose modification if renal impairment exists.

Drug Preparation:
- Oral tablets should be stored in tight, light-resistant containers; vials of powder for injection and suspension should be stored at 15–30°C (59–86°F).

Drug Administration:
- Oral: Administer with full (8 oz or 240 mL) glass of water.
- IV: Add each 5 mL of drug to 125 mL of 5% dextrose in water ONLY. Stable for 6 hours. If patient is fluid restricted, can mix each 5 mL in 75 mL of 5% dextrose immediately prior to administration and give within 2 hours. DO NOT REFRIGERATE. Administer over 60–90 minutes.

Drug Interactions:
- Warfarin: increases PT. Monitor PT closely and decrease dose of warfarin as needed.
- Sulfonylureas: increases hypoglycemic effect. Monitor blood glucose closely and reduce sulfonylurea dose as needed.

COMPLICATIONS

- Phenytoin: increases and prolongs serum levels. Monitor serum phenytoin level closely and reduce dose as needed.
- Thiazide diuretics (in elderly): increases toxicity (thrombocytopenia with purpura). AVOID CONCURRENT USE.
- Cyclosporine: decreases cyclosporine effect; increases risk of nephrotoxicity. AVOID CONCURRENT USE when possible.
- Methotrexate: increases methotrexate level and potential toxicity (e.g., bone marrow depression). Monitor levels or decrease methotrexate dose as needed.
- Oral contraceptives: decreases contraceptive effect. Monitor for breakthrough bleeding and counsel patient to use barrier contraceptive in addition during antibiotic therapy.
- Ammonium chloride or ascorbic acid: causes antibiotic drug precipitation in kidneys. AVOID CONCURRENT USE.

Lab Effects/Interference:
- Jaffe alkaline picrate reaction overestimation of creatinine by 10%.

Special Considerations:
- Drug is teratogenic, so should not be used in pregnant women if avoidable.
- Drug is excreted in breastmilk and can cause kernicterus in infants. Alternative drug should be used or mother should interrupt breastfeeding during drug use.
- Contraindicated if patient has porphyria.
- Contraindicated in patients with hypersensitivity to sulfites, sulfonamides, or to trimethoprim.
- Contraindicated if severe renal failure (creatinine clearance < 15 mL/minute).
- Use with caution at reduced dosage in patients with glucose-6-phosphate dehydrogenase deficiency (G6PD); hemolysis may occur. Also, use with caution in patients with impaired renal or hepatic function, severe allergy, bronchial asthma, and blood dyscrasias.
- Use cautiously in patients with known hypersensitivity to sulfonamide-derivative drugs such as thiazides, acetazolamide, tolbutamide.
- Increased incidence of adverse side effects in AIDS patients, especially allergic, hematologic reactions. Monitor closely for toxicity.
- Drug is first-line treatment for *P. carinii* pneumonia; it is at least as effective as pentamidine, with a cure rate of 70–80%.
- Send specimen for culture and sensitivity prior to initial drug dose, as appropriate.

Potential Toxicities/Side Effects and the Nursing Process

I.   ALTERATION IN SKIN INTEGRITY related to HYPERSENSITIVITY REACTION

Defining Characteristics: Skin reactions ranging from mild maculopapular rash with urticaria, pruritus to erythema multiforme, exfoliative dermatitis, and Stevens-Johnson syndrome. Risk for rash is increased in AIDS patients; usually occurs 7–14 days after beginning drug. Other allergic manifestations include fever, chills, photosensitivity, angioedema, and anaphylaxis.

Nursing Implications: Assess for prior hypersensitivity to drug. Assess for signs/symptoms of drug allergy. Instruct patient to report rash, allergic reaction immediately. Discuss any drug continuance with physician if rash appears. Teach patient symptomatic management of discomfort and skin irritation. Be prepared to treat severe acute hypersensitivity reactions with airway management, oxygen, epinephrine, corticosteroids, antihistamines as ordered.

II. POTENTIAL FOR INFECTION, BLEEDING, AND FATIGUE related to HEMATOLOGIC TOXICITY

Defining Characteristics: Leukopenia, neutropenia, and thrombocytopenia are common in AIDS patients. Agranulocytosis, aplastic and megaloblastic anemia, thrombocytopenia, hemolytic anemia, neutropenia, hypoprothrombinemia, and eosinophilia may occur less commonly. Increased risk exists in folate-deficient patients: elderly, alcoholic, malnourished; also, patients receiving folate antimetabolites, e.g., phenytoin, methotrexate, or thiazide diuretics; or in patients with renal dysfunction.

Nursing Implications: Assess baseline risk, CBC, and monitor CBC periodically during treatment. Assess for and teach patient to monitor signs/symptoms of infection, bleeding, fatigue, and to report these. If side effects occur, discuss with physician use of folinic acid (leucovorin).

III. ALTERATION IN NUTRITION, LESS THAN BODY REQUIREMENTS, related to GI TOXICITY

Defining Characteristics: Nausea, vomiting, and anorexia are most common; pseudomembranous colitis, glossitis, stomatitis, abdominal pain, diarrhea may occur.

Nursing Implications: Assess GI function. Teach patient to assess for and instruct to report GI side effects, and to administer prescribed antiemetics or antidiarrheals as needed. Assess oral mucosa, and if stomatitis develops, discuss with physician use of leucovorin (folinic acid). Teach patient oral hygiene. Take drug with 8 oz (240 mL) water to prevent esophageal ulcerations. Discuss food preferences, use of spices, and suggest small, frequent meals if anorexia develops.

IV. SENSORY/PERCEPTUAL DYSFUNCTION related to FATIGUE, WEAKNESS

Defining Characteristics: Headache, vertigo, insomnia, fatigue, weakness, mental depression, seizures, and hallucinations may occur.

Nursing Implications: Assess baseline neurologic function and comfort and monitor during treatment. Instruct patient to report any changes. Discuss any abnormalities with physician.

V. ALTERATION IN URINARY ELIMINATION related to RENAL TOXICITY

Defining Characteristics: Increased BUN and creatinine, crystal and stone formation in urine, interstitial nephritis, and renal failure may occur.

COMPLICATIONS

Nursing Implications: Assess baseline renal function; expect that drug dose will be decreased in presence of renal dysfunction. Instruct patient to take drug with at least 8 oz water and to increase oral fluids to 2–3 qt/day.

VI.   ALTERATION IN COMFORT related to IV ADMINISTRATION

Defining Characteristics: Drug may cause pain, inflammation, and rare thrombophlebitis at IV site.

Nursing Implications: Change IV site q 48 h. Assess for phlebitis, discomfort, and IV patency prior to each administration. Administer drug slowly over 60–90 minutes in large volume of 5% dextrose (see Drug Administration). Apply heat to promote comfort.

VII.   FUNGAL SUPERINFECTION related to REDISTRIBUTION OF ENDOGENOUS MICROORGANISMS

Defining Characteristics: Vaginal candidiasis, vaginitis may occur as endogenous bacteria are eliminated and normal fungal population expands.

Nursing Implications: Instruct female patient to report vaginal itching or discharge. Discuss appropriate antifungal treatment with physician. Teach perineal hygiene and symptomatic management.

Drug: dalbavancin (Dalvance)

Class: Antibacterial (systemic).

Mechanism of Action: Semisynthetic lipoglycopeptide, interferes with cell wall synthesis, thereby preventing cross-linking. Dalbavancin is bactericidal in vitro against *Staphylococcus aureus* and *Streptococcus pyogenes.*

Metabolism: Drug is not a substrate, inhibitor, or inducer of CYP450 isoenzymes. A minor metabolite of dalbavancin (hydroxy-dalbavancin) has been observed in urine. A small percentage (20% of dose) is excreted in feces. An average 33% of the administered dose is excreted in urine as unchanged dalbavancin; 12% of administered dose is excreted in urine as metabolite hydroxy-dalbavancin.

Indications: Acute bacterial skin and skin structure infections (ABSSSI) caused by designated susceptible strains of gram-positive microorganisms—*Staphylococcus aureus* (including methicillin-susceptible and -resistant strains), *Streptococcus pyogenes*, *Streptococcus agalactiae*, and *Streptococcus anginosus* group (including *S. anginosus*, *S. intermedius*, and *S. constellatus*).

Dosage/Range:
- Two-dose regimen: 1,000 mg, followed one week later by 500 mg.
- Dosage adjustment for patients with creatinine clearance less than 30 mL/min and not receiving regularly scheduled hemodialysis: 750 mg, followed one week later by 375 mg.
- Administer by IV infusion over 30 minutes.

Drug Preparation:
- Reconstituted vials may be stored either refrigerated at 2–8°C (36–46°F), or at controlled room temperature (20–25°C [68–77°F]). Do not freeze.
- Aseptically transfer required dose of reconstituted dalbavancin solution from vial(s) to an IV bag or bottle containing 5% dextrose injection, USP. The diluted solution must have a final dalbavancin concentration of 1–5 mg/mL. Discard any unused portion of the reconstituted solution.
- Once diluted into an IV bag or bottle, drug may be stored either refrigerated at 2–8°C (36–46°F) or at controlled room temperature (20–25°C [68–77°F]). Do not freeze.
- Total time from reconstitution to dilution to administration should not exceed 48 hours.
- Inspect visually for particulate matter prior to infusion. If particulate matter is identified, do not use.
- Administered via IV infusion, using a total infusion time of 30 minutes.
- Do not co-infuse with other medications or electrolytes. Saline-based infusion solutions may cause precipitation and should not be used. Compatibility with intravenous medications, additives, or substances other than 5% dextrose injection, USP has not been established.
- If a common IV line is being used to administer other drugs, line should be flushed with 5% dextrose injection, USP before and after each dalbavancin infusion.

Drug Interaction: No clinical drug–drug interaction studies have been conducted. There is minimal potential for drug–drug interactions between dalbavancin and cytochrome P450 (CYP450) substrates, inhibitors, or inducers.

Lab Effects/Interference: Drug–lab test interactions have not been reported.

Special Considerations:
- Most common adverse reactions in patients treated with dalbavancin were nausea (5.5%), headache (4.7%), and diarrhea (4.4%).
- Hypersensitivity to dalbavancin is possible.
- Serious hypersensitivity (anaphylactic) and skin reactions have been reported with glycopeptide antibacterial agents, including dalbavancin; exercise caution in patients with known hypersensitivity to glycopeptides.
- Rapid IV infusion of glycopeptide antibacterial agents can cause reactions.
- ALT elevations with dalbavancin treatment were reported in clinical trials.
- *Clostridium difficile*–associated diarrhea (CDAD) is reported with nearly all systemic antibacterial agents, including dalbavancin. Evaluate if diarrhea occurs.

COMPLICATIONS

Potential Toxicities/Side Effects and the Nursing Process

I.   POTENTIAL FOR INJURY related to HYPERSENSITIVITY REACTION

Defining Characteristics: Urticaria, pruritus, rash (maculopapular or erythematous), fever and chills, eosinophilia, myalgia, edema, erythema, and angioedema.

Nursing Implications: Assess allergy to cephalosporin antibiotics and penicillin; if patient states "yes," determine actual response (e.g., "swollen lips angioedema"). If angioedema is present, patient *should not* receive drug. Discuss other patient responses with physician to determine whether drug should be given. Assess baseline skin condition, including integrity, and allergy history to drugs. Instruct patient to report rash, itching, and other skin changes. Teach patient skin care and symptomatic measures as appropriate. If skin rash develops, discuss drug discontinuance with physician. If rash progresses, drug should be discontinued, as fatal Stevens-Johnson syndrome may develop. Be prepared to treat severe acute hypersensitivity reactions with airway management, oxygen, epinephrine, corticosteroids, and antihistamines as ordered.

II.   ALTERATION IN NUTRITION, LESS THAN BODY REQUIREMENTS, related to GI SIDE EFFECTS

Defining Characteristic: Nausea, vomiting, diarrhea, and anorexia may occur; rarely, pseudomembranous colitis caused by *C. difficile* resistant to the antibiotic occurs.

Nursing Implications: Assess baseline nutritional status. Instruct patient to report GI disturbances. Administer, and teach patient to self-administer, antiemetics as needed and as ordered. Teach patient importance of a nutritious diet; suggest small, frequent, high-calorie, high-protein meals as appropriate. Assess baseline LFTs and monitor periodically during treatment. Discuss abnormalities and drug interruption with physician.

III.   FUNGAL SUPERINFECTION related to REDISTRIBUTION OF ENDOGENOUS MICROORGANISMS

Defining Characteristics: Vaginal candidiasis and vaginitis may occur as endogenous bacteria are eliminated and normal fungal population expands.

Nursing Implications: Instruct female patients to report vaginal itching or discharge. Discuss appropriate antifungal treatment with physician. Teach perineal hygiene and symptomatic management.

IV.   ALTERATIONS IN COMFORT related to LOCAL INJECTION-SITE IRRITATION

Defining Characteristics: Pain and phlebitis may develop in IV sites.

Nursing Implications: Change IV sites every 48 hours, and assess for signs and symptoms of phlebitis prior to each administration. Administer drug slowly. Apply warm packs to increase comfort.

V. ALTERATIONS IN COMFORT related to HEADACHE

Defining Characteristics: Headache has occurred in some patients.

Nursing Implications: Assess baseline hearing (ability to hear spoken voice) and continue to assess during therapy. Teach patient potential side effects, and instruct patient to report any hearing/perceptual problems (e.g., tinnitus, vertigo, decreased hearing). Discuss drug discontinuance and audiogram with physician to confirm hearing dysfunction if symptoms arise. Assess for increased risk if given concurrently with other ototoxic medications (e.g., cisplatin, furosemide).

Drug: daptomycin (Cubicin)

Class: Cyclic lipopeptide antibiotic.

Mechanism of Action: This antibiotic is the first in a new structural class. It is derived from the fermentation of *Streptomyces roseosporus*. The mechanism of action is not fully understood. Daptomycin binds to bacterial membranes and causes a rapid depolarization of membrane potential. This loss of membrane potential leads to inhibition of protein, DNA, and RNA synthesis resulting in bacterial cell death. It acts against gram-positive bacteria, and retains in vitro potency against isolates resistant to methicillin, vancomycin, and linezolid.

Metabolism: Excreted by the kidney. Renal excretion is primary route of elimination.

Indication: For treatment of complicated skin and skin structure infections (cSSSI) and septicemias including right-sided endocarditis.

Dosage/Range:
Adult:
• 4 mg/kg by IV infusion q d for 7–14 days.
• Drug dose should be reduced or adjusted in patients with severe renal insufficiency.

Drug Preparation:
• 0.9% sodium chloride injection.
• Administer over 30 minutes.

Drug Interactions:
• Tobramycin: interaction between daptomycin and tobramycin is unknown. Caution is warranted when daptomycin is coadministered with tobramycin.
• Warfarin: anticoagulant activity in patients receiving daptomycin and warfarin should be monitored for the first several days.

Lab Effects/Interference:
• No reported drug-laboratory test interactions.

COMPLICATIONS

Special Considerations:
- Contraindicated in patients with known hypersensitivity to daptomycin.
- Obtain ordered specimen and send for culture and sensitivity prior to first antibiotic dose.
- Consider alternative antibiotic therapy if anemia, drug rash or fever, arthralgia, or unexplained rise in BUN and serum creatinine occur.

Potential Toxicities/Side Effects and the Nursing Process

I. ALTERATION IN NUTRITION, LESS THAN BODY REQUIREMENTS, related to GI SIDE EFFECTS

Defining Characteristics: Constipation, nausea, diarrhea, vomiting, dyspepsia.

Nursing Implications: Assess baseline nutritional status, preexisting nausea/vomiting, anorexia. Assess baseline bowel pattern. Administer symptomatic interventions if side effects occur; discuss with physician use of alternative drug(s).

II. POTENTIAL FOR INJURY related to HYPERSENSITIVITY REACTION

Defining Characteristics: Rash, urticaria, pruritus, and fever can occur in individuals with hypersensitivity to daptomycin.

Nursing Implications: Assess for drug allergies prior to drug administration. Instruct patient to report any allergic reactions. Assess for signs/symptoms of allergic reaction after drug dose.

III. SENSORY/PERCEPTUAL ALTERATIONS related to CNS EFFECTS OF DIZZINESS AND HEADACHE

Defining Characteristics: Dizziness, headache, and insomnia may occur.

Nursing Implications: Assess baseline neurologic status. Teach patient about side effects and to report dizziness or headache. If signs/symptoms arise, discuss drug discontinuance with physician.

Drug: demeclocycline hydrochloride (Declomycin)

Class: Antibacterial (systemic); tetracycline; antiprotozoal.

Mechanism of Action: Bacteriostatic but may be bactericidal at high concentrations. Binds to bacterial ribosomes and prevents protein synthesis.

Metabolism: Absorbed from the GI tract. Widely distributed into body tissues and fluids. Crosses placenta and is excreted in breastmilk. Concentrated in the liver, excreted into the bile. The rate of demeclocycline hydrochloride clearance is less than half that of tetracycline.

Indication: For treatment of a broad range of gram-negative and gram-positive organisms. Demeclocycline hydrochloride may also be used in special cases of fluid retention (SIADH). A syndrome of polyuria, polydipsia, and weakness has been shown to be nephrogenic, dose-dependent, and reversible on discontinuation of therapy.

Dosage/Range:
Adult:

- Oral: 150 mg q 6 hours or 300 mg q 12 hours.
- Duration of therapy depends on indication.
- As treatment for hyponatremia: 600–1,200 mg daily.
- Drug dose should be reduced or adjusted in patients with hepatic or renal insufficiency.

Drug Preparation:

- Oral: Take 1 hour before meals or 2 hours after meals. Dose-reduce in patients with renal and liver impairment.

Drug Interactions:

- Oral anticoagulants: increase PT. Monitor patient closely and decrease anticoagulant dose as needed.
- Concurrent use of tetracyclines with oral contraceptives may render oral contraceptives less effective. Advise patient to use barrier contraceptive as well during a course of tetracycline therapy.
- Methoxyflurane: fatal renal toxicity has been reported with concurrent use.
- Iron preparations: decreases oral absorption. Administer iron preparations 3 hours after or 2 hours before any tetracycline.
- Antacids and antidiarrheals: may decrease absorption of tetracyclines. Avoid concurrent use.

Lab Effects/Interference:

- No reported drug-laboratory test interactions.
- SGPT, alk phos, amylase, SGOT, and bilirubin: serum concentrations may be increased.

Special Considerations:

- Avoid use in pregnant or lactating women.
- Contraindicated in patients with known hypersensitivity to tetracyclines.
- Obtain ordered specimen and send for culture and sensitivity prior to first antibiotic dose.

Potential Toxicities/Side Effects and the Nursing Process

I.   ALTERATION IN NUTRITION related to GI SIDE EFFECTS

Defining Characteristics: Anorexia, nausea, vomiting, diarrhea, glossitis, dysphagia, enterocolitis, pancreatitis.

Nursing Implications: Assess baseline nutritional status. Assess for and teach patient to report any symptoms. Administer and teach patient self-administration of prescribed antiemetic or antidiarrheal medication as appropriate. Administer and teach to self-administer oral dose with at least 8 oz of water at least 1 hour before or 2 hours after a meal or sleep.

II.   ALTERATION IN SKIN INTEGRITY related to RASH, PHOTOSENSITIVITY

Defining Characteristics: Maculopapular and erythematous rash may occur. Photosensitivity risk (exaggerated sunburn) persists 1–2 days after completion of drug therapy.

Nursing Implications: Teach patient about potential side effects, to avoid sunlight during drug therapy, and to report rash and other abnormalities. Teach symptomatic skin care as appropriate.

III.   INJURY related to HYPERSENSITIVITY

Defining Characteristics: Urticaria, angioneurotic edema, anaphylaxis may occur; also fever, arthralgias, eosinophilia, and pericarditis.

Nursing Implications: Assess drug allergy history. Assess baseline allergy history. Assess baseline skin integrity. Teach patient to report rash, pruritus. Teach patient symptomatic management of rash, pruritus. Assess for hypersensitivity reaction; if it occurs, monitor VS, discontinue drug, notify physician, and institute supportive measures.

IV.   FUNGAL SUPERINFECTION related to REDISTRIBUTION OF ENDOGENOUS MICROORGANISMS

Defining Characteristics: Vaginal moniliasis, vaginitis may occur as endogenous bacteria are eliminated and normal fungal population expands.

Nursing Implications: Teach female patient to report vaginal itching or discharge. Discuss appropriate antifungal treatment with physician. Teach perineal hygiene and symptom management.

Drug: dicloxacillin sodium (Dycill, Dynapen, Pathocil)

Class: Penicillin antibacterial.

Mechanism of Action: Semisynthetic antibiotic prepared from fungus *Penicillium*. Contains β-lactam ring and is bactericidal by inhibiting cell wall synthesis.

Metabolism: Well-absorbed from GI tract, but food decreases rate and extent of absorption. Widely distributed through body tissues and fluids; crosses placenta and is excreted in breastmilk; 95–99% bound to serum proteins. Excreted in urine and bile.

Indication: For treatment of, and active against, penicillin-resistant staphylococci that produce penicillinase. Used to treat upper and lower respiratory tract and skin infections.

Dosage/Range:
- Adult: 125–500 mg PO q 6 h × 14 days (depends on severity of infection).

Drug Preparation:
- Store in tight containers at < 40°C (104°F).

Drug Administration:
- Oral: administer at least 1 hour before or 2 hours after meals.

Drug Interactions:
- Aminoglycosides: synergism.
- Rifampin: possible antagonism, only at high doses of penicillin.
- Probenecid: increased serum level of penicillin; may be coadministered to exert this effect.

Lab Effects/Interference:
Major clinical significance:
- Urine glucose: high urinary concentrations of a penicillin may produce false-positive or falsely elevated test results with copper sulfate tests (Benedict's, Clinitest, or Fehling's); glucose enzymatic tests (Clinistix or Testape) are not affected.

Clinical significance:
- Coombs' (direct antiglobulin) test: false-positive result may occur during therapy with any penicillin.
- ALT, alk phos, AST, serum LDH values may be increased.
- WBC: leukopenia or neutropenia is associated with the use of all penicillins; the effect is more likely to occur with prolonged therapy and severe hepatic function impairment.

Special Considerations:
- Contraindicated in patients with prior hypersensitivity to penicillins. Use with caution in patients sensitive to other β-lactams (e.g., cephalosporins) since partial cross-allergenicity exists.
- Obtain ordered specimen and send for culture and sensitivity prior to first antibiotic dose.
- Consider alternative antibiotic therapy if eosinophilia, drug fever or rash, arthralgia, hematuria, or unexplained rise in BUN and serum creatinine occur.
- Monitor electrolytes and renal, hepatic, and hematologic laboratory parameters during extended treatment periods.
- Use with caution in pregnancy or with nursing women.

Potential Toxicities/Side Effects and the Nursing Process

I. POTENTIAL FOR INJURY related to HYPERSENSITIVITY REACTION

Defining Characteristics: Urticaria, pruritus, rash (maculopapular or erythematous), fever and chills, eosinophilia, myalgia, edema, erythema, angioedema, Stevens-Johnson syndrome, and exfoliative skin reactions occur in 5% of patients. Increased risk exists in individuals allergic to cephalosporin antibiotics.

COMPLICATIONS

Nursing Implications: Assess allergy to cephalosporin antibiotics and penicillin: if patient states "yes," determine actual response (e.g., "swollen lips = angioedema"). If angioedema, patient SHOULD NOT receive drug. Discuss other patient responses with physician to determine whether drug should be given. Assess baseline skin condition including integrity and allergy history to drugs. Instruct patient to report rash, itching, and other skin changes. Teach patient skin care and symptomatic measures as appropriate. If skin rash develops, discuss drug discontinuance with physician. If rash progresses, drug should be discontinued, as fatal Stevens-Johnson syndrome may develop. Be prepared to treat severe acute hypersensitivity reactions with airway management, oxygen, epinephrine, corticosteroids, antihistamines as ordered.

II.   ALTERATION IN NUTRITION, LESS THAN BODY REQUIREMENTS, related to GI SIDE EFFECTS

Defining Characteristics: Nausea, vomiting, diarrhea may occur; rarely, pseudomembranous colitis caused by *C. difficile* resistant to the antibiotic occurs. Rarely, transient increases in LFTs—AST, ALT, alk phos, bili—may occur.

Nursing Implications: Assess baseline nutritional status. Instruct patient to report GI disturbances. Administer and teach patient to self-administer antiemetics as needed and as ordered. Teach patient importance of nutritious diet and suggest small, frequent, high-calorie, high-protein meals as appropriate. Assess baseline LFTs, and monitor periodically during treatment. Discuss abnormalities and drug interruption with physician.

III.   FUNGAL SUPERINFECTION related to REDISTRIBUTION OF ENDOGENOUS MICROORGANISMS

Defining Characteristics: Vaginal candidiasis, vaginitis may occur as endogenous bacteria are eliminated and normal fungal population expands.

Nursing Implications: Instruct female patient to report vaginal itching or discharge. Discuss appropriate antifungal treatment with physician. Teach perineal hygiene and symptomatic management.

IV.   ALTERATIONS IN PROTECTIVE MECHANISMS (RARE) related to TRANSIENT LEUKOPENIA

Defining Characteristics: Rarely, transient leukopenia, lymphocytosis, anemia, eosinophilia may occur. Prolonged PT, prolonged aPTT, and hypoprothrombinemia have occurred rarely, especially in elderly or debilitated patients, or in individuals with vitamin K deficiency.

Nursing Implications: Assess baseline laboratory parameters, and monitor periodically during treatment. Assess patient for response to antibiotics. Discuss abnormalities with physician.

V.   KNOWLEDGE DEFICIT related to SELF-ADMINISTRATION OF MEDICATION

Defining Characteristics: Increased compliance when patient is instructed in self-care activities.

Nursing Implications: Assess knowledge about infection and planned treatment. Teach about drug action, potential side effects, and when and how to take drug (take medication as directed, 1 hour before or 2 hours after food). Instruct patient to report any possible drug side effects that occur.

Drug: doripenem (Doribax)

Class: Antibacterial. Doripenem is a β-lactam antibiotic, carbapenem type.

Mechanism of Action: Bactericidal through inhibition of cell wall synthesis, with resulting cell wall instability and cell lysis.

Metabolism: Metabolized to an inactive ring-opened metabolite by dehydropeptidase-I. Doripenem is not a substrate for hepatic CYP450 enzymes. Within 48 hours, approximately 70% is excreted unchanged by the kidneys and 15% as the ring-opened metabolite. Less than 1% excreted in feces after 1 week. Pharmacokinetics are linear over a dose range of 500 to 1,000 mg IV over 1 h. Following a single 1-hour IV infusion of 500 mg, the mean plasma C_{max} and AUC are 23 µg/mL and 36.3 µg h/mL, respectively. Dosage adjustment is necessary in patients with moderate and severe renal function impairment. Hepatic function impairment: Not established; however, because doripenem does not undergo hepatic *metabolism,* the pharmacokinetics are not expected to be affected by hepatic function impairment.

Indication: For treatment of complicated intra-abdominal infections and complicated urinary tract infections, including pyelonephritis, caused by susceptible strains of specific microorganisms. Active against most anaerobic and aerobic gram-positive and gram-negative organisms. Doripenem demonstrates more potent activity against *P. aeruginosa* than imipenem.

Dosage/Range:
Adult:
- Complicated intra-abdominal infection: IV 500 mg, infused over 1 h, every 8 h for 5 to 14 days.
- Complicated UTI, including pyelonephritis: IV 500 mg, infused over 1 h, every 8 h for 10 days. Duration may be extended to 14 days for patients with concurrent bacteremia.
- Renal function impairment: IV CrCl 30 to 50 mL/min or less: 250 mg, infused over 1 h, every 8 h; CrCl greater than 10 to less than 30 mL/min: 250 mg, infused over 1 h, every 12 h.

COMPLICATIONS

Drug Preparation:
- Store vial at 59–86°F. Constituted suspension in vial may be stored for 1 hour prior to dilution in infusion bag. Infusion solution prepared in normal saline may be stored at room temperature for 8 hours (includes infusion time) or under refrigeration for 24 hours (includes infusion time). Infusion solution prepared in dextrose 5% may be stored at room temperature for 4 hours (includes infusion time) or under refrigeration for 24 hours (includes infusion time).
- Product does not contain a bacteriostatic preservative.
- To prepare 500-mg dose: constitute with 10 mL of sterile water for injection or sodium chloride 0.9% injection, gently shaking vial to form a suspension (concentration, 50 mg/mL). Withdraw suspension and add to infusion bag containing normal saline 100 mL or dextrose 5%, gently shaking until clear (concentration, 4.5 mg/mL).
- To prepare 250-mg dose: constitute with 10 mL of sterile water for injection or sodium chloride 0.9% injection, gently shaking vial to form a suspension (concentration, 50 mg/mL). Withdraw suspension and add to infusion bag containing normal saline 100 mL or dextrose 5%, gently shaking until clear (concentration, 4.5 mg/mL). Remove 55 mL of this solution from bag and discard. Infuse remaining solution (concentration, 4.5 mg/mL).
- Do not mix product with or physically add to solutions containing other drugs.
- Consider a switch to appropriate oral therapy after at least 3 days of parenteral therapy, once clinical improvement has been demonstrated.

Drug Interactions:
- Probenecid: Doripenem plasma levels may be increased and prolonged because of interference with active tubular secretion by probenecid.
- Valproic acid: Valproic acid serum concentrations may be reduced to subtherapeutic levels, resulting in loss of seizure control. If serum valproic acid levels cannot be maintained in the therapeutic range or if seizures occur, consider alternative antibacterial or anticonvulsant therapy.

Lab Effects/Interference:
- None well-documented.

Special Considerations:
- Lactation: Undetermined.
- Hypersensitivity: Serious and occasionally fatal anaphylactic and serious skin reactions have been reported in patients receiving β-lactam antibiotics. These reactions are more likely to occur in individuals with a history of sensitivity to multiple allergens.
- Superinfection: May result in bacterial or fungal overgrowth of nonsusceptible organisms.
- Pseudomembranous colitis: Consider possibility in patients with diarrhea.
- **Contraindicated in patients hypersensitive to doripenem,** and serious skin reactions have been reported in patients receiving β-lactam antibiotics. Use cautiously in patients sensitive to penicillin or other β-lactams, as partial cross-allergenicity exists.
- Drug dosage needs to be reduced if moderate to severe renal insufficiency.

Potential Toxicities/Side Effects and the Nursing Process

I. POTENTIAL FOR INJURY related to HYPERSENSITIVITY REACTION

Defining Characteristics: Urticaria, pruritus, rash (maculopapular or erythematous), fever and chills, eosinophilia, myalgia, edema, erythema, angioedema, Stevens-Johnson syndrome, and exfoliative skin reactions occur in 5% of patients. Increased risk in individuals allergic to penicillin.

Nursing Implications: Assess allergy to cephalosporin antibiotics and penicillin: if patient states "yes," determine actual response (e.g., "swollen lips = angioedema"). If angioedema, discuss with physician risk versus benefit prior to drug administration, as there is partial cross-allergenicity. Discuss other patient responses with physician to determine whether drug should be given. Assess baseline skin condition, including integrity and allergy history to drugs. Instruct patient to report rash, itching, other skin changes. Teach patient skin care and symptomatic measures as appropriate. If skin rash develops, discuss drug discontinuance with physician. If rash progresses, drug should be discontinued, as fatal Stevens-Johnson syndrome may develop. Be prepared to treat severe acute hypersensitivity reactions with airway management, oxygen, epinephrine, corticosteroids, antihistamines as ordered.

II. ALTERATION IN NUTRITION, LESS THAN BODY REQUIREMENTS, related to GI SIDE EFFECTS

Defining Characteristics: Nausea, vomiting occurs more frequently than diarrhea, anorexia; rarely, pseudomembranous colitis caused by *C. difficile* resistant to the antibiotic occurs. Rarely, transient increases in LFTs—AST, ALT, alk phos, bili—may occur.

Nursing Implications: Assess baseline nutritional status. Instruct patient to report GI disturbances. Administer and teach patient to self-administer antiemetics as needed and as ordered. Teach patient importance of nutritious diet and suggest small, frequent, high-calorie, high-protein meals as appropriate. Assess baseline LFTs and monitor periodically during treatment. Discuss abnormalities and drug interruption with physician.

III. FUNGAL SUPERINFECTION related to REDISTRIBUTION OF ENDOGENOUS MICROORGANISMS

Defining Characteristics: Vaginal candidiasis, vaginitis may occur as endogenous bacteria are eliminated and normal fungal population expands.

Nursing Implications: Instruct female patient to report vaginal itching or discharge. Discuss appropriate antifungal treatment with physician. Teach perineal hygiene and symptomatic management.

COMPLICATIONS

IV.   ALTERATIONS IN PROTECTIVE MECHANISMS (RARE) related to ANEMIA

Defining Characteristics: Rarely, anemia may occur.

Nursing Implications: Assess baseline laboratory parameters, and monitor periodically during treatment. Assess patient for response to antibiotics. Discuss abnormalities with physician.

V.   ALTERATIONS IN SENSORY/PERCEPTUAL PATTERNS related to HEADACHE AND SEIZURES

Defining Characteristics: Headache, somnolence, seizures occur rarely. Most seizures have occurred in patients with preexisting CNS problems, those who had received higher-than-recommended IV doses, the elderly, and patients with impaired renal function.

Nursing Implications: Assess baseline neurologic function and comfort, and monitor during treatment. Instruct patient to report any changes. Discuss any abnormalities with physician. Institute seizure precautions. If seizures occur, discuss with physician anticonvulsant therapy or discontinuance of antibiotic.

VI.   ALTERATIONS IN COMFORT related to LOCAL INJECTION IRRITATION

Defining Characteristics: Phlebitis may develop in IV sites.

Nursing Implications: Change IV sites q 48 h, and assess for signs/symptoms of phlebitis prior to each administration. Administer drug slowly. Apply warm packs to increase comfort.

Drug: doxycycline hyclate (Vibramycin, Doryx, MonoDox)

Class: Antibacterial (systemic); antiprotozoal.

Mechanism of Action: Bacteriostatic but may be bactericidal at high concentrations. Binds to bacterial ribosomes and prevents protein synthesis.

Metabolism: Absorbed (60–80%) from GI tract. Widely distributed into body tissues and fluids. Crosses placenta and is excreted in breastmilk. Excreted unchanged in urine.

Indication: Drug is used for treatment of a broad range of gram-positive and gram-negative bacteria, *Chlamydia,* and *Mycoplasma.* It may be used to treat acne, certain amoeba infections, and as a preventive for malaria and anthrax.

Dosage/Range:
Adult:
- Oral: 100 mg q 12 hours for the first day, then 100–200 mg once daily, or 50–100 mg q 12 hours. Duration of therapy depends on indication.
- IV: 200 mg daily or 100 mg q 12 hours for the first day, then 100–200 mg daily or 50–100 mg q 12 hours. Duration of therapy depends on indication.

Drug Preparation:
- Oral: may be taken with food, water, milk, or carbonated beverages.
- IV: add 10 mL sterile water for injection to 100-mg vial or 20 mL to each 200-mg vial. Further dilute in 100–1,000 mL or in 200–2,000 mL, respectively, of lactated Ringer's injection or 5% dextrose and lactated Ringer's injection. Infuse over 1 to 4 hours.
- CONCENTRATIONS LESS THAN 100 MICROGRAMS/ML OR GREATER THAN 1 MG/ML ARE NOT RECOMMENDED.
- AVOID RAPID ADMINISTRATION.
- Solution stable for 6 hours, so use after mixing. Avoid exposure to heat or sunlight. Convert to oral preparation as soon as possible, as there is risk of thrombophlebitis.
- DO NOT ADMINISTER INTRAMUSCULARLY OR SUBCUTANEOUSLY.

Drug Interactions:
- Hepatotoxic drugs: may increase hepatotoxicity if given concurrently. Assess baseline and periodically during treatment.
- Iron preparations: decrease oral and possibly IV absorption. Administer iron preparations 3 hours after or 2 hours before any tetracycline.
- Oral anticoagulants: increase PT. Monitor patient closely and decrease anticoagulant dose as needed.
- Antidiarrheals (containing kaolin, pectate, or bismuth): may decrease absorption of tetracyclines. Avoid concurrent use.
- Oral contraceptives: decreased effectiveness of contraceptive and increased incidence of breakthrough bleeding. Advise patient to use barrier contraceptive as well during a course of tetracycline therapy.
- Lithium: may decrease lithium levels. Monitor serum levels and increase dose as needed.

Lab Effects/Interference:
- Urine catecholamine determinations: may produce false elevations of urinary catecholamines because of interfering fluorescence in the Hingerty method.
- SGPT, alk phos, amylase, SGOT, and bilirubin: serum concentrations may be increased.

Special Considerations:
- Use cautiously in patients with myasthenia gravis: may increase muscle weakness.
- Avoid use in pregnant or lactating women.
- Obtain ordered specimen for culture and sensitivity prior to first dose.
- IV preparation contains ascorbic acid and may cause false-positive result using Clinitest, or false-negative result when using Clinistix and Testape.
- Drug has affinity for ischemic, necrotic tissue, and may localize in tumors.

COMPLICATIONS

Potential Toxicities/Side Effects and the Nursing Process

I.   ALTERATION IN NUTRITION related to GI SIDE EFFECTS

Defining Characteristics: Nausea, vomiting, diarrhea, anorexia, abdominal discomfort, epigastric burning and distress, glossitis, black hairy tongue may occur.

Nursing Implications: Assess baseline nutritional status. Assess for and teach patient to report any symptoms. Administer and teach patient self-administration of prescribed antiemetic or antidiarrheal medication as appropriate. Administer and teach patient to self-administer oral dose with at least 8 oz of water taken at least 1 hour before lying down for sleep.

II.   ALTERATION IN SKIN INTEGRITY related to RASH, PHOTOSENSITIVITY

Defining Characteristics: Maculopapular and erythematous rashes may occur. Rarely, exfoliative dermatitis, onycholysis, and nail discoloration. Photosensitivity risk (exaggerated sunburn) persists 1–2 days after completion of drug therapy.

Nursing Implications: Teach patient about potential side effects, to avoid sunlight during drug therapy, and to report rash, other abnormalities. Teach symptomatic skin care as appropriate.

III.   INJURY related to HYPERSENSITIVITY

Defining Characteristics: Urticaria, angioneurotic edema, anaphylaxis may occur; also, fever, rash, arthralgias, eosinophilia, and pericarditis.

Nursing Implications: Assess drug allergy history. Assess baseline allergy history. Assess baseline skin integrity. Teach patient to report rash, pruritus. Teach patient symptomatic management of rash, pruritus. Assess for hypersensitivity reaction; if it occurs, monitor VS, discontinue drug, notify physician, and institute supportive measures.

IV.   FUNGAL SUPERINFECTION related to REDISTRIBUTION OF ENDOGENOUS MICROORGANISMS

Defining Characteristics: Vaginal moniliasis, vaginitis may occur as endogenous bacteria are eliminated and normal fungal population expands.

Nursing Implications: Teach female patient to report vaginal itching or discharge. Discuss appropriate antifungal treatment with physician. Teach perineal hygiene and symptomatic management.

V.   ALTERATION IN HEPATIC FUNCTION

Defining Characteristics: Associated with high IV doses (> 2 g/day): hepatotoxicity and cholestasis may occur.

Nursing Implications: Assess baseline LFTs and monitor during therapy.

VI. INFECTION AND BLEEDING related to NEUTROPENIA, THROMBOCYTOPENIA

Defining Characteristics: Neutropenia, leukocytosis, leukopenia, atypical lymphocytes, thrombocytopenia, thrombocytopenic purpura, hemolytic anemia occur rarely with long-term therapy.

Nursing Implications: Assess baseline WBC, hematocrit, and platelets, and monitor periodically during long-term therapy.

VII. ALTERATIONS IN COMFORT related to LOCAL ADMINISTRATION EFFECTS

Defining Characteristics: IM administration may cause pain, induration due to muscle injury. IV administration may cause erythema, pain, swelling, and thrombophlebitis.

Nursing Implications: Rotate sites. Apply ice as ordered to painful buttock. Assess IV site prior to each dose for phlebitis or swelling and change site at least q 48 hours. Apply heat to painful IV sites as ordered.

VIII. SENSORY/PERCEPTUAL ALTERATION

Defining Characteristics: Lightheadedness, dizziness, headache may occur.

Nursing Implications: Assess baseline neurologic status. Teach patient to report any changes and discuss them with physician.

Drug: ertapenem sodium (Invanz)

Class: Antibiotic, carbapenem.

Mechanism of Action: The bactericidal activity results from the inhibition of cell wall synthesis. Penetrates the cell wall of most gram-positive and gram-negative bacteria to reach penicillin-binding protein (PBP) targets.

Metabolism: Widely distributed in body tissues and fluids, excreted in urine.

Indication: For treatment of gynecologic infections (*Streptococcus agalactiae* [group B streptococci], *E. coli, B. fragilis, Porphyromonas asaccharolytica, Peptostreptococcus*, or *Prevotella bivia*); intra-abdominal infections (*E. coli, Clostridium clostridioforme, Eubacterium lentum, Peptostreptococcus, B. fragilis, B. distasonis, B. ovatus, B. thetaiotamicron, B. uniformis*); respiratory tract infections (penicillin-susceptible *S. pneumoniae*, non-beta-lactamase–producing strains of *H. influenzae, Moraxella catarrhalis*); skin and skin structures (oxacillin-susceptible [methicillin-susceptible] strains of *S. aureus, S. agalactiae*, group A beta-hemolytic *S. pyogenes, E. coli, Klebsiella pneumoniae, P. mirabilis, B. fragilis, Peptostreptococcus* species, *Porphyromonas asaccharolytica*, or *Prevotella bivia*); urinary tract infections (*E. coli, Klebsiella pneumoniae*).

COMPLICATIONS

Dosage/Range:

Adult:

• Acute pelvic infection: 1 g IV/IM once a day for 3–10 days.
• Community-acquired pneumonia: 1 g IV/IM once a day for 10–14 days.
• Intra-abdominal infection: 1 g IV/IM once a day for 5–14 days.
• Skin/skin structure infections: 1 g IV/IM once a day for 7–14 days.
• Urinary tract infections: 1 g IV/IM once a day for 10–14 days.
• Adjust dose in patients with renal impairment and on hemodialysis.

Drug Administration:
• IV infusion for up to 14 days.
• IM injection for up to 7 days.
• DO NOT DILUTE WITH diluents containing dextrose.

Drug Interactions:
• Probenecid competes with ertapenem for active tubular secretion; increasing AUC by 25% and reducing the plasma and renal clearances by 20% and 35%, respectively.

Lab Effects/Interference:
• Ertapenem possess the characteristic low toxicity of the β-lactam group of antibiotics.
• Periodically assess organ system function: renal, hepatic, and hematopoietic.

Potential Toxicities/Side Effects and the Nursing Process

I.   POTENTIAL FOR INJURY related to HYPERSENSITIVITY REACTION AND LOCAL REACTIONS (pain at injection site)

Defining Characteristics: Urticaria, pruritus, rash (maculopapular or erythematous), fever and chills, eosinophilia, myalgia, edema, erythema, angioedema.

Nursing Implications: Assess allergy to cephalosporin antibiotics and penicillin; if patient states "yes," determine actual response (e.g., "swollen lips = angioedema"). If angioedema, patient SHOULD NOT receive drug. Discuss other patient responses with physician to determine whether drug should be given. Assess baseline skin condition including integrity and allergy history to drugs. Instruct patient to report rash, itching, and other skin changes. Teach patient skin care and symptomatic measures as appropriate. If skin rash develops, discuss drug discontinuance with physician. Be prepared to treat severe acute hypersensitivity reactions with airway management, oxygen, epinephrine, corticosteroids, antihistamines as ordered.

II.   ALTERATION IN NUTRITION, LESS THAN BODY REQUIREMENTS, related to GI SIDE EFFECTS

Defining Characteristics: Nausea, vomiting, diarrhea may occur; rarely, pseudomembranous colitis caused by antibiotic resistance occurs.

Nursing Implications: Assess baseline nutritional status. Instruct patient to report GI disturbances. Administer and teach patient to self-administer antiemetics as needed and as ordered. Teach patient importance of nutritious diet and suggest small, frequent, high-calorie, high-protein meals as appropriate. Assess baseline LFTs, and monitor periodically during treatment. Discuss abnormalities and drug interruption with physician.

III. FUNGAL SUPERINFECTION related to REDISTRIBUTION OF ENDOGENOUS MICROORGANISMS

Defining Characteristics: Vaginal candidiasis, vaginitis may occur as endogenous bacteria are eliminated and normal fungal population expands.

Nursing Implications: Instruct female patient to report vaginal itching or discharge. Discuss appropriate antifungal treatment with physician. Teach perineal hygiene and symptomatic management.

Drug: erythromycin (ERYC, E-Mycin, Ilotycin, Erythrocin)

Class: Antibacterial (macrolide).

Mechanism of Action: Erythromycin is a bacteriostatic macrolide antibiotic. It may be bactericidal in high concentrations or when used against highly susceptible organisms. It is thought to penetrate the bacterial cell membrane and to reversibly bind to the 50S ribosomal subunit. It does not directly inhibit peptide formation; rather, it inhibits the translocation of peptides from the acceptor site on the ribosome to the donor site, inhibiting subsequent protein synthesis. Effective against actively dividing organisms.

Metabolism: 90% of the drug is metabolized by the liver; may accumulate in patients with severe hepatic disease. Primarily excreted into the bile. Between 2% and 5% is excreted unchanged by the kidneys following oral administration; 12–15% excreted unchanged following IV administration. Erythromycins cross the placental barrier in pregnancy; can be found in breastmilk.

Indication: For treatment of bacterial infections, such as bronchitis, diphtheria, Legionnaires' disease, pertussis, pneumonia, rheumatic fever, veneral disease, and ear, intestine, lung, urinary tract, and skin infections. Erythromycin is a broad-spectrum antibiotic with activity against gram-positive and gram-negative bacteria, and other infectious agents, including *Chlamydia trachomatis,* mycoplasmas (*Mycoplasma pneumoniae* and *Ureaplasma urealyticum*), and spirochetes (*Treponema pallidum* and *Borrelia* species). Erythromycin has good activity against *S. pyogenes, S. pneumoniae* (group A beta-hemolytic streptococci*)*, and *S. aureus.*

Dosage/Range:
• Oral: 250 mg once q 6 h for 10 days; or 500 mg q 6 h for 10 days; or 333 mg q 8 h.
• IV: 500 mg q 6 h; up to 1,000 mg q 6 h (Legionnaires' disease).

COMPLICATIONS

Drug Preparation:
- Further dilute in 0.9% sodium chloride to a concentration of 1–5 mg/mL (500 mg/100 mL, 1,000 mg/250 mL).
- Reconstitute 500-mg or 1-g vials with 10 or 20 mL, respectively, of sterile water for injection only (no preservatives).

Drug Administration:
- Must not be given IV push.
- Intermittent IV infusion over 1 hour is appropriate.

Drug Interactions:
- Use of alcohol concurrently with IV erythromycin increases peak blood alcohol concentrations by 40%; this is thought to be related to rapid gastric emptying, less exposure to alcohol dehydrogenase in the gastric mucosa, and slower small intestine transit time.
- Concurrent use of astemizole or terfenadine with erythromycins is contraindicated and may increase risk of cardiotoxicity, such as torsades de pointes, ventricular tachycardia, and death.
- Erythromycins may inhibit carbamazepine and valproic acid metabolism, resulting in increased anticonvulsant plasma concentration and toxicity.
- Concurrent use of chloramphenicol, lincomycins, and erythromycins is not recommended due to their antagonizing effects. It is best to avoid concurrent use of bactericidal and bacteriostatic drugs until culture and sensitivity results are determined.
- Erythromycin can increase cyclosporin plasma concentrations and may increase the risk of nephrotoxicity.
- Erythromycins inhibit the metabolism of ergotamine and increase the vasospasm associated with ergotamines.
- Simultaneous administration of erythromycin and lovastatin should be used with caution since concurrent use may increase the risk of rhabdomyolysis.
- Concurrent use of midazolam and triazolam with erythromycins can increase the pharmacologic effect of these drugs.
- Erythromycins may cause prolonged prothrombin time and increased risk of hemorrhage, especially in the elderly.
- Use of erythromycins and xanthines (i.e., aminophylline, caffeine, oxtriphylline, and theophylline) may lead to increased serum levels of xanthines and toxicity.

Lab Effects/Interference:
- Serum SGPT, serum SGOT, serum bilirubin, and alkaline phosphatase—values may be increased by all erythromycins.
- Urinary catecholamines may produce false-positive results when patient is on erythromycin.

Special Considerations:
- Do not use when there is a known hypersensitivity to erythromycins.
- Use with caution in patients with impaired hepatic function.
- Patients with a history of hearing loss may be at risk of further hearing loss, especially if hepatic or renal function is present, or if on high-dose erythromycins, or if patient is elderly.

Potential Toxicities/Side Effects and the Nursing Process

I.   ALTERATION IN NUTRITION related to GI SIDE EFFECTS

Defining Characteristics: Nausea, vomiting, anorexia have occurred frequently. Also, transient increase LFTs—AST (SGOT), ALT (SGPT), LDH, alk phos, bili—has occurred. Hepatotoxicity (fever, nausea, skin rash, stomach pain, severe and unusual tiredness or weakness, yellow eyes or skin, and vomiting) has occurred less frequently. Pancreatitis (severe abdominal pain, nausea, and vomiting) has occurred but is rare.

Nursing Implications: Assess baseline nutritional status, preexisting nausea/vomiting, anorexia. Assess baseline LFTs and monitor periodically during treatment. Teach patient to report side effects. Provide symptomatic interventions if side effects occur; discuss with physician use of alternative drug(s).

II.   POTENTIAL FOR INJURY related to HYPERSENSITIVITY REACTION

Defining Characteristics: Urticaria, pruritus, rash (maculopapular or erythematous), fever and chills, eosinophilia, myalgia, edema, erythema, angioedema.

Nursing Implications: Assess for drug allergies to erythromycin or macrolide antibiotic prior to drug administration. Teach patient to report any allergic reactions. Assess for signs/symptoms of allergic reaction after drug dose. Assess baseline skin integrity and presence of drug allergies; monitor patient closely during drug infusions. Teach patient to report immediately signs/symptoms of rash, pruritus, shortness of breath, any adverse sensation. Teach patient skin care and symptomatic measures as appropriate. If skin rash develops, discuss drug discontinuance with physician. If rash progresses, especially in human immunodeficiency virus (HIV)-infected patients, drug should be discontinued, as fatal Stevens-Johnson syndrome may develop. Be prepared to treat severe acute hypersensitivity reactions with airway management, oxygen, epinephrine, corticosteroids, antihistamines as ordered.

III.   ALTERATIONS IN COMFORT related to LOCAL INJECTION IRRITATION

Defining Characteristics: Incidence of phlebitis, thrombophlebitis, and pain when administering IV.

Nursing Implications: Change IV sites q 48 hours, and assess for signs/symptoms of phlebitis prior to each administration. Administer drug slowly. Apply warm packs to increase comfort.

IV.   ALTERATIONS IN CARDIAC OUTPUT related to CARDIOVASCULAR CHANGES

Defining Characteristics: Rare incidence of cardiac arrhythmias, EKG changes (e.g., QT prolongation), torsades de pointes (irregular or slow heart rate, recurrent fainting, sudden death).

COMPLICATIONS

Nursing Implications: Assess baseline heart rate and blood pressure; monitor during therapy, at least with initial dose.

V.   SENSORY/PERCEPTUAL ALTERATIONS related to OTOTOXICITY

Defining Characteristics: Damage to eighth cranial nerve (auditory) may result in dizziness, nystagmus, vertigo, ataxia (vestibular damage), and more commonly tinnitus, roaring sound in ears, and impaired hearing (auditory damage). Hearing loss usually begins with high-frequency loss, followed by clinical hearing loss, then permanent hearing loss if damage continues. Increased risk in elderly, renally, hepatically impaired patients.

Nursing Implications: Assess baseline hearing (ability to hear spoken voice) and continue to assess during therapy. Teach patient potential side effects, and instruct patient to report any hearing/perceptual problems (e.g., tinnitus, vertigo, decreased hearing). Discuss drug discontinuance and audiogram with physician to confirm hearing dysfunction if symptoms arise. Assess for increased risk if given concurrently with other ototoxic medications (e.g., cisplatin, furosemide).

VI.   FUNGAL SUPERINFECTION related to REDISTRIBUTION OF ENDOGENOUS MICROORGANISMS

Defining Characteristics: Vaginal candidiasis (sore mouth or tongue; white patches in mouth and/or tongue); vaginitis (vaginal candidiasis); vaginal itching and discharge may occur as endogenous bacteria are eliminated and normal fungal population expands.

Nursing Implications: Teach female patient to report vaginal itching or discharge. Discuss appropriate antifungal treatment with physician. Teach perineal hygiene and symptomatic management.

Drug: fidaxomicin (Dificid)

Class: Antibacterial (macrolide).

Mechanism of Action: Fidaxomicin is a fermentation product obtained from the Actinomycete *Dactylosporangium aurantiacum*. Active primarily against species of clostridia, including *C. difficile*. Bactericidal against *C. difficile* in vitro, inhibiting RNA synthesis by RNA polymerases. Bactericidal for *C. difficile*–associated diarrhea (CDAD). Since there is minimal systemic absorption of fidaxomicin, Dificid is not effective for treatment of systemic infections. Demonstrates no in-vitro cross-resistance with other classes of antibacterial drugs. Fidaxomicin and its main metabolite OP-1118 do not exhibit any antagonistic interaction with other classes of antibacterial drugs.

Metabolism: Fidaxomicin is primarily transformed by hydrolysis at the isobutyryl ester to form its main and microbiologically active metabolite, OP-1118. Metabolism of fidaxomicin and formation of OP-1118 are not dependent on cytochrome P450 (CYP) enzymes. Fidaxomicin acts locally in the gastrointestinal tract on *C. difficile*. Fidaxomicin has minimal systemic absorption following oral administration, with plasma concentrations of fidaxomicin and OP-1118 in the ng/mL range at the therapeutic dose. Fidaxomicin is mainly confined to the gastrointestinal tract following oral administration. Mainly excreted in feces.

Indication: For treatment of diarrhea caused by *Clostridium difficile* (*C. difficile*–associated diarrhea).

Dosage/Range:
- The recommended dose is one 200-mg Dificid tablet orally twice daily for 10 days with or without food.

Drug Interactions:
- Fidaxomicin and its main metabolite, OP-1118, are substrates of the efflux transporter, P-glycoprotein (P-gp), which is expressed in the gastrointestinal tract.
- Cyclosporine: is an inhibitor of multiple transporters, including P-gp. Plasma concentrations of fidaxomicin and OP-1118 were significantly increased but remained in the ng/mL range. Concentrations of fidaxomicin and OP-1118 may decrease at the site of action (i.e., gastrointestinal tract) via P-gp inhibition; however, concomitant P-gp inhibitor use had no attributable effect on safety or treatment outcome of fidaxomicin-treated patients in controlled clinical trials. Fidaxomicin may be coadministered with P-gp inhibitors, and no dose adjustment is recommended.

Lab Effects/Interference:
- None.

Special Considerations:
- Do not use when there is a known hypersensitivity to erythromycins or other macrolides.
- Use during pregnancy only if clearly needed.
- It is not known whether fidaxomicin is excreted in breastmilk. Because many drugs are excreted in breastmilk, caution should be exercised when Dificid is administered to a nursing woman.
- The safety and effectiveness of Dificid in patients less than 18 years of age have not been established.

Potential Toxicities/Side Effects and the Nursing Process

I. ALTERATION IN NUTRITION related to GI SIDE EFFECTS

Defining Characteristics: Nausea (11%), vomiting (7%), abdominal pain (6%), gastrointestinal hemorrhage (4%).

Nursing Implications: Assess baseline nutritional status, preexisting nausea/vomiting, anorexia. Assess baseline LFTs and monitor periodically during treatment. Teach patient to report side effects. Provide symptomatic interventions if side effects occur; discuss with physician use of alternative drug(s).

II.   INFECTION, BLEEDING related to BONE MARROW DEPRESSION (rare)

Defining Characteristics: Neutropenia and anemia occur in 2% of patients, respectively.

Nursing Implications: Assess baseline WBC, ANC, and platelet count; monitor throughout therapy (every other day initially, then 3 times per week). Hold ganciclovir if ANC < 500/mm^3, platelet count < 25,000/mm^3. Assess for signs/symptoms of infection or bleeding; instruct patient in signs/symptoms of infection and bleeding, and instruct to report these immediately. Teach patient self-care measures to minimize risk of infection, bleeding, including avoidance of OTC aspirin-containing medicines. Administer or teach patient to self-administer prescribed G-CSF or GM-CSF. Assess Hgb/HCT and signs/symptoms of fatigue. Instruct patient to alternate rest and activity periods.

III.   FUNGAL SUPERINFECTION related to REDISTRIBUTION OF ENDOGENOUS MICROORGANISMS

Defining Characteristics: Vaginal candidiasis (sore mouth or tongue; white patches in mouth and/or tongue); vaginitis (vaginal candidiasis); vaginal itching and discharge may occur as endogenous bacteria are eliminated and normal fungal population expands.

Nursing Implications: Teach female patient to report vaginal itching or discharge. Discuss appropriate antifungal treatment with physician. Teach perineal hygiene and symptomatic management.

Drug: gatifloxacin (Tequin)

Class: Quinolone.

Mechanism of Action: Acts intracellularly by inhibiting DNA gyrase (bacterial topoisomerase IV).

Metabolism: Widely distributed to most body fluids and tissues with highest concentrations in organs such as kidneys, gallbladder, lungs, liver, gynecologic tissue, prostatic tissue, phagocytic cells, urine, sputum, and bile. Well-absorbed from GI tract. Metabolized in liver; excreted in urine and feces. Crosses placenta and is excreted in breastmilk.

Indication: For treatment of bacterial infections of the lungs, sinuses, skin, and urinary tract.

Gatifloxacin is a broad-spectrum anti-infective, active against a wide range of aerobic gram-positive and gram-negative organisms.

Dosage/Range:
• 400 mg PO or IV daily.

Drug Preparation:
• Oral: Take drug with large glass of water; preferably 2 hours after meal/food. Encourage oral fluids of 2–3 qt/day.

- IV: Further dilute drug in 0.9% sodium chloride or 5% dextrose in water to final concentration of 2 mg/mL.

Drug Interactions:
- Antacids (containing magnesium, aluminum, or calcium) and iron decrease absorption of serum level of gatifloxacin; do not administer concurrently. If must administer antacids or iron, administer at least 4 hours apart. The administration of antacids containing aluminum, magnesium, calcium, sucralfate, zinc, or iron may substantially reduce the absorption of gatifloxacin; do not administer concurrently.
- Serum digoxin concentrations should be monitored; gatifloxacin may raise serum levels in some patients.
- Probenecid: decreases the renal tubular secretion of gatifloxacin resulting in a prolonged elimination half-life and increased risk of toxicity.
- Gatifloxacin may have the potential to prolong the QT interval of the EKG in some patients. Gatifloxacin should not be used in patients with prolonged QT interval; patients with uncorrected hypokalemia; and patients taking quinidine, procainamide, amiodarone, and sotalol (antiarrhythmic agents).
- Increased intracranial pressure and psychosis have been reported along with CNS stimulation.
- Hypersensitivity reactions have been reported.

Lab Effects/Interference:
- Serum SGPT, serum alk phos, serum SGOT, and serum LDH: values may be increased

Special Considerations:
- Used in treatment of infections of urinary and lower respiratory tracts, skin, bone and joint, and GI tract, as well as gonorrhea.
- Contraindicated in pregnancy or in women who are breastfeeding.
- Obtain ordered specimen for culture and sensitivity prior to first drug dose.
- Use cautiously in patients with seizure disorders.
- Used in the treatment of infections or most bacterial infections.

COMPLICATIONS

Potential Toxicities/Side Effects and the Nursing Process

I.   ALTERATION IN NUTRITION related to GI SIDE EFFECTS

Defining Characteristics: Incidence of nausea, vomiting, abdominal discomfort, diarrhea, anorexia.

Nursing Implications: Assess baseline nutritional and elimination status. Teach patient to report GI disturbances. Administer and teach patient to self-administer antiemetics and antidiarrheals as needed and as ordered. Teach patient importance of nutritious diet and suggest small, frequent, high-calorie, high-protein meals as appropriate. Assess baseline LFTs and monitor periodically during treatment. Discuss abnormalities and drug interruption with physician. Assess taking other hepatotoxic drugs (see Special Considerations).

II.   SENSORY/PERCEPTUAL ALTERATIONS related to CNS EFFECTS

Defining Characteristics: Incidence of headache, restlessness. Dizziness, hallucinations, and scizures may also occur. Exacerbated by caffeine, as quinolones delay caffeine excretion.

Nursing Implications: Assess baseline neurologic function and comfort, and monitor during treatment. Teach patient to report any changes. Discuss any abnormalities with physician. Teach patient to limit or restrict all medications and caffeine-containing fluids (e.g., tea, coffee, caffeinated soft drinks).

III.   ALTERATION IN SKIN INTEGRITY related to ALLERGY/HYPERSENSITIVITY

Defining Characteristics: Incidence of rash; other manifestations include eosinophilia, urticaria, flushing, fever, chills, photosensitivity, angioedema. Fatal hypersensitivity reactions have occurred rarely. Direct exposure to sunlight can cause sunburn (moderate-to-severe phototoxicity).

Nursing Implications: Assess baseline skin condition, including integrity and drug allergy history. Teach patient to report rash, itching, other skin changes. Teach patient skin care and symptomatic measures as appropriate. If skin rash develops, discuss drug discontinuance with physician. Be prepared to treat severe acute hypersensitivity reactions with airway management, oxygen, epinephrine, corticosteroids, antihistamines as ordered. Teach patient to avoid excessive sun exposure and to use skin protection factor (SPF) 15 or higher. If rash progresses, especially in HIV-infected patients, drug should be discontinued, as fatal Stevens-Johnson syndrome may develop.

IV.   FUNGAL SUPERINFECTION related to REDISTRIBUTION OF ENDOGENOUS MICROORGANISMS

Defining Characteristics: Vaginal moniliasis, vaginitis may occur as endogenous bacteria are eliminated and normal fungal population expands.

Nursing Implications: Teach female patient to report vaginal itching or discharge. Discuss appropriate antifungal treatment with physician. Teach perineal hygiene and symptomatic management.

V.   ALTERATION IN URINARY ELIMINATION related to RENAL TOXICITY

Defining Characteristics: Increased BUN and creatinine, crystal and stone formation in urine, interstitial nephritis, and renal failure may occur.

Nursing Implications: Assess baseline renal function; expect that drug dose will be decreased in presence of renal dysfunction. Teach patient to take drug with at least 8 oz of water, and to increase oral fluids to 2–3 qt/day.

VI.   ALTERATIONS IN COMFORT related to IV ADMINISTRATION

Defining Characteristics: Drug may cause pain, inflammation, and rare thrombophlebitis at IV site.

Nursing Implications: Change IV site q 48 hours. Assess for phlebitis, discomfort, and IV patency prior to each administration. Administer drug slowly over 60–90 minutes in large volume of 5% dextrose (see Drug Preparation). Apply heat to promote comfort.

Drug: gemifloxacin mesylate (Factive)

Class: Quinolone.

Mechanism of Action: Acts inhibiting DNA synthesis through the inhibition of DNA gyrase and topoisomerase IV, which are essential for bacterial growth.

Metabolism: Widely distributed to most body fluids and tissues after oral administration. Gemifloxacin penetrates well into lung tissues and fluids. Well-absorbed from GI tract. Metabolized to a limited extent in the liver; excreted in urine and feces. The safety in pregnant women has not been established. The drug is excreted in breastmilk in animal studies.

Indication: Used in acute bacterial exacerbations of chronic bronchitis (*S. pneumoniae*, *H. influenza*, *H. parainfluenzae*, *Moraxella catarrhalis*) and mild to moderate community-acquired pneumonia caused by susceptible strains of designated microorganisms, including multidrug–resistant strains of *S. pneumoniae*, *H. influenza*, *M. catarrhalis*, *Mycoplasma pneumoniae*, *Chlamydophila pneumoniae*, or *Klebsiella pneumoniae*. Gemifloxacin is a broad-spectrum anti-infective, active against a wide range of aerobic gram-positive and gram-negative organisms.

Dosage/Range:
* 320 mg orally once a day for 5–7 days.

Drug Preparation:
* Oral: Take drug with or without food. Take with large glass of water; encourage oral fluids of 2–3 qt/day.

Drug Interactions:
* Antacids (containing magnesium, aluminum, or calcium) and iron decrease absorption of serum level of gemifloxacin; do not administer concurrently. If must administer antacids or iron, administer at least 3 hours before or 2 hours after. The administration of antacids containing aluminum, magnesium, calcium, sucralfate, zinc, or iron may substantially reduce the absorption of gemifloxacin; do not administer concurrently.
* Probenecid: decreases the renal tubular secretion of gemifloxacin resulting in a prolonged elimination half-life and increased risk of toxicity.
* Gemifloxacin may have the potential to prolong the QT interval of the EKG in some patients. Gemifloxacin should not be used in patients with prolonged QT interval; patients

with uncorrected hypokalemia or hypomagnesemia; and patients taking quinidine, procainamide, amiodarone, and sotalol (Class 1A antiarrhythmic agents).
- Increased intracranial pressure and psychosis have been reported along with CNS stimulation.
- Hypersensitivity reactions have been reported.
- Fluoroquinolones have been shown to cause arthropathy and osteochondrosis in animal studies. Discontinue if patient experiences pain, inflammation, or rupture of a tendon. Elderly patients, athletes, and patients taking corticosteroids are more prone to tendonitis.
- Pseudomembranous colitis has been reported and may range from mild to life-threatening.

Lab Effects/Interference:
- Serum SGPT, serum alk phos, serum SGOT, and serum LDH: values may be increased.

Special Considerations:
- Used in treatment of infections of lower respiratory tracts.
- Contraindicated in pregnancy or in women who are breastfeeding.
- Obtain ordered specimen for culture and sensitivity prior to first drug dose.
- Use cautiously in patients with seizure disorders.
- Used in the treatment of infections or most bacterial infections.

Potential Toxicities/Side Effects and the Nursing Process

I.   ALTERATION IN NUTRITION related to GI SIDE EFFECTS

Defining Characteristics: Incidence of nausea, vomiting, abdominal discomfort, diarrhea, anorexia.

Nursing Implications: Assess baseline nutritional and elimination status. Teach patient to report GI disturbances. Administer and teach patient to self-administer antiemetics and antidiarrheals as needed and as ordered. Teach patient importance of nutritious diet, and suggest small, frequent, high-calorie, high-protein meals as appropriate. Assess baseline LFTs and monitor periodically during treatment. Discuss abnormalities and drug interruption with physician. Assess taking other hepatotoxic drugs.

II.   SENSORY/PERCEPTUAL ALTERATIONS related to CNS EFFECTS

Defining Characteristics: Incidence of headache, restlessness. Dizziness, hallucinations, and seizures may also occur. Exacerbated by caffeine, as quinolones delay caffeine excretion.

Nursing Implications: Assess baseline neurologic function and comfort, and monitor during treatment. Teach patient to report any changes. Discuss any abnormalities with physician. Teach patient to limit or restrict all medications and caffeine-containing fluids (e.g., tea, coffee, caffeinated soft drinks).

III.   ALTERATION IN SKIN INTEGRITY related to ALLERGY/HYPERSENSITIVITY

Defining Characteristics: Incidence of rash; other manifestations include eosinophilia, urticaria, flushing, fever, chills, photosensitivity, angioedema. Fatal hypersensitivity reactions have occurred rarely. Direct exposure to sunlight can cause sunburn (moderate-to-severe phototoxicity).

Nursing Implications: Assess baseline skin condition, including integrity and drug allergy history. Teach patient to report rash, itching, and other skin changes. Teach patient skin care and symptomatic measures as appropriate. If skin rash develops, discuss drug discontinuance with physician. Be prepared to treat severe acute hypersensitivity reactions with airway management, oxygen, epinephrine, corticosteroids, antihistamines as ordered. Teach patient to avoid excessive sun exposure and to use skin protection factor (SPF) 15 or higher. If rash progresses, especially in HIV-infected patients, drug should be discontinued, as fatal Stevens-Johnson syndrome may develop.

IV.   FUNGAL SUPERINFECTION related to REDISTRIBUTION OF ENDOGENOUS MICROORGANISMS

Defining Characteristics: Vaginal moniliasis, vaginitis may occur as endogenous bacteria are eliminated and normal fungal population expands.

Nursing Implications: Teach female patient to report vaginal itching or discharge. Discuss appropriate antifungal treatment with physician. Teach perineal hygiene and symptomatic management.

V.   ALTERATION IN URINARY ELIMINATION related to RENAL TOXICITY

Defining Characteristics: Increased BUN and creatinine, crystal and stone formation in urine, interstitial nephritis, and renal failure may occur.

Nursing Implications: Assess baseline renal function; expect that drug dose will be decreased in presence of renal dysfunction. Teach patient to take drug with at least 8 oz of water, and to increase oral fluids to 2–3 qt/day.

Drug: gentamicin sulfate (Garamycin, Gentamicin)

Class: Aminoglycoside antibacterial.

Mechanism of Action: Derived from *Micromonospora;* bactericidal, most probably by inhibition of protein synthesis.

Metabolism: Well-absorbed following IV administration, but variability in absorption after IM injection (peak serum level 0.5–2 hours, duration 8–12 hours). Widely distributed into body fluids. Minimally protein-bound. Readily crosses placenta and into breastmilk. Drug excreted unchanged in the urine.

Indication: For treatment of serious infections caused by susceptible bacteria. Active against aerobic microorganisms: many sensitive gram-negative organisms (including *Acinetobacter, Brucella, Citrobacter, Enterobacter, E. coli, Klebsiella, Proteus, Pseudomonas, Salmonella, Serratia,* and *Shigella*) and some sensitive gram-positive organisms (*S. aureus* and *S. epidermidis*). Over time, bacterial resistance may develop, either naturally or acquired.

Dosage/Range:
- IM, IV: Loading dose, 2 mg/kg, then 3–6 mg/kg/day in one daily dose, two equal doses in split 8-hour dosing.
- IT: 4–8 mg (preservative-free).
- Desired peak serum concentration 4–10 mg/mL, and trough serum concentration is 1–2 mg/mL.
- DOSE REDUCTION IF RENAL DYSFUNCTION.

Drug Preparation:
- Store injectable at < 40°C (104°F). Stable for 24 hours at room temperature in 0.9% sodium chloride or 5% dextrose.

Drug Administration:
- Do not mix with other drugs.
- IV: Mix in 50–200 mL 0.9% sodium chloride or 5% dextrose injection and infuse over 30 minutes to 2 hours. Can also be given IM.

Drug Interactions:
- Increased risk of toxicity with other ototoxic drugs: acyclovir, other aminoglycosides, amphotericin B, bacitracin, cephalosporins, colistin, cisplatin, ethacrynic acid, furosemide, vancomycin.
- Potentiation of neuromuscular blockade when given concurrently with general anesthetics (succinylcholine, tubocurarine); use cautiously, observe for signs/symptoms of respiratory depression.
- Synergism with extended-spectrum penicillins, but must be administered separately.

Lab Effects/Interference:
- Serum ALT, serum alk phos, serum AST, serum bili, and serum LDH values may be increased.
- BUN and serum creatinine concentrations may be increased.
- Serum Ca++, serum Mg++, serum K+, and serum Na+ concentrations may be decreased.

Special Considerations:
- Used as first-line treatment in short-term treatment of serious gram-negative infections (e.g., septicemia, respiratory tract infections).
- Use against gram-positive organisms only as second-line treatment.
- Use in pregnancy only if infection is life-threatening and no safer drug exists; drug crosses placenta and may cause fetal toxicity.

Potential Toxicities/Side Effects and the Nursing Process

I. ALTERATIONS IN SENSORY/PERCEPTUAL PATTERNS related to OTOTOXICITY

Defining Characteristics: Damage to eighth cranial nerve (auditory) may result in dizziness, nystagmus, vertigo, ataxia (vestibular damage), and more commonly tinnitus, roaring sound in ears, and impaired hearing (auditory damage). Hearing loss usually begins with high-frequency loss, followed by clinical hearing loss, then permanent hearing loss if damage continues. Increased risk in elderly or renally impaired patients.

Nursing Implications: Assess baseline hearing (ability to hear spoken voice) and continue to access during therapy. Teach patient potential side effects and instruct patient to report any hearing/perceptual problems (e.g., tinnitus, vertigo, decreased hearing). Discuss drug discontinuance and audiogram with physician to confirm hearing dysfunction if symptoms arise. Assess for increased risk if given concurrently with other ototoxic medications (e.g., cisplatin, furosemide).

II. ALTERATION IN URINARY ELIMINATION related to NEPHROTOXICITY

Defining Characteristics: Renal damage characterized by tubular necrosis with increased serum BUN, creatinine; decreased urine creatinine clearance and specific gravity; proteinuria and casts in urine. Azotemia usually not associated with oliguria. Rarely, electrolyte wasting with hypomagnesemia, hypocalcemia, and hypokalemia may occur. Renal dysfunction is usually reversible after drug discontinuance. Increased risk exists in elderly and if preexisting renal dysfunction. Risk low in well-hydrated patients with normal renal function when normal doses given.

Nursing Implications: Assess baseline renal function and electrolytes, and monitor periodically during therapy. Discuss any abnormalities with physician, as drug should be dose-reduced or discontinued if renal dysfunction develops. Assess baseline total body fluid balance, weight, and monitor periodically during antibiotic therapy. Monitor hydration status to keep patient well hydrated. Assess drug peak and trough levels as ordered so that drug dosage is correctly titrated. Increased risk of toxicity if peak serum concentration > 10–12 mg/mL. Draw blood for peak drug concentration 30 minutes after end of 30-minute infusion or at the end of a 60-minute infusion; draw trough immediately before next dose.

III. ALTERATIONS IN SENSORY/PERCEPTUAL PATTERNS related to CNS EFFECTS, NEUROMUSCULAR BLOCKADE

Defining Characteristics: Headache, tremor, lethargy may occur. Peripheral neuropathy or encephalopathy (numbness, skin tingling, muscle twitching) may occur rarely. Neuromuscular blockade is dose-related, self-limiting, and uncommon; risk is greater with topical application or when drug is administered to patient with neuromuscular disease (myasthenia gravis) or hypocalcemia.

COMPLICATIONS

Nursing Implications: Assess baseline neurologic status. Assess coexisting risk factors, neuromuscular blockade medications. Teach patient about side effects and to report headache, tremor, lethargy. Observe for respiratory depression. If signs/symptoms arise, discuss drug discontinuance with physician.

IV.   POTENTIAL FOR INJURY related to HYPERSENSITIVITY

Defining Characteristics: Rash, urticaria, pruritus, fever, eosinophilia have occurred rarely. CROSS-SENSITIVITY between AMINOGLYCOSIDES exists.

Nursing Implications: Assess for drug allergies to any aminoglycoside—amikacin, gentamicin, kanamycin, neomycin, netilmicin, streptomycin, tobramycin—prior to drug administration. Instruct patient to report any allergic reactions. Assess for signs/symptoms of allergic reaction after drug dose.

V.   ALTERATION IN NUTRITION, LESS THAN BODY REQUIREMENTS, related to GI SIDE EFFECTS

Defining Characteristics: Nausea, vomiting, anorexia have occurred rarely. Also, transient hepatomegaly with increased LFTs—AST, ALT, LDH, alk phos, bili—has occurred.

Nursing Implications: Assess baseline nutritional status, preexisting nausea/vomiting, anorexia. Assess baseline LFTs and monitor periodically during treatment. Instruct patient to report side effects. Provide symptomatic interventions if side effects occur; discuss with physician use of alternative drug(s).

VI.   POTENTIAL FOR FATIGUE, INFECTION, AND BLEEDING related to BONE MARROW INJURY

Defining Characteristics: Anemia, leukopenia, granulocytopenia, and thrombocytopenia may occur. Also, patients receiving antibiotics are at risk for overgrowth of nonsusceptible microorganisms, such as fungi (superinfection). Rare.

Nursing Implications: Assess baseline CBC, differential, and monitor periodically during treatment. Instruct patient to report signs/symptoms of fatigue, infection, or bleeding immediately. Assess for signs/symptoms of superinfection. Discuss any adverse effects with physician.

Drug: imipenem/cilastatin sodium (Primaxin)

Class: Antibacterial. Imipenem is a β-lactam antibiotic, carbapenem type; cilastatin inhibits an enzyme in the kidneys that breaks down imipenem, increasing drug potency and protecting kidneys.

Mechanism of Action: Semisynthetic derivative of cephalosporin C (produced by fungus); contains β-lactam ring and is related to penicillins and cephamycins (e.g., cefoxitin). Bactericidal through inhibition of cell wall synthesis, with resulting cell wall instability and cell lysis.

Metabolism: Not well-absorbed from GI tract, so must be given IV. Incompletely absorbed after IM injection. Widely distributed in body tissues and fluids, including bile; does not result in significant CSF drug levels. Crosses placenta and is excreted in breastmilk. Cilastatin decreases renal metabolism of imipenem; both drugs are excreted in urine, and to a lesser degree in feces.

Indication: For treatment of serious infections of lower respiratory tract and urinary tract, intra-abdominal and gynecologic infections, bacterial septicemia, bone and joint infections, skin and skin structure infections, endocarditis, and polymicrobic infections due to susceptible microorganisms. Active against most anaerobic and aerobic gram-positive and gram-negative organisms. These include *Staphylococcus, Streptococcus, E. coli, P. aeruginosa, Proteus, Klebsiella, Enterobacter*. Some activity against *Mycobacterium*. Resists hydrolysis by β lactamase enzymes produced by microorganisms, so resistance to these organisms is much less than other β-lactam antibiotics (e.g., cephalosporins, penicillins). Used in treatment of serious infections of lower respiratory tract, urinary tract, abdomen, female pelvis, skin, bone, and joint, as well as polymicrobial infections and infections resistant to other antibiotics.

Dosage/Range:
Adult:
- IV: 250 mg–1 g q 6–8 h (maximum 50 mg/kg or 4 g/day, whichever is less).
- IM (if unable to give IV): 500–750 mg q 12 h (maximum 1.5 g/day). Reduce dose if renal insufficiency, according to manufacturer's package insert.

Drug Preparation:
- Store vial of sterile powder at < 30°C (86°F).
- IV: Reconstitute according to manufacturer's package insert and further dilute in 100 mL 0.9% sodium chloride or 5% dextrose injection. Infuse over 60 minutes for each gram of drug administered. Slow infusion if nausea/vomiting develop.
- IM: Reconstitute drug with lidocaine HCl 1% injection (without epinephrine) as directed by package insert. Administer deep IM in large muscle mass (e.g., gluteus maximus). Assess allergy to lidocaine. IM preparation SHOULD NOT BE USED FOR IV ADMINISTRATION.

Drug Interactions:
- Probenecid: increases serum concentrations of imipenem. DO NOT USE CONCURRENTLY.
- Aminoglycosides: may have synergistic antimicrobial effect.
- β-lactam antibiotics (cephalosporins, extended-spectrum penicillins): Antagonism. Imipenem stimulates production of β-lactamase enzymes by the bacteria that inactivate the cephalosporins and penicillins. DO NOT USE CONCURRENTLY.

COMPLICATIONS

- Ganciclovir: may decrease seizure threshold. Do not use concurrently unless critical for life-saving treatment.
- Co-trimoxazole: possible synergy against *Nocardia asteroides*.
- Chloramphenicol: possible antagonism. Consider chloramphenicol administration 2+ hours after imipenem (requires clinical study).

Lab Effects/Interference:
- Serum ALT, serum alk phos, and serum AST values may be transiently increased.

Clinical significance:
- Coombs' (direct antiglobulin) tests: may occur during therapy.
- Serum LDH values may be transiently increased.
- Serum bili, BUN concentrations, and serum creatinine concentrations may be transiently increased.
- HCT and Hgb concentrations may be decreased.

Special Considerations:
- Contraindicated in patients hypersensitive to imipenem or cilastatin. Use cautiously in patients sensitive to penicillin or other β-lactams, as partial cross-allergenicity exists.
- Do not give IM preparation reconstituted with 1% lidocaine if hypersensitive to lidocaine.
- Drug may cause false-positive glucose determination when using Clinitest.
- Ensure specimen sent for culture and sensitivity prior to first antibiotic dose.
- Drug has significantly broad antibacterial properties.
- Drug dosage needs to be reduced if severe renal insufficiency.
- Slow IV infusion if nausea/vomiting develop.

Potential Toxicities/Side Effects and the Nursing Process

I.   POTENTIAL FOR INJURY related to HYPERSENSITIVITY REACTION

Defining Characteristics: Urticaria, pruritus, rash (maculopapular or erythematous), fever and chills, eosinophilia, myalgia, edema, erythema, angioedema, Stevens-Johnson syndrome, and exfoliative skin reactions occur in 5% of patients. Increased risk in individuals allergic to penicillin.

Nursing Implications: Assess allergy to cephalosporin antibiotics and penicillin: if patient states "yes," determine actual response (e.g., "swollen lips = angioedema"). If angioedema, discuss with physician RISK versus benefit prior to drug administration, as there is partial cross-allergenicity. Discuss other patient responses with physician to determine whether drug should be given. Assess baseline skin condition, including integrity and allergy history to drugs. Instruct patient to report rash, itching, other skin changes. Teach patient skin care and symptomatic measures as appropriate. If skin rash develops, discuss drug discontinuance with physician. If rash progresses, drug should be discontinued, as fatal Stevens-Johnson syndrome may develop. Be prepared to treat severe acute hypersensitivity reactions with airway management, oxygen, epinephrine, corticosteroids, antihistamines as ordered.

II. ALTERATION IN NUTRITION, LESS THAN BODY REQUIREMENTS, related to GI SIDE EFFECTS

Defining Characteristics: Nausea, vomiting occurs more frequently than diarrhea, anorexia; rarely, pseudomembranous colitis caused by *C. difficile* resistant to the antibiotic occurs. Rarely, transient increases in LFTs—AST, ALT, alk phos, bili—may occur.

Nursing Implications: Assess baseline nutritional status. Instruct patient to report GI disturbances. Administer and teach patient to self-administer antiemetics as needed and as ordered. Teach patient importance of nutritious diet and suggest small, frequent, high-calorie, high-protein meals as appropriate. Assess baseline LFTs and monitor periodically during treatment. Discuss abnormalities and drug interruption with physician.

III. FUNGAL SUPERINFECTION related to REDISTRIBUTION OF ENDOGENOUS MICROORGANISMS

Defining Characteristics: Vaginal candidiasis, vaginitis may occur as endogenous bacteria are eliminated and normal fungal population expands.

Nursing Implications: Instruct female patient to report vaginal itching or discharge. Discuss appropriate antifungal treatment with physician. Teach perineal hygiene and symptomatic management.

IV. ALTERATIONS IN PROTECTIVE MECHANISMS (RARE) related to TRANSIENT LEUKOPENIA

Defining Characteristics: Rarely, transient leukopenia, lymphocytosis, anemia, eosinophilia may occur. Prolonged PT, prolonged aPTT, and hypoprothrombinemia have occurred rarely, especially in elderly or debilitated patients, or in individuals with vitamin K deficiency.

Nursing Implications: Assess baseline laboratory parameters, and monitor periodically during treatment. Assess patient for response to antibiotics. Discuss abnormalities with physician.

V. ALTERATIONS IN SENSORY/PERCEPTUAL PATTERNS related to DIZZINESS, SOMNOLENCE

Defining Characteristics: Dizziness, headache, somnolence, seizures occur rarely. Most seizures have occurred in patients with preexisting CNS problems, those who had received higher-than-recommended IV doses, the elderly, and patients with impaired renal function.

Nursing Implications: Assess baseline neurologic function and comfort, and monitor during treatment. Instruct patient to report any changes. Discuss any abnormalities with

COMPLICATIONS

physician. Institute seizure precautions. If seizures occur, discuss with physician anticonvulsant therapy or discontinuance of antibiotic.

VI.   ALTERATIONS IN COMFORT related to LOCAL INJECTION IRRITATION

Defining Characteristics: Pain, induration, sterile abscesses may form in IM injection
sites; phlebitis may develop in IV sites.

Nursing Implications: Rotate IM injection sites, and administer drug deep IM in large
muscle mass (e.g., gluteus maximus). Use IM injection when IV administration is not
possible. Change IV sites q 48 h, and assess for signs/symptoms of phlebitis prior to each
administration. Administer drug slowly. Apply warm packs to increase comfort.

Drug: kanamycin sulfate (Kantrex)

Class: Aminoglycoside antibacterial.

Mechanism of Action: Synthetic antibiotic derived from *Streptomyces*; bactericidal, most
probably by inhibition of protein synthesis.

Metabolism: Well-absorbed following parenteral administration, but variable absorption
after IM injection (peak serum level 0.5–2 hours, duration 8–12 hours). Widely distributed
into body fluids. Minimally protein-bound. Readily crosses placenta and into breastmilk.
Drug excreted unchanged in the urine.

Indication: For short-term treatment of serious infections caused by susceptible strains of
microorganisms and for short-term adjunctive therapy for supressions of intestinal bacteria; treatment of hepatic coma. Active against aerobic microorganisms: many sensitive
gram-negative organisms (including *Acinetobacter, Citrobacter, Enterobacter, E. coli,
Klebsiella, Proteus, Salmonella, Serratia,* and *Shigella*) and some sensitive gram-positive
organisms (*S. aureus* and *S. epidermidis*). Over time, bacterial resistance may develop,
either naturally or acquired.

Dosage/Range:
- IM, IV: 15 mg/kg/day in equally divided doses at 8- or 12-hour intervals.
- Desired peak serum concentration 15–30 mg/mL, and trough serum concentration is
  5–10 mg/mL.
- DOSE REDUCTION IF RENAL IMPAIRMENT.

Drug Preparation:
- Store capsules in tight containers at temperature < 40°C (104°F).
- Injection should be stored at < 40°C (104°F), preferably 15–30°C (59–86°F).
- Mix 500 mg in 100–200 mL of IV infusion solution. Stable for 24 hours at room
  temperature in 0.9% sodium chloride or 5% dextrose. DO NOT MIX WITH OTHER
  MEDICATIONS.

Drug Administration:
- Deep IM: upper outer quadrant of buttock.
- IV: Infuse over 30–60 minutes.
- Orally (preoperative bowel sterilization): 1 g PO qh × four doses, then q 4 h × four doses.
- Wound irrigation: 2–2.5 mg/mL in 0.9% sodium chloride irrigant.

Drug Interactions:
- Increased risk of toxicity with other ototoxic drugs: acyclovir, other aminoglycosides, amphotericin B, bacitracin, cephalosporins, colistin, cisplatin, ethacrynic acid, furosemide, vancomycin.
- Potentiation of neuromuscular blockade when given concurrently with general anesthetics (succinylcholine, tubocurarine); use cautiously, observe for signs/symptoms of respiratory depression.
- Synergism with extended-spectrum penicillins, but must be administered separately.

Lab Effects/Interference:
- Serum ALT, serum alk phos, serum AST, serum bili, and serum LDH values may be increased.
- BUN and serum creatinine concentrations may be increased.
- Serum Ca++, serum Mg++, serum K+, and serum Na+ concentrations may be decreased.

Special Considerations:
- Used as first-line treatment in short-term treatment of serious gram-negative infections (e.g., septicemia, respiratory tract infections).
- Use against gram-positive organisms only as second-line treatment.
- Use in pregnancy only if infection is life-threatening and no safer drug exists; drug crosses placenta and may cause fetal toxicity.

Potential Toxicities/Side Effects and the Nursing Process

I. ALTERATION IN SENSORY/PERCEPTUAL PATTERNS related to OTOTOXICITY

Defining Characteristics: Damage to eighth cranial nerve (auditory) may result in dizziness, nystagmus, vertigo, ataxia (vestibular damage), and less commonly tinnitus, roaring sound in ears, and impaired hearing (auditory damage). Hearing loss usually begins with high-frequency loss, followed by clinical hearing loss, then permanent hearing loss if damage continues. Increased risk in elderly or renally impaired patients.

Nursing Implications: Assess baseline hearing (ability to hear spoken voice) and continue during therapy. Teach patient potential side effects, and instruct patient to report any hearing/perceptual problems (e.g., tinnitus, vertigo, decreased hearing). Discuss drug discontinuance and audiogram with physician to confirm hearing dysfunction if symptoms arise. Assess for increased risk if given concurrently with other ototoxic medications (e.g., cisplatin, furosemide).

COMPLICATIONS

II.   ALTERATION IN URINARY ELIMINATION related to NEPHROTOXICITY

Defining Characteristics: Renal damage characterized by tubular necrosis with increased serum BUN, creatinine; decreased urine creatinine clearance and specific gravity; proteinuria and casts in urine. Azotemia usually not associated with oliguria. Rarely, electrolyte wasting with hypomagnesemia, hypocalcemia, and hypokalemia may occur. Renal dysfunction usually reversible after drug discontinuance. Increased risk exists in elderly and if there is preexisting renal dysfunction. Risk is low in well-hydrated patients with normal renal function when normal doses given.

Nursing Implications: Assess baseline renal function and electrolytes, and monitor periodically during therapy. Discuss any abnormalities with physician, as drug should be dose-reduced or discontinued if renal dysfunction develops. Assess baseline total body fluid balance, weight, and monitor periodically during antibiotic therapy. Monitor hydration status to keep patient well hydrated. Assess drug peak and trough levels as ordered so that drug dosage is correctly titrated. Increased risk of toxicity if peak serum concentration > 30–35 mg/mL. Draw blood for peak drug concentration 30 minutes after end of 30-minute infusion or at the end of a 60-minute infusion; draw trough immediately before next dose.

III.   ALTERATIONS IN SENSORY/PERCEPTUAL PATTERNS related to CNS EFFECTS, NEUROMUSCULAR BLOCKADE

Defining Characteristics: Headache, tremor, lethargy may occur. Peripheral neuropathy or encephalopathy (numbness, skin tingling, muscle twitching) may occur rarely. Neuromuscular blockade is dose-related, self-limiting, and uncommon; risk is greater with topical application or when drug is administered to patient with neuromuscular disease (myasthenia gravis) or hypocalcemia.

Nursing Implications: Assess baseline neurologic status. Assess coexisting risk factors, neuromuscular blockade medications. Teach patient about side effects, and instruct to report headache, tremor, lethargy. Observe for respiratory depression. If signs/symptoms arise, discuss drug discontinuance with physician.

IV.   POTENTIAL FOR INJURY related to HYPERSENSITIVITY

Defining Characteristics: Rash, urticaria, pruritus, fever, eosinophilia have occurred rarely. CROSS-SENSITIVITY between AMINOGLYCOSIDES exists!

Nursing Implications: Assess for drug allergies to any aminoglycoside—amikacin, gentamicin, kanamycin, neomycin, netilmicin, streptomycin, tobramycin—prior to drug administration. Instruct patient to report any allergic reactions. Assess for signs/symptoms of allergic reaction after drug dose.

V.   ALTERATION IN NUTRITION, LESS THAN BODY REQUIREMENTS, related to GI SIDE EFFECTS

Defining Characteristics: Nausea, vomiting, anorexia have occurred rarely. Also, transient hepatomegaly with increased LFTs—AST, ALT, alk phos—has occurred.

Nursing Implications: Assess baseline nutritional status, preexisting nausea/vomiting, anorexia. Assess baseline LFTs and monitor periodically during treatment. Instruct patient to report side effects. Provide symptomatic interventions if side effects occur; discuss with physician use of alternative drug(s).

VI.   POTENTIAL FOR FATIGUE, INFECTION, AND BLEEDING related to BONE MARROW INJURY

Defining Characteristics: Anemia, leukopenia, granulocytopenia, and thrombocytopenia may occur. Also, patients receiving antibiotics are at risk for overgrowth of nonsusceptible microorganisms, such as fungi (superinfection). Rare.

Nursing Implications: Assess baseline CBC, differential, and monitor periodically during treatment. Instruct patient to report signs/symptoms of fatigue, infection, or bleeding immediately. Assess for signs/symptoms of superinfection. Discuss any adverse effects with physician.

Drug: levofloxacin (Levaquin)

Class: Fluoroquinolone antibiotic.

Mechanism of Action: Drug is a synthetic, broad-spectrum antibacterial agent. Inhibits DNA gyrase (bacterial topoisomerase II), which is necessary for DNA replication, transcription, and repair. Has activity against a wide range of gram-negative and gram-positive bacteria, as well as against some bacteria resistant to β-lactam antibiotics.

Metabolism: Drug is well-absorbed from the GI tract without regard to food, with 99% bioavailability; peak serum levels occur in 1–2 hours. Steady state is reached in 48 hours. Drug is not extensively metabolized, with 87% of drug excreted largely unchanged in the urine at 48 hours. Terminal half-life is 6–8 hours.

Indication: For treatment of bacterial infections such as pneumonia, chronic bronchitis and sinus, urinary tract, kidney, prostate, and skin infections.

Dosage/Range:
- 500 mg daily × 7 days (acute bacterial exacerbation of chronic bronchitis), × 7–14 days (community-acquired pneumonia), × 7–10 days (uncomplicated skin and skin structure

infection), × 10–14 days (acute maxillary sinusitis), × 10 days (uncomplicated UTI, acute pyelonephritis).

Drug Preparation:
- Oral, available in 250-mg and 500-mg tablets.
- IV: Administer over 60 min to prevent hypotension; IV available in premixed 250-mg or 500-mg bags, or 20-mL vial containing 500 mg that is further diluted in 5% dextrose, 0.9% sodium chloride.

Drug Administration:
- Administer without regard to food.
- Dose-reduce if renal compromise (see Special Considerations section).
- Administer oral doses at least 2 hours before or 2 hours after antacids containing magnesium or aluminum, as well as sucralfate, medications such as iron, and multivitamins containing zinc.

Drug Interactions:
- Antacids containing magnesium or aluminum, sucralfate, iron, multivitamins containing zinc: may decrease serum levels of levofloxacin; take any of these agents at least 2 hours before or 2 hours after levofloxacin.
- Theophylline: possible increase in theophylline serum levels; monitor levels and change dose accordingly.
- Warfarin: theoretically could enhance effects of oral anticoagulants; monitor INR closely and modify dose accordingly.
- NSAIDs: possible increase in the risk of CNS stimulation and seizures; assess patient risk for seizures, and use cautiously if at all in patients at risk.
- Anti-diabetic agents: changes in glucose (hyper- or hypoglycemia); monitor blood sugar closely, and modify dose accordingly.

Lab Effects/Interference:
- Decreased glucose, decreased lymphocytes.

Special Considerations:
- Indicated for the treatment of acute maxillary sinusitis due to *Streptococcus pneumoniae, Haemophilus influenzae, Moraxella catarrhalis*; acute bacterial exacerbation of chronic bronchitis due to *Staphylococcus aureus, Streptococcus pneumoniae, H. influenzae, H. parainfluenzae,* or *Moraxella catarrhalis;* community-acquired pneumonia due to *Staphylococcus aureus, Streptococcus pneumoniae, H. influenzae, H. parainfluenzae, Klebsiella pneumoniae, Moraxella catarrhalis, Chlamydia pneumoniae, Legionella pneumonophila,* or *Mycoplasma pneumoniae.*
- Active against the above as well as aerobic gram-positive *Enterococcus faecalis* and *S. pyogenes* and aerobic gram-negative microorganisms *Enterobacter cloacae, E. coli, P. mirabilis,* and *P. aeruginosa.*
- Dose modifications for renal dysfunction:

Acute Bacterial Exacerbation of:	Chronic Bronchitis, Community-Acquired	Pneumonia, Acute Maxillary Sinusitis, Uncomplicated Skin Infections
Renal status	Initial dose	Subsequent dose
Cr cl 20–49 mL/min	500 mg	250 mg q 24 h
Cr cl 10–19 mL/min	500 mg	250 mg q 48 h
Hemodialysis	500 mg	250 mg q 48 h
CAPD	500 mg q 48 h	250 mg q 48 h
Uncomplicated UTI/Acute Pyelonephritis		
Cr cl 10–19 mL/min	250 mg	250 mg q 48 h

- Use drug cautiously, if at all, in the following patients: (1) known or suspected CNS or seizure disorder (e.g., severe cerebral arteriosclerosis or epilepsy); (2) possess factors lowering seizure threshold (e.g., renal dysfunction, other drug therapy); (3) pregnant or nursing mothers; (4) children < 18 years old.
- Obtain ordered specimen for culture and sensitivity prior to first drug dose.

Potential Toxicities/Side Effects and the Nursing Process

I. ALTERATION IN NUTRITION related to GI SIDE EFFECTS

Defining Characteristics: 0.1–3.0% incidence of nausea, vomiting, abdominal discomfort, diarrhea, anorexia. As with all antibiotics, pseudomembranous colitis may occur, ranging in severity from mild to life-threatening. Treatment with antibiotics changes the intestinal microflora, so *C. difficile* bacteria may overgrow. Once diagnosis is made, mild diarrhea may stop with cessation of drug; if moderate to severe, it will require hydration, electrolyte replacement, nutritional support, and antibacterial coverage against *C. difficile*.

Nursing Implications: Assess baseline nutritional and elimination status. Teach patient to report GI disturbances. Teach patient to report diarrhea immediately, and consider whether this is pseudomembranous colitis and send stool specimen for *C. difficile*; if positive, discuss drug discontinuance with physician. Administer and teach patient to self-administer antiemetics, antidiarrheals as needed and as ordered. Teach patient importance of nutritious diet, and suggest small, frequent, high-calorie, high-protein meals as appropriate. Assess baseline LFTs and monitor periodically during treatment. Discuss abnormalities and drug interruption with physician.

II. SENSORY/PERCEPTUAL ALTERATIONS related to CNS EFFECTS

Defining Characteristics: 1–2% incidence of insomnia, dizziness, taste perversion, headache, nervousness, anxiety, tremors, and seizures may also occur.

COMPLICATIONS

Nursing Implications: Assess baseline neurologic function and comfort, and monitor during treatment. Teach patient to report any changes. Discuss any abnormalities with physician. Teach patient to avoid caffeine-containing fluids, medications (e.g., tea, coffee, soft drinks).

III.   ALTERATION IN SKIN INTEGRITY related to ALLERGY/HYPERSENSITIVITY

Defining Characteristics: 1–4% incidence of rash; other manifestations include eosinophilia, urticaria, flushing, fever, chills, photosensitivity, angioedema. Fatal hypersensitivity reactions have occurred rarely. Direct exposure to sunlight can cause sunburn (moderate-to-severe phototoxicity).

Nursing Implications: Assess baseline skin condition, including integrity and drug allergy history. Teach patient to report rash, itching, other skin changes. Teach patient skin care and symptomatic measures as appropriate. If skin rash develops, discuss drug discontinuance with physician. If rash progresses, especially in HIV-infected patients, drug should be discontinued, as fatal Stevens-Johnson syndrome may develop. Be prepared to treat severe acute hypersensitivity reactions with airway management, oxygen, epinephrine, corticosteroids, antihistamines as ordered. Teach patient to avoid excessive sun exposure and to use skin protection factor (SPF) 15 or higher.

IV.   FUNGAL SUPERINFECTION related to REDISTRIBUTION OF ENDOGENOUS MICROORGANISMS

Defining Characteristics: Vaginal moniliasis, vaginitis may occur as endogenous bacteria are eliminated and normal fungal population expands.

Nursing Implications: Teach female patient to report vaginal itching or discharge. Discuss appropriate antifungal treatment with physician. Teach perineal hygiene and symptomatic management.

Drug: linezolid (Zyvox)

Class: Oxazolidinone class of antibiotic.

Mechanism of Action: Linezolid inhibits initiation of protein synthesis by preventing the formation of the fmet-tRNA:mRNA:30S subunit ternary complex. Oxazolidinones bind to the 50S subunit in a region shared with the peptidyl transferase inhibitor chloramphenicol. Oxazolidinones are not peptidyl transferase inhibitors, and it is not known which specific ribosome reaction is inhibited by 50S subunit binding.

Metabolism: Primarily metabolized by oxidation of the morpholine ring, resulting in two inactive carboxylic acid metabolites. Only about 30% of a dose is excreted unchanged in the urine.

Indication: Linezolid has a specific mechanism of action against bacteria resistant to other antibiotics, including methicillin-resistant *Staphylococcus aureus* (MRSA), multiresistant strains of *S. pneumoniae*, and vancomycin-resistant *enterococcus faecium* (VRE). The drug is used to treat nosocomial and community-acquired pneumonia, septicemias, and complicated and uncomplicated skin and skin structure infections caused by susceptible strains of specific organisms.

Dosage/Range:
- Oral: 400–600 mg q 12 h for 10 to 14 days; up to 28 days for VRE.
- IV: 600 mg q 12 h for 10–14 days; up to 28 days for VRE.

Drug Preparation:
- Available in single-use, ready-to-use infusion bags.

Drug Administration:
- IV infusion over 30–120 minutes.
- Linezolid has the potential to interact with adrenergic (phenylpropanolamine, pseudoephedrine) and serotonergic agents since it is a reversible, nonselective monoamine oxidase inhibitor.
- Large quantities of foods or beverages with high tyramine content should be avoided.

Lab Effects/Interference:
- Thrombocytopenia has been seen when this drug is administered long-term (up to 28 days).

Special Considerations:
- IV and PO doses are the same.

Potential Toxicities/Side Effects and the Nursing Process

I.   ALTERATION IN NUTRITION related to GI SIDE EFFECTS

Defining Characteristics: Nausea, vomiting, anorexia have occurred frequently.

Nursing Implications: Assess baseline nutritional status, preexisting nausea/vomiting, anorexia. Teach patient to report side effects. Provide symptomatic interventions if side effects occur; discuss with physician use of alternative drug(s).

II.   POTENTIAL FOR INJURY related to HYPERSENSITIVITY REACTION

Defining Characteristics: Urticaria, pruritus, rash (maculopapular or erythematous), fever and chills, eosinophilia, myalgia, edema, erythema, angioedema.

Nursing Implications: Assess for drug allergies to erythromycin or macrolide antibiotic prior to drug administration. Teach patient to report any allergic reactions. Assess for signs/symptoms of allergic reaction after drug dose. Assess baseline skin integrity and presence of drug allergies; monitor patient closely during drug infusions. Teach patient to report immediately signs/symptoms of rash, pruritus, shortness of breath, any adverse sensation. Teach patient skin care and symptomatic measures as appropriate. If skin rash develops, discuss drug discontinuance with physician. If rash progresses, especially in human immunodeficiency virus (HIV)-infected patients, drug should be discontinued, as fatal Stevens-Johnson syndrome may develop. Be prepared to treat severe acute hypersensitivity reactions with airway management, oxygen, epinephrine, corticosteroids, antihistamines as ordered.

III.   ALTERATIONS IN COMFORT related to HEADACHE

Defining Characteristics: Headache has occurred in some patients.

Nursing Implications: Assess baseline hearing (ability to hear spoken voice) and continue to assess during therapy. Teach patient potential side effects, and instruct patient to report any hearing/perceptual problems (e.g., tinnitus, vertigo, decreased hearing). Discuss drug discontinuance and audiogram with physician to confirm hearing dysfunction if symptoms arise. Assess for increased risk if given concurrently with other ototoxic medications (e.g., cisplatin, furosemide).

IV.   FUNGAL SUPERINFECTION related to REDISTRIBUTION OF ENDOGENOUS MICROORGANISMS

Defining Characteristics: Vaginal or oral candidiasis (sore mouth or tongue; white patches in mouth and/or tongue); vaginitis (vaginal candidiasis); vaginal itching and discharge may occur as endogenous bacteria are eliminated and normal fungal population expands.

Nursing Implications: Teach female patient to report vaginal itching or discharge. Discuss appropriate antifungal treatment with physician. Teach perineal hygiene and symptomatic management.

Drug: meropenem (Merrem)

Class: Antibiotic, carbapenem.

Mechanism of Action: The bactericidal activity results from the inhibition of cell wall synthesis. Penetrates the cell wall of most gram-positive and gram-negative bacteria to reach penicillin-binding protein (PBP) targets.

Metabolism: Widely distributed in body tissues and fluids, excreted in urine.

Indication: Drug is used as empiric anti-infective therapy of presumed bacterial infections in febrile neutropenia patients. It is also used to treat severe infections of the skin and skin structures (beta-lactamase–producing strains [but not oxacillin-resistant (methicillin-resistant) strains of *S. aureus*; group A beta-hemolytic streptococci of *S. pyogenes*; group B streptococci of *S. agalactiae*; *viridans streptococci*; non-vancomycin-resistant strains of

Enterococcus faecalis; *P. aeruginosa*; *E. coli*; *P. mirabilis*; *B. fragilis*; *Peptostreptococcus*), respiratory tract (CAP caused by *S. pneumoniae*, *P. aeruginosa, Klebiella*, or other gram-negative bacteria; nosocomial pneumonia), gastrointestinal tract (susceptible *viridans streptococci*; *E. coli*; *Klebsiella pneumoniae*; *P. aeruginosa*; *B. fragilis*; *B. thetaiotamicron;* *Peptostreptococcus*), bacterial meningitis (*S. pneumoniae*; *H. influenzae*; *Enterobacter;* *Citrobacter; Serratia marcescens*). Other infections include urinary tract infections, acinebacter infections, anthrax, and bacillus, burkholderia, vampylobacter, capnocytophaga, nocardia and rhodococcus infections.

Dosage/Range:
Adult:
- Intra-abdominal infection: 1 g IV every 8 hours.
- Meningitis: bacterial 2 g IV every 8 hours.

Drug Preparation:
- IV bolus, dilute with 5–20 mL. Sterile water for injection and give over 3–5 minutes.
- IV infusion dilute with D₅W or normal saline, infuse over 15–30 minutes, maximum concentration 50 mg/mL.

Drug Interactions:
- Probenecid competes with meropenem for active tubular secretion and thus inhibits the renal excretion of meropenem.
- Meropenem may reduce serum levels of valproic acid to subtherapeutic levels.

Lab Effects/Interference:
- Meropenem possesses the characteristic low toxicity of the β-lactam group of antibiotics.
- Periodically assess organ system function; renal, hepatic, and hematopoietic.

Potential Toxicities/Side Effects and the Nursing Process

I.   POTENTIAL FOR INJURY related to HYPERSENSITIVITY REACTION AND LOCAL REACTIONS (pain at injection site)

Defining Characteristics: Urticaria, pruritus, rash (maculopapular or erythematous), fever and chills, eosinophilia, myalgia, edema, erythema, angioedema.

Nursing Implications: Assess allergy to cephalosporin antibiotics and penicillin: if patient states "yes," determine actual response (e.g., "swollen lips = angioedema"). If angioedema, patient SHOULD NOT receive drug. Discuss other patient responses with physician to determine whether drug should be given. Assess baseline skin condition, including integrity and allergy history to drugs. Instruct patient to report rash, itching, and other skin changes. Teach patient skin care and symptomatic measures as appropriate. If skin rash develops, discuss drug discontinuance with physician. Be prepared to treat severe acute hypersensitivity reactions with airway management, oxygen, epinephrine, corticosteroids, antihistamines as ordered.

II. ALTERATION IN NUTRITION, LESS THAN BODY REQUIREMENTS, related to GI SIDE EFFECTS

Defining Characteristics: Nausea, vomiting, diarrhea may occur; rarely, pseudomembranous colitis caused by antibiotic resistance occurs.

Nursing Implications: Assess baseline nutritional status. Instruct patient to report GI disturbances. Administer and teach patient to self-administer antiemetics as needed and as ordered. Teach patient importance of nutritious diet, and suggest small, frequent, high-calorie, high-protein meals as appropriate. Assess baseline LFTs, and monitor periodically during treatment. Discuss abnormalities and drug interruption with physician.

III. FUNGAL SUPERINFECTION related to REDISTRIBUTION OF ENDOGENOUS MICROORGANISMS

Defining Characteristics: Vaginal candidiasis, vaginitis may occur as endogenous bacteria are eliminated and normal fungal population expands.

Nursing Implications: Instruct female patient to report vaginal itching or discharge. Discuss appropriate antifungal treatment with physician. Teach perineal hygiene and symptomatic management.

Drug: metronidazole hydrochloride (Flagyl)

Class: Antibacterial (systemic); antiprotozoal.

Mechanism of Action: Disrupts DNA, inhibits nucleic acid synthesis in susceptible organisms.

Metabolism: Well-absorbed after oral administration; rate affected by food, but not amount absorbed. Oral and IV serum levels are similar. Widely distributed in body tissues and fluids, including CSF, placenta, breastmilk. Excreted in urine (60–80%) and feces.

Indication: For treatment of parasitic and bacterial infections. This drug is active against anaerobic gram-negative (*Bacteroides*) and gram-positive bacilli (*Clostridium*), and protozoa (*Trichomonas, Giardia*).

Dosage/Range:
Adult:
- Oral: 250–750 mg PO tid × 7–10 days or single dose of 2 g PO (trichomoniasis).
- Pseudomembranous colitis: 250 mg PO qid × 7–14 days or 500 mg PO tid × 7–14 days.
- IV: Loading dose of 15 mg/kg IV over 1 hour (1 g); then maintenance dose of 7.5 mg/kg IV (500 mg) q 8 h (maximum 4 g/day).

Drug Preparation:
- Oral: Store in light-resistant container at < 30°C (86°F).

- IV: Protect from light and freezing. Reconstitute according to manufacturer's package insert. Further dilute with 0.9% sodium chloride or 5% dextrose to concentration of ≤ 8 mg/mL. Do not use aluminum needles. Administer over 30–60 minutes. May be given as continuous or intermittent infusion.

Drug Interactions:
- Coumarin anticoagulants: increase anticoagulant effect. Avoid concurrent use if possible; otherwise, monitor PT closely and decrease anticoagulant drug dose as needed.
- Alcohol: inhibits alcohol metabolism, causing a disulfiram-like reaction (flushing, headache, nausea, vomiting, abdominal cramps, diaphoresis). Avoid alcohol and alcohol-containing medications for 48 hours after last metronidazole dose.
- Disulfiram: causes acute psychoses and confusion. Avoid concurrent use and separate use by 2 weeks.
- Phenobarbital/phenytoin: decrease metronidazole activity. Monitor effectiveness and increase metronidazole dose as needed.
- Cimetidine: increases metronidazole levels with potential for increased toxicity. Avoid concurrent administration.

Lab Effects/Interference:
- Serum ALT, serum AST, and LDH: metronidazole has a high absorbance at the wavelength at which NADH is determined; therefore, elevated liver enzyme concentrations may appear to be suppressed by metronidazole when measured by continuous-flow methods based on endpoint decrease.

Special Considerations:
- Carcinogenic in rodents, so drug is used only when necessary.
- Contraindicated in first trimester of pregnancy and administered only as salvage therapy in second and third trimesters when other agents have failed; lactating mothers should interrupt breastfeeding during treatment with drug.
- Use with caution in patients with a history of blood dyscrasias, CNS disorders/dysfunction, hepatic dysfunction, or alcoholism.
- May interfere with laboratory determinations of LFTs (AST, ALT, LDH).

Potential Toxicities/Side Effects and the Nursing Process

I. ALTERATION IN NUTRITION, LESS THAN BODY REQUIREMENTS, related to GI SIDE EFFECTS

Defining Characteristics: Nausea (with/without headache), anorexia, dry mouth, metallic taste in mouth have occurred; less frequently, vomiting, diarrhea, epigastric distress, or constipation. Rare pseudomembranous colitis.

Nursing Implications: Assess baseline nutritional and elimination status. Instruct patient to report GI disturbances. Administer and teach patient to self-administer antiemetics, antidiarrheals as needed and as ordered. Teach patient importance of nutritious diet, and suggest small, frequent, high-calorie, high-protein meals as appropriate. Assess baseline

LFTs and monitor periodically during treatment. Discuss abnormalities and drug interruption with physician. Assess whether taking other hepatotoxic drugs (see Special Considerations section). Instruct patient to avoid alcohol and alcohol-containing medications for 48 hours after last drug dose.

II.   ALTERATIONS IN SENSORY/PERCEPTUAL PATTERNS related to PERIPHERAL NEUROPATHY

Defining Characteristics: Peripheral neuropathy (numbness, tingling, paresthesia) is reversible with drug discontinuance. Headache, dizziness, ataxia, confusion, mood changes have also occurred.

Nursing Implications: Assess baseline neurologic function and comfort, and monitor during treatment. Instruct patient to report any changes. Discuss abnormalities and drug discontinuance with physician.

III.   ALTERATIONS IN SKIN INTEGRITY related to SENSITIVITY REACTIONS

Defining Characteristics: Urticaria, erythematous rash, pruritus, flushing, transient joint pain may occur.

Nursing Implications: Assess drug allergy history. Assess baseline skin integrity. Instruct patient to report rash, pruritus. Teach patient symptomatic management of rash, pruritus.

IV.   ALTERATIONS IN URINARY ELIMINATION related to DYSURIA

Defining Characteristics: Urethral burning, dysuria, cystitis, polyuria, incontinence, sensation of pelvic pressure may occur with oral dose. Urine may be dark or reddish-brown.

Nursing Implications: Assess baseline elimination status. Instruct patient to report side effects, and to increase oral fluids to 2–3 qt/day. Reassure patient urine color change is related to drug and will disappear when drug therapy is completed.

V.   ALTERATIONS IN SEXUALITY related to DECREASED LIBIDO, DYSPAREUNIA

Defining Characteristics: Decreased libido, dyspareunia, dryness of vagina and vulva may occur.

Nursing Implications: Assess pattern of sexuality. Inform patient and partner that these effects, if they occur, are temporary. Suggest frequent perineal hygiene as needed to relieve dryness and use of lubricants during intercourse.

VI. FUNGAL SUPERINFECTION related to REDISTRIBUTION OF ENDOGENOUS MICROORGANISMS

Defining Characteristics: Vaginal candidiasis, vaginitis may occur as endogenous bacteria are eliminated and normal fungal population expands.

Nursing Implications: Instruct female patient to report vaginal itching or discharge. Discuss appropriate antifungal treatment with physician. Teach perineal hygiene and symptomatic management.

VII. ALTERATIONS IN COMFORT related to PHLEBITIS

Defining Characteristics: Phlebitis and thrombophlebitis may occur with IV administration.

Nursing Implications: Assess IV site prior to each dose for phlebitis, erythema, and swelling, and change site at least q 48 h. Apply heat to painful IV site as ordered.

Drug: mezlocillin sodium (Mezlin)

Class: Antibacterial (extended-spectrum penicillin).

Mechanism of Action: Semisynthetic antibiotic prepared from fungus *Penicillium*. Contains β-lactam ring and is bactericidal by inhibiting cell wall synthesis.

Metabolism: Poorly absorbed from GI tract, so must be given parenterally. Widely distributed in body tissues and fluids. Crosses placenta and is excreted in breastmilk. Excreted via urine and bile.

Indication: For treatment of infections of the lower respiratory tract, urinary tract, skin or skin structures, intra-abdominal infections, uncomplicated gonorrhea, gynecological infections, septicemia, streptococcal infections, severe infections, and *Pseudomonas* infections caused by susceptible strains of specific microorganisms. Active against most gram-positive (except penicillinase-producing strains) and most gram-negative bacilli. Used in the treatment of serious gram-negative infections, especially *P. aeruginosa*–related infections of lower respiratory tract, urinary tract, and skin.

Dosage/Range:
Adult:
- IV: 200–300 mg/kg/day in four to six divided doses (usual dose 3 g q 4–6 h).
- Dose modification if severe renal insufficiency; refer to manufacturer's package insert.

Drug Preparation:
- IV: Reconstitute each gram with at least 10 mL sterile water for injection. Further dilute in 50–100 mL 0.9% sodium chloride or 5% dextrose injection. Administer over 30 minutes.

COMPLICATIONS

- IM: Reconstitute each gram with 3–4 mL sterile water for injection or 0.5–1% lidocaine HCl (without epinephrine). Maximum dose is 2 g. Divide dose into two injections, as needed, and administer deep IM in large muscle mass. Administer slowly. Make certain patient is NOT ALLERGIC to lidocaine.

Drug Interactions:
- Aminoglycosides: synergism.
- Aminoglycosides (e.g., gentamicin): incompatible when mixed together; administer at separate sites at different times. Also, penicillinase-resistant penicillins can inactivate aminoglycoside serum samples from patients receiving both drugs.
- Clavulanic acid (inhibits β-lactamase): increases antibacterial action.
- Probenecid: increased serum level of mezlocillin; may be coadministered to exert this effect.

Lab Effects/Interference:
Major clinical significance:
- Urine glucose: high urinary concentrations of a penicillin may produce false-positive or falsely elevated test results with copper sulfate tests (Benedict's, Clinitest, or Fehling's); glucose enzymatic tests (Clinistix or Testape) are not affected.

Clinical significance:
- Coombs' (direct antiglobulin) test: false-positive result may occur during therapy with any penicillin.
- Urine protein: high urinary concentrations of mezlocillin may produce false-positive protein reactions (pseudoproteinuria) with the sulfosalicylic acid and boiling test, the acetic acid test, the biuret reaction, and the nitric acid test; bromophenol blue reagent test strips (Multistix) are reportedly unaffected.
- ALT, alk phos, AST, serum LDH values may be increased.
- Serum bili: an increase has been associated with mezlocillin.
- BUN and serum creatinine: an increase has been associated with mezlocillin.
- Serum K+: hypokalemia may occur following the administration of parenteral mezlocillin, which may act as a non-reabsorbable anion in the distal renal tubules; this may cause an increase in pH and result in increased urinary K+ loss. The risk of hypokalemia increases with the use of larger doses.
- Serum Na+: hypernatremia may occur following administration of large doses of parenteral mezlocillin because of the high Na+ content of these medications.
- WBC: leukopenia or neutropenia is associated with the use of all penicillins; the effect is more likely to occur with prolonged therapy and severe hepatic function impairment.

Special Considerations:
- Contraindicated in patients with prior hypersensitivity to penicillins. Use with caution in patients sensitive to other β-lactams (e.g., cephalosporins) since partial cross-allergenicity exists.
- Obtain ordered specimen, and send for culture and sensitivity test prior to first antibiotic dose.
- Consider alternative antibiotic therapy if eosinophilia, drug fever or rash, arthralgia, hematuria, or unexplained rise in BUN and serum creatinine occur.

- Monitor electrolytes and renal, hepatic, and hematologic laboratory parameters during extended treatment periods.
- Use with caution in pregnancy or with nursing women.
- Na content is 1.85 mEq/g of drug.

Potential Toxicities/Side Effects and the Nursing Process

I. POTENTIAL FOR INJURY related to HYPERSENSITIVITY REACTION

Defining Characteristics: Urticaria, pruritus, rash (maculopapular or erythematous), fever and chills, eosinophilia, myalgia, edema, erythema, angioedema, Stevens-Johnson syndrome, and exfoliative skin reactions occur in 5% of patients. Increased risk in individuals allergic to cephalosporin antibiotics.

Nursing Implications: Assess allergy to cephalosporin antibiotics and penicillin: if patient states "yes," determine actual response (e.g., "swollen lips = angioedema"). If angioedema, patient SHOULD NOT receive drug. Discuss other patient responses with physician to determine whether drug should be given. Assess baseline skin condition, including integrity and allergy history to drugs. Instruct patient to report rash, itching, and other skin changes. Teach patient skin care and symptomatic measures as appropriate. If skin rash develops, discuss drug discontinuance with physician. If rash progresses, drug should be discontinued, as fatal Stevens-Johnson syndrome may develop. Be prepared to treat severe acute hypersensitivity reactions with airway management, oxygen, epinephrine, corticosteroids, antihistamines as ordered.

II. ALTERATION IN NUTRITION, LESS THAN BODY REQUIREMENTS, related to GI SIDE EFFECTS

Defining Characteristics: Nausea, vomiting, diarrhea may occur; rarely, pseudomembranous colitis caused by *C. difficile* resistant to the antibiotic occurs. Rarely, transient increases in LFTs—AST, ALT, alk phos, bili—may occur.

Nursing Implications: Assess baseline nutritional status. Instruct patient to report GI disturbances. Administer and teach patient to self-administer antiemetics as needed and as ordered. Teach patient importance of nutritious diet, and suggest small, frequent, high-calorie, high-protein meals as appropriate. Assess baseline LFTs, and monitor periodically during treatment. Discuss abnormalities and drug interruption with physician.

III. FUNGAL SUPERINFECTION related to REDISTRIBUTION OF ENDOGENOUS MICROORGANISMS

Defining Characteristics: Vaginal candidiasis, vaginitis may occur as endogenous bacteria are eliminated and normal fungal population expands.

COMPLICATIONS

Nursing Implications: Instruct female patient to report vaginal itching or discharge. Discuss appropriate antifungal treatment with physician. Teach perineal hygiene and symptomatic management.

IV. ALTERATIONS IN PROTECTIVE MECHANISMS (RARE) related to TRANSIENT LEUKOPENIA

Defining Characteristics: Rarely, transient leukopenia, lymphocytosis, anemia, eosinophilia may occur. Prolonged PT, prolonged aPTT, and hypoprothrombinemia have occurred rarely, especially in elderly or debilitated patients, or in individuals with vitamin K deficiency.

Nursing Implications: Assess baseline laboratory parameters, and monitor periodically during treatment. Assess patient for response to antibiotics. Discuss abnormalities with physician. Assess for signs/symptoms of bleeding.

V. ALTERATIONS IN SENSORY/PERCEPTUAL PATTERNS related to DIZZINESS, SOMNOLENCE

Defining Characteristics: Dizziness, headache, somnolence occur rarely. Neuromuscular irritability and seizures may occur with high drug serum levels.

Nursing Implications: Assess baseline neurologic function and comfort, and monitor during treatment. Instruct patient to report any changes. Discuss any abnormalities with physician. Institute seizure precautions.

VI. ALTERATIONS IN COMFORT related to LOCAL INJECTION IRRITATION

Defining Characteristics: Vein irritation (pain, erythema), phlebitis, and thrombophlebitis may occur at IV administration site.

Nursing Implications: Change IV sites q 48 h, and assess for signs/symptoms of phlebitis prior to each administration. Administer drug slowly. Apply warm packs to increase comfort. Discuss central line with patient and physician to facilitate administration.

VII. ALTERATION IN FLUID AND ELECTROLYTE BALANCE related to HYPOKALEMIA AND INCREASED SODIUM INTAKE

Defining Characteristics: Prolonged therapy may cause hypokalemia; also, drug is prepared as sodium salt. Frequent IV infusions increase fluid intake.

Nursing Implications: Assess baseline electrolytes, fluid balance, weight, and monitor throughout therapy. Monitor renal function studies, especially if patient has preexisting renal dysfunction.

Drug: minocycline hydrochloride (Minocin, Vectrin, Dynacin)

Class: Antibacterial (systemic); antiprotozoal.

Mechanism of Action: Bacteriostatic, but may be bactericidal at high concentrations. Binds to bacterial ribosomes and prevents protein synthesis.

Metabolism: Absorbed (60–80%) from GI tract. Widely distributed into body tissues and fluids. Crosses placenta and is excreted in breastmilk. Excreted unchanged in urine.

Indication: For treatment of a broad range of gram-positive and gram-negative bacteria and a variety of bacterial infections.

Dosage/Range:
Adult:
- Oral: 200 mg initially, then 100 mg q 12 h for 5–15 days; or 100–200 mg initially, then 50 mg q 6 h for 5–15 days.
- IV: 200 mg initially, then 100 mg q 12 h for 5–15 days (depends on indication).
- Dose modification necessary if renal dysfunction exists.

Drug Preparation:
- Oral: may be taken with food, water, or milk.
- IV: add 5–10 mL sterile water for injection to 100-mg vial. Further dilute in 500 to 1,000 mL of 0.9% sodium chloride injection, dextrose injection, dextrose and sodium chloride injections, Ringer's injection, or lactated Ringer's injection. Do not use other calcium-containing solutions, since precipitate may form.
- AVOID RAPID ADMINISTRATION.
- Solution stable for 24 hours at room temperature. Avoid exposure to heat or sunlight. Convert to oral preparation as soon as possible, as there is risk of thrombophlebitis.
- DO NOT ADMINISTER INTRAMUSCULARLY OR SUBCUTANEOUSLY.

Drug Interactions:
- Hepatotoxic drugs: may increase hepatotoxicity if given concurrently. Assess baseline and periodically during treatment.
- Iron preparations: decrease oral and possibly IV absorption. Administer iron preparations 3 hours after or 2 hours before any tetracycline.
- Oral anticoagulants: increase PT. Monitor patient closely and decrease anticoagulant dose as needed.
- Antidiarrheals (containing kaolin, pectate, or bismuth): may decrease absorption of tetracyclines. Avoid concurrent use.
- Oral contraceptives: decreased effectiveness of contraceptive and increased incidence of breakthrough bleeding. Advise patient to use barrier contraceptive as well during a course of tetracycline therapy.
- Lithium: may decrease lithium levels. Monitor serum levels and increase dose as needed.

Lab Effects/Interference:
- Urine catecholamine determinations: may produce false elevations of urinary catecholamines because of interfering fluorescence in the Hingerty method.

- SGPT, alk phos, amylase, SGOT, and bilirubin: serum concentrations may be increased.

Special Considerations:

- May cause dizziness, lightheadedness, or unsteadiness (CNS toxicity).
- Pigmentation of skin and mucous membranes may occur.
- Use cautiously in patients with myasthenia gravis: may increase muscle weakness.
- Avoid use in pregnant or lactating women.
- Obtain ordered specimen for culture and sensitivity prior to first dose.
- IV preparation contains ascorbic acid and may cause false-positive result using Clinitest, or false-negative when using Clinistix and Testape.
- Drug has affinity for ischemic, necrotic tissue, and may localize in tumors.

Potential Toxicities/Side Effects and the Nursing Process

I.   ALTERATION IN NUTRITION related to GI SIDE EFFECTS

Defining Characteristics: Nausea, vomiting, diarrhea, anorexia, abdominal discomfort, epigastric burning and distress, glossitis, black hairy tongue may occur.

Nursing Implications: Assess baseline nutritional status. Assess for and teach patient to report any symptoms. Administer and teach patient self-administration of prescribed antiemetic or antidiarrheal medication as appropriate. Administer and teach patient to self-administer oral dose with at least 8 oz of water taken at least 1 hour before lying down for sleep.

II.   ALTERATION IN SKIN INTEGRITY related to RASH, PHOTOSENSITIVITY

Defining Characteristics: Maculopapular and erythematous rashes may occur. Rarely, exfoliative dermatitis, onycholysis, and nail discoloration. Photosensitivity risk (exaggerated sunburn) persists 1–2 days after completion of drug therapy.

Nursing Implications: Teach patient about potential side effects, to avoid sunlight during drug therapy, and to report rash, other abnormalities. Teach symptomatic skin care as appropriate.

III.   INJURY related to HYPERSENSITIVITY

Defining Characteristics: Urticaria, angioneurotic edema, anaphylaxis may occur; also, fever, rash, arthralgias, eosinophilia, and pericarditis.

Nursing Implications: Assess drug allergy history. Assess baseline allergy history. Assess baseline skin integrity. Teach patient to report rash, pruritus. Teach patent symptomatic management of rash, pruritus. Assess for hypersensitivity reaction; if it occurs, monitor VS, discontinue drug, notify physician, and institute supportive measures.

IV. FUNGAL SUPERINFECTION related to REDISTRIBUTION OF ENDOGENOUS MICROORGANISMS

Defining Characteristics: Vaginal moniliasis, vaginitis may occur as endogenous bacteria are eliminated and normal fungal population expands.

Nursing Implications: Teach female patient to report vaginal itching or discharge. Discuss appropriate antifungal treatment with physician. Teach perineal hygiene and symptomatic management.

V. ALTERATION IN HEPATIC FUNCTION

Defining Characteristics: Associated with high IV doses (> 2 g/day): hepatotoxicity and cholestasis may occur.

Nursing Implications: Assess baseline LFTs and monitor during therapy.

VI. INFECTION AND BLEEDING related to NEUTROPENIA, THROMBOCYTOPENIA

Defining Characteristics: Neutropenia, leukocytosis, leukopenia, atypical lymphocytes, thrombocytopenia, thrombocytopenic purpura, hemolytic anemia occur rarely with long-term therapy.

Nursing Implications: Assess baseline WBC, HCT, and platelets, and monitor periodically during long-term therapy.

VII. ALTERATION IN COMFORT related to LOCAL ADMINISTRATION EFFECTS

Defining Characteristics: IM administration may cause pain, induration due to muscle injury. IV administration may cause erythema, pain, swelling, and thrombophlebitis.

Nursing Implications: Rotate sites. Apply ice as ordered to painful buttock. Assess IV site prior to each dose for phlebitis or swelling, and change site at least q 48 h. Apply heat to painful IV sites as ordered.

VIII. SENSORY/PERCEPTUAL ALTERATION

Defining Characteristics: Lightheadedness, dizziness, headache may occur.

Nursing Implications: Assess baseline neurologic status. Teach patient to report any changes and discuss them with physician.

COMPLICATIONS

Drug: moxifloxacin (ABC Pack; Avelox)

Class: Antibiotic; quinolone.

Mechanism of Action: Acts intracellularly by inhibiting DNA gyrase and bacterial topoisomerase IV. DNA gyrase is required for DNA replication and transcription, DNA repair, recombination, and transposition; inhibition is bactericidal.

Metabolism: Widely distributed to most body fluids and tissues with highest concentrations in organs, such as kidneys, gallbladder, lungs, liver, gynecologic tissue, prostatic tissue, phagocytic cells, urine, sputum, and bile. Well-absorbed from GI tract. Metabolized in liver; excreted in urine and feces. Crosses placenta and is excreted in breastmilk.

Indication: For treatment of different types of bacterial infections of the complicated and uncomplicated skin and skin structures, sinuses, lungs (bronchitis and CAP), and complicated intra-abdominal infections. Moxifloxacin is a broad-spectrum anti-infective, active against a wide range of aerobic gram-positive and gram-negative organisms.

Dosage/Range:
- 400 mg PO or IV daily.

Drug Preparation:
- Oral: Take drug with large glass of water, preferably 2 hours after meal/food. Encourage oral fluids of 2–3 qt/day.
- IV: Further dilute drug in 0.9% sodium chloride or 5% dextrose in water to final concentration of 2 mg/mL. Administer over 60 minutes; do not infuse by rapid or bolus IV infusion.
- Do not refrigerate.

Drug Interactions:
- Antacids (containing magnesium, aluminum, or calcium) and iron decrease absorption of serum level of moxifloxacin; do not administer concurrently. If must administer antacids or iron, administer at least 4 hours apart. The administration of antacids containing aluminum, magnesium, calcium, sucralfate, zinc, or iron may substantially reduce the absorption of moxifloxacin; do not administer concurrently.
- Serum digoxin concentrations should be monitored; moxifloxacin may raise serum levels in some patients.
- Probenecid: decreases the renal tubular secretion of moxifloxacin, resulting in a prolonged elimination half-life and increased risk of toxicity.
- Moxifloxacin may have the potential to prolong the QT interval of the EKG in some patients. Moxifloxacin should not be used in patients with prolonged QT interval; patients with uncorrected hypokalemia; and patients on quinidine, procainamide, amiodarone, and sotalol (antiarrhythmic agents).
- Increased intracranial pressure and psychosis has been reported along with CNS stimulation.
- Hypersensitivity reactions have been reported.

Lab Effects/Interference:
- Serum SGPT, serum alk phos, serum SGOT, and serum LDH—values may be increased.

Special Considerations:
- Used in the treatment of respiratory tract infections (acute bacterial exacerbation of chronic bronchitis, acute bacterial sinusitis, and commonly acquired pneumonia).
- Used in the treatment of uncomplicated infections of the skin and skin structures.
- Contraindicated in pregnancy or women who are breastfeeding.
- Obtain ordered specimen for culture and sensitivity prior to first drug dose.
- Use cautiously in patients with seizure disorders.

Potential Toxicities/Side Effects and the Nursing Process

I. ALTERATION IN NUTRITION related to GI SIDE EFFECTS

Defining Characteristics: Incidence of nausea, vomiting, abdominal discomfort, diarrhea, anorexia.

Nursing Implications: Assess baseline nutritional and elimination status. Teach patient to report GI disturbances. Administer and teach patient to self-administer antiemetics, antidiarrheals as needed and as ordered. Teach patient importance of nutritious diet, and suggest small, frequent, high-calorie, high-protein meals as appropriate. Assess baseline LFTs and monitor periodically during treatment. Discuss abnormalities and drug interruption with physician.

II. SENSORY/PERCEPTUAL ALTERATIONS related to CNS EFFECTS

Defining Characteristics: Incidence of headache, restlessness. Dizziness, hallucinations, and seizures may also occur. Exacerbated by caffeine as quinolones delay caffeine excretion.

Nursing Implications: Assess baseline neurologic function and comfort, and monitor during treatment. Teach patient to report any changes. Discuss any abnormalities with physician. Teach patient to limit or restrict all caffeine-containing fluids, medications, e.g., tea, coffee, soft drinks.

III. ALTERATION IN SKIN INTEGRITY related to ALLERGY/HYPERSENSITIVITY

Defining Characteristics: Incidence of rash; other manifestations include eosinophilia, urticaria, flushing, fever, chills, photosensitivity, angioedema. Fatal hypersensitivity reactions have occurred rarely. Direct exposure to sunlight can cause sunburn (moderate-to-severe phototoxicity).

Nursing Implications: Assess baseline skin condition, including integrity and drug allergy history. Teach patient to report rash, itching, and other skin changes. Teach patient skin care and symptomatic measures as appropriate. If skin rash develops, discuss drug discontinuance with physician. Be prepared to treat severe acute hypersensitivity reactions with

COMPLICATIONS

airway management, oxygen, epinephrine, corticosteroids, antihistamines as ordered. Teach patient to avoid excessive sun exposure and to use skin protection factor (SPF) 15 or higher. If rash progresses, especially in HIV-infected patients, drug should be discontinued, as fatal Stevens-Johnson syndrome may develop.

IV.   FUNGAL SUPERINFECTION related to REDISTRIBUTION OF ENDOGENOUS MICROORGANISMS

Defining Characteristics: Vaginal moniliasis, vaginitis may occur as endogenous bacteria are eliminated and normal fungal population expands.

Nursing Implications: Teach female patient to report vaginal itching or discharge. Discuss appropriate antifungal treatment with physician. Teach perineal hygiene and symptomatic management.

V.   ALTERATION IN URINARY ELIMINATION related to RENAL TOXICITY

Defining Characteristics: Increased BUN and creatinine, crystal and stone formation in urine, interstitial nephritis, and renal failure may occur.

Nursing Implications: Assess baseline renal function; expect that drug dose will be decreased in presence of renal dysfunction. Teach patient to take drug with at least 8 oz of water, and to increase oral fluids to 2–3 qt/day.

VI.   ALTERATION IN COMFORT related to LOCAL ADMINISTRATION

Defining Characteristics: Drug may cause pain, inflammation, and rare thrombophlebitis at IV site.

Nursing Implications: Change IV site q 48 hours. Assess for phlebitis, discomfort, and IV patency prior to each administration. Administer drug slowly over 60–90 minutes in large volume of 5% dextrose (see Drug Preparation). Apply heat to promote comfort.

Drug: nafcillin sodium (Unipen)

Class: Antibacterial (systemic).

Mechanism of Action: Semisynthetic antibiotic. Contains β-lactam ring and is bactericidal by inhibiting cell wall synthesis. Penicillinase-resistant penicillin; active against penicillin-resistant staphylococci that produce the enzyme penicillinase.

Metabolism: Incompletely absorbed from GI tract; rapidly absorbed when given IM or IV. Widely distributed in body tissues and fluid, including bile. Crosses placenta and is excreted in breastmilk; 70–90% bound to serum proteins. Metabolized in liver, excreted in bile, and to a lesser degree in the urine.

Indication: For treatment of infections caused by, or suspected of being caused by, susceptible penicillinase-producing staphlocci, including respiratory tract; skin and skin structures; bone and joint; urinary tract infections; meningitis; and bacteremia.

Dosage/Range:
Adult:
- Oral: 500 mg–1 g PO q 6 h.
- IM/IV: 500 mg–2 g q 4 h.

Drug Preparation:
- Oral: Reconstitute per manufacturer's recommendation or by capsules or tablets. Administer 1 hour before meals or 2 hours after meals.
- IM: Reconstitute with sterile or bacteriostatic water for injection, and give deep IM in large muscle (e.g., gluteus maximus).
- IV: Reconstitute with sterile water for injection or 0.9% sodium chloride for injection according to manufacturer's package insert. Further dilute in 100 mL IV solution and infuse over 40–60 minutes.

Drug Interactions:
- Aminoglycosides: synergism.
- Aminoglycosides (e.g., gentamicin): incompatible when mixed together; administer at separate sites at different times. Also, penicillinase-resistant penicillins can inactivate aminoglycoside serum samples from patients receiving both drugs.
- Rifampin: possible antagonism, only at high doses of penicillin.
- Probenecid: increased serum level of nafcillin; may be coadministered to exert this effect.

Lab Effects/Interference:
Major clinical significance:
- Urine glucose: high urinary concentrations of a penicillin may produce false-positive or falsely elevated test results with copper sulfate tests (Benedict's, Clinitest, or Fehling's); glucose enzymatic tests (Clinistix or Testape) are not affected.

Clinical significance:
- Coombs' (direct antiglobulin) test: false-positive result may occur during therapy with any penicillin.
- ALT, alk phos, AST, serum LDH: values may be increased.
- WBC: leukopenia or neutropenia is associated with the use of all penicillins; the effect is more likely to occur with prolonged therapy and severe hepatic function impairment.

Special Considerations:
- Contraindicated in patients with prior hypersensitivity to penicillins. Use with caution in patients sensitive to other β-lactams (e.g., cephalosporins) since partial cross-allergenicity exists.
- Obtain ordered specimen and send for culture and sensitivity prior to first antibiotic dose.
- Consider alternative antibiotic therapy if eosinophilia, drug fever or rash, arthralgia, hematuria, or unexplained rise in BUN and serum creatinine occur.
- Monitor electrolytes and renal, hepatic, and hematologic laboratory parameters during extended treatment periods.
- Use with caution in pregnancy or with nursing women.

COMPLICATIONS

Potential Toxicities/Side Effects and the Nursing Process

I.   POTENTIAL FOR INJURY related to HYPERSENSITIVITY REACTION

Defining Characteristics: Urticaria, pruritus, rash (maculopapular or erythematous), fever and chills, eosinophilia, myalgia, edema, erythema, angioedema, Stevens-Johnson syndrome, and exfoliative skin reactions occur in 5% of patients. Increased risk in individuals allergic to cephalosporin antibiotics.

Nursing Implications: Assess allergy to cephalosporin antibiotics and penicillin: if patient states "yes," determine actual response (e.g., "swollen lips = angioedema"). If angioedema, patient SHOULD NOT receive drug. Discuss other patient responses with physician to determine whether drug should be given. Assess baseline skin condition, including integrity and allergy history to drugs. Instruct patient to report rash, itching, other skin changes. Teach patient skin care and symptomatic measures as appropriate. If skin rash develops, discuss drug discontinuance with physician. If rash progresses, drug should be discontinued, as fatal Stevens-Johnson syndrome may develop. Be prepared to treat severe acute hypersensitivity reactions with airway management, oxygen, epinephrine, corticosteroids, antihistamines as ordered.

II.   ALTERATION IN NUTRITION, LESS THAN BODY REQUIREMENTS, related to GI SIDE EFFECTS

Defining Characteristics: Nausea, vomiting, diarrhea may occur; rarely, pseudomembranous colitis caused by *C. difficile* resistant to the antibiotic occurs. Rarely, transient increases in LFTs—AST, ALT, alk phos, bili—may occur.

Nursing Implications: Assess baseline nutritional status. Instruct patient to report GI disturbances. Administer and teach patient to self-administer antiemetics, antidiarrheals as needed and as ordered. Teach patient importance of nutritious diet, and suggest small, frequent, high-calorie, high-protein meals as appropriate. Assess baseline LFTs and monitor periodically during treatment. Discuss abnormalities and drug interruption with physician.

III.   FUNGAL SUPERINFECTION related to REDISTRIBUTION OF ENDOGENOUS MICROORGANISMS

Defining Characteristics: Vaginal candidiasis, vaginitis may occur as endogenous bacteria are eliminated and normal fungal population expands.

Nursing Implications: Instruct female patient to report vaginal itching or discharge. Discuss appropriate antifungal treatment with physician. Teach perineal hygiene and symptomatic management.

IV. ALTERATIONS IN PROTECTIVE MECHANISMS (RARE) related to TRANSIENT LEUKOPENIA

Defining Characteristics: Rarely, transient leukopenia, lymphocytosis, anemia, eosinophilia may occur. Prolonged PT, prolonged aPTT, and hypoprothrombinemia have occurred rarely, especially in elderly or debilitated patients, or in individuals with vitamin K deficiency.

Nursing Implications: Assess baseline laboratory parameters, and monitor periodically during treatment. Assess patient for response to antibiotics. Discuss abnormalities with physician.

V. ALTERATIONS IN COMFORT related to PHLEBITIS

Defining Characteristics: Phlebitis and thrombophlebitis may occur with IV administration. Increased risk in elderly.

Nursing Implications: Assess IV site prior to each dose for phlebitis, erythema, and swelling, and change site at least q 48 h. Apply heat to painful IV site as ordered.

Drug: norfloxacin (Noroxin)

Class: Fluoroquinolone.

Mechanism of Action: Acts intracellularly by inhibiting DNA gyrase (bacterial topoisomerase IV).

Metabolism: Widely distributed to most body fluids and tissues. Well-absorbed from GI tract. Metabolized in liver; excreted in urine and feces and crosses the placenta.

Indication: For treatment of certain types of infections of the urinary tract and prostate. Norfloxacin is a broad-spectrum anti-infective, active against a wide range of aerobic gram-positive and gram-negative organisms.

Dosage/Range:
• 400–800 mg PO daily.

Drug Preparation:
• Oral: Take drug with large glass of water; preferably 2 hours after meal/food. Encourage oral fluids of 2–3 qt/day.

Drug Interactions:
• Antacids, didanosine, iron salts, multivitamins, sucralfate, zinc salts may decrease oral absorption of norfloxacin; do not administer concurrently. If must administer antacids or iron, administer at least 4 hours apart.
• Anticoagulants: Anticoagulant effect of warfarin may be increased.

COMPLICATIONS

- Antineoplastic agents may decrease serum norfloxacin levels.
- Caffeine plasma concentrations may be elevated and the half-life may be prolonged.
- Cyclosporine: Norfloxacin may elevate serum cyclosporine levels.
- CYP1A2 substrates (e.g., caffeine, clozapine, ropinirole, tacrine, theophylline, tizanidine): Plasma concentrations of these agents may be elevated, increasing the pharmacologic effects and adverse reactions.
- Nitrofurantoin: The antimicrobial effect of norfloxacin may be reduced; coadministration is not recommended.
- NSAIDs: Risk of CNS convulsions and convulsive seizures may be increased.
- Probenecid: Norfloxacin urinary elimination may be reduced.
- Sulfonylureas (e.g., glyburide): Severe hypoglycemia has been reported. Monitor blood glucose during coadministration of these agents.
- Theophylline: Decreased Cl and increased plasma levels of theophylline may result in toxicity.

Lab Effects/Interference:
- None well-documented.

Special Considerations:
- **Black Box Warning—Tendonitis: Norfloxacin has been associated with an increased risk of tendonitis and tendon rupture in patients of all ages. The risk is increased in patients older than 60 years of age, in patients taking corticosteroids, and in patients with kidney, heart, or lung transplants.**
- Contraindicated in pregnancy or in women who are breastfeeding.
- Prolonged QT interval and ventricular arrhythmias may occur.
- Obtain ordered specimen for culture and sensitivity prior to first drug dose.

Potential Toxicities/Side Effects and the Nursing Process

I.   ALTERATION IN NUTRITION related to GI SIDE EFFECTS

Defining Characteristics: Incidence of nausea, vomiting, abdominal discomfort, diarrhea, anorexia. Hepatic failure, including death; hepatitis; jaundice, including cholestatic jaundice and elevated LFTs has been documented.

Nursing Implications: Assess baseline nutritional and elimination status. Teach patient to report GI disturbances. Administer and teach patient to self-administer antiemetics and antidiarrheals as needed and as ordered. Teach patient importance of nutritious diet, and suggest small, frequent, high-calorie, high-protein meals as appropriate. Assess baseline LFTs and monitor periodically during treatment. Discuss abnormalities and drug interruption with physician. Assess taking other hepatotoxic drugs.

II.   SENSORY/PERCEPTUAL ALTERATIONS related to CNS EFFECTS

Defining Characteristics: Incidence of headache, restlessness. Dizziness, hallucinations, and seizures may also occur. Exacerbated by caffeine, as quinolones delay caffeine excretion.

Nursing Implications: Assess baseline neurologic function and comfort, and monitor during treatment. Teach patient to report any changes. Discuss any abnormalities with physician. Teach patient to limit or restrict all medications and caffeine-containing fluids (e.g., tea, coffee, caffeinated soft drinks).

III. ALTERATION IN SKIN INTEGRITY related to ALLERGY/HYPERSENSITIVITY

Defining Characteristics: Incidence of rash; other manifestations include eosinophilia, urticaria, flushing, fever, chills, photosensitivity, angioedema. Fatal hypersensitivity reactions have occurred rarely. Direct exposure to sunlight can cause sunburn (moderate to severe phototoxicity).

Nursing Implications: Assess baseline skin condition, including integrity and drug allergy history. Teach patient to report rash, itching, other skin changes. Teach patient skin care and symptomatic measures as appropriate. If skin rash develops, discuss drug discontinuance with physician. Be prepared to treat severe acute hypersensitivity reactions with airway management, oxygen, epinephrine, corticosteroids, antihistamines as ordered. Teach patient to avoid excessive sun exposure and to use skin protection factor (SPF) 15 or higher. If rash progresses, especially in HIV-infected patients, drug should be discontinued, as fatal Stevens-Johnson syndrome may develop.

IV. FUNGAL SUPERINFECTION related to REDISTRIBUTION OF ENDOGENOUS MICROORGANISMS

Defining Characteristics: Vaginal moniliasis, vaginitis may occur as endogenous bacteria are eliminated and normal fungal population expands.

Nursing Implications: Teach female patient to report vaginal itching or discharge. Discuss appropriate antifungal treatment with physician. Teach perineal hygiene and symptomatic management.

V. ALTERATION IN URINARY ELIMINATION related to RENAL TOXICITY

Defining Characteristics: Increased BUN and creatinine, crystal and stone formation in urine, interstitial nephritis, and renal failure may occur.

Nursing Implications: Assess baseline renal function; expect that drug dose will be decreased in presence of renal dysfunction. Teach patient to take drug with at least 8 oz of water, and to increase oral fluids to 2–3 qt/day.

VI. ALTERATIONS IN CARDIAC OUTPUT related to CARDIOVASCULAR CHANGES

Defining Characteristics: Rare, ~1% incidence of hypotension, transient EKG changes (e.g., premature ventricular contractions), bradycardia, flushing, and chest pain.

Nursing Implications: Assess baseline heart rate and BP; monitor during therapy, at least with initial dose.

Drug: oritavancin (Orbactiv)

Class: Antibacterial.

Mechanism of Action: Lipoglycopeptide antibacterial drug indicated for treatment of adult patients with acute bacterial skin and skin structure infections caused, or suspected to be caused, by gram-positive microorganisms.

Metabolism: Oritavancin is bound to plasma proteins and is excreted unchanged in feces and urine.

Indications: Treatment of adult patients with acute bacterial skin and skin structure infections (ABSSSI) caused by susceptible gram-positive microorganisms—*Staphylococcus aureus* (including methicillin-susceptible and -resistant isolates), *Streptococcus pyogenes*, *Streptococcus agalactiae*, *Streptococcus dysgalactiae*, *Streptococcus anginosus* group (including *S. anginosus*, *S. intermedius*, and *S. constellatus*), and *Enterococcus faecalis* (vancomycin-susceptible isolates only).

Dosage/Range: A 1,200-mg single dose is administered by IV infusion over 3 hours.

Drug Preparation:
* Oritavancin is intended for IV infusion, only after reconstitution and dilution.
* Aseptic technique should be used to reconstitute oritavancin vials. Reconstitute per manufacturer package insert instructions with sterile water for injection.
* Gently swirl to avoid foaming and ensure powder is completely reconstituted in solution. Inspect vial visually for particulate matter after reconstitution. Fluid should be clear, colorless to pale yellow solution.
* Dilution: Use *only* 5% dextrose in sterile water (D_5W) for dilution. Do *not* use normal saline for dilution, as it is incompatible with oritavancin and may cause precipitation of drug.
* Because no preservative or bacteriostatic agent is present in this product, aseptic technique must be used in preparing the final IV solution.
* Diluted IV solution in an infusion bag should be used within 6 hours when stored at room temperature, or used within 12 hours when refrigerated at 2–8°C (36–46°F). Combined storage time (reconstituted solution in vial and diluted solution in bag) and 3-hour infusion time should not exceed 6 hours at room temperature or 12 hours if refrigerated.

Drug Interaction: In vitro studies with human liver microsomes showed that oritavancin inhibited the activities of cytochrome P450 (CYP) enzymes 1A2, 2B6, 2D6, 2C9, 2C19, and 3A4. The observed inhibition of multiple CYP isoforms by oritavancin in vitro is likely to be reversible, and the mechanism of inhibition is probably noncompetitive. In vitro studies indicate that oritavancin is neither a substrate nor an inhibitor of the efflux transporter P-glycoprotein (P-gp).

Lab Effects/Interference:
- Concomitant warfarin use: Coadministration of oritavancin and warfarin may result in higher exposure of warfarin, which may increase risk of bleeding. Use oritavancin in patients on chronic warfarin therapy only when the benefits can be expected to outweigh the risk of bleeding.
- Coagulation test interference: Oritavancin has been shown to artificially prolong aPTT for up to 48 hours, and may prolong PT and INR for up to 24 hours.
- Use of intravenous unfractionated heparin sodium is contraindicated for 48 hours after oritavancin administration.

Special Considerations:
- Hypersensitivity reactions have been reported with use of antibacterial agents including oritavancin. Discontinue infusion if signs of acute hypersensitivity occur. Monitor patients with known hypersensitivity to glycopeptides.
- Infusion-related reactions have been reported. Slow infusion rate or interrupt infusion if an infusion reaction develops.
- *Clostridium difficile*–associated colitis: Evaluate patients if diarrhea occurs.
- Osteomyelitis: Institute appropriate alternative antibacterial therapy in patients with confirmed or suspected osteomyelitis.

Potential Toxicities/Side Effects and the Nursing Process

I. POTENTIAL FOR INJURY related to HYPERSENSITIVITY REACTION

Defining Characteristics: Urticaria, pruritus, rash (maculopapular or erythematous), fever and chills, eosinophilia, myalgia, edema, erythema, and angioedema.

Nursing Implications: Assess allergy to cephalosporin antibiotics and penicillin; if patient states "yes," determine actual response (e.g., "swollen lips = angioedema"). If angioedema is present, patient *should not* receive drug. Discuss other patient responses with physician to determine whether drug should be given. Assess baseline skin condition, including integrity, and allergy history to drugs. Instruct patient to report rash, itching, and other skin changes. Teach patient skin care and symptomatic measures as appropriate. If skin rash develops, discuss drug discontinuance with physician. If rash progresses, drug should be discontinued, as fatal Stevens-Johnson syndrome may develop. Be prepared to treat severe acute hypersensitivity reactions with airway management, oxygen, epinephrine, corticosteroids, and antihistamines as ordered.

II. ALTERATION IN NUTRITION, LESS THAN BODY REQUIREMENTS, related to GI SIDE EFFECTS

Defining Characteristics: Nausea, vomiting, diarrhea, and anorexia may occur; rarely, pseudomembranous colitis caused by *C. difficile* resistant to the antibiotic occurs.

COMPLICATIONS

Nursing Implications: Assess baseline nutritional status. Instruct patient to report GI disturbances. Administer, and teach patient to self-administer, antiemetics as needed and as ordered. Teach patient about importance of a nutritious diet; suggest small, frequent, high-caloric, high-protein meals as appropriate. Assess baseline LFTs and monitor periodically during treatment. Discuss abnormalities and drug interruption with physician.

III.   FUNGAL SUPERINFECTION related to REDISTRIBUTION OF ENDOGENOUS MICROORGANISMS

Defining Characteristics: Vaginal candidiasis and vaginitis may occur as endogenous bacteria are eliminated and normal fungal population expands.

Nursing Implications: Instruct female patients to report vaginal itching or discharge. Discuss appropriate antifungal treatment with physician. Teach perineal hygiene and symptomatic management.

IV.   ALTERATIONS IN PROTECTIVE MECHANISMS (RARE) related to TRANSIENT LEUKOPENIA

Defining Characteristics: Rarely, transient leukopenia, lymphocytosis, anemia, and eosinophilia may occur. Prolonged PT, prolonged aPTT, and hypoprothrombinemia have occurred rarely, especially in elderly or debilitated patients, or in individuals with vitamin K deficiency.

Nursing Implications: Assess baseline laboratory parameters, and monitor periodically during treatment. Assess patient for response to antibiotics. Discuss abnormalities with physician. Assess for signs and symptoms of bleeding. If they occur, especially in elderly or debilitated patients, discuss vitamin K administration with physician. Instruct patient to avoid aspirin. If taking oral anticoagulants, assess for increased PT and signs and symptoms of bleeding.

V.   ALTERATIONS IN COMFORT related to LOCAL INJECTION-SITE IRRITATION

Defining Characteristics: Pain and phlebitis may develop in IV sites.

Nursing Implications: Change IV sites every 48 hours, and assess for signs and symptoms of phlebitis prior to each administration. Administer drug slowly. Apply warm packs to increase comfort.

Drug: oxacillin sodium (Bactocill, Prostaphlin)

Class: Antibacterial (systemic).

Mechanism of Action: Semisynthetic antibiotic. Contains β-lactam ring and is bactericidal by inhibiting cell wall synthesis. Penicillinase-resistant penicillin and active against penicillin-resistant staphylococci, which produce the enzyme penicillinase.

Metabolism: Incompletely absorbed from GI tract; rapidly absorbed when given IM or IV. Widely distributed in body tissues and fluid, including bile. Crosses placenta and is excreted in breastmilk; 89–94% bound to serum proteins. Metabolized in liver, excreted in urine.

Indication: For treatment of infections caused by penicillinase-producing staphylococci; initial therapy of suspected staphylococcal infections eliminating bacteria that cause infections, including pneumonia, meningitis, urinary tract, skin, bone, joint, blood, and heart valve infections.

Dosage/Range:
Adult:
• Oral: 500 mg–1 g PO q 6 h.
• IM/IV: 500 mg–2 g q 4 h.

Drug Preparation:
• Oral: Reconstitute per manufacturer's package insert or by capsules or tablets. Administer 1 hour before meals or 2 hours after meals.
• IM: Reconstitute with sterile or bacteriostatic water for injection, and give deep IM in large muscle (e.g., gluteus maximus).
• IV: Reconstitute with sterile water for injection or 0.9% sodium chloride for injection according to manufacturer's package insert. Further dilute in 100-mL IV solution and infuse over 40–60 minutes.

Drug Interactions:
• Aminoglycosides: synergism.
• Aminoglycosides (e.g., gentamicin): incompatible when mixed together; administer at separate sites at different times. Also, penicillinase-resistant penicillins can inactivate aminoglycoside serum samples from patients receiving both drugs.
• Rifampin: possible antagonism, only at high doses of oxacillin.
• Probenecid: increased serum level of oxacillin; may be coadministered to exert this effect.

Lab Effects/Interference:
Major clinical significance:
• Urine glucose: high urinary concentrations of a penicillin may produce false-positive or falsely elevated test results with copper sulfate tests (Benedict's, Clinitest, or Fehling's); glucose enzymatic tests (Clinistix or Testape) are not affected.

Clinical significance:
• Coombs' (direct antiglobulin) test: false-positive result may occur during therapy with any penicillin.
• ALT, alk phos, AST, serum LDH values may be increased.
• WBC: leukopenia or neutropenia is associated with the use of all penicillins; the effect is more likely to occur with prolonged therapy and severe hepatic function impairment.

Special Considerations:
• Contraindicated in patients with prior hypersensitivity to penicillins. Use with caution in patients sensitive to other β-lactams (e.g., cephalosporins) since partial cross-allergenicity.

COMPLICATIONS

- Obtain ordered specimen and send for culture and sensitivity prior to first antibiotic dose.
- Consider alternative antibiotic therapy if eosinophilia, drug fever or rash, arthralgia, hematuria, or unexplained rise in BUN and serum creatinine occur.
- Monitor electrolytes and renal, hepatic, and hematologic laboratory parameters during extended treatment periods.
- Use with caution in pregnant or nursing women.

Potential Toxicities/Side Effects and the Nursing Process

I.   POTENTIAL FOR INJURY related to HYPERSENSITIVITY REACTION

Defining Characteristics: Urticaria, pruritus, rash (maculopapular or erythematous), fever and chills, eosinophilia, myalgia, edema, erythema, angioedema, Stevens-Johnson syndrome, and exfoliative skin reactions occur in 5% of patients. Increased risk in individuals allergic to cephalosporin antibiotics.

Nursing Implications: Assess allergy to cephalosporin antibiotics and penicillin: if patient states "yes," determine actual response (e.g., "swollen lips = angioedema"). If angioedema, patient SHOULD NOT receive drug. Discuss other patient responses with physician to determine whether drug should be given. Assess baseline skin condition, including integrity and allergy history to drugs. Instruct patient to report rash, itching, and other skin changes. Teach patient skin care and symptomatic measures as appropriate. If skin rash develops, discuss drug discontinuance with physician. If rash progresses, drug should be discontinued, as fatal Stevens-Johnson syndrome may develop. Be prepared to treat severe acute hypersensitivity reactions with airway management, oxygen, epinephrine, corticosteroids, antihistamines as ordered.

II.   ALTERATION IN NUTRITION, LESS THAN BODY REQUIREMENTS, related to INCREASED LFTs

Defining Characteristics: Oral lesions may occur, as may hepatitis (rare) and increased LFTs.

Nursing Implications: Assess baseline oral mucosa, and LFTs—AST, ALT, alk phos, bili. Teach patient to practice oral hygiene after meals and at bedtime, and instruct to report any oral lesions. Monitor LFTs periodically during treatment, and discuss abnormalities with physician.

III.   FUNGAL SUPERINFECTION related to REDISTRIBUTION OF ENDOGENOUS MICROORGANISMS

Defining Characteristics: Vaginal candidiasis, vaginitis may occur as endogenous bacteria are eliminated and normal fungal population expands.

Nursing Implications: Instruct female patient to report vaginal itching or discharge. Discuss appropriate antifungal treatment with physician. Teach perineal hygiene and symptomatic management.

IV. ALTERATIONS IN PROTECTIVE MECHANISMS (RARE) related to TRANSIENT LEUKOPENIA

Defining Characteristics: Rarely, transient leukopenia, lymphocytosis, anemia, eosinophilia may occur. Prolonged PT, prolonged aPTT, and hypoprothrombinemia have occurred rarely, especially in elderly or debilitated patients, or in individuals with vitamin K deficiency.

Nursing Implications: Assess baseline laboratory parameters, and monitor periodically during treatment. Assess patient for response to antibiotics. Discuss abnormalities with physician.

V. ALTERATIONS IN COMFORT related to PHLEBITIS

Defining Characteristics: Phlebitis and thrombophlebitis may occur with IV administration. Increased risk in elderly.

Nursing Implications: Assess IV site prior to each dose for phlebitis, erythema, and swelling, and change site at least q 48 h. Apply heat to painful IV site as ordered.

VI. ALTERATIONS IN URINARY ELIMINATION related to RENAL DAMAGE

Defining Characteristics: Interstitial nephritis, transient proteinuria, hematuria may occur.

Nursing Implications: Assess baseline liver, renal function tests (e.g., serum BUN, creatinine, and urinalysis), and monitor during therapy.

VII. ALTERATIONS IN SENSORY/PERCEPTUAL PATTERNS related to NEUROPATHY

Defining Characteristics: Neuropathy, seizures, neuromuscular irritability may occur rarely.

Nursing Implications: Assess baseline neurologic function and comfort, and monitor during treatment. Instruct patient to report any changes. Discuss any abnormalities with physician.

COMPLICATIONS

Drug: penicillin G (PenG potassium, PenG sodium, intravenous; PenVK, oral preparation)

Class: Natural penicillin.

Mechanism of Action: Produced by fermentation of *Penicillium chrysogenum*.

Metabolism: Decreased oral absorption, but IM or IV absorption is quite rapid and complete. Widely distributed in body tissues and fluids; 45–68% bound to proteins. Eliminated in urine and bile.

Indication: This drug is used to treat a variety of bacterial infections. Active against many gram-positive bacteria (streptococci, staphylococci) but resistant to *S. aureus* and *S. epidermidis* strains that produce penicillinases. Also active against some gram-negative bacteria (*Neisseria, H. influenzae*), and spirochetes.

Dosage/Range:
- Oral: 250–500 mg qid.
- IV: 200,000–4 million U q 4 h.
- Dose modification may be necessary in patients with renal impairment.

Drug Preparation:
- Oral: Administer at least 1 hour before or 2 hours after meals.
- IM: Reconstitute drug as directed. Administration of greater than 100,000 U is likely to result in some discomfort. Give IM deep in large muscle mass.
- IV: Reconstitute drug as directed. Further dilute in 0.9% sodium chloride or 5% dextrose in water, and administer over 1–2 hours.

Drug Interactions:
- Aminoglycosides: synergism.
- Aminoglycosides (e.g., gentamicin): incompatible when mixed together; administer at separate sites at different times. Also, penicillinase-resistant penicillins can inactivate aminoglycoside serum samples from patients receiving both drugs.
- Rifampin: possible antagonism, only at high doses of penicillin.
- Probenecid: increased serum level of penicillin; may be coadministered to exert this effect.

Lab Effects/Interference:
Major clinical significance:
- Urine glucose: high urinary concentrations of a penicillin may produce false-positive or falsely elevated test results with copper sulfate tests (Benedict's, Clinitest, or Fehling's); glucose enzymatic tests (Clinistix or Testape) are not affected.

Clinical significance:
- Coombs' (direct antiglobulin) test: false-positive result may occur during therapy with any penicillin.
- ALT, alk phos, AST, serum LDH values may be increased.
- Serum K+: hyperkalemia may occur following administration of parenteral penicillin G potassium because of the high potassium content.

- Serum Na+: hypernatremia may occur following administration of large doses of parenteral penicillin G sodium because of the high sodium content.
- WBC: leukopenia or neutropenia is associated with the use of all penicillins; the effect is more likely to occur with prolonged therapy and severe hepatic function impairment.

Special Considerations:

- Contraindicated in patients with prior hypersensitivity to penicillins. Use with caution in patients sensitive to other β-lactams (e.g., cephalosporins) since partial cross-allergenicity exists.
- Obtain ordered specimen and send for culture and sensitivity test prior to first antibiotic dose.
- Consider alternative antibiotic therapy if eosinophilia, drug fever or rash, arthralgia, hematuria, or unexplained rise in BUN and serum creatinine occur.
- Monitor electrolytes and renal, hepatic, and hematologic laboratory parameters during extended treatment periods.
- Hyperkalemia may occur with high-dose therapy: monitor serum K+.
- Use with caution in pregnant or nursing women.
- Penicillin G benzathine should never be given IV (suspension); give IM only.

Potential Toxicities/Side Effects and the Nursing Process

I.   POTENTIAL FOR INJURY related to HYPERSENSITIVITY REACTION

Defining Characteristics: Urticaria, pruritus, rash (maculopapular or erythematous), fever and chills, eosinophilia, myalgia, edema, erythema, angioedema, Stevens-Johnson syndrome, and exfoliative skin reactions occur in 5% of patients. Increased risk exists in individuals allergic to cephalosporin antibiotics.

Nursing Implications: Assess allergy to cephalosporin antibiotics and penicillin: if patient states "yes," determine actual response (e.g., "swollen lips = angioedema"). If angioedema, patient SHOULD NOT receive drug. Discuss other patient responses with physician to determine whether drug should be given. Assess baseline skin condition, including integrity and allergy history to drugs. Instruct patient to report rash, itching, and other skin changes. Teach patient skin care and symptomatic measures as appropriate. If skin rash develops, discuss drug discontinuance with physician. If rash progresses, drug should be discontinued, as fatal Stevens-Johnson syndrome may develop. Be prepared to treat severe acute hypersensitivity reactions with airway management, oxygen, epinephrine, corticosteroids, antihistamines as ordered.

II.   ALTERATION IN NUTRITION, LESS THAN BODY REQUIREMENTS, related to GI SIDE EFFECTS

Defining Characteristics: Rarely, nausea, vomiting, diarrhea, and pseudomembranous colitis caused by *C. difficile* resistant to the antibiotic may occur. Rarely, transient increases in LFTs—AST, ALT, alk phos, bili—may occur.

COMPLICATIONS

Nursing Implications: Assess baseline nutritional status. Instruct patient to report GI disturbances. Administer and teach patient to self-administer antiemetics as needed and as ordered. Teach patient importance of nutritious diet, and suggest small, frequent, high-calorie, high-protein meals as appropriate. Assess baseline LFTs and monitor periodically during treatment. Discuss abnormalities and drug interruption with physician.

III. **FUNGAL SUPERINFECTION related to REDISTRIBUTION OF ENDOGENOUS MICROORGANISMS**

Defining Characteristics: Vaginal candidiasis, vaginitis may occur as endogenous bacteria are eliminated and normal fungal population expands.

Nursing Implications: Instruct female patient to report vaginal itching or discharge. Discuss appropriate antifungal treatment with physician. Teach perineal hygiene and symptomatic management.

IV. **ALTERATIONS IN PROTECTIVE MECHANISMS (RARE) related to RARE LEUKOPENIA**

Defining Characteristics: Rarely, hemolytic anemia, leukopenia, thrombocytopenia may occur.

Nursing Implications: Assess baseline laboratory parameters, and monitor periodically during treatment. Assess patient for response to antibiotics. Discuss abnormalities with physician.

V. **ALTERATIONS IN SENSORY/PERCEPTUAL PATTERNS related to NEUROPATHY**

Defining Characteristics: Neuropathy, seizures may occur with high doses.

Nursing Implications: Assess baseline neurologic function and comfort, and monitor during treatment. Instruct patient to report any changes. Discuss any abnormalities with physician.

VI. **ALTERATIONS IN COMFORT related to LOCAL INJECTION IRRITATION**

Defining Characteristics: Pain, induration may form in IM injection sites; phlebitis may develop in IV sites.

Nursing Implications: Rotate IM injection sites, and administer drug deep IM in large muscle mass (e.g., gluteus maximus). Use IM injection when IV administration is not possible. Change IV sites q 48 h, and assess for signs/symptoms of phlebitis prior to each administration. Administer drug slowly. Apply warm packs to increase comfort.

Drug: piperacillin sodium (Pipracil); combined with tazobactam sodium (Zosyn)

Class: Antibacterial (systemic) (extended-spectrum penicillin).

Mechanism of Action: Semisynthetic antibiotic prepared from fungus *Penicillium*. Contains β-lactam ring and is bactericidal by inhibiting cell wall synthesis.

Metabolism: Poorly absorbed from GI tract, so must be given parenterally. Widely distributed in body tissues and fluids. Crosses placenta and is excreted in breastmilk. Excreted via urine and bile.

Indication: For treatment of intra-abdominal, urinary tract, gynecologic, lower respiratory tract infections; septicemia; skin and skin structures infections; bone and joint infections; gonococcal urethritis; surgical prophylaxis; and treatment of infections caused by susceptible microorganisms. Active against most gram-positive (except penicillinase-producing strains) and most gram-negative bacilli. Used in the treatment of serious gram-negative infections, especially *P. aeruginosa*–related infections of lower respiratory tract, urinary tract, and skin. When combined with tazobactam sodium, which inhibits β-lactamases, piperacillin sodium is effective against resistant bacteria.

Dosage/Range:
- IV route preferred.

Adult:
Piperacillin sodium:
- IV: 3–4 g q 4–6 h (maximum 24 g, but higher doses may be used in severe infection); IM: maximum 2 g/per dose.

Zosyn:
- 3 g piperacillin and 0.375 g tazobactam (3.375 g)–4 g piperacillin and 0.50 g tazobactam (4.50 g) q 6 h IV × 7–10 days.
- Moderate-to-severe pneumonia caused by piperacillin-resistant *S. aureus* that produces β-lactamase: 3.375 g IV q 6 h plus aminoglycoside × 7–10 days.
- Dose modification necessary if severe renal insufficiency exists.

Drug Preparation:
- IV: Reconstitute each gram of drug with at least 5 mL of sterile or bacteriostatic water. Further dilute in 50–100 mL 0.9% sodium chloride or 5% dextrose injection and infuse over 30 minutes.
- IM: Reconstitute with 2 mL of sterile or bacteriostatic water, or 0.5–1.0% lidocaine HCl (without epinephrine), with final concentration 1 g/2.5 mL. Administer as deep IM injection in large muscle mass (e.g., gluteus maximus). Make certain patient is NOT ALLERGIC to lidocaine.

Drug Interactions:
- Aminoglycosides: synergism.

COMPLICATIONS

• Aminoglycosides (e.g., gentamicin): incompatible when mixed together; administer at separate sites at different times. Also, penicil-linase-resistant penicillins can inactivate aminoglycoside serum samples from patients receiving both drugs.
• Clavulanic acid (inhibits β-lactamase): increases antibacterial action.
• Probenecid: increased serum level of piperacillin; may be coadministered to exert this effect.
• Tazobactam: inhibits β-lactamase, thus broadening drug's antimicrobial effectiveness.

Lab Effects/Interference:
Major clinical significance:
• Urine glucose: high urinary concentrations of a penicillin may produce false-positive or falsely elevated test results with copper sulfate tests (Benedict's, Clinitest, or Fehling's); glucose enzymatic tests (Clinistix or Testape) are not affected.
• PTT and PT: an increase has been associated with IV piperacillin.

Clinical significance:
• Coombs' (direct antiglobulin) test: false-positive result may occur during therapy with any penicillin.
• Urine protein: high urinary concentrations of piperacillin may produce false-positive protein reactions (pseudoproteinuria) with the sulfosalicylic acid and boiling test; bromophenol blue reagent test strips (Multistix) are reportedly unaffected.
• ALT, alk phos, AST, serum LDH values may be increased.
• Serum bili: an increase has been associated with piperacillin.
• BUN and serum creatinine: increased concentrations have been associated with piperacillin.
• Serum K+: hypokalemia may occur following administration of parenteral piperacillin, which may act as a non-reabsorbable anion in the distal tubals; this may cause an increase in pH and result in increased urinary potassium loss: the risk of hypokalemia increases with use of larger doses.
• WBC: leukopenia or neutropenia is associated with the use of all penicillins; the effect is more likely to occur with prolonged therapy and severe hepatic function impairment.

Special Considerations:
• Contraindicated in patients with prior hypersensitivity to penicillins. Use with caution in patients sensitive to other β-lactams (e.g., cephalosporins), since partial cross-allergenicity exists.
• Obtain ordered specimen and send for culture and sensitivity test prior to first antibiotic dose.
• Consider alternative antibiotic therapy if eosinophilia, drug fever or rash, arthralgia, hematuria, or unexplained rise in BUN and serum creatinine occur.
• Monitor electrolytes and renal, hepatic, and hematologic laboratory parameters during extended treatment periods.
• Use with caution in pregnant or nursing women.
• Low Na content: 1.98 mEq/g of drug.
• Increased activity against *P. aeruginosa*.

Potential Toxicities/Side Effects and the Nursing Process

I.   POTENTIAL FOR INJURY related to HYPERSENSITIVITY REACTION

Defining Characteristics: Urticaria, pruritus, rash (maculopapular or erythematous), fever and chills, eosinophilia, myalgia, edema, erythema, angioedema, Stevens-Johnson syndrome, and exfoliative skin reactions occur in 5% of patients. Increased risk exists in individuals allergic to cephalosporin antibiotics.

Nursing Implications: Assess allergy to cephalosporin antibiotics and penicillin: if patient states "yes," determine actual response (e.g., "swollen lips = angioedema"). If angioedema, patient SHOULD NOT receive drug. Discuss other patient responses with physician to determine whether drug should be given. Assess baseline skin condition, including integrity and allergy history to drugs. Instruct patient to report rash, itching, other skin changes. Teach patient skin care and symptomatic measures as appropriate. If skin rash develops, discuss drug discontinuance with physician. If rash progresses, drug should be discontinued, as fatal Stevens-Johnson syndrome may develop. Be prepared to treat severe acute hypersensitivity reactions with airway management, oxygen, epinephrine, corticosteroids, antihistamines as ordered.

II.   ALTERATION IN NUTRITION, LESS THAN BODY REQUIREMENTS, related to GI SIDE EFFECTS

Defining Characteristics: Nausea, vomiting, diarrhea may occur; rarely, pseudomembranous colitis caused by *C. difficile* resistant to the antibiotic occurs. Rarely, transient increases in LFTs—AST, ALT, alk phos, bili—may occur.

Nursing Implications: Assess baseline nutritional status. Instruct patient to report GI disturbances. Administer and teach patient to self-administer antiemetics as needed and as ordered. Teach patient importance of nutritious diet, and suggest small, frequent, high-calorie, high-protein meals as appropriate. Assess baseline LFTs and monitor periodically during treatment. Discuss abnormalities and drug interruption with physician.

III.   FUNGAL SUPERINFECTION related to REDISTRIBUTION OF ENDOGENOUS MICROORGANISMS

Defining Characteristics: Vaginal candidiasis, vaginitis may occur as endogenous bacteria are eliminated and normal fungal population expands.

Nursing Implications: Instruct female patient to report vaginal itching or discharge. Discuss appropriate antifungal treatment with physician. Teach perineal hygiene and symptomatic management.

COMPLICATIONS

IV.   ALTERATIONS IN PROTECTIVE MECHANISMS (RARE) related to
HEMATOLOGIC ABNORMALITIES

Defining Characteristics: Rarely, transient leukopenia, lymphocytosis, anemia, eosinophilia may occur. Prolonged PT, prolonged aPTT, and hypoprothrombinemia have occurred rarely, especially in elderly or debilitated patients, or in individuals with vitamin K deficiency.

Nursing Implications: Assess baseline laboratory parameters, and monitor periodically during treatment. Assess patient for response to antibiotics. Discuss abnormalities with physician. Assess for signs/symptoms of bleeding.

V.   ALTERATIONS IN SENSORY/PERCEPTUAL PATTERNS related to
DIZZINESS, SOMNOLENCE

Defining Characteristics: Dizziness, headache, somnolence occur rarely. Neuromuscular irritability and seizures may occur with high drug serum levels.

Nursing Implications: Assess baseline neurologic function and comfort, and monitor during treatment. Instruct patient to report any changes. Discuss any abnormalities with physician. Institute seizure precautions.

VI.   ALTERATIONS IN COMFORT related to LOCAL INJECTION IRRITATION

Defining Characteristics: Vein irritation (pain, erythema), phlebitis, and thrombophlebitis may occur at IV administration site.

Nursing Implications: Change IV sites q 48 h, and assess for signs/symptoms of phlebitis prior to each administration. Administer drug slowly. Apply warm packs to increase comfort. Discuss central line with patient and physician to facilitate administration.

VII.   ALTERATION IN FLUID AND ELECTROLYTE BALANCE related to
HYPOKALEMIA AND INCREASED SODIUM INTAKE

Defining Characteristics: Prolonged therapy may cause hypokalemia; also, drug is prepared as sodium salt. Frequent IV infusions increase fluid intake.

Nursing Implications: Assess baseline electrolytes, fluid balance, weight, and monitor throughout therapy. Monitor renal function studies, especially if patient has preexisting renal dysfunction.

Drug: quinupristin and dalfopristin (Synercid)

Class: Macrolide-lincoasmide-streptogram (MLS) class of antibiotic.

Mechanism of Action: Synercid inhibits bacterial protein synthesis by each component irreversibly binding to different sites on the 50S bacterial ribosome subunit to form stable quinupristin-ribosome-dalfopristin tertiary complex. Quinupristin inhibits peptide chain formation and results in early termination, while dalfopristin directly interferes with peptidyl transferase and inhibits peptide chain elongation.

Metabolism: Quinupristin and dalfopristin are rapidly converted in the liver to several active metabolites. Quinupristin is broken down into two active metabolites: one glutathione-conjugated metabolite and one cysteine-conjugated metabolite. Dalfopristin has one active metabolite formed by drug hydrolysis. Elimination half-life is approximately 0.9 and 0.75 hours for quinupristin and dalfopristin, respectively. Protein binding for quinupristin ranges from 55–78%, and from 11–26% for dalfopristin. Excreted in feces (75–77%) and urine (15% of quinupristin and 19% dalfopristin).

Indication: For treatment of serious or life-threatening infections associated with VREG; treatment of complicated skin and skin structure infections caused by *Staplococcus aureus* (methicillin-susceptible) or *S. pyogenes*. Active against gram-positive aerobic microorganisms (e.g., *Enterococcus faecium*), including vancomycin- and teicoplanin-resistant organisms and vancomycin-resistant, but teicoplanin-susceptible organisms; staphylococci; streptococci; some anaerobes and respiratory pathogens.

Dosage/Range:
- Recommended dose is 7.5 mg/kg of actual body weight in D_5W over 60 minutes q 8–12 h, depending upon the type and severity of infection.

Drug Preparation:
- Reconstitute single-dose vial by slowly adding 5 mL of solution or preservative-free sterile water for injection. CAUTION: FURTHER DILUTION IS REQUIRED PRIOR TO ADMINSTRATION.
- According to patient weight, Synercid solution should be added to 250 mL of D_5W solution within 30 minutes of initial reconstitution.
- Stability of the prepared infusate is 5 h at room temperature or 54 h under refrigeration at 2–8°C (36–46°F).
- Drug is NOT compatible with 0.9% sodium chloride or heparin-containing solutions.
- Desired dose should be administered IV over 60 minutes. If drug is administered through a common IV line, flush with 5% dextrose prior to and following administration.

Drug Interactions:
- Synercid should not be physically mixed with or added to other drugs since compatibility has not been established.
- Drugs metabolized by CYP3A4 isoenzyme system: drug is metabolized by CYP3A4 isoenzymes and is an inhibitor of CYP3A4, and thus may increase the serum

concentrations of drugs metabolized by this isoenzyme, e.g., nifedipine, cyclosporin. Use together with caution and assess for toxicity.

Lab Effects/Interference:
* Eosinophils, BUN, GGT (gamma glutamyl transferase), LDH, CPK, AST, ALT, blood glucose, alk phos, and creatinine: concentrations may be increased.
* Hemoglobin and hematocrit: may be decreased.
* Serum K+ and platelet count: may be increased or decreased.

Special Considerations:
* Infusion via central line preferred to decrease incidence of local infusion reactions.

Potential Toxicities/Side Effects and the Nursing Process

I.   ALTERATION IN NUTRITION related to GI SIDE EFFECTS

Defining Characteristics: Nausea, vomiting, diarrhea, constipation, abdominal pain, dyspepsia, stomatitis, and pseudomembranous enterocolitis may occur.

Nursing Implications: Assess elimination and nutrition pattern, baseline and during therapy. Teach patient to report diarrhea and/or abdominal pain immediately. Discuss drug discontinuance with physician if diarrhea occurs. Guaiac stool for occult blood, and notify physician if positive. If severe diarrhea develops, discuss management plan, including endoscopy, fluid and electrolyte replacement. Assess for nausea/vomiting, and administer prescribed antiemetic medications. Encourage small, frequent feedings as tolerated.

II.   ALTERATION IN SKIN INTEGRITY related to HYPERSENSITIVITY

Defining Characteristics: Maculopapular rash and urticaria may occur. Allergic reactions (anaphylactic-like) may rarely occur.

Nursing Implications: Assess baseline allergy history. Assess baseline skin integrity. Teach patient to report rash, pruritus. Teach patient symptomatic management of rash, pruritus. Assess for hypersensitivity reaction; if it occurs, monitor VS, discontinue drug, notify physician, and institute supportive measures.

III.   ALTERATION IN COMFORT related to LOCAL ADMINISTRATION EFFECTS

Defining Characteristics: IV administration may cause erythema, pain, swelling, and thrombophlebitis.

Nursing Implications: Assess IV site prior to each dose for phlebitis or swelling, and change site at least q 48 hours. Administer dose slowly over 60 minutes. Apply heat to painful IV sites as ordered. Infuse via central line if possible.

IV. ALTERATION IN COMFORT

Defining Characteristics: Myalgias and arthralgias may occur.

Nursing Implications: Assess baseline T, VS, neurologic status, and comfort level, and monitor q 4–6 hours if patient in hospital. Teach patient self-care measures, including use of prescribed medications, as well as use of heat or cold for myalgias and arthralgias.

V. ALTERATION IN HEPATIC FUNCTION

Defining Characteristics: Transient increases in serum BR, AST (SGOT), alk phos have occurred.

Nursing Implications: Assess baseline LFTs and monitor during therapy.

VI. FUNGAL SUPERINFECTION related to REDISTRIBUTION OF ENDOGENOUS MICROORGANISMS

Defining Characteristics: Vaginal moniliasis, vaginitis, and oral moniliasis may occur as endogenous bacteria are eliminated and normal fungal population expands.

Nursing Implications: Teach female patient to report vaginal itching or discharge. Discuss appropriate antifungal treatment with physician. Teach perineal hygiene and symptomatic management.

Drug: rifaximin (Xifaxan)

Class: Anti-infective, antidiarrheals, gastrointestinal, rifamycin.

Mechanism of Action: Acts by binding to the beta-subunit of bacterial DNA-dependent RNA polymerase resulting in inhibition of bacterial RNA synthesis. Structural analog of rifampin.

Metabolism: Well-absorbed following PO administration. Poorly absorbed from the gastrointestinal tract. Drug excreted unchanged in the feces.

Indication: For treatment of bacterial infections only in the intestines. Active against *E. coli* (enterotoxigenic and enteroaggregative strains).

Dosage/Range:
- Traveler's diarrhea: 200 mg orally three times daily for 3 days.

Drug Preparation:
- Oral preparation.

Drug Administration:
- May be taken with or without food.

COMPLICATIONS

Drug Interactions:
- Rifaximin has not been shown to significantly affect intestinal or hepatic CYP3A4 activity.
- Rifaximin has not been shown to affect contraceptives containing ethinyl estradiol and norgestimate.

Lab Effects/Interference:
- None reported.

Special Considerations:
- Rifaximin was teratogenic in animal studies. There are no adequate and well-controlled studies in pregnant women.

Potential Toxicities/Side Effects and the Nursing Process

I.   ALTERATION IN NUTRITION related to GI SIDE EFFECTS

Defining Characteristics: Gas, abdominal pain, nausea, vomiting, constipation, and pseudomembranous enterocolitis may occur.

Nursing Implications: Assess elimination and nutrition pattern, baseline and during therapy. Teach patient to report changes in diarrhea and/or abdominal pain immediately. Guaiac stool for occult blood, and notify physician if positive. Discuss management plan, including fluid and electrolyte replacement. Assess for nausea/vomiting, and administer prescribed antiemetic medications. Encourage small, frequent feedings as tolerated.

Drug: streptomycin sulfate

Class: Antibacterial; antimycobacterial (systemic).

Mechanism of Action: Synthetic antibiotic derived from *Streptomyces*; bactericidal, most probably by inhibition of protein synthesis; active against *Mycobacterium tuberculosis*.

Metabolism: Well-absorbed following IM administration. Widely distributed into body fluids; 35% bound to plasma proteins. Readily crosses placenta and into breastmilk. Drug excreted unchanged in the urine.

Indication: This drug is used to treat moderate to severe infections caused by susceptible strains of *Mycobacterium tuberculosis* and nontuberculosis infections. Active as second-line agent against sensitive microorganisms (including *Brucella, Nocardia, M. avium-intracellulare*).

Dosage/Range:
- Antituberculosis regimen: Adults: 15 mg/kg/day or 1 g/day IM × 2–3 months, then 1 g 2–3 × per week. Elderly: dose may be limited to 10 mg/kg (or 750 mg). Desired serum peak is 5–25 mg/mL, and trough < 5 mg/mL.

Drug Preparation:
- Prepare a solution with concentration of ≤ 500 mg/mL, using sterile water for injection or 0.9% sodium chloride. Use within 2 days if kept at room temperature, or within 2 weeks if refrigerated at 2–8°C (36–46°F).

Drug Administration:
- Deep IM: into large muscle mass; rotate sites as sterile abscesses may form. DO NOT GIVE IV.

Drug Interactions:
- Increased risk of toxicity with other ototoxic drugs: acyclovir, other aminoglycosides, amphotericin B, bacitracin, cephalosporins, colistin, cisplatin, ethacrynic acid, furosemide, vancomycin.
- Potentiation of neuromuscular blockade when given concurrently with general anesthetics (succinylcholine, tubocurarine)—use cautiously, observe for signs/symptoms of respiratory depression.
- Synergism with extended-spectrum penicillins, but must be administered separately.

Lab Effects/Interference:
- Serum ALT, serum alk phos, serum AST, serum bili, and serum LDH values may be increased.
- BUN and serum creatinine concentrations may be increased.
- Serum Ca++, serum Mg++, serum K+, and serum Na+ concentrations may be decreased.

Special Considerations:
- Used parenterally with at least one other agent in treatment of tuberculosis.
- Use in pregnancy only if infection is life-threatening and no safer drug exists; drug crosses placenta and may cause fetal toxicity.

Potential Toxicities/Side Effects and the Nursing Process

I.   ALTERATIONS IN SENSORY/PERCEPTUAL PATTERNS related to OTOTOXICITY

Defining Characteristics: Damage to eighth cranial nerve (auditory) may result in dizziness, nystagmus, vertigo, ataxia (vestibular damage), and more commonly, tinnitus, roaring sound in ears, and impaired hearing (auditory damage). Hearing loss usually begins with high-frequency loss, followed by clinical hearing loss, then permanent hearing loss if damage continues. Increased risk in elderly or renally impaired patients.

Nursing Implications: Assess baseline hearing (ability to hear spoken voice) and continue during therapy. Teach patient potential side effects, and instruct patient to report any hearing/perceptual problems (e.g., tinnitus, vertigo, decreased hearing). Discuss drug discontinuance and audiogram with physician to confirm hearing dysfunction if symptoms arise. Assess for increased risk if given concurrently with other ototoxic medications (e.g., cisplatin, furosemide).

COMPLICATIONS

II.   ALTERATION IN URINARY ELIMINATION related to NEPHROTOXICITY

Defining Characteristics: Risk of nephrotoxicity is less than with other aminoglycosides. Renal damage characterized by tubular necrosis with increased serum BUN, creatinine; decreased urine creatinine clearance and specific gravity; proteinuria and casts in urine. Azotemia usually not associated with oliguria. Rarely, electrolyte wasting with hypomagnesemia, hypocalcemia, and hypokalemia may occur. Renal dysfunction is usually reversible after drug discontinuance. Increased risk exists in elderly and if there is preexisting renal dysfunction. Risk is low in well-hydrated patients with normal renal function when normal doses are given.

Nursing Implications: Assess baseline renal function and electrolytes, and monitor periodically during therapy. Discuss any abnormalities with physician, as drug should be dose-reduced or discontinued if renal dysfunction develops. Assess baseline total body fluid balance, weight, and monitor periodically during antibiotic therapy. Monitor hydration status to keep patient well hydrated. Assess drug peak and trough levels as ordered so that drug dosage is correctly titrated. Increased risk of toxicity if peak serum concentration > 40 mg/mL. Draw blood for peak drug concentration 30 minutes after end of 30-minute infusion or at the end of a 60-minute infusion; draw trough immediately before next dose.

III.   ALTERATIONS IN SENSORY/PERCEPTUAL PATTERNS related to CNS EFFECTS, NEUROMUSCULAR BLOCKADE

Defining Characteristics: Headache, tremor, lethargy may occur. Peripheral neuropathy or encephalopathy (numbness, skin tingling, muscle twitching) may occur rarely. Neuromuscular blockade is dose-related, self-limiting, and uncommon. Risk is greater with topical application or when drug is administered to patient with neuromuscular disease (myasthenia gravis) or hypocalcemia.

Nursing Implications: Assess baseline neurologic status. Assess coexisting risk factors, neuromuscular blockade medications. Teach patient about side effects and instruct to report headache, tremor, lethargy. Observe for respiratory depression. If signs/symptoms arise, discuss drug discontinuance with physician.

IV.   POTENTIAL FOR INJURY related to HYPERSENSITIVITY

Defining Characteristics: Rash, urticaria, pruritus, fever, eosinophilia have occurred rarely. CROSS-SENSITIVITY between AMINOGLYCOSIDES exists! Handling of drug can cause sensitization to the drug.

Nursing Implications: Assess for drug allergies to any aminoglycoside—amikacin, gentamicin, kanamycin, neomycin, netilmicin, streptomycin, tobramycin—prior to drug administration. Instruct patient to report any allergic reactions. Assess for signs/symptoms of allergic reaction after drug dose. Take special care in preparing drug or wear gloves.

V. ALTERATION IN NUTRITION, LESS THAN BODY REQUIREMENTS, related to GI SIDE EFFECTS

Defining Characteristics: Nausea, vomiting, anorexia have occurred rarely. Also, transient hepatomegaly with increased LFTs—AST, ALT, LDH, alk phos—has occurred.

Nursing Implications: Assess baseline nutritional status, preexisting nausea/vomiting, anorexia. Assess baseline LFTs and monitor periodically during treatment. Instruct patient to report side effects. Provide symptomatic interventions if side effects occur; discuss with physician use of alternative drug(s).

VI. POTENTIAL FOR FATIGUE, INFECTION, AND BLEEDING related to BONE MARROW INJURY

Defining Characteristics: Anemia, leukopenia, granulocytopenia, and thrombocytopenia may occur. Also, patients receiving antibiotics are at risk for overgrowth of nonsusceptible microorganisms, such as fungi (superinfection). Rare.

Nursing Implications: Assess baseline CBC, differential, and monitor periodically during treatment. Instruct patient to report signs/symptoms of fatigue, infection, or bleeding immediately. Assess for signs/symptoms of superinfection. Discuss any adverse effects with physician.

VII. ALTERATION IN SKIN INTEGRITY related to IRRITATION AT INJECTION SITE, EXFOLIATIVE DERMATITIS

Defining Characteristics: Exfoliative dermatitis rarely occurs; may develop pain, irritation, and sterile abscesses at injection site.

Nursing Implications: Assess skin integrity and presence of lesions. Monitor for changes during treatment, and instruct patient to report them. Rotate injection sites and give injection deeply into large muscle mass, e.g., upper outer quadrant of buttock. Administer solutions of ≤ 500 mg/mL.

COMPLICATIONS

Drug: tedizolid phosphate (Sivextro)

Class: Antibacterial; tedizolid belongs to the oxazolidinone class of antibacterial drugs.

Mechanism of Action: Tedizolid phosphate, a phosphate prodrug, is converted to tedizolid in the presence of phosphatases. Tedizolid is mediated by binding to the 50S subunit of the bacterial ribosome, resulting in inhibition of protein synthesis. Tedizolid inhibits bacterial protein synthesis through a mechanism of action different from that of non-oxazolidinone antibacterial agents.

Metabolism: Tedizolid accounts for approximately 95% of the total circulating metabolites in plasma. The majority of its elimination occurs via the liver, 82% recovered in feces and 18% in urine.

Indications: Oxazolidinone-class antibacterial drugs are indicated in adults for treatment of acute bacterial skin and skin structure infections (ABSSSI) caused by susceptible grampositive microorganisms—*Staphylococcus aureus* (including methicillin-resistant [MRSA] and methicillin-susceptible [MSSA] isolates), *Streptococcus pyogenes*, *Streptococcus agalactiae*, *Streptococcus anginosus* group (including *S. anginosus*, *S. intermedius*, and *S. constellatus*), and *Enterococcus faecalis*.

Dosage/Range:

• Recommended dosage is 200 mg administered once daily for 6 days either orally (with or without food) or as an IV infusion in patients 18 years or older.
• No dose adjustment is necessary when changing from IV to oral formulation.
• If patients miss a dose, they should take it as soon as possible, anytime up to 8 hours prior to their next scheduled dose. If less than 8 hours remains before the next dose, wait until the next scheduled dose to resume administration.

Drug Preparation:

• Supplied as a sterile, lyophilized powder for injection in single-use vials.
• Reconstitute with sterile water for injection, USP and subsequently dilute only with 0.9% sodium chloride injection, USP. Vials contain no antimicrobial preservatives and are intended for single use only. Vials should be reconstituted using aseptic technique. Reconstitute the tedizolid phosphate with sterile water for injection.
• Minimize foaming. *Avoid* vigorous agitation or shaking of vial during or after reconstitution. Gently swirl contents, then let vial stand until powder is completely dissolved and any foam disperses.
• Inspect vial to ensure solution contains no particulate matter and no cake or powder remains. If necessary, invert vial to dissolve any remaining powder and swirl gently to prevent foaming. Reconstituted solution should be clear and colorless to pale yellow in color. Total storage time should not exceed 24 hours at either room temperature or under refrigeration at 2–8°C (36–46°F).
• Reconstituted solution must be further diluted in 0.9% sodium chloride injection, USP. Invert the bag gently to mix contents. Do *not* shake bag, as this may cause foaming.
• Administer as IV infusion only. Do not administer as IV push or bolus. Do not mix tedizolid phosphate with other drugs when administering. Drug is not intended for intra-arterial, intramuscular, intrathecal, intraperitoneal, or subcutaneous administration.
• The IV bag containing reconstituted and diluted IV solution should be inspected visually for particulate matter prior to administration. Discard if visible particles are observed. Resulting solution should be clear and colorless to pale yellow in color.
• After reconstitution and dilution, administer via IV infusion using a total time of 1 hour.
• Total time from reconstitution to administration should not exceed 24 hours at room temperature or under refrigeration at 2–8°C (36–46°F).

Drug Interaction:
- Neither tedizolid phosphate nor tedizolid detectably inhibited or induced the metabolism of selected CYP enzyme substrates. No potential drug interactions with tedizolid were identified in in vitro CYP inhibition or induction studies. These results suggest that drug–drug interactions based on oxidative metabolism are unlikely.
- Drug combination studies with tedizolid and aztreonam, ceftriaxone, ceftazidime, imipenem, rifampin, trimethoprim/sulfamethoxazole, minocycline, clindamycin, ciprofloxacin, daptomycin, vancomycin, gentamicin, amphotericin B, ketoconazole, and terbinafine demonstrated neither synergy nor antagonism.

Lab Effects/Interference: Has not been documented in prescribing materials.

Special Considerations: Most common adverse reactions in patients treated with tedizolid phosphate were nausea (8%), headache (6%), diarrhea (4%), vomiting (3%), and dizziness (2%)

Potential Toxicities/Side Effects and the Nursing Process

I. ALTERATION IN NUTRITION related to GI SIDE EFFECTS

Defining Characteristics: Nausea, vomiting, and anorexia have occurred frequently.

Nursing Implications: Assess baseline nutritional status, preexisting nausea/vomiting, and anorexia. Teach patient to report side effects. Provide symptomatic interventions if side effects occur; discuss with physician use of alternative drug(s).

II. ALTERATIONS IN COMFORT related to HEADACHE AND DIZZINESS

Defining Characteristics: Headache has occurred in some patients.

Nursing Implications: Assess baseline hearing (ability to hear spoken voice) and continue to assess during therapy. Teach patient about potential side effects, and instruct patient to report any hearing/perceptual problems (e.g., tinnitus, vertigo, decreased hearing). Discuss drug discontinuance and audiogram with physician to confirm hearing dysfunction if symptoms arise. Assess for increased risk if drug is given concurrently with other ototoxic medications (e.g., cisplatin, furosemide).

III. FUNGAL SUPERINFECTION related to REDISTRIBUTION OF ENDOGENOUS MICROORGANISMS

Defining Characteristics: Vaginal or oral candidiasis (sore mouth or tongue; white patches in mouth and/or tongue), vaginitis (vaginal candidiasis), and vaginal itching and discharge may occur as endogenous bacteria are eliminated and normal fungal population expands.

COMPLICATIONS

Nursing Implications: Teach female patients to report vaginal itching or discharge. Discuss appropriate antifungal treatment with physician. Teach perineal hygiene and symptomatic management.

Drug: telavancin (Vibativ)

Class: Lipopeptide antibiotic.

Mechanism of Action: Inhibits bacterial cell wall synthesis by interfering with the polymerization and cross-linking of peptidoglycan. Telavancin binds to the bacterial membrane and disrupts membrane barrier function.

Metabolism: Excreted by the kidney. Renal excretion is primary route of elimination.

Indication: Is used to treat severe skin infections, hospital-acquired, and ventilator-acquired pneumonia. It acts against gram-positive bacteria, including *Staphylococcus aureus* (methicillin-susceptible and methicillin-resistant isolates) and *Enterococcus faecalis* (vancomycin-susceptible isolates only).

Dosage/Range:
Adult:
- IV: 10 mg/kg administered over a 60-min period by IV infusion once every 24 h for 7 to 14 days.
- Drug dose should be reduced or adjusted in patients with severe renal insufficiency.
- Renal function impairment: CrCl 30–50 mL/min, give 7.5 mg/kg every 24 h. CrCl 30–10 mL/min, give 10 mg/kg every 48 h.

Drug Preparation:
- Reconstitute 250-mg vial with 15 mL of dextrose 5% injection, sterile water for injection, or sodium chloride 0.9% injection; reconstitute the 750-mg vial with 45 mL of dextrose 5% injection, sterile water for injection, sodium chloride 0.9% injection. The resultant solution has a concentration of 15 mg/mL.
- Administer over a period of no less than 60 min by IV infusion.
- Discard the vial if the vacuum did not pull the diluent into the vial.
- If the same IV line is used for sequential infusion of additional medications, the line should be flushed before and after infusion of telavancin with dextrose 5% injection, sodium chloride 0.9% injection, or lactated Ringer's injection.

Drug Interactions:
- Drugs affecting kidney function (e.g., ACE inhibitors, loop diuretics, NSAIDs): risk of renal adverse events may be increased. Use with caution. Observe the patient for adverse renal events. Monitor renal function.
- QT-prolonging drugs (e.g., amiodarone, pimozide, ziprasidone): possible additive effects with other drugs that prolong the QT interval. Use with caution.

Lab Effects/Interference:
- Telavancin does not interfere with coagulation; however, it interferes with certain tests used to monitor coagulation, including activated *clotting* time, aPTT, coagulation-based

factor Xa tests, INR, and PT. No evidence of increased risk of bleeding has been observed. Telavancin interferes with urine qualitative dipstick protein assays and quantitative dye methods (e.g., pyrogallol red-molybdate). However, micro albumin assay is not affected and can be used to monitor urinary protein excretion during telavancin treatment.

Special Considerations:
- Contraindicated in patients with known hypersensitivity to telavancin.
- Obtain ordered specimen and send for culture and sensitivity prior to first antibiotic dose.
- Consider alternative antibiotic therapy if anemia, drug rash or fever, arthralgia, or unexplained rise in BUN and serum creatinine occur.

Potential Toxicities/Side Effects and the Nursing Process

I.   ALTERATION IN NUTRITION, LESS THAN BODY REQUIREMENTS, related to GI SIDE EFFECTS

Defining Characteristics: Constipation, nausea, diarrhea, vomiting, dyspepsia.

Nursing Implications: Assess baseline nutritional status, preexisting nausea/vomiting, anorexia. Assess baseline bowel pattern. Administer symptomatic interventions if side effects occur; discuss with physician use of alternative drug(s).

II.   POTENTIAL FOR INJURY related to HYPERSENSITIVITY REACTION

Defining Characteristics: Rash, urticaria, pruritus, and fever can occur in individuals with hypersensitivity to telavancin.

Nursing Implications: Assess for drug allergies prior to drug administration. Instruct patient to report any allergic reactions. Assess for signs/symptoms of allergic reaction after drug dose.

III.   SENSORY/PERCEPTUAL ALTERATIONS related to CNS EFFECTS OF DIZZINESS AND HEADACHE

Defining Characteristics: Dizziness, headache, and insomnia may occur.

Nursing Implications: Assess baseline neurologic status. Teach patient about side effects and to report dizziness or headache. If signs/symptoms arise, discuss drug discontinuance with physician.

IV.   ALTERATIONS IN COMFORT related to LOCAL INJECTION IRRITATION

Defining Characteristics: Pain or phlebitis may develop in IV sites.

Nursing Implications: Change IV sites q 48 h, and assess for signs/symptoms of phlebitis prior to each administration. Administer drug slowly. Apply warm packs to increase comfort.

COMPLICATIONS

Drug: telithromycin (Ketek)

Class: Antimicrobial agent. This antibiotic is a new structural class called ketolides.

Mechanism of Action: Similar to that of macrolides and is related to the 50S-ribosomal subunit binding with inhibition of bacterial protein synthesis. Telithromycin appears to have greater affinity for the ribosomal binding site than macrolides. Demonstrated efficacy against *Staphylococcus aureus, Streptococcus aureus, Streptococcus pneumoniae, H. influenzae, Moraxella catarrhalis, Chlamydia pneumoniae,* and *Mycoplasma pneumoniae.*

Metabolism: Absorbed from the GI tract. Eliminated by multiple pathways: 7% of the dose is excreted unchanged by biliary and/or intestinal secretion; 13% of the dose is excreted unchanged in urine; and 37% of the dose is metabolized by the liver. May accumulate in patients with severe hepatic disease.

Indication: For treatment of bacterial infections in the lungs and sinuses and mild to moderate community-acquired pneumonia caused by *S. pneumoniae,* including multidrug-resistant isolates. Demonstrated efficacy against *Staphylococcus aureus, Streptococcus aureus, Streptococcus pneumoniae, H. influenzae, Moraxella catarrhalis, Chlamydia pneumoniae,* and *Mycoplasma pneumoniae.*

Dosage/Range:
- Adult: oral: 800 mg daily for 5–10 days. Duration of therapy depends on indication. Drug dose should be reduced or adjusted in patients with hepatic or renal insufficiency.

Drug Preparation:
- Oral: administration of telithromycin with food had no significant effect on extent or rate of oral absorption in healthy subjects.

Drug Interactions:
- Class I, IA, and III antiarrhythmic agents: concomitant use is contraindicated as it may lead to QT prolongation. Serum levels may be increased.
- CYP3A4 inhibitors: itraconazole and ketoconazole: increase telithromycin levels and AUC by ~54% and 95%, respectively.
- CYP3A4 substrates: cisapride, simvastin, and midazolam: increase serum concentration of cisapride by 95%; significantly increase serum concentration of simvastin and midazolam. These drugs SHOULD NOT be used when a patient is taking telithromycin.
- CYP2D6 substrates: metoprolol: increase serum concentrations. Administer with caution. Rifampin decreases serum concentrations. Digoxin increases serum concentration. Theophylline increases serum concentrations. Take 1 hour apart to decrease the gastrointestinal side effects. Sotalol decreases serum concentrations.

Lab Effects/Interference:
- No reported drug-laboratory test interactions. SGPT, alk phos, amylase, SGOT, and bilirubin: serum concentrations may be increased in patients with preexisting hepatic disease.

Special Considerations:
- Avoid use in pregnant or lactating women.
- Contraindicated in patients with known hypersensitivity, patients with previous history of hepatitis and/or jaundice associated with the use of this drug or any macrolide antibiotic, such as azithromycin (Zithromax), erythromycin, clarithromycin (Biaxin), or dirithromycin (Dynabac).
- Acute hepatic failure and severe liver injury (in some cases fatal) have been reported in patients immediately during or immediately after receiving this drug. Monitor closely (for jaundice, hyperbilirubinuria, acholic stools, liver tenderness, or hepatomegaly), and teach patient to report signs/symptoms (fatigue, malaise, anorexia, nausea, jaundice, dark amber urine). If patient has any signs or symptoms, drug must be stopped and the patient evaluated for this (LFTs, physical exam). The drug should be discontinued if hepatitis or transaminase elevations plus symptoms occur.
- Use with caution, if at all, in patients with myasthenia gravis, as they may have worsening symptoms of the disease (such as death and life-threatening breathing difficulties within a few hours of the first dose).
- Obtain ordered specimen and send for culture and sensitivity prior to first antibiotic dose.

Potential Toxicities/Side Effects and the Nursing Process

I.   ALTERATION IN NUTRITION related to GI SIDE EFFECTS

Defining Characteristics: Anorexia, nausea, vomiting, diarrhea, glossitis, dysphagia, gastroenteritis, gastritis, constipation.

Nursing Implications: Assess baseline nutritional status. Assess for and teach patient to report any symptoms. Administer and teach patient self-administration of prescribed antiemetic or antidiarrheal medication as appropriate.

II.   ALTERATION IN PROTECTIVE MECHANISMS

Defining Characteristics: Prolonged PT, prolonged INR, cardiac arrhythmias, including atrial arrhythmias, bradycardia, and hypotension.

Nursing Implications: Monitor and teach patient about potential side effects and to report abnormalities, such as fainting and dizziness.

III.   POTENTIAL FOR INJURY related to VISUAL DISTURBANCES

Defining Characteristics: Blurred vision and difficulty focusing.

Nursing Implications: Assess baseline visual and neurologic status. Teach patient to report any changes in vision. If signs/symptoms arise, discuss discontinuance with physician, and institute supportive measures.

COMPLICATIONS

IV.   FUNGAL SUPERINFECTION related to REDISTRIBUTION OF ENDOGENOUS MICROORGANISMS

Defining Characteristics: Vaginal moniliasis, vaginitis may occur as endogenous bacteria are eliminated and normal fungal population expands.

Nursing Implications: Teach female patient to report vaginal itching or discharge. Discuss appropriate antifungal treatment with physician. Teach perineal hygiene and symptom management.

Drug: ticarcillin disodium (Ticar); combined with clavulanate potassium (Timentin)

Class: Antibacterial (systemic) (extended-spectrum penicillin).

Mechanism of Action: Semisynthetic antibiotic prepared from fungus *Penicillium*. Contains β-lactam ring and is bactericidal by inhibiting cell wall synthesis.

Metabolism: Poorly absorbed from GI tract, so must be given parenterally. Widely distributed in body tissues and fluids. Crosses placenta and is excreted in breastmilk. Excreted via urine and bile.

Indication: For treatment of bacterial septicemia, skin and skin structure infections, lower respiratory infections, bone and joint infections, GU and gynecologic infections, and intra-abdominal infections caused by susceptible strains of bacteria. Active against most gram-positive (except penicillinase-producing strains) and most gram-negative bacilli. Used in the treatment of serious gram-negative infections, especially *P. aeruginosa*–related infections of lower respiratory tract, urinary tract, and skin. When combined with clavulanate potassium, the drug is protected from breakdown by bacterial β-lactamase enzymes, thus keeping therapeutic antibiotic serum levels.

Dosage/Range:
• IV dosing preferred but drug can be given IM or IV.

Adult:
Ticarcillin disodium:
• 3 g q 4–6 h (200–300 mg/kg/day in divided doses).
• Dosage modification required if renal insufficiency exists; refer to manufacturer's package insert.

Timentin:
• 3 g ticarcillin plus 0.1 g clavulanic acid (3.1 g) IV q 4–6 h × 10–14 days if weight < 60 kg: 200–300 mg ticarcillin/kg/d in divided doses q 4–6 h IV.

Drug Preparation:
• IV: reconstitute each gram with 4 mL 0.9% sodium chloride or 5% dextrose injection. Further dilute in 50–100 mL IV solution and infuse over 30 minutes to 2 hours.

- IM: reconstitute each gram with 2 mL sterile water for injection or 1% lidocaine HCl (without epinephrine). Ensure patient is NOT ALLERGIC to lidocaine. Inject drug deep IM in large muscle mass (e.g., gluteus maximus). Maximum 2 g at one site.

Drug Interactions:
- Aminoglycosides: synergism.
- Aminoglycosides (e.g., gentamicin): incompatible when mixed together; administer at separate sites at different times. Also, penicillinase-resistant penicillins can inactivate aminoglycoside serum samples from patients receiving both drugs.
- Probenecid: increased serum level of penicillin; may be coadministered to exert this effect.
- Clavulanic acid (β-lactamase inhibitor): Synergistic bacterial effect.

Lab Effects/Interference:
Major clinical significance:
- Urine glucose: high urinary concentrations of a penicillin may produce false-positive or falsely elevated test results with copper sulfate tests (Benedict's, Clinitest, or Fehling's); glucose enzymatic tests (Clinistix or Testape) are not affected.
- PTT and PT: an increase has been associated with ticarcillin.

Clinical significance:
- Coombs' (direct antiglobulin) test: false-positive result may occur during therapy with any penicillin.
- Urine protein: high urinary concentrations of ticarcillin may produce false-positive protein reactions (pseudoproteinuria) with the sulfosalicylic acid and boiling test; bromophenol blue reagent test strips (Multistix) are reportedly unaffected.
- ALT, alk phos, AST, serum LDH values may be increased.
- Serum bili: an increase has been associated with ticarcillin.
- BUN and serum creatinine: increased concentrations have been associated with ticarcillin.
- Serum K+: hypokalemia may occur following administration of parenteral ticarcillin, which may act as a non-reabsorbable anion in the distal tubules; this may cause an increase in pH and result in increased urinary potassium loss. The risk of hypokalemia increases with use of larger doses.
- WBC: leukopenia or neutropenia is associated with the use of all penicillins; the effect is more likely to occur with prolonged therapy and severe hepatic function impairment.

Special Considerations:
- Contraindicated in patients with prior hypersensitivity to penicillins. Use with caution in patients sensitive to other β-lactams (e.g., cephalosporins) since partial cross-allergenicity exists.
- Obtain ordered specimen, and send for culture and sensitivity test prior to first antibiotic dose.
- Consider alternative antibiotic therapy if eosinophilia, drug fever or rash, arthralgia, hematuria, or unexplained rise in BUN and serum creatinine occur.
- Monitor electrolytes and renal, hepatic, and hematologic laboratory parameters during extended treatment periods.
- Use with caution in pregnant or nursing women.

COMPLICATIONS

• Decreased incidence of hypokalemia, and less salt load, than other extended-spectrum penicillins.

Potential Toxicities/Side Effects and the Nursing Process

I.   POTENTIAL FOR INJURY related to HYPERSENSITIVITY REACTION

Defining Characteristics: Urticaria, pruritus, rash (maculopapular or erythematous), fever and chills, eosinophilia, myalgia, edema, erythema, angioedema, Stevens-Johnson syndrome, and exfoliative skin reactions occur in 5% of patients. Increased risk in individuals allergic to cephalosporin antibiotics.

Nursing Implications: Assess allergy to cephalosporin antibiotics and penicillin: if patient states "yes," determine actual response (e.g., "swollen lips = angioedema"). If angioedema, patient SHOULD NOT receive drug. Discuss other patient responses with physician to determine whether drug should be given. Assess baseline skin condition, including integrity and allergy history to drugs. Instruct patient to report rash, itching, other skin changes. Teach patient skin care and symptomatic measures as appropriate. If skin rash develops, discuss drug discontinuance with physician. If rash progresses, drug should be discontinued, as fatal Stevens-Johnson syndrome may develop. Be prepared to treat severe acute hypersensitivity reactions with airway management, oxygen, epinephrine, corticosteroids, antihistamines as ordered.

II.   ALTERATION IN NUTRITION, LESS THAN BODY REQUIREMENTS, related to GI SIDE EFFECTS

Defining Characteristics: Nausea, vomiting, diarrhea may occur; rarely, pseudomembranous colitis caused by *C. difficile* resistant to the antibiotic occurs. Rarely, transient increases in LFTs—AST, ALT, alk phos, bili—may occur.

Nursing Implications: Assess baseline nutritional status. Instruct patient to report GI disturbances. Administer and teach patient to self-administer antiemetics, antidiarrheals as needed and as ordered. Teach patient importance of nutritious diet, and suggest small, frequent, high-calorie, high-protein meals as appropriate. Assess baseline LFTs, and monitor periodically during treatment. Discuss abnormalities and drug interruption with physician.

III.   FUNGAL SUPERINFECTION related to REDISTRIBUTION OF ENDOGENOUS MICROORGANISMS

Defining Characteristics: Vaginal candidiasis, vaginitis may occur as endogenous bacteria are eliminated and normal fungal population expands.

Nursing Implications: Instruct female patient to report vaginal itching or discharge. Discuss appropriate antifungal treatment with physician. Teach perineal hygiene and symptomatic management.

IV.　ALTERATIONS IN PROTECTIVE MECHANISMS (RARE) related to TRANSIENT LEUKOPENIA

Defining Characteristics: Rarely, transient leukopenia, lymphocytosis, anemia, eosinophilia may occur. Prolonged PT, prolonged aPTT, and hypoprothrombinemia have occurred rarely, especially in elderly or debilitated patients, or in individuals with vitamin K deficiency.

Nursing Implications: Assess baseline laboratory parameters, and monitor periodically during treatment. Assess patient for response to antibiotics. Discuss abnormalities with physician. Assess for signs/symptoms of bleeding.

V.　ALTERATIONS IN SENSORY/PERCEPTUAL PATTERNS related to DIZZINESS, SOMNOLENCE

Defining Characteristics: Dizziness, headache, somnolence occur rarely. Neuromuscular irritability and seizures may occur with high drug serum levels.

Nursing Implications: Assess baseline neurologic function and comfort, and monitor during treatment. Instruct patient to report any changes. Discuss any abnormalities with physician. Institute seizure precautions.

VI.　ALTERATIONS IN COMFORT related to LOCAL INJECTION IRRITATION

Defining Characteristics: Vein irritation (pain, erythema), phlebitis, and thrombophlebitis may occur at IV administration site.

Nursing Implications: Change IV sites q 48 h, and assess for signs/symptoms of phlebitis prior to each administration. Administer drug slowly. Apply warm packs to increase comfort. Discuss central line with patient and physician to facilitate administration.

VII.　ALTERATION IN FLUID AND ELECTROLYTE BALANCE related to HYPOKALEMIA AND INCREASED SODIUM INTAKE

Defining Characteristics: Prolonged therapy may cause hypokalemia; also, drug is prepared as sodium salt. Frequent IV infusions increase fluid intake.

Nursing Implications: Assess baseline electrolytes, fluid balance, weight, and monitor throughout therapy. Monitor renal function studies, especially if patient has preexisting renal dysfunction.

Drug: tigecycline (Tygacil)

Class: Antimicrobial agent. This antibiotic is the first in a new class called glycylcyclines. This novel IV antibiotic has a broad spectrum of antimicrobial activity, including activity against the drug-resistant bacteria methicillin-resistant *Staphylococcus aureus* (MRSA).

Mechanism of Action: Inhibits protein transplantation in bacteria by binding to the 30S ribosomal subunit and blocking entry of amino-acyl tRNA molecules into the A site of the ribosome.

Metabolism: Is not extensively metabolized. Eliminated by multiple pathways: 7% of the dose is excreted unchanged by biliary and/or intestinal secretion; 59% of the dose is excreted unchanged in bile/feces and 33% of the dose is excreted in the urine. May accumulate in patients with severe hepatic disease.

Indication: For treatment of community-acquired bacterial pneumonia, complicated skin and skin structure infections, and complicated intra-abdominal infections caused by susceptible strains of specific microorganisms. Demonstrated efficacy against methicillin-susceptible and -resistant *Staphylococcus aureus* (MRSA), *E. coli, Enterococcus faecalis* (vancomycin-resistant isolates), *Streptococcus anginosus, Streptococcus intermedius, Streptococcus constellatus, B. fragilis, B. thetaiotaomicron, B. uniformis, B. vulgatus, Clostridium perfringens*, and *Peptostreptococcus micros*.

Dosage/Range:
Adult:
- Initial dose 100 mg IV, followed by 50 mg every 12 hours.
- Duration of therapy depends on indication.
- Drug dose should be reduced or adjusted in patients with severe hepatic insufficiency.

Drug Preparation:
- IV injection should be administered over 30–60 minutes every 12 hours.

Drug Interactions:
- Monitor prothrombin time if administered with warfarin.
- Concurrent use of antibacterial drugs with oral contraceptives may render the oral contraceptives less effective.

Lab Effects/Interference:
- No reported drug-laboratory test interactions. SGPT, alk phos, amylase, SGOT, and bilirubin: serum concentrations may be increased in patients with preexisting hepatic disease.

Special Considerations:
- Avoid use in pregnant or lactating women.
- Contraindicated in patients with known hypersensitivity.
- Obtain ordered specimen and send for culture and sensitivity prior to first antibiotic dose.

Potential Toxicities/Side Effects and the Nursing Process

I.   ALTERATION IN NUTRITION related to GI SIDE EFFECTS

Defining Characteristics: Anorexia, nausea, vomiting, diarrhea, glossitis, dysphagia, gastroenteritis, gastritis, constipation.

Nursing Implications: Assess baseline nutritional status. Assess for and teach patient to report any symptoms. Administer and teach patient self-administration of prescribed anti-emetic or antidiarrheal medication as appropriate.

II.   POTENTIAL FOR INJURY related to HYPERSENSITIVITY REACTION

Defining Characteristics: Urticaria, pruritus, rash (maculopapular or erythematous), fever and chills, eosinophilia, myalgia, edema, erythema, angioedema, Stevens-Johnson syndrome, and exfoliative skin reactions occur.

Nursing Implications: Assess allergy to antibiotics: if patient states "yes," determine actual response (e.g., "swollen lips = angioedema"). If angioedema, patient SHOULD NOT receive drug. Discuss other patient responses with physician to determine whether drug should be given. Assess baseline skin condition, including integrity and allergy history to drugs. Instruct patient to report rash, itching, and other skin changes. Teach patient skin care and symptomatic measures as appropriate. If skin rash develops, discuss drug discontinuance with physician. If rash progresses, drug should be discontinued, as fatal Stevens-Johnson syndrome may develop. Be prepared to treat severe acute hypersensitivity reactions with airway management, oxygen, epinephrine, corticosteroids, and antihistamines as ordered.

III.   ALTERATIONS IN COMFORT related to LOCAL INJECTION IRRITATION

Defining Characteristics: Vein irritation (pain, erythema), phlebitis, and thrombophlebitis may occur at IV administration site.

Nursing Implications: Change IV sites q 48 h, and assess for signs/symptoms of phlebitis prior to each administration. Administer drug slowly. Apply warm packs to increase comfort. Discuss central line with patient and physician to facilitate administration.

IV.   FUNGAL SUPERINFECTION related to REDISTRIBUTION OF ENDOGENOUS MICROORGANISMS

Defining Characteristics: Vaginal moniliasis, vaginitis may occur as endogenous bacteria are eliminated and normal fungal population expands.

Nursing Implications: Teach female patient to report vaginal itching or discharge. Discuss appropriate antifungal treatment with physician. Teach perineal hygiene and symptom management.

COMPLICATIONS

Drug: tobramycin sulfate (Nebcin)

Class: Aminoglycoside antibacterial (systemic).

Mechanism of Action: Synthetic antibiotic derived from *Streptomyces*; bactericidal, most probably by inhibition of protein synthesis.

Metabolism: Well-absorbed following parenteral administration, but variability in absorption after IM injection (peak serum level 0.5–2 hours, duration 8–12 hours). Widely distributed into body fluids. Minimally protein-bound. Readily crosses placenta and into breastmilk. Drug excreted unchanged in the urine.

Indication: For treatment of a variety of bacterial infections, including bone and joint infections, bacterial meningitis and other central nervous system infections, respiratory tract infections, septicemia, skin and skin structure infections, urinary tract infections, and empiric treatment of febrile neutropenia. Active against aerobic microorganisms: many sensitive gram-negative (including *Acinetobacter, Citrobacter, Enterobacter, E. coli, Klebsiella, Proteus, Pseudomonas, Salmonella, Serratia,* and *Shigella*) and some sensitive gram-positive organisms (*S. aureus* and *S. epidermidis*). Over time, bacterial resistance may develop, either naturally or acquired.

Dosage/Range:
- 3 mg/kg/day given in equally divided doses q 8 h.
- Desired peak serum concentration is 4–10 mg/mL, and trough serum concentration is 1–2 mg/mL.
- May use 5–6 mg/kg/day in three equally divided doses to treat life-threatening infections.
- If loading dose required, 2 mg/kg; usual dosing q 8 h, but q 12 or q 24 dosing may also be used.
- DOSE-REDUCE IF RENAL IMPAIRMENT.

Drug Preparation:
- Store unreconstituted vials at 15–30°C (59–86°F).
- Store injections at 25°C (77°F).
- Store reconstituted solution (using sterile water for injection, with final concentration 40 mg/mL) at room temperature (stable 24 hours) or in refrigerator at 2–8°C (36–46°F) (stable 96 hours).

Drug Administration:
- IV: further dilute by adding dose to 50–100 mL in 0.9% sodium chloride and administer over 30–60 minutes.

Drug Interactions:
- Increased risk of toxicity with other ototoxic drugs: acyclovir, other aminoglycosides, amphotericin B, bacitracin, cephalosporins, colistin, cisplatin, ethacrynic acid, furosemide, vancomycin.
- Potentiation of neuromuscular blockade when given concurrently with general anesthetics (succinylcholine, tubocurarine); use cautiously; observe for signs/symptoms of respiratory depression.
- Synergism with extended-spectrum penicillins, but must be administered separately.

Lab Effects/Interference:
- Serum ALT, serum alk phos, serum AST, serum bili, and serum LDH values may be increased.
- BUN and serum creatinine concentrations may be increased.
- Serum Ca++, serum Mg++, serum K+, and serum Na+ concentrations may be decreased.

Special Considerations:
- Used as first-line treatment in short-term treatment of serious gram-negative infections (e.g., septicemia, respiratory tract infections).
- Use against gram-positive organisms only as second-line treatment.
- Use in pregnancy only if infection is life-threatening and no safer drug exists; drug crosses placenta and may cause fetal toxicity.

Potential Toxicities/Side Effects and the Nursing Process

I.   ALTERATIONS IN SENSORY/PERCEPTUAL PATTERNS related to OTOTOXICITY

Defining Characteristics: Damage to eighth cranial nerve (auditory) may result in dizziness, nystagmus, vertigo, ataxia (vestibular damage), and more commonly, tinnitus, roaring sound in ears, and impaired hearing (auditory damage). Hearing loss usually begins with high-frequency loss, followed by clinical hearing loss, then permanent hearing loss if damage continues. Increased risk in elderly or renally impaired patients.

Nursing Implications: Assess baseline hearing (ability to hear spoken voice) and continue during therapy. Teach patient potential side effects, and instruct patient to report any hearing/perceptual problems (e.g., tinnitus, vertigo, decreased hearing). Discuss drug discontinuance and audiogram with physician to confirm hearing dysfunction if symptoms arise. Assess for increased risk if given concurrently with other ototoxic medications (e.g., cisplatin, furosemide).

II.   ALTERATION IN URINARY ELIMINATION related to NEPHROTOXICITY

Defining Characteristics: Risk of nephrotoxicity is less than with other aminoglycosides. Renal damage characterized by tubular necrosis with increased serum BUN, creatinine; decreased urine creatinine clearance and specific gravity; proteinuria and casts in urine. Azotemia usually not associated with oliguria. Rarely, electrolyte wasting with hypomagnesemia, hypocalcemia, and hypokalemia may occur. Renal dysfunction is usually reversible after drug discontinuance. Increased risk exists in elderly and if there is preexisting renal dysfunction. Risk is low in well-hydrated patients with normal renal function when normal doses given.

Nursing Implications: Assess baseline renal function and electrolytes, and monitor periodically during therapy. Discuss any abnormalities with physician, as drug should be dose-reduced or discontinued if renal dysfunction develops. Assess baseline total body fluid balance, weight, and monitor periodically during antibiotic therapy. Monitor hydration status to keep patient well hydrated. Assess drug peak and trough levels as ordered so that drug dosage is correctly titrated. Increased risk of toxicity if peak serum concentration > 10–12 mg/mL. Draw blood for peak drug concentration 30 minutes after end of 30-minute infusion or at the end of a 60-minute infusion; draw trough immediately before next dose.

COMPLICATIONS

III.   ALTERATIONS IN SENSORY/PERCEPTUAL PATTERNS related to CNS
        EFFECTS, NEUROMUSCULAR BLOCKADE

Defining Characteristics: Headache, tremor, lethargy may occur. Peripheral neuropathy or encephalopathy (numbness, skin tingling, muscle twitching) may occur rarely. Neuromuscular blockade is dose-related, self-limiting, and uncommon. Risk is greater with topical application or when drug is administered to patient with neuromuscular disease (myasthenia gravis) or hypocalcemia.

Nursing Implications: Assess baseline neurologic status. Assess coexisting risk factors, neuromuscular blockade medications. Teach patient about side effects, and instruct to report headache, tremor, lethargy. Observe for respiratory depression. If signs/symptoms arise, discuss drug discontinuance with physician.

IV.   POTENTIAL FOR INJURY related to HYPERSENSITIVITY

Defining Characteristics: Rash, urticaria, pruritus, fever, eosinophilia have occurred rarely. CROSS-SENSITIVITY between AMINOGLYCOSIDES exists!

Nursing Implications: Assess for drug allergies to any aminoglycoside—amikacin, gentamicin, kanamycin, neomycin, netilmicin, streptomycin, tobramycin—prior to drug administration. Instruct patient to report any allergic reactions. Assess for signs/symptoms of allergic reaction after drug dose.

V.   ALTERATION IN NUTRITION, LESS THAN BODY REQUIREMENTS, related to
      GI SIDE EFFECTS

Defining Characteristics: Nausea, vomiting, anorexia have occurred rarely. Also, transient hepatomegaly with increased LFTs—AST, ALT, LDH, alk phos—has occurred.

Nursing Implications: Assess baseline nutritional status, preexisting nausea/vomiting, anorexia. Assess baseline LFTs and monitor periodically during treatment. Instruct patient to report side effects. Provide symptomatic interventions if side effects occur; discuss with physician use of alternative drug(s).

VI.   POTENTIAL FOR FATIGUE, INFECTION, AND BLEEDING related to BONE
       MARROW INJURY

Defining Characteristics: Anemia, leukopenia, granulocytopenia, and thrombocytopenia may occur. Also, patients receiving antibiotics are at risk for overgrowth of nonsusceptible microorganisms, such as fungi (superinfection). Rare.

Nursing Implications: Assess baseline CBC, differential, and monitor periodically during treatment. Instruct patient to report signs/symptoms of fatigue, infection, or bleeding immediately. Assess for signs/symptoms of superinfection. Discuss any adverse effects with physician.

Drug: vancomycin hydrochloride (Vancocin)

Class: Antibacterial (systemic).

Mechanism of Action: Derived from cultures of *Streptomyces orientalis*; drug is bactericidal by binding to bacterial cell wall, thus blocking protein polymerization and cell wall synthesis. Also damages cell membrane and acts at a different site than the penicillins. Bacteriostatic for enterococci.

Metabolism: Not well-absorbed from the GI tract—except in those patients with colitis—especially if patient has renal compromise. Effective when administered IV and is widely distributed in body tissues and fluid, including bile. Crosses placenta; unknown whether drug is excreted in breastmilk; 52–60% bound to plasma proteins. IV dose excreted primarily by kidneys and, to a small degree, in bile; oral dose excreted in feces.

Indication: For treatment of *C. difficile*–associated diarrhea and staphylococcal enterocolitis. Active against many gram-positive organisms (staphylococci, group A b-hemolytic streptococci, *S. pneumoniae, C. difficile,* enterococci, *Corynebacterium, Clostridium*).

Dosage/Range:
Adult:
- Oral (for use in pseudomembranous colitis): capsules or powder: 0.5–1 g/day in four divided doses × 7–10 days.
- IV: 500 mg or 1 g q 12 h.
- Desired peak serum concentration is 20 to 40 mg/mL; and trough serum concentration is 5–15 mg/mL.
- Dose reduction necessary if renal dysfunction; see manufacturer's package insert.

Drug Preparation:
- Oral dose for treatment of *C. difficile* pseudomembranous colitis. Oral dose not recommended for treating systemic infections.
- Reconstituted by adding 10 mL of sterile water to 500-mg vial (20 mL to 1-g vial). Further dilute in at least 100 mL 0.9% sodium chloride or 5% dextrose in water, and infuse over 1 hour (central line).
- For peripheral lines, further dilution in 250 mL is recommended.
- Causes tissue necrosis if given IM; DO NOT ADMINISTER IM.

Drug Interactions:
- Nephrotoxic drugs (aminoglycoside antibiotics, amphotericin B, cisplatin, colistin): increased risk of nephrotoxicity; avoid concurrent use if possible.

Lab Effects/Interference:
- BUN concentrations may be increased.

Special Considerations:
- Use cautiously in patients with renal dysfunction.
- DO NOT USE in patients with hearing loss—or use at reduced doses if necessary in life-threatening infections.
- Contraindicated in patients with known hypersensitivity.
- Obtain ordered specimen for culture and sensitivity prior to first antibiotic dose.
- Use with caution in pregnancy, as fetal effects are unknown, and in lactating mothers, as drug may be excreted in breastmilk.

Potential Toxicities/Side Effects and the Nursing Process

I.   ALTERATIONS IN SENSORY PERCEPTUAL PATTERNS related to OTOTOXICITY

Defining Characteristics: IV drug appears to damage eighth cranial nerve (auditory). First symptom of ototoxicity is tinnitus and may progress to deafness; may also be associated with vertigo and dizziness (vestibular branch). High risk exists in patients with renal impairment who are receiving concurrent ototoxic drugs (e.g., cisplatin) or prolonged therapy, or those whose age > 60 years old.

Nursing Implications: Assess baseline hearing (ability to hear spoken voice) or audiogram if patient is at high risk—both at baseline and throughout therapy. Monitor serum drug concentrations during therapy if at high risk. Teach patient potential side effects, and instruct patient to report any hearing/perceptual problems (e.g., tinnitus, decreased hearing, vertigo). Discuss drug discontinuance with physician if symptoms arise.

II.   ALTERATION IN URINARY ELIMINATION related to NEPHROTOXICITY

Defining Characteristics: Renal damage may occur, characterized by transient increases in serum BUN or creatinine, hyaline casts, and albuminuria. May cause acute interstitial nephritis. High risk in patients with renal impairment who are receiving concurrent nephrotoxic drugs (e.g., cisplatin) or prolonged therapy, or those whose age > 60 years.

Nursing Implications: Assess baseline renal function and electrolytes, and monitor periodically during therapy. Discuss any abnormalities with physician, as drug should be dose-reduced or discontinued if renal dysfunction develops. Assess baseline hydration status, including urinary output, total body balance, daily weights; keep patient well hydrated.

III.   ALTERATION IN COMFORT related to LOCAL TISSUE EFFECTS

Defining Characteristics: Vesicant if given IM (causing tissue necrosis). Irritating to veins when given IV, causing pain and thrombophlebitis.

Nursing Implications: Administer drug IV, *NOT* IM. Assess IV site prior to each dose and at completion of dose; instruct patient to report pain or burning; change IV site if irritation, phlebitis develop. Change site at least q 48 h and consider central line for prolonged therapy. AVOID EXTRAVASATION.

IV. ALTERATION IN CARDIAC OUTPUT related to RAPID IV INFUSION

Defining Characteristics: Rapid IV administration may cause histamine release and "red-neck" syndrome, characterized by rapid onset of hypotension, flushing, and erythematous or maculopapular rash of neck, face, chest. May be associated with wheezing, dyspnea, angioedema, urticaria, pruritus. Rarely, seizures and cardiac arrest may occur. Syndrome occurs minutes after beginning infusion, but may occur at end; usually resolves spontaneously over 2+ hours, but may require antihistamines, corticosteroids, or IV fluids. Rare when drug is administered over 1 hour.

Nursing Implications: Monitor temperature, VS at baseline, 5 minutes into IV administration, and at end of infusion, at least with the initial dose, infuse over at least 1 hour, using infusion controller if necessary. Observe patient during first 5 minutes, and instruct patient to report rash, wheezing, itching immediately. If reaction occurs, stop infusion, assess VS, and notify physician. Patient may be treated with antihistamine or IV fluids, or both. Completion of dose and subsequent doses may be ordered at very slow rate. Document episode in medical record and update care plan/medication sheet to reflect change in drug administration.

V. INJURY related to BONE MARROW SUPPRESSION

Defining Characteristics: Rarely, leukopenia, thrombocytopenia, agranulocytosis may occur, especially with cumulative doses > 25 g.

Nursing Implications: Monitor baseline and periodic WBC, differential, platelet count, especially if receiving other bone marrow-suppressive drugs. Discuss abnormalities with physician.

VI. INFECTION related to OVERGROWTH OF NONSUSCEPTIBLE MICROORGANISMS

Defining Characteristics: Normal microflora populations altered by drug, with possible overgrowth by nonsusceptible microorganisms, i.e., fungi, gram-negative bacteria.

Nursing Implications: Assess for signs/symptoms of other infections of skin, mucous membranes. Instruct patient to report signs/symptoms. Discuss further antimicrobial therapy with physician.

COMPLICATIONS

ANTIFUNGALS

Drug: amphotericin B (deoxycholate) (Fungizone); amphotericin B lipid complex (Abelcet); amphotericin B cholesteryl sulfate complex (Amphotec); liposomal amphotericin B (AmBisome)

Class: Antifungal (systemic); antiprotozoal.

Mechanism of Action: Produced by *Streptomyces*; binds to sterol molecule in fungal membrane, causing disruption and leakage of intracellular ions. Is fungistatic (prevents replication at normal doses) and fungicidal (kills fungi at high doses).

Metabolism: Poorly absorbed from GI tract so must be given IV. Crosses BBB and the placenta; 90–95% bound to serum proteins. Single-dose elimination half-life is 24 hours, while following long-term administration is 15 days.

Indication: For treatment of progressive and potentially life-threatening fungal infections. It may be used to treat protozoal infections. Active against systemic fungal infections (*Aspergillus, Candida, Cryptococcus, Histoplasma capsulatum*); used to treat fungal meningitis and *Leishmania* (protozoan) infections.

Dosage/Range:
Adult:
Amphotericin B (deoxycholate):
- Initial: 0.25 mg/kg IV (or first dose of 1 mg IV) over 6-hour period (may use 2–4 hours). Gradual increase in daily dosage (e.g., over 1 week) to dose of 0.5 mg/kg/day to 1 mg/kg/day or 1.5 mg/kg on alternate days (maximum 1.5 mg/kg/day).
- If dose is interrupted for > 1 week, reinstitute at 0.25 mg/kg/day and titrate up.
- Intrathecal: 25 mg (0.1 mL diluted with 10–20 mL CSF) biw–tiw.
- Oral: oral candida: amphotericin B oral suspension: 1 mL (100 mg) qid.

Lipid-based amphotericin B (infection refractory or pt has renal impairment):
- Amphotec: test dose 1.6–8.3 mg/10 mL IV over 15–30 min, 3–4 mg/kg/d prepared as a 0.6 mg/mL infusion IV at 1 mg/kg/hr.
- Abelcet: 5 mg/kg/day (1–2 mg/mL) IV at 2.5 mg/kg/hr; if infusion time > 2 h shake to remix q 2 h.
- AmBisome: 3–5 mg/kg/day IV (1–2 mg/mL) over 1–2 hours.
- Bladder irrigation: 50 mg/mL solution given into bladder intermittently or as a continuous irrigation × 5–20 days.

Drug Preparation:
Amphotericin B deoxycholate:
- Use sterile water for injection (NO PRESERVATIVES) to reconstitute drug; for peripheral line only further dilute to a concentration of 0.1 mg/mL using 500 mL of 5% dextrose injection. Manufacturer recommends protecting from light but appears to be stable for 24 hours in room light.

Drug Administration:
- Administer slowly over 2–6 hours.
- If an inline filter is used, it must have a mean pore diameter of ≥ 1 mm or drug will be filtered out; no filter for Amphotec, Abelcet.
- Protect from light during infusion.

Drug Interactions:
- Norfloxacin: possible enhanced antifungal action.
- Additive nephrotoxic effects when combined with other nephrotoxic drugs: aminoglycosides, cisplatin, cyclosporine, pentamidine, vancomycin, so concurrent administration should be avoided.
- Enhanced hypokalemic effects when combined with other drugs that lower serum potassium: corticosteroids.
- Enhanced digitoxin: toxicity related to amphotericin-induced hypokalemia.
- Synergism with flucytosine with increased drug effect.
- Antagonism with miconazole: do not use together.
- Nitrogen mustard: increases toxicity (renal, bronchospasm, hypotension)—avoid concurrent administration.
- Granulocyte transfusions: acute pulmonary dysfunction may occur if given concurrently or close together. Time administration far apart and monitor pulmonary function.

Lab Effects/Interference:
- Increased AST, ALT, alk phos, creatinine, BUN.
- Hypomagnesemia, hypokalemia, hypocalcemia.
- Hypoglycemia, hyperglycemia.

Special Considerations:
- Use with caution in patients with renal dysfunction.
- Contraindicated if hypersensitive to amphotericin.
- Safety in pregnancy has not been established—use with caution and only if benefits outweigh risks.
- Drug encapsulation in liposome decreases toxicity, including renal toxicity. Amphotericin B lipid complex injection is approved for the treatment of aspergillosis in patients refractory or intolerant to conventional amphotericin B.

Potential Toxicities/Side Effects and the Nursing Process

I.   POTENTIAL FOR INJURY related to DRUG ADMINISTRATION

Defining Characteristics: Headache, hypotension, malaise, myalgias, tachypnea, cramping, nausea, and vomiting may occur. Fever and chills usually begin 1–3 hours after infusion is started, and tolerance develops with subsequent doses. Rapid IV administration may cause hypertension and shock, hypokalemia, and arrhythmias.

COMPLICATIONS

Nursing Implications: Assess baseline comfort level, temperature, VS. Teach patient potential side effects, and instruct to report any changes. Discuss premedication with physician, such as ibuprofen (inhibits prostaglandin PGE_2) and/or hydrocortisone. Discuss with physician use of IV meperidine HCl (Demerol) for management of rigor if it develops. Administer test dose (e.g., 1 mg/250 mL 5% dextrose IV over 1–4 hours) and monitor temperature, heart rate, BP, respiratory rate during infusion. Administer drug slowly (over 2–6 hours) and escalate dose slowly. Administer antiemetic agents as needed, then prophylactically.

II.   ALTERATION IN URINARY ELIMINATION related to NEPHROTOXICITY

Defining Characteristics: 80% incidence; multiple toxic effects (vasoconstriction, lytic action on renal tubular cell membranes, calcium deposits in distal nephron); hypokalemia may precede azotemia with increased BUN and creatinine, decreased creatinine clearance, and increased excretion of K+, uric acid, and protein. Renal tubular acidosis may occur. Renal impairment usually diminishes after drug discontinuance, but some degree of impairment may be permanent.

Nursing Implications: Assess baseline renal function and electrolytes; monitor every other day during dosage escalation, then at least weekly. Discuss any abnormalities with physician. Drug should be dose-reduced if renal dysfunction develops. Slowly administer initial test dose, then gradually increase doses over first week. Assess fluid status and total body balance closely to keep patient well hydrated. Assess for signs/symptoms of hypokalemia: arthralgia, myalgia, muscle weakness. Administer potassium and magnesium replacements as ordered.

III.   FATIGUE related to ANEMIA

Defining Characteristics: High incidence of reversible normocytic, normochromic anemia that rarely requires transfusion.

Nursing Implications: Assess baseline CBC, HCT; monitor Hgb and HCT during treatment. Instruct patient to report fatigue, shortness of breath, headache. Transfuse red blood cells as needed and ordered by physician.

IV.   ALTERATION IN COMFORT, PAIN related to PAIN AT INJECTION SITE

Defining Characteristics: Drug may cause pain at injection site, phlebitis, thrombophlebitis; extravasation causes local irritation.

Nursing Implications: Select veins for IV administration distally and then more proximally, avoiding phlebitic veins or small veins. Apply heat to increase comfort. Administer drug slowly.

V.   ALTERATION IN CARDIAC OUTPUT related to CARDIOPULMONARY DYSFUNCTION

Defining Characteristics: Rarely, hypertension, ventricular fibrillation, cardiac arrest, failure, pulmonary edema may occur. Pulmonary hypersensitivity may occur with bronchospasm, wheezing, or pulmonary pneumonitis.

Nursing Implications: Monitor VS closely, noting heart rate and rhythm, BP, breath sounds at baseline and during infusion. Instruct patient to report dyspnea, other changes in breathing pattern, or general feeling state ASAP. Discuss any changes, abnormalities with physician. Administer granulocyte transfusions as far apart from amphotericin administration as possible, and monitor pulmonary status closely. Be prepared to provide basic life support/resuscitation if needed.

VI.   ALTERATIONS IN SENSORY/PERCEPTUAL PATTERNS related to PERIPHERAL AND CNS DYSFUNCTION

Defining Characteristics: Rarely, hearing loss, tinnitus, transient vertigo, blurred vision or diplopia, peripheral neuropathy, and seizures may occur. Following intrathecal drug administration: headache, lumbar nerves, arachnoiditis, and visual changes may occur.

Nursing Implications: Assess baseline neurologic function and monitor during drug administration and over time, especially when drug is given intrathecally. Notify physician if abnormalities occur. Discuss with physician coadministration of small doses of intrathecal corticosteroids to decrease CNS irritation.

VII.   ALTERATION IN NUTRITION, LESS THAN BODY REQUIREMENTS related to GI TOXICITY

Defining Characteristics: Anorexia, nausea, vomiting, dyspepsia, cramping, epigastric pain, and diarrhea may occur. Rarely, melena and hemorrhagic gastroenteritis may occur. Elevated LFTs may occur.

Nursing Implications: Assess baseline nutritional status, including weight and usual weight. Administer antiemetics as ordered and needed, then prophylactically prior to infusion if nausea and/or vomiting develop. Administer antidiarrheal medicine as ordered and needed. Instruct patient to report any symptoms; teach/reinforce importance of high-calorie, high-protein diet; suggest family/significant other bring in favorite foods from home as appropriate. Assess LFT results at baseline and periodically during treatment as elevated serum aminotransferase, bili, and alk phos may occur. Discuss abnormalities with physician. Encourage patient to eat favorite foods, especially those high in calories, protein, potassium, and magnesium. Monitor daily weight during treatment, and discuss weight loss with dietitian, patient, and physician to revise nutritional plan.

COMPLICATIONS

VIII. ALTERATION IN PROTECTIVE MECHANISMS related to BONE MARROW INJURY

Defining Characteristics: Rarely, thrombocytopenia, leukopenia, agranulocytosis, and coagulation defects may occur.

Nursing Implications: Assess baseline CBC, differential. Assess for any signs/symptoms of bleeding or infection, and discuss with physician if they occur. Teach patient general self-assessment guidelines, such as taking temperature and reporting any changes from baseline condition.

Drug: anidulafungin (Eraxis)

Class: Antifungal.

Mechanism of Action: Semisynthetic lipopeptide synthesized from fermentation products of *Aspergillus nidulans*. Fungistatic by damaging fungal cell membrane increasing permeability, altering cell metabolism, and inhibiting cell growth. Fungicidal at high concentrations. Inhibits the synthesis of β(1,3)-D-glucan synthase, resulting in selective inhibition of the synthesis of glucan, an integral component of the fungal cell wall.

Metabolism: Unique among echinocandins because it slowly degrades in human plasma, undergoing a process of biotransformation rather than metabolism. Degradation products pass into the feces via the biliary tree.

Indication: For treatment of certain types of fungal infections, including esophageal candidiasis, candemia, and other forms of *Candida* infections (intra-abdominal abscess and peritonitis).

Dosage/Range:
- Esophageal candidiasis: 100 mg/day (loading dose), followed by 50 mg/day × 14 days or × 7 days after resolution of symptoms.
- Candidemia and other deep-tissue *Candida* infections: 200 mg on day 1, followed by 100 mg/day × 14 days after the last positive blood culture.

Drug Preparation:
- Do not mix or co-infuse with other medications.
- No dose adjustment is required in patients based on age, sex, weight, disease state, concomitant drug therapy, or renal or hepatic insufficiency.
- IV: Use manufacturer's suggested dilution guideline.
- Infuse slowly; histamine-mediated reactions have been observed related to infusion rate.

Drug Interactions:
- Contraindications: hypersensitivity to anidulafungin, other echinocandins, or any component of the formulation.
- Anidulafungin was found to be safe and was not affected by concomitant treatment with substrates, inhibitors, or inducers of the cytochrome P450 metabolic pathway, including rifampin and cyclosporine in clinical trials.

Lab Effects/Interference:
Major clinical significance:
• Elevated liver function tests, hepatitis, and worsening hepatic failure have been reported.

Special Considerations:
• Used in treatment of fungal infections.
• On the basis of a lack of interactions with amphotericin B and voriconazole, anidulafungin is well suited to be used in combination with other antifungal agents.
• Histamine-mediated reactions (urticaria, flushing, hypotension) have been observed related to infusion rate.

Potential Toxicities/Side Effects and the Nursing Process

I. POTENTIAL FOR INJURY related to INFUSION-RELATED ADVERSE EVENTS

Defining Characteristics: Infusion-related adverse events occurred in 1.3% (N = 6) of the patients in clinical trials. Hypotension with tachycardia, dyspnea, rash, urticaria, flushing, pruritus, dyspnea, hypotension, and dizziness may occur.

Nursing Implications: Assess baseline VS and monitor throughout infusion. Instruct patient to report signs/symptoms immediately. Assess for signs/symptoms: nausea, generalized itching, crampy abdominal pain, chest tightness, anxiety, agitation, sense of impending doom, wheezing, and dizziness.

II. ALTERATION IN NUTRITION, LESS THAN BODY REQUIREMENTS, related to GI SIDE EFFECTS

Defining Characteristics: Nausea, vomiting, diarrhea, and anorexia may occur.

Nursing Implications: Assess baseline nutritional and elimination status. Instruct patient to report GI disturbances. Administer and teach patient to self-administer antiemetics, antidiarrheals as needed and as ordered. Teach patient importance of nutritious diet, and suggest small, frequent, high-calorie, high-protein meals as appropriate.

III. ALTERATIONS IN SENSORY/PERCEPTUAL PATTERNS related to CNS, ENDOCRINE EFFECTS

Defining Characteristics: Dizziness, headache, and somnolence may occur. Hypokalemia occurs in 3% of patients.

Nursing Implications: Assess baseline neurologic function and comfort, and monitor during treatment. Instruct patient to report any changes. Discuss any abnormalities with physician.

COMPLICATIONS

Drug: caspofungin (Cancidas)

Class: Echinocandin; glucan synthesis inhibitor.

Mechanism of Action: Caspofungin inhibits the synthesis of β(1,3)-D-glucan, an integral component of the fungal cell wall of susceptible filamentous fungi.

Metabolism: Caspofungin is slowly metabolized by hydrolysis and N-acetylation. Elimination route is via feces and urine.

Indication: For treatment of invasive aspergillosis in patients refractory to or intolerant of other antifungal therapies; empirical treatment for presumed fungal infections in febrile neutropenia, treatment of esophageal candidiasis, and treatment of candidemia and the following *Candida* infections: intra-abdominal abscess, peritonitis and pleural space infections. Drug has demonstrated activity in regions of active cell growth of *Aspergillus fumigatus*.

Dosage/Range:
- The recommended dose of caspofungin is a 70-mg loading dose on the first day, followed by 50 mg/daily.
- No dosage adjustment is necessary for the elderly.
- No dosage adjustment is necessary for patients with renal insufficiency. Caspofungin is not dialyzable.
- No dosage adjustment is recommended for patients with mild hepatic insufficiency (Child-Pugh score 5 to 6). In those with moderate hepatic insufficiency (Child-Pugh score 7 to 9), a daily dose of 35 mg after the 70-mg loading dose is recommended.

Drug Administration:
- Caspofungin should be given as a slow IV infusion in 250 mL 0.9% sodium chloride over 1 hour.
- Caspofungin is not compatible with dextrose-containing solutions.

Drug Interactions:
- Transient increase in AST and ALT have been observed when caspofungin and cyclosporine are coadministered. Therefore, concomitant use of these two agents is not recommended unless the potential benefit outweighs the potential risk.

Potential Toxicities/Side Effects and the Nursing Process

I.   ALTERATIONS IN COMFORT related to LOCAL VEIN IRRITATION (IV ADMINISTRATION)

Defining Characteristics: Erythema, irritation, pain, swelling, phlebitis may occur at injection site. Consider use of central line.

Nursing Implications: Assess IV site for patency, irritation prior to each dose. Change IV site at least q 48 hours. Apply warmth/heat to painful area as needed.

II. POTENTIAL FOR INJURY related to HYPERSENSITIVITY REACTION

Defining Characteristics: Fever and erythema. Increased risk in allergic individuals.

Nursing Implications: Assess allergy/allergic potential to drug. Discuss other patient responses with physician to determine whether drug should be given. Assess baseline skin condition including integrity and allergy history to drugs. Teach patient to report rash, itching, and other skin changes. Teach patient skin care and symptomatic measures as appropriate. If reaction occurs, discuss drug discontinuance with physician.

III. ALTERATION IN NUTRITION, LESS THAN BODY REQUIREMENTS, related to GI SIDE EFFECTS

Defining Characteristics: Nausea and vomiting may occur. Rarely, transient increases in LFTs—AST (SGOT), ALT (SGPT), alk phos, bili—may occur with coadministration of cyclosporine.

Nursing Implications: Assess baseline nutritional status. Teach patient to report GI disturbances. Administer and teach patient to self-administer antiemetics as needed and as ordered. Teach patient importance of nutritious diet and suggest small, frequent, high-caloric, high-protein meals as appropriate. Assess baseline LFTs and monitor periodically during treatment. Discuss abnormalities and drug interruption with physician.

IV. SENSORY/PERCEPTUAL ALTERATIONS

Defining Characteristics: Headache.

Nursing Implications: Assess baseline neurologic function and comfort and monitor during treatment. Teach patient to report any changes. Discuss any abnormalities with physician.

Drug: fluconazole (Diflucan)

Class: Azole, antifungal (systemic).

Mechanism of Action: Fungistatic; causes increased permeability of fungal cell membrane, so intracellular nutrients leak out (potassium, amino acids) and cell is unable to take in nutrients to make DNA (precursors for purine, pyrimidines).

Metabolism: Drug is rapidly and highly absorbed from GI tract, with > 90% of drug bioavailable. GI absorption is unaffected by food or gastric pH. Steady-state plasma levels achieved in 5–10 days, or by second day if loading dose given. Widely distributed in body tissues and fluids, including CSF. There is minimal protein binding. It is unknown whether drug crosses the placenta or is excreted in human milk; 60–80% of drug is excreted unchanged in the urine. Renal dysfunction results in higher circulating serum levels with

COMPLICATIONS

prolonged drug effect and potential toxicity. Drug elimination in elderly clients may be decreased.

Indication: For treatment of most fungi, including yeast.

Dosage/Range:
- Oral and parenteral dosages are the same; IV dosage recommended for patients unable to take oral form. Dose is a single daily dose.
- Dosage depends on fungal infection. Candidiasis (oropharyngeal or esophageal): 200 mg day 1, followed by 100 mg/day (may titrate based on patient's response up to 400 mg/day) × 2 weeks (oropharyngeal); × 3 weeks or at least × 2 weeks after symptoms resolve (esophageal). Candidiasis (systemic): 400 mg day 1, followed by 200 mg/day × 4 weeks at least, then × 2 weeks after symptoms resolve (esophageal). Cryptococcal infections: Initial: 400 mg day 1, followed by 200–400 mg/day × 10–12 weeks after CSF cultures for *Cryptococcus* are negative. Maintenance (AIDS patients): 200 mg/day indefinitely.
- DOSE-REDUCE AFTER LOADING DOSE IF RENAL COMPROMISE based on creatinine clearance (e.g., 21–50 mL/min, dose-reduce 50%; if 11–20 mL/min, dose-reduce 75%).

Drug Preparation:
- Oral: store in tight containers at < 30°C (86°F).
- Parenteral: glass vials for injection should be stored at 5–30°C (41–86°F); protect from freezing. Plastic containers should be stored at 5–25°C (41–77°F). Inspect for any discoloration, particulate matter, or leaks in plastic bags. If found, do not use.

Drug Administration:
- Oral: once daily without regard to food intake.
- IV: once daily at a rate ≤ 200 mg/hour. DO NOT ADD ADDITIVES. DO NOT ADMINISTER IV IN SERIES THAT COULD INTRODUCE AIR EMBOLISM.

Drug Interactions:
- Coumarin anticoagulants: increased PT; monitor PT closely.
- Cyclosporine: increased cyclosporine serum levels; monitor closely and adjust dose.
- Phenytoin: increased phenytoin serum level; monitor closely and reduce phenytoin dose as needed.
- Rifampin: decreased fluconazole serum level; increase fluconazole dose when given concurrently.
- Sulfonylurea antidiabetic agents (tolbutamide, glyburide, glipizide): increased drug serum levels; monitor blood glucose levels closely and decrease dose as needed.
- Thiazide diuretics: increased fluconazole serum level; do not appear to increase fluconazole toxicity so dose adjustment not necessary.
- Rifampin, isoniazid, phenytoin, valproic acid, oral sulfonylurea: increased risk of elevated hepatic transaminases exists.

Lab Effects/Interference:
Major clinical significance:
- ALT, alk phos, AST, and serum bili values may be elevated.

Special Considerations:
* Drug is being studied as a prophylactic antifungal agent in patients at risk for neutropenia and fungal infections (cancer patients receiving myelosuppressive chemotherapy, bone marrow transplant patients).
* Use cautiously in patients with renal dysfunction; dose reduction based on creatinine clearance (see Dosage/Range section).
* Absorption NOT affected by gastric pH or food intake.
* Risk of drug toxicity may be higher in patients with HIV infection.

Potential Toxicities/Side Effects and the Nursing Process

I. ALTERATION IN NUTRITION, LESS THAN BODY REQUIREMENTS, related to GI SIDE EFFECTS

Defining Characteristics: 2–8% incidence of mild-to-moderate nausea, vomiting, abdominal pain, diarrhea is seen; anorexia, dyspepsia, dry mouth, flatus, bloating occur rarely; 5–7% incidence of mild, transient increases in LFTs, which are reversible with drug discontinuance.

Nursing Implications: Assess baseline nutritional and elimination status. Instruct patient to report GI disturbances. Administer and teach patient to self-administer antiemetics, antidiarrheals as needed and as ordered. Teach patient importance of nutritious diet and suggest small, frequent, high-calorie, high-protein meals as appropriate. Assess baseline LFTs and monitor periodically during treatment. Discuss abnormalities and drug interruption with physician. Assess whether patient is taking other hepatotoxic drugs (see Special Considerations section).

II. ALTERATION IN SKIN INTEGRITY related to ALLERGY/HYPERSENSITIVITY

Defining Characteristics: 5% incidence is seen of rash, often diffuse, associated with eosinophilia and pruritus; rarely, exfoliative dermatitis and Stevens-Johnson syndrome may occur in patients receiving multiple drugs.

Nursing Implications: Assess baseline skin condition, including integrity and drug allergy history. Instruct patient to report rash, itching, and other skin changes. Teach patient skin care and symptomatic measures as appropriate. If skin rash develops, discuss drug discontinuance with physician. If rash progresses, especially in HIV-infected patients, drug should be discontinued, as fatal Stevens-Johnson syndrome may develop. Be prepared to treat severe acute hypersensitivity reactions with airway management, oxygen, epinephrine, corticosteroids, antihistamines as ordered.

III. ALTERATIONS IN SENSORY/PERCEPTUAL PATTERNS related to CNS EFFECTS

Defining Characteristics: Dizziness and headache occur in 2% of patients. Rarely, somnolence, delirium/coma, dysesthesia, malaise, fatigue, seizure, and psychiatric disturbance may occur.

COMPLICATIONS

Nursing Implications: Assess baseline neurologic function and comfort, and monitor during treatment. Instruct patient to report any changes. Discuss any abnormalities with physician.

Drug: flucytosine (Ancobon)

Class: Antifungal (systemic).

Mechanism of Action: Nonantibiotic antifungal; enters fungal cell and undergoes deamination to fluorouracil, which acts as an antimetabolite, preventing RNA and protein synthesis; may also interfere with DNA synthesis.

Metabolism: Oral preparation well-absorbed from GI tract; decreased rate of absorption when taken with food. Widely distributed into body tissues and fluids, including CSF; 75–90% of dose excreted unchanged by kidneys, with increased serum levels and toxicity in patients with renal dysfunction.

Indication: For treatment of *Candida* and *Cryptococcus*.

Dosage/Range:
* Oral: 50–150 mg/kg/day in four equally divided doses given q 6 h × weeks or months until fungal studies are negative. Dose may be 150–250 mg/kg/day in *Cryptococcus* meningitis.
* Dose must be reduced in patients with renal dysfunction.
* Dose must be determined by flucytosine levels (therapeutic range is 25–120 mg/mL).
* Dose may be determined by creatinine clearance. Individual dose of 12.5–37.5 mg/kg given:
* q 12 h if creatinine clearance is 20–40 mL/min.
* q 24 h if creatinine clearance is 10–20 mL/min.
* q 24–48 h if creatinine clearance is < 10 mL/min.

Drug Preparation:
* Store in tight, light-resistant container at < 40°C (104°F).
* Oral.

Drug Interactions:
* Amphotericin B: theoretic synergism.
* Norfloxacin: theoretic synergism.

Lab Effects/Interference:
* Rare anemia, leukopenia, agranulocytosis, thrombocytopenia, pancytopenia, eosinophilia.

Special Considerations:
* Use only in severe infections, as drug is toxic.
* Theoretically synergistic with amphotericin, but some studies do not show significant benefit of combination.
* Therapeutic response (negative fungal cultures) may take weeks to months.
* Drug has no antineoplastic activity.

• Drug is teratogenic, capable of causing fetal malformations when given to pregnant women. Risks and benefits should be carefully considered before drug is used in a pregnant patient.

Potential Toxicities/Side Effects and the Nursing Process

I. POTENTIAL FOR INFECTION, BLEEDING, AND FATIGUE related to BONE MARROW DEPRESSION

Defining Characteristics: Anemia, leukopenia, thrombocytopenia may occur; agranulocytosis and aplastic anemia occur rarely. Increased risk exists with increased serum flucytosine levels (100 mg/mL), especially in patients with renal compromise or those receiving concurrent amphotericin B.

Nursing Implications: Assess baseline CBC, differential, BUN, and creatinine, and monitor closely during therapy, especially if receiving concurrent amphotericin B. Assess for signs/symptoms of bleeding, fatigue, infection during therapy. Teach patient to self-assess for signs/symptoms of infection, bleeding, and instruct to report them immediately. Discuss dose with physician; dose modification is needed if renal dysfunction occurs. Monitor flucytosine therapeutic levels (to maintain level of 25–100 mg/mL).

II. ALTERATION IN NUTRITION, LESS THAN BODY REQUIREMENTS, related to MUCOSITIS, NAUSEA, VOMITING

Defining Characteristics: Frequently dividing epithelial cells of GI mucosa are damaged, leading to diarrhea and possible bowel perforation (rare). Nausea, vomiting, anorexia, abdominal bloating may also occur. Elevated LFTs may occur, but are dose-related and reversible; liver enlargement may occur.

Nursing Implications: Assess elimination and nutritional status, baseline and throughout treatment. Assess baseline LFTs. Instruct patient to report diarrhea, nausea, vomiting immediately, and teach self-administration of prescribed antiemetics and antidiarrheal medication. Monitor weight, and teach patient importance of high-protein, high-calorie diet. Instruct patient to administer dose over 15 minutes to decrease nausea and vomiting. If weight loss occurs/persists, refer to dietitian/nutritionist. Monitor LFTs during treatment: AST, ALT, bili, and alk phos.

III. INJURY related to ANAPHYLAXIS

Defining Characteristics: Rare anaphylaxis has occurred in patients with AIDS, characterized by diffuse erythema, pruritus, injection of conjunctiva, fever, tachycardia, hypotension, edema, and abdominal pain.

Nursing Implications: Instruct AIDS patients to report any signs/symptoms of rash, pruritus, conjunctivitis, abdominal pain immediately. Use drug cautiously in AIDS patients. Monitor any adverse sensations over time. Assess for signs/symptoms.

COMPLICATIONS

IV.   ALTERATION IN SENSORY/PERCEPTUAL PATTERNS related to CNS CHANGES

Defining Characteristics: Confusion, sedation, hallucinations, and headaches occur infrequently.

Nursing Implications: Assess baseline mental status. Instruct patient to report headaches, abnormal thoughts, mental status changes. Discuss alternative drug if mental status changes occur.

Drug: isavuconazonium sulfate (Cresemba)

Class: Isavuconazonium sulfate is an azole antifungal indicated for patients 18 years of age and older.

Mechanism of Action: Prodrug of isavuconazole, an azole antifungal drug.

Metabolism: Isavuconazole is extensively distributed and is highly protein bound (greater than 99%), predominantly to albumin. Isavuconazonium sulfate was recovered in both feces and urine. Renal excretion of isavuconazole itself was less than 1% of the dose administered.

Indications: Treatment of invasive aspergillosis and invasive mucomycosis.

Dosage/Range:
- Loading dose: 372 mg isavuconazonium sulfate (equivalent to 200 mg of isavuconazole) every 8 hours for 6 doses (48 hours) via oral or IV administration.
- Maintenance dose: 372 mg isavuconazonium sulfate (equivalent to 200 mg of isavuconazole) once daily via oral or IV administration starting 12–24 hours after the last loading dose.
- Capsules can be taken with or without food; swallow capsules whole. Do not chew, crush, dissolve, or open capsules.
- Switching between intravenous and oral formulations of isavuconazonium sulfate is acceptable as bioequivalence has been demonstrated; a loading dose is not required when switching between formulations.

Drug Preparation:
- Aseptic technique must be strictly observed in all handling, no preservative or bacteriostatic agent is present in isavuconazonium sulfate or in materials specified for its reconstitution.
- Isavuconazonium sulfate is water soluble, preservative free, sterile, and nonpyrogenic.
- Reconstitute drug by adding water for injection, USP per package insert. Gently shake to dissolve powder completely. Visually inspect reconstituted solution for particulate matter and discoloration.
- Reconstituted isavuconazonium sulfate should be clear and free of visible particulates. Reconstituted solution may be stored below 25°C for a maximum of 1 hour prior to preparation of patient infusion solution.

- IV formulation may form insoluble particulates following reconstitution. Isavuconazonium sulfate for injection must be administered via an infusion set with an in-line filter (pore size, 0.2–1.2 micron). Flush IV lines with 0.9% sodium chloride injection, USP or 5% dextrose injection, USP prior to and after infusion of isavuconazonium sulfate.
- Infuse IV formulation over a minimum of 1 hour in 250 mL of a compatible diluent, to reduce risk of infusion-related reactions. Do not administer as an IV bolus injection. Do not infuse isavuconazonium sulfate with other IV medications.
- After dilution of IV formulation, avoid unnecessary vibration or vigorous shaking of solution. Do not use a pneumatic transport system.

Drug Interaction:
- Review patient's concomitant medications.
- CYP3A4 inhibitors or inducers may alter plasma concentrations of isavuconazole. Appropriate therapeutic drug monitoring and dose adjustment of immunosuppressants (i.e., tacrolimus, sirolimus, and cyclosporine) may be necessary when coadministered with isavuconazonium sulfate. Drugs with a narrow therapeutic window that are P-gp substrates, such as digoxin, may require dose adjustment when administered concomitantly with isavuconazonium sulfate.
- Several drugs may significantly alter isavuconazole concentrations. Coadministration of strong CYP3A4 inhibitors, such as ketoconazole or high-dose ritonavir (400 mg every 12 hours), with isavuconazonium sulfate is contraindicated because strong CYP3A4 inhibitors can increase plasma concentration of isavuconazole.
- Isavuconazole may alter concentrations of several drugs. Coadministration of strong CYP3A4 inducers, such as rifampin, carbamazepine, St. John's wort, or long-acting barbiturates, with isavuconazonium sulfate is contraindicated because strong CYP3A4 inducers can decrease plasma concentration of isavuconazole.

Lab Effects/Interference: Serious hepatic reactions have been reported. Evaluate liver-related lab tests at beginning and during course of isavuconazonium sulfate therapy.

Special Considerations:
- Infusion-related reactions have been reported during IV administration of isavuconazonium sulfate. Discontinue infusion if an infusion-related reaction occurs.
- Do not administer drug to pregnant women unless the benefit to the mother outweighs the risk to the fetus. Inform pregnant patients of potential hazards.
- Isavuconazonium sulfate is contraindicated in persons with known hypersensitivity to isavuconazole. Serious hypersensitivity and severe skin reactions, such as anaphylaxis and Stevens-Johnson syndrome, have been reported during treatment with other azole antifungal agents. Discontinue isavuconazonium sulfate if patient develops an exfoliative cutaneous reaction.
- Isavuconazonium sulfate has been shown to shorten the QTc interval. It is contraindicated in patients with familial short QT syndrome.

Potential Toxicities/Side Effects and the Nursing Process

I.   ALTERATION IN SKIN INTEGRITY related to ALLERGY/HYPERSENSITIVITY

Defining Characteristics: Rash, often diffuse, associated with eosinophilia and pruritus, has been reported. Rarely, exfoliative dermatitis and Stevens-Johnson syndrome may occur in patients receiving multiple drugs.

Nursing Implications: Assess patient's baseline skin condition, including integrity, and drug allergy history. Instruct patient to report rash, itching, and other skin changes. Teach patient skin care and symptomatic measures as appropriate. If skin rash develops, discuss drug discontinuance with physician. If rash progresses, drug should be discontinued, as fatal Stevens-Johnson syndrome may develop. Be prepared to treat severe acute hypersensitivity reactions with airway management, oxygen, epinephrine, corticosteroids, and antihistamines, as ordered. Assess baseline VS. Instruct patient to report signs and symptoms immediately. Assess for nausea, generalized itching, crampy abdominal pain, chest tightness, anxiety, agitation, sense of impending doom, wheezing, and dizziness.

II.   ALTERATION IN COMFORT related to PRURITUS, PHLEBITIS, SKIN
      ERUPTIONS, AND FEVER

Defining Characteristics: Phlebitis and pruritus with or without rash may occur.

Nursing Implications: Assess temperature, skin integrity, and comfort prior to drug administration, and monitor throughout treatment. Discuss with physician use of diphenhydramine to decrease itching. Change IV sites every 48 hours to decrease phlebitis, or discuss use of a central line with patient and physician. If rash and pruritus worsen, discuss drug discontinuance with physician.

III. ALTERATION IN NUTRITION, LESS THAN BODY REQUIREMENTS, related to
      GI SIDE EFFECTS

Defining Characteristics: Nausea, vomiting, diarrhea, constipation and anorexia; mild, transient increases in LFTs.

Nursing Implications: Assess patient's baseline nutritional and elimination status. Instruct patient to report GI disturbances. Administer, and teach patient to self-administer, antiemetics and antidiarrheals as needed and as ordered. Teach patient importance of a nutritious diet; suggest small, frequent, high-calorie, high-protein meals as appropriate. Assess baseline LFTs and monitor periodically during treatment. Discuss abnormalities and drug interruption with physician. Assess whether patient is taking other hepatotoxic drugs.

Drug: itraconazole (Sporanox)

Class: Azole; antifungal.

Mechanism of Action: Fungistatic; may be fungicidal, depending on concentration; azole antifungals interfere with cytochrome P450 activity, which is necessary for the demethylation of 14-a-methylsterols to ergosterol. Ergosterol, the principal sterol in the fungal cell membrane, becomes depleted. This damages the cell membrane, producing alterations in membrane function and permeability. In *Candida albicans,* azole antifungals inhibit transformation of blastospores into invasive mycelial form.

Metabolism: Rapidly absorbed from GI tract in acid environment. Decreased absorption in patients with gastric hypochlorhydria or achlorhydria or in patients taking medications that raise pH (antacids, H_2 antagonists).

Indication: For treatment of fungal infections.

Dosage/Range:
- Oral: 100–200 mg/day × 7–14 days (candidiasis); longer for other infections (400 mg/ day in severe infections).
- Although studies did not provide a loading dose, in life-threatening situations a loading dose of 200 mg three times a day (600 mg/day) for the first 3 days is recommended, based on pharmacokinetic data.
- Doses above 200 mg/day should be given in two divided doses.
- IV: 200 mg bid × 4 doses followed by 200 mg daily; give each dose over 1 hour—do not use for more than 14 days.

Drug Preparation:
- Store in tightly closed container at < 40°C (104°F).
- Itraconazole injection must be diluted prior to IV infusion. The entire 250-mg ampule should be diluted in the 50-mL bag of 0.9% sodium chloride provided by the manufacturer. The final concentration of the solution is 3.33 mg/mL (250 mg/75 mL).

Drug Administration:
- Orally in single or split dose, depending on total daily dose.
- Should take with meals to increase absorption of medication.
- Oral solution should be taken on an empty stomach to increase absorption of the medication.
- To administer a 200-mg dose of itraconazole, 60 mL should be given by IV infusion over 60 minutes. The infusion should be given using a controlled infusion device, the manufacturer-provided infusion set, and a dedicated IV line. When the infusion is complete, the manufacturer recommends that the infusion set be flushed via the two-way stopcock using 15–20 mL of 0.9% sodium chloride over 30 seconds to 15 minutes. The entire IV line should then be discarded.

Drug Interactions:
- Drugs that increase gastric pH: antacids, anticholinergics/antispasmodics, histamine H_2-receptor antagonists, or omeprazole will decrease the absorption of itraconazole.

COMPLICATIONS

- Didanosine contains a buffer to increase its absorption; this will decrease the absorption of itraconazole, since itraconazole needs an acidic environment.
- Use with oral antidiabetic agents has increased the plasma concentration of these sulfonylurea agents, leading to hypoglycemia.
- Use with carbamazepine may decrease itraconazole plasma concentrations, leading to clinical failure or relapse.
- Itraconazole may increase digoxin concentrations, leading to digoxin toxicity.
- Use with lovastatin or simvastatin may increase the plasma concentrations of these cholesterol-lowering agents and may increase the risk of rhabdomyolysis.
- Use with midazolam or triazolam may potentiate the hypnotic and sedative effects of these benzodiazepines.

Lab Effects/Interference:
Major clinical significance:
- ALT, alk phos, AST, serum bili values may be elevated.
- Serum K+: hypokalemia has occurred in approximately 2–6% of patients treated with itraconazole and has resulted in ventricular fibrillation, especially in higher doses.

Special Considerations:
- High failure rate in HIV-infected patients due to achlorhydria.

Potential Toxicities/Side Effects and the Nursing Process

I.   ALTERATION IN NUTRITION, LESS THAN BODY REQUIREMENTS, related to GI SIDE EFFECTS

Defining Characteristics: Increased LFTs may occur: AST, ALT, alk phos. Hepatotoxicity is less common, is usually reversible, and is rarely fatal.

Nursing Implications: Assess baseline nutritional and elimination status. Instruct patient to report GI disturbances. Administer and teach patient to self-administer antiemetics, antidiarrheals as needed and as ordered. Teach patient importance of nutritious diet, and suggest small, frequent, high-calorie, high-protein meals as appropriate. Assess baseline LFTs and monitor periodically during treatment. Discuss abnormalities and drug interruption with physician. Assess whether taking other hepatotoxic drugs (see Special Considerations section). Assess for increased fatigue, jaundice, dark urine, pale stools (signs of hepatotoxicity), and discuss drug discontinuance immediately with physician.

II.   ALTERATION IN SKIN INTEGRITY related to ALLERGIC REACTION

Defining Characteristics: Rash, dermatitis, purpura, urticaria occur; rarely, anaphylaxis may occur.

Nursing Implications: Assess baseline skin condition and integrity. Instruct patient to report itch, rash, and other skin changes. Teach patient skin care and symptomatic measures. If rash or dermatitis progresses, discuss drug discontinuance with physician. Assess for signs/symptoms of anaphylaxis.

Drug: ketoconazole (Nizoral)

Class: Azole; antifungal (systemic).

Mechanism of Action: Fungistatic by damaging fungal cell membrane and increasing permeability, altering cell metabolism, and inhibiting cell growth. Fungicidal in high concentrations.

Metabolism: Rapidly absorbed from GI tract in acid environment. Decreased absorption in patients with gastric hypochlorhydria (25% of all AIDS patients) or in patients taking medications that raise pH (antacids, H_2 antagonists). Distributed widely but cerebrospinal penetration is unpredictable. Drug is ~90% protein-bound. Partially metabolized in liver and mostly excreted in the feces via bile.

Indication: For treatment of mucocutaneous candidiasis, histoplasmosis, coccidioidomycosis, and blastomycosis.

Dosage/Range:
- Oral: 200 mg/day × 7–14 days (candidiasis); longer for other infections (400 mg/day in severe infections).

Drug Preparation:
- Store in tightly closed container at < 40°C (104°F).

Drug Administration:
- Orally in single dose.
- May take with meals to decrease GI side effects (unclear if food increases absorption).
- In patients with gastric achlorhydria, patient may be instructed to dissolve ketoconazole in 4-mL aqueous solution of 0.2 N hydrochloric acid and drink through a straw; follow with 4 oz (120 mL) water.

Drug Interactions:
- Drugs that increase gastric pH: antacids, cimetidine, ranitidine, famotidine, sucralfate decrease ketoconazole absorption; give these drugs at least 2 hours after ketoconazole.
- Other hepatotoxic drugs: use cautiously and monitor liver function studies closely.
- Rifampin or rifampin plus isoniazid: decreased ketoconazole levels especially if isoniazid is taken as well. Increase ketoconazole dose.
- Acyclovir: synergism and increased antiviral action against herpes simplex virus.
- Norfloxacin: theoretically increases antifungal action of ketoconazole but studies are inconsistent.
- Coumarin anticoagulants: increased PT; monitor patient closely and decrease anticoagulant dose accordingly.
- Cyclosporine: increased cyclosporine serum level; monitor serum level and decrease cyclosporine dose accordingly.
- Phenytoin: may have altered serum levels of phenytoin or ketoconazole; monitor serum levels of each and adjust dosages accordingly.
- Theophylline: may decrease theophylline serum concentrations; monitor serum levels and increase dosage accordingly.
- Corticosteroids: may increase corticosteroid serum level; may need to decrease dosage.

COMPLICATIONS

Lab Effects/Interference:
Major clinical significance:
- ALT, alk phos, AST, serum bili values may be elevated.
- ACTH-induced serum corticosteroid concentrations and serum testosterone concentrations may be decreased by doses of 800 mg/day of ketoconazole; serum testosterone concentrations are abolished by values of 1.6 g/day of ketoconazole but return to baseline values when ketoconazole is discontinued.

Special Considerations:
- Monitor liver function studies.
- High failure rate in HIV-infected patients due to achlorhydria.

Potential Toxicities/Side Effects and the Nursing Process

I.   ALTERATION IN NUTRITION, LESS THAN BODY REQUIREMENTS, related to GI SIDE EFFECTS

Defining Characteristics: Nausea, vomiting is seen in 3–10% of patients. Diarrhea, abdominal pain, flatulence, constipation may occur less frequently. Increased LFTs may occur: AST, ALT, alk phos. Hepatotoxicity is less common, is usually reversible, and is rarely fatal.

Nursing Implications: Assess baseline nutritional and elimination status. Instruct patient to report GI disturbances. Administer and teach patient to self-administer antiemetics, antidiarrheals as needed and as ordered. Teach patient importance of nutritious diet, and suggest small, frequent, high-calorie, high-protein meals as appropriate. Assess baseline LFTs and monitor periodically during treatment. Discuss abnormalities and drug interruption with physician. Assess whether taking other hepatotoxic drugs (see Special Considerations section). Assess for increased fatigue, jaundice, dark urine, pale stools (signs of hepatotoxicity), and discuss drug discontinuance immediately with physician.

II.   ALTERATION IN COMFORT related to GYNECOMASTIA AND BREAST TENDERNESS

Defining Characteristics: Breast enlargement and tenderness may occur in some men, lasting weeks to duration of therapy.

Nursing Implications: Assess for occurrence in male patients. Assess comfort level, degree of tenderness, and self-care measures used to increase comfort. Assess impact on body image.

III.   ALTERATION IN SKIN INTEGRITY related to ALLERGIC REACTION

Defining Characteristics: Rash, dermatitis, purpura, urticaria occur in 1% of patients; rarely, anaphylaxis may occur.

Nursing Implications: Assess baseline skin condition and integrity. Teach patient to report itch, rash, and other skin changes. Teach patient skin care and symptomatic measures. If rash or dermatitis progresses, discuss drug discontinuance with physician. Assess for signs/symptoms of anaphylaxis.

IV. ALTERATIONS IN SENSORY/PERCEPTUAL PATTERNS related to CNS EFFECTS

Defining Characteristics: Dizziness, headache, nervousness, insomnia, lethargy, somnolence, and paresthesia have occurred in ~1% of patients.

Nursing Implications: Assess baseline neurologic function and comfort and monitor during treatment. Instruct patient to report any changes. Discuss any abnormalities with physician.

Drug: micafungin sodium (Mycamine)

Class: Antifungal.

Mechanism of Action: Fungistatic by damaging fungal cell membrane, increasing permeability, altering cell metabolism, and inhibiting cell growth. Inhibits the synthesis of 1,3-β-D-glucan, an integral component of the fungal cell wall.

Metabolism: Metabolized by liver and excreted in urine.

Indication: For treatment of fungal infections in cancer patients; it is fungicidal at high concentrations.

Dosage/Range:
- Esophageal candidiasis: 150 mg/day × 15 days.
- Prophylaxis of candida infections in HSCT recipients 50 mg/day × 19 days.

Drug Preparation:
- Do not mix or co-infuse with other medications. Mycafungin has been shown to precipitate when mixed directly with a number of other commonly used medications.
- No dose adjustment is required with concomitant use of mycophenolate mofetil, cyclosporine, tacrolimus, prednisolone, sirolimus, nifedipine, fluconazole, ritonavir, or rifampin.
- A loading dose is not required; typically, 85% of the steady state is achieved after three daily doses.
- IV: Dilute in 0.9% sodium chloride, USP (without a bacteriostatic agent) or 5% dextrose injection, USP.
- Infuse over 1 hour. Stable × 24 hours at room temperature.

Drug Interactions:
- Coumarin anticoagulants: increased PT. Monitor patient closely and decrease anticoagulant dose accordingly.
- Norfloxacin: may increase antifungal action.

COMPLICATIONS

- Cyclosporine: increased cyclosporine serum level. Monitor serum level and decrease cyclosporine dose accordingly.

Lab Effects/Interference:
Major clinical significance:
- ALT, alk phos, AST, serum bili values may be elevated.

Special Considerations:
- Used in treatment of fungal infections.
- Monitor HCT, Hgb, serum electrolytes, and lipids, as changes may occur during treatment.

Potential Toxicities/Side Effects and the Nursing Process

I.   POTENTIAL FOR INJURY related to ANAPHYLAXIS

Defining Characteristics: Anaphylaxis with tachycardia, arrhythmias, and cardiac arrest may occur.

Nursing Implications: Assess baseline VS and monitor throughout infusion. Instruct patient to report signs/symptoms immediately. Assess for signs/symptoms: nausea, generalized itching, crampy abdominal pain, chest tightness, anxiety, agitation, sense of impending doom, wheezing, and dizziness.

II.   ALTERATION IN COMFORT related to PRURITUS, PHLEBITIS, SKIN ERUPTIONS, FEVER

Defining Characteristics: Phlebitis, pruritus with or without rash may occur.

Nursing Implications: Assess temperature, skin integrity, and comfort prior to drug administration, and monitor throughout treatment. Discuss with physician use of diphenhydramine to decrease itching. Change IV sites q 48 h to decrease phlebitis, or discuss with patient and physician use of central line. If rash and pruritus worsen, discuss with physician drug discontinuance.

III.   ALTERATION IN NUTRITION, LESS THAN BODY REQUIREMENTS, related to GI SIDE EFFECTS

Defining Characteristics: Nausea, vomiting, diarrhea, and anorexia may occur.

Nursing Implications: Assess baseline nutritional and elimination status. Instruct patient to report GI disturbances. Administer and teach patient to self-administer antiemetics, antidiarrheals as needed and as ordered. Teach patient importance of nutritious diet, and suggest small, frequent, high-calorie, high-protein meals as appropriate.

IV. ALTERATIONS IN SENSORY/PERCEPTUAL PATTERNS related to CNS, ENDOCRINE EFFECTS

Defining Characteristics: Dizziness, headache, and somnolence may occur.

Nursing Implications: Assess baseline neurologic function and comfort and monitor during treatment. Instruct patient to report any changes. Discuss any abnormalities with physician.

Drug: miconazole nitrate (Monistat)

Class: Azole; antifungal (systemic).

Mechanism of Action: Fungistatic by damaging fungal cell membrane and increasing permeability, altering cell metabolism, and inhibiting cell growth.

Metabolism: Limited (50%) oral absorption so usually given parenterally; 91–93% protein-bound to plasma proteins. Unpredictable penetration into CSF, so must be given intrathecally to achieve therapeutic levels. Metabolized by liver and excreted in urine.

Indication: For treatment of fungal infections in cancer patients. It is fungicidal at high concentrations. Active against most fungi, especially candidiasis, coccidioidomycosis, cryptococcosis.

Dosage/Range:
IV:
- Coccidioidomycosis: 1.8–3.6 g/day × 3–20+ weeks.
- Cryptococcosis: 1.2–2.4 g/day × 3–12+ weeks.
- Candidiasis: 600 mg–1.8 g/day × 1–20+ weeks.
- Intrathecal: refer to protocol; usually 20 mg q 1–2 days, or q 3–7 days if given by lumbar puncture.
- Intravesical: 200 mg in dilute solution 2–4 × day or by continuous bladder irrigation.

Drug Preparation:
- IV: dilute in 200 mL of 0.9% sodium chloride (preferred) or 5% dextrose injection and infuse over 30–60 min; daily dosage usually given in three divided doses q 8 h. Stable × 24 hours at room temperature.
- Intrathecal: is administered undiluted.
- Intravesical: as above (dosage) in conjunction with IV drug as well.

Drug Interactions:
- Coumarin anticoagulants: increased PT. Monitor patient closely and decrease anticoagulant dose accordingly.
- Norfloxacin: may increase antifungal action.
- Oral sulfonylureas: increased hypoglycemia effect. Monitor blood glucose and decrease dose of oral sulfonylurea.

COMPLICATIONS

- Rifampin or rifampin plus isoniazid: decreased miconazole levels, especially if isoniazid taken as well. Increase miconazole dose.
- Phenytoin: may have altered serum levels of phenytoin or miconazole. Monitor serum levels of each and adjust dosages accordingly.
- Cyclosporine: increased cyclosporine serum level. Monitor serum level and decrease cyclosporine dose accordingly.

Lab Effects/Interference:

Major clinical significance:

- ALT, alk phos, AST, serum bili values may be elevated.

Clinical significance:

- Serum lipid profile: hyperlipidemia has occurred in patients receiving IV miconazole; this is reportedly due to the vehicle in the miconazole solution, PEG 40 castor oil (Cremophor EL).

Special Considerations:

- Used in treatment of severe fungal infections.
- Initial dose should be in hospital with resuscitation equipment available to determine hypersensitivity (cardiac arrest has occurred with initial dose). Drug is suspended in castor oil base, which stimulates allergic reaction. Subsequent dosing can be safely given to selected patients in ambulatory settings.
- IV push injection of drug may cause arrhythmias, so drug must be diluted (200+ mL) and administered over 30–60 minutes.
- Monitor HCT, Hgb, serum electrolytes, and lipids, as changes may occur during treatment.

Potential Toxicities/Side Effects and the Nursing Process

I.   POTENTIAL FOR INJURY related to ANAPHYLAXIS

Defining Characteristics: Anaphylaxis with tachycardia, arrhythmias, and cardiac arrest may occur on first IV dose, probably related to suspension medium of drug (castor oil).

Nursing Implications: Ensure first dose is given in inpatient setting with resuscitation equipment and physician available. Assess baseline VS and monitor throughout infusion. Instruct patient to report signs/symptoms immediately. Assess for signs/symptoms: nausea, generalized itching, crampy abdominal pain, chest tightness, anxiety, agitation, sense of impending doom, wheezing, and dizziness.

II.   ALTERATION IN COMFORT related to PRURITUS, PHLEBITIS, SKIN ERUPTIONS, FEVER

Defining Characteristics: Phlebitis, pruritus with or without rash may occur.

Nursing Implications: Assess temperature, skin integrity, and comfort prior to drug administration and monitor throughout treatment. Discuss with physician use of diphenhydramine to decrease itching. Change IV sites q 48 h to decrease phlebitis, or discuss with patient and physician use of central line. If rash and pruritus worsen, discuss with physician drug discontinuance.

III. ALTERATION IN NUTRITION, LESS THAN BODY REQUIREMENTS, related to GI SIDE EFFECTS

Defining Characteristics: Nausea, vomiting, diarrhea, anorexia, and bitter taste may occur.

Nursing Implications: Assess baseline nutritional and elimination status. Instruct patient to report GI disturbances. Administer and teach patient to self-administer antiemetics, antidiarrheals as needed and as ordered. Teach patient importance of nutritious diet and suggest small, frequent, high-calorie, high-protein meals as appropriate.

IV. ALTERATIONS IN SENSORY/PERCEPTUAL PATTERNS related to CNS, ENDOCRINE EFFECTS

Defining Characteristics: Dizziness, flushing, anxiety, increased libido, blurred vision, eye dryness, headache may occur.

Nursing Implications: Assess baseline neurologic function and comfort and monitor during treatment. Instruct patient to report any changes. Discuss any abnormalities with physician.

Drug: nystatin (Mycostatin, Nilstat)

Class: Antifungal.

Mechanism of Action: Binds to sterol molecule in fungi cell membrane, increasing permeability so that potassium and other intracellular ions are lost.

Metabolism: Drug is not absorbed from intact skin, mucous membranes, and is poorly absorbed from GI tract. Excreted as unchanged drug in feces.

Indication: Active against yeast and fungi, especially *Candida*.

Dosage/Range:
- Oral (for treatment of oral or intestinal candidiasis): 500,000–1 million U tid; continue therapy for 48 hours after clinical remission to prevent recurrence.
- Powder: topical for *Candida* rash infections.
- Vaginal: 100,000 U as vaginal tablet, inserted into vagina daily or bid × 14 days.

Drug Preparation:
- Oral suspension and tablets should be stored in tight, light-resistant containers < 40°C (104°F).

COMPLICATIONS

Drug Administration:
• Oral suspension. Instruct patient to:
  • Rinse mouth with oral hygiene solution to clean food debris.
  • Hold suspension in mouth and swish for 1–2 minutes, then swallow or spit solution.
  • Do not rinse mouth or eat for 15–30 minutes

Drug Interactions:
• None.

Lab Effects/Interference:
• None known.

Special Considerations:
• For patients with oral thrush who have difficulty taking oral suspension:
  • Oral suspension can be frozen in medicine cups so it is easier to administer if the patient has stomatitis.
  • Vaginal suppository may be sucked, as this increases mucosal contact with drug.
  • Cannot be used to treat systemic infections.
  • Adverse effects are infrequent.

Potential Toxicities/Side Effects and the Nursing Process

I.   ALTERATION IN NUTRITION, LESS THAN BODY REQUIREMENTS, related to GI SIDE EFFECTS

Defining Characteristics: High oral doses may cause nausea, vomiting, diarrhea.

Nursing Implications: Assess baseline nutritional status. Instruct patient to report GI disturbances. Administer and teach patient to self-administer antiemetics, antidiarrheals as needed and as ordered. Teach patient importance of nutritious diet and suggest small, frequent, high-calorie, high-protein meals as appropriate.

II.   KNOWLEDGE DEFICIT related to SELF-ADMINISTRATION OF MEDICATION

Defining Characteristics: Increased compliance when patient is instructed in self-care activities.

Nursing Implications: Assess knowledge about infection and planned treatment. Teach about drug action, potential side effects, and when and how to take drug. Instruct patient to rinse mouth with saline gargle (or other rinse) to remove food debris prior to taking nystatin suspension; solution should be swished in mouth 1–2 minutes, then swallowed or spit out. Patient should not eat or rinse mouth for 15–30 minutes.

Drug: posaconazole (Noxafil)

Class: Triazole; antifungal (systemic).

Mechanism of Action: Fungistatic; inhibits fungi by blocking ergosterol synthesis through inhibition of the enzyme lanosterol 14 alpha-demethylase (CYP51). Ergosterol depletion coupled with accumulation of methylated sterol precursors results in inhibition of fungal cell growth, fungal death by damaging fungal cell membrane and increasing permeability, altering cell metabolism, and inhibiting cell growth. Fungicidal at high concentrations.

Metabolism: Absorbed from GI tract when administered as an oral suspension. Partially metabolized in liver and mostly excreted in the feces via bile.

Indication: Active against invasive *Candida* species, *Aspergillus* species, non-*Aspergillus* hyalohypho-mycetes, phaeohyphomycetes, zygomycetes, and endemic fungi.

Dosage/Range:
- Oral: 200 mg q 6 hours for 7 days (loading dose) and then 400 mg q 12 hours daily (maintenance therapy) dose may be increased if there is an inadequate response to infections.

Drug Preparation:
- Drug is given orally.

Drug Administration:
- Orally. May take 1 hour before meals or 1 hour after meals.
- Absorption enhanced by coadministration with food and nutritional supplements.

Drug Interactions:
- Drugs that increase gastric pH: antacids, cimetidine, ranitidine, and sucralfate have minor or no significant effect on posaconazole.
- Hepatotoxic drugs: use cautiously, and monitor liver function studies closely.
- Coumarin anticoagulants: increases PT; monitor patient closely and decrease anticoagulant dose accordingly.
- Potential interactions could occur with concomitant use of posaconazole and cisapride, astemizole, terfenadine, quinidine, pimozide, bepridil, sertindole, dofetilide, and halofantrine.
- Well-tolerated in pediatric and elderly patients.

Lab Effects/Interference:
Major clinical significance:
- ALT, alk phos, AST, serum bili values may be elevated.

Special Considerations:
- Monitor liver function studies.

Potential Toxicities/Side Effects and the Nursing Process

I.   ALTERATION IN NUTRITION, LESS THAN BODY REQUIREMENTS, related to GI SIDE EFFECTS

Defining Characteristics: Nausea, vomiting is seen in 18% of patients. Diarrhea, abdominal pain, flatulence, constipation may occur less frequently. Increased LFTs may occur: AST, ALT, alk phos. Hepatotoxicity is less common, is usually reversible, and is rarely fatal.

Nursing Implications: Assess baseline nutritional and elimination status. Instruct patient to report GI disturbances. Administer and teach patient to self-administer antiemetics, antidiarrheals as needed and as ordered. Teach patient importance of nutritious diet and suggest small, frequent, high-calorie, high-protein meals as appropriate. Assess baseline LFTs and monitor periodically during treatment. Discuss abnormalities and drug interruption with physician. Assess whether taking other hepatotoxic drugs (see Special Considerations section). Assess for increased fatigue, jaundice, dark urine, pale stools (signs of hepatotoxicity), and discuss drug discontinuance immediately with physician.

II.   ALTERATION IN SENSORY/PERCEPTUAL PATTERNS related to HEADACHE

Defining Characteristics: Treatment-related disturbances are common (17%). Generally mild and rarely result in discontinuing treatment.

Nursing Implications: Assess for occurrence. Assess comfort level. Educate patient about this side effect. Assess impact on body image.

III.   ALTERATION IN COMFORT related to PRURITUS, DRY SKIN, AND FLUSHING

Defining Characteristics: Rash, dry skin, and flushing.

Nursing Implications: Assess temperature, skin integrity, and comfort before drug administration and monitor throughout course of treatment. Discuss with physician use of diphenhydramine to decrease itching and cream or lotions to smooth skin and maintain skin integrity. If rash and skin condition worsens, discuss with physician drug discontinuance.

Drug: voriconazole (VFEND)

Class: Triazole; antifungal (systemic).

Mechanism of Action: Fungistatic by damaging fungal cell membrane and increasing permeability, altering cell metabolism, and inhibiting cell growth.

Metabolism: Rapidly absorbed from GI tract in acid environment. Partially metabolized in liver and mostly excreted in the feces via bile.

Indication: For treatment of fungal infections in cancer patients. It is fungicidal at high concentrations. Active against invasive *Aspergillus fumigatus, Fusarium* spp. infection, and *Scedosporium apiospermum* infection.

Dosage/Range:
- Oral: 200 mg q 12 hours for 7–14 days; dose may be increased if there is an inadequate response to infections (300 mg q 12 hours).
- IV preparation is available. The final voriconazole preparation must be infused over 1–2 hours at a maximum rate of 3 mg/kg per hour.

Drug Preparation:
- Once reconstituted, drug should be used immediately, or it can be stored for no longer than 24 hours at 2–8°C (37–46°F).

Drug Administration:
- Orally. May take 1 hour before meals or 1 hour after meals.
- The final voriconazole preparation must be infused over 1–2 hours at a maximum rate of 3 mg/kg per hour.

Drug Interactions:
- Drugs that increase gastric pH: antacids, cimetidine, ranitidine have minor or no significant effect on voriconazole.
- Hepatotoxic drugs: use cautiously, and monitor liver function studies closely.
- Rifampin decreases the steady state of voriconazole.
- Coumarin anticoagulants: increases PT; monitor patient closely and decrease anticoagulant dose accordingly.
- Cyclosporine: increases cyclosporine serum level; monitor serum level and decrease cyclosporine dose accordingly.
- Phenytoin: may have altered serum levels of phenytoin or ketoconazole; monitor serum levels of each and adjust dosages accordingly.
- Carbamazepine and long-acting barbiturates and macrolide antibiotics reduce the efficacy of voriconazole.

Lab Effects/Interference:
Major clinical significance:
- ALT, alk phos, AST, serum bili values may be elevated.

Special Considerations:
- Monitor liver function studies.

Potential Toxicities/Side Effects and the Nursing Process

I.   ALTERATION IN NUTRITION, LESS THAN BODY REQUIREMENTS, related to GI SIDE EFFECTS

Defining Characteristics: Nausea, vomiting is seen in 3–10% of patients. Diarrhea, abdominal pain, flatulence, constipation may occur less frequently. Increased LFTs may occur: AST, ALT, alk phos. Hepatotoxicity is less common, is usually reversible, and is rarely fatal.

COMPLICATIONS

Nursing Implications: Assess baseline nutritional and elimination status. Instruct patient to report GI disturbances. Administer and teach patient to self-administer antiemetics, antidiarrheals as needed and as ordered. Teach patient importance of nutritious diet, and suggest small, frequent, high-calorie, high-protein meals as appropriate. Assess baseline LFTs and monitor periodically during treatment. Discuss abnormalities and drug interruption with physician. Assess whether taking other hepatotoxic drugs (see Special Considerations section). Assess for increased fatigue, jaundice, dark urine, pale stools (signs of hepatotoxicity), and discuss drug discontinuance immediately with physician.

II.   ALTERATION IN SENSORY/PERCEPTUAL PATTERNS related to VISUAL DISTURBANCES

Defining Characteristics: Treatment-related visual disturbances are common (30%). Generally mild and rarely result in discontinuing treatment.

Nursing Implications: Assess for occurrence. Assess comfort level. Educate patient about this side effect. Assess impact on body image.

III.   ALTERATION IN SKIN INTEGRITY related to ALLERGIC REACTION

Defining Characteristics: Rash, dermatitis, purpura, urticaria occur in 6% of patients.

Nursing Implications: Assess baseline skin condition and integrity. Teach patient to report itch, rash, and other skin changes. Teach patient skin care and symptomatic measures. If rash or dermatitis progresses, discuss drug discontinuance with physician. Assess for signs/symptoms of anaphylaxis.

ANTIVIRALS

Drug: acyclovir (Zovirax)

Class: Antiviral (systemic).

Mechanism of Action: Interferes with DNA synthesis so that viral replication cannot occur.

Metabolism: Variable GI absorption; unaffected by food. Widely distributed in body tissue and fluids, including CSF. Variable protein-binding (9–33%). Crosses placenta and is excreted in breastmilk.

Indication: Active against herpes simplex virus (HSV-1, HSV-2), varicella-zoster virus (VZV) (shingles), Epstein-Barr virus (EBV), and cytomegalovirus (CMV).

Dosage/Range:
Adult:
- Oral: 200 mg PO q 4 h (genital herpes) to 800 mg PO 5 ×/day (acute herpes zoster).
- IV (initial/recurrent infections in immunocompromised patients): 5–10 mg/kg q 8 h × 7 days; 5 mg/kg q 8 h × 7–14 days (herpes simplex); 10 mg/kg q 8 h × 7–14 days (herpes zoster, herpes encephalitis).
- Use ideal body weight for dose calculation.
- Avoid doses greater than 1,000 mg/dose.
- Dose modification is required if renal dysfunction is present.

Drug Preparation:
- Oral: store in tight, light-resistant containers at 15–25°C (59–77°F).
- IV: reconstitute with sterile water for injection per manufacturer's directions and further dilute in 50–100 mL IV fluid; a final concentration of 7 mg/mL or less is recommended to minimize the incidence of phlebitis; infuse over 1 hour.

Drug Interactions:
- Zidovudine: potentiates antiretroviral activity of zidovudine but may cause increased neurotoxicity (drowsiness, lethargy) in AIDS patients. Monitor for increased neurotoxicity.
- Probenecid: may increase plasma half-life. Monitor for increased acyclovir toxicity.
- Antifungals: potential antiviral synergy.
- Interferon: potential synergistic antiviral effect, potential increased neurotoxicity. Use together with caution.
- Methotrexate (intrathecal): possible increased neurotoxicity. Use together with caution.

Lab Effects/Interference:
Major clinical significance:
- BUN and serum creatinine concentrations required prior to and during therapy, since IV acyclovir may be nephrotoxic; if acyclovir is given by rapid IV injection or its urine solubility is exceeded, precipitation of acyclovir crystals may occur in renal tubules; renal tubular damage may occur and may progress to acute renal failure.

Clinical significance:
- Pap test: although clear association has not been shown to date, patients with genital herpes may be at increased risk of developing cervical cancer. Pap test should be done at least once a year to detect early cervical changes.

Special Considerations:
- Use cautiously in patients with preexisting renal dysfunction or dehydration; underlying neurologic dysfunction or neurologic reactions to cytotoxic drugs, intrathecal methotrexate, or interferon and in patients with hepatic dysfunction.
- It is imperative that patients be well hydrated, with adequate urine output prior to and for up to 2 hours after IV dosing.
- Administer with caution if patient is receiving other nephrotoxic drugs.
- Contraindicated in patients hypersensitive to drug.
- Minimal injury to normal cells, so few adverse effects exist.

COMPLICATIONS

Potential Toxicities/Side Effects and the Nursing Process

I.   ALTERATION IN URINARY ELIMINATION related to RENAL TOXICITY

Defining Characteristics: Transient increase is seen in renal function tests (serum BUN, creatinine) and decreased urine creatinine clearance, as drug may precipitate in renal tubules during dehydration or rapid IV drug administration. Increased risk exists if pre-existing renal disease or concurrent administration of nephrotoxic drugs.

Nursing Implications: Assess baseline renal function and monitor periodically during therapy. Notify physician of any abnormalities before administering next dose. Ensure adequate hydration and urine output prior to and for 2 hours after IV drug administration. Administer IV drug slowly over 1 hour.

II.   ALTERATIONS IN SENSORY/PERCEPTUAL PATTERNS related to ENCEPHALOPATHY

Defining Characteristics: IV administration: encephalopathy (lethargy, tremors, confusion, agitation, seizures, dizziness) may occur rarely. Oral: headache occurs in 13% of patients receiving chronic suppressive treatment.

Nursing Implications: Assess baseline neurologic function and comfort, and monitor during treatment. Instruct patient to report any changes. Discuss any abnormalities with physician.

III.   ALTERATIONS IN COMFORT related to LOCAL VEIN IRRITATION (IV ADMINISTRATION)

Defining Characteristics: Erythema, irritation, pain, swelling, phlebitis may occur at injection site.

Nursing Implications: Assess IV site for patency, irritation prior to each dose. Change IV site at least q 48 h. Apply warmth/heat to painful area as needed.

IV.   ALTERATION IN NUTRITION, LESS THAN BODY REQUIREMENTS, related to GI SIDE EFFECTS (ORAL DOSAGE)

Defining Characteristics: Nausea, vomiting, and diarrhea occur in 2–5% of patients receiving chronic therapy.

Nursing Implications: Assess history of nausea/vomiting, diarrhea, and instruct patient to report any occurrence. Teach patient self-medication of prescribed antinausea or antidiarrheal medicines. Discuss drug discontinuance with physician if symptoms are severe.

V.   ALTERATION IN SKIN INTEGRITY related to RASH

Defining Characteristics: Rash, urticaria, pruritus may occur.

Nursing Implications: Assess baseline history of drug allergy and skin integrity. Instruct patient to report any occurrence of rash, pruritus. Teach symptomatic management measures unless severe; if severe, discuss drug discontinuance with physician.

VI.   KNOWLEDGE DEFICIT related to (ORAL) DRUG ADMINISTRATION

Defining Characteristics: Patient may not realize drug does not cure viral infection; nor does it prevent spread of virus to others. Prodrome of tingling, itching, or pain can herald mucocutaneous herpes.

Nursing Implications: Teach patient about herpetic infection and goal of therapy to suppress infection. When used to treat recurrent episodes of chronic infection, teach patient to recognize prodromal symptoms and to take prescribed drug then or within 2 days of onset of lesions. Teach patient about routes of viral spread and instruct to avoid contacts with others that may lead to viral spread.

Drug: cidofovir (Vistide)

Class: Antiviral (systemic).

Mechanism of Action: Suppresses CMV replication by selective inhibition of viral DNA synthesis.

Metabolism: Less than 6% bound to plasma proteins. Renal clearance is reduced with the concomitant administration of probenecid.

Indication: For treatment of viral infections in cancer patients.

Dosage/Range:
- Weekly induction regimen: 5 mg/kg infused every week × 2 weeks.
- Twice-monthly maintenance regimen: 5 mg/kg infused every other week.

Drug Preparation:
- Requires chemotherapy safety handling (drug is mutagenic, tumorigenic, embryotoxic).
- Reconstitute drug (single use, nonpreserved); vial contains 75 mg/mL.
- Further dilute in 100 mL 0.9% sodium chloride.

Drug Administration:
- Administer 2 g probenecid (four 500-mg tabs) 3 hours prior to drug infusion.
- Infuse 1 L of 0.9% sodium chloride over 1–2 hours immediately prior to drug infusion.
- Infuse IV drug over 1 hour.
- As ordered by physician, may administer second liter of 0.9% sodium chloride at the start of the drug infusion and continue for 1–3 hours.
- Two hours after end of drug infusion, administer 1 g probenecid (two 500-mg tabs).

- Eight hours after end of the drug infusion, administer 1 g probenecid (two 500-mg tabs).

Drug Interactions:
- Probenecid: interacts with the metabolism or renal tubular excretion of acetaminophen, acyclovir, angiotensin-converting enzyme (ACE) inhibitors, barbiturates, NSAIDs, theophylline, zidovudine.
- Increased nephrotoxicity when combined with other nephrotoxic drugs.

Lab Effects/Interference:
- Serum creatinine levels may be elevated.

Special Considerations:
- Indicated for the treatment of AIDS patients who have newly diagnosed or relapsed CMV retinitis.
- Dose-limiting toxicity is nephrotoxicity evidenced by proteinuria and increased serum creatinine.
- Treatment requires prehydration and posthydration use of concomitant probenecid.
- Drug contraindicated in patients with baseline serum creatinine > 1.5 mg/dL, creatinine clearance ≤ 55 mL/min, proteinuria ≥ 3+, past severe hypersensitivity to probenecid or other sulfa-containing medications, hypersensitivity to cidofovir, and patients who are pregnant or breastfeeding.

DOSE REDUCTIONS:
(a) Patients with baseline normal renal function:

Renal Abnormality	Cidofovir Dosage
Serum creatinine 0.3–0.4 mg/dL > baseline	3 mg/kg
Serum creatinine = 0.5 mg/dL above baseline	discontinue cidofovir
Proteinuria ≥ 3+	discontinue cidofovir

(b) Patients with baseline renal impairment:

Creatinine Clearance (mL/min)	Induction (once a week × 2 weeks)	Maintenance (once every 2 weeks)
41–55	2.0 mg/kg	2.0 mg/kg
30–40	1.5 mg/kg	1.1 mg/kg
20–29	1.0 mg/kg	1.0 mg/kg
≤ 19	0.5 mg/kg	0.1 mg/kg

- Patient teaching:
    - Encourage increased oral intake of fluids to 1–3 L as tolerated.
    - Return to clinic for appointments (induction: weekly × 2 weeks, maintenance every other week).

- Report side effects immediately.
- Ophthalmologic appointments as scheduled for intraocular pressure (IOP), visual acuity monitoring.

Potential Toxicities/Side Effects and the Nursing Process

I.   POTENTIAL FOR INJURY related to NEUTROPENIA

Defining Characteristics: Neutropenia (< 750/mm^2) may occur in 28% of patients, and < 500/mm^3 occurred in 20% of patients. Infections occurred in 25% of patients.

Nursing Implications: Monitor WBC and ANC prior to each drug dose, and hold treatment if neutropenic. Discuss with physician use of G-CSF. If the patient is receiving zidovudine, the zidovudine should be temporarily discontinued or dose decreased by 50% on days of probenecid therapy. Instruct patient to monitor temperature and to report fever > 101°F immediately. Discuss use of G-CSF with physician as needed (up to 34% required G-CSF in clinical trials).

II.   ALTERATION IN NUTRITION, LESS THAN BODY REQUIREMENTS, related to NAUSEA/VOMITING

Defining Characteristics: Nausea/vomiting occurs in about 65% of patients

Nursing Implications: Encourage patients to eat food prior to each dose of probenecid. Discuss antiemetic prior to the first dose of probenecid and then during period of probenecid therapy.

III.   ALTERATION IN COMFORT related to FEVER, CHILLS, RASH, HEADACHE FROM PROBENECID

Defining Characteristics: Fever occurs in up to 57% of patients, rash in 30%, headache in 27%, chills in 24%. Asthenia (46% incidence), diarrhea (27%), alopecia (25%), anorexia (22%), dyspnea (22%), abdominal pain (17%), and anemia (20%). In clinical trials, 25% of patients withdrew from treatment due to adverse events.

Nursing Implications: Assess baseline comfort, and instruct patient to report symptoms. Discuss symptom management with physician, such as antihistamine and/or antipyretic (acetaminophen) for fever, and then use prophylactically in subsequent doses.

IV.   ALTERATION IN ELIMINATION related to RENAL TOXICITY

Defining Characteristics: Creatinine elevations to > 1.5 mg/dL occur in approximately 17% of patients, proteinuria in 80% of patients, and decreased serum bicarbonate in > 5% of patients.

COMPLICATIONS

Nursing Implications: Encourage patients to increase their daily oral fluid intake to 2–3 L. Closely monitor renal function; patients who have received foscarnet are at increased risk for nephrotoxicity. Ensure that patient receives prehydration and posthydration, and is able to take oral fluids. Discuss dose reductions based on alterations in renal function with physician. Check urine for protein. If positive, discuss additional hydration and rechecking of urine for blood with physician.

V.   ALTERATIONS IN SENSORY/PERCEPTUAL PATTERNS related to OCULAR HYPOTONY

Defining Characteristics: OCULAR HYPOTONY occurs rarely, may be increased risk for patients with concomitant diabetes mellitus.

Nursing Implications: Patients should see ophthalmologist for IOP assessments and visual acuity periodically.

VI.   METABOLIC ACIDOSIS related to DECREASED SERUM BICARBONATE

Defining Characteristics: Occurs rarely (2%).

Nursing Implications: Assess for decreases in serum bicarbonate < 16 mEq/L associated with evidence of renal tubular damage (incidence 9%). Serious metabolic acidosis in association with liver failure, mucormycosis, aspergillus, and disseminated MAC has occurred, with subsequent death in one patient. Monitor baseline chemistries, and review results prior to each treatment.

Drug: famciclovir (Famvir)

Class: Antiviral (systemic).

Mechanism of Action: Rapidly transformed into antiviral penciclovir, which inhibits herpes simplex types HSV-1, HSV-2, or VZV by inhibiting HSV-2 polymerase. Herpes viral DNA synthesis and viral replication are selectively inhibited.

Metabolism: Oral bioavailability is 77%, with peak plasma levels 30–90 minutes after dosing. Plasma half-life is 2.3 hours. In the virus, the active form of the drug has a long intracellular half-life. Low protein binding and rapid and complete elimination in the urine (73%) and feces (27%).

Indication: For treatment of viral infections in cancer patients.

Dosage/Range:
- Herpes zoster: 500 mg q 8 h × 7 days.
- Genital herpes: 125 mg bid × 5 days.

Drug Preparation:
- Available in 125-, 250-, 500-mg tablets.

Drug Administration:
- Oral, without regard to meals.

Drug Interactions:
- None.

Lab Effects/Interference:
- None known.

Special Considerations:
- Treatment of herpes zoster: viral shedding stopped 50% faster than with placebo, with full crusting in < 1 week, and shorter time to relief from acute pain. In addition, drug significantly reduces the duration of postherpetic neuralgia by 2 months compared to placebo.
- Dose should be reduced in patients with renal impairment according to the table below:

Condition	Creatinine Clearance (cc/min)	Dose
Herpes zoster	40–59	500 mg q 12 h
	20–39	500 mg q 24 h
	< 20	250 mg q 48 h
Recurrent genital herpes	20–39	125 mg q 24 h
	< 20	125 mg q 48 h

Potential Toxicities/Side Effects and the Nursing Process

I.   ALTERATION IN COMFORT related to HEADACHE, NAUSEA

Defining Characteristics: Headache occurred in approximately 22% of patients. Nausea occurred in 12% of patients.

Nursing Implications: Teach patient that side effects may occur and are usually mild. Instruct patient to report headache that does not resolve with acetaminophen, or nausea that does not resolve with diet modification.

Drug: foscarnet sodium (Foscavir)

Class: Antiviral (systemic).

Mechanism of Action: Inhibits binding sites on virus-specific DNA polymerases and reverse transcriptases without affecting cellular DNA polymerases. Thus, prevents viral replication of all known herpes viruses: CMV, HSV-1, HSV-2, EBV, and VZV.

COMPLICATIONS

Metabolism: 14–17% bound to plasma proteins and excreted into urine 80–90% unchanged by kidneys. Variable penetration into CSF.

Indication: For treatment of CMV retinitis in AIDS patients. Foscarnet sodium is active against resistant herpes simplex viruses that are resistant via thymidine kinase deficiency.

Dosage/Range:
Adult (normal renal function):
- IV induction: 60 mg/kg IV over 1 hour q 8 h × 2–3 weeks.
- Maintenance: 90–120 mg/kg/day IV over 2 hours.
- Dose modification is necessary if renal insufficiency. See manufacturer's package insert.

Drug Preparation:
- Add drug solution (24 mg/mL) to 0.9% sodium chloride or 5% dextrose to achieve a final concentration = 12 mg/mL.

Drug Administration:
- Administer via rate controller or infusion pump over 1 hour (induction) or 2 hours (maintenance) via peripheral or central vein.
- Do not administer or give concurrently with other drugs or solutions.

Drug Interactions:
- Incompatible with D30W, amphotericin B, lactated Ringer's, total parenteral nutrition (TPN), acyclovir, ganciclovir, trimetrexate, pentamidine, vancomycin, trimethoprim/sulfamethoxazole, diazepam, digoxin, phenytoin, leucovorin, prochlorperazine.
- Pentamidine: potentially fatal HYPOCALCEMIA; seizures have occurred; AVOID CONCURRENT USE.
- Nephrotoxic drugs (amphotericin B, aminoglycosides): additive nephrotoxicity; AVOID CONCURRENT USE.
- Hypocalcemic agents: additive hypocalcemia; AVOID CONCURRENT USE.
- Zidovudine: increased anemia; monitor patient closely and transfuse with red blood cells as ordered.

Lab Effects/Alterations:
Major clinical significance:
- Serum calcium (ionized), serum calcium (total), and serum phosphate: concentrations of phosphate may be increased or decreased; concentrations of total calcium may be decreased; although the total calcium concentration may also appear normal, the level of ionized calcium may be decreased and result in symptomatic hypocalcemia.
- Serum creatinine concentrations may be increased.
- Serum Mg++ concentrations may be decreased.

Clinical significance:
- ALT, alk phos, AST, and serum bili values may be increased.
- Serum K+ concentrations may be decreased.

Special Considerations:
- Contraindicated in patients hypersensitive to foscarnet.
- DO NOT administer concomitantly with IV pentamidine.

- Avoid use during pregnancy; lactating women should interrupt breastfeeding while receiving the drug.
- Regular monitoring of renal function IMPERATIVE; dose modifications must be made if renal insufficiency exists.
- Use measures for safe handling of cytotoxic drugs (see *Appendix 1*).

Potential Toxicities/Side Effects and the Nursing Process

I. ALTERATION IN URINARY ELIMINATION related to RENAL TOXICITY

Defining Characteristics: Abnormal renal function occurs commonly; increased serum creatinine, decreased creatinine clearance, acute renal failure may occur.

Nursing Implications: Assess baseline elimination pattern and renal function studies, and monitor closely throughout treatment. Manufacturer suggests creatinine clearance be calculated biw–tiw (induction) and q 1–2 weeks (maintenance). Creatinine clearance can be calculated from modified Cockcroft and Gault equation:

$$\text{For male: } \frac{140-\text{age}}{\text{serum creatinine} \times 72}$$

$$\text{For female: } \frac{140-\text{age}}{\text{serum creatinine} \times 72} \times 0.085$$

Discuss dose modifications with physician if renal dysfunction occurs. Ensure adequate hydration and urinary output prior to and following dose; administer drug slowly over 1–2 hours, at no more than 1 mg/kg/min. Teach patient to increase oral fluids as tolerated to clear drug from kidneys.

II. ALTERATION IN ELECTROLYTE BALANCE related to METABOLIC ABNORMALITIES

Defining Characteristics: Hypocalcemia, hypophosphatemia, hyperphosphatemia, hypomagnesemia, and hypokalemia occur. Transient decreased ionized calcium may not appear in serum total calcium value. Tetany and seizures may occur, especially in patients receiving foscarnet and IV pentamidine. Increased risk exists if renal impairment or neurologic impairment.

Nursing Implications: Assess baseline calcium, phosphorus, magnesium, potassium, and concurrent drugs that might affect these values. Assess patient for signs/symptoms of hypocalcemia, such as perioral tingling, numbness, or paresthesias during or after infusion. Instruct patient to report these signs/symptoms immediately. If signs/symptoms occur, stop infusion, notify physician, and evaluate serum electrolyte, renal studies. Administer ordered electrolyte repletion.

COMPLICATIONS

III.   ALTERATIONS IN SENSORY/PERCEPTUAL PATTERNS related to NEUROLOGIC CHANGES

Defining Characteristics: Headache, paresthesia, dizziness, involuntary muscle contractions, hypoesthesia, neuropathy, and seizurcs (including grand mal) have occurred. Increased risk exists of hypocalcemia (ionized Ca++) and renal insufficiency.

Nursing Implications: Assess baseline risk factors and neurologic status, and monitor during treatment. Assess for and instruct patient to report signs/symptoms. Discuss abnormalities with physician, and possible drug discontinuance.

IV.   FATIGUE related to ANEMIA

Defining Characteristics: Anemia occurs in 33% of patients and in 60% of patients receiving concomitant zidovudine.

Nursing Implications: Assess baseline HCT/Hgb, activity tolerance, cardiopulmonary status, and monitor during therapy. Instruct patient to report increasing fatigue, headache, irritability, shortness of breath, chest pain. Transfuse RBCs as ordered by physician. Discuss with clinic patient self-care ability; refer for home health assistance as needed.

V.   ALTERATION IN NUTRITION, LESS THAN BODY REQUIREMENTS, related to GI SIDE EFFECTS

Defining Characteristics: Nausea, vomiting, diarrhea are common; anorexia, abdominal pain may also occur.

Nursing Implications: Assess baseline nutrition and liver function, and monitor during therapy. Instruct patient to report GI side effects. Administer or teach patient to self-administer prescribed antiemetic or antidiarrheal medications. Encourage adequate oral or IV hydration. Notify physician of abnormal LFTs. If anorexia occurs, encourage favorite foods and small, frequent meals as tolerated.

VI.   INFECTION related to NEUTROPENIA

Defining Characteristics: May occur in 17% of patients; increased risk when receiving concurrent zidovudine.

Nursing Implications: Assess baseline WBC, ANC, and temperature; monitor during therapy. Assess for signs/symptoms of infection and discuss these with physician. Instruct patient to report signs/symptoms of infection.

VII. ALTERATIONS IN COMFORT related to LOCAL VEIN IRRITATION (IV ADMINISTRATION)

Defining Characteristics: Erythema, irritation, pain, swelling, phlebitis may occur at injection site. Consider use of central line.

Nursing Implications: Assess IV site for patency, irritation prior to each dose. Change IV site at least q 48 h. Apply warmth/heat to painful area as needed.

VIII. ALTERATION IN SKIN INTEGRITY related to RASH

Defining Characteristics: Rash, sweating may occur. Also, rarely, local irritation and ulcerations of penile epithelium in males, and vulvo-vaginal mucosa in females has occurred—perhaps related to drug in urine.

Nursing Implications: Assess skin integrity baseline and during treatment. Instruct patient to report any irritation or lesions. Teach patient to perform frequent perineal hygiene.

Drug: ganciclovir (Cytovene)

Class: Antiviral (systemic).

Mechanism of Action: Interferes with DNA synthesis so that viral replication cannot occur.

Metabolism: Poorly absorbed from GI tract. Appears to be widely distributed, concentrates in kidneys, and is well distributed to the eyes. Crosses BBB. Drug crosses placenta and is excreted in breastmilk in animals. Excreted unchanged in urine.

Indication: Active against CMV infections, especially in the retina.

Dosage/Range:
Adult:
- IV induction: 5 mg/kg IV q 12 h × 14–21 days.
- Maintenance: 5 mg/kg IV 7 days/week or 6 mg/kg/day × 5 days/week.
- Intravitreous by ophthalmologist (investigational).
- DOSE MUST BE REDUCED IN RENAL IMPAIRMENT.

Drug Preparation:
- Drug is CARCINOGENIC and TERATOGENIC: use chemotherapy handling precautions (see *Appendix 1*) when preparing and administering ganciclovir.
- Administer only if ANC is > 500 cells/mm³ and platelet count > 25,000/mm³.
- Add 10 mL of sterile water for injection to 500-mg vial. Further dilute dose in 50–250 mL of IV fluid and infuse over at least 1 hour.

Drug Interactions:
- Zidovudine: increased hematologic toxicity (neutropenia, anemia); do not use together if possible.
- Consider didanosine (ddI) instead of zidovudine (AZT) or concomitant use of neutrophil growth factor (e.g., G-CSF or GM-CSF).
- Foscarnet: additive or synergistic antiviral activity.
- Probenecid: may increase ganciclovir serum levels. Monitor closely and decrease ganciclovir dose as needed.
- Immunosuppressant (corticosteroids, cyclosporine, azathioprine): increased bone marrow suppression; dose-reduce or hold immunosuppressants during ganciclovir treatment.
- Interferon: potent synergism against herpes virus, VZV.
- Imipenem/cilastatin: increase neurotoxicity with seizures. AVOID CONCURRENT USE.
- Cytotoxic antineoplastic agents: additive toxicity in bone marrow, gonads, GI epithelium/mucosa.
- Other cytotoxic drugs (dapsone, pentamidine, flucytosine, amphotericin B, trimethoprim-sulfamethoxazole): increase toxicity. Use cautiously if unable to avoid concurrent use.

Lab Effects/Interference:
- Serum ALT, serum alk phos, serum AST, and serum bili values may be increased.
- BUN and serum creatinine values may be increased.

Special Considerations:
- Do not use in pregnancy.
- Patient should be well hydrated; use with caution at reduced doses if renal insufficiency exists.
- Drug is mutagenic; patient should use barrier contraceptive.
- CMV retinitis patient should see ophthalmologist at least every 6 weeks during ganciclovir therapy.
- Administer over at least 1 hour.
- Monitor blood counts frequently.

Potential Toxicities/Side Effects and the Nursing Process

I.   INFECTION, BLEEDING related to BONE MARROW DEPRESSION

Defining Characteristics: Neutropenia ($< 1,000/mm^3$) occurs in 25–50% of patients, especially in patients with AIDS or those undergoing bone marrow transplant. Thrombocytopenia ($< 50,000/mm^3$) occurs in 20% of patients. Anemia occurs in 1% of patients.

Nursing Implications: Assess baseline WBC, ANC, and platelet count; monitor throughout therapy (every other day initially, then 3 × per week). Hold ganciclovir if ANC < 500/mm³, platelet count < 25,000/mm³. Assess for signs/symptoms of infection or bleeding; instruct patient in signs/symptoms of infection and bleeding, and instruct to report these immediately. Teach patient self-care measures to minimize risk of infection, bleeding, including avoidance of OTC aspirin-containing medicines. Administer or teach patient to self-administer prescribed G-CSF or GM-CSF. Assess Hgb/HCT and signs/symptoms of fatigue. Instruct patient to alternate rest and activity periods.

II. ALTERATIONS IN SENSORY/PERCEPTUAL PATTERNS related to SENSORY CHANGES

Defining Characteristics: Retinal detachment may occur in 30% of patients treated for CMV retinitis. Local reactions (foreign body sensation, conjunctival or vitreal hemorrhage) may occur with intravitreal injection. CNS effects include headache, confusion, altered dreams, ataxia, and dizziness, affecting 5–17% of patients.

Nursing Implications: Assess baseline neurologic status, including vision, and monitor during treatment. Patient should see ophthalmologist at least every 6 weeks. Instruct patient to report any abnormalities and discuss them with physician.

III. ALTERATION IN NUTRITION, LESS THAN BODY REQUIREMENTS, related to GI SIDE EFFECTS

Defining Characteristics: Nausea, vomiting, diarrhea, anorexia may occur in 2% of patients. Elevated LFTs may occur due to drug, but may be difficult to distinguish from CMV infection of liver or biliary tree.

Nursing Implications: Assess baseline nutrition, liver function, and monitor during therapy. Instruct patient to report GI side effects. Administer or teach patient to self-administer prescribed antiemetic or antidiarrheal medications. Encourage adequate oral or IV hydration. Notify physician of abnormal LFTs. If anorexia occurs, encourage favorite foods and small, frequent meals as tolerated.

IV. ALTERATION IN URINARY ELIMINATION related to RENAL TOXICITY

Defining Characteristics: 2% of patients have increased serum BUN, creatinine, hematuria. Increased risk exists in elderly or patients with renal insufficiency.

Nursing Implications: Ensure adequate hydration with urinary output prior to drug administration and infuse drug over at least 1 hour. Dose should be reduced in patients with decreased renal function.

V. ALTERATIONS IN COMFORT related to LOCAL VEIN IRRITATION (IV ADMINISTRATION)

Defining Characteristics: Inflammation, phlebitis, pain occur often at IV infusion site due to high pH of drug.

COMPLICATIONS

Nursing Implications: Assess IV site for patency, irritation, prior to each dose. Change IV site at least q 48 h. Apply warmth/heat to painful area as needed. Assess need for tunneled central line. Avoid drug extravasation.

VI.   ALTERATION IN CARDIAC OUTPUT related to CHANGES IN BP

Defining Characteristics: Rarely, hypotension, or hypertension, arrhythmia, myocardial infarction, arrest occur.

Nursing Implications: Assess baseline VS and monitor throughout treatment. Notify physician of any changes from baseline.

VII.   ALTERATION IN SEXUALITY/REPRODUCTIVE PATTERNS related to REPRODUCTIVE HAZARD

Defining Characteristics: Drug is carcinogenic, mutagenic, and teratogenic; may produce infertility in males. It is unknown whether drug crosses placenta and is excreted in breastmilk.

Nursing Implications: Assess sexuality/reproductive patterns. Teach patient and partner about reproductive hazards; offer contraceptive counseling or refer for counseling as barrier contraceptive should be used by patient.

Drug: valacyclovir hydrochloride (Valtrex)

Class: Antiviral (systemic).

Mechanism of Action: Drug is well-absorbed and rapidly converted to acyclovir. Drug interferes with DNA synthesis so that viral replication cannot occur.

Metabolism: Widely distributed in body tissues and fluids including the CNS.

Indication: For treatment of viral infections in cancer patients. It is active against HSV-1, HSV-2, VZV (shingles), EBV, and CMV.

Dosage/Range:
- Herpes zoster: 1 g tid × 7 days.

Drug Preparation:
- Available in 500-mg caplets.
- Oral, without regard to meals.

Drug Interactions:
- Cimetidine and probenecid decrease renal clearance of valacyclovir.

Lab Effects/Interference:
- None known.

Special Considerations:
• Dose-reduce for renal impairment:

Creatinine Clearance (cc/min)	Dose
≥ 50	1 g q 8 h
30–49	1 g q 12 h
10–29	1 g q 24 h
< 10	500 mg q 24 h

• Treatment should be started within 48 hours of rash onset.
• AVOID DRUG IN IMMUNOCOMPROMISED PATIENTS, as patients with advanced HIV infection, and those undergoing bone marrow and renal transplants, have developed thrombotic thrombocytopenic purpura/hemolytic uremic syndrome (TTP/HUS).

Potential Toxicities/Side Effects and the Nursing Process

I. ALTERATION IN COMFORT related to HEADACHE, NAUSEA

Defining Characteristics: Headache occurred in approximately 22% of patients. Nausea occurred in 12% of patients.

Nursing Implications: Teach patient that side effects may occur and are usually mild. Patient should report headache that does not resolve with acetaminophen or nausea that does not resolve by diet modification.

Drug: valganciclovir hydrochloride (Valcyte)

Class: Antiviral (systemic)

Mechanism of Action: Valganciclovir is an antiviral drug. Interferes with DNA synthesis so that viral replication cannot occur. Valganciclovir is a cytomegalovirus (CMV) nucleoside analogue DNA polymerase inhibitor. Valganciclovir is metabolized to ganciclovir. There are pediatric indications for use also; see package insert for the specific pediatric indications.

Metabolism: Appears to be widely distributed, concentrates in kidneys, and is well-distributed to the eyes. Crosses BBB. Drug crosses placenta and is excreted in breastmilk in animals. Excreted unchanged in urine. The bioavailability of ganciclovir from valganciclovir is significantly higher than from ganciclovir capsules. Valganciclovir tablets cannot be substituted for ganciclovir capsules on a one-to-one basis.

Indication: Active against CMV retinitis in patients with acquired immunodeficiency syndrome (AIDS) and prevention of CMV disease in kidney, heart, or kidney–pancreas transplant in adults. It is also active against CMV infections, especially in the retina.

COMPLICATIONS

Contraindications:
- Valganciclovir is not indicated for use in either adult or pediatric liver transplant patients.
- The safety and efficacy of valganciclovir has not been established for:
  - Prevention of CMV disease in solid organ transplants other than those indicated and prevention of CMV disease in pediatric solid organ transplant patients less than 4 months of age.
  - Treatment of congenital CMV disease.

Dosage/Range:
Adult:
- Tablets: 450 mg and tablets should be taken with food.
- Oral solution: 50 mg/mL and must be prepared by the pharmacist prior to dispensing to the patient.
- DOSE MUST BE REDUCED IN RENAL IMPAIRMENT.

Drug Preparation:
- Drug is CARCINOGENIC, TERATOGENIC, IMPAIRS FERTILITY, and is TOXIC to the blood forming organs; use chemotherapy handling precautions (see *Appendix 1*) when preparing and administering ganciclovir.
- Valganciclovir tablets should not be broken or crushed.
- Valganciclovir for oral solution and tablets cannot be substituted for ganciclovir capsules on a one-to-one basis.
- Adult patients should use valganciclovir tablets, not valganciclovir for oral solution.
- Administer only if ANC is > 500 cells/mm^3 and platelet count > 25,000/mm^3.
- Add 10 mL of sterile water for injection to 500-mg vial. Further dilute dose in 50–250 mL of IV fluid and infuse over at least 1 hour.

Drug Administration:
- Adult dosage - Treatment of CMV retinitis.
  - Induction: 900 mg (two 450-mg tablets) twice a day for 21 days.
- Maintenance: 900 mg (two 450-mg tablets) once a day.
- Prevention of CMV disease in heart or kidney–pancreas transplant patients.
  - 900 mg (two 450-mg tablets) once a day within 10 days of transplantation until 100 days posttransplantation.
  - Prevention of CMV disease in kidney transplant patients.
  - 900 mg (two 450-mg tablets) once a day within 10 days of transplantation until 200 days posttransplantation.

Drug Interactions:
- Zidovudine: increased hematologic toxicity (neutropenia, anemia); do not use together if possible. Monitor with frequent tests of white blood cell counts with differential and hemoglobin levels.
- Didanosine: may increase didanosine concentrations. Monitor for didanosine (ddI) toxicity.

- Probenecid: may increase ganciclovir serum levels. Monitor closely for ganciclovir toxicity; decrease dose as needed.
- Mycophenolate mofetil (MMF): may increase ganciclovir concentrations and levels of MMF metabolites in patients with renal impairment. Monitor for ganciclovir and MMF toxicity.

Special Considerations:
- Hypersensitivity to valganciclovir or ganciclovir.
- Most common adverse events and laboratory abnormalities (reported in at least one indication by > 20% of patients) are diarrhea, pyrexia, nausea, tremor, neutropenia, graft rejection, thrombocytopenia, and vomiting.
- Do not use in pregnancy.
- Patient should be well-hydrated.
- Drug is mutagenic; patient should use barrier contraceptive for 90 days.
- Monitor blood counts frequently.
- Black Box Warning:
    - WARNING: HEMATOLOGIC TOXICITY, CARCINOGENICITY, TERATOGE-NICITY, AND IMPAIRMENT OF FERTILITY
- Clinical toxicity of valganciclovir, which is metabolized to ganciclovir, includes granulocytopenia, anemia, and thrombocytopenia.
- In animal studies, ganciclovir was carcinogenic, teratogenic, and caused aspermatogenesis.

Potential Toxicities/Side Effects and the Nursing Process

I.   INFECTION, BLEEDING related to BONE MARROW DEPRESSION

Defining Characteristics: Severe leukopenia, neutropenia, anemia, thrombocytopenia, pancytopenia, bone marrow aplasia, and aplastic anemia have been reported in patients treated with valganciclovir or ganciclovir. Valganciclovir should not be administered if the absolute neutrophil count is less than 500 cells/μL, the platelet count is less than 25,000/μL, or the hemoglobin is less than 8 g/dL. Valganciclovir should also be used with caution in patients with preexisting cytopenias, or who have received or who are receiving myelosuppressive drugs or irradiation.

Nursing Implications: Assess baseline WBC, ANC, and platelet count; monitor throughout therapy (every other day initially, then 3 times per week). Hold valganciclovir if ANC < 500/mm^3, platelet count < 25,000/mm^3. Assess for signs/symptoms of infection or bleeding; instruct patient in signs/symptoms of infection and bleeding, and instruct to report these immediately. Teach patient self-care measures to minimize risk of infection, bleeding, including avoidance of OTC aspirin-containing medicines. Administer or teach patient to self-administer prescribed G-CSF or GM-CSF. Assess Hgb/HCT and signs/symptoms of fatigue. Instruct patient to alternate rest and activity periods.

COMPLICATIONS

II.   ALTERATION IN NUTRITION, LESS THAN BODY REQUIREMENTS, related to GI SIDE EFFECTS

Defining Characteristics: Nausea, vomiting, diarrhea, anorexia may occur in 2% of patients. Elevated LFTs may occur due to drug, but may be difficult to distinguish from CMV infection of liver or biliary tree.

Nursing Implications: Assess baseline nutrition, liver function, and monitor during therapy. Instruct patient to report GI side effects. Administer or teach patient to self-administer prescribed antiemetic or antidiarrheal medications. Encourage adequate oral or IV hydration. Notify physician of abnormal LFTs. If anorexia occurs, encourage favorite foods and small, frequent meals as tolerated.

III.   ALTERATION IN URINARY ELIMINATION related to RENAL TOXICITY

Defining Characteristics: 2% of patients have increased serum BUN, creatinine, hematuria. Increased risk of acute renal failure may occur in elderly patients with or without reduced renal function, patients who have concomitant nepthrotoxic drugs, or inadequately hydrated patients.

Nursing Implications: Ensure adequate hydration with urinary output prior to drug administration. Dose should be reduced in patients with decreased renal function. Use with caution in elderly patients or those taking nephrotoxic drugs, reduce dosage in patients with renal impairment, and monitor renal function.

IV.   ALTERATION IN CARDIAC OUTPUT related to CHANGES IN BP

Defining Characteristics: Rarely, hypotension, or hypertension, arrhythmia, myocardial infarction, arrest occur.

Nursing Implications: Assess baseline VS and monitor throughout treatment. Notify physician of any changes from baseline.

V.   ALTERATION IN SEXUALITY/REPRODUCTIVE PATTERNS related to REPRODUCTIVE HAZARD

Defining Characteristics: Drug is carcinogenic, mutagenic, and teratogenic; may produce temporary or permanent inhibition of spermatogenesis and infertility in males. It is unknown whether drug crosses placenta and is excreted in breastmilk.

Nursing Implications: Assess sexuality/reproductive patterns. Teach patient and partner about reproductive hazards; offer contraceptive counseling or refer for counseling, as barrier contraceptive should be used by patient.

Chapter *12*
Constipation

Constipation is a decreased frequency of defecation that is difficult or uncomfortable (Walsh, 1989). Constipation is multifactorial, and can be related to diet and nutrition, changes in routine, metabolic and endocrine conditions, or problems in the colon and rectum, to name a few. Drugs can frequently cause constipation, such as opioids, anticholinergics (e.g., H1 antihistamines), antihypertensives, the serotonin (5-HT3) receptor antagonist antiemetics (e.g., ondansetron), and chemotherapeutic drugs such as vincristine. Levy (1992) reports five causes of constipation in cancer patients:

- Disease itself: primary bowel cancers, paraneoplastic autonomic neuropathy.
- Disease sequelae: dehydration, paralysis, immobility, alterations in bowel elimination patterns.
- Prior history of laxative abuse, hemorrhoids/anal fissures, other diseases.
- Cancer therapy: chemotherapy (vinca alkaloids, e.g., vincristine, vinblastine); bowel surgery.
- Medications used to manage symptoms: opioids, antihistamines, tricyclic antidepressants, aluminum antacids.

Complications of constipation can be severe (i.e., bowel perforation), extremely painful, and compromise quality of life. Nurses play an enormous role in preventing morbidity from constipation in patients with cancer. Assessment of the patient's previous and current nutrition and elimination patterns, along with assessment of probable etiology of constipation, are critical, as is patient/family teaching about constipation management and prevention. Teaching should include dietary modifications to include high-fiber intake (fruits, vegetables, or nutritional supplements high in fiber); fluid intake of 3 L/day; and moderate exercise as tolerated. Patients receiving drugs (i.e., opioids) that are likely to be constipating should also receive a bowel regimen to prevent constipation. Available laxatives include the following types:

- *Bulk-forming laxatives* cause the stool to retain water, and thus increase peristalsis (fiber, bran, psyllium, methylcellulose).
- *Lubricants* coat and soften the stool so it can move more smoothly through the intestines (mineral oil).
- *Saline laxatives* pull water into the gut and into the stool, increasing peristalsis (magnesium citrate, sodium biphosphate, magnesium hydroxide).
- *Osmotic laxatives* work through colonic bacteria that metabolize osmotic laxatives causing increased osmotic pressure gradient, pulling water into the gut and then into the stool, thus increasing peristalsis (lactulose, sorbitol, polyethylene glycol).
- *Detergent laxatives* reduce surface tension of the colonic cells, so water and fats enter the stool; in addition, electrolyte and water absorption is decreased (docusate salts).

- *Stimulant laxatives* irritate the gut, increasing gut motility (bisacodyl).
- *Anthraquinone laxatives* are activated by gut bacteria degradation (senna, casanthrol, cascara).
- *Suppositories* cause local irritation and stimulate rectal emptying (glycerin, bisacodyl, senna).

New approaches to opioid-induced constipation prevention and management include the use of opioid antagonists, such as methylnaltrexone (Relistor) and naloxegol (Movantik).

References

AstraZeneca Pharmaceuticals, LP. Movantik (naloxegol) [package insert]. Wilmington, DE, January 2015.

Levy MH. 1992; *Prim. Care Cancer* 12 (4) 11–18 Constipation and Diarrhea in Cancer Patients, Part I.

Walsh TD. Constipation. Walsh TD, ed. *Symptom Control.* Cambridge, MA: Blackwell Scientific Publications Inc., 1989; 331–381.

Drug: bisacodyl (Dulcolax)

Class: Stimulant laxative.

Mechanism of Action: Stimulates/irritates smooth muscle of intestines, increasing peristalsis; increases fluid accumulation in colon and small intestines. Indicated for relief of constipation and bowel preparation prior to bowel surgery.

Metabolism: Minimal oral absorption. Evacuation occurs in 6–10 hours when taken orally, or within 15 minutes to 1 hour when administered rectally.

Indication: For relief of constipation, preparation for diagnostic procedures (e.g., colonoscopy), and in preoperative and postoperative treatment when constipation occurs.

Dosage/Range:
Adult:
- Oral: 5–15 mg at bedtime or early morning. Bowel preparation may use up to 30 mg.
- Suppository: 10 mg PR.

Drug Preparation:
- Administer oral tablet > 1 hour after antacids or milk.
- Insert suppository as high as possible against wall of rectum.

Drug Interactions:
- None.

Lab Effects/Interference:
- None known.

Special Considerations:
- Contraindicated in patients with signs/symptoms of acute abdomen (nausea, vomiting, abdominal pain), intestinal obstruction, fecal impaction, or ulcerative bowel lesions.

Potential Toxicities/Side Effects and the Nursing Process

I.   ALTERATIONS IN BOWEL ELIMINATION related to CHRONIC USE

Defining Characteristics: Removes defecation reflexes when used chronically (laxative dependence). Narcotic analgesics and vinca alkaloid chemotherapy may predispose to constipation.

Nursing Implications: Assess baseline elimination pattern. Teach patient how to self-administer laxative. Encourage patient to normalize bowel habits through adequate fluid intake (2–3 L/day), diet high in fiber and bulk (bran, cereals, fruits, and vegetables), and exercise as tolerated. Teach patient bowel regimen when on narcotics or vinca alkaloids to promote regular evacuation.

II.   ALTERATION IN NUTRITION, LESS THAN BODY REQUIREMENTS, related to GI SIDE EFFECTS

Defining Characteristics: Constipation or drug may cause nausea, vomiting, abdominal pain; rectal suppository may cause burning in rectum as it is absorbed.

Nursing Implications: Assess comfort level and GI distress related to constipation. Encourage patient to drink cold fluids or ginger ale as tolerated. Encourage patient to try resting in different positions; warm packs may decrease abdominal pain. Teach patient to expect burning sensation with suppository use; reassure that it will resolve in 5–10 minutes.

III.   ALTERATION IN FLUID AND ELECTROLYTE BALANCE related to LAXATIVE ABUSE

Defining Characteristics: Diarrhea resulting from laxative abuse can deplete fluid volume, nutrients, and electrolytes.

Nursing Implications: Teach patient regular bowel regimen when receiving constipating drugs (narcotics, vinca alkaloids). Teach patient to replace lost fluids and electrolytes (encourage chicken soup, sports drink).

Drug: docusate calcium, docusate potassium, docusate sodium (Dioctyl Calcium Sulfosuccinate, Dioctyl Potassium Sulfosuccinate, Dioctyl Sodium Sulfosuccinate, Colace, Diocto-K, Diosuccin, DOK-250, Doxinate, Duosol, Laxinate 100, Regulax SS, Stulex)

Class: Stool softener.

Mechanism of Action: The calcium, sodium, and potassium salts of docusate soften stool by decreasing surface tension, emulsification, and wetting action, thus increasing stool absorption of water in the bowel.

COMPLICATIONS

Metabolism: Appears to be absorbed somewhat in the duodenum and jejunum, and excreted in bile. Stool softening occurs in 1–3 days.

Indication: To soften stool.

Dosage/Range:
Adult:
• Oral: 50–360 mg/day, in single or divided doses, depending on stool-softening response.

Drug Preparation:
• Oral: store gelatin capsule in tight container; store syrup in light-resistant containers.
• Rectal: according to manufacturer's package insert.

Drug Interactions:
• Mineral oil: increased mineral oil absorption; AVOID CONCURRENT USE.

Lab Effects/Interference:
• None known.

Special Considerations:
• Useful in prevention of straining-at-stool in patients receiving narcotics; when combined with other agents/laxatives, prevents constipation in these patients.
• Does not increase intestinal peristalsis; stop drug if severe abdominal cramping occurs.
• Is effective only in prevention of constipation, not in treating constipation.

Potential Toxicities/Side Effects and the Nursing Process

I.   KNOWLEDGE DEFICIT related to BOWEL ELIMINATION

Defining Characteristics: Oncology patients who are receiving narcotic analgesics, vinca alkaloid chemotherapy (vincristine, vinblastine, vindesine), or who are dehydrated or hypercalcemic are at increased risk of constipation.

Nursing Implications: Assess baseline elimination pattern. Teach patient need for bowel movement at least every other day, depending on usual pattern. Teach patient importance of adequate fluid intake (2–3 L/day), diet high in fiber and bulk (bran, cereals, fruits, vegetables, and supplements with fiber), and exercise as tolerated. Teach self-administration of stool softeners and prescribed laxatives.

Drug: glycerin suppository (Fleet Babylax, Sani-Supp)

Class: Hyperosmotic laxative.

Mechanism of Action: Local irritant, with hyperosmotic action, drawing water from tissues into feces and stimulating fecal evacuation within 15–30 minutes.

Metabolism: Poorly absorbed from rectum.

Indication: To relieve constipation.

Dosage/Range:
Adult:
- Rectal suppository: 2–3 g PR.
- Enema: 5–15 mL PR.

Drug Preparation:
- Rectal administration must be retained for 15 minutes.

Drug Interactions:
- None.

Lab Effects/Interference:
- None known.

Special Considerations:
- Contraindicated in patients with undiagnosed abdominal pain, intestinal obstruction.

Potential Toxicities/Side Effects and the Nursing Process

I.   ALTERATIONS IN BOWEL ELIMINATION related to CHRONIC USE

Defining Characteristics: Removes defecation reflexes when used chronically (laxative dependence). Narcotic analgesics and vinca alkaloid chemotherapy may predispose to constipation.

Nursing Implications: Assess baseline elimination pattern. Teach patient how to self-administer laxative. Encourage patient to normalize bowel habits through adequate fluid intake (2–3 L/day), diet high in fiber and bulk (bran, cereals, fruits, and vegetables), and exercise as tolerated. Teach patient bowel regimen when on narcotics or vinca alkaloids to promote regular evacuation.

II.   ALTERATION IN FLUID AND ELECTROLYTE BALANCE related to LAXATIVE ABUSE

Defining Characteristics: Diarrhea resulting from laxative abuse can deplete fluid volume, nutrients, and electrolytes.

Nursing Implications: Teach patient regular bowel regimen when receiving constipating drugs (narcotics, vinca alkaloids). Teach patient to replace lost fluids and electrolytes (encourage chicken soup, sports drink).

III.   ALTERATION IN COMFORT related to CRAMPING PAIN, RECTAL IRRITATION, OR DISCOMFORT

Defining Characteristics: Cramping pain, rectal irritation, and inflammation or discomfort may occur.

Nursing Implications: Teach patient this may occur. If discomfort is not self-limited, suggest sitz bath, warm or cold packs, and position changes.

COMPLICATIONS

Drug: magnesium citrate

Class: Saline laxative.

Mechanism of Action: Draws water into small intestinal lumen, stimulating peristalsis and evacuation in 3–6 hours.

Metabolism: 15–30% absorbed, excreted in urine.

Indication: For relief of occasional constipation (generally produces bowel movement in 1/2–6 hrs).

Dosage/Range:
Adult:
• Oral: 11–25 g (5–10 oz or 150–300 mL)/day as single or divided dose at bedtime.

Drug Preparation:
• Refrigerate and serve with ice. Taste can be masked by adding small amount of juice.

Drug Interactions:
• None.

Lab Effects/Interference:
• None known.

Special Considerations:
• Contraindicated in patients with signs/symptoms of acute abdomen (nausea, vomiting, abdominal pain), intestinal obstruction, fecal impaction, or ulcerative bowel lesions.
• Contraindicated in patients with rectal fissures, myocardial infarction, renal disease.

Potential Toxicities/Side Effects and the Nursing Process

I.   ALTERATIONS IN BOWEL ELIMINATION related to CHRONIC USE

Defining Characteristics: Removes defecation reflexes when used chronically (laxative dependence). Narcotic analgesics and vinca alkaloid chemotherapy may predispose to constipation.

Nursing Implications: Assess baseline elimination pattern. Teach patient how to self-administer laxative. Encourage patient to normalize bowel habits through adequate fluid intake (2–3 L/day), diet high in fiber and bulk (bran, cereals, fruits, and vegetables), and exercise as tolerated. Teach patient bowel regimen when on narcotics or vinca alkaloids to promote regular evacuation.

II.   ALTERATION IN NUTRITION, LESS THAN BODY REQUIREMENTS, related to GI SIDE EFFECTS

Defining Characteristics: Constipation or drug may cause nausea and abdominal pain.

Nursing Implications: Assess comfort level and GI distress related to constipation. Encourage patient to drink cold fluids or ginger ale as tolerated. Encourage patient to try resting in different positions; warm packs may decrease abdominal pain.

III. ALTERATION IN FLUID AND ELECTROLYTE BALANCE
related to LAXATIVE ABUSE

Defining Characteristics: Diarrhea resulting from laxative abuse can deplete fluid volume, nutrients, and electrolytes.

Nursing Implications: Teach patient regular bowel regimen when receiving constipating drugs (narcotics, vinca alkaloids). Teach patient to replace lost fluids and electrolytes (encourage chicken soup, sports drink).

Drug: methylcellulose (Citrucel)

Class: Bulk-producing laxative.

Mechanism of Action: Absorbs water; bulk expansion stimulates peristalsis and evacuation in 12–24 hours. May also be used to slow diarrhea.

Metabolism: Not absorbed by GI tract.

Indication: For relief of constipation.

Dosage/Range:
Adult:
• Oral: up to 6 g/day PO in 2–3 divided doses.

Drug Preparation:
• Administer each dose with at least 250 mL of water or juice.

Drug Interactions:
• None.

Lab Effects/Interference:
• None known.

Special Considerations:
• Safest and most physiologically normal laxative.

Potential Toxicities/Side Effects and the Nursing Process

I. ALTERATIONS IN BOWEL ELIMINATION related to CHRONIC USE

Defining Characteristics: Removes defecation reflexes when used chronically (laxative dependence). Narcotic analgesics and vinca alkaloid chemotherapy may predispose to constipation.

Nursing Implications: Assess baseline elimination pattern. Teach patient how to self-administer laxative. Encourage patient to normalize bowel habits through adequate fluid intake (2–3 L/day), diet high in fiber and bulk (bran, cereals, fruits, and vegetables), and exercise as tolerated. Teach patient bowel regimen when on narcotics or vinca alkaloids to promote regular evacuation.

COMPLICATIONS

II. ALTERATION IN NUTRITION, LESS THAN BODY REQUIREMENTS, related to GI SIDE EFFECTS

Defining Characteristics: Constipation or drug may cause nausea, vomiting, cramps.

Nursing Implications: Assess comfort level and GI distress related to constipation. Encourage patient to drink cold fluids or ginger ale as tolerated. Encourage patient to try resting in different positions; warm packs may decrease abdominal pain. Teach patient laxative effect may take 12–24 hours, and assess need for other cathartic(s).

Drug: methylnaltrexone bromide (Relistor)

Class: Selective, peripherally acting opioid antagonist.

Mechanism of Action: Mu opioid antagonist that competes with opioid analgesics for opioid receptors in the periphery, such as in the gut, but not in the CNS, as it is unable to cross the blood–brain barrier. Thus, it does not interfere with opioid pain relief, which is centrally mediated. Drug inhibits opioid-induced delayed intestinal transit time.

Metabolism: Absorbed rapidly with peak serum level in 30 minutes. Drug is metabolized in the liver and is excreted by the kidneys (about 50%) and in the feces; 85% of the drug is excreted intact. The terminal half-life is 8 hours.

Indication: For treatment of opioid-induced constipation in patients with advanced illness who are receiving palliative care when response to laxative therapy has not been sufficient.

Contraindication: Patients with known or suspected mechanical GI obstruction.

Dosage Range:
- 8 mg SQ every other day (weight 38–62 kg [84–136 lbs]) or 12 mg for patients weighing 62–114 kg (136–251 lbs), as needed. For patients weighing more or less: (1) dose at 0.15 mg/kg; and (2) calculate injection volume by multiplying weight in kg by 0.0075, and round up the volume to the nearest 0.1 mL.
- If needed more frequently than every other day, maximum frequency is once every 24 hours.
- Dose-reduce 50% if patient has renal impairment (creatinine clearance < 30 mL/min). Adult patients with severe renal impairment should only be prescribed single-use vials to ensure correct dosing.
- If severe or persistent diarrhea occurs during treatment, advise patients to discontinue therapy and contact their physician.
- Use cautiously in patients with known or suspected lesions of GI tract, as drug may rarely cause GI perforation.
- Drug is contraindicated in patients with known or suspected mechanical GI obstruction.
- Safety and efficacy of drug in pediatric patients has not been established.

Drug Preparation:
- Drug is available as
  - Single-use vials containing (1) 12 mg in 0.6 mL for subcutaneous administration, **for use** with a 27-gauge × ½-inch needle and 1-mL syringe, and

(2) 12 mg in 0.6 mL for subcutaneous administration with one 1-mL syringe with retractable 27-gauge × ½ -inch needle, 2 alcohol swabs; aseptically draw up ordered amount.
- Single-use **prefilled syringe** containing (1) 8 mg in 0.4-mL solution for subcutaneous administration, with a 29-gauge × ½-inch fixed needle and a needle guard, and (2) 12 mg in 0.6-mL solution for subcutaneous administration with a 29-gauge × ½-inch fixed needle and needle guard. Select prefilled syringe for exact dose.
- Once drawn up, if not used right away, may be stored at ambient room temperature for 24 hours.
- Store vial at controlled room temperature and protect from light.

Drug Administration:
- Subcutaneous injection (8-mg dose is 0.4 mL, and 12-mg dose is 0.6 mL) in upper arm, abdomen, or thigh.

Drug Interactions:
- Weak inhibitor of cytochrome P450 isozyme CYP2D6 activity, but did not interact with dextromethorphan.

Special Considerations:
- Approved only for adult use. Drug has not been studied in patients with peritoneal catheters.
- Most common side effects are abdominal pain, flatulence, nausea, dizziness, diarrhea, and hyperhidrosis.

Warnings and Precautions:
- GI perforation has been reported. Use drug cautiously in patients with known or suspected lesions of the GI tract. Teach patients to notify provider right away if they develop severe, persistent, or worsening abdominal symptoms.
- Severe or persistent diarrhea; discontinue therapy and discuss with physician.
- Post-marketing reports include cramping, perforation, vomiting, diaphoresis, flushing, malaise, pain.
- No difference in efficacy or safety profile in older patients.
- Thirty percent of patients have laxation within 30 minutes of drug administration, and 48–62% have laxation within 4 hours of first dose.

Potential Toxicities/Side Effects and the Nursing Process

I.   ALTERATION IN NUTRITION, POTENTIAL, related to GI SIDE EFFECTS

Defining Characteristics: Drug may cause nausea (11.5%), abdominal pain (28.5%), flatulence (13.3%), and diarrhea (5.5%).

Nursing Implications: Assess comfort level and GI distress related to constipation. Encourage patient to drink cold fluids or ginger ale as tolerated. Encourage patient to try resting in different positions; warm packs may decrease abdominal pain. Teach patient to call nurse or physician if abdominal pain, nausea, or vomiting become more severe or if new symptoms develop. If patient develops persistent or severe diarrhea, stop drug and discuss with physician.

Drug: mineral oil (Fleet Mineral Oil)

Class: Lubricant laxative.

Mechanism of Action: Lubricates intestine, preventing fecal fluid from being absorbed in colon; water retention distends colon, stimulating peristalsis and evacuation in 6–8 hours.

Metabolism: Minimal GI absorption occurs following oral or rectal administration.

Indication: For relief of constipation.

Dosage/Range:
Adult:
• Oral: 15–45 mL PO in single or divided doses.
• Rectal enemas: 120 mL PR as a single dose.

Drug Preparation:
• Administer plain mineral oil at bedtime on an empty stomach.
• Administer mineral oil emulsion with food if desired at bedtime.
• May mix with juice to mask taste.

Drug Interactions:
• Docusate salts: increase mineral oil absorption; DO NOT ADMINISTER CONCURRENTLY.
• Fat-soluble vitamins: decrease absorption with chronic mineral oil administration.

Lab Effects/Interference:
• Decreased fat-soluble vitamins (e.g., vitamins A, D, E, K) with chronic drug administration.

Special Considerations:
• Contraindicated in patients with signs/symptoms of acute abdomen (nausea, vomiting, abdominal pain), intestinal obstruction, fecal impaction, or ulcerative bowel lesions.
• Do not use for more than 1 week.

Potential Toxicities/Side Effects and the Nursing Process

I.   ALTERATIONS IN BOWEL ELIMINATION related to CHRONIC USE

Defining Characteristics: Removes defecation reflexes when used chronically (laxative dependence). Narcotic analgesics and vinca alkaloid chemotherapy may predispose to constipation.

Nursing Implications: Assess baseline elimination pattern. Teach patient how to self-administer laxative. Encourage patient to normalize bowel habits through adequate fluid intake (2–3 L/day), diet high in fiber and bulk (bran, cereals, fruits, and vegetables), and exercise as tolerated. Teach patient bowel regimen when on narcotics or vinca alkaloids to promote regular evacuation.

II. ALTERATION IN NUTRITION, LESS THAN BODY REQUIREMENTS, related to GI SIDE EFFECTS

Defining Characteristics: Constipation or drug may cause nausea, vomiting, cramps.

Nursing Implications: Assess comfort level and GI distress related to constipation. Encourage patient to drink cold fluids or ginger ale as tolerated. Encourage patient to try resting in different positions; warm packs may decrease abdominal pain. Teach patient to expect burning sensation with suppository use; reassure that it will resolve in 5–10 minutes.

Drug: naloxegol (Movantik)

Class: Opioid antagonist.

Mechanism of Action: Naloxegol is mu-opioid receptor antagonist, and blocks GI mu-opioid receptor binding, thereby decreasing the constipating effect of opioid analgesics. It results in slowed GI motility and transit time. The drug does not cross the blood–brain barrier at recommended doses due to PEGylation, although it is a naloxone derivative.

Metabolism: Following oral administration, peak concentration occurs in less than 2 hours, with a secondary peak occurring 0.4–3 hours after the first peak. Consuming a high-fat meal increases the extent and rate of absorption. Naloxegol is metabolized by the CYP3A microenzyme system. The rug is primarily excreted in the feces (68%), and to a lesser degree in the urine (16%). Half-life of therapeutic doses ranges from 6 to 11 hours.

Indication: Treatment of opioid-induced constipation in adults with chronic noncancer pain. The drug has shown efficacy in patients receiving opioids for at least 4 weeks.

Contraindications:
• Known or suspected GI obstruction, or patient at increased risk of recurrent obstruction.
• Concomitant use with strong CYP3A4 inhibitors (e.g., clarithromycin, ketoconazole).
• Known serious or severe hypersensitivity reaction to naloxegol or its excipients.

Dosage/Range:
• 25 mg PO once daily; if not tolerated, reduce dose to 12.5 mg once daily.
• If renal impairment (Cr Cl < 60 mL/min): 12.5 mg once daily, increase to 25 mg once daily if tolerated and monitor for adverse reactions.
• Stop maintenance laxative therapy before starting naloxegol; may resume if the patient develops opioid-induced constipation symptoms after taking naloxegol for 3 days.
• Discontinue treatment if opioid analgesic is also discontinued.

Drug Preparation: Available in 12.5- and 25-mg tablets.

COMPLICATIONS

Drug Administration:
- Teach the patient to take the tablet on an empty stomach at least 1 hour before the first meal of the day or 2 hours after the meal.
- The patient should swallow the tablets whole; do not crush or chew them.
- Avoid grapefruit juice or eating grapefruit.

Drug Interactions:
- Naloxegol is metabolized primarily by CYP3A and is a substrate of the P-glycoprotein transporter. It is contraindicated in patients who must take strong CYP3A4 inhibitors.
- Moderate CYP3A4 inhibitors (e.g., diltiazem, erythromycin, verapamil): Increased naloxegol concentrations. Avoid coadministration; if it is unavoidable, reduce the naloxegol dose to 12.5 mg once daily, and monitor for adverse reactions.
- Strong CYP3A4 inducers (e.g., rifampin, carbamazepine, St. John's wort): Decreased concentration of naloxegol. Do not use concomitantly. Teach patients not to take St. John's wort when receiving naloxegol.
- Other opioid antagonists: There is a potential for an additive effect and increased risk of opioid withdrawal. Do not use concomitantly.

Lab Effects/Interference: None known.

Special Considerations:
- Most common adverse reactions in clinical trials with an incidence of 3% or greater: abdominal pain, diarrhea, nausea, flatulence, vomiting, headache.
- Warnings and precautions:
  - **GI perforation** may occur rarely, in patients with loss of structural integrity (e.g., peptic ulcer disease, Ogilvie's syndrome, diverticular disease, infiltrative GI malignancies or peritoneal metastases). Weigh the relative risk against the potential benefit. Monitor the patient closely for development of severe, persistent, or worsening abdominal pain, and discontinue the drug immediately if it occurs.
  - **Opioid withdrawal** may occur rarely (<1%); it is characterized by hyperhidrosis, chills, diarrhea, abdominal pain, anxiety, irritability, and yawning. Risk for opioid withdrawal may be higher in patients (1) receiving methadone for pain or (2) having a disruption of the blood–brain barrier, in which case they may also be at risk for reduced analgesia. Weigh the relative risk against the potential benefit. Monitor the patient closely for opioid withdrawal.
  - Use in pregnancy may precipitate opioid withdrawal in the fetus.
  - Nursing mothers should make a decision to discontinue nursing or the drug, taking into account the importance to the mother.

Potential Toxicities/Side Effects and the Nursing Process

I.   ALTERATION IN NUTRITION, LESS THAN BODY REQUIREMENTS, related to GI SIDE EFFECTS, HEADACHE

Defining Characteristics: Incidence of symptoms in patients in the clinical trials (for opioid-induced constipation and noncancer pain) at doses of 25 mg and 12.5 mg naloxegol, respectively, was as follows: abdominal pain (21%, 21%; 7% placebo), diarrhea (9%, 6%;

5% placebo), nausea (8%, 7%; 5% placebo), flatulence (6%, 3%; 3% placebo), vomiting (5%, 3%; 4% placebo), and headache (4%, 4%; 3% placebo).

Nursing Implications: Assess the patient's comfort level and GI distress related to constipation as well as the potential side effects of naloxegol. Teach the patient strategies to manage symptoms, and to report symptoms that persist. Encourage the patient to drink cold fluids or ginger ale as tolerated. Encourage the patient to try resting in different positions; warm packs may decrease abdominal pain.

Drug: polyethylene glycol 3350, NF powder (Miralax)

Class: Osmotic cathartic.

Mechanism of Action: Drug is an osmotic agent that pulls water into the intestines with the stool, softening the stool and causing peristalsis and evacuation in 2–4 days.

Metabolism: Is not fermented by colonic microflora and does not affect intestinal absorption or secretion of glucose or electrolytes.

Indication: For relief of constipation.

Dosage/Range:
• 17 g (1 heaping T) (product comes with a measuring cup).

Drug Preparation:
• Mix in 8 oz of water and take orally once a day.

Drug Administration:
• Oral. Available in 14-oz and 26-oz containers.
• Store at room temperature.

Drug Interactions:
• None.

Lab Effects/Interference:
• None.

Special Considerations:
• Contraindicated in patients with bowel obstruction.
• Indicated for the treatment of occasional constipation for up to 2 weeks.
• Use during pregnancy only if clearly needed.
• Excessive or frequent use or use > 2 weeks may result in electrolyte imbalance and dependence on laxatives.

Potential Toxicities/Side Effects and the Nursing Process

I.   ALTERATIONS IN BOWEL ELIMINATION related to CHRONIC USE

Defining Characteristics: Removes defecation reflexes when used chronically (laxative dependence). Narcotic analgesics and vinca alkaloid chemotherapy may predispose to constipation.

Nursing Implications: Assess baseline elimination pattern. Teach patient how to self-administer laxative. Encourage patient to normalize bowel habits through adequate fluid intake (2–3 L/day), diet high in fiber and bulk (bran, cereals, fruits, and vegetables), and exercise as tolerated. Teach patient bowel regimen when on narcotics or vinca alkaloids to promote regular evacuation.

II.   ALTERATION IN NUTRITION related to GI SIDE EFFECTS

Defining Characteristics: Constipation or drug may cause nausea, cramps, abdominal bloating, flatulence. High doses may cause diarrhea, especially in the elderly. Continued use beyond 2 weeks may cause electrolyte imbalance.

Nursing Implications: Assess comfort level and GI distress related to constipation. Encourage patient to drink cold fluids or ginger ale as tolerated. Encourage patient to try resting in different positions; warm packs may decrease abdominal pain. Teach patient laxative effect may take 2–4 days, and assess need for other cathartic(s).

Drug: senna (Senexon, Senokot)

Class: Irritant/stimulant laxative.

Mechanism of Action: Stimulates/irritates smooth muscle of intestines, increasing peristalsis; increases fluid accumulation in colon and small intestines. Indicated for relief of constipation or bowel preparation prior to bowel surgery.

Metabolism: Minimal oral absorption occurs. Evacuation occurs in 6–10 hours when taken orally.

Indication: For the relief of, and prevention of, constipation.

Dosage/Range:
- Senexon: 2 tablets at bedtime (187 mg senna).
- Senokot: 2–4 tablets bid (187 mg senna); 1–2 tsp granules bid (326 mg senna); 1 suppository at bedtime, repeat PRN in 2 hours (652 mg senna).
- Black-Draught: 2 tablets (600 mg senna) or ¼ to ½ level tsp granules (1.65 gm senna).

Drug Preparation:
- Store in a tightly closed bottle.

Drug Interactions:
- None.

Lab Effects/Interference:
- None known.

Special Considerations:
- Contraindicated in patients with signs/symptoms of acute abdomen (nausea, vomiting, abdominal pain), intestinal obstruction, fecal impaction, or ulcerative bowel lesions.
- Senna is very effective as part of bowel regimen for patients receiving narcotic analgesic medication.

Potential Toxicities/Side Effects and the Nursing Process

I.   ALTERATIONS IN BOWEL ELIMINATION related to CHRONIC USE

Defining Characteristics: Removes defecation reflexes when used chronically (laxative dependence). Narcotic analgesics and vinca alkaloid chemotherapy may predispose to constipation.

Nursing Implications: Assess baseline elimination pattern. Teach patient how to self-administer laxative. Encourage patient to normalize bowel habits through adequate fluid intake (2–3 L/day), diet high in fiber and bulk (bran, cereals, fruits, and vegetables), and exercise as tolerated. Teach patient bowel regimen when on narcotics or vinca alkaloids to promote regular evacuation.

II.   ALTERATION IN NUTRITION, LESS THAN BODY REQUIREMENTS, related to GI SIDE EFFECTS

Defining Characteristics: Constipation or drug may cause nausea, vomiting, abdominal pain; rectal suppository may cause burning in rectum as it is absorbed.

Nursing Implications: Assess comfort level and GI distress related to constipation. Encourage patient to drink cold fluids or ginger ale as tolerated. Encourage patient to try resting in different positions; warm packs may decrease abdominal pain. Teach patient to expect burning sensation with suppository use; reassure that it will resolve in 5–10 minutes.

III.   ALTERATION IN FLUID AND ELECTROLYTE BALANCE related to LAXATIVE ABUSE

Defining Characteristics: Diarrhea resulting from laxative abuse can deplete fluid volume, nutrients, and electrolytes.

Nursing Implications: Teach patient regular bowel regimen when receiving constipating drugs (narcotics, vinca alkaloids). Teach patient to replace lost fluids and electrolytes (encourage chicken soup, sports drink).

COMPLICATIONS

Drug: sorbitol

Class: Hyperosmotic laxative.

Mechanism of Action: Local irritant, with hyperosmotic action, drawing water from tissues into feces and stimulating fecal evacuation within 15–30 minutes.

Metabolism: Poorly absorbed from GI tract.

Indication: For the relief of constipation.

Dosage/Range:
Adult:
• Oral: 15 mL of 70% solution repeated until diarrhea starts.
• Rectal: 120 mL if a 25–30% solution is used.

Drug Preparation:
• Keep stored in tightly closed bottle.

Drug Interactions:
• None.

Lab Effects/Interference:
• None known.

Special Considerations:
• Contraindicated in patients with undiagnosed abdominal pain, intestinal obstruction.
• Oral 70% sorbitol may be as effective as lactulose in relieving constipation.

Potential Toxicities/Side Effects and the Nursing Process

I.   ALTERATIONS IN BOWEL ELIMINATION related to CHRONIC USE

Defining Characteristics: Removes defecation reflexes when used chronically (laxative dependence). Narcotic analgesics and vinca alkaloid chemotherapy may predispose to constipation.

Nursing Implications: Assess baseline elimination pattern. Teach patient how to self-administer laxative. Encourage patient to normalize bowel habits through adequate fluid intake (2–3 L/day), diet high in fiber and bulk (bran, cereals, fruits, and vegetables), and exercise as tolerated. Teach patient bowel regimen when on narcotics or vinca alkaloids to promote regular evacuation.

II.   ALTERATION IN FLUID AND ELECTROLYTE BALANCE related to LAXATIVE ABUSE

Defining Characteristics: Diarrhea resulting from laxative abuse can deplete fluid volume, nutrients, and electrolytes.

Nursing Implications: Teach patient regular bowel regimen when receiving constipating drugs (narcotics, vinca alkaloids). Teach patient to replace lost fluids and electrolytes (encourage chicken soup, sports drink).

III.   ALTERATION IN COMFORT related to CRAMPING PAIN, RECTAL IRRITATION, OR DISCOMFORT

Defining Characteristics: Cramping pain, rectal irritation, and inflammation or discomfort may occur.

Nursing Implications: Teach patient this may occur. If discomfort is not self-limited, suggest sitz bath, warm or cold packs, and position changes.

Chapter *13*
Diarrhea

Rutledge and Engleking (1998) define diarrhea as an abnormal increase in liquidity and frequency, occurring as acute (within 24–48 hours of a stimulus, resolving in 7–14 days) or chronic (late onset, lasting > 2–3 weeks). Diarrhea occurring in patients with cancer is most often related to osmotic, absorptive, secretory, exudative, or motility dysfunction, or is chemotherapy-induced (Muehlbauer & Christine-Lopez, 2014).

- *Osmotic diarrhea* occurs as a result of hyperosmolar or nonabsorbable substances, which draw large volumes of fluid into the intestines, producing watery stools that usually resolve with removal of the cause. Causative factors include high-osmolality tube feedings, lactulose or sorbitol, and gastrointestinal hemorrhage.
- *Malabsorptive diarrhea* results from changes in mucosal integrity, causing changes in membrane permeability; or loss of absorptive surfaces, resulting in diarrhea that is large-volume, frothy, and foul-smelling (steatorrhea). Causes include deficiency of an enzyme responsible for digestion of fats (lactose intolerance, pancreatic insufficiency) or surgical resection or removal of the intestines.
- *Secretory diarrhea* results from intestinal hypersecretion of large volumes (> 1 L/day) of watery stool with an osmolality equal to that in the plasma. Causes are endocrine tumors (VIPoma and carcinoid), enterotoxin-producing pathogens such as *C. difficile*, acute graft-versus-host disease, and short gut syndrome.
- *Exudative diarrhea* is caused by inflammation or ulceration of the bowel mucosa, resulting in stools containing mucus, blood, and serum protein; the patient experiences frequent stooling, although the total volume is usually < 1 L/day. Unfortunately, this type of diarrhea is associated with hypoalbuminemia and anemia. Causes are radiation to the bowel (radiation enteritis) or opportunistic infection in the denuded bowel, such as with neutropenic typhlitis.
- *Dysmotility-associated diarrhea* is related to factors that increase or decrease normal peristalsis, such as with irritable bowel syndrome, the ingestion of food or medication that affects peristalsis, or psychological factors such as anxiety or fear that cause parasympathetic stimulation. Diarrhea of this type is usually semisolid to liquid, small, and frequent.
- *Chemotherapy-induced diarrhea* occurs as a result of chemotherapy-induced cell death of the intestinal mucosa, causing overstimulation of intestinal water and electrolyte secretion. The patient experiences frequent watery to semisolid stools within 24–96 hours of chemotherapy administration. With irinotecan chemotherapy, acute diarrhea occurs initially during or soon after administration related to cholinergic stimulation, and then delayed diarrhea occurs about 9–12 days later. In combination with 5-fluorouracil, the delayed diarrhea can lead to dehydration, and together with neutropenia, sepsis. Some of the most common drugs causing diarrhea are capecitabine,

5-FU, methotrexate, lapatinib, Interleukin-2, erlotinib, sorafenib, sunitinib, imatinib, and ipilumumab. Nurses play a very important role in teaching patients about the potential life-threatening diarrhea that may occur from this chemotherapy, self-administration of antidiarrheal medicines, increased fluid and diet modifications, and triage if these efforts are not effective.

Nurses are key in the management of diarrhea. Nurses play a significant role in patient assessment and patient/family teaching. Assessment of the patient's previous and current nutrition and elimination patterns, as well as assessment of probable etiology of diarrhea, are critical, as is patient/family teaching about the management and prevention of diarrhea. If the patient has no likely cause for diarrhea and it is persistent, then the nurse needs to discuss ruling out a micro-organism cause, such as *C. difficile* in a patient who is receiving antibiotics.

Patient teaching includes (Muehlbauer & Christine-Lopez, 2014):

- Fluids: Increase fluid intake to at least 8 oz fluid replacement per episode of diarrhea; goal is at least 8–10 (8-oz) glasses of fluid per day. Drink fluids at room temperature.
- Diet modification:
  - Eat 5–6 small, frequent meals instead of 3 large meals.
  - Eat foods high in soluble fiber (e.g., applesauce, oatmeal, bananas, cooked carrots, peeled potatoes, rice); foods low in insoluble fiber (e.g., rice, noodles, well-cooked eggs, bananas, white toast, canned or cooked fruit without skin, skinned turkey or chicken, fish, mashed potatoes); foods and fluids that are high in electrolytes (e.g., sodium and potassium) to replace those lost in diarrhea (broths and soups, bananas, peach nectar, oranges, peeled potatoes).
  - Avoid foods high in insoluble fiber (e.g., raw fruit and vegetables, whole grain bread, nuts, popcorn, skins, seeds, legumes), greasy, fried, and/or high-fat foods; spicy foods; foods and beverages containing lactose or supplements with lactase enzyme; hyperosmotic liquids (e.g., fruit juice, sweetened fruit drinks); caffeinated beverages; alcohol.
- Care of irritated skin, mucosa in perirectal area; critical in neutropenic or immunocompromised patients.
- Self-administration of prescribed antidiarrheal medication(s).
- Need for blood tests to assess electrolyte imbalance and hydration if diarrhea is severe. Diarrhea can lead to severe fluid and electrolyte imbalance, as well as significant patient discomfort. Common electrolyte imbalances related to diarrhea include metabolic acidosis, hypokalemia, hyperchloremia, hypocalcemia, and hypomagnesemia. Signs and symptoms of dehydration include fever; poor skin turgor; pallor; dry mucous membranes; thick saliva; lethargy; confusion; dizziness; rapid, weak, thready pulse; hypotension; and decreased urinary output. These increase the patient's risk of injury and should be prevented.

Ippoliti (1998) describes antidiarrheal agents as:

- *Intraluminal agents*: Decrease water in gut by absorption, increasing bulk of the stool, and protecting intestinal mucosa; includes absorbents such as activated charcoal and mucilloid preparations, and adsorbents such as psyllium, kaolin, and pectate; less commonly used as more effective agents available without possible drug interactions or difficulty ingesting them.

- *Intestinal transit inhibitors*: Primarily anticholinergic (atropine sulfate and scopolamine) and opiate agonists (DTO and the synthetic opioids diphenoxylate and loperamide), which slow down intestinal peristalsis and increase fluid absorption.
- *Proabsorptive agents*: Intraluminal absorbent agents as above.
- *Antisecretory agents*: Octreotide (Sandostatin) is a synthetic somatostatin analogue that inhibits the secretion of gut hormones like serotonin and motilin, and thus slows transit time and improves regulation of water and electrolyte movement in the gut. Bismuth subsalicylate (Pepto-Bismol) also works to decrease gut mucosal inflammation and hypermotility by binding to toxins and inhibiting prostaglandin synthesis.

References

Muehlbauer PM, Christine-Lopez R. (2014). Diarrhea. Chapter 10 in Yarbro CH, Wujuk D, Gobel BH (Eds.), *Cancer Symptom Management*, 4th ed. Burlington, MA: Jones & Bartlett Learning, 185–213.

Novartis Pharmaceuticals Corporation. Sandostatin LAR Depot (octreotide acetate for injectable suspension) [package insert]. East Hanover, NJ: Novartis Pharmaceuticals Corporation, July 2014.

Rutledge D, Engleking C. Cancer-related Diarrhea: Selected Findings of a National Survey of Oncology Nurse Experiences. *Oncol Nurs Forum* 1998; 25 861–878.

Drug: deodorized tincture of opium (DTO, Laudanum)

Class: Opium antidiarrheal agent.

Mechanism of Action: Increases GI smooth muscle tone and inhibits GI motility, delaying movement of intestinal contents; water is absorbed from fecal contents, decreasing diarrhea.

Metabolism: Variable absorption from GI tract; metabolized by liver and excreted in urine.

Indication: For the relief of diarrhea in adults.

Dosage/Range:
Adult:
- Oral: 0.3–1 mL qid (maximum 6 mL/day).

Drug Preparation:
- Store in tight, light-resistant bottle. Administer with water or juice.

Drug Interactions:
- None.

Lab Effects/Interference:
- None known.

Special Considerations:
- DTO contains 25 times more morphine than paregoric.
- Physical dependence may develop if drug is used chronically (e.g., colitis).

- Controlled substance.
- May be used in combination with kaolin and pectin mixtures.
- Do not use in diarrhea that results from poisoning until poison is removed (e.g., by lavage or cathartics).

Potential Toxicities/Side Effects and the Nursing Process

I. ALTERATION IN NUTRITION, LESS THAN BODY REQUIREMENTS, related to GI SIDE EFFECTS

Defining Characteristics: Nausea, vomiting may occur.

Nursing Implications: Assess baseline nutrition, GI status. If nausea/vomiting appears to follow dose administration, administer DTO with juice to disguise taste.

Drug: diphenoxylate hydrochloride and atropine (Lomotil)

Class: Antidiarrheal agent.

Mechanism of Action: Diphenoxylate is a synthetic opiate agonist that inhibits intestinal smooth muscle activity, thereby slowing peristalsis so that excess water is absorbed from feces. Atropine discourages deliberate overdosage.

Metabolism: Well absorbed from GI tract. Metabolized in liver. Excreted principally via feces in bile. Onset of action 45 minutes to 1 hour; duration 3–4 hours.

Indication: For the relief of diarrhea.

Dosage/Range:
Adult:
- Oral: 5 mg PO qid then titrate to response × 2 days (if no response in 48 hours, drug ineffective).

Drug Preparation:
- Oral: one tablet contains 2.5 mg diphenoxylate HCl and 0.025 mg atropine sulfate.

Drug Interactions:
- CNS depressants (alcohol, barbiturates): potentiate CNS depressant action; use together cautiously.
- MAOIs: may cause hypertensive crisis (similar structure to meperidine); use together cautiously.

Lab Effects/Interference:
- None known.

Special Considerations:
- May be habit-forming when used in high doses (40–60 mg); physical dependence.
- Use with extreme caution in patients with hepatic cirrhosis, as drug may precipitate hepatic coma, and in patients with acute ulcerative colitis.
- Contraindicated in patients with jaundice, diarrhea resulting from poisoning or pseudomembranous colitis caused by antibiotics.

COMPLICATIONS

Potential Toxicities/Side Effects and the Nursing Process

I.   ALTERATION IN NUTRITION, LESS THAN BODY REQUIREMENTS, related to GI SIDE EFFECTS

Defining Characteristics: Nausea, vomiting, abdominal distension or discomfort, anorexia, mouth dryness, and (rarely) paralytic ileus may occur.

Nursing Implications: Assess baseline nutrition and elimination status. Instruct patient to report signs and symptoms. Discuss drug discontinuance with physician. Instruct patient that drug should be used for 2 days and physician notified if diarrhea persists.

II.   ALTERATIONS IN SENSORY/PERCEPTUAL PATTERNS related to SEDATION

Defining Characteristics: Sedation, dizziness, lethargy, restlessness or insomnia, headache, paresthesia occur rarely with higher doses and prolonged therapy. Blurred vision may occur due to mydriasis.

Nursing Implications: Teach patient that drug is for short-term relief of diarrhea. Assess for and instruct patient to report signs/symptoms. Discuss drug discontinuance with physician if symptoms are severe.

III.   ALTERATION IN SKIN INTEGRITY related to RASH, SENSITIVITY

Defining Characteristics: Pruritus, angioedema (swelling of lips, face, gums), giant urticaria may occur.

Nursing Implications: Assess for and instruct patient to report signs/symptoms immediately. Drug should be discontinued if angioedema or giant urticaria occurs.

Drug: kaolin/pectin (Kaodene, K-P, Kaopectate, K-Pek)

Class: Antidiarrheal agent.

Mechanism of Action: Drug acts as absorbent and protectant; decreases stool fluidity but not total amount of fluid excreted.

Metabolism: Not absorbed from GI tract and excreted in stool.

Indication: For the relief of diarrhea.

Dosage/Range:
Adult:
- Oral: 60–120 mL regular or 45–90 mL concentrated suspension after each loose bowel movement < 48 hours.

Drug Preparation:
- Shake well prior to administration.

Drug Interactions:
* Oral lincomycin: decreases lincomycin absorption; administer kaolin/pectin at least 2 hours before or 3–4 hours after lincomycin dose.
* Oral digoxin: decreases digoxin absorption; administer kaolin/pectin 2 hours after digoxin dose.

Lab Effects/Interference:
* None known.

Special Considerations:
* Few adverse effects.
* Used for temporary relief of diarrhea.

Potential Toxicities/Side Effects and the Nursing Process

I. KNOWLEDGE DEFICIT related to SELF-ADMINISTRATION

Defining Characteristics: Transient constipation may occur.

Nursing Implications: Assess understanding of medication and self-administration schedule. Instruct patient in self-administration and to notify nurse/physician if diarrhea persists beyond 48 hours or fever develops. Reinforce need to drink fluids, especially in elderly or debilitated patients, to prevent constipation.

Drug: loperamide hydrochloride (Imodium)

Class: Antidiarrheal agent.

Mechanism of Action: Slows intestinal motility by inhibiting peristalsis (direct effect on circular and longitudinal intestinal muscles); increases stool bulk and viscosity.

Metabolism: Well absorbed from GI tract. Metabolized and small amounts are excreted in urine and feces as intact drug.

Dosage/Range:
Adult:
* Oral: 4 mg followed by 2 mg after each unformed stool (maximum 16 mg or higher if under direction of a physician; 8 mg per 24-hour period if self-medicating).

Indication: For the relief of diarrhea.

Drug Preparation:
* Oral.

Drug Interactions:
* None.

Lab Effects/Interference:
* None known.

COMPLICATIONS

Special Considerations:
- Reduces electrolyte and fluid loss from intestines; may be used to reduce volume of ileostomy drainage. 2–3 times more potent than diphenoxylate.
- Use cautiously in patients with acute ulcerative colitis; drug should be discontinued if abdominal distension occurs (risk of megacolon).
- Intended for self-medication × 48 hours; patients should be taught to notify nurse/physician if symptoms persist or fever occurs.
- Contraindicated in diarrhea due to pseudomembranous colitis (antibiotic-related), in acute diarrhea caused by mucosal-penetrating organisms (*Shigella, E. coli, Salmonella*), or if hypersensitivity to drug exists.
- Use cautiously in pregnant or nursing women.

Potential Toxicities/Side Effects and the Nursing Process

I.   ALTERATION IN NUTRITION, LESS THAN BODY REQUIREMENTS, related to GI SIDE EFFECTS

Defining Characteristics: Less frequent adverse reactions occur than with diphenoxylate/atropine. Nausea, vomiting, abdominal pain, and distension may occur.

Nursing Implications: Assess baseline nutrition and elimination status. Instruct patient to report signs and symptoms. Discuss drug discontinuance with physician. Instruct patient that drug should be used for 2 days and physician notified if diarrhea persists.

II.   ALTERATIONS IN SENSORY/PERCEPTUAL PATTERNS related to DROWSINESS

Defining Characteristics: Drowsiness, dizziness, fatigue may occur.

Nursing Implications: Teach patient that drug is for short-term relief of diarrhea. Assess for and instruct patient to report signs/symptoms. Discuss drug discontinuance with physician if symptoms are severe.

III.   ALTERATION IN SKIN INTEGRITY related to RASH, SENSITIVITY

Defining Characteristics: Rarely, rash may develop.

Nursing Implications: Assess baseline skin integrity. Instruct patient to report rash. Discuss drug discontinuance with physician.

Drug: octreotide acetate (Sandostatin)

Class: Cyclic octapeptide that mimics the pharmacologic actions of the natural hormone somatostatin and is long-acting. It is a somatostatin analogue.

Mechanism of Action: Drug is a more potent inhibitor than somatostatin of growth hormone, glucagon, insulin; also suppresses LH (luteinizing hormone) response to GnRH (gonadotropin-releasing hormone); decreases splanchnic blood flow; and inhibits release of serotonin, gastrin, vasoactive intestinal peptide (VIP), secretin, motilin, and pancreatic-polypeptide–like somatostatin. Stimulates fluid and electrolyte absorption from GI tract, and lengthens transit time of intestinal contents. Controls symptoms associated with carcinoid syndrome (e.g., flushing, levels of serotonin metabolite 5-HIAA), and VIP-secreting adenomas (e.g., watery diarrhea).

Metabolism: Absorbed rapidly and completely after injection, with peak concentrations after 24 minutes. Protein binding 65%, and eliminated from plasma with a half-life of 1.7 hours (natural hormone is 1–3 minutes). Duration of action approximately 12 hours, depending upon tumor type. Excreted in urine, with decreased clearance by 26% in the elderly. LAR Depot consists of biodegradable microspheres that slowly release octreotide from the injection site over 4 weeks. After IM injection, serum octreotide concentration reaches a transient initial peak within 1 hour, then declines over the next 3–5 days, then slowly increases to plateau 2–3 weeks post-injection. Steady state is reached by the third monthly injection.

Indication: (1) Reduce blood levels of growth hormone and IGF-I (somatomedin C) in acromegaly patients who have had an inadequate response to or cannot be treated with surgical resection, pituitary irradiation, and bromocriptine mesylate at maximally tolerated doses; (2) symptomatic treatment of patients with metastatic carcinoid tumors where it suppresses or inhibits the severe diarrhea and flushing episodes associated with the disease; (3) treatment of profuse, watery diarrhea associated with vasoactive intestinal peptide tumors (VIPomas).

Dosage/Range:
Indicated Usage (patients not currently receiving Sandostatin injection subcutaneously):
- Acromegaly: 50 micrograms three times daily Sandostatin injection subcutaneously for 2 weeks, followed by Sandostatin LAR Depot 20 mg intragluteally every 4 weeks for 3 months.
- Carcinoid tumors and VIPomas: Sandostatin injection subcutaneously 100–600 micrograms/day in 2–4 divided doses for 2 weeks, followed by Sandostatin LAR Depot 20 mg intragluteally every 4 weeks for 2 months.
- Vasoactive intestinal peptide tumors (VIPoma).
Indicated Usage (patients currently receiving Sandostatin injection subcutaneously):
- Acromegaly: 20 mg Sandostatin LAR intragluteally every 4 weeks for 3 months.
- Carcinoid and VIPomas: 20 mg Sandostatin LAR intragluteally every 4 weeks for 2 months.
- Renal impairment, patients on dialysis: 10 mg Sandostatin LAR every 4 weeks.
- Hepatic impairment, cirrhosis: 10 mg Sandostatin LAR every 4 weeks.
Other Usage (octreotide) (Sandostatin LAR Depot):
- Renal failure: drug half-life may be increased, requiring dosage adjustment.
Carcinoid Tumors and VIPomas:
- If patient is not currently on octreotide acetate, begin therapy with immediate-release dosing for 2 weeks: Carcinoid: 100–600 µg/d SQ in 2–4 divided doses (mean daily dose 300 µg), although some patients may require up to 1,500 µg/d; VIPoma: 200–300 µg/d SQ in 2–4 divided doses (range 150–750 µg), and dosage may be individualized to control symptoms, but usually does not exceed 450 µg/d.

COMPLICATIONS

- For patients who respond to the initial 2-week therapy, switch to Sandostatin LAR Depot 20 mg IM q 4 weeks × 2 months. In addition, since it will take at least 2 weeks to achieve steady state, the patient should ALSO continue to receive Sandostatin immediate-release dosing SQ for at least 2 weeks at the same dose as in the first 2 weeks. After 2 months of Sandostatin LAR Depot 20 mg, the dose may be increased to 30 mg q 4 weeks if symptoms are not controlled. Some patients who have their symptoms controlled on 20 mg q 4 weeks may be decreased to 10 mg q 4 weeks. Do not exceed a 30-mg dose.
- Some patients may have exacerbation of symptoms and require temporary additional immediate release, in addition to the LAR Depot, to control the increase in symptoms.

Acromegaly:

- If patient is not currently on octreotide acetate, begin therapy with immediate-release dosing q 8 h at an initial dose of 50 µg tid, and gradually increase as needed (based on growth hormone [GH] levels), as the goal is to normalize GH and IGF-1 (somatomedin C) levels. After 2 weeks, tolerability and response should be evident, so that patient can be changed to LAR Depot at a dose of 20 mg q 4 weeks if effective and well tolerated.
- For patients currently on octreotide, they can be changed directly to LAR Depot q 4 weeks, and at the end of 3 months, the LAR Depot dose should be titrated based on growth hormone level:
  - GH ≤ 2.5 ng/mL, IGF-1 (somatomedin C) normal and controlled symptoms, 20 mg IM (intragluteally) q 4 weeks.
  - GH > 2.5 ng/mL, IGF-1 elevated and/or uncontrolled symptoms, increase dose to 30 mg IM q 4 weeks.
  - GH ≤ 1 ng/mL, IGF-1 normal and controlled symptoms, reduce dose to 10 mg IM q 4 weeks.

Drug Preparation:
- Available in 1-mL (50-µg, 100-µg, 500-µg) ampules, and 5-mL (200-micrograms/mL and 1,000-micrograms/mL) multidose vials. Stable in solution in 0.9% sodium chloride or 5% dextrose in water for 24 hours; dilute drug in 50–200 mL of 0.9% sodium chloride or 5% dextrose for IV infusions over 15–30 minutes.
- Patient may develop pain, stinging, tingling, or burning sensation at injection site, with redness and swelling.

LAR Depot:
- Available in (5-mL) vials containing 10-, 20-, or 30-mg octreotide-free peptide; injection kit includes a syringe containing 2.5 mL of diluent, two sterile 1.5-inch 19-gauge needles, and two alcohol wipes, as well as instruction booklet.
- Allow drug vial and diluent-filled syringe to reach room temperature (30–60 minutes) prior to preparation of drug suspension.
- Drug must be administered immediately after mixing.
- Tap vial to ensure drug has settled to bottom of vial; aseptically inject diluent slowly down the inside wall of the vial while rotating the vial to evenly distribute the diluent using one of the needles. Allow to sit for 5 minutes or longer to assure full saturation of the drug powder; once saturated, swirl the vial gently for 30–60 seconds until a milky uniform suspension appears (DO NOT shake vigorously or invert the vial). Aseptically withdraw the ordered dose, holding the vial at 45 degrees. There will be some remaining suspension as the vial has overfill. Add a small amount of air into the syringe, and gently

rock back and forth until the patient is given the injection (DO NOT invert syringe). Eliminate air from the syringe.
- Replace needle with second needle, and aseptically administer drug immediately.

Administration:
- Immediate-release injection: administer SQ, IV over 15–30 minutes, or IVP over 3 minutes.
- LAR: Administer IM in gluteal muscle, as other sites are too painful (never give IV or SC) q 28 days.
- Record injection site and rotate sites.
- Teach patients the importance of adhering closely to scheduled return visits for next injection so symptoms do not become exacerbated.

Drug Interactions:
- May affect absorption of orally administered drugs.
- Cyclosporine: decreased serum levels of cyclosporine, resulting in transplant rejection.
- Insulin, oral hypoglycemic agents: octreotide inhibits insulin and glucagon secretion. Monitor serum glucose level and adjust antidiabetic therapy dose PRN.
- Beta-blockers: ↓ heart rate; assess patient response and need for dosage adjustment of these drugs.
- Bromocriptine: bromocriptine availability.
- Drugs metabolized by CYP3A4 with narrow therapeutic window (e.g., quinidine): use together cautiously and monitor closely.

Lab Effects/Interference:
- Hypoglycemia or hyperglycemia; monitor during therapy.
- Suppression of TSH may result in hypothyroidism and decreased total/free T_4.
- Decreased vitamin B_{12} levels (Shilling's test); monitor during therapy.

Special Considerations:
- Sandostatin LAR Depot is indicated for patients in whom initial treatment with Sandostatin Injection has been shown to be effective and tolerated: (1) carcinoid tumors: the long-term treatment of severe diarrhea and flushing episodes, (2) VIPomas: long-term treatment of profuse watery diarrhea, (3) acromegaly: long-term maintenance therapy that requires medical treatment.
- Octreotide acetate is appropriate when other conventional antidiarrheal medications have failed, and other treatable causes of diarrhea have been excluded (e.g., obstruction, infection).
- Patient should be taught sterile SQ injection technique for immediate-release preparations.
- Laboratory test monitoring (efficacy) based on treatment intent:
  - Carcinoid: 5-HIAA (urinary 5-hydroxyindoleacetic acid), plasma substance P, and serotonin.
  - VIPoma: VIP (plasma vasoactive intestinal peptide) baseline and periodic total and/or free T_4.
  - Acromegaly: growth hormone, IGF-1 (somatomedin C).
- Adverse reactions of diabetes mellitus, hypothyroidism, and cardiovascular disease occur in patients treated for acromegaly.

COMPLICATIONS

- May change to long-acting depot if already controlled on immediate-release preparation, or in a new patient, after response is assessed after 2 weeks of immediate-release dosing.
- Drug inhibits gallbladder contraction and decreases bile secretion, which may lead to gallstones and biliary sludge. Monitor periodically.
- Drug may rarely cause alterations in hormonal levels, so patients receiving long-term therapy should be monitored baseline and periodically during treatment: glucose, glucose tolerance in patients receiving antidiabetic drugs, thyroid function (TSH, total and/ or free T_4), B_{12} level, and zinc level in patients receiving TPN.
- Hypoglycemia or hyperglycemia may occur. Monitor glucose closely, and antidiabetic treatment may need to be adjusted.
- Drug may significantly suppress thyroid-stimulating hormone (TSH), causing hypothyroidism; monitor thyroid levels periodically.
- In patients with acromegaly or carcinoid, drug may rarely cause cardiac abnormalities such as bradycardia (HR < 50 bpm), QT prolongation, nonspecific ST segment changes, and worsening of CHF; use drug cautiously in patients with cardiac risk factors. Drug may cause visual field defects in patients with growth-hormone–secreting tumors.

Potential Toxicities/Side Effects (dose- and schedule-dependent) and the Nursing Process

I.   ALTERATION IN NUTRITION, LESS THAN BODY REQUIREMENTS, related to CARBOHYDRATE METABOLISM

Defining Characteristics: Rarely, transient hypoglycemia or hyperglycemia due to altered balance between hormones regulating serum glucose (insulin, glucagon, growth hormone). Rarely, diarrhea, nausea and vomiting, abdominal pain, or discomfort. Incidence 3–10%. Drug may alter absorption of dietary fats.

Nursing Implications: Assess baseline nutritional balance. Instruct patient to report any changes, and assess for hyperglycemia (drowsiness, dry mouth, flushing, dry skin, fruity breath, polyuria, polydipsia, polyphagia, weight loss, stomach ache, nausea/vomiting, fatigue), hypoglycemia (anxiety, chills, cool/pale skin, difficulty concentrating, headache, hunger, shakiness, diaphoresis, fatigue, weakness, nausea). If patient is hypoglycemic, teach patient to carry candy. Monitor serum glucose, and discuss alterations with physician. Treat nausea and vomiting symptomatically, and discuss need for antiemetic if significant.

II.   ALTERATION IN COMFORT related to HEADACHE, FLUSHING

Defining Characteristics: Rarely (1–3%) patient may experience lightheadedness, dizziness, fatigue, pedal edema, headache, flushing of the face, weakness. Back and abdominal pain may also occur, as can injection-site pain.

Nursing Implications: Assess baseline comfort, and instruct patient to report any changes. Assess safety, and manage symptoms symptomatically. If unrelieved or significant, discuss with physician. Rotate injection sites, and teach patient local comfort measures at injection site.

Appendix 1
Occupational Exposure to Hazardous Drugs

A. Introduction

In response to numerous inquiries,[1] the Occupational Safety and Health Administration (OSHA) published guidelines for the management of cytotoxic (antineoplastic) drugs in the workplace in 1986.[106] At that time, surveys indicated little standardization in the use of engineering controls and personal protective equipment (PPE).[56, 73] Although practices have improved in subsequent years, problems still exist.[111] In addition, the occupational management of these chemicals has been further clarified. These trends, in conjunction with many information requests, have prompted OSHA to revise its recommendations for hazardous drug handling. In addition, some of these agents are covered under the Hazard Communication Standard (HCS) (29 CFR 1910.1200).[107] In order to provide recommendations consistent with current scientific knowledge, this informational guidance document has been expanded to cover hazardous drugs (HDs), in addition to the cytotoxic drugs (CDs) that were covered in the 1986 guidelines. The recommendations apply to all settings where employees are occupationally exposed to HDs, such as hospitals, physicians' offices, and home healthcare agencies. This review will:

- Provide criteria for classifying drugs as hazardous.
- Summarize the evidence supporting the management of HDs as an occupational hazard.
- Discuss the equipment and worker education recommended, as well as the legal requirements of standards, for the protection of workers exposed and potentially exposed to HDs.
- Update the important aspects of medical surveillance.
- List some common HDs currently in use.

Anesthetic agents have not been considered in this review. However, exposure to some of these agents is a recognized health hazard,[104] and they have been considered in a separate Technical Manual Chapter.

B. Categorization of Drugs as Hazardous

The purpose of this section is to describe the biologic effects of those pharmaceuticals that are considered hazardous. A number of pharmaceuticals in the healthcare setting may pose occupational risk to employees through acute and chronic workplace exposure. Past attention focused on drugs used to treat cancer. However, it is clear that many other agents also have toxicity profiles of concern. This recognition prompted the American Society of Hospital Pharmacists (ASHP) to define a class of agents as "hazardous drugs."[3] That report specified concerns about antineoplastic and nonantineoplastic hazardous drugs in use in most institutions throughout the country. OSHA shares this concern. The ASHP Technical

Assistance Bulletin (TAB) described four drug characteristics, each of which could be considered hazardous:

- Genotoxicity.
- Carcinogenicity.
- Teratogenicity or fertility impairment.
- Serious organ or other toxic manifestation at low doses in experimental animals or treated patients.

Table A.1 lists some common drugs that are considered hazardous by the above criteria. There is no standardized reference for this information, nor is there complete consensus on all agents listed. Professional judgment by personnel trained in pharmacology/ toxicology is essential in designating drugs as hazardous, and Reference 65 provides information regarding the development of such a list at one institution. Some drugs, which have a long history of safe use in humans despite in vitro or animal evidence to toxicity, may be excluded by the institution's experts by considerations such as those used to formulate GRAS (generally regarded as safe) lists by the FDA under the Food, Drug, and Cosmetics Act.

Table A.1   Some Common Drugs Considered Hazardous

Chemical/Generic Name	Source*
ALTRETAMINE	C
AMINOGLUTETHIMIDE	A
AZATHIOPRINE	ACE
L-ASPARAGINASE	ABC
BLEOMYCIN	ABC
BUSULFAN	ABC
CARBOPLATIN	ABC
CARMUSTINE	ABC
CHLORAMBUCIL	ABCE
CHLORAMPHENICOL	E
CHLOROTRIANISENE	B
CHLOROZOTOCIN	E
CISPLATIN	ABCE
CYCLOSPORIN	E
CYCLOPHOSPHAMIDE	ABCE

(continued)

Table A.1 *(Continued)*

Chemical/Generic Name	Source*
CYTARABINE	ABC
DACARBAZINE	ABC
DACTINOMYCIN	ABC
DAUNORUBICIN	ABC
DIETHYLSTILBESTROL	BE
DOXORUBICIN	ABCE
ESTRADIOL	B
ESTRAMUSTINE	AB
ETHINYL ESTRADIOL	B
ETOPOSIDE	ABC
FLOXURIDINE	AC
FLUOROURACIL	ABC
FLUTAMIDE	BC
GANCICLOVIR	AD
HYDROXYUREA	ABC
IDARUBICIN	AC
IFOSFAMIDE	ABC
INTERFERON-α	BC
ISOTRETINOIN	D
LEUPROLIDE	BC
LEVAMISOLE	C
LOMUSTINE	ABCE
MECHLORETHAMINE	BC
MEDROXYPROGESTERONE	B
MEGESTROL	BC
MELPHALAN	ABCE
MERCAPTOPURINE	ABC
METHOTREXATE	ABC
MITOMYCIN	ABC
MITOTANE	ABC
MITOXANTRONE	ABC

(continued)

Table A.1   *(Continued)*

Chemical/Generic Name	Source*
NAFARELIN	C
PIPOBROMAN	C
PLICAMYCIN	BC
PROCARBAZINE	ABCE
RIBAVIRIN	D
STREPTOZOCIN	AC
TAMOXIFEN	BC
TESTOLACTONE	BC
THIOGUANINE	ABC
THIOTEPA	ABC
URACIL MUSTARD	ACE
VIDARABINE	D
VINBLASTINE	ABC
VINCRISTINE	ABC
ZIDOVUDINE	D

*Sources:
A The National Institutes of Health, Clinical Center Nursing Department
B Antineoplastic drugs in the *Physicians' Desk Reference*
C American Hospital Formulary, Antineoplastics
D Johns Hopkins Hospital
E International Agency for Research on Cancer

Table A.1 is not all-inclusive, should not be construed as complete, and represents an assessment of some, but not all, marketed drugs at a fixed point in time. Table A.1 was developed through consultation with institutions that have assembled teams of pharmacists and other healthcare personnel to determine which drugs should be used with caution. These teams reviewed product literature and drug information when considering each product.

Sources for this appendix are the *Physicians' Desk Reference,* Section 10:00 in the American Hospital Formulary Service Drug Information,[68] IARC publications (particularly Volume 50),[43] the Johns Hopkins Hospital, and the National Institutes of Health, Clinical Center Nursing Department. No attempt to include investigational drugs was made, but they should be prudently handled as hazardous drugs until adequate information becomes available to exclude them. Any determination of the hazard status of drugs should be periodically reviewed and updated as new information becomes available. Importantly, new drugs should routinely undergo a hazard assessment.

List of Abbreviations

ANSI	American National Standards Institute
ASHP	American Society of Hospital Pharmacists
BSC	Biological safety cabinet
CD	Cytotoxic drug
EPA	Environmental Protection Agency
HCS	Hazard communication standard
HD	Hazardous drug
HEPA	High-efficiency particulate air
IARC	International Agency for Research on Cancer
MSDS	Material safety data sheet
NIOSH	National Institute for Occupational Safety and Health
NTP	National Toxicology Program
OSHA	Occupational Safety and Health Administration
PPE	Personal protective equipment

In contrast, investigational drugs are new chemicals for which there is often little information on potential toxicity. Structure or activity relationships with similar chemicals and in vitro data can be considered in determining potential toxic effects. Investigational drugs should be prudently handled as HDs unless adequate information becomes available to exclude them.

Some major considerations by professionals trained in pharmacology/toxicology[65] in designating a drug as hazardous are:

- Is the drug designated as Therapeutic Category 10:00 (Antineoplastic Agent) in the American Hospital Formulary Service Drug Information?[68]
- Does the manufacturer suggest the use of special isolation techniques in its handling, administration, or disposal?
- Is the drug known to be a human mutagen, carcinogen, teratogen, or reproductive toxicant?
- Is the drug known to be carcinogenic or teratogenic in animals? (Drugs known to be mutagenic in multiple bacterial systems or animals should also be considered hazardous.)
- Is the drug known to be acutely toxic to an organ system?

C. Background: Hazardous Drugs as Occupational Risk

Preparation, administration, and disposal of HDs may expose pharmacists, nurses, physicians, and other healthcare workers to potentially significant workplace levels of these chemicals. The literature establishing these agents as occupational hazards deals primarily with CDs; however, documentation of adverse exposure effects from other HDs is rapidly accumulating.[15,40–43,59] The degree of absorption that takes place during work and the significance of secondary early biologic effects on each individual encounter are difficult to assess and may vary depending on the HD. As a result, it is difficult to set safe levels of exposure on the basis of current scientific information.

However, there are several lines of evidence supporting the toxic potential of these drugs if handled improperly. Therefore, it is essential to minimize exposure to all HDs. Summary tables of much of the data presented below can be found in Sorsa[95] and Rogers.[84]

1. Mechanism of Action

Most HDs either bind directly to genetic material in the cell nucleus or affect cellular protein synthesis. Cytotoxic drugs may not distinguish between normal and cancerous cells. The growth and reproduction of the normal cells are often affected during treatment of cancerous cells.

2. Animal Data

Numerous studies document the carcinogenic, mutagenic, and teratogenic effects of HD exposure in animals. They are well summarized in the pertinent IARC publications.[37–43] Alkylating agents present the strongest evidence of carcinogenicity (e.g., cyclophosphamide, mechlorethamine hydrochloride [nitrogen mustard]). However, other classes, such as some antibiotics, have been implicated as well. Extensive evidence for mutagenic and reproductive effects can be found in all antineoplastic classes. The antiviral agent *ribavirin* has additionally been shown to be teratogenic in all rodent species tested.[31,49] The ASHP recommends that all pharmaceutical agents that are animal carcinogens be handled as if human carcinogens.

3. Human Data at Therapeutic Levels

Many HDs are known human carcinogens, for which there is no safe level of exposure. The development of secondary malignancies is a well-documented side effect of chemotherapy treatment.[52,86,90,115] Leukemia has been most frequently observed. However, other secondary malignancies, such as bladder cancer and lymphoma, have been documented in patients treated for other, usually solid, primary malignancies.[52,114] Chromosomal aberrations can result from chemotherapy treatment as well. One study, on *chlorambucil,* reveals chromosomal damage in recipients to be cumulative and related to both dose and duration of therapy.[77]

Numerous case reports have linked chemotherapeutic treatment to adverse reproductive outcomes.[7,88,91,98] Testicular and ovarian dysfunction, including permanent sterility, have occurred in male and female patients who have received CDs either singly or in combination.[14] In addition, some antineoplastic agents are known or suspected to be transmitted to infants through breastmilk.[79]

The literature also documents the effects of these drugs on other organ systems. Extravasation of some agents can cause severe soft-tissue injury, consisting of necrosis and sloughing of exposed areas.[23,78,87] Other HDs, such as *pentamidine* and *zidovudine* (formerly

AZT), are known to have significant side effects (i.e., hematologic abnormalities) in treated patients.[4,33] Serum transaminase elevation has also been reported in treated patients.[4,33]

4. Occupational Exposure—Airborne Levels

Monitoring efforts for cytotoxic drugs have detected measurable air levels when exhaust biological safety cabinets (BSCs) were not used for preparation or when monitoring was performed inside the BSC.[50,73]

Concentrations of *fluorouracil* ranging from 0.12 to 82.26 ng/m^3 have been found during monitoring of drug preparation without a BSC implying an opportunity for respiratory exposure.[73] Elevated concentrations of *cyclophosphamide* were found by these authors as well. Cyclophosphamide has also been detected on the HEPA filters of flow hoods used in HD preparation, demonstrating aerosolization of the drug and an exposure opportunity mitigated by effective engineering controls.[81]

A recent study has reported wipe samples of cyclophosphamide, one of the Class I IARC carcinogens, on surfaces of work stations in an oncology pharmacy and outpatient treatment areas (sinks and countertops). Concentrations ranged from 0.005 to 0.03 µg/cm^2, documenting opportunity for dermal exposure.[60]

Administration of drugs via aerosolization can lead to measurable air concentrations in the breathing zone of workers providing treatment. Concentrations up to 18 µg/m^3 have been found by personal air sampling of workers administering *pentamidine*.[67] Similar monitoring for *ribavirin* has found concentrations as high as 316 µg/m.[3,31]

5. Occupational Exposure—Biologic Evidence of Absorption
Urinary Mutagenicity
Falck et al. were the first to note evidence of mutagenicity in the urine of nurses who handled cytotoxic drugs.[26] The extent of this effect increased over the course of the work week. With improved handling practices, a decrease in mutagenic activity was seen.[27] Researchers have also studied pharmacy personnel who reconstitute antineoplastic drugs. These employees showed increasingly mutagenic urine over the period of exposure; when they stopped handling the drugs, activity fell within 2 days to the level of unexposed controls.[5,76] They also found mutagenicity in workers using horizontal laminar flow BSCs that decreased to control levels with the use of vertical flow containment BSCs.[76] Other studies have failed to find a relationship between exposure and urine mutagenicity.[25] Sorsa[95] summarizes this information and discusses the factors, such as differences in urine collection timing and variations in the use of PPE, which could lead to disparate results. Differences may also be related to smoking status; smokers exposed to CDs exhibit greater urine mutagenicity than exposed nonsmokers or control smokers, suggesting contamination of the work area by CDs and some contribution of smoking to their mutagenic profile.[9]

Urinary Thioethers
Urinary thioethers are glutathione-conjugated metabolites of alkylating agents that have been evaluated as an indirect means of measuring exposure. Workers who handle cytotoxic drugs have been reported to have increased levels compared to controls and also have

increasing thioether levels over a 5-day work week.[44,48] Other studies of nurses who handle CDs and of treated patients have yielded variable results that could be due to confounding by smoking, PPE, and glutathione-S-transferase activity.[11]

Urinary Metabolites

Venitt[112] assayed the urine of pharmacy and nursing personnel handling cisplatin and found platinum concentrations at or below the limit of detection for both workers and controls. Hirst[35] found *cyclophosphamide* in the urine of two nurses who handled the drug, documenting worker absorption. (Hirst also documented skin absorption in human volunteers by using gas chromatography after topical application of the drug.) Urinary *pentamidine* recovery has also been reported in exposed healthcare workers.[94]

6. Occupational Exposure—Human Effects

Cytogenetic Effects

A number of studies have examined the relationship of exposure to CDs in the workplace to chromosomal aberrations. These studies have looked at a variety of markers for damage, including sister chromatid exchanges (SCE), structural aberrations (e.g., gaps, breaks, translocations), and micronuclei in peripheral blood lymphocytes. The results have been somewhat conflicting. Several authors found increases in one or more markers.[74,75,88,113] Increased mutilation frequency has been reported as well.[17] Other studies have failed to find a significant difference between workers and controls.[99,101] Some researchers have found higher individual elevations[28] or a relationship between number of drugs handled and SCEs.[8] These disparate results are not unexpected. The difficulties in quantitating exposure have resulted in different exposure magnitudes between studies; workers in several negative studies appear to have a lower overall exposure.[10] In addition, differences in the use of PPE and work technique will alter absorption of CDs and resultant biologic effects.

Finally, techniques for SCE measurement may not be optimal. A recent study that looked at correlation of phosphoramide-induced SCE levels with duration of anticancer drug handling found a statistically significant correlation coefficient of 0.[63,66]

Taken together, the evidence indicates an excess of markers of mutagenic exposure in unprotected workers.

Reproductive Effects

Reproductive effects associated with occupational exposure to CDs have been well documented. Hemminki et al.[32] found no difference in exposure between nurses who had spontaneous abortions and those who had normal pregnancies. However, the study group consisted of nurses who were employed in surgical or medical floors of a general hospital. When the relationship between CD exposure and congenital malformations was explored, the study group was expanded to include oncology nurses, among others, and an odds ratio of 4:7 was found for exposures of more than once per week. This observed odds ratio is statistically significant. Selevan et al.[39] found a relationship between CD exposure and spontaneous abortion in a case-control study of Finnish nurses. This well-designed study reviewed the reproductive histories of 568 women (167 cases) and found a statistically significant odds ratio of 2:3. Similar results were obtained in another large case-control study of French nurses,[102] and a study of Baltimore area nurses found a significantly higher proportion of adverse pregnancy outcomes when exposure to antineoplastic agents occurred during the pregnancy.[85] The nurses involved in these studies usually prepared and administered the drugs. Therefore, workplace exposure of these groups of professionals to such products has been associated with adverse reproductive outcomes in several investigations.

Other Effects

Hepatocellular damage has been reported in nurses working in an oncology ward; the injury appeared to be related to intensity and duration of work exposure to CDs.[96] Symptoms such as lightheadedness, dizziness, nausea, headache, and allergic reactions have also been described in employees after the preparation and administration of antineoplastic drugs in unventilated areas.[22,96] In occupational settings, these agents are known to be toxic to the skin and mucous membranes, including the cornea.[69,82]

Pentamidine has been associated with respiratory damage in one worker who administered the aerosol. The injury consisted of a decrease in diffusing capacity that improved after exposure ceased.[29] The onset of bronchospasm in a pentamidine-exposed worker has also been reported.[22] Employees involved in the aerosol administration of *ribavirin* have noted symptoms of respiratory tract irritation.[55] A number of medications including *psyllium* and various antibiotics are known respiratory and dermal sensitizers. Exposure in susceptible individuals can lead to asthma or allergic contact dermatitis.

D. Work Areas

Risks to personnel working with HDs are a function of the drugs' inherent toxicity and the extent of exposure. The main routes of exposure are: inhalation of dusts or aerosols, dermal absorption, and ingestion. The primary means of ingestion is contact with contaminated food or cigarettes. Opportunity for exposure to HDs may occur at many points in the handling of these drugs.

1. Pharmacy or Other Preparation Areas

In large oncology centers, HDs are usually prepared in the pharmacy. However, in small hospitals, outpatient treatment areas, and physicians' offices they have been prepared by physicians or nurses without appropriate engineering controls and protective apparel.[16,20] Many HDs must be reconstituted, transferred from one container to another, or manipulated before administration to patients. Even if care is taken, opportunity for absorption through inhalation or direct skin contact can occur.[35,36,73,116] Examples of manipulations that can cause splattering, spraying, and aerosolization include:

- Withdrawal of needles from drug vials.
- Drug transfer using syringes and needles or filter straws.
- Breaking open of ampoules.
- Expulsion of air from a drug-filled syringe.

Evaluation of these preparation techniques, using fluorescent dye solutions, has shown contamination of gloves and the sleeves and chest of gowns.[97]

Horizontal airflow workbenches provide an aseptic environment for the preparation of injectable drugs. However, these units provide a flow of filtered air originating at the back of the workspace and exiting toward the employee using the unit. Thus, they increase the likelihood of drug exposure for both the preparer and other personnel in the room. As a result, the use of horizontal BSCs is contraindicated in the preparation of HDs. Smoking, drinking, applying cosmetics, and eating where these drugs are prepared, stored, or used also increase the chance of exposure.

2. Administration of Drugs to Patients

Administration of drugs to patients is generally performed by nurses or physicians. Drug injection into the IV line, clearing of air from the syringe or infusion line, and leakage at the tubing, syringe, or stopcock connection present opportunities for skin contact and aerosol generation. Clipping used needles and crushing used syringes can produce considerable aerosolization as well.

Such techniques where needles and syringes are contaminated with blood or other potentially infectious material are prohibited by the Bloodborne Pathogens Standard.[109] Prohibition of clipping or crushing of any needle or syringe is sound practice.

Excreta from patients who have received certain antineoplastic drugs may contain high concentrations of the drug or its hazardous metabolites. For example, patients receiving *cyclophosphamide* excrete large amounts of the drug and its mutagenic metabolites.[46,92] Patients treated with *cisplatin* have been shown to excrete potentially hazardous amounts of the drug.[112] Unprotected handling of urine or urine-soaked sheets by nursing or housekeeping personnel poses a source of exposure.

3. Disposal of Drugs and Contaminated Materials

Contaminated materials used in the preparation and administration of HDs, such as gloves, gowns, syringes, and vials, present a hazard to support and housekeeping staff. The use of properly labeled, sealed, and covered disposal containers, handled by trained and protected personnel, should be routine and is required under the Bloodborne Pathogens Standard[109] if such items are contaminated with blood or other potentially infectious materials. HDs and contaminated materials should be disposed of in accordance with federal, state, and local laws. Disposal of some of these drugs is regulated by the EPA. Those drugs that are unused commercial chemical products and are considered by the EPA to be toxic wastes must be disposed of in accordance with 40 CFR Part 261.33.[24] Spills can also represent a hazard; the employer should ensure that all employees are familiar with appropriate spill procedures.

4. Survey of Current Work Practices

Surveys of U.S. cancer centers and oncology clinics reveal wide variation in work practices, equipment, or training for personnel preparing CDs.[56,73] This lack of standardization results in a high prevalence of potential occupational exposure to CDs. One survey found that 40% of hospital pharmacists reported a skin exposure to CDs at least once a month, and only 28% had medical surveillance programs in their workplace.[16] Nurses, particularly those in outpatient settings, were found to be even less well protected than pharmacists.[111] Such findings emphasize current lack of protection for all personnel who risk potential exposure to HDs.

E. Prevention of Employee Exposure

1. Hazardous Drug Safety and Health Plan

Where hazardous drugs, as defined in this review, are used in the workplace, sound practice would dictate that a written Hazardous Drug Safety and Health Plan be developed. Such a plan assists in:

- Protecting employees from health hazards associated with HDs.
- Keeping exposures as low as reasonably achievable.

When a Hazardous Drug Safety and Health Plan is developed, it should be readily available and accessible to all employees, including temporary employees, contractors, and trainees.

The ASHP recommends that the plan include each of the following elements and indicate specific measures that the employer is taking to ensure employee protection:[3]

- Standard operating procedures relevant to safety and health considerations to be followed when healthcare workers are exposed to hazardous drugs.
- Criteria that the employer uses to determine and implement control measures to reduce employee exposure to hazardous drugs including engineering controls, the use of PPE, and hygiene practices.
- A requirement that ventilation systems and other protective equipment function properly, and specific measures to ensure proper and adequate performance of such equipment.
- Provision for information and training.
- The circumstances under which the use of specific HDs (i.e., FDA investigational drugs) require prior approval from the employer before implementation.
- Provision for medical examinations of potentially exposed personnel.
- Designation of personnel responsible for implementation of the Hazardous Drug Safety and Health Plan, including the assignment of a Hazardous Drug Officer (who is an industrial hygienist, nurse, or pharmacist health and safety representative); and, if appropriate, establishment of a Hazardous Drug Committee or a joint Hazardous Drug Committee/ Chemical Committee.

The ASHP further recommends that specific consideration of the following provisions be included where appropriate:

- Establishment of a designated HD handling area.
- Use of containment devices such as BSCs.
- Procedures for safe removal of contaminated waste.
- Decontamination procedures.

The ASHP recommends that the Hazardous Drug Safety and Health Plan be reviewed and its effectiveness reevaluated at least annually and updated as necessary.

A comparison of OSHA 200 log entries to employee medical clinic appointment or visit rosters can be made[3] to establish if there is evidence of disorders that could be related to hazardous drug.

Previous health and safety inspections by local health departments, fire departments, regulatory or accrediting agencies may be helpful for the facility's planning purposes, as well as any OSHA review of hazards and programs in the facility. Joint Commission on Accreditation of Healthcare Organizations (JCAHO) or College of American Pathologists (CAP) review of facilities may contain information on hazardous drugs used in the facility.

2. Drug Preparation Precautions

Work Area

The ASHP recommends that HD preparation be performed in a restricted, preferably centralized, area. Signs restricting the access of unauthorized personnel are to be prominently displayed. Eating, drinking, smoking, chewing gum, applying cosmetics, and storing food in the preparation area should be prohibited.[71] The ASHP recommends that procedures for spills and emergencies, such as skin or eye contact, be available to workers, preferably posted in the area.[3]

Biological Safety Cabinets

Class II or III BSCs that meet the current National Sanitation Foundation Standard 49[70,72] should minimize exposure to HDs during preparation. Although these cabinets are designed for biohazards, several studies have documented reduced urine mutagenicity in CD-exposed workers or reduce environmental levels after the institution of BSCs.[5,51,61] If a BSC is unavailable—for example, in a private practice office—accepted medical practice is the sharing of a cabinet (e.g., several medical offices share a cabinet) or sending the patient to a center where HDs can be prepared in a BSC. Alternatively, preparation can be performed in a facility with a BSC and the drugs transported to the area of administration. Use of a dedicated BSC, where only HDs are prepared, is prudent medical practice.

Types of BSCs

Four main types of Class II BSCs are available. They all have downward airflow and HEPA filters. They are differentiated by the amount of air recirculated within the cabinet, whether this air is vented to the room or the outside, and whether contaminated ducts are under positive or negative pressure. These four types are:

- Type A cabinets recirculate approximately 70% of cabinet air through HEPA filters back into the cabinet; the rest is discharged through a HEPA filter into the preparation room. Contaminated ducts are under positive pressure.
- Type B1 cabinets have higher velocity air inflow, recirculate 30% of the cabinet air, and exhaust the rest to the outside through HEPA filters. They have negative pressure contaminated ducts and plenums.
- Type B2 systems are similar to type B1 except that no air is recirculated.

- Type B3 cabinets are similar to type A in that they recirculate approximately 70% of cabinet air. However, the other 30% is vented to the outside and the ducts are under negative pressure.

Class III cabinets are totally enclosed with gas-tight construction. The entire cabinet is under negative pressure, and operations are performed through attached gloves. All air is HEPA-filtered.

Class II, type B, or Class III BSCs are recommended since they vent to the outside.[3] Those without air recirculation are the most protective. If the BSC has an outside exhaust, it should be vented away from air intake units.

The blower on the vertical airflow hood should be on at all times. If the BSC is turned off, it should be decontaminated and covered in plastic until airflow is resumed.[3,72] Each BSC should be equipped with a continuous monitoring device to allow confirmation of adequate air flow and cabinet performance. The cabinet should be in an area with minimal air turbulence; this will reduce leakage to the environment.[6,70] Additional information on design and performance testing of BSCs can be found in papers by Avis and Levchuck,[6] Bryan and Marback,[10] and the National Sanitation Foundation.[70] Practical information regarding space needs and conversion possibilities is contained in the ASHP's 1990 technical assistance bulletins.[3]

Ventilation and BSCs installed should be maintained and evaluated for proper performance in accordance with the manufacturer's instructions.

Decontamination

The cabinet should be cleaned according to the manufacturer's instructions. Some manufacturers have recommended weekly decontamination as well as whenever spills occur or when the cabinet requires moving, service, or certification.

Decontamination should consist of surface cleaning with water and detergent, followed by thorough rinsing. The use of detergent is recommended because there is no single accepted method of chemical deactivation for all agents involved.[13,45] Quaternary ammonium cleaners should be avoided due to the possibility of vapor buildup in recirculated air.[3] Ethyl alcohol or 70% isopropyl alcohol may be used with the cleaner if the contamination is soluble only in alcohol.[3] Alcohol vapor buildup has also been a concern, so the use of alcohol should be avoided in BSCs where air is recirculated.[3] Spray cleaners should also be avoided due to the risk of spraying the HEPA filter. Ordinary decontamination procedures, which include fumigation with a germicidal agent, are inappropriate in a BSC used for HDs because such procedures do not remove or deactivate the drugs.

Removable work trays, if present, should be lifted in the BSC, so the back and the sump below can be cleaned. During cleaning, the worker should wear PPE similar to that used for spills. *Ideally, the sash should remain down during cleaning; however, a NIOSH-approved respirator appropriate for the hazard must be worn by the worker if the sash will be lifted during the process.* The exhaust fan/blower should be left on. Cleaning should proceed from least to most contaminated areas. The drain spillage trough area should be cleaned twice since it can be heavily contaminated. All materials from the decontamination process should be handled as HDs and disposed of in accordance with federal, state, and local laws.

Service and Certification

The ASHP recommends that BSCs be serviced and certified by a qualified technician every 6 months or any time the cabinet is moved or repaired.[3,71] Technicians servicing these cabinets or changing the HEPA filters should be aware of HD risk through hazard communication training from their employers and should use the same PPE as recommended for large spills. Certification of the BSC includes performance testing as outlined in the procedures of the National Sanitation Foundation's Standard Number 49.[70] Helpful information on such testing can be found in the ASHP 1990 technical assistance bulletins,[3] the BSC manufacturer's equipment manuals, and Bryan and Marback's paper.[10] HEPA filters should be changed when they restrict air flow or if they are contaminated by an accidental spill. They should be bagged in plastic and disposed of as HDs. Any time the cabinet is turned off or transported, it should be sealed with plastic.

Personal Protective Equipment

1. Gloves

Research indicates that the thickness of gloves used in handling HDs is more important than the type of material, since all materials tested have been found to be permeable to some HDs.[3,19,53] The best results are seen with latex gloves. Therefore, latex gloves should be used for the preparation of HDs unless the drug-product manufacturer specifically stipulates that some other glove provides better protection.[19,53,72,93,100] Thicker, longer latex gloves that cover the gown cuff are recommended for use with HDs. *Individuals with latex allergy should consider the use of vinyl or nitrile gloves or glove liners.* Gloves with minimal or no powder are preferred since the powder may absorb contamination.[3,104]

The sources referenced here have noted great variability in permeability within and between glove lots. Therefore, double gloving is recommended if it does not interfere with an individual's technique.[3] Because all gloves are permeable to some extent and their permeability increases with time, they should be changed regularly (hourly) or immediately if they are torn, punctured, or contaminated with a spill. Hands should always be washed before gloves are put on and after they are removed. Employees need thorough training in proper methods for contaminated glove removal.

2. Gowns

A protective disposable gown made of lint-free, low-permeability fabric with a closed front, long sleeves, and elastic or knit closed cuff should be worn. The cuffs should be tucked under the gloves. If double gloves are worn, the outer glove should be over the gown cuff and the inner glove should be under the gown cuff. When the gown is removed, the inner glove should be removed last. Gowns and gloves in use in the HD preparation area should not be used outside the HD preparation area.[3]

As with gloves, there is no ideal material. Research has found nonporous Tyvek and Kaycel to be more permeable than Saranex-laminated Tyvek and polyethylene-coated Tyvek after 4 hours of exposure to the CDs tested.[54] However, little airflow is allowed with the latter materials. As a result, manufacturers have produced gowns with Saranex or polyethylene reinforced sleeves and front in an effort to decrease permeability in the most exposure-prone areas, but little research exists on decreasing exposure.

3. Respiratory Protection

A BSC is essential for the preparation of HDs. Where a BSC is not currently available, a *NIOSH-approved respirator* appropriate for the hazard must be worn to afford protection until the BSC is installed.* The use of respirators must comply with OSHA's Respiratory Protection Standard,[105] which outlines the aspects of a respirator program, including selection, fit testing, and worker training. Surgical masks are *not appropriate*, since they *do not prevent* aerosol inhalation. Permanent respirator use, in lieu of BSCs, is imprudent practice and should not be a substitute for engineering controls.

4. Eye and Face Protection

Whenever splashes, sprays, or aerosols of HDs may be generated, which can result in eye, nose, or mouth contamination, chemical barrier face and eye protection must be provided and used in accordance with 29 CFR 1910.133. Eyeglasses with temporary side shields are inadequate protection.

When a respirator is used to provide temporary protection as described here, and splashes, sprays, or aerosols are possible, employee protection should be either:

- A respirator with a full face piece, or
- A plastic face shield or splash goggles complying with ANSI standards[2] when using a respirator of less than full face piece design.
- Eyewash facilities should also be made available.

5. PPE Disposal and Decontamination

All gowns, gloves, and disposable materials used in preparation should be disposed of according to the hospital's hazardous drug waste procedures and as described under this review's section on Waste Disposal. Goggles, face shields, and respirators may be cleaned with mild detergent and water for reuse.

Work Equipment

NIH has recommended the work with HDs be carried out in a BSC on a disposable, plastic-backed paper liner. The liner should be changed after preparation is completed for the day, or after a shift, whichever comes first. Liners should also be changed after a spill.[103]

Syringes and IV sets with Luer-Lok fittings should be used for HDs. Syringe size should be large enough so that they are not full when the entire drug dose is present.

A covered disposable container should be used to contain excess solution. A covered sharps container should be in the BSC.

The ASHP recommends that HD-labeled plastic bags be available for all contaminated materials (including gloves, gowns, and paper liners), so that contaminated material can be immediately placed in them and disposed of in accordance with ASHP recommendations.[3]

---

*NIOSH recommendation at the time of this publication is for a respirator with a high-efficiency filter, preferably a powered air-purifying respirator.

Work Practices

Correct work practices are essential to worker protection. *Aseptic technique* is assumed as a standard practice in drug preparation. The general principles of aseptic technique, therefore, will not be detailed here. It should be noted, however, that BSC benches differ from horizontal flow units in several ways that require special precautions. Manipulations should not be performed close to the work surface of a BSC. Unsterilized items, including liners and hands, should be kept downstream from the working area. Entry and exit of the cabinet should be perpendicular to the front. Rapid lateral hand movements should be avoided. Additional information can be found in the National Sanitation Foundation Standard 49 for Class II (Laminar Flow) Biohazard Cabinetry[70] and Avis and Levchuck's paper.[6] All operators should be trained in these containment-area protocols.

All PPE should be donned before work is started in the BSC. All items necessary for drug preparation should be placed within the BSC before work is begun. Extraneous items should be kept out of the work area.

1. Labeling

In addition to standard pharmacy labeling practices, all syringes and IV bags containing HDs should be labeled with a distinctive warning label such as:

SPECIAL HANDLING/Disposal Precautions

In addition, those HDs covered under HCS must have labels in accordance with section (f) of the standard to warn employees handling the drug(s) of the hazards.

2. Disposing of Needles

The ASHP recommends that all syringes and needles used in the course of preparation be placed in medical waste-disposal (sharps) containers for disposal without being crushed, clipped, or capped.[3,103]

3. Priming

Prudent practice dictates that drug administration sets be attached and primed within the BSC prior to addition of the drug. This eliminates the need to prime the set in a less well-controlled environment and ensures that any fluid that escapes during priming contains no drug. If priming must occur at the site of administration, the intravenous line should be primed with nondrug-containing fluid, or a backflow closed system should be used.[3]

4. Handling Vials

Extremes of positive and negative pressure in medication vials should be avoided, for example, attempting to withdraw 10 mL of fluid from a 10-mL vial, or placing 10 mL of a fluid into an air-filled 10-mL vial. The use of large-bore needles, #18 or #20, avoids *high-pressure syringing* of solutions. However, some experienced personnel believe that large-bore needles are more likely to drip. Multi-use dispensing pins are recommended to avoid these problems.

Venting devices such as filter needles or dispensing pins permit outside air to replace the withdrawn liquid. Proper worker education is essential before using these devices.[3] Although venting devices are recommended, another technique is to add diluent slowly to the vial by alternately injecting small amounts and allowing displaced air to escape into the syringe. When all diluent has been added, a small amount of additional air may be withdrawn to create a slight negative pressure in the vial. This should not be expelled into room air because it may contain drug residue. It should either be injected into a vacuum vial or remain in the syringe to be discarded.

If any negative pressure must be applied to withdraw a dosage from a stoppered vial and handling safety is compromised, an air-filled syringe should be used to equalize pressure in the stoppered vial. The volume of drug to be withdrawn can be replaced by injecting small amounts of air into the vial and withdrawing equal amounts of liquid until the required volume is withdrawn. The drug should be cleared from the needle and hub (neck) of the syringe before separating to reduce spraying on separation.

5. Handling Ampules
Prudent practice requires that ampules with dry material should be *gently tapped down* before opening to move any material in the top of the ampule to the bottom quantity. A sterile gauze pad should be wrapped around the ampule neck before breaking the top.[3] This can protect against cuts and catch airborne powder or aerosol. If diluent is to be added, it should be injected slowly down the inside wall of the ampule. The ampule should be tilted gently to ensure that all the powder is wet before agitating it to dissolve the contents.

After the solution is withdrawn from the ampule with a syringe, the needle should be cleared of solution by holding it vertically with the point upwards; the syringe should be tapped to remove air bubbles. Any bubbles should be expelled into a closed container.

6. Packaging HDs for Transport
The outside of bags or bottles containing the prepared drug should be wiped with moist gauze.

Entry ports should be wiped with moist alcohol pads and capped. Transport should occur in sealed plastic bags and in containers designed to avoid breakage.

HDs that are shipped and that are subject to EPA regulation as hazardous waste are also subject to Department of Transportation (DOT) regulations as specified in 49 CFR Part 172.101.

7. Handling Nonliquid HDs
The handling of nonliquid forms of HDs requires special precautions as well. Tablets that may produce dust or potential exposure to the handler should be counted in a BSC. Capsules (i.e., gel caps or coated tablets) are unlikely to produce dust unless broken in handling.

These are counted in a BSC on equipment designated for HDs only, because even manual counting devices may be covered with dust from the drugs handled. Automated counting machines should not be used unless an enclosed process isolates the hazard from the employee(s).

Compounding should also occur in a BSC. A gown and gloves should be worn. *(If a BSC is unavailable, an appropriate NIOSH-approved respirator must be worn.)*

Drug Administration
1. Personal Protective Equipment
The National Study Commission on Cytotoxic Exposure has recommended that personnel administering HDs wear gowns, latex gloves, and chemical splash goggles or

equivalent safety glasses as described under the PPE Section, Preparation.[71] *NIOSH-approved respirators should be worn when administering aerosolized drugs.*

2. Administration Kit

Protective and administration equipment may be packaged together and labeled as an HD administration kit. Such a kit should include:

* Personal protective equipment.
* Gauze (4 × 4) for cleanup.
* Alcohol wipes.
* Disposable plastic-backed absorbent liner.
* Puncture-resistant container for needles and syringes.
* Thick sealable plastic bag (with warning label).
* Accessory warning labels.

3. Work Practices

Safe work practices when handling HDs should include:

* Hands should be washed before donning and after removing gloves. Gowns or gloves that become contaminated should be changed immediately. Employees should be trained in proper methods to remove contaminated gloves and gowns. After use, gloves and gowns should be disposed of in accordance with ASHP recommendations.
* Infusion sets and pumps, which should have Luer-Lok fittings, should be observed for leakage during use. A plastic-backed absorbent pad should be placed under the tubing during administration to catch any leakage. Sterile gauze should be placed around any push sites; IV tubing connection sites should be taped.
* Priming IV sets or expelling air from syringes should be carried out in a BSC. If done at the administration site, ASHP recommends that the line be primed with nondrug-containing solution or that a backflow closed system be used. IV containers with venting tubes should not be used.[3]
* Syringes, IV bottles and bags, and pumps should be wiped clean of any drug contamination with sterile gauze. Needles and syringes should not be crushed or clipped. They should be placed in a puncture-resistant container and then into the HD disposal bag with all other HD-contaminated materials. Administration sets should be disposed of intact. Disposal of the waste bag should follow HD disposal requirements. Unused drugs should be returned to the pharmacy.
* Protective goggles should be cleaned with detergent and properly rinsed. All protective equipment should be disposed of upon leaving the patient care area.
* Nursing stations where these drugs will be administered should have spill and emergency skin and eye decontamination kits available and relevant MSDSs for guidance. The HCS requires MSDSs to be readily available in the workplace to all employees working with hazardous chemicals.
* PPE should be used during the administration of oral HDs if splashing is possible.

A large number of investigational HDs are under clinical study in healthcare facilities. Personnel not directly involved in the investigation should not administer these drugs unless they have received adequate instructions regarding safe handling procedures. Literature regarding potential toxic effects of investigational drugs should be evaluated prior to the drug's introduction into the workplace.[65]

The increased use of HDs in the home environment necessitates special precautions. Employees involved in home care delivery should follow the above work practices, and employers should make administration and spill kits available. Home healthcare workers should have emergency protocols with them, as well as phone numbers and addresses, in the event emergency care becomes necessary.[3] Waste disposal for drugs delivered for home use and other home-contaminated material should also be considered by the employer and should follow applicable regulations.

4. Aerosolized Drugs

The administration of aerosolized HDs requires special engineering controls to prevent exposure to healthcare workers and others in the vicinity. In the case of *pentamidine,* these controls include treatment booths with local exhaust ventilation designed specifically for its administration. A variety of ventilation methods have also been used for the administration of *ribavirin.* These include isolation rooms with separate HEPA-filtered ventilation systems and administration via endotracheal tube.[30,47] Engineering controls used to manage employee exposure to anesthetic gases is a traditional example of occupational chemical management. Both isolation and ventilation are used for these volatile HDs.

Caring for Patients Receiving HDs

In accordance with the Bloodborne Pathogens Standard, universal precautions must be observed to prevent contact with blood or other potentially infectious materials. Under circumstances in which differentiation between body fluid types is difficult or impossible, all body fluids should be considered potentially infectious materials and must be managed as dictated in the Bloodborne Pathogens Standard.[109]

1. Personal Protective Equipment

Personnel dealing with excreta, primarily urine, from patients who have received HDs in the last 48 hours should be provided with and wear latex or other appropriate gloves and disposable gowns, to be discarded after each use or whenever contaminated, as detailed under Waste Disposal. Eye protection should be worn if splashing is possible. Such excreta contaminated with blood, or other potentially infectious materials as well, should be managed according to the Bloodborne Pathogen Standard. Hands should be washed after removal of gloves or after contact with the above substances.

2. Linen

Linen contaminated with HDs or excreta from patients who have received HDs in the past 48 hours is a potential source of exposure to employees. Linen soiled with blood or other potentially infectious materials, as well as contaminated with excreta, must also be managed according to the Bloodborne Pathogens Standard.[109] Linen contaminated with HDs should be placed in specially marked laundry bags and then placed in a labeled, impervious bag. The laundry bag and its contents should be prewashed, and then the linens added to other laundry for a second wash. Laundry personnel should wear latex gloves and gowns while handling prewashed material.

3. Reusable Items

Glassware or other contaminated reusable items should be washed twice with detergent by a trained employee wearing double latex gloves and a gown.

Waste Disposal

1. Equipment

Thick, leakproof plastic bags, colored differently from other hospital trash bags, should be used for routine accumulation and collection of used containers, discarded gloves, gowns, and any other disposable material. Bags containing hazardous chemicals (as defined by Section C of HCS), shall be labeled in accordance with Section F of the Hazard Communication Standard where appropriate. Where the Hazard Communication Standard does not apply, labels should indicate that bags contain HD-related wastes.

Needles, syringes, and breakable items not contaminated with blood or other potentially infectious materials should be placed in a waste-disposal (sharps) container before they are stored in the waste bag. Such items that are contaminated with blood or other potentially infectious material *must* be placed in a sharps container. Similarly, needles should not be clipped or capped nor syringes crushed. If contaminated by blood or other potentially infectious material, such needles/syringes *must not* be clipped, capped, or crushed (except in a rare instance where a *medical* procedure requires recapping). The waste bag should be kept inside a covered waste container clearly labeled "HD Waste Only." At least one such receptacle should be located in every area where the drugs are prepared or administered. Waste should not be moved from one area to another. The bag should be sealed when filled and the covered waste container taped.

2. Handling

Prudent practice dictates that every precaution be taken to prevent contamination of the exterior of the container. Personnel disposing of HD waste should wear gowns and protective gloves when handling waste containers with contaminated exteriors. Prudent practice further dictates that such a container with a contaminated exterior be placed in a second container in a manner that eliminates contamination of the second container. HD waste handlers should also receive hazard communication training as discussed in Section H.

3. Disposal

Hazardous drug-related wastes should be handled separately from other hospital trash and disposed of in accordance with applicable EPA, state, and local regulations for hazardous waste.[24,110] This disposal can occur at either an incinerator or a licensed sanitary landfill for toxic wastes, as appropriate. Commercial waste disposal is performed by a licensed company. While awaiting removal, the waste should be held in a secure area in covered, labeled drums with plastic liners.

Chemical inactivation traditionally has been a complicated process that requires specialized knowledge and training. The MSDS should be consulted regarding specific advice on cleanup (IARC[13]) and Lunn et al.[56] have validated inactivation procedures for specific agents that are effective. However, these procedures vary from drug to drug and may be impractical for small amounts. Care must be taken because of unique problems presented by the cleanup of some agents, such as byproduct formation.[57] Serious consideration should be given to alternative disposal methods.

Spills

Emergency procedures to cover spills or inadvertent release of hazardous drugs should be included in the facility's overall health and safety program.

Incidental spills and breakages should be cleaned up immediately by a properly protected person trained in the appropriate procedures. The area should be identified with a warning sign to limit access to the area. Incident reports should be filed to document the spill and those exposed.

1. Personnel Contamination

Contamination of protective equipment or clothing, or direct skin or eye contact should be treated by:

- Immediately removing the gloves or gown.
- Immediately cleansing the affected skin with soap and water.
- Flooding an affected eye at an eyewash fountain or with water or isotonic eyewash designated for that purpose for at least 15 minutes, for eye exposure.
- Obtaining medical attention. (Protocols for emergency procedures should be maintained at the designated sites for such medical care. Medical attention should also be sought for inhalation of HDs in powder form.)
- Documenting the exposure in the employee's medical record.

2. Cleanup of Small Spills

The ASHP considers small spills to be those less than 5 mL. The 5-mL volume of material should be used to categorize spills as large or small. Spills of less than 5 mL or 5 mg outside a BSC should be cleaned up immediately by personnel wearing gowns, double latex gloves, and splash goggles. *An appropriate NIOSH-approved respirator should be used for either powder or liquid spills where airborne powder or aerosol is or has been generated.*

- Liquids should be wiped with absorbent gauze pads; solids should be wiped with wet absorbent gauze. The spill areas should then be cleaned three times using a detergent solution followed by clean water.
- Any broken glass fragments should be picked up using a small scoop (never the hands) and placed in a sharps container. The container should then go into an HD disposal bag, along with used absorbent pads and any other contaminated waste.
- Contaminated reusable items (e.g., glassware and scoops) should be treated as outlined under Reusable Items.

3. Cleanup of Large Spills

When a large spill occurs, the area should be isolated and aerosol generation avoided. For spills larger than 5 mL, liquid spread is limited by gently covering with absorbent sheets or spill-control pads or pillows. If a powder is involved, damp cloths or towels should be used. Specific individuals should be trained to clean up large spills.

* As with small spills, protective apparel and respirators should be used when there is any suspicion of airborne powder or that an aerosol has been or will be generated. Most CDs are not volatile; however, this may not be true for all HDs. The volatility of the drug should be assessed in selecting the type of respiratory protection.
* As discussed under Waste Disposal, chemical inactivation should be avoided in this setting.
* All contaminated surfaces should be thoroughly cleaned three times with detergent and water.
* All contaminated absorbent sheets and other materials should be placed in the HD disposal bag.

4. Spills in BSCs

Extensive spills within a BSC necessitate decontamination of all interior BSC surfaces after completion of the spill cleanup. The ASHP[3] recommends this action for spills larger than 150 mL or the contents of one vial. If the HEPA filter of a BSC is contaminated, the unit should be labeled and sealed in plastic until the filter can be changed and disposed of properly by trained personnel wearing appropriate protective equipment.

5. Spill Kits

Spill kits, clearly labeled, should be kept in or near preparation and administrative areas. The MSDSs include sections on emergency procedures, including appropriate PPE. The ASHP recommends that kits include chemical splash goggles, two pairs of gloves, utility gloves, a low-permeability gown, two sheets ($12'' \times 12''$) of absorbent material, 250-mL and liter spill-control pillows, a waste-disposal (sharps) container, a small scoop to collect glass fragments, and two large HD waste-disposal bags.[3]

Prior to cleanup, appropriate protective equipment should be used. Absorbent sheets should be incinerable. Protective goggles and respirators should be cleaned with mild detergent and water after use.

Storage and Transport

1. Storage Areas

Access to areas where HDs are stored should be limited to authorized personnel with signs restricting entry.[72] A list of drugs covered by HD policies and information on spill and emergency contact procedures should be posted or easily available to employees. Facilities used for storing HDs should not be used for other drugs and should be designed to prevent containers from falling to the floor (e.g., bins with barrier fronts). Warning labels should be applied to all HD containers, as well as the shelves and bins where these containers are permanently stored.

2. Receipt of Damaged HD Packages

Damaged shipping cartons should be opened in an isolated area or a BSC by a designated employee wearing double gloves, a gown, goggles, and appropriate respiratory protection. Individuals must be trained to process damaged packages as well.

The ASHP recommends that broken containers and contaminated packaging mats be placed in a waste-disposal (sharps) container and then into HD disposal bags.[3] The bags should then be closed and placed in receptacles as described under Waste Disposal.

The appropriate protective equipment and waste-disposal materials should be kept in the area where shipments are received, and employees should be trained in their use and the risks of exposure to HDs.

3. Transport

HDs should be securely capped or sealed, placed in sealed clear plastic bags, and transported in containers designed to avoid breakage.

Personnel involved in transporting HDs should be trained in spill procedures, including sealing off the contaminated area and calling for appropriate assistance.

All HD containers should be labeled as noted in Drug Preparation Work Practices. If transport methods are used that produce stress on contents, such as the use of pneumatic tubes, guidance from the OSHA clarification of 1910.1030 with respect to transport (M.4.b.8[c]) should be followed. This clarification provides for use of packaging material inside the tube to prevent breakage. These recommendations that pertain to the Bloodborne Pathogens Standard are prudent practice for HDs (e.g., padded inserts for carriers).

F. Medical Surveillance

Workers who are potentially exposed to chemical hazards should be monitored in a systematic program or medical surveillance intended to prevent occupational injury and disease.[3,7] The purpose of surveillance is to identify the earliest reversible biologic effects so that exposure can be reduced or eliminated before the employee sustains irreversible damage. The occurrence of exposure-related disease or other adverse health effects should prompt immediate reevaluation of primary preventive measures (e.g., engineering controls, PPE). In this manner, medical surveillance acts as a check on the appropriateness of controls already in use.[62]

For detection and control of work-related health effects, *job-specific* medical evaluations should be performed:

- Before job placement.
- Periodically during employment.
- Following acute exposures.
- At the time of job termination or transfer (exit examination).

This information should be collected and analyzed in a systematic fashion to allow early detection of disease patterns in individual workers and groups of workers.

1. Preplacement Medical Examinations

Sound medical practice dictates that employees who will be working with HDs in the workplace have an initial evaluation consisting of a history, physical exam, and laboratory studies.

The employer should make the following information available to the examining physician:

- Description of the employee's duties as they relate to the employee's exposure.
- Employee's exposure levels or anticipated exposure levels.
- Description of any PPE used or to be used.
- Information from previous medical examinations of the employee that is not readily available to the examining physician.

The history details the individual's medical and reproductive experience with emphasis on potential risk factors, such as past hematopoietic, malignant, or hepatic disorders. It also includes a complete occupational history with information on extent of past exposures (including environmental sampling data, if possible) and use of protective equipment. Surrogates for worker exposure, in the absence of environmental sampling data, include:

- Records of drugs and quantities handled.
- Hours spent handling these drugs per week.
- Number of preparations/administrations per week.

The physical examination should be complete, but the skin, mucous membranes, cardiopulmonary, lymphatic system, and liver should be emphasized. An evaluation for respirator use must be performed in accordance with 29 CFR 1910.134, if the employee will wear a respirator. The laboratory assessment may include a complete blood count with differential, liver function tests, blood urea nitrogen, creatinine, and a urine dipstick. Other aspects of the physical and laboratory evaluation should be guided by known toxicities of the HD of exposure. Due to poor reproducibility, interindividual variability, and lack of prognostic value regarding disease development, no biologic monitoring tests (e.g., genotoxic markers) are currently recommended for routine use in employee surveillance. Biologic marker testing should be performed only within the context of a research protocol.

2. Periodic Medical Examinations

Recognized occupational medicine experts in the HD area recommend these exams to update the employee's medical, reproductive, and exposure histories. They are recommended on a yearly basis or every 2–3 years. The interval between exams is a function of the opportunity for exposure, duration of exposure, and possibly the age of the worker at the discretion of the occupational medicine physician, guided by the worker's history. Careful documentation of an individual's routine exposure and any acute accidental exposures are made. The physical examination and laboratory studies follow the format outlined in the preplacement examination.[54]

3. Postexposure Examinations

Postexposure evaluation is tailored to the type of exposure (e.g., spills or needle sticks from syringes containing HDs). An assessment of the extent of exposure is made and included in the confidential database (discussed in the Exposure/Health Outcome Linkage section) and in an incident report. The physical examination focuses on the involved area as well as other organ systems commonly affected (i.e., for CDs the skin and mucous membranes; for aerosolized HDs the pulmonary system). Treatment and laboratory studies follow as indicated and should be guided by emergency protocols.

4. Exit Examinations

The exit examination completes the information on the employee's medical, reproductive, and exposure histories. Examination and laboratory evaluation should be guided by the individual's history of exposures and follow the outline of the periodic evaluation.

5. Exposure/Health Outcome Linkage

Exposure assessment of all employees who have worked with HDs is important, and the maintenance of records is required by 29 CFR 1910.20. The use of previously outlined exposure surrogates is acceptable, although actual environmental or employee monitoring data are preferable. An MSDS can serve as an exposure record. Details of the use of PPE and engineering controls present should be included. A confidential database should be maintained with information regarding the individual's medical and reproductive history, with linkage to exposure information to facilitate epidemiologic review.

6. Reproductive Issues

The examining physician should consider the reproductive status of employees and inform them regarding relevant reproductive issues. The reproductive toxicity of hazardous drugs should be carefully explained to all workers who will be exposed to these chemicals, and is required for those chemicals covered by the HCS. Unfortunately, no information is available regarding the reproductive risks of HD handling with the current use of BSCs and PPE. However, as discussed earlier, both spontaneous abortion and congenital malformation excesses have been documented among workers handling some of these drugs without currently recommended engineering controls and precautions. The facility should have a policy regarding reproductive toxicity of HDs and worker exposure in male and female employees and should follow that policy.

G. Hazard Communication

> *This section is for informational purposes only and is not a substitute for the requirements of the Hazard Communication Standard.*

The Hazard Communication Standard (HCS),[107] is applicable to some drugs. It defines a hazardous chemical as *any chemical that is a physical hazard or a health hazard.*
Physical hazard refers to characteristics such as combustibility or reactivity. A health hazard is defined as *a chemical for which there is statistically significant evidence based on at least one study conducted in accordance with established scientific principles that acute or chronic health effects may occur in exposed employees.* Appendixes A and B of the HCS outline the criteria used to determine whether an agent is hazardous.

According to HCS Appendix A, agents with any of the following characteristics would be considered hazardous:

- Carcinogens.
- Corrosives.
- Toxic or highly toxic agents (defined on the basis of median lethal doses).
- Irritants.
- Sensitizers.
- Target organ effectors, including reproductive toxins, hepatotoxins, nephrotoxins, neurotoxins, agents that act on the hematopoietic system, and agents that damage the lungs, skin, eyes, or mucous membranes.

Both human and animal data are to be used in this determination. HCS Appendix C lists sources of toxicity information.

As a result of the February 21, 1990 Supreme Court decision,[21] all provisions of the Hazard Communication Standard (29 CFR 1910.1200)[107] are now in effect for all industrial segments. This includes the coverage of drugs and pharmaceuticals in the nonmanufacturing sector. On February 9, 1994, OSHA issued a revised Hazard Communication Final Rule with technical clarification regarding drugs and pharmaceutical agents.

The Hazard Communication Standard (HCS) requires that drugs posing a health hazard (with the exception of those in solid, final form for direct administration to the patient, i.e., tablets or pills) be included on lists of hazardous chemicals to which employees are exposed.[107] Their storage and use locations can be confirmed by reviewing purchasing office records of currently used and past used agents such as those in Table A.1. Employee exposure records, including workplace monitoring, biologic monitoring, and MSDSs, as well as employee medical records related to drugs posing a health hazard, must be maintained and access to them provided to employees in accordance with 29 CFR 1910.20. Training required under the HCS should include all employees potentially exposed to these agents, not only healthcare professional staff, but also physical plant, maintenance, or support staff.

MSDSs are required to be prepared and transmitted with the initial shipment of all hazardous chemicals including covered drugs and pharmaceutical products. This excludes drugs defined by the Federal Food, Drug, and Cosmetic Act, which are in solid, final form for direct administration to the patient (e.g., tablets, pills, or capsules) or which are packaged for sale to consumers in a retail establishment. Package inserts and the *Physicians' Desk Reference* are not acceptable in lieu of requirements of MSDSs under the Standard. Items mandated by the Standard will use the term *shall* instead of *should.*

1. Written Hazard Communication Program

Employers shall develop, implement, and maintain at the workplace, a written hazard communication program for employees handling or otherwise exposed to chemicals, including drugs that represent a health hazard to employees. The written program will describe how the criteria specified in the Standard concerning labels and other forms of warning, MSDSs, and employee information and training will be met. This also includes the following:

- List of the covered hazardous drugs known to be present using an identity that is referenced on the appropriate MSDS.

- Methods the employer will use to inform employees of the hazards of nonroutine tasks in their work areas.
- Methods the employer will use to inform employees of other employers of hazards at the worksite.

The employer shall make the written hazard communication program available, upon request, to employees, their designated representatives, and the Assistant Secretary of OSHA in accordance with requirements of the HCS.

2. MSDSs

In accordance with requirements in the Hazard Communication Standard, the employer must maintain MSDSs accessible to employees for all covered HDs used in the hospital. Specifics regarding MSDS content are contained in the Standard. Essential information includes health hazards, primary exposure routes, carcinogenic evaluations, acute exposure treatment, chemical inactivators, solubility, stability, volatility, PPE-required, and spill procedures for each covered HD. MSDSs shall also be made readily available upon request to employees, their designated representatives, or the Assistant Secretary of OSHA.

H. Training and Information Dissemination

In compliance with the Hazard Communication Standard, all personnel involved in any aspect of the handling of covered HDs (physicians, nurses, pharmacists, housekeepers, employees involved in receiving, transport, or storage) must receive information and training to apprise them of the hazards of HDs present in the work area.[71] Such information should be provided at the time of an employee's initial assignment to a work area where HDs are present and prior to assignments involving new hazards. The employer should provide annual refresher information and training.

The National Study Commission on Cytotoxic Exposure has recommended that knowledge and competence of personnel be evaluated after the first orientation or training session, and then yearly, or more often if a need is perceived.[71] Evaluation may involve direct observation of an individual's performance on the job. In addition, non-HD solutions should be used for evaluation of preparation technique; quinine, which will fluoresce under ultraviolet light, provides an easy mechanism for evaluation of technique.

1. Employee Information

Employees must be informed of the requirements of the Hazard Communication Standard, 29 CFR 1910.1200:

- Any operation/procedure in their work area where drugs that present a hazard are present.
- The location and availability of the written hazard communication program.

In addition, they should be informed regarding:

- Any operations or procedure in their work area where other HDs are present.
- The location and availability of any other plan regarding HDs.

2. Employee Training

Employee training must include at least:

- Methods of observations that may be used to detect the presence or release of an HCS-covered hazardous drug in the work area (such as monitoring conducted by the employer, continuous monitoring devices, visual appearance, or odor of covered HDs being released).
- Physical and health hazards of the covered HDs in the area.
- Measures employees can take to protect themselves from these hazards, including specific procedures that the employer has implemented to protect the employees from exposure to such drugs, such as identification of covered drugs and those to be handled as hazardous, appropriate work practices, emergency procedures (for spills or employee exposure), and PPE.
- Details of the hazard communication program developed by the employer, including an explanation of the labeling system and the MSDS, and how employees can obtain and use the appropriate hazard information.

It is essential that workers understand the carcinogenic potential and reproductive hazards of these drugs. Both females and males should understand the importance of avoiding exposure, especially early in pregnancy, so they can make informed decisions about the hazards involved. In addition, the facility's policy regarding reproductive toxicity of HDs should be explained to workers. Updated information should be provided to employees on a regular basis and whenever their jobs involve new hazards. Medical staff and other personnel who are not hospital employees should be informed of hospital policies and of the expectation that they will comply with these policies.

I. Record Keeping

Any workplace-exposure record created in connection with HD handling shall be kept, transferred, and made available for at least 30 years, and medical records shall be kept for the duration of employment plus 30 years in accordance with the Access to Employee Exposure and Medical Records Standard (29 CFR 1910.20).[108] In addition, sound practice dictates that training records should include the following information:

- Dates of the training sessions.
- Contents or a summary of the training sessions.
- Names and qualifications of the persons conducting the training.
- Names and job titles of all persons attending the training sessions.

Training records should be maintained for 3 years from the date on which the training occurred.

Position Statement

For the handling of cytotoxic agents by women who are pregnant, attempting to conceive, or breastfeeding, there are substantial data regarding the mutagenic, teratogenic, and abortifacient properties of certain cytotoxic agents both in animals and humans who have received therapeutic doses of these agents. Additionally, the scientific literature suggests a possible association of occupational exposure to certain cytotoxic agents during the first trimester of pregnancy with fetal loss or malformation. These data suggest the need for caution when women who are pregnant, or attempting to conceive, handle cytotoxic agents. Incidentally, there is no evidence relating male exposure to cytotoxic agents with adverse fetal outcome. There are no studies that address the possible risk associated with the occupational exposure to cytotoxic agents and the passage of these agents into breastmilk. Nevertheless, it is prudent that women who are breastfeeding should exercise caution in handling cytotoxic agents.

If all procedures for safe handling, such as those recommended by the Commission, are complied with, the potential for exposure will be minimized. Personnel should be provided with information to make an individual decision. This information should be provided in written form, and it is advisable that a statement of understanding be signed. It is essential to refer to individual state right-to-know laws to ensure compliance.

Approved by the National Study Commission on Cytotoxic Exposure, September 1987.

References

1. American Medical Association Council on Scientific Affairs. Guidelines for handling parenteral antineoplastics. *JAMA* 1985; 253 1590–1592.
2. American National Standards Institute. Occupational and educational eye and face protection. *ANSI* 1968; Z87 1.
3. American Society of Hospital Pharmacists. ASHP technical assistance bulletin on handling cytotoxic and hazardous drugs. *Am. J. Hosp. Pharm.* 1990; 47 1033–1049.
4. Andersen R, Boedicker M, Ma M, Goldstein HJC. Adverse reactions associated with pentamidine isethionate in AIDS patients: recommendations for monitoring therapy. *Drug Intell. Clin. Pharm.* 1986; 20 862–868.
5. Anderson RW, Puckett WH, Dana WJ, et al. Risk of handling injectable antineoplastic agents. *Am. J. Hosp. Pharm.* 1982; 39 1881–1887.
6. Avis KE, Levchuck JW. Special considerations in the use of vertical laminar flow workbenches. *Am. J. Hosp. Pharm.* 1984; 41 81–87.
7. Barber RK. Fetal and neonatal effects of cytotoxic agents. *Obstet. Gynecol.* 1981; 51 41S–47S.
8. Benhamou S, Pot-Deprun J, Sancho-Garnier H, Chouroulinkov I. Sister chromatid exchanges and chromosomal aberrations in lymphocytes of nurses handling cytostatic drugs. *Int. J. Cancer* 1988; 41 350–353.
9. Bos RP, Leenars AO, Theuws JL, Henderson PT. Mutagenicity of urine from nurses handling cytostatic drugs, influence of smoking. *Int. Arch. Occ. Envir. Health* 1982; 50 359–369.
10. Bryan D, Marback RC. Laminar-airflow equipment certification: what the pharmacist needs to know. *Am. J. Hosp. Pharm.* 1984; 41 1343–1349.
11. Burgaz S, Ozdamar YN, Karakaya AE. A signal assay for the detection of toxic compounds: application on the urines of cancer patients on chemotherapy and of nurses handling cytotoxic drugs. *Human Toxicol.* 1988; 7 557–560.
12. California Department of Health Services Occupational Health Surveillance and Evaluation Program. *Health Care Worker Exposure to Ribavirin Aerosol: Field Investigation FI-86-009.* Berkeley: California Department of Health Services, 1986.
13. Castegnaro M, Adams J, Armour MA, eds, et al. Laboratory decontamination and destruction of carcinogens in laboratory wastes: some antineoplastic agents. International Agency for Research on Cancer. Scientific Publications No. 73. Lyons, France: IARC 1985.

14. Chapman RM. Effect of cytotoxic therapy on sexuality and gonadal function. Perry MC, Yarbro JW, (eds), *Toxicity of Chemotherapy.* Orlando: Grune & Stratton, 1984: 343–363.

15. Chen CH, Vazquez-Padua M, Cheng YC. Effect of antihuman immunodeficiency virus nucleoside analogs on mDNA and its implications for delayed toxicity. *Mol. Pharm.* 1990; 39 625–628.

16. Christensen CJ, Lemasters GK, Wakeman MA. Work practices and policies of hospital pharmacists preparing antineoplastic agents. *J. Occup. Med.* 1990; 32 508–512.

17. Chrysostomou A, Morley AA, Seshadri R. Mutation frequency in nurses and pharmacists working with cytotoxic drugs. *Aust. N. Z. J. Med.* 1984; 14 831–834.

18. Connor JD, Hintz M, Van Dyke R. Ribavirin pharmacokinetics in children and adults during therapeutic trials. Smith RA, Knight V, Smith JAD, (eds), In *Clinical Applications of Ribavirin.* Orlando: Academic Press, 1984.

19. Connor TH, Laidlaw JL, Theiss JC, et al. Permeability of latex and polyvinyl chloride gloves to carmustine. *Am. J. Hosp. Pharm.* 1984; 41 676–679.

20. Crudi CB. A compounding dilemma: I've kept the drug sterile but have I contaminated myself? *Nat. Intra. Therapy J.* 1980; 3 77–80.

21. Dole V. United Steelworkers. 1990; 494 U.S.26.

22. Doll C. Aerosolised pentamidine. *Lancet* 1989; ii 1284–1285.

23. Duvall E, Baumann B. An unusual accident during the administration of chemotherapy. *Cancer Nurse.* 1980; 3 305–306.

24. Environmental Protection Agency. *Discarded commercial chemical products, off specification species, container residues, and spill residues thereof.* 40 CFR 1991; 261.33(f).

25. Everson RB, Ratcliffe JM, Flack PM, et al. Detection of low levels of urinary mutagen excretion by chemotherapy workers, which was not related to occupational drug exposures. *Cancer Res.* 1985; 45 6487–6497.

26. Falck K, Grohn P, Sorsa M, et al. Mutagenicity in urine of nurses handling cytostatic drugs. *Lancet* 1979; i 1250–1251.

27. Falck K, Sorsa M, Vainio H. Use of the bacterial fluctuation test to detect mutagenicity in urine of nurses handling cytostatic drugs (abstract). *Mutat. Res.* 1981; 85 236–237.

28. Ferguson LR, Everts R, Robbie MA, et al. The use within New Zealand of cytogenetic approaches to monitoring of hospital pharmacists for exposure to cytotoxic drugs: report of a pilot study in Auckland. *Aust. J. Hosp Pharm.* 1988; 18 228–233.

29. Gude JK. Selective delivery of pentamidine to the lung by aerosol. *Am. Rev. Resp. Dis.* 1989; 139 1060.

30. Guglielmo BJ, Jacobs RA, Locksley RM. The exposure of healthcare workers to ribavirin aerosol. *JAMA* 1989; 261 1880–1881.

31. Harrison R, Bellows J, Rempel D, et al. Assessing exposures of healthcare personnel to aerosols of ribavirin-California. *Morbidity & Mortality Weekly Rep.* 1988; 37 560–563.

32. Hemminki K, Kyyronen P, Lindbohm ML. Spontaneous abortions and malformations in the offspring of nurses exposed to anaesthetic gases, cytostatic drugs, and other potential hazards in hospitals, based on registered information of outcome. *J. Epidem. Comm. Health* 1985; 39 141–147.

33. Henderson DK, Gerberding JL. Prophylactic zidovudine after occupational exposure to the human immunodeficiency virus: An interim analysis. *J. Infectious Dis.* 1989; 160 321–327.

34. Hillyard IW. The preclinical toxicology and safety of ribavirin. Smith RA, Kirkpatrick W, (eds), *In Ribavirin: a broad spectrum antiviral agent.* New York: Academic Press 1980.

35. Hirst M, Tse S, Mills DG, et al. Occupational exposure to cyclophosphamide. *Lancet* 1984; i 186–188.

36. Hoy RH, Stump LM. Effect of an air-venting filter device on aerosol production from vials. *Am. J. Hosp. Pharm.* 1984; 41 324–326.

37. International Agency for Research on Cancer. *IARC Monographs on the Evaluation of the Carcinogenic Risk of Chemicals to Man: Some Aziridines, N-, S-, and O-mustards and selenium.* Lyons, France. 1975; Vol. 9.

38. International Agency for Research on Cancer. *IARC Monographs on the Evaluation of the Carcinogenic Risk of Chemicals to Man: Some naturally occurring substances.* Lyons, France: IARC. 1976; Vol. 10.

39. International Agency for Research on Cancer. *IARC Monographs on the Evaluation of the Carcinogenic Risk of Chemicals to Humans: Some Antineoplastic and Immunosuppressive Agents.* Lyons, France: IARC. 1981; Vol. 26.

40. International Agency for Research on Cancer. *IARC Monographs on the Evaluation of the Carcinogenic Risk of Chemicals to Humans: Chemicals, Industrial Processes and Industries Associated with Cancer in Humans.* Lyons, France: IARC. 1982; Vol. 1–29 (Suppl. 4).

41. International Agency for Research on Cancer. *IARC Monographs on the Evaluation of the Carcinogenic Risk of Chemicals to Humans: Genetic and related effects: An updating of selected IARC Monographs from Volumes 1–42.* Lyons, France: IARC. 1987; Vol. 1–42 (Suppl. 6).

42. International Agency for Research on Cancer. *IARC Monographs on the Evaluation of the Carcinogenic Risk of Chemicals to Humans; Overall evaluations of carcinogenicity: An updating of IARC Monographs Volumes 1 to 42.* Lyons, France: IARC. 1987; Vol. 1–42 (Suppl. 7).

43. International Agency for Research on Cancer. *IARC Monographs on the Evaluation of the Carcinogenic Risk of Chemicals to Humans: Pharmaceutical Drugs,* Lyons, France: IARC.

44. Jagun O, Ryan M, Waldron HA. Urinary thioether excretion in nurses handling cytotoxic drugs. *Lancet* 1982; i 443–444.

45. Johnson EG, Janosik JE. Manufacturer's recommendations for handling spilled antineoplastic agents. *Am. J. Hosp. Pharm.* 1989; 46 318–319.

46. Juma FD, Rogers HJ, Trounce JR, Bradbrook ID. Pharmacokinetics of intravenous cyclophosphamide in man, estimated by gas liquid chromatography. *Cancer Chemother. Pharmacol.* 1978; 1 229–231.

47. Kacmarek RM. Ribavirin and pentamidine aerosols: caregiver beware! *Respiratory Care* 1990; 35 1034–1036.

48. Karakaya AE, Burgaz S, Bayhan A. The significance of urinary thioethers as indicators of exposure to alkylating agents. *Arch. Toxicol.* 1989; 13 (suppl) 117–119.

49. Kilham L, Ferm VH. Congenital anomalies induced in hamster embryos with ribavirin. *Science* 1977; 195 413–414.

50. Kleinberg ML, Quinn MJ. Airborne drug levels in a laminar-flow hood. *Am. J. Hosp. Pharm.* 1981; 38 1301–1303.

51. Kolmodin-Hedman B, Hartvig P, Sorsa M, Falck K. Occupational handling of cytostatic drugs. *Arch. Toxicol.* 1983; 54 25–33.

52. Kyle RA. Second malignancies associated with chemotherapy. Perry MC, Yarbro JW, (eds), *Toxicity of Chemotherapy.* Orlando: Grune & Stratton, 1984: 479–506.

53. Laidlaw JL, Connor TH, Theiss JC, et al. Permeability of latex and polyvinyl chloride gloves to 20 antineoplastic drugs. *Am. J. Hosp. Pharm.* 1984; 41 2618–2623.

54. Laidlaw JL, Connor TH, Theiss JC, et al. Permeability of four disposable protective clothing materials to seven antineoplastic drugs. *Am. J. Hosp. Pharm.* 1985; 42 2449–2454.

55. Lee SB. Ribavirin-exposure to healthcare workers. *Am. Ind. Hyg. Assoc.* 1988; 49 A13–A14.

56. LeRoy ML, Roberts MJ, Theisen JA. Procedures for handling antineoplastic injections in comprehensive cancer centers. *Am. J. Hosp. Pharm.* 1983; 40 601–603.

57. Lunn G, Sansone EB. Validated methods for handling spilled antineoplastic agents. *Am. J. Hosp. Pharm.* 1989; 46 1131.

58. Lunn G, Sansone EB, Andrews AW, Hellwig LC. Degradation and disposal of some antineoplastic drugs. *J. Pharm. Sciences* 1989; 78 652–659.
59. Matthews T, Boehme R. Antiviral activity and mechanism of action of ganciclovir. *Rev. Infect. Diseases* 1988; 10 (suppl 3) S490–94.
60. McDevitt JJ, Lees PSJ, McDiarmid MA. Exposure of hospital pharmacists and nurses to antineoplastic agents. *J. Occup. Med.* 1993; 35 57–60.
61. McDiarmid MA, Egan T, Furio M, et al. Sampling for airborne fluorouracil in a hospital drug preparation area. *Am. J. Hosp. Pharm.* 1988; 43 1942–1945.
62. McDiarmid MA, Emmett EA. Biological monitoring and medical surveillance of workers exposed to antineoplastic agents. *Seminars in Occup. Med.* 1987; 2 109–117.
63. McDiarmid MA, Jacobson-Kram D. Aerosolized pentamidine and public health. *Lancet* 1989; ii 863.
64. McDiarmid MA. Medical surveillance for antineoplastic-drug handlers. *Am. J. Hosp. Pharm.* 1990; 47 1061–1066.
65. McDiarmid MA, Gurley HT, Arrington D. Pharmaceuticals as hospital hazards: Managing the risks. *J. Occup. Med.* 1991; 33 155–158.
66. McDiarmid MA, Kolodner K, Humphrey F, et al. Baseline and phosphoramide mustard-induced sister chromatid exchanges in pharmacists handling anti-cancer drugs. *Mutat. Res.* 1992; 279 199–204.
67. McDiarmid MA, Schaefer J, Richard CL, Chaisson RE, Tepper BS. Efficacy of engineering controls in reducing occupational exposure to aerosolized pentamidine. *Chest* 1992; 102 1764–1766.
68. McEvoy GK, ed. *American Hospital Formulary Service Drug Information*. Bethesda: American Society of Hospital Pharmacists, 1993.
69. McLendon BF, Bron AF. Corneal toxicity from vinblastine solution. *Br. J. Ophthalmol.* 1978; 62 97–99.
70. National Sanitation Foundation. *Standard No. 49 for Class II (Laminar Flow) Biohazard Cabinetry*. Ann Arbor: National Sanitation Foundation, 1990.
71. National Study Commission on Cytotoxic Exposure. Louis P Jeffrey Sc. D, Chairman, (ed), *Recommendations for Handling Cytotoxic Agents*. Providence, Rhode Island: Rhode Island Hospital, 1983.
72. National Study Commission on Cytotoxic Exposure. Louis P Jeffrey Sc. D, (ed), *Consensus Responses to Unresolved Questions Concerning Cytotoxic Agents*. Providence, Rhode Island: Chairman, Rhode Island Hospital, 1984.
73. Neal AD, Wadden RA, Chiou WL. Exposure of hospital workers to airborne antineoplastic agents. *Am. J. Hosp. Pharm.* 1983; 40 597–601.
74. Nikula E, Kiviniitty K, Leisti J, Taskinen P. Chromosome aberrations in lymphocytes of nurses handling cytostatic agents. *Scand. J. Work Environ. Health* 1984; 10 71–74.
75. Norppa H, Sorsa M, Vainio H, et al. Increased sister chromatid exchange frequencies in lymphocytes of nurses handling cytostatic drugs. *Scand. J. Work Environ. Health* 1980; 6 299–301.
76. Nguyen TV, Theiss JC, Matney TS. Exposure of pharmacy personnel to mutagenic antineoplastic drugs. *Cancer Res.* 42 4792–4796.
77. Palmer RG, Dore CJ, Denman AM. Chlorambucil-induced chromosome damage to human lymphocytes is dose-dependent and cumulative. *Lancet* 1984; i 246–249.
78. Perry MC, Yarbro JW, eds. *Toxicity of Chemotherapy*. Orlando, FL: Grune & Stratton, 1984.
79. Physicians' Desk Reference.Barnhart ER, (eds), *Physicians' Desk Reference,* 45th ed. Oradell, New Jersey: Medical Economics Data, 1991: 730.
80. Pohlova H, Cerna M, Rossner P. Chromosomal aberrations, SCE and urine mutagenicity in workers occupationally exposed to cytostatic drugs. *Mutat. Res.* 1986; 174 213–217.

81. Pyy L, Sorsa M, Hakala E. Ambient monitoring of cyclophosphamide in manufacture and hospitals. *Am. Ind. Hyg. Assoc. J.* 1988; 49 314–317.

82. Reich SD, Bachur NR. Contact dermatitis associated with adriamycin (NSC-123127) and daunorubicin (NSC-82151). *Cancer Chemotherap. Rep.* 1975; 59 677–678.

83. Reynolds RD, Ignoffo R, Lawrence J, et al. Adverse reactions to AMSA in medical personnel. *Cancer Treat. Rep.* 1982; 66 1885.

84. Rogers B. Health hazards to personnel handling antineoplastic agents. *Occupational Med. State Art Rev.* 1987; 2 513–524.

85. Rogers B, Emmett EA. Handling antineoplastic agents: urine mutagenicity in nurses. *IMAGE J. Nurs. Scholarship.* 1987; 19 108–113.

86. Rosner F. Acute leukemia as a delayed consequence of cancer chemotherapy. *Cancer* 1976; 37 1033–1036.

87. Rudolph R, Suzuki M, Luce JK. Experimental skin necrosis produced by adriamycin. *Cancer Treat. Rep.* 1979; 63 529–537.

88. Schafer AI. Teratogenic effects of antileukemic therapy. *Arch. Int. Med.* 1981; 141 514–515.

89. Selevan SG, Lindbolm ML, Homung RW, Hemminki K. A study of occupational exposure to antineoplastic drugs and fetal loss in nurses. *New Engl. J. Med.* 1985; 313 1173–1178.

90. Sieber SM. Cancer chemotherapeutic agents and carcinogenesis. *Cancer Chemotherapy Rep.* 1975; 59 915–918.

91. Sieber SM, Adamson RH. Toxicity of antineoplastic agents in man: chromosomal aberrations, antifertility effects, congenital malformations, and carcinogenic potential. *Adv. Cancer Res.* 1975; 22 57–155.

92. Siebert D, Simon U. Cyclophosphamide: pilot study of genetically active metabolites in the urine of a treated human patient. *Mutat. Res.* 1973; 19 65–72.

93. Slevin ML, Ang LM, Johnston A, Turner P. The efficiency of protective gloves used in the handling of cytotoxic drugs. *Cancer Chemo. Pharmacol.* 1984; 12 151–153.

94. Smaldone GC, Vincicuerra C, Marchese J. Detection of inhaled pentamidine in healthcare workers. *New Engl. J. Med.* 1991; 325 891–892.

95. Sorsa M, Hemminki K, Vanio H. Occupational exposure to anticancer drugs—potential and real hazards. *Mutat. Res.* 1985; 154 135–149.

96. Sotaniemi EA, Sutinen S, Arranto AJ, et al. Liver damage in nurses handling cytostatic agents. *Acta Med. Scand.* 1983; 214 181–189.

97. Stellman JM. The spread of chemotherapeutic agents at work: assessment through stimulation. *Cancer Invest.* 1987; 5 75–81.

98. Stephens JD, Golbus MS, Miller TR, et al. Multiple congenital abnormalities in a fetus exposed to 5-fluorouracil during the first trimester. *Am. J. Obstet. Gynecol.* 1980; 137 747–749.

99. Stiller A, Obe G, Bool I, Pribilla W. No elevation of the frequencies of chromosomal aberrations as a consequence of handling cytostatic drugs. *Mutat. Res.* 1983; 121 253–259.

100. Stoikes ME, Carlson JD, Farris FF, Walker PR. Permeability of latex and polyvinyl chloride gloves to fluorouracil and methotrexate. *Am. J. Hosp. Pharm.* 1987; 44 1341–1346.

101. Stucker I, Hirsch A, Doloy T, et al. Urine mutagenicity, chromosomal abnormalities, and sister chromatid exchanges in lymphocytes of nurses handling cytostatic drugs. *Int. Arch. Occup. Environ. Health* 1986; 57 195–205.

102. Stucker I, Caillard JF, Collin R, et al. Risk of spontaneous abortion among nurses handling antineoplastic drugs. *Scand. J. Work Environ. Health* 1990; 16 102–107.

103. U.S. Department of Health and Human Services. Public Health Service. National Institutes of Health. *Recommendations for the Safe Handling of Cytotoxic Drugs.* NIH Publication No. 92-2621. 1992.

104. U.S. Department of Health and Human Services. Public Health Service. Centers for Disease Control. National Institute for Occupational Safety and Health. *Guidelines for Protecting the Safety and Health of Health Care Workers.* DHHS (NIOSH) Publication No. 88–119. 1988.

105. U.S. Department of Labor, Occupational Safety and Health Administration. Respiratory Protection Standard. 1984; 29 CFR 1910.134.

106. U.S. Department of Labor, Occupational Safety and Health Administration. Work practice guidelines for personnel dealing with cytotoxic (antineoplastic) drugs. OSHA Publication #8-1.1. 1986.

107. U.S. Department of Labor, Occupational Safety and Health Administration. *Hazard Communication Standard.* 1989; 29 CFR 1910.1200, as amended February 9, 1994.

108. U.S. Department of Labor, Occupational Safety and Health Administration. *Access to Employee and Medical Records Standard.* 1990; 29 CFR 1910. 20.

109. U.S. Department of Labor, Occupational Safety and Health Administration. *Occupational Exposure to Bloodborne Pathogens Standard.* 1991; 29 CFR 1910. 1030.

110. Vaccari FL, Tonat K, DeChristoforo R, et al. Disposal of antineoplastic waste at the NIH. *Am. J. Hosp. Pharm.* 1984; 41 87–92.

111. Valanis B, Vollmer WM, Labuhn K, Glass A, Corelle C. Antineoplastic drug handling protection after OSHA guidelines: comparison by profession, handling activity, and work site. *J. Occup. Med.* 1992; 34 149–155.

112. Venitt S, Crofton-Sleigh C, Hunt J, et al. Monitoring exposure of nursing and pharmacy personnel to cytotoxic drugs. Urinary mutation assays and urinary platinum as markers of absorption. *Lancet* 1984; i: 74 6.

113. Waksvik H, Klepp O, Brogger A. Chromosome analyses of nurses handling cytostatic agents. *Cancer Treat. Rep.* 1981; 65 607–610.

114. Wall RL, Clausen KP. Carcinoma of the urinary bladder in patients receiving cyclophosphamide. *New Engl. J. Med.* 1975; 293 271–273.

115. Weisburger JH, Griswold DP, Prejean JD, et al. Tumor induction by cytostatics. The carcinogenic properties of some of the principal drugs used in clinical cancer chemotherapy. *Recent Results Cancer Res.* 1975; 52 1–17.

116. Zimmerman PF, Larsen RK, Barkley EW, Gallelli JF. Recommendations for the safe handling of injectable antineoplastic drug products. *Am. J. Hosp. Pharm.* 1981; 38 1693–1695.

Appendix 2
Common Terminology Criteria for Adverse Events (CTCAE)

Rather than include the entire CTCAE, the following gives the highlights of the resource. The CTCAE can be found online at http://evs.nci.nih.gov/ftp1/CTCAE/CTCAE_4.03_2010-06-14_QuickReference_5x7.pdf

Version 4.0
Published: May 28, 2009 (v4.03: June 14, 2010)
U.S. DEPARTMENT OF HEALTH AND HUMAN SERVICES
National Institutes of Health
National Cancer Institute

Common Terminology Criteria for Adverse Events v4.0 (CTCAE)

Publish Date: May 28, 2009 (v4.03 June 14, 2010)

Quick Reference

The NCI Common Terminology Criteria for Adverse Events is a descriptive terminology that can be utilized for Adverse Event (AE) reporting. A grading (severity) scale is provided for each AE term.

Components and Organization
CTCAE Terms

An Adverse Event (AE) is any unfavorable and unintended sign (including an abnormal laboratory finding), symptom, or disease temporally associated with the use of a medical treatment or procedure that may or may *not* be considered related to the medical treatment or procedure. An AE is a term that is a unique representation of a specific event used for medical documentation and scientific analyses. Each CTCAE v4.0 term is a MedDRA LLT (Lowest Level Term).

Definitions

A brief definition is provided to clarify the meaning of each AE term.

Grades

Grade refers to the severity of the AE. The CTCAE displays Grades 1 through 5 with unique clinical descriptions of severity for each AE based on this general guideline:

Grade 1:

Mild; asymptomatic or mild symptoms; clinical or diagnostic observations only; intervention not indicated.

Grade 2:

Moderate; minimal, local, or noninvasive intervention indicated; limiting age-appropriate instrumental ADL (e.g., preparing meals, shopping for groceries or clothes, using the telephone, managing money).

Grade 3:

Severe or medically significant but not immediately life-threatening; hospitalization or prolongation of hospitalization indicated; disabling; limiting self-care ADL (e.g., bathing, dressing and undressing, feeding self, using toilet, taking medications, and not bedridden).

Grade 4:

Life-threatening consequences; urgent intervention indicated.

Grade 5:

Death related to AE.

Not all Grades are appropriate for all AEs. Therefore, some AEs are listed with fewer than five options for Grade selection.

Index

Generic names are indicated by boldface type.
Figures and tables are indicated by *f* and *t*, respectively, following the page number.